PN Adult Medical Surgical Nursing
REVIEW MODULE EDITION 12.0

W9-BKJ-764

Contributors

Alissa Althoff, Ed.D, MSN, RN

Brenda S. Ball, MEd, BSN, RN

Michelle E. Cawley, MSN, RN

Shannon Davis, MSN, BSN, RN

Sharon M Falk, MSN, RN, CCCTM, CHSE

Laurie Fontenot, MSN, RN

Lori Grace, MSN, RN

Norma Jean Henry, MSN/Ed., RN

Honey C. Holman, MSN, RN

Janean Johnson, DNP, RN, CNE

Terri Lemon DNP, MSN, RN

Beth Cusatis Phillips, PhD,
RN, CNE, CHSE

Pamela Roland, MSN, MBA, RN

LaKeisha Wheless, MSN, RN

Debborah Williams, MSN, RN

Consultants

Maureen Abraham, MSN,
RNC, CNE, LCCE

Tracey Bousquet, BSN, RN

Lois Churchill, MN, RN

Mary Davis-James, MSN/Ed., RN

Melissa Duckett, DNP, MSN, RN, CCRN

Margaret Hendrix, DNP RN

Donna Russo, RN, MSN, CCRN, CNE

Justin T. Schneider, DNP,
RN, AGPCNP–BC, CNE

Melanie A. Schock, DNP, RN, CNE, CPN

Tameka Scott, DNP, RN

Natalie Selover, DNP, RN

Gale Sewell, PhD., MSN, RN, CNE

Tracey Siegel, EdD, MSN RN CNE FAADN

Virginia Tufano, EdD, MSN, RN

Sarah Veal, MSN, RN, CNE

Director of content review: Kristen Lawler

Director of development: Derek Prater

Project management: Meri Ann Mason

Coordination of content review: Alissa Althoff, Honey C. Holman

Copy editing: Kelly Von Lunen, Tricia Lunt, Bethany Robertson,
Kya Rodgers, Rebecca Her, Sam Shiel, Alethea Surland, Graphic World

Layout: Bethany Robertson, Maureen Bradshaw, Haylee Hedge, scottie. o

Illustrations: Randi Hardy, Graphic World

Online media: Brant Stacy, Ron Hanson, Britney Frerking, Trevor Lund

Interior book design: Spring Lenox

IMPORTANT NOTICE TO THE READER

Welcome to the Assessment Technologies Institute® PN Adult Medical Surgical Nursing Review Module Edition 12.0. The mission of ATI's Content Mastery Series® Review Modules is to provide user-friendly compendiums of nursing knowledge that will:
- Help you locate important information quickly.
- Assist in your learning efforts.
- Provide exercises for applying your nursing knowledge.
- Facilitate your entry into the nursing profession as a newly licensed nurse.

ORGANIZATION

This Review Module is organized into units covering the foundations of nursing care (Unit 1), body systems and physiological processes (Units 2 to 13), and perioperative nursing care (Unit 14). Chapters within these units conform to one of three organizing principles for presenting the content.
- Nursing concepts
- Procedures
- System disorders

Nursing concepts chapters begin with an overview describing the central concept and its relevance to nursing. Subordinate themes are covered in outline form to demonstrate relationships and present the information in a clear, succinct manner.

Procedures chapters include an overview describing the procedure(s) covered in the chapter. These chapters provide nursing knowledge relevant to each procedure, including indications, nursing considerations, interpretation of findings, and complications.

System disorders chapters include an overview describing the disorder(s) and/or disease process. These chapters address assessments, including risk factors, expected findings, laboratory tests, and diagnostic procedures. Next, you will focus on patient-centered care, including nursing care, medications, therapeutic procedures, interprofessional care, and client education. Finally, you will find complications related to the disorder, along with nursing actions in response to those complications.

ACTIVE LEARNING SCENARIOS AND APPLICATION EXERCISES

Each chapter includes opportunities for you to test your knowledge and to practice applying that knowledge. Active Learning Scenario exercises pose a nursing scenario and then direct you to use an ATI Active Learning Template (included both in the chapter and in the Appendix) to record the important knowledge a nurse should apply to the scenario. An example is then provided to which you can compare your completed Active Learning Template. Application exercises throughout the chapters include NCLEX-style questions, such as multiple-choice and multiple-select items, providing you with opportunities to practice answering the kinds of questions you might expect to see on ATI assessments or the NCLEX. Answers and rationales are provided to further your learning.

NCLEX® CONNECTIONS

To prepare for the NCLEX-PN, it is important to understand how the content in this Review Module is connected to the NCLEX-PN test plan. You can find information on the detailed test plan at the National Council of State Boards of Nursing's website, www.ncsbn.org. When reviewing content in this Review Module, regularly ask yourself, "How does this content fit into the test plan, and what types of questions related to this content should I expect?"

To help you in this process, we've included NCLEX Connections at the beginning of each section and with the rationales for application exercises. The NCLEX Connections at the beginning of each unit point out areas of the test plan that relate to the content within that unit. The NCLEX Connections included with application exercises demonstrate how each exercise fits within the content outline. These NCLEX Connections will help you understand how the content outline is organized, starting with major client needs categories and subcategories and followed by related content areaa. The major client needs categories are:
- Safe and Effective Care Environment
  - Management of Care
  - Safety and Infection Control
- Health Promotion and Maintenance
- Psychosocial Integrity
- Physiological Integrity
  - Basic Care and Comfort
  - Pharmacological and Parenteral Therapies
  - Reduction of Risk Potential
  - Physiological Adaptation

An NCLEX Connection might, for example, alert you that content within a unit is related to:
- Reduction of Risk Potential
  - Diagnostic Tests
    - Monitor the results of diagnostic testing and intervene as needed.

QSEN COMPETENCIES

As you use the Review Modules, you will note the integration of the Quality and Safety Education for nurses (QSEN) competencies throughout the chapters. These competencies are integral components of the curriculum of many nursing programs in the United States and prepare you to provide safe, high-quality care as a newly licensed nurse. Icons appear to draw your attention to the six QSEN competencies.

Safety: The minimization of risk factors that could cause injury or harm while promoting quality care and maintaining a secure environment for clients, self, and others.

Patient-Centered Care: The provision of caring and compassionate, culturally sensitive care that addresses clients' physiological, psychological, sociological, spiritual, and cultural needs, preferences, and values.

Evidence-Based Practice: The use of current knowledge from research and other credible sources, on which to base clinical judgment and client care.

Informatics: The use of information technology as a communication and information-gathering tool that supports clinical decision-making and scientifically based nursing practice.

Quality Improvement: Care related and organizational processes that involve the development and implementation of a plan to improve health care services and better meet clients' needs.

Teamwork and Collaboration: The delivery of client care in partnership with multidisciplinary members of the health care team to achieve continuity of care and positive client outcomes.

ICONS

Icons are used throughout the Review Module to draw your attention to particular areas. Keep an eye out for these icons.

(N) This icon is used for NCLEX Connections.

(G) This icon indicates gerontological considerations, or knowledge specific to the care of older adult clients.

Qs This icon is used for content related to safety and is a QSEN competency. When you see this icon, take note of safety concerns or steps that nurses can take to ensure client safety and a safe environment.

Qpcc This icon is a QSEN competency that indicates the importance of a holistic approach to providing care.

Qebp This icon, a QSEN competency, points out the integration of research into clinical practice.

Qi This icon is a QSEN competency and highlights the use of information technology to support nursing practice.

Qqi This icon is used to focus on the QSEN competency of integrating planning processes to meet clients' needs.

Qtc This icon highlights the QSEN competency of care delivery using an interprofessional approach.

SDoH This icon highlights content related to social determinants of health.

M◇ This icon appears at the top-right of pages and indicates availability of an online media supplement, such as a graphic, animation, or video. If you have an electronic copy of the Review Module, this icon will appear alongside clickable links to media supplements. If you have a hard copy version of the Review Module, visit www.atitesting.com for details on how to access these features.

FEEDBACK

ATI welcomes your feedback. Please submit to comments@atitesting.com. Changes to the text are made for subsequent printings of the book and for subsequent releases of the electronic version. For the printed books, print runs are based on when existing stock is depleted. For the eBook, updates are made routinely depending on the volume of changes. As such, ATI encourages faculty and students to refer to the Review Module addendums for information on what updates have been made. These addendums, which are available in the Help/FAQs on the student site and the Resources/eBooks & Active Learning on the faculty site, are updated regularly and always include the most current information on updates to the Review Modules.

Table of Contents

NCLEX® Connections   1

UNIT 1   *Foundations of Nursing Care for Adult Clients*   *3*

CHAPTER 1	Health, Wellness, and Illness	3
CHAPTER 2	LGBTQIA Populations	7
CHAPTER 3	Emergency Nursing Principles and Management	15

NCLEX® Connections   23

UNIT 2   *Neurologic Disorders*   *25*

SECTION: *Diagnostic and Therapeutic Procedures*   25

| CHAPTER 4 | Neurologic Diagnostic Procedures | 25 |
| CHAPTER 5 | Pain Management | 33 |

NCLEX® Connections   39

SECTION: *Central Nervous System Disorders*   41

CHAPTER 6	Meningitis	41
CHAPTER 7	Seizures and Epilepsy	45
CHAPTER 8	Parkinson's Disease	51
CHAPTER 9	Delirium and Dementia	55

CHAPTER 10	Multiple Sclerosis	61
CHAPTER 11	Headaches	65
CHAPTER 12	Increased Intracranial Pressure Disorders	69
CHAPTER 13	Stroke	77

NCLEX® Connections   85

| SECTION: *Sensory Disorders* | 87 |

| CHAPTER 14 | Disorders of the Eye | 87 |
| CHAPTER 15 | Middle and Inner Ear Disorders | 93 |

NCLEX® Connections   99

UNIT 3 — *Respiratory Disorders*   101

| SECTION: *Diagnostic and Therapeutic Procedures* | 101 |

| CHAPTER 16 | Respiratory Diagnostic and Therapeutic Procedures | 101 |
| CHAPTER 17 | Respiratory Management and Mechanical Ventilation | 109 |

NCLEX® Connections   117

| SECTION: *Respiratory System Disorders* | 119 |

CHAPTER 18	Acute Respiratory Disorders	119
CHAPTER 19	Asthma	127
CHAPTER 20	Chronic Obstructive Pulmonary Disease	131
CHAPTER 21	Tuberculosis	137

NCLEX® Connections 143

SECTION: *Respiratory Emergencies*   *145*

CHAPTER 22   Pulmonary Embolism   145

CHAPTER 23   Pneumothorax, Hemothorax, and Flail Chest   151

CHAPTER 24   Respiratory Failure   157

NCLEX® Connections 165

UNIT 4   *Cardiovascular Disorders*   *167*

SECTION: *Diagnostic and Therapeutic Procedures*   *167*

CHAPTER 25   Cardiovascular Diagnostic and Therapeutic Procedures   167

CHAPTER 26   Electrocardiography and Dysrhythmia Monitoring   175

CHAPTER 27   Invasive Cardiovascular Procedures   181

NCLEX® Connections 191

SECTION: *Cardiac Disorders*   *193*

CHAPTER 28   Angina and Myocardial Infarction   193

CHAPTER 29   Heart Failure and Pulmonary Edema   201

CHAPTER 30   Valvular Heart Disease and Inflammatory Disorders   209

              Inflammatory Disorders   *212*

NCLEX® Connections 217

SECTION: *Vascular Disorders*   *219*

CHAPTER 31   Peripheral Vascular Diseases   219

CHAPTER 32   Hypertension   229

CHAPTER 33   Shock   235

CHAPTER 34   Aneurysms   243

NCLEX® Connections   249

UNIT 5   *Hematologic Disorders*   *251*

SECTION: *Diagnostic and Therapeutic Procedures*   *251*

CHAPTER 35   Hematologic Diagnostic Procedures   251

CHAPTER 36   Blood and Blood Product Transfusions   255

NCLEX® Connections   261

SECTION: *Hematologic Disorders*   *263*

CHAPTER 37   Anemias   263

NCLEX® Connections   269

UNIT 6   *Fluid/Electrolyte/Acid-Base Imbalances*   *271*

CHAPTER 38   Fluid Imbalances   271

CHAPTER 39   Electrolyte Imbalances   277

Sodium Imbalances   277

Potassium Imbalances   279

Other Electrolyte Imbalances   282

CHAPTER 40   Acid-Base Imbalances   287

NCLEX® Connections   293

UNIT 7   *Gastrointestinal Disorders*   *295*

SECTION: *Diagnostic and Therapeutic Procedures*   *295*

CHAPTER 41   Gastrointestinal Diagnostic Procedures   295

CHAPTER 42   Gastrointestinal Therapeutic Procedures   303

NCLEX® Connections   311

	SECTION: *Upper Gastrointestinal Disorders*	*313*
CHAPTER 43	Esophageal Disorders	313
CHAPTER 44	Peptic Ulcer Disease	321
CHAPTER 45	Acute and Chronic Gastritis	327

NCLEX® Connections   331

	SECTION: *Lower Gastrointestinal Disorders*	*333*
CHAPTER 46	Noninflammatory Bowel Disorders	333
CHAPTER 47	Inflammatory Bowel Disease	341

NCLEX® Connections   349

	SECTION: *Gallbladder and Pancreas Disorders*	*351*
CHAPTER 48	Cholecystitis and Cholelithiasis	351
CHAPTER 49	Pancreatitis	355

NCLEX® Connections   361

	SECTION: *Liver Disorders*	*363*
CHAPTER 50	Hepatitis and Cirrhosis	363

NCLEX® Connections   371

CHAPTER 51	Obesity	373

NCLEX® Connections 379

UNIT 8   *Renal Disorders*   *381*

SECTION: *Diagnostic and Therapeutic Procedures*   *381*

CHAPTER 52   **Renal Diagnostic Procedures**   381

CHAPTER 53   **Hemodialysis and Peritoneal Dialysis**   387

NCLEX® Connections 393

SECTION: *Renal System Disorders*   *395*

CHAPTER 54   **Polycystic Kidney Disease, Acute Kidney Injury, and Chronic Kidney Disease** 395

CHAPTER 55   **Infections of the Renal and Urinary System**   403

CHAPTER 56   **Renal Calculi**   411

NCLEX® Connections 417

UNIT 9   *Reproductive Disorders*   *419*

SECTION: *Diagnostic and Therapeutic Procedures*   *419*

CHAPTER 57   **Diagnostic and Therapeutic Procedures for Reproductive Disorders**   419

NCLEX® Connections 435

SECTION: *REPRODUCTIVE PROCESSES AND DISORDERS*   *437*

CHAPTER 58   **Reproductive Physiologic Processes**   437

     Menstrual Disorders   *437*

     Conditions Related to Menses or Bleeding   *439*

CHAPTER 59   **Disorders of Reproductive Tissue**   445

CHAPTER 60   Infections of the Reproductive System   459

General Infections   459

Infections Identified by Type of Lesion if Present   461

Infections Identified by Type of Discharge if Present   464

Other Infections   466

NCLEX® Connections   471

UNIT 10   *Musculoskeletal Disorders*   **473**

SECTION: *Diagnostic and Therapeutic Procedures*   473

CHAPTER 61   Musculoskeletal Diagnostic Procedures   473

CHAPTER 62   Arthroplasty   479

CHAPTER 63   Amputations   485

NCLEX® Connections   489

SECTION: *Musculoskeletal Disorders*   491

CHAPTER 64   Osteoporosis   491

CHAPTER 65   Musculoskeletal Trauma   497

CHAPTER 66   Osteoarthritis and Low-Back Pain   507

NCLEX® Connections   513

UNIT 11   *Integumentary Disorders*   **515**

SECTION: *Diagnostic and Therapeutic Procedures*   515

CHAPTER 67   Integumentary Diagnostic Procedures   515

NCLEX® Connections 519

SECTION: *Integumentary Disorders* — 521

CHAPTER 68 — Skin Disorders — 521

CHAPTER 69 — Burns — 527

NCLEX® Connections 537

UNIT 12 — *Endocrine Disorders* — **539**

SECTION: *Diagnostic and Therapeutic Procedures* — 539

CHAPTER 70 — Endocrine Diagnostic Procedures — 539

NCLEX® Connections 547

SECTION: *Pituitary Disorders* — 549

CHAPTER 71 — Pituitary Disorders — 549

NCLEX® Connections 557

SECTION: *Thyroid Disorders* — 559

CHAPTER 72 — Hyperthyroidism — 559

CHAPTER 73 — Hypothyroidism — 567

NCLEX® Connections 571

SECTION: *Adrenal Disorders* — 573

CHAPTER 74 — Adrenal Disorders — 573

NCLEX® Connections 581

SECTION: *Diabetes Mellitus* — 583

CHAPTER 75 — Diabetes Mellitus Management and Complications — 583

UNIT 13   *Immune System and Connective Tissue Disorders*   **597**

SECTION: *Diagnostic and Therapeutic Procedures*   *597*

CHAPTER 76   Immune and Infectious Disorders Diagnostic Procedures   597

CHAPTER 77   Immunizations   601

NCLEX® Connections   607

SECTION: *Immune Disorders*   *609*

CHAPTER 78   HIV/AIDS   609

NCLEX® Connections   615

SECTION: *Connective Tissue Disorders*   *617*

CHAPTER 79   Lupus Erythematosus, Gout, and Fibromyalgia   617

CHAPTER 80   Rheumatoid Arthritis   625

NCLEX® Connections   629

SECTION: *Cancer-Related Disorders*   *631*

CHAPTER 81   General Principles of Cancer   631

CHAPTER 82   Cancer Screening and Diagnostic Procedures   637

CHAPTER 83   Cancer Treatment Options   643

CHAPTER 84   Cancer Disorders   653

CHAPTER 85   Pain Management for Clients Who Have Cancer   685

UNIT 14 · *Nursing Care of Perioperative Clients* · 695

CHAPTER 86 · Preoperative Nursing Care · 695

CHAPTER 87 · Postoperative Nursing Care · 701

References · *707*

Active Learning Templates · *A1*

Basic Concept · A1

Diagnostic Procedure · A3

Growth and Development · A5

Medication · A7

Nursing Skill · A9

System Disorder · A11

Therapeutic Procedure · A13

Concept Analysis · A15

NCLEX® Connections

When reviewing the following chapters, keep in mind the relevant topics and tasks of the NCLEX outline.

Health Promotion and Maintenance

HEALTH PROMOTION/DISEASE PREVENTION
Identify risk factors for disease/illness.

Assist client in disease prevention activities.

Physiological Adaptation

ALTERATIONS IN BODY SYSTEMS: Provide care to correct client alteration in body system.

MEDICAL EMERGENCIES
Respond and intervene to a client life-threatening situation.

Notify primary health care provider about client unexpected response/emergency situation.

UNIT 1   FOUNDATIONS OF NURSING
CARE FOR ADULT CLIENTS

CHAPTER 1 **Health, Wellness, and Illness**

Health and wellness combine to form a state of optimal physical functioning and a feeling of emotional and social contentment. Wellness involves the ability to adapt emotionally and physically to a changing state of health and environment.

Illness is an altered level of functioning in response to a disease process. Disease is a condition that results in the physiological alteration in the composition of the body.

Nurses must understand the variables affecting health, wellness, and illness, and how they relate to clients' individual perceptions of health needs.

Health and wellness

The level of health and wellness is unique to each individual and relative to the individual's usual state of functioning. For example, a person who has rheumatoid arthritis, a strong support system, and positive outlook might consider themselves healthy while functioning at an optimal level with minimal pain.

VARIABLES Qpcc
- **Modifiable:** Can be changed (smoking, nutrition, access to health education, sexual practices, exercise)
- **Non-modifiable:** Cannot be changed (sex, age, developmental level, genetic traits)

ASPECTS OF HEALTH AND WELLNESS

- **Physical:** Able to perform activities of daily living
- **Emotional:** Adapts to stress; expresses and identifies emotions
- **Social:** Interacts successfully with others
- **Intellectual:** Effectively learns and disseminates information
- **Spiritual:** Adopts a belief that provides meaning to life
- **Occupational:** Balances occupational activities with leisure time
- **Environmental:** Creates measures to improve standards of living and quality of life

ENVIRONMENT

- A client's state of health and wellness is constantly changing and adapting to a continually fluctuating external and internal environment.
- THE EXTERNAL ENVIRONMENT
  - **Social:** Crime vs. safety, poverty vs. prosperity, peace vs. social unrest, and presence vs. absence of support from social networks
  - **Physical:** Access to health care, sanitation, availability of clean water, and geographic location
- THE INTERNAL ENVIRONMENT includes cumulative life experiences, cultural and spiritual beliefs, age, developmental stage, sex, emotional factors, and perception of physical functioning.

DESIRED OUTCOMES

- Desired outcomes are to obtain and maintain optimal state of wellness and function through access to and use of health promotion, wellness, and illness prevention strategies.
- Health and wellness can be achieved through health education and positive action (stress management, smoking cessation, weight loss, immunizations, seeking health care).

ILLNESS-WELLNESS CONTINUUM

The Illness–Wellness Continuum is a data collection tool used to measure the level of wellness to premature death.
- It can be useful as a data collection guide or tool to set goals and find ways to improve a client's state of health or to have the client return to a previous state of health, which can include an illness within optimal wellness. The health care professional can assist the client to see where they are at on the continuum and seek ways to move toward optimal wellness.
- At the center of the continuum is the client's normal state of health.
- The range of wellness to illness runs from optimal wellness to severe illness.
- The degree of wellness is relative to the usual state of wellness for a client and is achieved through awareness, education, and personal growth.

Illness

- Illness is the impairment of a client's physical, social, emotional, spiritual, developmental, or intellectual functioning.
- Illness encompasses the effects of a disease on a client. However, illness and disease are not synonymous.

Response to illness can be influenced by:
- Degree of physical changes as a result of a disease process
- Perceptions by self and others of the illness, which can be influenced by various reliable and unreliable sources of information (friends, magazines, TV, internet)
- Cultural values and beliefs
- Denial or fear of illness
- Social demands, time constraints, economic resources, and health care access

HEALTH PROMOTION AND DISEASE PREVENTION

Use health education and awareness to reduce risk factors and promote health care.

HEALTH/WELLNESS DATA COLLECTION

- Physical data collection
- Evaluating health perceptions
- Identifying risks to health/wellness
- Identifying access to health care

Identifying social determinants of health

Neighborhood and Built Environment
- Air pollutants from factories exacerbate manifestations of asthma.
- Lack of sidewalks causes lack of safe places to walk for exercise.
- Limited public transportation affects ability to commute and less options for employment.

Social and Community Context
- Sole caregiver for family member neglects primary care for self.
- Health education materials about diet and exercise are not in the primary language of the client.
- Cultural or religious beliefs may impact decision about health care.

Economic Stability
- Prescription medication costs prohibit use of medications for chronic conditions.
- Lack of health insurance may cause delay in seeking care for symptoms.
- Financial difficulties prohibit client from completing prescribed treatments.

Health and Health Care
- Lack of primary care resources in community affects preventative care.
- Lack of providers in community may lead to lack of follow-up for chronic conditions.
- Lack of access to telehealth resources.

Education
- Lack of education leads to lower-paying jobs.
- Level of health literacy affects understanding of educational materials.
- Lower levels of education are associated with chronic medical conditions.

Food and Nutrition
- Lack of affordable, nutritious foods contributes to undernutrition or overnutrition.
- Food insecurity increases risk for chronic illnesses.
- Contaminated food causes foodborne illnesses.

NURSING CARE

Assist with determining the health needs of a client and create strategies to meet those needs QPCC

INTERVENTIONS

- Recommend resources to strengthen coping abilities. QPCC
- Identify and encourage use of support systems during times of illness and stress.
- Identify obstacles to health and wellness and create strategies to reduce these obstacles.
- Identify ways to reduce health risks and improve compliance.
- Assist with the development of health education methods to improve health awareness and reduce health risks.

Application Exercises

1. A nurse is assisting with the development of a plan of care for a client. The client is 50 years old. Their height is 63 inches (160 cm), and their BMI is 28. The client smokes 4 to 5 cigarettes daily. They exercise once every week. They have a family history of hypertension and diabetes. Describe the characteristics of this client that are modifiable variables and nonmodifiable variables.

2. A nurse is collecting data with a client during their first appointment in a clinic. Match each characteristic to the aspect of health and wellness for which the nurse is collecting data.

   A. Environmental
   B. Occupational
   C. Spiritual
   D. Intellectual
   E. Social
   F. Emotional
   G. Physical

   1. Able to perform activities of daily living
   2. Expresses emotions
   3. Interacts successfully with others
   4. Able to effectively learn information
   5. Adopts beliefs that provide meaning to life
   6. Balances work time with leisure time
   7. Creates measures to improve quality of life

3. A nurse in a health care clinic is assisting with the evaluation of the level of wellness for clients using the illness-wellness continuum tool. Sort the following clients by whether the nurse should measure them within the center of the continuum or within the range of optimal wellness to severe illness.

   A. A school-age client who is up-to-date on their immunizations
   B. An adult client who has influenza
   C. An adult client who has a new diagnosis of type 2 diabetes mellitus
   D. An adult client who has a long history of well-controlled rheumatoid arthritis
   E. An adolescent client who has a urinary tract infection

4. A nurse is caring for a client who was just informed of a new diagnosis of breast cancer. Which of the following statements by the client represents the SDOH of health and health care?

   A. "I do not have a family history of breast cancer."
   B. "I need a second opinion. There is no lump."
   C. "I wish we lived closer to the big medical centers in the city."
   D. "I hope I have enough sick leave to get paid for the time I will be off work."

5. A nurse is caring for a client who has a new diagnosis of type 2 diabetes mellitus and reports difficulty following the diet and remembering to take the prescribed medication. Which of the following actions should the nurse take to promote client compliance? (Select all that apply.)

   A. Recommend a referral to the dietitian to assist with meal planning.
   B. Contact the client's support system.
   C. Collect data regarding age-related cognitive awareness.
   D. Encourage the use of a daily medication dispenser.
   E. Review provided educational materials for home use.

Active Learning Scenario

A nurse is caring for a client who has a family history of cardiovascular disease and continues to smoke despite numerous attempts to quit. What nursing interventions should the nurse use to meet the health needs of this client? Use the ATI Active Learning Template: Basic Concept to complete this item.

RELATED CONTENT: Include one statement identifying the goal.

UNDERLYING PRINCIPLES: Include one statement regarding health promotion and disease prevention.

NURSING INTERVENTIONS: Include a minimum of four.

Active Learning Scenario Key

Using the ATI Active Learning Template: Basic Concept

RELATED CONTENT: Identifying obstacles for compliance and adherence

UNDERLYING PRINCIPLES: Health promotion and disease prevention are influenced by many factors that a nurse should address for a client's success.

NURSING INTERVENTIONS
- Assist with providing the client with resources to strengthen coping abilities.
- Encourage use of support systems (family, support group).
- Identify ways to improve adherence.
- Assist with the development of health education methods to reduce health risks.
- Identify the client's obstacles to health and wellness.
- Assist with the creation of strategies to reduce the client's obstacles.

Ⓝ *NCLEX® Connection: Health Promotion and Maintenance, High-Risk Behaviors*

Application Exercises Key

1. When generating solutions, the nurse should recognize that age, height, and family history of hypertension and diabetes are all non-modifiable variables. Smoking, BMI, and exercise are modifiable variables.

   Ⓝ *NCLEX® Connection: Health Promotion and Maintenance, Health Promotion/Disease Prevention*

2. A, 7; B, 6; C, 5; D, 4; E, 3; F, 2; G, 1

   When recognizing cues about health and wellness, the nurse collects data about physical aspects, such as activities of daily living. The nurse collects data about emotional aspects, such as expressing emotions. The nurse collects data about social aspects, such as interacting successfully with others. The nurse collects data about intellectual aspects, such as ability to effectively learn information. The nurse collects data about spiritual aspects, such as adopting a belief that provides meaning to life. The nurse collects data about occupational aspects, such as balancing work time with leisure time. The nurse collects data about environmental a

   Ⓝ *NCLEX® Connection: Health Promotion and Maintenance, Health Promotion/Disease Prevention*

3. **WITHIN THE RANGE OF OPTIMAL WELLNESS TO SEVERE ILLNESS:** B, C, E

   WITHIN THE CENTER OF THE CONTINUUM: A, D

   When recognizing cues, the nurse should recognize that the adult client who has a long history of well-controlled rheumatoid arthritis and the school-age client who is up-to-date on their immunizations are measured within the center of the continuum, which is the normal state of health for the client. Clients who have acute illness, such as influenza or a urinary tract infection, are measured within the range of optimal wellness to severe illness. A client who has a new diagnosis of a chronic disease, such as type 2 diabetes mellitus, is also meas.

   Ⓝ *NCLEX® Connection: Health Promotion and Maintenance, Health Promotion/Disease Prevention*

4. C. **CORRECT:** When evaluating the response of the client, the nurse recognizes that the statement "I wish we lived closer to the big medical centers in the city" represents the SDOH of health and health care, which include the availability of health care services.

   Ⓝ *NCLEX® Connection: Health Promotion and Maintenance, Community Resources*

5. A, B, D, E. **CORRECT:** When taking actions, the nurse should recognize that recommending the dietitian as a resource will promote client adherence by strengthening coping abilities. Contacting the client's support system will promote client adherence by encouraging the client to use the support system during times of illness and stress. Encouraging the use of a daily medication dispenser will promote medication adherence. Reviewing provided educational materials will promote client adherence by improving health awareness and reducing health risks after discharge. There is no indication that the nurse should collect data regarding the client's age-related cognitive awareness.

   Ⓝ *NCLEX® Connection: Health Promotion and Maintenance, Health Promotion/Disease Prevention*

CHAPTER 2

LGBTQIA Populations

The lesbian, gay, bisexual, transgender, queer, intersex, asexual (LGBTQIA) population is a diverse group that includes various races, ethnicities, ages, and socioeconomic statuses.

All health care professionals should establish a trusting relationship that is conducive for clients to discuss gender identity and sexual orientation. This will allow health care professionals to assist with planning care that is culturally sensitive, compassionate, and individualized while respecting the dignity of LGBTQIA population.

TERMINOLOGY

Multiple terms can be used to identify gender and sexual orientation. Some common terminology includes the following.

Sexuality: An individual's personal expression and experience of intimacy (not limited to sexual organs)

Sexual orientation: An individual's preferences based on sexual attraction, behaviors, identity, or combination of factors
- **Heterosexual:** Attracted to people of a different gender
- **Gay:** Attracted to people of the same gender
- **Lesbian:** Woman who is attracted to people of the same gender
- **Bisexual:** Attracted to more than one gender
- **Queer:** Identifying as a sexual orientation or gender identity outside of heterosexual norms

Gender identity: An individual's personal self-concept of gender, which can differ from sex assigned at birth. This is not the same as sexual orientation.
- **Cisgender:** Gender that aligns with sex assigned at birth
- **Gender-nonconforming:** Gender identity, expression, or role that differs from binary cultural norms of sex and gender
  - **Transgender:** Identifying as a gender that does not align with sex assigned at birth
    - **Trans woman:** An individual assigned male at birth who identifies as female
    - **Trans male:** An individual assigned female at birth who identifies as male
  - **Nonbinary:** Gender other than male or female (e.g., genderfluid, genderqueer, agender)

Gender dysphoria: The discomfort or distress that can be caused by a discrepancy between an individual's gender identity and sex assigned at birth.

Transition: Changing gender presentation or characteristics to align with one's gender identity.

> ! Language regarding identity can shift rapidly. Refer to current literature and LGBTQIA populations for updates as needed.

GENDER DYSPHORIA

Not all gender-nonconforming individuals have gender dysphoria. According to the *Diagnostic and Statistical Manual of Mental Disorders* (DSM-5-TR), children must experience at least six diagnostic criteria findings for at least 6 months to have gender dysphoria. The DSM-5-TR criteria for gender dysphoria for adolescents and adults include having at least two of the criteria findings for a least 6 months. **(2.1)**

2.1 Characteristics of gender dysphoria

CHILDREN	ADOLESCENTS AND ADULTS
• An ambition to be a gender other than the gender that matches assigned sex at birth	• An ambition to be a gender other than the gender that matches assigned sex at birth
• A strong preference for wearing clothing of or role-playing a gender other than the gender that matches assigned sex at birth	• A sentiment of having general emotions and reactions of a gender other than gender that matches assigned sex at birth
• A strong preference for playing with children of a gender other than the gender that matches assigned sex at birth	• An ambition to be treated as another gender
• A dislike of the child's own sexual anatomy	• An ambition to be rid of primary/secondary sex traits due to incongruence with one's experienced or expressed gender
• An ambition of primary/secondary sex traits that match the child's identified gender	• An ambition to stop development of anticipated secondary sex traits
• A strong rejection of traditionally masculine or feminine toys/activities/games	• An ambition for primary/secondary sex traits of a gender other than the gender that matches assigned sex at birth

American Psychiatric Association Publishing. (2022). Diagnostic and Statistical Manual of Mental Disorders (DSM-5-TR)

Health care professionals can assist individuals who have gender dysphoria with affirming their gender identity by reviewing various options for the expression of that identity and guiding decisions about treatment options for alleviating gender dysphoria.

- Discuss differences in gender roles and expression, which may involve living temporarily or full-time in a gender role that is consistent with the client's gender identity.
- Review social affirmation, which includes the use of pronouns that align with the client's gender identity.
- Discuss medical affirmation, use of hormones, and gender-affirming therapeutic procedures to change primary and/or secondary sex characteristics (e.g., breast/chest, external or internal genitalia, facial anatomy, body shape).
- Assist with referral for psychotherapy (individual, partner, family, or group) to allow an individual to explore their gender role, identity, and expression. Topics can include the impact of gender dysphoria and stigma on mental health; enhancing peer and social support; and alleviating internalized phobias.
- Discuss legal affirmation, including legally changing name and gender on forms of identification.

Transition may be done socially (disclosing to friends or family), legally (changing name and gender on legal documents), and/or medically (hormone therapy or surgical intervention). Clients in all stages of transition should be made to feel comfortable. Using the client's correct pronouns (e.g., he/him, she/her, they/them) is an easy way to build rapport with clients.

HEALTH PROMOTION AND DISEASE PREVENTION

SEXUALLY TRANSMITTED INFECTIONS

- Clients who are sexually active should receive annual screening for chlamydia, gonorrhea, syphilis, and HIV. The screening sites for chlamydia and gonorrhea can vary depending upon the client's sexual behavior.
- Examinations can be difficult or uncomfortable for clients who experience gender dysphoria. The provider should explain the process for examinations and screenings.
- Encourage clients to participate in their plan of care.

- Encourage consistent use of condoms to decrease risk of HIV.
- Reinforce education with at-risk clients about the use of pre-exposure prophylaxis (PreP) medication to prevent HIV infection.
- Reinforce education with clients who use sex toys about proper care. (Wash items with hot soapy water or other cleaners as recommended between each use, or cover items with new condom prior to each use.)
- Reinforce education with clients that condoms provide a barrier protection against STIs that are transmitted by infected secretions (e.g., HIV, gonorrhea, chlamydia, trichomoniasis). However, condoms are less effective against STIs transmitted via skin and mucous membrane contact (e.g., herpes simplex virus, human papillomavirus [HPV], syphilis).

CANCER

- Encourage clients to receive the recommended schedule of screenings for cancer.
- Reinforce education for transgender clients about their risk factors and encourage the continuation of recommended screenings for breast, cervical, uterine, or prostate cancer. (2.2)

HEALTHY PEOPLE 2030

According to the Healthy People 2030, the overall goal is to "improve the health, safety and well-being of lesbian, gay, bisexual, and transgender people." The focus is to collect data on the health conditions and improve health of LGBTQIA populations with a primary focus on adolescents. To accomplish this, the Healthy People 2030 has created the following objectives:

ADOLESCENTS

- Decrease bullying of LGBTQIA high school students.
- Decrease the proportion of LGBTQIA high school students who have used illicit drugs.
- Decrease suicidal thoughts in LGBTQIA high school students.

2.2 STI screening recommendations

CHLAMYDIA/GONORRHEA	Adapt screening recommendations based on the client's anatomy. (Extend annual, routine screening for chlamydia and gonorrhea in cisgender women younger than 25 to all clients who have a cervix).
	Screen at the rectum and pharynx for gonorrhea, depending upon the client's reported sexual behaviors and exposure.
SYPHILIS	At least annually, dependent upon the client's reported sexual behaviors and exposure
HIV	Discuss and offer to all transgender clients. Frequency of repeat screenings should be based on the client's level of risk.
HUMAN PAPILLOMAVIRUS (HPV), CERVICAL AND ANAL CANCER	Screening for clients who have a cervix should follow current screening guidelines for cervical cancer (women 21 to 29 years of age every 3 years with cytology, women 30 to 65 years of age every 3 years with cytology, or every 5 years with a combination of cytology and HPV testing).

Obtained from: https://www.cdc.gov/std/treatment-guidelines/screening-recommendations.htm

DATA COLLECTION

- Add additional surveys that collect data on LGBTQIA populations.
- Add additional states, territories, and the District of Columbia that use the standard module on sexual orientation and gender identity in the Behavioral Risk Factor Surveillance System.

SEXUALLY TRANSMITTED INFECTIONS

- Decrease the rate of syphilis in men who have sex with men.
- Decrease the number of new HIV infections.
- Promote knowledge of HIV status.
- Decrease number of new HIV diagnoses.
- Increase access to HIV medical care.
- Increase viral suppression.

SOCIAL DETERMINANTS OF HEALTH SDoH

Economic stability

Financial concerns possibly related to employment discrimination

Neighborhood and physical environment

- Unsafe environments can lead to isolation and violence.
- Rejection by family can lead to homelessness.

Education

School climates that are non-supporting increase the risk for bullying and violence among LGBTQIA adolescents.

Food

Potential lower socioeconomic status due to other factors can lead to financial instability and inability to purchase food.

Community and social context

- Increased social isolation
- Lack of family support can lead to decreased health outcomes.
- Stigma related to gender nonconformity can lead to prejudice and discrimination. This can contribute to abuse and neglect in relationships with peers and family members, which can lead to psychological distress.

Health care

- Discrimination and fear of disclosure of personal information can lead to client not seeking health care services.
- Limited access to health insurance
- Limited access to health care services (physical and mental health services)
- Decreased provider knowledge and comfort can lead to health disparities.

DATA COLLECTION

HEALTH RISK FACTORS

- Mental health conditions: depression, anxiety, eating disorders
- Suicidality
- BMI greater than 30
- Cardiovascular conditions
- STIs (HIV)

PATIENT-CENTERED CARE

CHILDREN

Prior to puberty, many children experiment with cross-gender play and expression. Sexual exploration, experimentation, and discovery are part of the normal process of incorporating sexuality into one's sexual identity. Cross-gender interests and expression in the prepubertal years are neither necessarily nor predictably associated with adolescent or adult sexual orientation. Children who are gender-nonconforming before puberty experience less gender dysphoria and more often identify as gay or lesbian than transgender in adolescence and adulthood.

NURSING INTERVENTIONS: During routine health care visits for toddlers and young children, assist with asking the child's guardians/parents about their child's gender play and preference, body image, self-esteem concerns, and expressions of femininity and masculinity. This allows for normalizing the child's ongoing and evolving sexuality, a universal developmental experience.

ADOLESCENTS

The American Academy of Pediatrics, American Academy of Family Physicians, American College of Obstetricians and Gynecologists, and Society for Adolescent Health and Medicine encourage health care professionals to routinely review concerns of sexuality with adolescent clients. Due to stigmas and discrimination, LGBTQIA adolescents are at an increased risk for depression and suicide, using alcohol and drugs, and experiencing bullying. Adolescents are at high risk for victimization, harassment, assault, and physical and sexual abuse, which can occur at home, school, or in the community.

NURSING INTERVENTIONS
- Provide compassionate care. Be knowledgeable and accepting.
- Ask the adolescent questions about their sexual identity, sexual attraction, sexual behaviors, and gender identity.
- Collect data about gender dysphoria in a direct, respectful manner.
- Assist with collaborating with school nurse (anti-bullying policies, school connectedness, opportunities for student engagement, academic support).

- School nurses can advocate for professional development activities among staff to increase the awareness of LGBTQIA adolescents to build a culture of inclusiveness. (Work with counselors and teachers to ensure policies. Offer support and safety. Ensure nondisclosure of adolescents' health records.)
- Offer the client and family counseling and psychotherapy.
- Address coexisting mental health concerns.
- Provide the client and family with information for peer support groups.

OLDER ADULTS

- There are approximately 217,000 to 700,000 transgender adults in the U.S. who are older than 65. Ⓖ
- There will be more than 7 million LGBTQIA adults age 65 or older by 2030.
- LGBTQIA populations are vulnerable to the stressors of lifelong discrimination and victimization, external and internalized stigma, and lack of access to quality physical and emotional support due to their sexual orientation or gender identity. These factors can result in poor outcomes for these populations.

NURSING INTERVENTIONS

- Respect the individual's sexual orientation and gender identification.
- Older adults may encounter issues such as increased social isolation and limited physical and mental health access, often caused by mistrust of these systems in terms of their sensitivity, a lack of expanded caregiver support, financial issues due employment discrimination, and legal issues connected to partner status and decision-making.
- Due to the stigma of the AIDS epidemic and fear of discrimination, older adults may withhold personal information about their sexual orientation or gender identity.

NURSING ACTIONS

Health care professionals should provide gender-affirming care to decrease stigmas and biases. Other actions include:
- Promote welcoming, therapeutic, and inclusive relationship with all clients.
- Use inclusive terms and language.
- Avoid assumptions about a client's identity.
- Ask the client their name and pronouns. Identify and include any request for name changes on client's health records.
- Assist with obtaining the client's health history: genetic background, support individuals, previous interventions for transitioning (medications, therapeutic procedures).

PHYSICAL EXAMINATION: Review client's health record prior to physical exam. Reinforce procedures and their importance. (Genitalia may not align with outward gender presentation.)

INTERPROFESSIONAL CARE

The interprofessional team can include providers, mental health professionals (psychologists, psychiatrists), endocrinologists, pediatricians, social workers, case managers, and school nurses.

Gender-affirming care

There are several types of gender-affirming surgeries (GAS) and gender-affirming procedures that can assist the client with transition to their identified gender. Some procedures produce feminizing or masculinizing effects that involve changes to the client's primary and secondary sex traits.

All adolescents and adults who desire gender-affirming therapeutic management should receive education and counseling on options for fertility preservation (sperm banking, oocyte or embryo freezing) prior to initiating the suppression of puberty or initiating hormonal therapy.

Therapies can be fully or partially reversible, or irreversible.
- **Fully reversible**: Use of gonadotropin-releasing hormone (GnRH) analogs
- **Partially reversible**: Hormone therapy to masculinize or feminize the body
- **Irreversible**: Surgical procedures

DATA COLLECTION

The Endocrine Society recommendations for individuals desiring hormonal therapy include the following.

ADOLESCENTS

- Interprofessional team of medical and mental health providers manage therapy, and confirm the adolescent's gender dysphoria and mental health capacity for informed consent.
- After the adolescent experiences physical changes in puberty, hormonal therapy can be initiated by gradually increasing the dose schedule.
- GnRH analogs are recommended to suppress puberty hormones.
- Clinical pubertal development should be monitored every 3 to 6 months and laboratory parameters every 6 to 12 months during sex hormone treatment.
- Depending on the state, surgery can be initiated in adolescents who 16 years or older with parental consent.

ADULTS

- Clinicians confirm the diagnostic criteria of gender dysphoria and the criteria for the endocrine phase of transition before beginning treatment.
- Clinicians should evaluate and address medical conditions that can be exacerbated by hormone depletion and treatment with sex hormones of the affirmed gender before beginning therapy.
- Endocrinologists provide education to clients undergoing therapy about the onset and time course of physical changes induced by sex hormone treatment.

The Endocrine Society recommendations for individuals desiring gender-affirming surgery include the following.

- Providers can approve GAS after a client completes at least 1 year of consistent adherence to hormone therapy (unless hormone therapy is not desired or medical contraindication is present).
- The clinician responsible for endocrine treatment and the primary care provider ensure appropriate medical clearance for genital gender-affirming surgery and collaborate with the surgeon regarding hormone use during and after surgery.
- Clinicians can refer clients who have undergone hormonal therapy for GAS when:
  - The client has had a satisfactory social role change.
  - The client is satisfied about the hormonal effects.
  - The client desires definitive surgical changes.
- Clients should pursue genital gender-affirming surgery only after the mental health provider and clinician responsible for endocrine transition therapy both agree that surgery is medically necessary and would benefit the client's overall health and/or well-being.

PATIENT-CENTERED CARE

THERAPEUTIC MANAGEMENT

HORMONE THERAPY GOALS
- Stimulate development of secondary gender characteristics.
- Possibly stop menstruation.

Gonadotropin-releasing hormone analogs

In adolescent clients, GnRH analogues are the preferred treatment for puberty suppression; however, they are very expensive.
- Adolescents who have a penis: GnRH prevents luteinizing hormone secretion and testosterone secretion.
- Adolescents who have a vagina: GnRH prevents the production of estrogens. Continuous oral contraceptives (or depot medroxyprogesterone) may be used to suppress menses.

Testosterone

An androgen hormone that converts to estrogen in oral form and promotes erythropoiesis

THERAPEUTIC EFFECTS
- Deepened voice
- Reduction in breast tissue
- Change in hair growth and distribution pattern
- Enlargement of the clitoris
- Increased muscle mass
- Vaginal dryness and cessation of menses

FORMS: Available for administration in topical gels, topical patch, IM injections, or oral form.
- PO is least effective and not used as first-line therapy.
- IM: Initiated at low dose and can increase dosage every 1 to 2 weeks as prescribed. Testosterone blood levels will vary.

- Sub-dermal: Pellets are implanted in the hip or lateral abdominal wall to umbilicus at least every 3 months.
- Buccal: Tablets are placed on the gums above the incisor tooth. Alternate sides of the oral cavity for placement. Replace within 8 hr if tablet accidentally falls out.
- Nasal: Gel is administered via metered dose pump; can cause rhinorrhea and epistaxis. The client should avoid blowing their nose or sniffing for at least 1 hr after administration.
- Topical gel or patch: Expensive; provides consistent results but at a decreased rate. Apply patch to upper arm, thigh, back, or abdomen. Wash hands and cover area with clothing after gel has dried. Wait at least 5 to 6 hr after application for swimming or showering because medication can be removed from skin.
- Axillary: Topical solution that is alcohol-based; flammable. Apply same time each morning. Wait at least 2 hr if desire to swim

NURSING INTERVENTIONS
- Reinforce with clients that it could take 1 year to see results.
- Monitor for adverse effects (weight gain, headaches, seborrhea, acne, edema, psychosis, polycythemia, hypercholesterolemia, liver impairment).
- Check for history of heart and liver disease (increased risk for heart attack and stroke and can cause increase liver enzymes and low-density lipoproteins [LDLs]).
- Monitor hemoglobin, hematocrit, and cholesterol levels during therapy and testosterone levels at least every 3 months.
- Monitor weight, intake, and output.

Progesterone/Progestins

Medroxyprogesterone can be prescribed early during therapy and used short-term as a part feminizing therapy (assists with menstrual cessation).

NURSING CONSIDERATIONS: Monitor for adverse effects (depressed mood, weight gain).

Estrogen/Estradiol

Hormone that can be used for feminization therapy. There is a risk for prostate and breast cancer. Administered PO, transdermal, or as injection. If taken orally, there is an increased risk for venous thromboembolism (VTE). Therefore, transdermal or injectable estrogen is preferred.

THERAPEUTIC EFFECTS
- Breast tissue development
- Decrease testicular size and erectile function
- Decreased hair growth and muscle mass
- Softening of skin
- Emotional changes

NURSING CONSIDERATIONS
- Monitor estrogen and testosterone levels during therapy.
- Risk of prostate cancer, breast cancer.
- Monitor for adverse effects (headaches, nausea, vomiting, weight gain/loss, breast tenderness).

Spironolactone

Considered an antiandrogen; potassium-sparing diuretic that binds with androgen receptors that can inhibit testosterone secretion. Causes the adverse effects of gynecomastia, irregular menses, voice deepening, impotence, and hirsutism.

NURSING CONSIDERATIONS
- Monitor blood pressure (hypotension).
- Polyuria and polydipsia are common.
- Monitor potassium levels (hyperkalemia).

5-alpha-reductase inhibitors

Finasteride and dutasteride are considered an antiandrogen; prevents the conversion of testosterone; decreases size of prostate tissue.

NURSING CONSIDERATIONS: Monitor for adverse effects (dizziness, cold sweats, chills).

SURGICAL PROCEDURES

Gender-affirming surgeries are generally the last option in the transition process. The nurse should assist with collaborating with the interprofessional team, client, and family to promote positive outcomes for the client's transition. The general requirements for GAS include:
- Client should take continuous hormonal therapy for 1 year.
- Client should live in their desired role for at least 1 year.
- Client should be greater than 18 years of age and capable of making informed decisions and providing consent.

PROCEDURES
- **Hair removal** (electrolysis/laser/waxing) to remove facial hair or other areas of hair growth
- **Voice/communication therapy** to assist with the development of the client's verbal and nonverbal communication skills, which promotes comfort with their gender identity. A referral to a speech-language pathologist can be indicated.
- **Liposuction** to remove fatty tissue
- The client may also desire other noninvasive practices, such as breast binding or padding, genital tucking or prostheses, and padding of hips or buttocks.

Face/neck

- **Hair transplantation**
- **Facial reconstruction** to reshape the client's facial features
- **Chondrolaryngoplasty** reduction of the thyroid cartilage to minimize the prominent appearance of the Adam's apple

Breast

- **Augmentation** simulates breast tissue by use of implant (gel, saline, silicone).
  - Client may experience soreness and bruising after surgery.
- **Mastectomy** removes breast tissue.

Genitals

- **Orchiectomy** involves removal of one or both testicles.
- **Hysterectomy** removes the uterus.
- **Salpingo-oophorectomy** removes ovaries.
- **Penectomy** removes the penis.
- **Vaginectomy** removes the vagina.
- **Scrotoplasty** inserts prosthetic testes for the creation of a scrotum.
- **Vaginoplasty** creates a vagina.
- **Phalloplasty** creates a penis.

NURSING INTERVENTIONS

PREOPERATIVE CARE

- Ensure the client has provided informed consent.
- Ensure the client receives written/verbal instructions about procedure.
- Reinforce instructions with the client about the preparation of the bowels (clear liquids, laxatives, enemas if prescribed).
- Encourage the client to increase intake of fluids.
- Reinforce with the client about lab tests (hemoglobin and hematocrit).
- Assist with preparing the client for surgery.
  - Insert peripheral IV.
  - Administer prescribed antimicrobials on the day of surgery.

PERIOPERATIVE CARE

- Ensure the client is positioned properly. Lithotomy position is often used, depending on type of surgery.
- Assist with monitoring for adverse effects of general or epidural anesthesia.

POSTOPERATIVE CARE

- Check for pain. Administer prescribed analgesics.
- Monitor vital signs.
- Provide care for catheters or drains.
- Monitor operative site for bleeding or infection. Provide wound care as prescribed (cleansing/packing).
- Administer hormone medication as prescribed.
- Apply ice to affected area to decrease swelling and discomfort.
- Monitor neurovascular status. Encourage movement of lower limbs to prevent compartment syndrome.
- Administer anticoagulants to prevent VTE.
- Encourage client to adhere to activity level (bed rest).
- Remove urinary catheter (postoperative day 7 to 12) and drains (drainage less than 20 mL in 24 hr) as prescribed, depending on type of surgical procedure.
- Apply breast binders as indicated for breast surgeries.
- Monitor for unexpected findings or complications (VTE, vaginal/rectal fistulas, perforation, compartment syndrome of lower limbs, bleeding, surgical wound infection, urinary incontinence, hematomas).

POSTOPERATIVE CLIENT EDUCATION

- Encourage the client to keep follow-up appointments.
- Report leakage of stool may indicate fistula.
- Provide social support by referring to support groups and other community resources.

VAGINOPLASTY

- Do not take submersion baths for at least 8 weeks.
- Avoid strenuous activities for at least 6 weeks.
- Avoid activities such as swimming or bike riding for at least 3 months.
- Scant vaginal bleeding or brownish drainage is expected for at least 6 weeks.
- Take stool softeners as prescribed.
- Follow recommended instructions for wound care (vaginal packing/dilators).

Active Learning Scenario

A nurse is assisting with providing an education session to a group of newly licensed nurses about nursing interventions for adolescents who experience gender dysphoria. Discuss at least four interventions that the nurse should take. Use the ATI Active Learning Template: Basic Concept to complete this.

Application Exercises

1. A nurse is reinforcing teaching about STI prevention for a group of clients who identify as LGBTQIA. Which of the following statements by the clients indicates understanding? (Select all that apply.)

   A. "Condoms are effective against herpes when lesions are present."

   B. "I should receive yearly screenings for chlamydia and gonorrhea."

   C. "Condoms should be used consistently."

   D. "The sites for STI screening can vary depending on my preference for sexual activity."

   E. "It's considered a low risk if I have more than one partner."

2. A nurse is discussing the care of LGBTQIA populations with a group of newly licensed nurses. Which of the following statements should the nurse include in their discussion? (Select all that apply.)

   A. "Adolescents who identify as LGBTQIA have an increased risk for experiencing bullying."

   B. "Older adults who identify as LGBTQIA are at risk for social isolation."

   C. "The nurse should ask clients about their gender identity."

   D. "The nurse should respect the client's gender identity."

   E. "The nurse should discuss the client's gender identity with other relatives."

3. A nurse is reinforcing teaching with a client who has a new prescription for testosterone gel. Which of the following statements should the nurse make? (Select all that apply.)

   A. "You should have your testosterone level checked within 1 month after starting therapy and then every 3 months."

   B. "This medication can cause headaches, swelling, and weight gain."

   C. "You will notice results within 1 month of therapy."

   D. "After the gel has dried, you should cover the area with clothing."

   E. "This medication can cause your cholesterol level to increase."

4. A nurse is reviewing the EMR of a client who is desiring gender-affirming surgery. Which of the following information from the client's record should the nurse identify as required criteria for surgery?

   A. The client has lived alone for at least 6 months.

   B. The client is at least 16 years of age.

   C. The client has taken continuous hormonal therapy for at least 1 year.

   D. The client's partner gives informed consent.

5. A nurse is assisting with planning care for a client following gender-affirming surgery (GAS) of the genitalia. Which of the following actions should the nurse recommend implementing? (Select all that apply.)

   A. Remove urinary catheter within 24 hr.

   B. Apply ice to affected area.

   C. Remove drains when output is greater than 20 mL/hr.

   D. Administer anticoagulants.

   E. Perform frequent neurovascular checks.

Active Learning Scenario Key

Using the ATI Active Learning Template: Basic Concept
- Provide compassionate care. Be knowledgeable and accepting.
- Ask the adolescent questions about their sexual identity, sexual attraction, sexual behaviors, and gender identity.
- Collect data about gender dysphoria in a direct, respectful manner.
- Assist with collaborating with school nurse (anti-bullying policies, school connectedness, opportunities for student engagement, academic support).
- School nurses can advocate for professional development activities among staff to increase the awareness of LGBTQIA population/adolescents to build culture of inclusiveness (work with counselors and teachers to ensure policies offer support and safety and ensure non-disclosure of the adolescents' health record).
- Offer counseling and psychotherapy to the client and family.
- Address coexisting mental health concerns.
- Provide the client and family with information for peer support groups.

ⓝ *NCLEX® Connection: Management of Care, Advocacy*

Application Exercises Key

1. A. Condoms are least effective at preventing the transmission of STIs such as genital herpes because this condition is spread by contact with active lesions as well.
    B. **CORRECT:** The screening recommendations for clients who are sexually active include yearly screenings for chlamydia and gonorrhea. This would allow early identification of these conditions and prevent the possible transmission to others.
    C. **CORRECT:** Condoms serve as a barrier of protection against certain STIs and should be used consistently to prevent the transmission of STIs such as gonorrhea, chlamydia, HIV, and trichomoniasis.
    D. **CORRECT:** The screening sites for STIs can vary depending on the client's preference for sexual activity.
    E. The client is considered high risk if they have multiple sex partners.

ⓝ *NCLEX® Connection: Health Promotion and Maintenance, Health Promotion/Disease Prevention*

2. A, B, C, D. **CORRECT:** The nurse should also discuss risk factors for LGBTQIA populations such as adolescents being bullied and older adults at increased risk for social isolation. Information about LGBTQIA populations should include the nurse respecting the client's gender identity, asking questions about the client's gender identity, and maintaining the client's confidentiality.

ⓝ *NCLEX® Connection: Health Promotion and Maintenance, Health Promotion/Disease Prevention*

3. A. **CORRECT:** The client should have their testosterone level checked within 1 month of starting therapy and then at least every 3 months.
    B. **CORRECT:** Testosterone can cause adverse effects of headache, weight gain, edema, psychosis, and hypercholesterolemia.
    C. After client takes testosterone, it can take at least 1 year to see the expected results.
    D. **CORRECT:** The nurse should inform the client to wash their hands before and after application and apply to dry skin as prescribed. After the gel has dried, cover the area with clothing.
    E. **CORRECT:** Testosterone is an androgen hormone that can be taken as part of gender-affirming care to produce masculinizing effects. The nurse should inform the client about administration and adverse effects of therapy.

ⓝ *NCLEX® Connection: Pharmacological Therapies, Expected Actions/Outcomes*

4. C. **CORRECT:** General requirements for gender-affirming surgery include that the client must be at least 18 years of age, has taken continuous hormonal therapy for at least 1 year, has lived in their identified gender identity for at least 1 year, and gives informed consent for surgery.

ⓝ *NCLEX® Connection: Reduction of Risk Potential, Therapeutic Procedures*

5. B, D, E. **CORRECT:** When assisting with planning care for a client following GAS, the nurse should recommend to apply ice to the affected area, administer anticoagulants, and perform frequent neurovascular checks. Applying ice will decrease swelling to affected area, administering anticoagulants will prevent VTE, and performing frequent neurovascular checks will assist with identifying unexpected findings such as compartment syndrome.
    A, C. If a client has an indwelling urinary catheter, the nurse should plan to remove it 7 to 12 days following GAS, and remove drains when output is less than 20 mL/day.

ⓝ *NCLEX® Connection: Physiological Adaptation, Alterations in Body Systems*

UNIT 1   FOUNDATIONS OF NURSING
CARE FOR ADULT CLIENTS

CHAPTER 3   *Emergency Nursing Principles and Management*

Emergency nursing principles are the guidelines that nurses follow to identify and manage emergency situations for a client or multiple clients. The emergency department (ED) can be a tedious environment that requires the nurse to use clinical judgment to care for clients with various conditions. Nurses must have the ability to identify and report emergent situations and assist with intervening when life-threatening conditions exist.

Overcrowding and increased wait times in the ED are major concerns in the health care setting. Nurses and all members of the interprofessional team must do their part to ensure that client care is managed effectively in the ED.

A Goal of Healthy People 2030 is to decrease emergency department visits with a longer wait time rather than recommend for a client to see a provider in the emergency care setting. Q EBP

The Joint Commission updated their Core Measures to make facilities accountable for wait times in the ED to time of transfer to inpatient hospital admission bed. This would improve quality care by improving the client's access to recommended treatments. Overall, this will allow the facility to evaluate their processes and determine how to improve their services to ensure quality of care in the emergency care setting.

Emergency nursing principles: triage, primary survey (ABCDE principles), secondary survey

Emergency nursing care management: cold/heat injuries, poisoning/bites, substance use disorder, drug overdose, trauma, maltreatments, human trafficking, psychiatric emergencies, cardiac emergencies Q EBP

TRIAGE

Triage is known as setting priorities. Time and experience are required for the nurse to become an effective member of the triage team. The nurse, provider, and other members of the health care team work together in the triage area to determine the needs of the client.

EDs can use either a three- or five-level system (such as the Emergency Severity Index [ESI] or the Canadian Triage and Acuity Scale [CTAS]) to triage and categorize clients' conditions.
- The three-level system of triage consist of these categories: emergent (life-threatening), urgent (treat within 2 hr), and nonurgent (can delay treatment).
- The CTAS categorizes client conditions (with the inclusion of time parameters) as: resuscitation (level one), emergent (level two), urgent (level three), less urgent (level four), and nonurgent (level five). Resuscitation triage requires immediate treatment to prevent death. Nonurgent is a non-life-threatening condition requiring simple evaluation and care management.

PRIMARY SURVEY

A primary survey is a rapid data collection to detect life-threatening conditions.
- The primary survey should be completed systematically so life-threatening conditions are not missed.
- Standard precautions (gloves, gowns, eye protection, face masks, and shoe covers) must be worn to prevent contamination with bodily fluids.
- The ABCDE can be used to as a method of triage by the nurse to guide the primary survey.

ABCDE PRINCIPLE

AIRWAY/CERVICAL SPINE

This is the most important step in performing the primary survey. If a patent airway is not established, subsequent steps of the primary survey are futile. As a result of hypoxia, brain injury or death will occur within 3 to 5 min if the airway is not patent. Q s

NURSING ACTIONS

- Determine airway patency. (If airway is partially obstructed, speech could be potentially coarse or muffled.)
- If a client is awake and responsive, the airway is open.
- If the client is unresponsive without suspicion of trauma, the airway should be opened with a head-tilt/chin-lift maneuver. Qs
  - Do NOT perform this technique on clients who have a potential cervical spine injury.
  - To perform the head-tilt/chin-lift maneuver, the nurse should assume a position at the head of the client, place one hand on the forehead, and place the other hand underneath the client's chin. The head should be tilted while the chin is lifted upward and forward. This maneuver lifts the tongue away from the laryngopharynx and provides for a patent airway. Qs
- If the client is unresponsive with suspicion of trauma, the airway should be opened with a modified jaw thrust maneuver.
  - The nurse should assume a position at the head of the client and place both hands on either side of the client's head. Locate the connection between the maxilla and the mandible. Lift the jaw superiorly while maintaining alignment of the cervical spine.
- Inspect the airway for blood, broken teeth, vomitus, and secretions. If present, obstructions should be cleared with suction or a finger-sweep method if the object is clearly visible.
- The open airway can be maintained with airway adjuncts, such as an oropharyngeal or nasopharyngeal airway.
- A bag valve mask with a 100% oxygen source is indicated for clients who need additional support during resuscitation until an advanced airway is established.
- A non-rebreather mask with 100% oxygen source is indicated for clients who are spontaneously breathing.

BREATHING

Once a patent airway is achieved, the nurse should check for the presence and effectiveness of breathing.

DATA COLLECTION

- Auscultation of breath sounds
- Observation of chest expansion and respiratory effort
- Notation of rate and depth of respirations
- Identification of chest trauma
- Determination of tracheal position
- Oxygen saturation level

NURSING ACTIONS: If a client is not breathing or is breathing inadequately, manual ventilation should be performed by a bag valve mask with supplemental oxygen or mouth-to-mask ventilation until a bag valve mask can be obtained.

CIRCULATION

- Once adequate ventilation is accomplished, circulation is determined.
- Nurses should check heart rate, blood pressure, peripheral pulses, and capillary refill for adequate perfusion.
- Check for bleeding. Control bleeding if present.
- Nurses should consider cardiac arrest, myocardial dysfunction, and hemorrhage as precursors to shock and leading to ineffective circulation.
- Shock can develop if circulation is compromised. Shock is the body's response to inadequate tissue perfusion and oxygenation. It manifests with an increased heart rate and hypotension and can result in tissue ischemia and necrosis.

NURSING ACTIONS

- **Interventions for restoring effective circulation**
  - Perform CPR. Qpcc
  - Hemorrhage control: Apply direct pressure to visible, significant external bleeding.
    - If bleeding is not controlled with direct pressure, apply a tourniquet distal to injured area.
  - Ensure client has IV access (large-bore IV catheters are inserted into the antecubital fossa of both arms unless there is obvious injury to the extremity).
  - Assist with infusion isotonic IV fluids, such as lactated Ringer's and 0.9% sodium chloride, and/or blood products.
- **Interventions to alleviate shock** Qpcc
  - Administer oxygen.
  - Apply pressure to obvious bleeding.
  - Monitor client receiving IV fluids and blood products.
  - Monitor vital signs and intake and urinary output.
  - Remain with the client and provide reassurance and support for anxiety.

3.1 AVPU mnemonic

A Alert
V Responsive to **v**oice
P Responsive to **p**ain
U Unresponsive

3.2 Glasgow Coma Scale

EYE-OPENING RESPONSE		+ VERBAL RESPONSE		+ MOTOR RESPONSE	
Spontaneous	4	Oriented	5	Obeys commands	6
To voice	3	Confused	4	Localizes pain	5
To pain	2	Inappropriate words	3	Withdraws	4
None	1	Incomprehensible sounds	2	Flexion	3
		None	1	Extension	2
				None	1

A score less than 8 indicates severe brain injury. A score of 15 is expected for a client who has neurological function within expected limits.

DISABILITY

Disability is a quick check to determine the client's level of consciousness.

- The nurse can use various tools, such as the AVPU mnemonic. Q_EBP
- The Glasgow Coma Scale is another widely-used method. Q_EBP

NURSING ACTIONS: Neurologic checks must be repeated at frequent intervals to ensure immediate response to any change.

EXPOSURE

The nurse collects further data and looks for injuries that are not visibly apparent. The nurse must maintain the client's privacy and remove clothing to look for any life-threatening injuries.

NURSING ACTIONS

- The nurse removes the client's clothing for a complete physical assessment. The nurse might need to cut off the client's clothing to accomplish this task.
- Clothing is always removed during a resuscitation situation to assess for additional injuries or those related to chemical and thermal burns involving the clothing.
- The nurse should preserve items of evidence (clothing, bullets, drugs, weapons).
- Cover client with blanket to keep warm.

SECONDARY SURVEY

The secondary survey is performed after the priorities are completed. Some of the responsibilities of the nurse include:

- Assist with obtaining comprehensive physical assessment and health history.
- Assist with performing diagnostic and laboratory testing and review the results.
- Provide wound care and insertion of drainage tubes.
- Provide comfort and emotional support to the client and family.
- Assist with crisis intervention.
- Assist with implementing appropriate referrals if needed.

Heat- and cold-related injuries

Hypothermia, heatstroke, and frostbite are some of the conditions that can occur because of exposure to heat and cold. **Hypothermia** occurs when the client's core temperature is 35° C (95° F) or less. **Heat exhaustion** occurs after prolonged exposure to elevated temperatures and causes excessive diaphoresis and tachycardia, leading to dehydration. Clients must receive rapid treatment for the dehydration and low sodium to prevent developing heat stroke. **Heat stroke** is a medical emergency, and clients must receive immediate treatment to prevent death. **Frostbite** is a skin condition that is caused by exposure of the skin to frigid temperatures and results in vascular and cellular damage.

DATA COLLECTION

RISK FACTORS

Hypothermia

- Victims of trauma are at risk for hypothermia due to exposure, unwarmed oxygen, and cold IV fluids.
- Clients who are without permanent housing
- Age (older adults, infants).

Heatstroke

- Clients who work in hot environments
- Age (older adults, younger children)

EXPECTED FINDINGS

Hypothermia

- Shivering
- Impaired judgment
- Dysarthria
- Drowsiness
- Unexpected body core temperature

Heatstroke

- Elevated temperature (greater than 40° C [104° F])
- Perspiration (present/absent)
- Increased heart rate
- Alterations in mental status
- Unexpected blood potassium or sodium levels

Frostbite

Extent of injury to exposed skin may not be evident for at least 24 hr after injury and is categorized as superficial (first degree), partial thickness (second degree), or full thickness (third and fourth degree).

- First degree: Least severe form. Only superficial layers of exposed skin are affected with hyperemia and edema.
- Second degree: Blisters with clear to milky fluid, swelling, discoloration of skin.
- Third degree: Blister dark in coloration and filled with dark fluid, necrosis, possible eschar. May require debridement.
- Fourth degree: Lack of blood supply to the affected area leads to necrosis that extends to tendons, bone, and muscle; presence of gangrene. May require amputation of affected part area.

PATIENT-CENTERED CARE

NURSING ACTIONS

Hypothermia

- Check the client's status by using ABCDE.
- Monitor and obtain the client's core temperature and vital signs.
- Remove wet clothing from the client.
- Cover the client with warm blankets.

- Increase the temperature of the room.
- Use a heat lamp to provide additional warmth.
- Assist with infusion of warmed IV fluids.
- Monitor for complications: hypoxemia, acidosis, and comatose state.

Heat stroke/exhaustion

- Administer oxygen as needed.
- Ensure client has large-gauge IV catheter.
- Insert indwelling urinary catheter if indicated.
- Apply cool wet towels, ice packs, and cooling blankets.

CLIENT EDUCATION

To prevent hyperthermia

- Wear lightweight, loose-fitting clothing.
- Avoid excessive sun exposure.
- Stay indoors with fans or air conditioning when outside temperatures are elevated.
- Limit consumption of alcohol and caffeine.
- If overheated, take a cool water shower or bath.

Frostbite

- Prepare to rewarm client. Bathing affected areas in warm bath (104° to 108° F [40° to 42° C]) will improve blood circulation and promote healing of damaged tissue. This rewarming process can increase pain as circulation improves to affected areas of skin.
- Avoid rubbing or massaging injured area.
- Collect data for pain. Administer prescribed analgesic if needed.
- Administer tetanus toxoid IM vaccine to prevent complications related to growth of tetanus in wounds.

Poisoning

Poisoning is exposure to a toxic agent (medication, illicit drug, or ingestion of toxic agent). Poisoning can be intentional or unintentional and is considered a medical emergency and requires rapid management therapy.

DATA COLLECTION

RISK FACTORS: Children less than 5 years of age are at risk for accidental poisoning.

EXPECTED FINDINGS: Sudden alteration in level of consciousness

PATIENT-CENTERED CARE

NURSING ACTIONS

Obtain a client history to identify the toxic agent. Treatment depends on the type of toxic agent.

- Implement supportive care.
- Contact the poison control center (800-222-1222).
- Monitor laboratory tests (blood toxin screen, electrolytes, ABGs, blood glucose levels, coagulation profile, kidney and liver function).
- Prevent further absorption of the toxin.
- Extract or remove the poison.
- Administer antidotes when necessary.
- Assist with providing measures for respiratory support (oxygen, airway management, mechanical ventilation).
- Monitor compromised circulation (resulting from excess perspiration, vomiting, diarrhea).
- Restore fluids with IV fluid therapy.
- Monitor blood pressure, cardiac monitoring, and ECG.
- Assist with procedures as indicated depending on type of poisoning: activated charcoal (given PO or by NGT), gastric lavage (if done within 1 hr of ingestion), and administration of cathartics, such as sorbitol. Syrup of ipecac is no longer recommended; vomiting increases the risk for aspiration.
- Other actions depending on the type of poisoning include dialysis and hemoperfusion to remove toxins.
- Administer diazepam if seizures occur.

Opioid poisoning (overdose)

CDC reports the incidence of opioid drug overdose is steadily increasing and is the leading cause of injury and death in the United States. Prescription and illegal opioid misuse and overdose are currently a national epidemic. A Healthy People 2030 goal is to decrease drug overdose deaths by increasing access to naloxone and to increase the proportion of people who get a referral for substance use treatment after an ED visit. The American Heart Association has developed new opioid-associated emergency guidelines for emergency responders and health care providers to use for clients who have suspected opioid poisoning. First responders are now equipped with naloxone for emergent injection if opioid poisoning is suspected. Ⓠ EBP

DATA COLLECTION

EXPECTED FINDINGS

- Pinpoint pupils
- Decreased blood pressure
- Respiratory depression
- Seizures
- Decreased LOC
- Hypoxia

PATIENT-CENTERED CARE

NURSING ACTIONS

- Monitor for expected findings.
- Check for responsiveness and breathing. If client is not breathing and has absent pulse, initiate CPR and use an AED.
- If the client is breathing and has a pulse, maintain open airway, and provide rescue breathing.
- Reverse heroin and other opiate toxicity with naloxone (antagonist).
- Initiate referral for substance use treatment and management.

Bites (animals/snakes/ spiders/bugs)

A snakebite from a venomous snake is a medical emergency. The nurse should be familiar with indigenous snakes in the community.

RISK FACTORS

Children ages 1 to 9 are at highest risk for snakebites.

EXPECTED FINDINGS

- Pain
- Nausea, vomiting
- Numbness
- Paresthesia

PATIENT-CENTERED CARE

NURSING ACTIONS

Snake/spider bite

- Check for tissue edema every 15 to 30 min if bitten by a snake or spider. Monitor circumference of affected extremity.
- Administer opioid medications for pain due to snake or spider bite.
- Generally, ice, tourniquets, heparin, and corticosteroids are contraindicated in the first 6 to 8 hr after the bite.
- Antivenom based on the type and severity of a snake bite is most effective if administered within 4 to 12 hr.

Animal bite

- Clean with soap and rinse with warm water for 5 to 10 minutes.
- Apply antibiotic ointment, clean bandage, and gauze dressing.
- Administer tetanus immunization if indicated.
- Administer rabies immunization if indicated (given days 3, 7, and 14).
- Administer antibiotics for deep puncture wounds if indicated.

Psychiatric emergencies

A psychiatric emergency is an urgent situation in which the client has disturbances of thought, affect, mood, and behavior that can result in the client being unable to cope. The CDC reports that the number of ED visits with clients who have behavioral disorders has increased.

DATA COLLECTION

EXPECTED FINDINGS

- Changes in mood
- Anxiety
- Stress
- Decreased self-esteem

PATIENT-CENTERED CARE

NURSING ACTIONS

- Be calm, supportive, and reassuring.
- Monitor for expected findings.
- Avoid restraints.
- Administer medications as indicated.
- Provide safe environment (suicidal).
- Refer for crisis intervention (suicidal).
- Initiate safety precautions (suicidal).

Violence (intimate partner violence), maltreatment (child/elder maltreatment), human trafficking

In the ED setting, nurses must be able to recognize cues of physical violence and maltreatment. It is mandated by law that these findings are reported. Human trafficking is the exploitation of individuals by coercion or force. Human trafficking is increasing globally and affects more than 20 million individuals per year. These individuals may have limited access to health care. The ED is often the setting in which the individual presents with injuries.

DATA COLLECTION

RISK FACTORS

- Vulnerable clients
- History of substance use and misuse

EXPECTED FINDINGS

- Bruising
- Hematomas
- Burns
- Lacerations
- Skeletal fractures

- Black eyes
- Blunt trauma to abdomen
- Injuries that are healing in various stages
- Frightened appearance
- Agitation
- May report dizziness, headache, rash, sores, abdominal pain (human trafficking)

PATIENT-CENTERED CARE

NURSING ACTIONS

- Be supportive.
- Ask questions (may need to ask when not around others).
- Preserve items of evidence (clothing, bullets, drugs, weapons).

Cardiac emergencies

The Joint Commission requires all health care facilities to implement an early warning system (EWS), which identifies a client's physiologic status based on scoring matrix. The client, their family, and staff can activate the EWS in the event of declining health.

A Rapid Response Team (RRT) can respond to the EWS incident. An RRT is an interprofessional team that can consist of a respiratory therapist, critical care nurse, hospitalists, and other health care providers. The RRT evaluates the client's condition and determines the plan of action to improve client outcomes.

EMERGENCY NURSE CERTIFICATIONS

- Basic Life Support (BLS), Advanced Cardiac Life Support (ACLS), and Pediatric Advanced Life Support (PALS) are certifications required for nurses practicing in United States emergency departments. Current BLS and ACLS guidelines are available from the American Heart Association (AHA) at www.heart.org.
- BLS involves a hands-on approach for assessment and management to restore airway, breathing, and circulation.
- ACLS builds on the BLS assessment and management skills to include advanced concepts.
  - Cardiac monitoring for specific resuscitation rhythms, airway management, defibrillation, cardioversion, IV access, administration of antidysrhythmic medications and management of post-resuscitation clients
- PALS is built on the BLS protocol for neonatal and pediatric assessment and management skills to include advanced concepts for resuscitation of children.
- Certification courses are based on evidence-based practice management theory and the basic concepts and techniques for cardiopulmonary resuscitation (CPR). Q EBP

PATIENT-CENTERED CARE

SUDDEN CARDIAC ARREST

NURSING ACTIONS

- If a client is not responsive, has no respirations, and has no pulse, call for help and initiate CPR.
- Obtain and use an automated external defibrillator, when available.
- Ensure the client has a patent IV access.
- Gather emergency resuscitative equipment.
- Assist with the transfer of client to a higher level of care post-resuscitation.

VENTRICULAR FIBRILLATION AND PULSELESS VENTRICULAR TACHYCARDIA

Ventricular fibrillation (VF) is the fluttering of the ventricles that causes a loss of consciousness, pulselessness, and apnea. This requires collaborative care to defibrillate immediately using ACLS protocol.

Pulseless ventricular tachycardia (pVT) is an irritable firing of ectopic ventricular beats at a rate of 140 to 180/min. The client may eventually become unconscious and deteriorate into VF.

AHA ACLS guidelines for VF or pulseless VT

- Initiate the CPR components of BLS. Q EBP
- Defibrillate according to AHA ACLS guidelines.
- Provide 2 minutes of high-quality CPR. (Ensure (IV/IO access is established if not already present.)
- Monitor heart rhythm to determine the need to defibrillate. If the rhythm is not shockable, reevaluate for post-resuscitation care.
- If the rhythm is shockable, shock should be delivered, followed by 2 minutes of high-quality CPR.
- Epinephrine is administered according to ACLS guidelines. Client may require advanced airway placement.

OTHER ACTIONS

- The client may receive amiodarone or lidocaine if not responding to epinephrine.
- Identify reversible causes and assist with treatment.

3.3 Common causes of pulseless electrical activity

5 H's	5 T's
Hypovolemia	Toxins (drug or medication toxicity)
Hypoxia	
Hydrogen ion accumulation, resulting in acidosis	Tamponade (cardiac)
	Tension pneumothorax
Hyperkalemia or hypokalemia	Thrombosis (coronary)
	Thrombosis (pulmonary)
Hypothermia	

PULSELESS ELECTRICAL ACTIVITY/ VENTRICULAR ASYSTOLE

Pulseless electrical activity (PEA) is a rhythm that appears to have electrical activity but is not sufficient to stimulate effective cardiac contractions and requires implementation of BLS and ACLS protocol.

Asystole: a complete absence of electrical activity and ventricular movement of the heart. The client is in complete cardiac arrest and requires implementation of BLS and ACLS protocol.

AHA ACLS Protocol for PEA/Asystole

- Assist with providing and initiating the CPR components of BLS.
- Perform high-quality CPR for 2 minutes. (Ensure (IV/IO access is established if not already present).
- Epinephrine is administered according to ACLS (may need advanced airway insertion), and capnography.
- Check heart rhythm. Determine the need to deliver shock.
- Determine common causes of condition.
- If the rhythm is shockable, shock should be delivered, followed by 2 minutes of high-quality CPR.

OTHER ACTIONS
- The client may receive amiodarone or lidocaine.
- Asystole is often the final rhythm as the electrical and mechanical activity of the heart has stopped. The provider should consider ceasing resuscitation if asystole persists.

Active Learning Scenario

A nurse newly hired to an emergency department (ED) is reviewing emergency triage. Use the ATI Active Learning Template: Basic Concept to complete this item.

RELATED CONTENT: Identify the most common categories of the ED triage system.

UNDERLYING PRINCIPLES: Define each of the three triage levels.

NURSING INTERVENTIONS: Describe a client who meets the criteria for each of the three triage levels.

Application Exercises

1. A nurse in the ED is assisting with the care of a group of clients. Which of the following clients should the nurse classify as urgent when using the three-level system of triage? (Select all that apply.)
   A. Client who reports nausea and insomnia
   B. Client who has a pressure injury and a blood glucose of 200 mg/dL (less than 200 mg/dL)
   C. Client who reports right calf pain and shortness of breath
   D. Client who has left-sided weakness and numbness
   E. Client who reports urinary frequency and fever

2. A nurse encounters an unresponsive client during a walk. The client's partner states, "He was pulling weeds in the yard and slumped to the ground." Which of the following techniques should the nurse use to open the client's airway?
   A. Head-tilt, chin-lift maneuver
   B. Modified jaw thrust
   C. Hyperextension of the head
   D. Flexion of the head

3. A nurse is assisting with caring for a client who has been exposed to freezing temperatures for several hours and is alert and talking. Which of the following actions should the nurse take? (Select all that apply.)
   A. Remove wet clothing.
   B. Maintain room temperature.
   C. Apply warm blankets.
   D. Assist with infusing warm IV fluids.
   E. Administer acetaminophen.

4. A nurse in the ED is assisting with the care of a client who is suspected of having opioid poisoning. While collecting data during the interview, the nurse notes that the client suddenly becomes unresponsive, and respirations and pulse are absent. Which of the following actions should the nurse take? (Select all that apply.)
   A. Monitor the client after receiving naloxone.
   B. Monitor the client after receiving lidocaine.
   C. Administer syrup of ipecac.
   D. Begin performing CPR.
   E. Obtain AED.

5. A nurse in the ED is assisting with the care for a client who suddenly becomes unresponsive and notes ventricular asystole on their monitor. Sort the actions the nurse should assist with taking in the correct order.
   A. Analyze heart rhythm with AED.
   B. Observe administration of epinephrine.
   C. Perform initial round of high-quality CPR.
   D. Identify cause of condition.

Active Learning Scenario Key

Using the ATI Active Learning Template: Basic Concept

RELATED CONTENT
- Emergent
- Urgent
- Nonurgent

UNDERLYING PRINCIPLES
- Emergent: The client requires immediate treatment.
- Urgent: The client requires treatment within 2 hr.
- Nonurgent: The client can wait for treatment without threat to life.

NURSING INTERVENTIONS
- Emergent: A client who has sustained a traumatic amputation, or head or neck injury.
- Urgent: A client who has a kidney stone, gallbladder colic, or fracture.
- Nonurgent: A client who has a rash, minor cut, or backache.

(N) *NCLEX® Connection: Physiological Adaptation, Medical Emergencies*

Application Exercises Key

1. B, E. **CORRECT:** When using the three-level system of triage, the nurse should identify those urgent conditions should be managed within 2 hours. The nurse should use the ABCDE when determining priority. Therefore, the client with the pressure injury and blood glucose of 200 mg/dL (less than 200 mg/dL) and the client who reports urinary frequency and fever have urgent conditions that can be managed within 2 hours. The emergent conditions are the right calf pain and shortness of breath, which could indicate embolus, and the left-sided weakness and numbness, which could indicate stroke. The nurse or provider should be notified immediately of these findings. The nonurgent condition is the client who has nausea and insomnia.

(N) *NCLEX® Connection: Coordinated Care, Establishing Priorities*

2. A. **CORRECT:** The nurse should open the client's airway by using the head-tilt, chin-lift maneuver because this method prevents further injury when the client is unresponsive without suspicion of trauma. The modified jaw thrust is used for a client who is unresponsive with suspected traumatic neck injury. Hyperextension of the head can close off the client's airway. Flexion of the head will not open the client's airway.

(N) *NCLEX® Connection: Physiological Adaptation, Medical Emergencies*

3. A, C, D. **CORRECT:** Clients who are experiencing hypothermia require rewarming and monitoring of their core temperature. The nurse should remove wet clothing, apply warm blankets, and prepare to infuse warm IV fluids. These measures would assist with increasing the client's temperature. Instead of maintaining the current room temperature, the nurse should increase it. A warm environment would assist with improving the client's temperature as well. Administering acetaminophen is not indicated for management of hypothermia. It could be used as an analgesic. However, it has antipyretic properties as well and could potentially decrease the client's temperature.

(N) *NCLEX® Connection: Physiological Adaptation, Alterations in Body Systems*

4. A, D, E. **CORRECT:** When taking action, the nurse should identify that a client who is suspected of having opioid poisoning/overdose requires emergent interventions. The client is currently unresponsive and is not breathing and has an absent pulse. The nurse should call for more help and obtain an AED and begin high-quality CPR. The antidote for opioid toxicity is naloxone. Therefore, the nurse should plan to monitor the client after receiving this medication to reverse the effects. Monitoring the client after they receive lidocaine is not indicated at this time. Lidocaine is indicated if the client has a ventricular dysrhythmia. Administering syrup of ipecac would induce vomiting, and this is indicated and no longer recommended for ingested poison because of the risk for aspiration.

(N) *NCLEX® Connection: Physiological Adaptation, Medical Emergencies*

5. A, 3; B, 2; C, 1; D, 4

When taking action while assisting with care for a client who is experiencing ventricular asystole, the nurse should identify that this is a medical emergency that requires immediate action. The initial action the nurse should take is to activate the emergency response system. This will ensure that additional help arrives to assist with the management of the client's condition. While help arrives, the nurse should immediately perform CPR according to BLS guidelines. According to the Adult Cardiac Arrest Algorithm, the nurse should observe the administration of epinephrine, next followed by another round of high-quality CPR. The nurse should ensure the AED is turned on so that it can analyze the client's heart rhythm. Lastly, the nurse should identify the cause of the client's condition and recommend actions to treat.

(N) *NCLEX® Connection: Physiological Adaptation, Medical Emergencies*

When reviewing the following chapters, keep in mind the relevant topics and tasks of the NCLEX outline.

Basic Care and Comfort

NONPHARMACOLOGICAL COMFORT INTERVENTIONS: Provide nonpharmacological comfort measures for pain relief.

Pharmacological Therapies

ADVERSE EFFECTS/CONTRAINDICATIONS/SIDE EFFECTS/ INTERACTIONS
Monitor client for actual and potential adverse effects of medications.

Monitor and document client response to management of medication side effects including prescribed, over-the-counter, and herbal supplement.

Reinforce client teaching on possible effects of medications.

EXPECTED ACTIONS/OUTCOMES: Monitor client use of medications over time.

PHARMACOLOGICAL PAIN MANAGEMENT: Identify client need for pain medication.

Reduction of Risk Potential

DIAGNOSTIC TESTS: Perform diagnostic testing (e.g., blood glucose, oxygen saturation, testing for occult blood).

POTENTIAL FOR COMPLICATIONS OF DIAGNOSTIC TESTS/ TREATMENTS/PROCEDURES
Use precautions to prevent injury and/or complications associated with a procedure or diagnosis.

Identify client risk, and implement interventions.

THERAPEUTIC PROCEDURES: Reinforce client teaching on treatments and procedures.

CHAPTER 4
Neurologic Diagnostic Procedures

Neurologic data collection and diagnostic procedures are used to evaluate neurologic function by testing indicators such as mental status, motor functioning, and electrical activity.

For diagnostic testing and procedures, the client must provide informed consent. It is the responsibility of the nurse to ensure that this is completed prior to the procedure or testing.

Neurologic data collection and diagnostic procedures that nurses should be knowledgeable about include cerebral angiography, cerebral computed tomography (CT) scan, electroencephalography (EEG), Glasgow Coma Scale (GCS), intracranial pressure monitoring, lumbar puncture (spinal tap), magnetic resonance imaging (MRI), positron emission tomography (PET), single-photon emission computed tomography (SPECT), and radiography (x-ray).

Cerebral angiography

Cerebral angiography provides visualization of the cerebral blood vessels.
- Digital subtraction angiography hides the bones and tissues from the images, providing x-rays with only the vessels apparent.
- The procedure detects defects, narrowing, or obstruction of arteries or blood vessels in the brain.
- The procedure is performed within the radiology department because iodine-based contrast dye is injected into an artery during the procedure.

INDICATIONS

Cerebral angiography is used to check the blood flow to and within the brain, identify aneurysms, and define the vascularity of tumors.

CONSIDERATIONS

PREPROCEDURE

If the client is pregnant, a determination of the risks to the fetus versus the benefits of the information obtained by this procedure should be made.

NURSING ACTIONS
- Instruct the client to refrain from consuming food or fluids at least 6 hr prior to the procedure. Some providers may allow clear fluids up to the time of the procedure.
- Check for history of allergies. If a client has an allergy to contrast media, they may be given a steroid or antihistamine prior to the procedure.
- Any history of bleeding or taking anticoagulant medication requires additional considerations and additional monitoring to ensure clotting after the procedure. Qs
- A mild sedative for relaxation is occasionally administered prior to and during the procedure, and vital signs are continuously monitored during the procedure.
- Check BUN and blood creatinine to determine the kidney's ability to excrete the dye.

CLIENT EDUCATION
- Void immediately prior to the procedure.
- Following dye injection, it is common to experience a metallic taste and feel a sensation of warmth.

INTRAPROCEDURE
- The client is placed on a radiography table, where the client's head is secured.
- A catheter is placed into an artery (usually in the groin or the neck), dye is injected, and x-ray pictures are taken.
- Once all pictures are taken, the catheter is removed and an arterial closure device is used, or pressure is held over the artery to control bleeding by thrombus formation sealing the artery.

POSTPROCEDURE

NURSING ACTIONS
- Closely monitor the area to ensure that clotting occurs.
- Movements are restricted depending on the type of procedure used to seal the artery to prevent rebleeding at the catheter site.
- Perform neurological checks, and monitor vital signs frequently.
- Place an ice pack on the insertion site.
- Encourage fluids to promote contrast clearance through the kidneys.

COMPLICATIONS

There is a risk for bleeding or hematoma formation at the entry site.

NURSING ACTIONS
- Check the insertion site frequently.
- Check the affected extremity distal to the puncture site for adequate circulation (color, temperature, pulses, capillary refill).
- If bleeding occurs, apply pressure over the artery and notify the provider. Q̧EBP

Cerebral computed tomography scan

A CT scan provides cross-sectional images of the cranial cavity. A contrast medium can be used to enhance the images.

INDICATIONS

CT scanning can be used to identify tumors and infarctions, detect abnormalities, monitor response to treatment, and guide needles used for biopsies.

CONSIDERATIONS

PREPROCEDURE

If the client is pregnant, a determination of the risks to the fetus versus the benefits of the information obtained by this procedure should be made.

NURSING ACTIONS
- If contrast media and/or sedation is expected:
  - Instruct the client to refrain from consuming food or fluids for 3 to 4 hr prior to the procedure.
  - Check for allergy to shellfish or iodine. Contrast media (iodine) may not always be a contraindication in clients who have a shellfish allergy. Further data collection may be needed.
  - Check BUN and creatinine because contrast media is excreted by the kidneys. Q̧s
- Because this procedure is performed with the client in a supine position, placing pillows in the small of the client's back can assist in preventing back pain. The head must be secured to prevent unnecessary movement during the procedure.
- Inform client that various clicking sounds will be heard as scanner moves around.
- Ensure that the client is not wearing any metal (hairpins, jewelry, clips, dentures) prior to the procedure. In general, clients wear a hospital gown to prevent any metals from interfering with the x-rays.

INTRAPROCEDURE
- The client must lie supine with the head stabilized during the procedure.
- Although CT scanning is painless, sedation can be provided.

POSTPROCEDURE

NURSING ACTIONS
- There is no follow-up care associated with a CT scan.
- If contrast media is injected, monitor for allergic reaction and changes in kidney function.
- If sedation is administered, monitor the client until stable.

Electroencephalography

An EEG is a noninvasive procedure that checks the electrical activity of the brain and is used to determine abnormalities in brain wave patterns. An EEG provides information about the ability of the brain to function and highlights areas of abnormality.

INDICATIONS

EEGs are most commonly performed to identify and determine seizure activity, but they are also useful for detecting sleep disorders and behavioral changes.

CONSIDERATIONS

PREPROCEDURE

NURSING ACTIONS: Review medications with the provider to determine if they should be continued prior to this procedure.

CLIENT EDUCATION
- Wash the hair to eliminate all oils, gels, and sprays.
- If testing is diagnostic for sleep condition, the client should sleep less prior to procedure.
- To stimulate electrical activity during the test, you might be exposed to bright flashing lights or asked to hyperventilate for 3 to 4 min.
- Avoid taking any stimulant or sedative medication as directed prior to the procedure.
- Avoid drinking caffeinated beverages the morning of the procedure.
- Meal fasting is not indicated.

INTRAPROCEDURE

- The procedure generally takes 45 to 120 min.
- There are no risks associated with this procedure.
- With the client resting in a chair or lying in bed, small electrodes are placed on the scalp and connected to a brain wave machine or computer.
- Electrical signals produced by the brain are recorded by the machine or computer in the form of wavy lines. This documents brain activity.
- Notations are made when stimuli are presented or when sleep occurs. (Flashes of light or pictures can be used during the procedure to check the client's response to stimuli.)

POSTPROCEDURE

CLIENT EDUCATION: Resume your normal activities and routine.

Glasgow Coma Scale

This data collection tool concentrates on neurologic function and is useful to determine the level of consciousness and monitor response to treatment. The Glasgow Coma Scale (GCS) is reported as a number that allows providers to immediately determine if neurologic changes have occurred.

INDICATIONS

GCS scores are helpful in determining changes in the level of consciousness for clients who have head injuries, space-occupying lesions or cerebral infarctions, and encephalitis. This is important because complications related to neurologic injuries can occur rapidly and require immediate treatment.

CONSIDERATIONS

GCS scores are calculated by using appropriate stimuli (a painful stimulus can be necessary) and then determining the client's response in three areas. ⓠEBP
- **Eye opening (E):** The best eye response, with responses ranging from 4 to 1
  - 4 = Eye opening occurs spontaneously.
  - 3 = Eye opening occurs secondary to sound.
  - 2 = Eye opening occurs secondary to pain.
  - 1 = Eye opening does not occur.
- **Verbal (V):** The best verbal response, with responses ranging from 5 to 1
  - 5 = Conversation is coherent and oriented.
  - 4 = Conversation is incoherent and disoriented.
  - 3 = Words are spoken but inappropriately.
  - 2 = Sounds are made but no words.
  - 1 = Vocalization does not occur.

- **Motor (M):** The best motor response, with responses ranging from 6 to 1
  - 6 = Commands are followed.
  - 5 = Local reaction to pain occurs.
  - 4 = General withdrawal from pain.
  - 3 = Decorticate posture (adduction of arms, flexion of elbows and wrists) is present.
  - 2 = Decerebrate posture (abduction of arms, extension of elbows and wrists) is present.
  - 1 = Motor response does not occur.

Responses within each subscale are added, with the total score quantitatively describing the client's level of consciousness. **E + V + M = Total GCS**

INTERPRETATION OF FINDINGS

- The highest GCS score is 15, indicating full consciousness. In general, total scores of the GCS correlate with the degree or level of coma.
- A score less than 8 is associated with severe head injury and coma.

Lumbar puncture (spinal tap)

A lumbar puncture is a procedure during which a small amount of cerebrospinal fluid (CSF) is withdrawn from the spinal canal and then analyzed to determine its constituents.

INDICATIONS

This procedure is used to detect the presence of some diseases (syphilis, meningitis), infection, and malignancies. A lumbar puncture may also be used to reduce CSF pressure, determine CSF pressure readings, instill a contrast medium or air for diagnostic tests, or administer medication or chemotherapy directly to spinal fluid.

CONSIDERATIONS

PREPROCEDURE

The risks versus benefits of a lumbar puncture should be discussed with the client prior to this procedure.
- A lumbar puncture can be associated with rare but serious complications, such as brain herniation, especially when performed in the presence of increased intracranial pressure (ICP).
- Lumbar punctures for clients who have bleeding disorders or who are taking anticoagulants can result in bleeding that compresses the spinal cord

NURSING ACTIONS

- Ensure that all of the client's jewelry is removed and that the client is wearing only a hospital gown.
- Instruct the client to void prior to the procedure.
- Obtain vital signs and perform a baseline neurological check of the client's legs.
- Clients should be positioned to stretch the spinal canal. This can be done by having the client assume a "cannonball," or fetal position while on one side or by having the client stretch over an overbed table, if sitting is preferred.

INTRAPROCEDURE

- Ensure that sterility is maintained during the procedure.
- The area of the needle insertion is cleansed, and a local anesthetic is injected.
- The needle is inserted, and the CSF is withdrawn, after which the needle is removed.
- A manometer can be used to determine the opening pressure of the spinal cord, which is useful if increased pressure is a consideration.

POSTPROCEDURE

CSF is sent to the pathology department for analysis.

NURSING ACTIONS

- Monitor the puncture site. The client should remain lying for several hours to ensure that the site clots and to decrease the risk of a post-lumbar puncture headache, caused by CSF leakage. Q EBP
- Obtain vital signs, perform neurological check of the client's legs.
- Collect pain data.
- Encourage fluid intake

CLIENT EDUCATION: Normal activities may be resumed after prescribed bed rest is complete as long as in stable condition.

COMPLICATIONS

If clotting does not occur to seal the dura puncture site, CSF can leak, resulting in a headache and increasing the potential for infection.

NURSING ACTIONS: Encourage the client to lie flat in bed. Provide fluids for hydration, and administer pain medication.

Magnetic resonance imaging scan

An MRI scan of the head provides cross-sectional images of the cranial cavity. A contrast medium may be used to enhance the images.

- Unlike CT scans, MRI images are obtained using magnets. Thus, the consequences associated with radiation are avoided. This makes this procedure safer for clients who are pregnant.
- The use of magnets precludes the ability to scan a client who has an artificial device (pacemakers, surgical clips, intravenous access port). Q s

! Use MRI-approved equipment to monitor vital signs and provide ventilator/oxygen assistance to clients undergoing MRI scans.

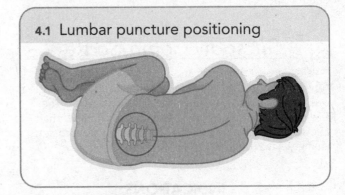

4.1 Lumbar puncture positioning

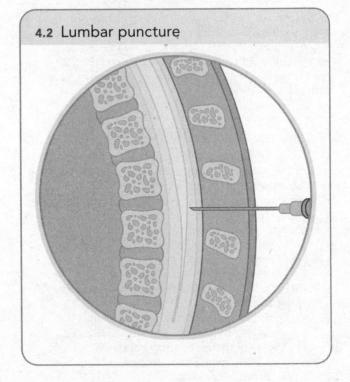

4.2 Lumbar puncture

INDICATIONS

- MRI scans are used to detect abnormalities, monitor response to treatment, and guide needles used for biopsies.
- MRIs are capable of discriminating soft tissue from tumor or bone. This makes the MRI scan effective in determining tumor size and blood vessel location.

CONSIDERATIONS

PREPROCEDURE

NURSING ACTIONS
- Remove any transdermal patches with a foil backing, as these can cause burn injuries. Qs
- Ensure that metal objects (dentures, jewelry, belts, hair accessories) are removed prior to this procedure. The client should wear a hospital gown to prevent any metals from interfering with the magnet.
- If sedation is expected, the client should refrain from food or fluids for 4 to 8 hr prior to the procedure.
- Determine if the client has a history of claustrophobia, and explain the tight space and noise.
- Ask the client about any implants containing metal (pacemaker, orthopedic joints, artificial heart valves, intrauterine devices, aneurysm clips).
- Ensure all people who will be in the scanning area while the magnet is on remove all jewelry, electronics, and phones to prevent damage to themselves or the magnet.
- Place pillows in the small of the client's back to prevent back pain from lying supine. The head must be secured to prevent unnecessary movement during the procedure.

INTRAPROCEDURE

- Ensure the client remains supine with the head stabilized.
- MRI scanning is noisy, and earplugs or sedation may be provided.

POSTPROCEDURE

NURSING ACTIONS
- If contrast media is injected, monitor the site to ensure that clotting has occurred and monitor for any indications of an allergic reaction.
- Sedation may be given, and the client should be monitored until stable.

PET and SPECT scans

Positron emission tomography and single-photon emission computed tomography scans are nuclear medicine procedures that produce three-dimensional images of the head. These images can be static (depicting vessels) or functional (depicting brain activity).
- A glucose-based tracer is injected into the blood stream prior to the PET scan. This initiates regional metabolic activity, which is then documented by the PET scanner. A radioisotope is used for SPECT scanning.
- A CT scan may be performed after a PET/SPECT scan, as this provides information regarding brain activity and pathological location (brain injury, death, neoplasm).

INDICATIONS

A PET/SPECT scan captures regional metabolic processes, which is most useful in determining tumor activity and/or response to treatment. PET/SPECT scans are also able to determine the presence of dementia, indicated by the inability of the brain to respond to the tracer.

CONSIDERATIONS

PREPROCEDURE

PET/SPECT scans use radiation. Thus, the risks and benefits to a client who might be pregnant must be discussed.

NURSING ACTIONS: Check for a history of diabetes mellitus. While this condition does not preclude a PET/SPECT scan, alterations in the client's medications can be necessary to avoid hyperglycemia or hypoglycemia before and after this procedure. Qs

INTRAPROCEDURE

- While the pictures are being obtained, the client must lie flat with the head restrained.
- This procedure is not painful, and sedation is rarely necessary.

POSTPROCEDURE

NURSING ACTIONS
- If radioisotopes are used, check for allergic reaction.
- There is no follow-up care after a PET/SPECT scan.
- Because the tracer is glucose-based and short-acting (less than 2 hr), it is broken down within the body as a sugar, not excreted.

Radiography (x-ray)

- An x-ray uses electromagnetic radiation to capture images of the internal structures of an individual.
- A structure's image is light or dark relative to the amount of radiation the tissue absorbs. The image is recorded on a radiograph, which is a black-and-white image that is held up to light for visualization. Some are recorded digitally and available immediately.

INDICATIONS

X-ray examinations of the skull and spine can reveal fractures, curvatures, bone erosion and dislocation, and possible soft tissue calcification, all of which can damage the nervous system.

CONSIDERATIONS

PREPROCEDURE

NURSING ACTIONS
- There is no specific preprocedure protocol for x-rays that do not use contrast. X-rays are often the first diagnostic tool used after an injury (to rule out cervical fracture in head trauma).
- Determine whether the client is pregnant.
- Ensure that the client's jewelry is removed and that no clothes cover the area.

CLIENT EDUCATION: The amount of radiation used in contemporary x-ray machines is very small.

INTRAPROCEDURE

The procedure is quick, but the client is to remain still during the procedure.

POSTPROCEDURE

NURSING ACTIONS: No postprocedure care is required.

Active Learning Scenario

A nurse is contributing to the plan of care for a client who is scheduled for a magnetic resonance imaging (MRI) scan with contrast media. What should the nurse include in the plan of care? Use the ATI Active Learning Template: Diagnostic Procedure to complete this item.

PROCEDURE NAME: Define this diagnostic test.

NURSING INTERVENTIONS (PRE, INTRA, POST): Identify three preprocedure actions, one intraprocedure action, and one postprocedure action.

Application Exercises

1. A nurse is reinforcing teaching for a client who is scheduled for a cerebral angiography. Which of the following statements by the client indicates understanding?
   - A. "I can eat as usual prior to the procedure."
   - B. "I will be standing up during the procedure."
   - C. "After the procedure, the urinary catheter will be removed."
   - D. "I will feel warm after that dye is injected."

2. A nurse is caring for a client who is scheduled for a cerebral computed tomography scan with contrast. Which of the following actions should the nurse take?
   - A. Hold the client in a left lateral position during the procedure.
   - B. Insert indwelling urinary catheter prior to procedure.
   - C. Ensure the client is not wearing any metal objects prior to procedure.
   - D. Administer an analgesic for pain after the procedure.

3. A nurse is reinforcing instructions with a client who is scheduled for an electroencephalogram (EEG) the next day. Which of the following statements should the nurse make?
   - A. "You should wash your hair prior to the procedure."
   - B. "You cannot eat or drink for at least 6 hours prior to the procedure."
   - C. "The procedure takes about 15 minutes to complete."
   - D. "They will apply small electrodes to your chest during the procedure."

4. A nurse is collecting data from a client for changes in their level of consciousness by using the Glasgow Coma Scale (GCS) tool. The nurse notes that the client opens their eyes when spoken to, speaks incoherently, and moves their extremities when pain is applied. What scores should the nurse suggest?

5. A nurse is assisting with the care for a client immediately following a lumbar puncture. Which of the following actions should the nurse take? (Select all that apply.)
   - A. Encourage the client to ambulate.
   - B. Administer analgesic for pain.
   - C. Encourage increased fluid intake.
   - D. Encourage to cough and deep breathe.
   - E. Monitor the puncture site for drainage.

Application Exercises Key

1. D. **CORRECT:** When evaluating outcomes after reinforcing teaching with a client about cerebral angiography procedure, the nurse should identify the client understands when the statement is made about feeling warm when the dye is injected. This is an expected reaction that is experienced after the injection of contrast dye. The nurse should reinforce teaching with the client not to eat for at least 6 hr prior to the procedure, lying on a radiology table is required, and there is no insertion of a urinary catheter.

   Ⓝ *NCLEX® Connection: Reduction of Risk Potential, Therapeutic Procedures*

2. C. **CORRECT:** A cerebral computed tomography scan with contrast requires the nurse to inform the client to remove any metal objects such as jewelry, hair accessories, hair clips, or belts from their body because these items can interfere with the scanning machine. An indwelling urinary catheter is not needed for this procedure. The client is positioned supine and is required to remain still during scanning. The procedure is painless, and an analgesic is not required.

   Ⓝ *NCLEX® Connection: Reduction of Risk Potential, Diagnostic Tests*

3. A. **CORRECT:** An EEG is a procedure that analyzes electrical activity of the brain. Therefore, the nurse should instruct the client to ensure that their hair is washed prior to the procedure, which will remove oils, gels, or sprays and allow for the placement of the scalp electrodes. Fasting is not indicated for this procedure because it can cause hypoglycemia, which can interfere with the results of testing. The procedure takes about 45-120 minutes to complete. The electrodes are applied to the client's scalp to determine the electrical activity of the brain.

   Ⓝ *NCLEX® Connection: Reduction of Risk Potential, Diagnostic Tests*

4. The client's GCS score should be 11. The client would receive E-3 for spontaneous eye-opening secondary to voice stimulation, V-4 for verbal conversation that is incoherent and disoriented, and M-4 for motor response as general withdrawal to pain.

   Ⓝ *NCLEX® Connection: Reduction of Risk Potential, Potential for Alterations in Body Systems*

5. B, C, E. **CORRECT:** When taking action while assisting with caring for a client immediately following a lumbar puncture, the nurse should administer an analgesic for pain, encourage the client to increase their fluid intake, and monitor the puncture site for CSF drainage or bleeding. These actions will provide comfort and prevent complications. The client may experience a mild headache following the procedure. Therefore, it is important for the nurse to collect data about the client's pain and provide interventions as needed. Administering a mild, prescribed analgesic such as acetaminophen should be sufficient. The nurse should encourage the client to increase their fluid intake to replace the loss of CSF and decrease the risk of postprocedure headache. Another action the nurse should take is monitoring the puncture site for drainage or bleeding. This is an unexpected finding that should be reported to the provider. The client should remain still or lie flat on their back after the procedure. Encouraging coughing and deep breathing can cause potential postprocedural complications such as increased ICP and should be avoided.

   Ⓝ *NCLEX® Connection: Reduction of Risk Potential, Potential for Complications From Diagnostic Tests/Treatments/Procedures*

Active Learning Scenario Key

Using the ATI Active Learning Template: Diagnostic Procedure

PROCEDURE NAME: Magnetic resonance imaging (MRI) scan relies on magnetic field to take multiple images of the body.

NURSING INTERVENTIONS (PRE, INTRA, POST)

- Preprocedure
  - Ensure that metal objects are removed from the client's body.
  - Remove any transdermal patches with a foil backing from the client's body.
  - Determine if the client has claustrophobia.
  - Question the client concerning implants containing metal.
  - Question the client regarding allergies.
- Intraprocedure: Stabilize the client's head.
- Postprocedure: Monitor for allergic reaction to the contrast media used during the MRI.

Ⓝ *NCLEX® Connection: Reduction of Risk Potential, Diagnostic Tests*

CHAPTER 5 *Pain Management*

Effective pain management includes the use of pharmacological and nonpharmacological pain management therapies.

Clients have a right to adequate data collection and management of pain. Nurses are accountable for the collection of data about pain and for effective pain management.

Nurses have a priority responsibility for the continual data collection of the client's pain level and to assist with the provision of individualized interventions. Depending on the setting and route of analgesia administration, the nurse should participate in evaluation of pain 10 to 60 min after administering medication. Qpcc

Data collection challenges can occur with clients who have cognitive impairment, who speak a different language than the nurse, or who receive prescribed mechanical ventilation.

PHYSIOLOGY

- Nociceptive pain involves transduction, transmission, perception, and modulation of impulses generated by nociceptors located throughout the body.
- Stimuli following tissue damage from cuts, burns, tumor growth, or chemicals trigger these nociceptors to send a message to the nervous system.
- Neuropathic pain is caused by changes in the peripheral or central nervous system.

DATA COLLECTION

Pain is whatever the person experiencing it says it is, and it exists whenever the person says it does. The client's report of pain is the most reliable diagnostic measure of pain. Self-report using standardized pain scales is useful for clients over the age of 7 years. Specialized pain scales are available for use with younger children and other clients who are unable to self-report pain. There are a variety of pain scales that feature images, numbers, intensity indicators, and descriptive words and are in various languages. Qpcc

- Collect data and document about pain (the fifth vital sign) according to the client's condition and agency guidelines.
- Use a focused data collection tool to obtain subjective data.

5.1 Pain categories

Acute pain

Acute pain is caused by tissue injury. The pain is temporary, usually self-limiting, and resolves with tissue healing.

Physiological responses (sympathetic nervous system) are fight-or-flight responses (tachycardia, hypertension, anxiety, diaphoresis, muscle tension).

Behavioral responses include grimacing, moaning, flinching, and guarding.

The nurse should be aware that a client not exhibiting physiological or behavioral responses does not mean that pain is absent.

Interventions include treatment of the underlying problem.

Surgical incisions and wounds from injury produce acute pain.

Chronic pain

Chronic pain is ongoing or recurs frequently, lasting longer than 3 months and persisting beyond tissue healing.

Physiological responses do not usually increase vital signs. The client's vital signs can actually be lower than normal in response to chronic pain. Clients can have depression, fatigue, decreased level of functioning, or disability.

Chronic pain might not have a known cause, and it might not respond to interventions.

Chronic pain can be classified as chronic cancer pain or chronic noncancer pain.

The pain associated with osteoarthritis and neuropathy are examples of chronic pain.

Nociceptive pain

Nociceptive pain arises from damage to or inflammation of tissue other than that of the peripheral and central nervous systems.

Nociceptive pain is the result of activation of normal processing of painful stimuli.

It is usually throbbing, aching, and localized.

This pain is managed using opioids and non-opioid medications.

TYPES OF NOCICEPTIVE PAIN

Somatic: in bones, joints, muscles, skin, or connective tissues.

Visceral: in internal organs such as the stomach or intestines. It can cause referred pain in other body locations separate from the stimulus.

Neuropathic pain

Neuropathic pain arises from abnormal or damaged pain nerves.

It differs from nociceptive pain as it is the abnormal processing of painful stimuli.

It includes phantom limb pain, pain below the level of a spinal cord injury, and diabetic neuropathy.

Neuropathic pain is usually intense, shooting, burning, or described as "pins and needles."

This pain typically is managed using adjuvant medications (antidepressants, antispasmodic agents, skeletal muscle relaxants).

5.2 Focused pain data collection

Location

USE ANATOMICAL TERMINOLOGY AND LANDMARKS TO DESCRIBE LOCATION.

Ask: *"Where is your pain?"*

Ask: *"Does it radiate anywhere else?"*

Ask clients to point to the location.

Quality

QUALITY REFERS TO HOW THE PAIN FEELS: sharp, dull, aching, burning, stabbing, pounding, throbbing, shooting, gnawing, tender, heavy, tight, tiring, exhausting, sickening, terrifying, torturing, nagging, annoying, intense, or unbearable.

Ask: *"What does the pain feel like?"* Give more than two choices (*"Is the pain throbbing, burning, or stabbing?"*).

Measures

INTENSITY, STRENGTH, AND SEVERITY ARE "MEASURES" OF THE PAIN. Use visual analog scales (description scale, number rating scale) to measure pain, monitor pain, and participate in evaluating the effectiveness of interventions.

Ask: *"How much pain do you have now?"*

Ask: *"What is the worst/best the pain has been?"*

Ask: *"Rate your pain on a scale of 0 to 10."*

Timing

ONSET, DURATION, FREQUENCY

Ask: *"When did it start?"*

Ask: *"How long does it last?"*

Ask: *"How often does it occur?"*

Ask: *"Is it constant or intermittent?"*

Setting

HOW THE PAIN AFFECTS DAILY LIFE OR HOW ACTIVITIES OF DAILY LIVING (ADLS) AFFECT THE PAIN

Ask: *"Where are you when the symptoms occur?"*

Ask: *"What are you doing when the symptoms occur?"*

Ask: *"How does the pain affect your sleep?"*

Ask: *"How does the pain affect your ability to work and do your job?"*

Associated manifestations

DOCUMENT ASSOCIATED MANIFESTATIONS: fatigue, depression, nausea, anxiety.

Ask: *"What other symptoms do you have when you are feeling pain?"*

Aggravating/relieving factors

Ask: *"What makes the pain better?"*

Ask: *"What makes the pain worse?"*

Ask: *"Are you currently taking any prescription, herbal, or over-the-counter medications?"*

TYPES OF PAIN

Pain can be categorized by duration (acute or chronic) or by pathology (nociceptive or neuropathic).

- Clients can experience mixed pain that is difficult to categorize. Conditions that cause mixed pain include fibromyalgia, HIV, and Lyme disease.
- Breakthrough pain occurs when a client experiences an exacerbation of acute pain. Clients who have chronic conditions can experience episodes of breakthrough pain requiring additional pain relief measures.

RISK FACTORS

Causes of acute and chronic pain

- Trauma
- Surgery
- Cancer (tumor invasion, nerve compression, bone metastases, associated infections, immobility)
- Arthritis
- Fibromyalgia
- Neuropathy
- Diagnostic or treatment procedures (injection, intubation, radiation)

Factors that affect the pain experience

- Age
  - Infants cannot verbalize or understand their pain.
  - Older adult clients can have multiple pathologies that cause pain and limit function. Ⓖ
- Fatigue can increase sensitivity to pain.
- Cognitive function: Clients who are cognitively impaired might not be able to report pain or report it accurately.
- Prior experiences can increase or decrease sensitivity depending on whether clients obtained adequate relief.
- Anxiety and fear can increase sensitivity to pain.
- Support systems can decrease sensitivity to pain.
- Culture can influence how clients express pain or the meaning they give to pain.

EXPECTED FINDINGS

- Behaviors complement self-reports and assist in pain data collection of nonverbal clients.
  - Facial expressions (grimacing, wrinkled forehead), body movements (restlessness, pacing, guarding)
  - Moaning, crying
  - Decreased attention span
- Blood pressure, pulse, and respiratory rate can temporarily increase with acute pain. Eventually, increases in vital signs will stabilize despite the persistence of pain. Therefore, physiologic indicators might not be an accurate measure of pain over time.

PATIENT-CENTERED CARE

NURSING CARE

- Use pharmacological and nonpharmacological strategies to relieve pain. Consider the client's preferences. Discuss the use of complementary and alternative practices. Qpcc
- Assist the client to set a pain-relief or comfort-function goal and refer back to the goal when determining pain interventions.
- Determine the client's need for scheduled analgesia, such as for chronic or postoperative pain.
- Premedicate the client prior to painful procedures (repositioning, wound care, invasive diagnostic testing).
- Refer to dosage charts that describe equianalgesia to compare the potency levels of various pain medications.

NONPHARMACOLOGICAL PAIN MANAGEMENT

- Nonpharmacological pain strategies help to improve coping by relieving stress associated with pain. These strategies can assist clients in reducing the amount of pharmacological interventions for pain and are particularly helpful when clients cannot take pain medication.
- Clients might choose nonpharmacological complementary and alternative measures to manage pain.
  ○ Mind-body practices (yoga, chiropractic manipulation, acupuncture)
  ○ Cognitive approaches (meditation, distraction)
  ○ Natural products (herbs, oils)

PHARMACOLOGICAL INTERVENTIONS

Analgesics are the mainstay for relieving pain.
- Treatment tools (the WHO analgesic ladder) suggest administering non-opioid analgesics first, progressing through weak opioids to stronger ones to manage pain.
- IV analgesia is used in the immediate postoperative period, and then clients are transitioned to oral medication as pain is managed properly through the postoperative period.
- Clients experiencing acute pain receive doses that are gradually titrated down until they can be comfortable without medication or at a minimal dose.
- The three classes of analgesics are non-opioids, opioids, and adjuvants.

Non-opioid analgesics are appropriate for treating mild to moderate pain, and are often added to opioids for treatment for more intense pain. Non-opioid analgesics also have antipyretic and anti-inflammatory properties.
- Non-opioid analgesics are often prescribed following painful procedures.
- Acetaminophen is most often used, alone or in combination with other mediations.
  ○ Ensure the total amount of acetaminophen a client consumes daily does not exceed 4 g for clients 50 kg (110 lb) or greater.
  ○ It is safe to administer acetaminophen concurrently with NSAIDs (ibuprofen, aspirin, celecoxib, naproxen, ketorolac) because the medications act in different ways.

Opioid analgesics are appropriate for treating moderate to severe pain.
- Opioid analgesics for moderate pain hydrocodone and codeine.
- Hydromorphone, fentanyl, morphine, or oxycodone are effective for more severe pain. Morphine is the opioid most used, and other opioid effects are compared with the effects of morphine.
- Meperidine is no longer recommended for use except in rare conditions at low doses.
- Check opioid formulations carefully to determine whether a short-acting or modified release (extended release) dose is indicated.
- For many opioids, the dose can be titrated upward progressively until the client experiences pain relief; however, upward titration increases the risk for adverse effects.
- Opioids are available in oral, intramuscular, intravenous, transdermal, transmucosal, and buccal routes.
- It is essential to monitor and intervene for adverse effects of opioid use.
  ○ Constipation: Use a preventative approach (monitoring of bowel movements, fluids, fiber intake, exercise, stool softeners, stimulant laxatives, enemas).
  ○ Nausea/vomiting: Administer antiemetics, advise clients to lie still and move slowly, and eliminate odors.
  ○ Sedation: Monitor level of consciousness and take safety precautions. Sedation usually precedes respiratory depression. Qs
  ○ Respiratory depression: Monitor respiratory rate prior to and following administration of opioids. Initial treatment of respiratory depression and sedation is generally a reduction in opioid dose. If necessary, administer naloxone to reverse opioid effects.

Adjuvant analgesics, or coanalgesics, enhance the effects of nonopioids, help alleviate other manifestations that aggravate pain (depression, seizures, inflammation), and are useful for treating neuropathic pain. Adjuvant medications include the following.
- Anticonvulsants: carbamazepine, gabapentin
- Tricyclic antidepressants: amitriptyline
- Glucocorticoids: dexamethasone
- Anesthetics: xylocaine, bupivacaine

Patient-controlled analgesia (PCA) is a medication delivery system that allows clients to self-administer safe doses of opioids.

- The nurse programs the pump so the client does not receive an overdose. Use of a PCA increases the client's sense of control and can decrease the amount of medication they need.
- Morphine and hydromorphone are typical opioids for PCA delivery.

Other pain management strategies
- Medication injections and short-term infusions
  - Local infusion into a wound
  - Regional infusion to block a group of nerves (epidural infusions)
- Spinal cord stimulator

Chronic pain interventions: Strategies specific for relieving chronic pain include the above interventions, plus:
- Administering long-acting or controlled-release opioid analgesics (including the transdermal route)
- Administering analgesics around the clock rather than PRN
- Recommending a referral to accredited pain management center, which offers a holistic approach to pain management

COMPLICATIONS

- Undertreatment of pain is a serious complication and can lead to increased anxiety with acute pain and depression with chronic pain. Collect data from clients for pain frequently, and intervene as appropriate.
- Sedation, respiratory depression, and coma can occur as a result of overdosing. Sedation always precedes respiratory depression. Qs
  - Identify high-risk clients (older adult clients). Ⓖ
  - Stop the opioid and give the antagonist naloxone if respiratory rate is below 8/min and shallow, or the client is difficult to arouse.
  - The nurse should closely monitor the client following administration of naloxone. The duration of the certain opioids can last longer than the effectiveness of the naloxone, creating a need for additional doses.

1. A nurse is collecting data on a client who had abdominal surgery. The client reports pain in the abdomen at 9 on a 0 to 10 scale. What type of pain is the client experiencing?
   - A. Acute
   - B. Chronic
   - C. Nociceptive
   - D. Neuropathic

2. A nurse is caring for a client who came into the emergency department after an injury to the right arm. The nurse is collecting data on the client's pain. Which question should the nurse ask first?
   - A. "Where is your pain?"
   - B. "What does it feel like?"
   - C. "How does it change with time?"
   - D. "How severe is your pain?"

3. A nurse is caring for a client who reports pain at 10 on a 0 to 10 scale. The nurse plans to administer morphine. Which of the following adverse effects should the nurse monitor for in the client? (Select all that apply.)
   - A. Confusion
   - B. Hypertension
   - C. Constipation
   - D. Bradypnea
   - E. Diarrhea

Active Learning Scenario

A nurse on a medical-surgical unit is reviewing with a group of newly licensed nurses the various types of pain the clients on the unit have. Use the ATI Active Learning Template: Basic Concept to complete this item.

UNDERLYING PRINCIPLES: List the four different types of pain, their definitions, and characteristics.

Active Learning Scenario Key

Using the ATI Active Learning Template: Basic Concept
UNDERLYING PRINCIPLES

Acute pain
- Definition: Protective, temporary, usually self-limiting, resolves with tissue healing
- Physiological responses: Tachycardia, hypertension, anxiety, diaphoresis, muscle tension
- Behavioral responses: Grimacing, moaning, flinching, guarding

Chronic pain
- Definition: Not protective; ongoing or recurs frequently, lasts longer than 3 months, persists beyond tissue healing, can be chronic cancer pain or chronic noncancer pain
- Physiological responses: No change in vital signs, depression, fatigue, decreased level of functioning, disability

Nociceptive pain
- Definition: Arises from damage to or inflammation of tissue other than that of the peripheral and central nervous systems, and is usually throbbing, aching, and localized; pain typically responds to opioids and non-opioid medications
- Types of nociceptive pain
  ○ Somatic: In bones, joints, muscles, skin, or connective tissues
  ○ Visceral: In internal organs such as the stomach or intestines, can cause referred pain

Neuropathic pain
- Definition: Arises from abnormal or damaged pain nerves (phantom limb pain, pain below the level of a spinal cord injury, diabetic neuropathy); usually intense, shooting, burning, or "pins and needles"
- Physiological responses to adjuvant medications (antidepressants, antispasmodic agents, skeletal muscle relaxants)

Ⓝ *NCLEX® Connection: Pharmacological Therapies, Pharmacological Pain Management*

Application Exercises Key

1. A. **CORRECT:** Postoperative pain is acute pain and must be managed to prevent long-term/chronic pain.

   Ⓝ *NCLEX® Connection: Reduction of Risk Potential: Changes/ Abnormalities in Vital Signs*

2. A. **CORRECT:** When performing a comprehensive pain assessment, it is important to first identify where the pain is located. The first question the nurse should ask is "Where is your pain located?" The second question the nurse should ask is "What does the pain feel like?" The third question is "How does the pain change with time?" The fourth question is for the nurse to ask the client to rate the severity of the pain.

   Ⓝ *NCLEX® Connection: Health Promotion and Maintenance, Data Collection Techniques*

3. A, C, D. **CORRECT:** A client receiving morphine is at risk for confusion, sedation, respiratory depression, hypotension, constipation, nausea, vomiting, and urinary retention.

   Ⓝ *NCLEX® Connection: Pharmacological Therapies, Pharmacological Pain Management*

When reviewing the following chapters, keep in mind the relevant topics and tasks of the NCLEX outline.

Physiological Adaptation

ALTERATIONS IN BODY SYSTEMS
Provide care to correct client alteration in body system.

Notify primary health care provider of a change in client status.

Pharmacological Therapies

ADVERSE EFFECTS/CONTRAINDICATIONS/SIDE EFFECTS/ INTERACTIONS
Monitor client for actual and potential adverse effects of medications.

Monitor and document client response to management of medication side effects including prescribed, over-the-counter, and herbal supplement.

Reinforce client teaching on possible effects of medications.

EXPECTED ACTIONS/OUTCOMES: Monitor client use of medications over time.

Safety and Infection Control

STANDARD PRECAUTIONS/TRANSMISSION-BASED PRECAUTIONS/SURGICAL ASEPSIS: Protect immunocompromised client from exposure to infectious diseases/organisms.

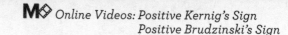

UNIT 2   NEUROLOGIC DISORDERS
SECTION: CENTRAL NERVOUS SYSTEM DISORDERS

CHAPTER 6 *Meningitis*

Meningitis is an inflammation of the meninges, which are the membranes that protect the brain and spinal cord.

Viral, or aseptic, meningitis is the most common form of meningitis and commonly resolves without treatment. Fungal meningitis is common in clients who have AIDS. Bacterial (or septic) meningitis is a contagious infection with a high mortality rate. The prognosis depends on how quickly care is initiated.

There are three vaccines for different pathogens that cause bacterial meningitis. One is available for high-risk populations, such as residential college students, which is required for college entrance.

HEALTH PROMOTION AND DISEASE PREVENTION

Haemophilus influenzae type b (Hib) vaccine

Ensure infants receive vaccine for bacterial meningitis on schedule. A series of four doses is recommended beginning at 2 months of age, with the final dose at 12 to 15 months.

Pneumococcal polysaccharide vaccine (PPSV)

Though primarily intended to prevent respiratory infection, this immunization also decreases the risk for CNS infections. Vaccinate adults who are immunocompromised, have a chronic disease, smoke cigarettes, or live in a long-term care facility. Follow CDC guidelines for reimmunization. Give one dose to adults older than 65 who have not previously been immunized nor have history of disease.

Meningococcal vaccine (MCV4) (Neisseria meningitidis)

Ensure that adolescents receive the vaccine on schedule and prior to living in a residential setting in college. Individuals in other communal living conditions (such as military) also should be immunized. An initial dose is recommended for healthy children between the ages of 11 to 12, with a booster administered at age 16.

DATA COLLECTION

RISK FACTORS

Viral meningitis
- Viral illnesses (mumps, measles, herpes, arboviruses [West Nile])
- There is no vaccine against viral meningitis.

Fungal meningitis: Fulminant fungal-based infection of the sinuses are from the organism *Cryptococcus neoformans.*

Bacterial meningitis: Bacterial-based infections (otitis media, pneumonia, sinusitis) in which the infectious micro-organism is *Neisseria meningitidis, Streptococcus pneumoniae,* or *Haemophilus influenzae*

Immunosuppression

Direct contamination of spinal fluid

Invasive procedures, skull fracture, or penetrating wound

Environment: Overcrowded or concentrated living conditions.

EXPECTED FINDINGS

SUBJECTIVE DATA
- Excruciating, constant headache
- Nuchal rigidity (stiff neck)
- Photophobia (sensitivity to light)

OBJECTIVE DATA: Physical data collection findings
- Fever and chills
- Nausea and vomiting
- Altered level of consciousness (confusion, disorientation, lethargy, difficulty arousing, coma)
- Positive Kernig's sign (resistance and pain with extension of the client's leg from a flexed position)
- Positive Brudzinski's sign (flexion of the knees and hips occurring with deliberate flexion of the client's neck)
- Hyperactive deep tendon reflexes
- Tachycardia
- Seizures
- Red macular rash (meningococcal meningitis)
- Restlessness, irritability

LABORATORY TESTS

Urine, throat, nose, and blood culture and sensitivity: Culture and sensitivity of various body fluids identify possible infectious bacteria and an appropriate broad-spectrum antibiotic. Not definitive for meningitis but can guide initial selection of antimicrobial.

CBC: Elevated WBC count

DIAGNOSTIC PROCEDURES

Cerebrospinal fluid (CSF) analysis
- CSF analysis is the most definitive diagnostic procedure. CSF is collected during a lumbar puncture performed by the provider.
- Results indicative of meningitis
  - Appearance of CSF: cloudy (bacterial) or clear (viral)
  - Elevated WBC
  - Elevated protein
  - Decreased glucose (bacterial)
  - Elevated CSF pressure

CT scan and MRI: A CT scan or an MRI can be performed to identify increased intracranial pressure (ICP) and/or an abscess.

PATIENT-CENTERED CARE

NURSING CARE

- Isolate the client as soon as meningitis is suspected.
- Maintain isolation precautions per hospital policy.
  - Initiate droplet precautions, which require a private room. Continue droplet precautions until antibiotics have been administered for 24 hr and oral and nasal secretions are no longer infectious. Clients who have bacterial meningitis might need to remain on droplet precautions continuously. Qs
  - Standard precautions are implemented for all clients who have meningitis.
- Implement fever-reduction measures, such as a cooling blanket, if necessary.
- Report meningococcal infections to the public health department.
- Decrease environmental stimuli.
- Provide a quiet environment.
- Minimize exposure to bright light (natural and electric).
- Maintain bed rest with the head of the bed elevated to 30°.
- Monitor for increased ICP.

- Tell the client to avoid coughing and sneezing, which increase ICP.
- Maintain client safety, such as seizure precautions. Qs
- Replace fluid and electrolytes as indicated by laboratory values.
- Older adult clients are at an increased risk for secondary complications, such as pneumonia. Ⓖ
- Monitor vital signs to check for septic shock.

MEDICATIONS

Ceftriaxone or cefotaxime in combination with vancomycin: Antibiotics given until culture and sensitivity results are available. Effective for bacterial infections.

Phenytoin: Anticonvulsants given if ICP increases or client experiences a seizure.

Acetaminophen, ibuprofen: Analgesics for headache and/or fever. Non-opioid to avoid masking changes in the level of consciousness.

Ciprofloxacin, rifampin, or ceftriaxone: Prophylactic antibiotics given to individuals in close contact with the client.

COMPLICATIONS

Increased ICP

Meningitis can cause ICP to increase, possibly to the point of brain herniation.

NURSING ACTIONS
- Monitor for indications of increasing ICP (decreased level of consciousness, pupillary changes, impaired extraocular movements).
- Provide interventions to reduce ICP (positioning with head of the bed elevation at 30° and avoidance of coughing and straining). Qs
- Mannitol can be administered via IV.

Application Exercises

1. A nurse is reviewing the use of the meningococcal vaccine (MCV4) for the prevention of meningitis with a newly licensed nurse. Which of the following information should the nurse include?

   A. The vaccine is indicated to reduce the risk of respiratory infection.

   B. The vaccine is administered in a series of four doses.

   C. The vaccine is recommended for adolescents before starting college.

   D. The vaccine is initially given at 2 months of age.

2. A nurse is collecting data from a client who has meningitis. Which of the following findings should the nurse expect? (Select all that apply.)

   A. Bradycardia

   B. Headache

   C. Nuchal rigidity

   D. Seizures

   E. Photophobia

3. A nurse is checking for the presence of Brudzinski's sign in a client who has suspected meningitis. Which of the following actions should the nurse take when performing this technique? (Select all that apply.)

   A. Place client in supine position.

   B. Flex client's hip and knee.

   C. Place hands behind the client's neck.

   D. Bend client's head toward chest.

   E. Straighten the client's flexed leg at the knee.

4. A nurse is assisting with care of a newly admitted client. The client has been identified as having bacterial meningitis. What is the priority nursing care for this client?

   A. Isolate the client.

   B. Provide a quiet environment.

   C. Initiate seizure precautions.

   D. Start IV fluids.

Active Learning Scenario

A nurse is reviewing the plan of care for a client who has bacterial meningitis. Use the ATI Active Learning Template: System Disorder to complete this item.

ALTERATION IN HEALTH (DIAGNOSIS): Define bacterial meningitis.

MEDICATIONS: Identify three medications, their actions, and the reason for administration.

COMPLICATIONS: Describe a complication of meningitis.

Active Learning Scenario Key

Using the ATI Active Learning Template: System Disorder

ALTERATION IN HEALTH (DIAGNOSIS): Bacterial meningitis is a bacterial infection that causes an inflammation of the meninges, the membranes that protect the brain and spinal cord.

MEDICATIONS

- Ceftriaxone with vancocin: antibiotics administered to treat the infection
- Acetaminophen: an antipyretic used to treat a fever
- Phenytoin: an anticonvulsant given to prevent the client from experiencing a seizure when at risk of ICP

COMPLICATIONS: Increased ICP, which can lead to seizures, coma, and death

Ⓝ *NCLEX® Connection: Physiological Adaptation, Alterations in Body Systems*

Application Exercises Key

1. C. **CORRECT:** When taking actions, the nurse should include in the teaching to the newly licensed nurse that the meningococcal vaccine is recommended for adolescents prior to starting college due to the increased risk for infection in communal living facilities.

   Ⓝ *NCLEX® Connection: Health Promotion and Maintenance, Health Promotion/Disease Prevention*

2. B, C, D, E. **CORRECT:** When recognizing cues, the nurse should expect a client who has meningitis to experience a headache, which can be related to increased intracranial pressure. The client can also exhibit nuchal rigidity (stiff neck), as well as experience seizures due to fever and increased intracranial pressure along with photophobia.

   Ⓝ *NCLEX® Connection: Physiological Adaptation, Basic Pathophysiology*

3. A, C, D. **CORRECT:** When recognizing cues to determine the presence of Brudzinski's sign for a client who has suspected meningitis, the nurse should place the client in the supine position and place hands behind the client's neck. While the nurse the client's head toward the chest, the lower extremities of the client will flex.

   Ⓝ *NCLEX® Connection: Physiological Adaptation, Alterations in Body Systems*

4. A. **CORRECT:** The nurse should analyze the findings and determine that the priority hypothesis is that the client who has been identified as having bacterial meningitis is at greatest risk for transmitting the infection; therefore, the nurse should initiate droplet precautions and place the client in a private room.

   Ⓝ *NCLEX® Connection: Physiological Adaptation, Alterations in Body Systems*

UNIT 2   NEUROLOGIC DISORDERS
SECTION: CENTRAL NERVOUS SYSTEM DISORDERS

CHAPTER 7 # Seizures and Epilepsy

Seizures are abrupt, abnormal, excessive, and uncontrolled electrical discharges of neurons within the brain that can cause alterations in the level of consciousness and/or changes in motor and sensory ability and/or behavior.

Epilepsy is the term used to define chronic recurring abnormal brain electrical activity resulting in two or more seizures. Seizures resulting from identifiable causes (substance withdrawal or fever) are not considered epilepsy.

The International League Against Epilepsy uses three broad categories to describe seizures: generalized, focal, and unknown

DATA COLLECTION

RISK FACTORS

- **Genetic predisposition**: Absence seizures are more common in children and tend to occur in families.
- **Acute febrile state**: Particularly among infants and children younger than 2 years old.
- **Head trauma**: Can be early or late onset (up to 9 months), and incidence is increased when the head trauma includes a skull fracture.
- **Cerebral edema:** Especially when it occurs acutely and seizure activity tends to disappear when the edema is successfully treated.
- **Abrupt cessation of antiepileptic drugs (AEDs)**: As a rebound activity.
- **Infection**: If intracranial, a result of increased intracranial pressure; if systemic, a result of the persistent febrile state.
- **Metabolic disorder:** A result of insufficient or excessive chemicals within the brain, such as occurring with hypoglycemia or hyponatremia.
- **Exposure to toxins:** Especially those associated with pesticides, carbon monoxide, and lead poisoning.
- **Stroke**: Most likely to occur within the first 24 hr following a stroke as a result of increased intracranial pressure.
- **Heart disease**: Common cause of new-onset seizures in older adults.
- **Brain tumor:** If benign, seizures caused by the increased bulk associated with the tumor; if malignant, associated with the ability of the brain tissue to function.

- **Hypoxia**: Results in a decreased oxygen level of the brain; necessary for neuronal activity.
- **Acute substance withdrawal**: Dehydration accompanies withdrawal, creating a toxic level of the substance in the body.
- **Fluid and electrolyte imbalances:** Results in abnormal levels of nutrients required for neuronal function.
- With older adult clients, increased seizure incidence is associated with cerebrovascular diseases. **Ⓖ**
- With clients who experience menses or pregnancy, changes in the incidence or pattern of seizure activity are associated with hormonal activity that alters the excitability of neurons in the cerebral cortex.

COMMON TRIGGERING FACTORS FOR SEIZURES
- Increased physical activity
- Excessive stress
- Hyperventilation
- Overwhelming fatigue
- Acute alcohol ingestion
- Excessive caffeine intake
- Exposure to flashing lights
- Substances such as cocaine, aerosols, and inhaled glue products

EXPECTED FINDINGS

Generalized seizures
Generalized seizure involves both cerebral hemispheres. Generalized seizures can begin with an aura (alteration in vision, smell, hearing, or emotional feeling). Clients can experience five types of generalized seizures.

Tonic-clonic seizure
- A tonic-clonic seizure begins for only a few seconds with a tonic episode (stiffening of muscles) and loss of consciousness.
- A 1- to 2-min clonic episode (rhythmic jerking of the extremities) follows the tonic episode.
- Breathing can stop during the tonic phase and become irregular during the clonic phase.
- Cyanosis can accompany breathing irregularities.
- Biting of the cheek or tongue can occur during clonic phase.
- Incontinence can also accompany a tonic-clonic seizure.
- During the postictal phase, a period of confusion and sleepiness follows the seizure.

Tonic seizure
Only the tonic phase is experienced.
Clients suddenly lose consciousness and experience sudden increased muscle tone, loss of consciousness, and autonomic manifestations (arrhythmia, apnea, vomiting, incontinence, salivation).
Tonic seizures generally last less than 30 seconds, but some sources indicate they can last several minutes.

Clonic seizure
- Only the clonic phase is experienced.
- The seizure lasts several minutes.
- During this type of seizure, the muscles contract and relax.

Myoclonic seizure
- Myoclonic seizures consist of brief jerking or stiffening of the extremities, which can be symmetrical or asymmetrical.
- This type of seizure lasts for seconds.

Atonic or akinetic seizure
- Atonic or akinetic seizures are characterized by a few seconds in which muscle tone is lost.
- The seizure is followed by a period of confusion.
- The loss of muscle tone frequently results in falling.

Absence
- Loss of consciousness for 10 to 30 seconds
- No motor activity or mild symmetrical activity such as blinking.
- May occur several hundred times daily
- Rare in adults, typically stop occurring during adolescence

Focal seizure: Partial or focal/local seizure involves only one cerebral hemisphere.
Clients can experience any of the following adverse effects.
- Client can have associated automatisms (behaviors that the client is unaware of, such as lip smacking or picking at clothes).
- The seizure can cause a loss of consciousness, blackout for several minutes, or consciousness may be maintained throughout the seizure.
- Consciousness is maintained throughout simple partial seizures.
- Seizure activity can consist of unusual sensations, a sense of déjà vu, autonomic abnormalities such as changes in heart rate and abnormal flushing, unilateral abnormal extremity movements, pain, or offensive smell.

Unknown seizures: Unclassified or idiopathic seizures do not fit into other categories. These types of seizures account for half of all seizure activity and occur for no known reason.

LABORATORY TESTS

Tests can include alcohol, illicit substance levels, HIV testing, and if suspected, screen for the presence of excessive toxins. Blood tests (CBC, electrolytes, BUN, and blood glucose) can be done to further address other causes of the seizure.

DIAGNOSTIC PROCEDURES

- Electroencephalogram (EEG) records electrical activity and can identify the origin of seizure activity.
- Magnetic resonance imaging (MRI), computed tomography (CT) imaging/computed axial tomography (CAT) scan, positron emission tomography (PET) scan, cerebrospinal fluid (CSF) analysis, and skull x-ray can be used to identify or rule out potential causes of seizures.

PATIENT-CENTERED CARE

NURSING CARE

During a seizure
- Protect the client's privacy and the client from injury (move furniture away, hold head in lap if on the floor). Qs
- Position the client to provide a patent airway.
- Be prepared to suction oral secretions.
- Turn the client to the side to decrease the risk of aspiration.
- Loosen restrictive clothing.
- Do not attempt to restrain the client.
- Do not attempt to open the jaw or insert airway during seizure activity (can damage teeth, lips, and tongue).
- Do not use padded tongue blades.
- Document onset and duration of seizure and findings (level of consciousness, apnea, cyanosis, motor activity, incontinence) prior to, during, and following the seizure.

After a seizure
- This is the postictal phase of the seizure episode.
- Maintain the client in a side-lying position to prevent aspiration and to facilitate drainage of oral secretions.
- Check vital signs.
- Check for injuries.
- Perform neurological checks.
- Allow the client to rest if necessary.
- Reorient and calm the client, who might be agitated or confused.
- Determine if client experienced an aura, which can indicate the origin of seizure in the brain.
- Try to determine possible trigger (such as fatigue).

7.1 Care of a client who has had a seizure

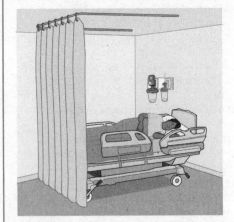

CLIENT: Client assisted to side-lying position

SIDE RAILS: Two to three side rails padded and raised

OXYGEN REGULATOR: Oxygen equipment available

SUCTION CANNISTER: Suction equipment available

CLIENT GOWN: Clothing loosened

PRIVACY CURTAIN: Privacy ensured as soon as possible

MEDICATIONS

- Administer prescribed antiepileptic drugs (AEDs), such as phenytoin.
- Initial goal is to control seizure activity using one medication. If the chosen medication is not effective, either the dose is increased, or another medication is added or substituted.
- Therapeutic levels are determined by blood tests. These are performed on a routine schedule to ensure compliance and effectiveness of the medication. ⓠEBP
- Allergic reactions to these medications are rare, yet can occur immediately or late in therapy. If the client is allergic, another medication may be substituted.

CLIENT EDUCATION
- Take medications at the same time every day to enhance effectiveness.
- The potential to develop tolerance to antiseizure medications over time can lead to an increase in seizures. Some clients develop sensitivity with age. If tolerance or sensitivity occurs, clients will need blood levels drawn frequently and medication dosages adjusted.
- Be aware of adverse effects and interactions with food or other medications. These are specific to the medication.
- Some antiepileptic medications cause oral gum overgrowth. Routine oral hygiene and dental visits can minimize this adverse effect.
- When using phenytoin, specific instructions should include avoidance of oral contraceptives, as this medication decreases their effectiveness. Warfarin should also not be given with this medication, as phenytoin can decrease absorption and increase metabolism of oral anticoagulants.

INTERPROFESSIONAL CARE

Provide the client with community resource information, including the Epilepsy Foundation.

THERAPEUTIC PROCEDURES

Vagal nerve stimulation and conventional surgical procedures can be helpful for clients whose seizures are not controlled with medication therapy.

Vagal nerve stimulator

- Vagal nerve stimulation is indicated for treatment of focal seizures.
- The vagal nerve stimulator is a device implanted into the left chest wall and connected to an electrode placed on the left vagus nerve.
- This procedure is performed under general anesthesia.
- The device is then programmed to administer intermittent stimulation of the brain via stimulation of the vagal nerve, at a rate specific to the client's needs.

Conventional surgical procedures

- Conventional surgical procedures are available for clients who experience partial or generalized seizures.
- Prior to surgery, AEDs are discontinued and the specific area of the seizure activity is identified through the use of EEG monitoring. Surgically implanted electrodes can also be used.
- The affected area of the brain can be excised if it is determined that vital brain function will not be affected.
- Partial corpus callosotomy can be used for clients who are not candidates for conventional surgical procedures. The procedure resects the corpus callosum, preventing neuronal discharges across hemispheres and reduces the severity and frequency of seizures.
- These procedures have associated morbidities, including infection, loss of cerebral function, and a lack of success in preventing seizures. ⓠs

Responsive neurostimulation system (RNS)

- Indicated for clients who have refractory seizures
- Electrodes are surgically implanted to sense, record, and interrupt seizure activity in the brain

NURSING ACTIONS

- Reinforce client education regarding seizure management.
  - Importance of monitoring AED levels and maintaining therapeutic medication levels
  - Possible medication interactions (decreased effectiveness of oral contraceptives)
- Encourage the client to wear a medical identification tag at all times.
- Reinforce instruction to clients who have a history of seizures to research state driving laws. Some states restrict or limit driving for individuals who have a recent history of seizures. ⓠs

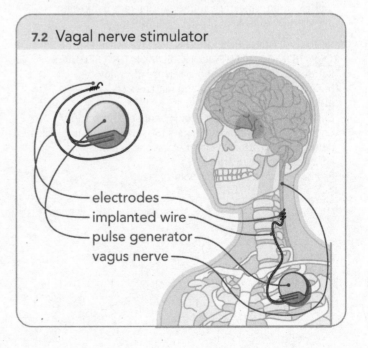

7.2 Vagal nerve stimulator

- electrodes
- implanted wire
- pulse generator
- vagus nerve

COMPLICATIONS

Status epilepticus

This is repeated seizure activity within a 30-min time frame or a single prolonged seizure lasting more than 5 min. The complications associated with this condition are related to decreased oxygen levels, inability of the brain to return to normal functioning, and continued assault on neuronal tissue. This acute condition requires immediate treatment to prevent permanent loss of brain function and death.

The usual causes are substance withdrawal, sudden withdrawal from AEDs, head injury, cerebral edema, infection, and metabolic disturbances. Qᴛᴄ

NURSING ACTIONS
- Maintain an airway, provide oxygen, establish IV access, perform ECG monitoring, and monitor vital signs, pulse oximetry, and ABG results.
- Assist with the administration of diazepam or lorazepam IV push, midazolam IM, or diazepam rectally, followed by IV phenytoin or fosphenytoin.

Sudden Unexpected Death in Epilepsy (SUDEP)

This is the sudden, expected death of an otherwise healthy individual who has epilepsy with no other known cause of death.

RISK FACTORS

- Most frequently occurs in clients aged 15 to 40 years
- Seizures of long duration
- Seizure clusters – increased frequency of seizures or multiple seizures within 8 hours
- Multiple antiepileptic medications
- Nonadherance to antiepileptic medication therapy
- Brain lesions
- Cardiac and respiratory abnormalities may be present
- Between 40 to 60% of SUDEP occur during sleep

NURSING ACTIONS FOR PREVENTION OF SUDEP – PROMOTION OF CONTROLLING/ELIMINATING SEIZURES
- Reinforce information about seizure alert devices, including watch monitors and mattress or pillow devices
- Encourage client to keep a journal of seizure activity
- Encourage avoidance of triggers for seizure activity
- Reinforce education to client about the benefits of adherence to medications
- Promote sleep hygiene for quality sleep

Application Exercises

1. A nurse is caring for clients who have seizure disorders. Match each manifestation the nurse observes with the type of seizure each client is experiencing.

   A. Atonic seizure
   B. Absence seizure
   C. Simple partial seizure
   D. Tonic-clonic seizure
   E. Myoclonic seizure

   1. The seizure lasted for several seconds.
   2. The client experienced incontinence.
   3. The client repeatedly experienced loss of consciousness with no motor activity.
   4. The client experienced flushing and an offensive smell.
   5. The client experienced loss of muscle tone.

2. A nurse is assisting a client who is ambulating to the bathroom. The client begins to have a seizure. Which actions should the nurse take? (Select all that apply.)

   A. Provide privacy.
   B. Ease the client to the floor if standing.
   C. Move furniture away from the client.
   D. Loosen the client's clothing.
   E. Protect the client's head.
   F. Restrain the client.

3. A nurse is reinforcing discharge instructions to a client who has a prescription for phenytoin. Which of the following information should the nurse include?

   A. Discontinue the medication if there is no seizure activity for 6 months.
   B. Watch for receding gums when taking the medication.
   C. Take the medication at the same time every day.
   D. Provide a urine sample to determine therapeutic levels of the medication.

4. A nurse is assisting with the preparation of information for a client about SUDEP and suggests including strategies to avoid seizure triggers and strategies to manage seizures. Sort each activity by whether the nurse should suggest including it as a Seizure trigger or a strategy for Seizure management.

   A. Flashing light therapy to regulate mood and promote relaxation
   B. Aerosol air fresheners for aromatherapy
   C. Moderate exercise
   D. Hot tub baths for relaxation
   E. Caffeinated beverages throughout the day

Application Exercises Key

1. A, 5; C, 3; E, 4, G, 2; I, 1

   When recognizing cues, the nurse identifies that jerking or stiffness for several seconds are manifestations of a myoclonic seizure. The nurse identifies that incontinence is a manifestation of a tonic-clonic seizure. The nurse identifies that loss of consciousness without motor activity is a manifestation of an absence seizure. The nurse identifies that unusual sensations, such as flushing and offensive smells are manifestations of a simple partial seizure. The nurse identifies that loss of muscle tone is a manifestation of an atonic seizure.

   Ⓝ *NCLEX Connections: Physiological Adaptation Alterations in Body Systems*

2. B, C, D, E. **CORRECT**: When taking actions to care for a client who is having a seizure, the nurse should ease the client to the floor to prevent injury from a fall. The nurse should move furniture away from the client when possible to protect the client from injury. The nurse should loosen the client's clothing to prevent restraining the client's movements. The nurse should protect the client's head from injury from a hard surface.

   Ⓝ *NCLEX Connections: Physiological Adaptation Alterations in Body Systems*

3. C. **CORRECT**: When taking actions to reinforce discharge instructions to a client who has a prescription for an antiseizure medication, the nurse should reinforce instructions to the client to adhere to the medication schedule as prescribed to maintain therapeutic levels of the medication.

   Ⓝ *NCLEX Connections: Pharmacological Therapies: Adverse Effects/Contraindications/Side Effects/Interactions*

4. **SEIZURE TRIGGER**: A, B, D, E; **SEIZURE MANAGEMENT**: C

   When generating solutions for education about prevention of SUDEP, the nurse should suggest instructing the client to avoid triggers such as chemical sprays, extreme temperatures, caffeine, and flashing lights. The nurse should suggest instructing the client to include moderate exercise in a temperature-controlled environment as a strategy for managing overall health and avoiding trigger such as extreme heat or hyperventilation.

   Ⓝ *NCLEX Connections: Physiological Adaptation Alterations in Body Systems*

Active Learning Scenario

A nurse is contributing to the plan of care for a client who is experiencing status epilepticus. What concepts should the nurse include in the plan of care? Use the ATI Active Learning Template: Basic Concept to complete this item.

RELATED CONTENT: Define the condition.

UNDERLYING PRINCIPLES: Describe four possible causes.

NURSING INTERVENTIONS: Describe five actions the nurse should plan to take.

Active Learning Scenario Key

Using the ATI Active Learning Template: Basic Concept

RELATED CONTENT: Status epilepticus is repeated seizure activity within a 30-min time frame or a single prolonged seizure lasting more than 5 min.

UNDERLYING PRINCIPLES
- Substance withdrawal
- Withdrawal from antiepileptic medication
- Infection
- Head injury
- Cerebral edema
- Metabolic disturbances

NURSING INTERVENTIONS
- Maintain a patent airway.
- Perform ECG monitoring.
- Review ABG results.
- Establish IV access.
- Provide oxygen.
- Monitor pulse oximetry.
- Administer lorazepam or diazepam.
- Administer phenytoin or fosphenytoin.

Ⓝ *NCLEX® Connection: Physiological Adaptation, Alterations in Body Systems*

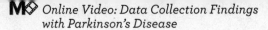

CHAPTER 8 *Parkinson's Disease*

Parkinson's disease (PD) is a progressively debilitating disease that grossly affects motor function. It is characterized by four primary findings: tremor, muscle rigidity, bradykinesia (slow movement), and postural instability. These findings occur due to overstimulation of the basal ganglia by acetylcholine.

The secretion of dopamine and acetylcholine in the body produce inhibitory and excitatory effects on the muscles respectively.

Overstimulation of the basal ganglia by acetylcholine occurs because degeneration of the substantia nigra results in decreased dopamine production. This allows acetylcholine to dominate, making smooth, controlled movements difficult.

Treatment of PD focuses on increasing the amount of dopamine or decreasing the amount of acetylcholine in a client's brain.

DATA COLLECTION

RISK FACTORS

- Onset of findings usually occur in clients over the age of 50
- Clients assigned male at birth
- Genetic predisposition
- Exposure to environmental toxins and chemical solvents
- Chronic use of antipsychotic medication

EXPECTED FINDINGS

- Bradykinesia (movement that is slow).
- Akinesia (no movement).

MANIFESTATIONS

- Stooped posture
- Slow, shuffling, and propulsive gait
- Slow, monotonous speech
- Tremors/pill-rolling tremor of the fingers
- Muscle rigidity (rhythmic interruption, mildly restrictive, total resistance to movement)
- Bradykinesia/akinesia
- Masklike expression
- Autonomic findings (orthostatic hypotension, flushing, diaphoresis)
- Difficulty chewing and swallowing
  - Drooling
  - Dysarthria
  - Progressive difficulty with ADLs
  - Mood swings
  - Cognitive impairment (dementia)

LABORATORY TESTS

- There are no definitive diagnostic procedures.
- Diagnosis is made based on manifestations, their progression, and by ruling out other diseases.

PATIENT-CENTERED CARE

NURSING CARE

- Administer medications at prescribed times. Monitor medication effectiveness, and make recommendations for changes in dosage and time of administration to provide best coverage.
- Monitor swallowing, and maintain adequate nutrition and weight. Consult speech and language therapist to determine swallowing if the client demonstrates a risk for choking. Qs
  - Consult the client's dietitian for appropriate diet, which often includes semisolid foods and thickened liquids.
  - Document the client's weight at least weekly.
  - Keep a diet intake log.
  - Encourage fluids and document intake.
  - Provide smaller, more frequent meals.
  - Sit the client upright to eat or drink.
  - Consult with an occupational therapist for adaptive eating devices. Qтc
  - Determine the need for high-calorie, high-protein supplements to maintain the client's weight.
- Maintain client mobility for as long as possible.
  - Encourage exercise, such as yoga (can also improve mental status).
  - Encourage use of assistive devices as disease progresses.
  - Encourage range-of-motion (ROM) exercises.
  - Reinforce with the client to stop occasionally when walking to slow down speed and reduce risk for injury.
  - Pace activities by providing rest periods.
  - Assist with ADLs as needed (hygiene, dressing).
- Promote client communication for as long as possible.
  - Reinforce teaching about facial muscle strengthening exercises.
  - Encourage the client to speak slowly and to pause frequently.
  - Assist with making a referral to a speech-language pathologist.
- Monitor mental and cognitive status.
  - Observe for manifestations of depression and dementia.
  - Provide a safe environment (no throw rugs, encourage the use of an electric razor). Qs

- Monitor personal and family coping with the client's chronic, degenerative disease.
- Provide a list of community resources (support groups) to the client and family.
- Assist with making a referral to a social worker or case manager as condition advances (financial issues, long-term home care, and respite care). Qᴛᴄ

MEDICATIONS

- Can take several weeks of use before improvement of manifestations is seen.
- While the client is taking a combination of medications, maintenance of therapeutic medication levels is necessary for adequate control.

Dopaminergics

- When given orally, levodopa is converted to dopamine in the brain, increasing dopamine levels in the basal ganglia.
- Dopaminergics may be combined with carbidopa to decrease peripheral metabolism of levodopa, requiring a smaller dose to make the same amount available to the brain. Adverse effects are subsequently less.
- Due to medication tolerance and metabolism, the dosage, form of medication, and administration times must be adjusted to avoid periods of poor mobility.

NURSING ACTIONS: Monitor for the "wearing-off" phenomenon and dyskinesias (problems with movement), which can indicate the need to adjust the dosage or time of administration or the need for a medication holiday.

Dopamine agonists

Dopamine agonists (bromocriptine, ropinirole, pramipexole) activate release of dopamine. May be used in conjunction with a dopaminergic for better results.

NURSING ACTIONS: Monitor for orthostatic hypotension, dyskinesias, and hallucinations. Qs

Anticholinergics

Anticholinergics (benztropine and trihexyphenidyl) help control tremors and rigidity.

NURSING ACTIONS: Monitor for anticholinergic effects (dry mouth, constipation, urinary retention, acute confusion).

Catechol O-methyltransferase (COMT) inhibitors

COMT inhibitors, such as entacapone, decrease the breakdown of levodopa, making more available to the brain as dopamine. Can be used in conjunction with a dopaminergic and dopamine agonist for better results.

NURSING ACTIONS
- Monitor for dyskinesia/hyperkinesia when used with levodopa.
- Monitor for diarrhea.
- Dark urine is a normal finding.

Monoamine oxidase type B (MAO-B) inhibitors

MAO-B inhibitors (selegiline and rasagiline) inhibit monoamine oxidase type B activity and increase dopamine levels. They reduce the wearing-off phenomenon when administered concurrently with levodopa.

NURSING ACTIONS: Severe reactions can occur when these medications are administered with sympathomimetics, meperidine, and fluoxetine.

CLIENT EDUCATION: Avoid foods high in tyramine, which can cause hypertensive crisis. Qs

Antivirals

Antivirals, such as amantadine, stimulate release of dopamine and prevent its reuptake.

NURSING ACTIONS
- Monitor for discoloration of the skin that subsides when amantadine is discontinued.
- Client might experience anxiety, confusion, and anticholinergic effects.

THERAPEUTIC PROCEDURES

Deep brain stimulation

An electrode is implanted in the thalamus and a small pulse generator is placed under the skin of the upper chest to block tremors.

NURSING ACTIONS: Monitor for infection, brain hemorrhage, or stroke-like findings.

INTERPROFESSIONAL CARE

- Because PD is a degenerative neurologic disorder, long-term treatment and care must be accommodated.
- During the later stages of the disorder, the client needs referrals to and support from disciplines such as speech therapists, occupational therapists, physical therapists, and social service/case management.

COMPLICATIONS

Aspiration pneumonia

As PD advances in severity, alterations in chewing and swallowing worsen, increasing the risk for aspiration.

NURSING ACTIONS
- Use swallowing precautions to decrease the risk for aspiration. Qs
- Contribute to develop a dietary plan based on the speech therapist's recommendations.
- Have a nurse in attendance when the client is eating.
- Encourage the client to eat slowly and chew thoroughly before swallowing. Qs
- Feed the client in an upright position and have suction equipment on standby.
- Participate in evaluating the need for enteral feedings to maintain weight and prevent aspiration as PD progresses.

Altered cognition (dementia, memory deficits)

Clients in advanced stages of PD can exhibit altered cognition in the form of dementia and memory loss.

NURSING ACTIONS
- Acknowledge the client's feelings.
- Provide for a safe environment.
- Contribute to develop a comprehensive plan of care with the family, client, and interprofessional team. Q℡

Urinary tract infection, depression, skin breakdown

Clients with PD can develop urinary problems, including urinary tract infections; depression and psychosis; and effects from immobility, such as skin breakdown.

NURSING ACTIONS
- Monitor for urinary incontinence and retention.
- Monitor for skin breakdown and provide skin care.
- Turn client frequently.
- Monitor client for manifestations of depression.
- Encourage client to set realistic and achievable goals.

Active Learning Scenario

A nurse is contributing to the plan of care for a client who has a new diagnosis of Parkinson's disease. What should the nurse include in the plan of care? Use the ATI Active Learning Template: System Disorder to complete this item.

ALTERATION IN HEALTH (DIAGNOSIS):
Define Parkinson's disease.

COMPLICATIONS: Identify four.

NURSING CARE: Describe six nursing actions.

Application Exercises

1. A nurse is caring for a client who has Parkinson's disease. Which of the following findings should the nurse anticipate the client to exhibit? (Select all that apply.)
   A. Decreased vision
   B. Pill-rolling tremor of the fingers
   C. Shuffling gait
   D. Drooling
   E. Lack of facial expression

2. A nurse is caring for a client who is taking benztropine and is reporting tremors and rigidity in the left hand and arm. Which of the following findings should the nurse identify as an adverse effect of benztropine? (Select all that apply.)
   A. Aspiration
   B. Diarrhea
   C. Dry mouth
   D. Dark urine
   E. Orthostatic hypotension

3. A nurse is assisting with the care of a client who has stage IV Parkinson's disease and has lost 20 lbs since their last checkup one month ago. The client presents with akinesia and rigidity. When contributing to the plan of care for the client's nutritional needs, which of the following actions should the nurse include? (Select all that apply.)
   A. Provide three large balanced meals daily
   B. Record diet and fluid intake daily
   C. Document weight every other week
   D. Offer cold fluids such as milk shakes
   E. Offer nutritional supplements between meals

Active Learning Scenario Key

Using the ATI Active Learning Template: System Disorder

ALTERATION IN HEALTH (DIAGNOSIS): Parkinson's disease is a debilitating condition that progresses to complete dependent care. The disease involves a decrease in dopamine production and an increase in secretion of acetylcholine, causing resting tremor, slowed movement, and muscular rigidity.

COMPLICATIONS
- Aspiration due to pharyngeal muscle involvement making swallowing difficult
- Orthostatic hypotension, slow movement, and muscle rigidity
- Change in speech pattern: slow, monotonous speech
- Altered emotional changes that can include depression and fear

NURSING CARE
- Add thickener to liquids to prevent aspiration.
- Consult with a dietitian about appropriate diet.
- Encourage periods of rest between activities.
- Allow adequate time to rise slowly from a sitting to standing position.
- Encourage slower speech when expressing thoughts.
- Observe for manifestations of depression and dementia.

ⓝ *NCLEX® Connection: Physiological Adaptation, Basic Pathophysiology*

Application Exercises Key

1. B, C, D, E. **CORRECT**: When recognizing cues, the nurse should identify that clients who have Parkinson's disease can manifest pill-rolling tremors of the fingers due to overstimulation of the basal ganglia by acetylcholine, making controlled movement difficult. Clients can also manifest a shuffling gait. The client who has Parkinson's disease can develop drooling, making the controlled movement of swallowing secretions difficult. Lack of facial expressions are also common, making controlled movement difficult. Bilateral ankle edema is not an expected finding in a client who has Parkinson's disease but can be an adverse effect of certain medications used for treatment. Decreased vision is not an expected finding in a client who has PD.

ⓝ *NCLEX Connections: Physiological Adaptation: Basic Pathophysiology*

2. C. **CORRECT**: When analyzing cues, the nurse should identify that anticholinergic effects, such as dry mount, are anticipated in clients who take benztropine. Benztropine does not cause drooling and does not increase the risk for aspiration. Diarrhea is not a clinical manifestation of benztropine. It is a potential side effect of catechol O-methyltransferase (COMT) inhibitors. Orthostatic hypotension is a side effect of dopamine agonists, not benztropine. Dark urine is an expected finding with catechol O-methyltransferase (COMT) inhibitors, not benztropine

ⓝ *NCLEX Connections: Pharmacological Therapies: Adverse Effects/Contraindications/Side Effects/Interactions*

3. B, D, E. **CORRECT**: When generating solutions, the nurse should record the client's diet and fluid intake daily to assess for dietary needs and to maintain adequate nutrition and hydration. The nurse should plan to provide cold fluids such as milkshakes. Thick and cold fluids are tolerated easier by the client. The nurse should offer nutritional supplements between meals to maintain the client's weight, provide small, frequent meals during the day to maintain adequate nutrition, and document the client's weight weekly to identify weight loss and intervene to maintain the client's weight.

ⓝ *NCLEX Connections: Basic Care and Comfort: Nutrition and Oral Hydration*

CHAPTER 9 # Delirium and Dementia

Alzheimer's disease (AD) is a nonreversible type of dementia that progressively develops over many years. AD is one of the leading causes of death in the United States, especially for adults over the age of 65. A framework made up of seven stages has been designed to categorize the disease and its manifestations. The framework is based on three general stages: early stage, middle stage, and late stage.

Dementia is defined as multiple cognitive deficits that impair memory and can affect language, motor skills, and/or abstract thinking. The percentage of dementia attributable to AD ranges from 60% to 90%.

The mean duration of survival after diagnosis is approximately 10 years, but some people can live with the disease for up to 20 years.

AD is most likely to occur in clients in their 60s and 70s. However, it can be diagnosed as early as 40. Age, sex, and genetics are known risk factors for AD, which usually occurs after the age of 65. ©

AD is characterized by memory loss, problems with judgment, and changes in personality. As the disease progresses, severe physical decline occurs along with deteriorating cognitive functions.

Delirium

Acute neurocognitive disorder experienced in more than 80% of clients in the intensive care unit and up to 50% of older adult hospitalized clients. Delirium is a medical emergency characterized by inattentiveness, disorganized thoughts, and an alteration in the client's level of consciousness, resulting in emotional manifestations, including psychotic behavior.

TYPES OF DELIRIUM

Hyperactive delirium

- Agitation
- Restlessness
- Aggressive behavior

Hypoactive delirium

- Lethargy
- Withdrawn behavior
- Subdued

Mixed delirium

A combination of both hyperactive and hypoactive delirium manifestations

ASSESSMENT

Confusion Assessment Method (CAM) and Delirium Index (DI) are used as screening methods.

RISK FACTORS

- Critical care settings
- Drug therapy, including anticholinergics, opioids, and antipsychotic medications
- Infections
- Alcohol toxicity
- Head trauma
- Acute and chronic illnesses
- Insomnia
- Sudden change in living environment
- Sensory deprivation or overload

PATIENT-CENTERED CARE

NURSING CARE

- Remove contributing factors causing the client's confusion.
- Collaborate with interdisciplinary team regarding client's plan of care.
- Reorient client frequently.
- Speak to client using a calm voice.
- Consider the use of calming music in the client's environment.

STAGES OF ALZHEIMER'S DISEASE

The progression of Alzheimer's disease can be different for each client. While there is no universal scale for the stages and manifestations, the following is an example of one scale.

Mild Alzheimer's (early stage)

- Memory lapses
- Losing or misplacing items
- Difficulty concentrating and organizing
- Unable to remember material just read
- Still able to perform ADLs
- Short-term memory loss noticeable to close relations
- Trouble remembering names when introduced to new people
- Greater difficulty performing tasks when under stress

Moderate Alzheimer's (middle stage)

- Forgetting events of one's own history
- Difficulty performing tasks that require planning and organizing (paying bills, managing money)
- Difficulty with complex mental arithmetic
- Personality and behavioral changes: appearing withdrawn or subdued, especially in social or mentally challenging situations; compulsive; repetitive actions
- Changes in sleep patterns
- Can wander and get lost
- Can be incontinent
- Clinical findings that are noticeable to others

Severe Alzheimer's (late stage)

- Losing ability to converse with others
- Assistance required for ADLs
- Incontinence
- Losing awareness of one's environment
- Progressing difficulty with physical abilities (walking, sitting, and eventually swallowing)
- Eventually losses all ability to move; can develop stupor and coma
- Death frequently related to choking or infection
- Vulnerable to infection, especially pneumonia, which can lead to death

DATA COLLECTION

Mini Mental State Examination (MMSE), set test using fruits, animals, colors, towns (FACT), Montreal Cognitive Assessment Test (MoCA), Brief Interview for Mental Status (BIMS), or Clock Drawing Test is used.

HEALTH PROMOTION

- Active lifestyle
- Mediterranean diet
- Management of chronic illnesses

RISK FACTORS

- Advanced age
- Chemical imbalances
- Family history of AD or Down syndrome
- Genetic predisposition, apolipoprotein E
- Environmental agents or virus (metal, or toxic waste)
- Previous head injury
- Assigned female at birth
- Ethnicity/race (African American and Hispanic people are at an increased risk for the development of AD more than non-Hispanic white people due to the APOE and ABCA7 genes.)
- Posttraumatic stress disorder (PTSD)

EXPECTED FINDINGS

The progression of Alzheimer's disease can be different for each client. There is no universal scale for the stages and manifestations.

For more information, see **PN MENTAL HEALTH NURSING CHAPTER 17: NEUROCOGNITIVE DISORDERS**.

LABORATORY TESTS

- No specific lab test can definitively diagnose AD.
- Several lab tests can rule out other causes of dementia.
- CBC, chemistry profile, vitamin B_{12}, thyroid hormone levels, and CSF examination may help in the diagnosis of AD.
- A genetic test for the presence of apolipoprotein can determine if there is an increased risk of AD, but it does not specifically diagnose AD. The presence of the protein increases the likelihood that dementia is due to AD.

DIAGNOSTIC PROCEDURES

- There is no definitive diagnostic procedure, except brain tissue examination upon death.
- Magnetic resonance imaging (MRI) computed tomography (CT) imaging/computed axial tomography (CAT) scan, positron emission tomography (PET) scan, and electroencephalogram (EEG) may be performed to rule out other possible causes of findings.
- A lumbar puncture may be performed for laboratory testing of cerebral spinal fluid for soluble beta protein precursor (sBPP). Beta amyloid protein normally assists in growth and protection of nerve cells. The presence of low levels of sBPP supports the diagnosis of AD.

PATIENT-CENTERED CARE

NURSING CARE

- Check cognitive status, memory, judgment, and personality changes.
- Initiate bowel and bladder program based on a set schedule.
- Encourage the client and family to participate in an AD support group.
- Provide a safe environment. Qs
  - Frequent monitoring/visual checks
  - Keep client from stairs, elevators, exits.
  - Remove or secure dangerous items in the client's environment.
- Provide frequent walks to reduce wandering.
- Maintain a sleeping schedule, and monitor for irregular sleeping patterns.
- Provide verbal and nonverbal ways to communicate with the client.
- Offer snacks or finger foods if the client is unable to sit for long periods of time.
- Check skin weekly for breakdown.
- Provide cognitive stimulation.
  - Offer varied environmental stimulations (walks, music, craft activities).
  - Keep a structured environment and introduce change gradually (client's daily routine or a room change).
  - Use a calendar to assist with orientation.
  - Use short directions when explaining an activity or care the client needs, such as a bath.
  - Be consistent and repetitive.
  - Use therapeutic touch.
- Provide memory training.
  - Reminisce with the client about the past.
  - Use memory techniques (making lists, rehearsing).
  - Stimulate memory by repeating the client's last statement.
- Avoid overstimulation. (Keep noise and clutter to a minimum, and avoid crowds.)
- Promote consistency by placing commonly used objects in the same location and using a routine schedule.
  - Reality orientation (early stages)
  - Easily viewed clock and single–day calendar
  - Pictures of family and pets
  - Frequent reorientation to time, place, and person
- Validation therapy (later stages)
  - Acknowledge the client's feelings.
  - Don't argue with the client; this will lead to the client becoming upset.
  - Reinforce and use repetitive actions or ideas cautiously.
- Promote self-care as long as possible. Assist with activities of daily living as needed.
- Speak directly to the client in short, concise sentences.
- Reduce agitation. (Use calm, redirecting statements. Provide a diversion. Use music therapy to calm or distract).
- Provide a routine toileting schedule.

9.1 Alzheimer's disease stages and manifestations

Mild Alzheimer's (early stage)

STAGE 1: No apparent manifestation
- Normal function
- Manifestation: No memory problems

STAGE 2: Forgetfulness
- (Can be normal age-related changes or very early manifestations of AD)
- Manifestations
  - Forgetfulness, especially of everyday objects (eyeglasses or wallet)
  - No memory problems evident to provider, friends, or coworkers

STAGE 3: Mild cognitive decline
- (Problems with memory or concentration can be measurable in clinical testing or during a detailed medical interview)
- Mild cognitive deficits, including losing or misplacing important objects
- Manifestations
  - Decreased ability to plan
  - Short-term memory loss noticeable to close relatives
  - Decreased attention span
  - Difficulty remembering words or names
  - Difficulty in social or work situations
  - Can get lost when driving

Moderate Alzheimer's (middle stage)

STAGE 4: Mild to moderate cognitive decline
- Medical interview will detect clear-cut deficiencies.
- Manifestations
  - Personality changes: appearing withdrawn or subdued, especially in social or mentally challenging situations
  - Obvious memory loss
  - Limited knowledge and memory of recent occasions, current events, or personal history
  - Difficulty performing tasks that require planning and organizing (paying bills or managing money)
  - Difficulty with complex mental arithmetic
  - Depression and social withdrawal can occur.

STAGE 5: Moderate cognitive decline
Manifestations
- Increasing cognitive deficits emerge.
- Inability to recall important details such as address, telephone number, or schools attended, but memory of information about self and family remains intact
- Assistance with ADLs becomes necessary.
- Disorientation and confusion as to time and place

Severe Alzheimer's (late stage)

STAGE 6: Moderate to severe cognitive decline
Manifestations
- Memory difficulties continue to worsen.
- Loss of awareness of recent events and surroundings
- Can recall own name but unable to recall personal history
- Significant personality changes are evident (delusions, hallucinations, and compulsive behaviors).
- Wandering behavior
- Requires assistance with ADLs such as dressing, toileting, and grooming
- Normal sleep/wake cycle is disrupted.
- Increased episodes of urinary and fecal incontinence

STAGE 7: Severe cognitive decline
Manifestations
- Ability to respond to environment, speak, and control movement is lost.
- Unrecognizable speech
- General urinary incontinence
- Inability to eat without assistance and impaired swallowing
- Gradual loss of all ability to move extremities (ataxia)

Refer to **REVIEW MODULE: MENTAL HEALTH NURSING: CHAPTER 17: NEUROCOGNITIVE DISORDERS**.

MEDICATIONS

- Most medications for clients who have dementia attempt to target behavioral and emotional problems (anxiety, agitation, combativeness, depression).
- These medications include antipsychotics, antidepressants, and anxiolytics. Closely monitor clients receiving these medications for adverse effects.
- AD medications temporarily slow the course of the disease and do not work for all clients.
  - Pharmacotherapeutics is based on the theory that AD is a result of depleted levels of the enzyme acetyltransferase, which is necessary to produce the neurotransmitter acetylcholine.
  - Benefits for clients who do respond to medication include improvements in cognition, behavior, and function.
- If a client fails to improve with one medication, a trial of one of the other medications is warranted.
  - **Donepezil** prevents the breakdown of acetylcholine (ACh), which increases the amount of ACh available. This results in increased nerve impulses at the nerve sites.
  - **Memantine** is the first of a new classification of medications with a low-to-moderate affinity. It blocks nerve cell damage caused by excess glutamate. It has shown to reduce client deterioration. Memantine may be given in conjunction with donepezil.
  - **Cholinesterase** inhibitors help slow this process.
  - **Pimavanserin** is an antipsychotic used to treat dementia-related psychosis.

NURSING ACTIONS

- Observe for frequent stools or upset stomach.
- Monitor for dizziness or headache. The client can feel lightheaded or have an unsteady gait.
- Use caution when administering this medication to clients who have asthma or COPD, as lung problems can worsen.

THERAPEUTIC PROCEDURES

Alternative Therapy: Ginkgo biloba, an herbal product taken to increase memory and blood circulation, can cause a variety of adverse effects and medication interactions. If a client is using ginkgo biloba or other nutritional supplements, that information should be shared with providers.

Complementary Medicine: Massage the client before bedtime to reduce stress and promote sleep.

9.2 Case study

Scenario introduction

Lilly is a nurse on the Alzheimer's Unit caring for Mrs. Roberts.

Scene 1

Lilly: "Good morning, Mrs. Roberts. How are you feeling today?"

Mrs. Roberts: "I have a terrible bruise on my arm, and I don't know how it got there."

Lilly: "You fell at home yesterday. Your daughter brought you to the emergency room. The fall caused that bruise on your arm and several other injuries as well."

Scene 2

Mrs. Roberts: "What day is it? Where's my daughter?"

Lilly: "Today is Thursday, October 6. Your daughter will be here within an hour."

Mrs. Roberts: "Okay. I really want to see my daughter. She takes care of me."

Scene 3

Mrs. Roberts: "What day is it? Where am I?"

Lilly: "Today is Thursday, October 6. You're in the hospital because you fell at home yesterday and the doctor wanted to keep you here due to your injuries."

Scenario conclusion

Mrs. Roberts' daughter arrives and plans on spending the day with her mother. Lilly completes her morning assessment.

Case study exercises

1. Lilly is contributing to the plan of care for Mrs. Roberts, who has mild Alzheimer's disease. Which of the following interventions should Lilly recommend for inclusion in the plan of care?

   A. Apply a waist restraint to reduce the risk of falls.

   B. Thicken all liquids.

   C. Provide protective undergarments.

   D. Reorient the client to self and current events.

2. Lilly is caring for Mrs. Roberts, who has Alzheimer's disease and fell at home prior to admission. Which of the following actions should the nurse take first to keep the client safe?

   A. Keep the call light near the client.

   B. Place the client in a room close to the nurses' station.

   C. Encourage the client to ask for assistance.

   D. Remind the client to walk with someone for support.

INTERPROFESSIONAL CARE

- Encourage the client and family to seek legal counsel regarding advanced directives, guardianship, or durable medical power of attorney.
- Refer the client and family to social services and case managers for possible adult day care facilities or long-term care facilities.
- Collaborate with the client and family for physical therapy to establish an individualized exercise regimen.
- Refer the client and family to the Alzheimer's Association and community outreach programs. This can include family support groups, in-home care, or respite care.
- Review the resources available to the family as the client's health declines. Include long-term care options. A variety of home care and community resources, such as respite care, can be available to the family in many areas of the country. Some respite care allows the client to remain at home rather than in a facility.

CLIENT EDUCATION

- Refer to social services and case managers for long-term/home management, Alzheimer's Association, community outreach programs, and support groups.
- Educate family/caregivers about illness, methods of care, medications, and adaptation of the home environment.
- Provide information about care for seizures that can happen late in the disease.
- Provide strategies to reduce caregiver stress.

Home safety measures Qs

- Remove scatter rugs.
- Install door locks that cannot be easily opened, and place alarms on doors.
- Keep a lock on the water heater and thermostat, and keep the water temperature at a safe level.
- Provide good lighting, especially on stairs.
- Install handrails on stairs, and mark step edges with colored tape.
- Place the mattress on the floor.
- Remove clutter, and clear hallways for walking.
- Secure electrical cords to baseboards.
- Keep cleaning supplies in locked cupboards.
- Install handrails in the bathroom, at bedside, and in the tub.
- Place a shower chair in the tub.
- Wear a medical identification bracelet if living at home with a caregiver.
- Enroll in Safe Return Home Program.
- Participate in an exercise program to maintain mobility.?

Application Exercises

1. A nurse is caring for a client who has Alzheimer's disease. A family member of the client asks the nurse about risk factors for the disease. Which of the following factors should be included in the nurse's response? (Select all that apply.)

   A. Exposure to metal

   B. Long-term estrogen therapy

   C. Sustained use of vitamin E

   D. Previous head injury

   E. History of herpes infection

2. A nurse is reinforcing teaching to the partner of a client who has Alzheimer's disease and has a new prescription for donepezil. Which of the following statements by the partner indicates the instruction is effective?

   A. "This medication should increase my spouse's appetite."

   B. "This medication should help my spouse sleep better."

   C. "This medication should help my spouse's daily function."

   D. "This medication should increase my spouse's energy level."

3. A nurse is assisting with a home visit to a client who has AD. The client's partner states that the client is often disoriented to time and place, is unsteady, and has a history of wandering. Which of the following safety measures should the nurse review with the partner? (Select all that apply.)

   A. Remove floor rugs.

   B. Have door locks that can be easily opened.

   C. Provide increased lighting in stairwells.

   D. Install handrails in the bathroom.

   E. Place the mattress on the floor.

Active Learning Scenario

A charge nurse in a long-term care facility is assisting with planning a program for assistive personnel about caring for a client who has Alzheimer's disease. What should be included in this program? Use the ATI Active Learning Template: System Disorder to complete this item.

NURSING CARE: Describe three nursing interventions for each of the following areas.

- Providing cognitive stimulation
- Providing memory training

Active Learning Scenario Key

Using the ATI Active Learning Template: System Disorder

NURSING CARE

- Providing cognitive stimulation
  - Offer varied environmental stimulations (walks, music, craft activities).
  - Keep a structured environment. Introduce change slowly.
  - Use a calendar to assist with orientation.
  - Use short directions when explaining care to be provided, such as a bath.
  - Be consistent and repetitive.
  - Use therapeutic touch.
- Providing memory training
  - Reminisce about the past.
  - Help the client make lists and rehearse.
  - Repeat the client's last statement to stimulate memory.

Ⓝ *NCLEX® Connection: Physiological Adaptation, Basic Pathophysiology*

Application Exercises Key

1. A, D, E. **CORRECT:** When taking actions, the nurse should identify that exposure to metal and toxic waste, a previous head injury, and a history of herpes infection are risk factors for Alzheimer's disease. Long-term estrogen therapy can prevent Alzheimer's disease. Long-term use of vitamin E is not a risk factor for Alzheimer's disease.

Ⓝ *NCLEX® Connection: Health Promotion and Maintenance, Health Promotion/Disease Prevention*

2. C. **CORRECT:** When evaluating outcomes, the nurse should identify that donepezil slows the progression of AD and can improve behavior and daily functions. Donepezil does not affect appetite, sleep or sleep patterns, or energy levels.

Ⓝ *NCLEX® Connection: Pharmacological Therapies, Medication Administration*

3. A, C, D, E. **CORRECT:** When taking actions, the nurse should identify that removing floor rugs; providing good lighting, especially in dark areas, such as stairways; installing handrails in the client's bathroom; and placing the client's mattress on the floor reduce the risk of falling or tripping. Easy-to-open door locks increase the risk for a client who wanders to get out of the home and get lost.

Ⓝ *NCLEX® Connection: Health Promotion and Maintenance, Developmental Stages and Transitions*

Case Study Exercises Key

1. D. **CORRECT:** When generating solutions, the nurse should identify that a client who has mild Alzheimer's can require reorientation to self and current events as cognitive function declines.

Ⓝ *NCLEX® Connection: Safety and Infection Control, Home Safety*

2. B. **CORRECT:** When prioritizing hypotheses, the nurse should identify that placing the client in close proximity to the nurses' station for close observation is the first action the nurse should take. The nurse keeping the call light within the client's reach is an appropriate action, but it is not the first action because the client might not remember to use it. The nurse should encourage the client to ask for assistance, but it is not the first action because the client might not remember to ask for assistance. The nurse should remind the client to walk with someone, but it is not the first action because the client might not remember to call for assistance.

Ⓝ *NCLEX® Connection: Safety and Infection Control, Home Safety*

UNIT 2 NEUROLOGIC DISORDERS
SECTION: CENTRAL NERVOUS SYSTEM DISORDERS

CHAPTER 10 *Multiple Sclerosis*

Multiple sclerosis (MS) is a chronic, progressive, irreversible, autoimmune neurologic disorder with an unknown etiology. MS affects about 1 million people in the United States. MS has no known cure and can progress in severity over time. An immune-mediated attack or infection destroys the myelin sheath (a fatty protein that surrounds nerve fibers). As a result, demyelination interrupts the conduction of nerve impulses. Plaques can form on the demyelinated axons, leaving them unable to regenerate and causing irreversible damage.

MS affects the nerve cells in the CNS (optic nerve, cerebrum, brainstem, cerebellum, and spinal cord), which can result in impaired and worsening function of voluntary muscles. The initial findings of MS can be vague so that diagnosis is not made for several years. Clients can experience acute exacerbations and remissions.

The 4 types of MS include:

- **Relapsing and remitting (RRMS):** The most common type of MS in which the client may report development of new findings and loss of function (relapse) and experience mild to moderate symptoms that resolve within a few weeks/months (remission)

- **Primary progressive (PPMS):** MS with a gradual and continuous reduction of CNS deterioration without remission

- **Secondary progressive (SPMS):** Begins as RRMS and becomes continuously progressive

- **Progressive relapsing (PRMS):** MS that includes frequent relapses with partial recovery without the return to baseline

DATA COLLECTION

RISK FACTORS

- Age 20-50 years (onset varies)
- Sex assigned at birth: female (occurs 2 to 3 times more often)
- Genetic predisposition (first-degree relative)
- Because MS is an autoimmune disease, there are factors that trigger relapses.
  - Viruses and infectious agents
  - Living in a cold climate
  - Physical injury
  - Emotional stress
  - Pregnancy
  - Fatigue
  - Overexertion
  - Temperature extremes
  - Hot shower/bath

EXPECTED FINDINGS

- Manifestations vary depending on area of CNS affected, but can include:
  - Fatigue
  - Pain
  - Coordination
    - Ataxia, intentional tremors
  - Cognitive
    - Memory loss, impaired judgment
  - Sensory deficits
    - Paresthesia, vertigo
    - Visual disturbances: diplopia, changes in peripheral vision, decreased visual acuity, scotomas (patches of blindness), periods of total blindness, nystagmus
    - Auricular: tinnitus, decreased hearing acuity
  - Dysphagia
  - Dysarthria
  - Motor
    - Muscle spasticity and muscle weakness
  - Bowel dysfunction (constipation, fecal incontinence)
  - Bladder dysfunction (incontinence)
  - Sexual dysfunction (decreased libido, impotence)

LABORATORY TESTS

- Cerebrospinal fluid (CSF) analysis: elevated protein, a slight increase in WBCs
- CSF electrophoresis: increased T lymphocytes and increased immunoglobulin G

DIAGNOSTIC PROCEDURES

- Magnetic resonance imaging (MRI) reveals plaques of the brain and spine, which is most diagnostic.
- Evoked potential testing (visual evoked response): optic nerve transmission deficits
- Urodynamics: evaluate bladder function

PATIENT-CENTERED CARE

NURSING CARE/CLIENT EDUCATION

- Monitor the following.
  - Visual acuity
  - Speech patterns: fatigue with talking
  - Swallowing
  - Activity tolerance
  - Skin integrity
- Discuss coping mechanisms and sources of support (family, friends, spiritual figures, support groups).
- Encourage fluid intake and other measures to decrease the risk of developing a urinary tract infection. Assist the client with bladder elimination: intermittent self-catheterization, bladder pacemaker, and Credé's maneuver (placing manual pressure on abdomen over the bladder to expel urine). Establish a voiding time schedule (every 1.5 to 2 hr initially) with gradual increase of the time interval for those experiencing incontinence. Qpcc
- Monitor cognitive changes and plan interventions to promote cognitive function. (Reorient the client. Place objects used daily in routine places.)
- Facilitate effective communication for dysarthria using a communication board.
- Exercise and stretch involved muscles. (Avoid overexertion and overheating).
- Promote energy conservation by grouping care and planning rest periods.
- Promote and maintain safe home and hospital environments to reduce the risk of injury (walking with wide base of support, assistive devices, skin precautions). Qs
- If experiencing diplopia, consider applying an eye patch to the client's eye. Instruct the client to frequently alternate patch placement (left/right eye). Inform client about scanning techniques. Instruct the client to visually scan their environment by moving the head from side to side.
- Educate client about medications (use, adverse effects, administration).
- Encourage the client to avoid crowded areas (infection risk).

MEDICATIONS

Disease-modifying therapies (immunomodulators)

Slow progression of MS and reduce the frequency and duration of relapses

Interferon beta-1a and beta-1b: Injectable agent that is used to manage the frequency of relapses and decrease physical disability. It should be started early in the course of the disease.
- Monitor for flu-like findings, which are an adverse effect.
- Educate client about self-administration, and alternate injection sites.
- Inform client to avoid crowded areas.

Glatiramer acetate: Injectable agent that is administered subcutaneously

Teriflunomide, fingolimod, dimethyl fumarate
- Pregnancy warning: Contraindicated; can cause fetal injury
- Lactation warnings: Contraindicated
- Reproductive warning: Use with caution in clients who might become pregnant.
- Oral alternatives for those who have experienced injection reactions.

NURSING EVALUATION OF MEDICATION EFFECTIVENESS: Decrease in episodes and severity of relapse

Mitoxantrone

Antineoplastic/anti-inflammatory medication that is administered as an IV Infusion at an outpatient facility

Risk of cardiotoxicity and leukemia

Natalizumab

Monoclonal antibody that binds to WBCs and is administered as an IV Infusion at an outpatient facility

Risk of developing opportunistic infections

OTHER MEDICATIONS

Prednisone, dexamethasone, methylprednisolone, and corticosteroids

- Lactation warnings: Risk is unknown; use with caution.
- Reproductive warning: Use with caution in clients who might become pregnant.
- Corticosteroids, prednisone, and dexamethasone or methylprednisolone are used to reduce inflammation in acute exacerbations and are administered in large doses over a 3- to 5-day period, followed by an oral taper with prednisone.

NURSING ACTIONS: Monitor for increased risk of infection, hypervolemia, hypernatremia, hypokalemia, hyperglycemia, gastrointestinal bleeding, and personality changes.

Dantrolene, tizanidine, baclofen, diazepam

- Pregnancy warning: Use with caution.
- Lactation warnings: Contraindicated
- Antispasmodics (dantrolene, baclofen) are used to manage muscle spasticity; baclofen can be used to improve bladder and bowel function.
- Intrathecal baclofen can be used for severe cases of MS.

NURSING ACTIONS
- Monitor for adverse effects: baclofen (dizziness, drowsiness, weakness, nausea).
- Monitor for liver damage with tizanidine or dantrolene.

CLIENT EDUCATION
- Report increased weakness and jaundice to the provider.
- Avoid stopping baclofen abruptly.

Carbamazepine

Anticonvulsants are used for paresthesia.

NURSING EVALUATION OF MEDICATION EFFECTIVENESS: Decrease in paresthesia

Docusate sodium

Stool softeners are used to manage constipation.

NURSING EVALUATION OF MEDICATION EFFECTIVENESS: Regular soft, formed bowel movements

Anticholinergics

Anticholinergics, oxybutynin, and urecholine are used to manage bladder dysfunction.

Propranolol and clonazepam

A beta blocker and a benzodiazepine are used for ataxia.

Amantadine, pemoline, dalfampridine, baclofen, tizanidine

Administered to combat fatigue that can interfere with ADLs

NURSING EVALUATION OF MEDICATION EFFECTIVENESS: Decrease in inflammation as evidenced by a decrease in manifestations (mobility, weakness, fatigue)

COMPLEMENTARY AND ALTERNATIVE THERAPIES

- Massage
- Yoga
- Aromatherapy
- Acupuncture
- Mediation/relaxation

INTERPROFESSIONAL CARE

- Interprofessional team: neurologist, ophthalmologist, speech–language pathologist, physical therapist, occupational therapist, mental health provider, case manager, social worker
- MS can cause psychosocial and financial concerns. Provide guidance and support, and assist with making appropriate referrals if needed.
- Plan for disease progression. Provide community resources and respite services for the client and family.
- Provide information about local MS support groups and National MS Society.
- Consider referral to occupational and physical therapy for home environment assessment to determine safety and ease of mobility. Use adaptive devices to assist with activities of daily living. Qᴛᴄ
- Recommend referral to speech language therapist for dysarthria and dysphagia.
- Emphasize need to avoid overexertion, stress, extremes of temperatures, humidity, and people who have infections.

COMPLICATIONS

- UTI
- Constipation
- Pressure injury, contracture deformities
- Pneumonia
- Osteoporosis

Active Learning Scenario

A nurse is reinforcing teaching with family members of a client who has a new diagnosis of multiple sclerosis. What information should the nurse include in the teaching? Use the ATI Active Learning Template: System Disorder to complete this item.

ALTERATION IN HEALTH (DIAGNOSIS)

LABORATORY TESTS

DIAGNOSTIC PROCEDURES

MEDICATIONS: Describe four medications and one teaching point for each.

Active Learning Scenario Key

Using the ATI Active Learning Template: System Disorder

ALTERATION IN HEALTH (DIAGNOSIS): MS is an autoimmune disorder characterized by the development of plaque in the white matter of the central nervous system. Plaque damages the myelin sheath and interferes with impulse transmission between the CNS and the body.

LABORATORY TESTS: Cerebrospinal fluid analysis

DIAGNOSTIC PROCEDURES: MRI of the brain and spine

MEDICATIONS
- Corticosteroids such as prednisone: Increased risk for infection, hypervolemia, hypernatremia, hypokalemia, GI bleeding, and personality changes
- Antispasmodics (dantrolene, tizanidine, baclofen, diazepam) are used to treat muscle spasticity. Report increased weakness and jaundice to provider. Avoid stopping baclofen abruptly.
- Immunomodulators such as interferon beta are used to prevent and treat relapses.
- Anticonvulsants such as carbamazepine are used for paresthesia.
- Stool softeners such as docusate sodium are used for constipation.
- Anticholinergics such as propantheline are used for bladder dysfunction.
- Propranolol and clonazepam, a beta blocker and a benzodiazepine, are used for tremors.

Ⓝ NCLEX® Connection: Physiological Adaptation, Alterations in Body Systems

Application Exercises

1. A nurse is preparing to collect data from a client who has multiple sclerosis (MS). Which of the following findings should the nurse expect?

    A. Elevated BP

    B. Client report of fatigue

    C. Client report of rhinitis

    D. Muscle rigidity

2. A nurse is reinforcing education with a client who has MS. Which of the following client statements indicates understanding?

    A. "I will plan to group my activities."

    B. "I won't be able to perform self-care."

    C. "I should have my partner do all of the housework."

    D. "I will perform vigorous exercising three times per day."

3. A nurse is assisting with the care of a client who has an acute exacerbation of MS. Which of the following actions should the nurse take? (Select all that apply.)

    A. Assist with ambulation 6 times daily.

    B. Monitor for dysphagia.

    C. Check skin integrity.

    D. Use a communication board.

    E. Encourage fluid intake.

4. A nurse is reinforcing teaching with a client who has multiple sclerosis and a new prescription for baclofen. Which of the following statements should the nurse include? (Select all that apply.)

    A. "This medication will help you with your tremors."

    B. "This medication will help you with your bladder function."

    C. "This medication can cause your skin to bruise easily."

    D. "This medication can cause you to experience dizziness."

    E. "Nasal congestion and drainage occur."

Application Exercises Key

1. B. **CORRECT:** When recognizing cues, the nurse should identify that the client report of fatigue is a common finding for a client who has MS. An elevated BP and client report of rhinitis are not expected findings with MS. A client who has MS may experience muscle spasms and weakness; therefore, rigid muscles are not an expected finding for a client who has MS.

    Ⓝ *NCLEX® Connection: Physiological Adaptation, Basic Pathophysiology*

2. A. **CORRECT:** A client who has MS should balance activity and rest and conserve their energy by grouping care and planning rest periods. Clients who are not in an acute MS flare should be able to perform self-care and participate in activities such as light housework and mild exercise. They should avoid fatigue and overexertion; therefore, vigorous exercising is not recommended.

    Ⓝ *NCLEX® Connection: Physiological Adaptation, Alterations in Body Systems*

3. B, C, D, E. **CORRECT:** The client with an acute exacerbation of MS may experience dysarthria and should be monitored for dysphagia, or difficulty swallowing. They are at risk of skin breakdown due to immobility, and this should be checked frequently. They may also need to utilize a communication board due to their dysarthria, or unclear speech. The nurse should encourage fluid intake to assist with preventing UTIs and constipation. At this time, it is unlikely the client will be able to ambulate several times per day.

    Ⓝ *NCLEX® Connection: Physiological Adaptation, Alterations in Body Systems*

4. B, D, E. **CORRECT:** Baclofen is an antispasmodic medication that is given to clients who have MS to treat muscle spasms. An adverse effect of this medication is drowsiness, dizziness, weakness, and nausea. Instruct the client to monitor for these findings, as they can lead to impaired safety. The client should be instructed not to discontinue baclofen abruptly. Propranolol is a beta blocker, and clonazepam is a benzodiazepine given to clients who have MS to treat tremors. Propantheline is an anticholinergic medication that is given to clients who have MS to treat bladder dysfunction, and baclofen can assist with improving bowel and bladder function. Prednisone is a corticosteroid medication that is given to clients who have MS to treat inflammation. An adverse effect of this medication is bruising of the skin.

    Ⓝ *NCLEX® Connection: Pharmacological Therapies, Expected Actions/Outcomes*

UNIT 2   NEUROLOGIC DISORDERS
SECTION: CENTRAL NERVOUS SYSTEM DISORDERS

CHAPTER 11 *Headaches*

Headaches can be acute or chronic, temporary, or life-threatening.

Headaches are a common occurrence and affect individuals of all ages. Headaches are associated with other conditions such as colds, allergies, and stress or muscle tension.

Primary headaches have no identifiable organic cause. They include migraine, tension, and cluster headaches. They can be managed in the primary care setting.

Secondary headaches are associated with an organic cause (a brain tumor or aneurysm) and warrant further investigation and medical management.

This chapter covers migraine headaches and cluster headaches.

HEALTH PROMOTION AND DISEASE PREVENTION

- Promote stress management strategies and recognition of triggers that cause the onset of a headache.
- Recommend use of a headache diary to help identify type of headache and response to interventions.
- Promote hand hygiene to prevent the spread of viruses that produce manifestations similar to the common cold.
- Review pain management to include over-the-counter medications and herbal remedies.

Migraine headaches

DATA COLLECTION

EXPECTED FINDINGS

- Photophobia and phonophobia (sensitivity to sounds)
- Nausea and vomiting
- Stress and anxiety
- Unilateral pain, often behind one eye or ear
- Health history and family history for headache patterns
- Alterations in ADLs for 4 to 72 hr
- Manifestations that are similar with each headache

Classified by categories

With aura
- Aura develops over minutes to an hour to include neurologic findings: numbness and tingling of mouth, lips, face, or hands; acute confusion; and visual disturbances (light flashes, bright spots).
- Severe, incapacitating, throbbing headache that is accompanied by nausea, vomiting, and drowsiness. A migraine with an aura lasts about 1 hr.
- Recovery with pain and aura subsiding. Muscle aches and contraction of head and neck muscles are common. Physical activity worsens pain, and client might sleep.

Without aura (common migraine)
- Pain is aggravated by physical activity.
- Unilateral, pulsating pain.
- One or more manifestations present: photophobia, phonophobia, nausea, and/or vomiting
- Persists for 4 to 72 hr. Often occurs in early morning, during periods of stress, or with premenstrual tension or fluid retention.

DIAGNOSTIC PROCEDURES

Neurologic imaging may be recommended if the client has positive findings on neurologic examination to determine the underlying cause.

PATIENT-CENTERED CARE

Nursing care focus during headache is pain management.
- Maintain a cool, dark, quiet environment.
- Elevate the head of the bed to 30°.
- Administer medications as prescribed.

MEDICATIONS

- **Abortive therapy** to alleviate pain during aura or soon after start of headache
  - For mild migraines: NSAIDs (ibuprofen, naproxen), acetaminophen, and over-the-counter anti-inflammatory medications in formulations for migraines
  - Antiemetics (metoclopramide) to relieve nausea and vomiting
  - Severe migraines
    - Triptan preparations (zolmitriptan, sumatriptan, eletriptan) to produce a vasoconstrictive effect
    - Ergotamine preparations with caffeine to narrow blood vessels and reduce inflammation
- **Preventive therapy** for frequent headaches or when other therapies are ineffective
  - NSAIDs with beta blocker (propranolol), calcium channel blocker, beta adrenergic blocker, or antiepileptic medications (divalproex, topiramate)
  - Client is instructed to check pulse when taking beta adrenergic blockers and calcium channel blockers.
  - Botulism toxin is approved for adults with chronic migraines. Injected into specific areas of the head and neck up to five treatment cycles

CLIENT EDUCATION

- Keep a diary to record headache patterns and triggers.
- Report changes in headache intensity or new visual or neurologic disturbances.
- Remain in a cool, dark, quiet environment.
- Elevate the head of the bed as desired.

Trigger avoidance and management Qᴘᴄᴄ

- Avoid foods with tyramine (pickles, caffeine, beer, wine, aged cheese, artificial sweeteners) and foods with preservatives.
- Medications known to induce migraines include estrogen, nitroglycerin, and nifedipine.
- Manage anger issues and handling conflict.
- Get adequate rest and sleep.
- Weather and altitude changes can trigger migraines for some clients.
- Avoid light glare or flickering lights.
- Monitor menstrual cycle pattern and hormone fluctuations. Hormone fluctuations during menstruation and ovulation can trigger migraines.
- Avoid intense environmental odors, perfumes, and tobacco smoke.

Complementary and alternative therapies Qᴘᴄᴄ

- Yoga, meditation, tai chi, exercise, biofeedback, and massage promote relaxation and alleviate muscle tension. Some might be offered at local community centers.
- Acupuncture and acupressure therapy can be helpful for pain management.
- Review herbal remedies and nutrition supplements with the provider because there is insufficient evidence to support their use in management of migraines. Qᴇʙᴘ
- Neurostimulator devices might be used to reduce migraine discomfort.

Cluster headaches

DATA COLLECTION

RISK FACTORS

- More frequent during spring and fall
- More common in males (sex assigned at birth) between 20 to 50 years of age

EXPECTED FINDINGS

- Brief episode of intense, unilateral, nonthrobbing pain lasting 15 min to 3 hr that can radiate to forehead, temple, or cheek
  - Occurring 1 to 8 times daily
  - Followed by period of remission
- No aura or preliminary manifestations
- Less common than migraines
- Tearing of the eye with runny nose and nasal congestion
- Facial sweating

- Drooping eyelid and eyelid edema
- Miosis (pupil constriction)
- Facial pallor or flushing
- Pacing, walking, or sitting and rocking activities
- Triggered by alcohol

PATIENT-CENTERED CARE

MEDICATIONS

(See medications for migraine headaches.)
- Triptans
- Ergotamine preparations
- Antiepileptic medications
- Calcium channel blockers
- Corticosteroids

THERAPEUTIC PROCEDURES

Home oxygen therapy at 12 L/min for 15 to 20 min at onset of headache can provide relief within 15 min.

CLIENT EDUCATION

- Remain in a cool, dark, quiet environment with head elevated.
- Remain in sitting position when using oxygen, and maintain safety precautions when using oxygen in the home. Qs
- Complementary and alternative therapies can promote relaxation.

Prevention strategies: Obtain adequate rest and sleep, exercise, and relaxation.

Risk factors (triggers) for headaches

- Anger outburst
- Anxiety and prolonged anticipation, or periods of stress
- Excessive physical activity, fatigue
- Altered sleep–wake cycles

Application Exercises

1. A nurse is obtaining a health history from a client who is being evaluated for the cause of frequent headaches. Which of the following questions should the nurse ask to identify the aura type of migraine headaches?

   A. "Do the headaches occur multiple times each day?"

   B. "Is your headache accompanied by profuse facial sweating?"

   C. "Does your headache occur on one side of your head?"

   D. "Do you have the same manifestations each time the headache occurs?"

2. A nurse in a clinic is reinforcing teaching with a client who has a history of migraine headaches about a new prescription for zolmitriptan. Which of the following statements by the client indicates understanding of the information provided?

   A. "This medication will relieve my symptoms by causing my blood vessels to dilate."

   B. "I should take this medication daily to prevent the headache from occurring."

   C. "I should expect facial flushing when I take this medication."

   D. "This medication will lower my sensitivity to food triggers."

3. A nurse is providing discharge instructions to a client who has a new diagnosis of migraine headaches. Which of the following instructions should the nurse include?

   A. Use music therapy for relaxation with the onset of the headache.

   B. Increase physical activity when a headache is present.

   C. Drink beverages that contain artificial sweeteners to prevent headaches.

   D. Apply a cool cloth to the face during a headache.

4. A nurse in a clinic is caring for a client who has frequent migraine headaches. The client asks about foods that can cause headaches. The nurse should instruct that which of the following foods can trigger a migraine headache?

   A. Baked salmon

   B. Chocolate

   C. Frozen strawberries

   D. Fresh asparagus

5. A nurse in a provider's office is obtaining a health history from a client who has cluster headaches. Which of the following are expected findings? (Select all that apply.)

   A. Pain is bilateral across the posterior occipital area.

   B. Client experiences altered sleep-wake cycle.

   C. Headache occurs approximately 1 to 8 times daily.

   D. Client describes headache pain as dull and throbbing.

   E. Nasal congestion and drainage occur.

Active Learning Scenario

A nurse in a clinic is interviewing a client who reports they think they are having migraine headaches. Use the ATI Active Learning Template: System Disorder and the ATI Pharmacology Review Module to complete this item.

EXPECTED FINDINGS: Identify three findings common to migraine headaches in general.

DIAGNOSTIC PROCEDURES: Describe guidelines for diagnosing migraine headache pain.

NURSING INTERVENTIONS: Identify three actions the nurse can take to assist the client with managing headaches.

Active Learning Scenario Key

Using the ATI Active Learning Template: System Disorder and the ATI Pharmacology Review Module

EXPECTED FINDINGS
- Throbbing, unilateral pain
- Family history of migraine headaches
- Associated manifestations last for 4 to 72 hr

DIAGNOSTIC PROCEDURES: Neurologic imaging recommended if the client has positive findings on neurologic examination to determine the underlying cause.

NURSING INTERVENTIONS
- Encourage the client to keep a journal to identify triggers (food, environment, hormone fluctuations).
- Reinforce teaching with the client about medications that can prevent or stop migraines.
- Discuss complementary strategies (yoga, tai chi) to promote relaxation.
- Urge the client to discuss herbal supplements that claim to provide migraine relief with the provider.

Ⓝ *NCLEX® Connection: Physiological Adaptation, Basic Pathophysiology*

Application Exercises Key

1. D. **CORRECT:** Clients who have aura-type migraines typically have the same manifestations each time the headache occurs. Cluster headaches typically occur 1 to 8 times each day. Profuse facial sweating is typical in the presence of cluster headaches. Unilateral headaches are associated with cluster headaches and common migraines.

Ⓝ *NCLEX® Connection: Reduction of Risk Potential, Potential for Alterations in Body Systems*

2. C. **CORRECT:** Zolmitriptan can cause facial flushing, tingling, and warmth. Zolmitriptan causes cranial arteries, the basilar arteries, and blood vessels in the dura mater to constrict. Zolmitriptan is used for abortive therapy in treating migraine headaches. It is not used for headache prevention. Zolmitriptan is used as a component of abortive therapy for treatment of migraine headaches and does not affect a client's sensitivity to food triggers.

Ⓝ *NCLEX® Connection: Pharmacological Therapies, Medication Administration*

3. D. **CORRECT:** A cool cloth placed over the client's eyes can provide comfort and relieve pain. A quiet, dark environment can provide comfort during a migraine headache. Increasing physical activity during a migraine headache can worsen the pain. Artificial sweeteners contain tyramine, which can trigger a migraine headache.

Ⓝ *NCLEX® Connection: Physiological Adaptation, Alterations in Body Systems*

4. B. **CORRECT:** The nurse understands that chocolate contains tyramine, which can trigger migraine headaches. The client should avoid fish that is smoked because it contains tyramine. Baked salmon does not contain tyramine and is not a trigger for migraine headaches. Fruits and vegetables are not a source of tyramine.

Ⓝ *NCLEX® Connection: Physiological Adaptation, Alterations in Body Systems*

5. B, C, E. **CORRECT:** Cluster headaches can be due to a lack of continuity in the sleep-wake cycle. Cluster headaches occur approximately 1 to 8 times daily. A client can have a runny nose and nasal congestion with a cluster headache. Cluster headaches typically cause pain on one side of the head and radiate to the forehead, temple, or cheek. Cluster headaches are described as unilateral, intense, and nonthrobbing.

Ⓝ *NCLEX® Connection: Physiological Adaptation, Basic Pathophysiology*

UNIT 2   NEUROLOGIC DISORDERS
SECTION: CENTRAL NERVOUS SYSTEM DISORDERS

CHAPTER 12 *Increased Intracranial Pressure Disorders*

Increased intracranial pressure occurs from lesions, brain tumors, or fluid accumulation from a brain injury in the cranium. The cranium is a closed bony structure that does not expand in an adult. The lesion or fluid takes up space in the cranium, resulting in increased intracranial pressure. Pressure increase beyond the expected levels increases edema and decreases brain tissue perfusion, leading to impaired neurologic function and possible death.

Brain tumors

- Brain tumors occur in any part of the brain, occupy space within the skull, and are classified according to the cell or tissue of origin. Cerebral tumors are the most common.
- Types of brain tumors include benign and malignant. Examples include malignant gliomas (neuroglial cells), benign meningiomas (meninges), pituitary adenomas, and acoustic neuromas (acoustic cranial nerve).
- A secondary classification, supratentorial tumors, occurs in the cerebral hemispheres above the tentorium cerebelli. Those below the tentorium cerebelli (tumors of the brainstem and cerebellum) are classified as infratentorial tumors.
- Brain tumors apply pressure to surrounding brain tissue, resulting in decreased outflow of cerebrospinal fluid, increased intracranial pressure, cerebral edema, and neurologic deficits. Tumors that involve the pituitary gland can cause endocrine dysfunction.
- Malignant brain tumors are associated with a high overall mortality rate. Primary malignant brain tumors originate from neuroglial tissue and rarely metastasize outside of the brain. Secondary malignant brain tumors are lesions that are metastases from a primary cancer located elsewhere in the body. Cranial metastatic lesions are most common from breast, kidney, lung, skin (melanomas), and gastrointestinal tract cancers.
- Benign brain tumors develop from the meninges or cranial nerves and do not metastasize. These tumors have distinct boundaries and cause damage either by the pressure they exert within the cranial cavity and/or by impairing the function of the cranial nerve.

HEALTH PROMOTION/ DISEASE PREVENTION

There are no routine screening procedures to detect brain tumors.

DATA COLLECTION

EXPECTED FINDINGS

PHYSICAL FINDINGS
- Dysarthria
- Dysphagia
- Change in coordination
- Change in gait
- Vertigo
- Hemiparesis
- Severe headache (worse upon awakening but improving over time; worsened by coughing or straining)
- Visual changes (blurring, visual field deficit)
- Focal or generalized seizures
- Loss of voluntary movement or the inability to control movement
- Change in cognitive function (memory loss, language impairment)
- Change in personality, inability to control emotions
- Nausea with or without vomiting
- Paralysis
- Hearing loss or ringing in the ear
- Facial drooping

DIAGNOSTIC PROCEDURES

- X-ray, computed tomography (CT) imaging scan, magnetic resonance imaging (MRI), brain scan, position emission tomography (PET) scan, and cerebral angiography are used to determine the size, location, and extent of the tumor.
- Lumbar puncture (LP) and electroencephalography (EEG) can provide additional information about the tumor.
- LP should not be done if the client has or shows manifestations of increasing intracranial pressure (ICP) to prevent brain herniation.
- Lab tests can be done to evaluate endocrine function, renal status, and electrolyte balance.
- Cerebral biopsy identifies cellular pathology.
  - This procedure can be performed in the surgical suite or in a radiology specialty suite.
  - Diagnostic procedure can be used to guide the biopsy, such as a CT or MRI scan. Image guiding systems, which use CT or MRI scan information, can be used in the surgical suite.
  - A piece of cerebral tissue that appears abnormal on the CT/MRI scan is obtained. This tissue is then sent to pathology, where diagnostic tests are performed.

CLIENT EDUCATION: Adhere to the specific instructions regarding medications.
- If on antiepileptic medications, these must be continued to prevent seizure activity. **Qs**
- If on aspirin products, these should be discontinued at least 72 hr prior to the procedure to minimize the risk of intracerebral bleeding.
- Other medications can be withheld prior to the procedure.
- Normally, preprocedure activities can be resumed after recovering from the general anesthetic. Care of the incision should include keeping the area clean and dry. If sutures are in place, they need to be removed 1 to 7 days later. Driving or other dangerous activities should be avoided until follow-up appointment occurs and diagnosis is known.

PATIENT-CENTERED CARE

NURSING CARE

- Maintain airway (monitor oxygen levels, administer oxygen as needed, and monitor lung sounds).
- Monitor neurologic status—in particular, monitoring for changes in level of consciousness, neurologic deficits, and occurrence of seizures.
- Maintain client safety. (Assist with transfers and ambulation; provide assistive devices as needed.) **Qs**
- Implement seizure precautions.
- Administer medications.

MEDICATIONS

- **Non-opioid analgesics** are used to treat headaches.
  - Opioid medications are avoided because they tend to decrease level of consciousness.
- **Corticosteroids** are used to reduce cerebral edema (relieving headaches, improving altered levels of consciousness).
  - Corticosteroid medications quickly reduce cerebral edema and can be rapidly administered to maximize their effectiveness.
  - Chronic administration is used to control cerebral edema associated with the presence or treatment of benign or malignant brain tumors.
- **Osmotic diuretics** decrease fluid content of the brain, resulting in a decrease in intracranial pressure.
- **Anticonvulsant medications** are used to control or prevent seizure activity.
  - Anticonvulsant medications suppress the neuronal activity within the brain, which prevents seizure activity.
  - There are several classifications of antiepileptic medications, each specifically designed to treat specific seizure behavior.

- **H2-antagonists** are used to decrease the acid content of the stomach, reducing the risk of stress ulcers.
  - H2-antagonists are administered during acute or stressful periods, such as after surgery, at the initiation of chemotherapy, or during the first several radiation therapy treatments.
  - The effect of these treatments, together with the necessity of corticosteroids, places the client at risk for stress ulcers. This is primarily preventative treatment.
- **Antiemetics** are used if nausea (with or without vomiting) is present.
  - Nausea and vomiting can be present as a result of the increased ICP, the site of the tumor, or the treatment required.
  - These medications are administered as prescribed, and can be provided as a preventative intervention, especially when the treatment is associated with nausea and vomiting.
- **Chemotherapy** can be given in conjunction with radiation. However, the blood-brain barrier can prevent adequate doses from reaching the tumor.

INTERPROFESSIONAL CARE

- Initiate appropriate referrals (social services; support groups; medical equipment; and physical, speech, and occupational therapy).
- Treatments include steroids, surgery, chemotherapy, conventional radiation therapy, stereotactic radiosurgery, and clinical trials. Chemotherapy and conventional radiation therapy can be administered prior to surgery to reduce the bulk of the tumor or after surgery to prevent tumor recurrence.
- In most cases when the tumor is benign, surgery is a curative treatment. However, these tumors can regrow. Radiation and chemotherapy can be provided to prevent recurrence.
- Some tumors can be malignant by location, meaning that while the pathology is benign, the location makes the mortality rate associated with them high.
- In cases where the tumor is a metastatic lesion from a primary lesion elsewhere in the body, treatments are palliative. These treatments can consist of surgery, radiation, and chemotherapy, in any combination, and are aimed at controlling intracerebral lesions.

THERAPEUTIC PROCEDURES

Craniotomy: complete or partial resection of brain tumor through surgical opening in the skull

PREOPERATIVE NURSING ACTIONS
- Explain the procedure to the client, answering all appropriate questions and providing emotional support.
- Questions regarding the surgery and its outcomes should be addressed in an effort to ensure all questions are answered.
- The client's partner should be present to hear the responses and avoid miscommunication.

- If the client takes aspirin, this medication needs to be stopped.
- No alcohol, tobacco, anticoagulants, or NSAIDs. Qpcc
- If the client uses alternative/complementary medications or treatments, make these known to the provider.
- Administer medications as prescribed. An anti-anxiety or muscle relaxant medication can be administered, if requested, and provided by the provider.

POSTOPERATIVE NURSING ACTIONS
- Closely monitor vital signs and neurologic status, including using the Glasgow Coma Scale.
- Treat pain adequately.
- Position client in the specified position related to the type of surgery. Turn client side to side, if not contraindicated.
- Straining activities (moving up in bed and attempting to have a bowel movement) should be avoided to prevent increased ICP. Postoperative bleeding and seizure activity are the greatest risks.
- Periorbital edema and ecchymosis are not unusual. Treat with cold compresses.
- Check head dressing every 1 to 2 hr for drainage.

COMPLICATIONS

Syndrome of inappropriate antidiuretic hormone

Syndrome of inappropriate antidiuretic hormone (SIADH) is a condition where fluid is retained as a result of an overproduction of vasopressin or antidiuretic hormone (ADH) from the posterior pituitary gland.
- SIADH occurs when the hypothalamus has been damaged and can no longer regulate the release of ADH.
- Treatment consists of fluid restriction, administration of oral conivaptan, and treatment of hyponatremia, with 3% hypertonic saline solution for severe cases.
- If SIADH is present, the client can have disorientation, headache, vomiting, muscle weakness, decreased LOC, irritability, loss of thirst, and weight gain.
- If severe or untreated, this condition can cause seizures and a coma.

Diabetes insipidus

Diabetes insipidus (DI) is seen most often after supratentorial surgery, especially when involving the pituitary gland or hypothalamus.
- This is a condition where large amounts of urine are excreted as a result of a deficiency of ADH from the posterior pituitary gland.
- The condition occurs when the hypothalamus has been damaged and can no longer regulate the release of ADH.
- Treatment of DI consists of massive fluid replacement, administration of synthetic vasopressin, careful attention to laboratory values, and replacement of essential nutrients as indicated.

Head injury

Head injuries are classified as open or closed. In an open head injury, the integrity of the skull is compromised by either a penetrating object or blunt force trauma. A closed head injury occurs from blunt trauma that causes acceleration of the head and then deceleration or hits a stationary object. Head injuries are also classified as mild, moderate, or severe, depending upon Glasgow Coma Scale ratings and the length of time the client was unconscious.

TYPES OF BRAIN INJURY
- Types of brain injury include concussion, contusion, diffuse axonal injury, and intracranial hemorrhage.
  - **A concussion, or mild traumatic brain injury,** occurs after head trauma that results in a change in the client's neurologic function but no identified brain damage and usually resolves within 72 hr. Post-concussion syndrome includes persistence of cognitive and physical manifestations for an unknown period of time.
  - **A contusion** occurs when the brain is bruised and the client has a period of unconsciousness associated with stupor and or confusion.
  - **Diffuse axonal injury** is a widespread injury to the brain that results in coma and is seen in severe head trauma.
  - **Intracranial hemorrhage** can occur in the epidural, subdural, or intracerebral space. It is a collection of blood following head trauma. There can be a delay of weeks to months in presenting manifestations for a subacute or chronic subdural hematoma.
- Open-head injuries pose a high risk for infection. Scalp injuries often result in profuse bleeding due to the poor vasoconstriction of the blood vessels of the scalp.
- Skull fractures can occur following forceful head injury. The brain might be damaged as a result. The client can have localized pain at the site of the fracture, and swelling can occur. The nurse should be alert for drainage from the ears or eyes (cerebral spinal fluid [CSF]).
- A cervical spine injury should always be suspected when a head injury occurs. A cervical spine injury must be ruled out prior to removing any devices used to stabilize the cervical spine. Qs

HEALTH PROMOTION AND DISEASE PREVENTION
- Wear helmets when skateboarding, riding a bike or motorcycle, skiing, and playing football or any other sport that could cause a head injury.
- Wear seat belts when driving or riding in a car.
- Avoid dangerous activities (speeding, driving under the influence of alcohol or drugs).
- Owners of firearms should lock all firearms.
- Avoid riding in the back of a pick-up truck.
- Promote programs directed at older adults to prevent falls, which are a major cause of neurologic injury in adults ages 65 to 75. Older adults who sustain head injuries are at greater risk for complications (hematomas) due to increased adherence of dura mater to skull and because of higher rates of anticoagulants prescribed to the older population. Ⓖ

DATA COLLECTION

RISK FACTORS

- Motor vehicle or motorcycle crashes
- Illicit drug and alcohol use
- Sports injuries
- Assault
- Gunshot wounds
- Falls

EXPECTED FINDINGS

- Amnesia (loss of memory) before or after the injury
- Loss of consciousness: Length of time the client is unconscious is significant.
- CSF leakage from the nose and ears can indicate a basilar skull fracture. Test for the "halo sign," clear or yellow-tinted ring surrounding a drop of blood when bloody drainage is placed on a piece of gauze.
- Manifestations of increased intracranial pressure
  - Severe headache, nausea, vomiting
  - Deteriorating level of consciousness, restlessness, irritability Q EBP
  - Dilated or pinpoint nonreactive pupils
  - Alteration in breathing pattern (Cheyne-Stokes respirations, central neurogenic hyperventilation, apnea)
  - Deterioration in motor function, abnormal posturing (decerebrate, decorticate, flaccidity)
  - Cushing's triad is a late finding characterized by severe hypertension with a widening pulse pressure (systolic – diastolic) and bradycardia
  - Seizures

LABORATORY TESTS

- ABGs
- CBC with differential
- Blood glucose level
- Electrolyte levels
- Blood and urine osmolarity
- Toxicology screen
- Monitor anti-seizure medication blood levels.

DIAGNOSTIC PROCEDURES

- Cervical spine films to diagnose a cervical spine injury
- Computerized tomography (CT) and/or a magnetic resonance imaging (MRI) of the head and/or neck (with and without contrast if indicated)
- Calculation of cerebral perfusion using the ICP monitor, if it is in place

PATIENT-CENTERED CARE

NURSING CARE

- Support of the family following head injury is of great importance. Effective coping can be very difficult to achieve without support from providers and community members. The Brain Injury Association of America provides families and clients with information needed to cope with this potentially devastating injury. Q PCC
- The family can face difficult decisions following head injury. If brain death has occurred, the family needs support when deciding whether to donate organs.
- Maintain cervical spine stability until cleared by an x-ray. Q s
- Report presence of CSF from nose or ears to the provider.
- Determine whether the client could possibly be under the influence of alcohol, illicit drugs, or medications, which could impair neurologic responsiveness and affect monitoring.
- Implement measures to prevent complications of immobility (turn every 2 hr, footboard, and splints). Specialty beds can be used.
- Monitor fluid and electrolyte values and osmolality to detect changes in sodium regulation, onset of diabetes insipidus, or severe hypovolemia.
- Provide adequate fluids to maintain cerebral perfusion and to minimize cerebral edema. When a large amount of IV fluids are prescribed, monitor for excess fluid volume, which could increase ICP.
- Maintain safety and seizure precautions (side rails up, padded side rails, call light within the client's reach). Q s
- Even if the level of consciousness is decreased, explain to the client the actions being taken and why. (Hearing is the last sense affected by a head injury.)

Monitor the client at regularly scheduled intervals

Respiratory status (the priority data collection): The brain is dependent upon oxygen to maintain function and has little reserve available if oxygen is deprived. Untreated hypoxia leads to brain injury or death if the brain has been denied adequate oxygenation for 3 to 5 min. Changes in level of consciousness, using the Glasgow Coma Scale (GCS), provide the earliest indication of neurologic deterioration.

Cranial nerve function: Eye blink response, gag reflex, tongue and shoulder movement

Check pupils for size, equality, and reaction to light: Pupils that are equal, round, and react to light and accommodation (PERRLA) are a normal finding.

Bilateral sensory and motor responses

Increased intracranial pressure (ICP): Monitored by placing a screw, catheter, or sensor through a burr hole into the ventricle, or the subarachnoid, epidural, or subdural space. Expected reference range is 10 to 15 mm Hg.

- ICP can be increased by:
  - Hypercarbia, which leads to cerebral vasodilation
  - Endotracheal or oral tracheal suctioning
  - Coughing
  - Extreme neck or hip flexion/extension
  - Maintaining the head of the bed at an angle less than 30°
  - Increasing intra-abdominal pressure (restrictive clothing, Valsalva maneuver)
- Implement actions that decrease ICP.
  - Elevate head at least 30° to reduce ICP and to promote venous drainage.
  - Avoid extreme flexion, extension, or rotation of the head, and maintain the body in a midline neutral position. Qpcc
  - Maintain a patent airway. Provide mechanical ventilation as indicated.
  - Administer oxygen as indicated to maintain PaO2 greater than 60 mm Hg.
  - The client should receive stool softeners and avoid the Valsalva maneuver with increased ICP.
  - Provide a calm, restful environment. (Limit visitors. Minimize noise.)
  - Use measures to maintain normal body temperature.
  - Brief periods of hyperventilation for the intubated client can be used after the first 24 hr following injury to help lower ICP. During the first 24 hr, hyperventilation can cause cerebral vasoconstriction, which can cause ischemia.

MEDICATIONS

Mannitol

Mannitol is an osmotic diuretic used to treat cerebral edema. When used for increased ICP, the medication draws fluid from the brain into the blood.

NURSING ACTIONS
- Administer IV to treat acute cerebral edema.
- Insert indwelling urinary catheter to monitor fluid and renal status.
- Monitor electrolytes and osmolality closely.

Barbiturates

Client can be placed in a coma (barbiturate coma) to decrease cellular metabolic demand until ICP can be decreased.

- Commonly used medications include pentobarbital and thiopental.
- When barbiturate coma is used, the ability to check neurologic function is made more difficult.
- Medication dosage is adjusted to keep the client completely unresponsive.
- Mechanical ventilation, cardiac and hemodynamic monitoring, and ICP monitoring are required.

Phenytoin

- Phenytoin is used prophylactically to prevent or treat seizures. It was the first medication used to suppress seizures that did not depress the entire CNS.
- Dosing for this medication is client-specific and based on therapeutic blood levels.

NURSING ACTIONS: Check for medication interactions.

Opioids

Morphine sulfate or fentanyl are analgesics used to control pain and restlessness.

NURSING ACTIONS
- Avoid opioid use with clients who are not mechanically ventilated due to CNS depressant effects.
  - Prevents accurate data collection of neurologic system
  - Can cause respiratory depression
- Administer naloxone, the reversal agent, if client becomes overmedicated or does not tolerate the opioids.

THERAPEUTIC PROCEDURES

Craniotomy

A craniotomy is the removal of nonviable brain tissue, which allows for expansion and/or removal of epidural or subdural hematomas. It is also used to decrease ICP and remove brain tumors. It involves drilling a burr hole or creating a bone flap to permit access to the affected area.

- Treatment of intracranial hemorrhages requires surgical evacuation.
- Burr holes are circular openings through the skull. The burr hole is used to check cerebral swelling, injury, size, and position of the ventricles.
- This is a life-saving procedure and is associated with many potential complications (severe neurologic impairment, infection, persistent seizures, neurologic deficiencies, and death).

NURSING ACTIONS
- Medications (mannitol and dexamethasone) can be administered every 6 hr for 24 to 72 hr postoperatively.
- Phenytoin or diazepam can be used to prevent seizure activity.
- Monitor ICP. Follow written protocols to check for changes in ICP.
- Position client in the specified position related to the type of surgery. Turn client side to side, if not contraindicated.
- Calm and reassure clients, clarifying misconceptions (brain surgery can be an extremely fearful procedure).

INTERPROFESSIONAL CARE

- Care should include professionals from other disciplines as indicated. This can include physical, occupational, recreational, and/or speech therapists due to neurologic deficits that can occur secondary to the area of the brain damaged.
- Contact social services or case manager to provide links to social service agencies and schools.
- Rehabilitation facilities are frequently used to compress the time required to recover from a head injury and support re-emergence into society.

COMPLICATIONS

Brain herniation

- A brain herniation is the downward shift of brain tissue due to cerebral edema. **(12.1)**
- The brain consists of brain tissue, cerebrospinal fluid, and blood. Due to the limited space within the skull, an alteration of any one of the components of the brain results in a compromise in the other components. When trauma creates a shift in these components, and the other components are unable to accommodate, the brain shifts from the cranial vault, or herniates. This can result in brain tissue moving downward through the foramen magnum.
- Findings include fixed dilated pupils, deteriorating level of consciousness, Cheyne–Stokes respirations, hemodynamic instability, and abnormal posturing.
- Recovery after this occurrence is rare, and urgent medical treatment (mannitol) and/or surgical (debulking) treatment is indicated.
- With treatment, severe neurologic impairment usually persists.

NURSING ACTIONS

- This situation should be prevented before treatment is needed.
- Close monitoring of vital signs and neurologic status allows early reporting of changes in the GCS score, an increase in the blood pressure, and an alteration in respiratory pattern and effort. Qs
- Frequently update family members on the health status of the client. Frequent updates and repeating medical information is often necessary to ensure comprehension among family members.

CLIENT EDUCATION

- The decision to surgically treat brain herniation is made in the presence of a critical situation.
- Social service workers and/or pastoral personnel can be helpful to support the family while reinforcing the medical situation. Qtc

Hematoma and intracranial hemorrhage

- Monitor for severe headache, rapid decline in level of consciousness, worsening neurologic function and herniation, and changes in ICP.
- Surgery is required to remove subdural and epidural hematoma.
- Intracranial hemorrhage is treated with osmotic diuretics.

Pulmonary edema

- Risk in clients receiving mannitol
- Findings mimic acute pulmonary edema without cardiac involvement.
- This is a life-threatening emergency. Immediate, aggressive treatment is used. Survival is rare.

Diabetes insipidus or syndrome of inappropriate antidiuretic hormone

Diabetes insipidus or syndrome of inappropriate antidiuretic hormone (SIADH) is a possible complication.

NURSING ACTIONS

- Monitor blood electrolytes and osmolality daily.
- Document strict intake and output.
- Weigh client daily.
- Treat electrolyte and fluid imbalance, as prescribed.
- Monitor for dehydration or fluid overload during treatment.

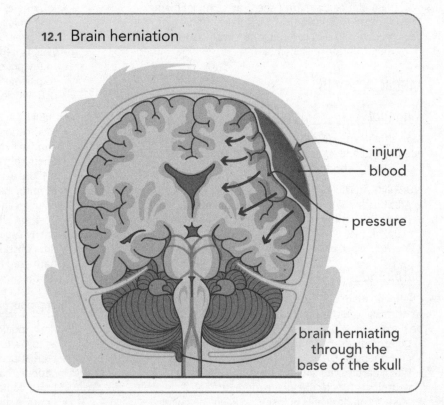

12.1 Brain herniation

injury
blood
pressure
brain herniating through the base of the skull

Application Exercises

1. A nurse is caring for a client who has a benign brain tumor. The client asks the nurse if this same type of tumor can occur in other areas of the body. Which of the following responses should the nurse make?

   A. "It can spread to breasts and kidneys."

   B. "It can develop in your gastrointestinal tract."

   C. "It is limited to brain tissue."

   D. "It probably started in another area of your body and spread to your brain."

2. A nurse is reviewing a new prescription for dexamethasone with a client who has an expanding brain tumor. Which of the following statements should the nurse make? (Select all that apply.)

   A. "It is given to reduce swelling of the brain."

   B. "You will need to monitor for low blood sugar."

   C. "You might notice weight gain."

   D. "Tumor growth will be delayed."

   E. "It can cause you to retain fluids."

3. A nurse is assisting with the care of a client who is having surgery for the removal of an encapsulated acoustic tumor. Which of the following potential complications should the nurse monitor for postoperatively? (Select all that apply.)

   A. Increased intracranial pressure

   B. Hemorrhagic shock

   C. Hydrocephalus

   D. Hypoglycemia

   E. Seizures

4. A nurse is caring for a client who has just undergone a craniotomy and has a respiratory rate of 12. Which of the following postoperative prescriptions should the nurse clarify with the provider?

   A. Dexamethasone 30 mg IV bolus BID

   B. Morphine sulfate 2 mg IV bolus PRN every 2 hr for pain

   C. Ondansetron 4 mg IV bolus PRN every 4 to 6 hr for nausea

   D. Phenytoin 100 mg IV bolus TID

5. A nurse is collecting data from a client who has increased intracranial pressure (ICP). Which of the following are expected findings? (Select all that apply.)

   A. Disoriented to time and place

   B. Restlessness and irritability

   C. Unequal pupils

   D. ICP 15 mm Hg

   E. Headache

Active Learning Scenario

A nurse is reinforcing preoperative teaching with a client who has a brain tumor and will undergo a craniotomy. What should be included in the teaching? Use the ATI Active Learning Template: Therapeutic Procedure to complete this item.

DESCRIPTION OF PROCEDURE

NURSING INTERVENTIONS: Describe three preoperative and three postoperative interventions.

Active Learning Scenario Key

Using the ATI Active Learning Template: Therapeutic Procedure

DESCRIPTION OF PROCEDURE: A craniotomy is a surgical opening in the skull to expose brain tissue. It involves a complete or partial resection of the brain tumor.

NURSING INTERVENTIONS

Preoperative
- Explain the procedure, answer appropriate questions, and provide emotional support.
- Provide written explanations.
- Include the client's partner when reinforcing teaching.
- Remind the client to stop taking aspirin at least 72 hr prior to the procedure, if appropriate.
- Review use of alternative/complementary therapies, and report their use to the provider.
- Review the need for a living will and durable power for health care decisions.
- Administer medications (anxiolytics, muscle relaxants) as prescribed.

Postoperative
- Monitor vital signs and neurologic status to include use of Glasgow Scale.
- Maintain client's head at the elevation of 30° and in a neutral position to prevent increased ICP.
- Monitor for postoperative bleeding and seizures.
- Prevent the client from performing any straining activities (moving up in bed, attempting to have a bowel movement).

Ⓝ *NCLEX® Connection: Reduction of Risk Potential, Potential for Complications From Surgical Procedures and Health Alterations*

Application Exercises Key

1. C. **CORRECT:** Benign brain tumors develop from the meninges or cranial nerves and do not metastasize and are not secondary to other types of tumors.

   Ⓝ *NCLEX® Connection: Physiological Adaptation, Basic Pathophysiology*

2. A, C, E. **CORRECT:** Dexamethasone is a common steroid prescribed to reduce cerebral edema. Weight gain and fluid retention are effects of dexamethasone. The client can experience hyperglycemia, not low blood sugar. Dexamethasone does not affect tumor growth.

   Ⓝ *NCLEX® Connection: Pharmacological Therapies, Expected Actions/Outcomes*

3. A, C, E. **CORRECT:** A client who has had a craniotomy should be monitored postoperatively for increased ICP. Following a craniotomy, the client should be monitored for the development of hydrocephalus. Seizures are a postoperative complication that should be monitored for following a craniotomy. Although hypovolemic shock can occur secondary to SIADH, hemorrhagic shock is not a concern. An alteration in glucose metabolism is not usually a postoperative concern following a craniotomy.

   Ⓝ *NCLEX® Connection: Reduction of Risk Potential, Potential for Complications From Surgical Procedures and Health Alterations*

4. B. **CORRECT:** The nurse should identify that the provider should be notified prior to administering morphine to a client who has a respiratory rate of 12 following a craniotomy. Morphine is a narcotic analgesic, which can cause CNS depressant effects such as respiratory depression. Dexamethasone is given to prevent cerebral edema and has no CNS depressant effects. Ondansetron is prescribed to manage nausea and has no CNS depressant effects. Phenytoin is prescribed to prevent seizures and has no CNS depressant effects.

   Ⓝ *NCLEX® Connection: Reduction of Risk Potential, Potential for Complications From Surgical Procedures and Health Alterations*

5. A, B, C, E. **CORRECT:** The nurse should identify that changes in level of consciousness are an early indicator of increased ICP. Increased ICP can cause behavioral changes, such as restlessness and irritability. Unequal pupils indicate pressure on the oculomotor nerve secondary to increased ICP. Additionally, a headache is a manifestation of increased ICP. An ICP of 15 mm Hg is within the expected reference range of 10 to 15 mm Hg.

   Ⓝ *NCLEX® Connection: Physiological Adaptation, Alterations in Body Systems*

CHAPTER 13 *Stroke*

Strokes, also known as cerebrovascular accidents or brain attacks, involve a disruption in the cerebral blood flow secondary to ischemia, hemorrhage, or embolism. Stroke is the fifth leading cause of death in the U.S. that affects > 795,000 people annually. Stroke is a medical emergency, and treatment should begin immediately to prevent or decrease permanent disability.

Classifications of strokes are hemorrhagic and ischemic.

Hemorrhagic strokes occur secondary to a ruptured artery or aneurysm. The prognosis for a client who has experienced a hemorrhagic stroke is poor due to the amount of ischemia and increased intracranial pressure (ICP) caused by the expanding collection of blood. If it is caught early and evacuation of the clot can be done with cessation of the active bleed, the prognosis of a hemorrhagic stroke improves significantly.

Ischemic is the most common type of stroke (further classified as thrombotic or embolic) that accounts for 87% of all strokes. This is caused by a blockage of circulation to the brain. It can be reversed with fibrinolytic therapy using alteplase, also known as tissue plasminogen activator (tPA), if given within 3 to 4.5 hr of the initial manifestations (unless contraindicated by factors [presence of active bleeding]).

- **Thrombotic** strokes occur secondary to the development of a blood clot on an atherosclerotic plaque in a cerebral artery that gradually shuts off the artery and causes ischemia distal to the occlusion. Manifestations of a thrombotic stroke evolve over a period of several hours to days.

- **Embolic** strokes are caused by an embolus traveling from another part of the body to a cerebral artery. Blood to the brain distal to the occlusion is immediately shut off, causing neurologic deficits or a loss of consciousness to instantly occur.

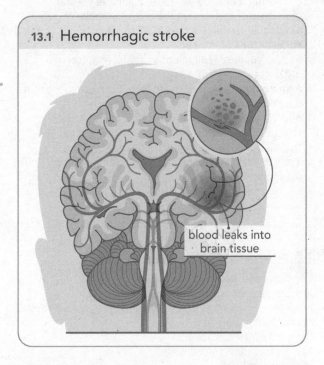

13.1 Hemorrhagic stroke

blood leaks into brain tissue

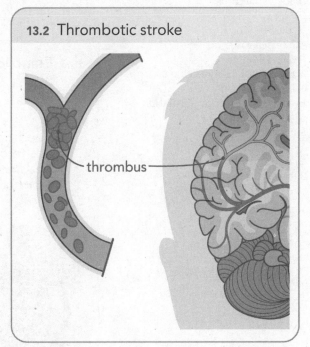

13.2 Thrombotic stroke

thrombus

HEALTH PROMOTION AND DISEASE PREVENTION

- Hypertension, diabetes mellitus, smoking, and other related disorders can increase a client's risk for a stroke. ⓠEBP
- Early treatment of hypertension, maintenance of blood glucose within expected range, and refraining from smoking will decrease these risk factors.
- Maintaining a healthy weight and getting regular exercise can also decrease the risk of a stroke.
- Educate clients about acting FAST to identify manifestations of stroke.
  - **F**acial drooping (Ask client to smile; look for unilateral facial drooping.)
  - **A**rm weakness (Ask client to raise both arms; look for downward drift.)
  - **S**peech impairment or difficulty speaking (Ask client to repeat simple phrases; listen for unexpected findings such as slurred speech.)
  - **T**ime to call 911. (If any of above findings present, call 911 immediately.)

DATA COLLECTION

RISK FACTORS

- Cerebral aneurysm
- Arteriovenous (AV) malformation
- Ethnicity: Black American, Hispanic, Indigenous Peoples, Alaska Native
- Family history of stroke
- Age greater than 65 (ischemic)
- Diabetes mellitus
- Obesity
- Hypertension
- Atherosclerosis
- Hyperlipidemia
- Hypercoagulability (sickle cell anemia)
- Heart disease (atrial fibrillation, cardiomyopathy)
- Smoking
- Alcohol consumption (more than 1–2 drinks per day)
- Substance use (cocaine)
- Use of oral contraceptives

EXPECTED FINDINGS

According to CDC 2021, the sudden signs of stroke include severe headache, vertigo, dizziness, gait impairment, vision impairment, confusion, trouble articulating, unilateral numbness and paresthesia.

- A transient episode of neurologic dysfunction caused by focal brain, spinal cord, or retinal ischemia without acute infarction is a condition that is known as a transient ischemic attack (TIA). During a TIA, there is brief interruption of cerebral blood flow. Manifestations of a TIA resolve within 1–24 hours without any permanent deficits.
- During a TIA, clients might report transient manifestations (visual disturbances, dizziness, slurred speech, a weak extremity), which can be a warning of an impending stroke.
- Antithrombotic medication and/or surgical removal of atherosclerotic plaques in the carotid artery can prevent the subsequent occurrence of a stroke.

PHYSICAL FINDINGS: Manifestations vary based on the area of the brain that is deprived of oxygenated blood. The left cerebral hemisphere of the brain is responsible for language, mathematical skills, and analytical thinking. The right hemisphere of the brain is responsible for visual and spatial awareness and proprioception. Clients experience contralateral findings depending on the side of the brain that is affected (ex: left hemisphere damage can cause right-sided deficits (hemiplegia [paralysis], hemiparesis [weakness]).

- Expressive and receptive aphasia (inability to speak and understand language)
- Agnosia (unable to recognize familiar objects)
- Alexia (reading difficulty)
- Agraphia (writing difficulty)

13.3 Embolic stroke

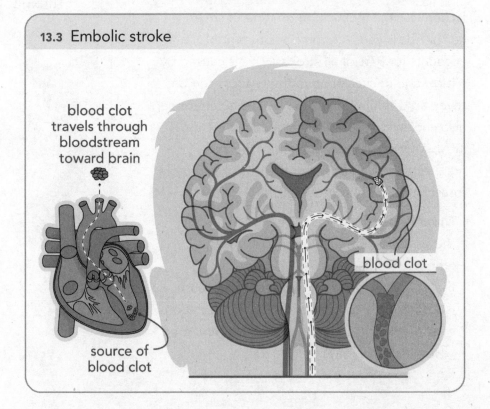

blood clot travels through bloodstream toward brain

blood clot

source of blood clot

- Right or left extremity hemiplegia (paralysis) or hemiparesis (weakness)
- Slow, cautious behavior
- Depression, anger, and quick to become frustrated
- Altered perception of deficits (overestimation of abilities)
- Ataxia (decreased coordination, loss of balance)
- Apraxia: inability to perform simple commands
- Unilateral neglect syndrome (ignore left side of the body: cannot see, feel, or move affected side, so client unaware of its existence). Can occur with left-hemispheric strokes but is more common with right-hemispheric strokes
- Loss of depth perception
- Poor impulse control and judgment
- Visual changes (hemianopsia: loss of visual field in one or both eyes)

LABORATORY AND DIAGNOSTIC PROCEDURES

CBC: Check hemoglobin, hematocrit, platelet, WBC, glucose.

Coagulation panel: Check PT, INR, aPTT: prior to initiation of fibrinolytic or anticoagulation medications.

12 lead ECG: Identify cardiac conditions such as atrial fibrillation or flutter.

Doppler ultrasound: (carotid) Determine perfusion; check for occlusion or blockage.

Computed tomography (CT) scan (without contrast): The initial diagnostic test and should be performed within 25 min from the time of client arrival to the emergency department. This will assist with the determination of type of stroke (ischemic versus hemorrhagic) and whether the client is a candidate for thrombolytic therapy.

Magnetic resonance imaging (MRI): can be used to identify edema, ischemia, and necrosis

Angiography: (cerebral CT or MRI) used to identify the presence of a cerebral hemorrhage, abnormal vessel structures (AV malformation, aneurysms), vessel ruptures, and regional perfusion of blood flow in the carotid arteries and brain

Dysphagia screening: The speech-language pathologist (SLP) can perform a swallowing study. The client swallows a barium substrate, and a radiograph is taken of peristaltic activity of the esophagus.

13.4 Hemianopsia

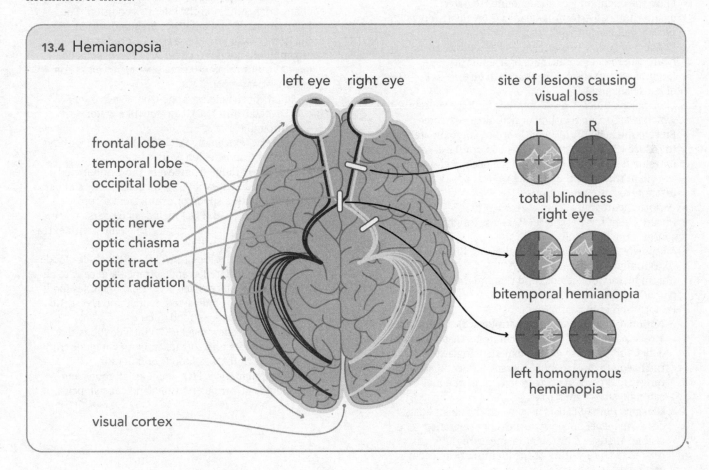

left eye   right eye

site of lesions causing visual loss

L   R

total blindness right eye

bitemporal hemianopia

left homonymous hemianopia

frontal lobe
temporal lobe
occipital lobe

optic nerve
optic chiasma
optic tract
optic radiation

visual cortex

PATIENT-CENTERED CARE

NURSING CARE

The Joint Commission core measures for stroke include actions to take for all clients who are experiencing a stroke. These include venous thromboembolism (VTE) prophylaxis, thrombolytic therapy as indicated, reevaluation of antithrombotic therapy, providing and documenting stoke education, and determining the need for rehabilitation. The nurse should be familiar with the core measures at their facility and ensure that appropriate actions are taken.

INITIAL CARE

- Priority actions for a client who is experiencing a stroke include assessing level of consciousness (LOC), maintaining airway patency, and checking vital signs and circulation.
- Monitor vital signs frequently (could be at least every 15 min to every 1 to 2 hr). Notify the provider immediately of unexpected findings such as increased blood pressure (greater than 185/110 mm Hg), which could indicate an ischemic stroke. A fever can cause an increase in intracranial pressure. Qs
- Provide oxygen therapy to maintain oxygen saturation level greater than 94% or if the client's level of consciousness is decreased.
- Place the client on a cardiac monitor to detect dysrhythmias. Perform 12-lead ECG (evaluate for presence of cardiac findings).
- Conduct a cardiac assessment and auscultate apical heart rate to detect murmurs or irregularity.
- Monitor for increased ICP (change in level of consciousness).
- Check blood glucose level (monitor for hyperglycemia, which is associated with poor neurologic outcome).
- Elevate the head of the client's bed to approximately 30° to reduce ICP and to promote venous drainage. Avoid extreme flexion or extension of the neck, and maintain the client's head in the midline neutral position. QEBP
- Institute seizure precautions.
- Perform neurological checks frequently.
- Ensure client has peripheral IV access (might need 2 large-bore IVs).
- Administer IV fluids (isotonic saline, no fluids containing dextrose).
- Obtain history of current condition (might need to ask partner or relatives).
- Perform screening assessments:
  - **National Institute of Health stroke scale (NIHSS):** a stroke scoring tool composed of items that determine deficits for clients who are experiencing a stroke and the need for thrombolytic therapy. The total score can range from 0–42. A score greater than or equal to 10 can indicate severe stroke.
  - **Glasgow Coma Scale** is used when the client has a decreased level of consciousness or orientation. The risk for increased intracranial pressure (ICP) exists related to the swelling of the brain that can occur secondary to ischemia.

CONTINUING CARE

- Assist with the client's communication skills if speech is impaired.
  - Assess the ability to understand speech by asking the client to follow simple commands.
  - Avoid using yes/no questions (in expressive aphasia).
  - Provide the client with alternate forms of communication: a communication board, computer, mobile device, or picture board of commonly requested items/needs.
  - For expressive and receptive aphasia, speak slowly and clearly; use one-step commands.
  - Collaborate with speech language pathologist (SLP) for communication concerns.
- Assist with safe feeding. Qs
  - Keep the client NPO until a thorough assessment of the client's swallowing is evaluated.
  - Monitor for dysphagia (drooling, choking, coughing, gagging, pocketing food, and taking longer than 10 seconds to swallow food).
  - Consult with SLP for possible evaluation of the client's swallowing and gag reflexes. The SLP may request further swallowing studies with radiography with barium substrate to check peristaltic activity of the esophagus.
  - Provide the client with their recommended food and liquid consistencies (determined by SLP) to minimize choking and aspiration. The recommendation can change depending on the client's condition. The International Dysphagia Diet Standardization Initiative (2019) provides a framework for dietary recommendation for a client who has dysphagia. **(REFER TO NUTRITION CHAPTER 8: MODIFIED DIETS FOR MORE INFORMATION.)**
    - Liquid consistencies range from levels 0–4.
      - Level 0 (thin/TNO): can flow like water through a straw
      - Level 4 (extremely thick/EX4): smooth with no lumps; can be eaten with a spoon
    - Food levels range from levels 3 to 7 and include:
      - 3: Liquidized level (LQ3) includes foods can be eaten with a spoon or drunk from a cup.
      - 4: Pureed level (PU4) includes no coarse textures with foods that are pureed in blender with extra gravy, sauce, milk.
      - 5: Minced and moist level (MM5) includes foods that are moistened and softened and easy to chew.
      - 6: Soft and bite-sized level (SB6) includes foods that are soft, bite-sized, tender and moist. No mixed textures of foods/liquids.
      - 7: Easy to chew level (EC7) include foods that have tender and soft texture; may include thin and thick textured foods and liquids.
      - 7: Regular level (RG7) includes all foods and liquids of various textures and consistencies.

- Have the client eat in an upright position and swallow with the head and neck flexed slightly forward.
- Provide the client with adaptive equipment for meals.
- Encourage the client to sip/drink liquids from a cup. Do not use a straw for liquids (risk for aspiration).
- Assist with feeding (if client has weakness on one side of the body, place food in the back of the mouth on the unaffected side). A RN should provide the initial feeding.
- Have suction on standby.
- Maintain a distraction-free environment during meals.
- Collaborate with dietitian to ensure adequate caloric intake, because weight loss is common following stroke. Qtc
- Prevent complications of immobility (atelectasis, pneumonia, pressure injury, and deep vein thrombosis [DVT]).
  - Assist with ambulation as soon as possible to reduce the risk for complications.
  - Provide preventive measures (applying SCDs, antiembolism, stockings).
  - Encourage range of motion exercises every 2 hr (active for unaffected extremities, passive for affected).
  - Elevate affected extremities to promote venous return and reduce swelling. An elastic glove can be placed on the affected hand if swelling is severe.
  - Instruct client to manage edema of extremities by massaging or stroking from the fingertips or toes back toward the body to encourage fluid movement.

13.5 Communication board

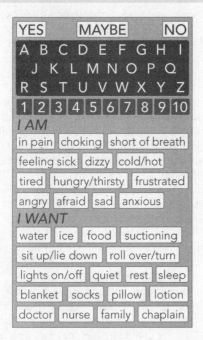

YES	MAYBE	NO

A B C D E F G H I
J K L M N O P Q
R S T U V W X Y Z
1 2 3 4 5 6 7 8 9 10

I AM
in pain | choking | short of breath
feeling sick | dizzy | cold/hot
tired | hungry/thirsty | frustrated
angry | afraid | sad | anxious

I WANT
water | ice | food | suctioning
sit up/lie down | roll over/turn
lights on/off | quiet | rest | sleep
blanket | socks | pillow | lotion
doctor | nurse | family | chaplain

- Maintain a safe environment to reduce the risk of falls and injuries.
  - Use assistive devices (transfer belts and sliding boards) during transfers. Sit-to-stand lifts can also facilitate transfers and reduce strain on the care provider's body. Qtc
  - If the client has one-sided neglect, reinforce with client how to protect and care for the affected extremity to avoid injury.
  - Shoulder subluxation can occur if the affected arm is not supported. The weight of the arm is such that it can cause a painful dislocation of the shoulder from its socket.
  - Encourage client to support their affected arm while in bed, in the wheelchair, or during ambulation with an arm sling or placed on pillows (if experiencing impaired balance, leaning to one side, or hemiparalysis).
  - Provide frequent rest periods from sitting in the wheelchair/chair by returning the client to bed after therapies and meals (if experiencing decreased endurance).
    - If the client has homonymous hemianopsia (loss of the same visual field in both eyes), instruct them to use a scanning technique (turning head from the direction of the unaffected side to the affected side) when eating and ambulating. Place personal supplies within reach on the unaffected side should be considered.
- Provide assistance with ADLs as needed.
  - Instruct the client to dress the affected side first and sit in a supportive chair that aids in balance. Have occupational therapy check the client for adaptive aids (a plate guard, utensils with built-up handles, a reaching tool to pick things up, and shirts and shoes that have hook and loop fasteners or tape instead of buttons and ties).
  - Use the unaffected side to exercise the affected side of the body.
- Support the client during periods of emotional lability and depression. Qpcc

MEDICATIONS

The Core Measures for The Joint Commission suggest that the client should discharged with prescription medications to manage and prevent strokes, such as anticoagulants (atrial fibrillation/flutter), thrombolytics, and statins.

Thrombolytic medications

Tissue plasminogen activator (Recombinant t-PA) alteplase
- A binder of fibrin that converts plasminogen to plasmin, which causes the fibrin in the clot to dissolve (fibrinolysis)
- Goal is to administer within 45 minutes after arrival to emergency department. Can give within 3-4.5 hr of initial manifestations for clients experiencing ischemic stroke due to embolic event as evidenced by CT scan results
- Contraindicated with active bleeding

- Do not administer with antiplatelets or anticoagulants within 24 hrs.
- An initial IV intermittent bolus is given, followed by an IV infusion.
- Monitor for adverse effects (hypotension, intracranial hemorrhage, bleeding, ecchymoses).

Anticoagulants

Warfarin
- Indicated for clients who have atrial fibrillation (or cardioembolic stroke) with a target international normalized ratio (INR) of 2 to 3 (secondary prevention)
- Anticoagulants should not be used in hemorrhagic stroke.

Direct oral anticoagulants

Dabigatran, apixaban, rivaroxaban: Alternative medications to warfarin therapy for clients experiencing atrial fibrillation (cardioembolic stroke)

Antiplatelets

Aspirin, dipyridamole, clopidogrel
- Low-dose aspirin is given within 24 to 48 hr following an ischemic stroke to prevent further clot formation.
- Platelet inhibitors (dipyridamole, clopidogrel) can be given to clients who have experienced thrombotic or embolic stroke.

Antiepileptics

Phenytoin, gabapentin
- These medications are not commonly given following a stroke unless the client develops seizures.
- Gabapentin can be given for paresthetic pain in an affected extremity.

Antihypertensives

ACE inhibitors, diuretics, calcium channel blockers (nimodipine)
- Nimodipine can be used to decrease vasospasms related to subarachnoid hemorrhage.
- Ace inhibitors, diuretics can be given after acute stroke to manage hypertension.

Cholesterol lowering agents

"Statins" (atorvastatin, simvastatin): Manage hyperlipidemia and prevent the formation of plaques

Other (stool softeners, analgesics, antianxiety)

- Stool softeners prevent constipation and straining when defecating (prevent increase in ICP).
- Analgesics: manage discomforts (headache)
- Antianxiety: promotes relaxation, decreases stress

THERAPEUTIC PROCEDURES

Systemic or catheter-directed thrombolytic therapy restores cerebral blood flow. It must be administered within 6 hr of the onset of manifestations. It is contraindicated for treatment of a hemorrhagic stroke and for clients who have an increased risk of bleeding due to anticoagulant therapy or other bleeding anomalies. Possibility of hemorrhagic stroke is ruled out with an MRI prior to the initiation of thrombolytic therapy.

- **Thrombectomy** (mechanical, endovascular, intra-arterial)
- **Carotid artery angioplasty with stenting (CAS)** involves inserting a catheter in the femoral artery and placing a distal/embolic protection device to catch clot debris during the procedure while a stent is being placed in the carotid artery to open a blockage. CAS is less invasive, blood loss is decreased, and length of hospitalization is shorter. Postoperative care is the same as carotid endarterectomy.
- **Extracranial-intracranial bypass** is a craniotomy performed to improve cerebral perfusion following a stroke or for clients who have had a TIA that is likely to progress to a stroke. It increases blood flow around a blocked artery and can help restore blood flow to affected areas of the brain.
- **Carotid endarterectomy:** Opens the artery by removing atherosclerotic plaque. This procedure is performed when the carotid artery is blocked or when the client is experiencing TIAs.
  - Assess for increased headache, neck swelling, and hoarseness of the voice.
  - Have emergency airway equipment available for use.

INTERPROFESSIONAL CARE

The interprofessional team for a client who is experiencing a stroke can consist of: neurologist, social worker, rehabilitation coordinators, psychologists, physical and occupational therapist, SLP, dietitian, and pharmacist.

- Speech and language therapists can be consulted for language therapy and swallowing exercises.
- Physical therapy can be consulted for assistance with reestablishment of ambulation with or without assistive devices (single or quad cane, walker) or wheelchair support. Wheelchair adaptations (an extended brake handle on the client's affected side of the wheelchair) can be necessary.
- Occupational therapy can be consulted for assistance with reestablishment of partial or full function of the affected hand and arm. If function does not return to the extremity, measures (massage and elastic gloves) will be prescribed by occupational therapy to prevent swelling of the extremity.
- Social services can be consulted to plan for rehabilitation services and temporary placement on a skilled rehabilitation unit or extended-care facility during provision of these services. Prior to discharge, the social worker can make a home visit with selected therapists and nurses to evaluate the need for environmental alterations in the home and adaptive equipment needed for ADLs.

COMPLICATIONS

Aspiration pneumonia

Dysphagia can result from neurologic involvement of the cranial nerves that innervate the face, tongue, soft palate, and throat. As a result, the client's risk of aspiration is great. Qs The client is at risk for developing aspiration pneumonia because of these findings.

Not all clients who have experienced a stroke have dysphagia, but all should be evaluated prior to reestablishing oral nutrition and hydration.

NURSING ACTIONS

- Keep the client completely NPO until evaluated by the SLP.
- When resuming intake, provide the client with the prescribed diet and liquid-consistency, and observe closely for choking.
- Have suction equipment available, but use with caution because nasotracheal suctioning increases ICP. QEBP
- An RN should provide the initial feeding and intervene if choking occurs. Some clients require an eating environment without distractions to prevent choking.

CLIENT EDUCATION

- Use recommended techniques for eating and adhere to instructions regarding prescribed consistency of liquids and solid foods.
- Sit upright and flex the head forward when swallowing to decrease the risk of choking. Qs

Unilateral neglect

Unilateral neglect is the loss of awareness of the side affected by the stroke. The client cannot see, feel, or move the affected side of the body; therefore, they forget that it exists. This lack of awareness poses a great risk for injury to the neglected extremities and creates a self-care deficit.

NURSING ACTIONS

- Observe affected extremities for injury (bruises and abrasions of the affected hand and arm, hyperflexion of the foot from it falling off the footrest on a wheelchair during transport).
- Apply an arm sling if the client is unable to remember to care for the affected extremity.
- Ensure that the footrest is on the wheelchair and that an ankle brace is on the affected foot.

CLIENT EDUCATION

- Dress the affected side first. QPCC
- Care for the affected side.
- Use the unaffected hand to pull the affected extremity to midline and out of danger from the wheel of the wheelchair or from hitting or smashing it against a doorway.
- Look over the affected side periodically.

Application Exercises

1. A nurse is providing teaching with a newly licensed nurse about the manifestations of stroke. Match the findings of stroke to the corresponding term.

   A. Inability to perform simple commands
   B. Loss of balance or coordination
   C. Difficulty writing
   D. Inability to speak or understand language
   E. Inability to recognize familiar objects by sight, hearing, or touch

   1. Agnosia
   2. Aphasia
   3. Agraphia
   4. Ataxia
   5. Apraxia

2. A nurse is caring for a client who has global aphasia (both receptive and expressive). Which of the following interventions should the nurse implement? (Select all that apply.)

   A. Speak slowly to the client.
   B. Assist the client to use cards with pictures.
   C. Speak to the client in a loud voice.
   D. Complete sentences that the client cannot finish.
   E. Give instructions to the client one step at a time.

3. A nurse is planning care for a client who had a stroke and is experiencing dysphagia. Which of the following actions should the nurse include in the plan? (Select all that apply.)

   A. Have suction equipment available for use.
   B. Eliminate distractions during mealtime.
   C. Place food on the unaffected side of the client's mouth.
   D. Assign assistive personnel to provide initial feeding.
   E. Inform client to swallow with the neck flexed forward.

4. A nurse is assisting with the care of a client who has left homonymous hemianopsia. Which of the following actions should the nurse take?

   A. Inform the client to scan to the right to see objects on the right side of the body.
   B. Place the client's bedside table on the right side of the bed.
   C. Orient the client to the food on the plate using the clock method.
   D. Place the wheelchair on the client's left side.

5. A nurse is caring for a client who is receiving an IV infusion of alteplase for the management of suspected ischemic stroke. Which of the following findings is an adverse effect of this medication?

   A. Hypertension
   B. Epistaxis
   C. Hypothermia
   D. Diplopia

Active Learning Scenario

A nurse is planning a health and wellness session about stroke prevention for a group of clients at a community health center. Which of the following information should the nurse include? Use the ATI Active Learning Template: Basic Concept to complete this item.

NURSING INTERVENTIONS: List 4 educational teaching points the nurse should discuss during this.

Active Learning Scenario Key

Using the ATI Active Learning Template: Basic Concept
NURSING INTERVENTIONS
- Hypertension, diabetes mellitus, smoking, and other related disorders can increase a client's risk for a stroke.
- Early treatment of hypertension, maintenance of blood glucose within expected range, and refraining from smoking will decrease these risk factors.
- Maintaining a healthy weight and getting regular exercise can also decrease the risk of a stroke.
- Educate clients about acting FAST to identify manifestations of stroke.
  - Facial drooping (Ask client to smile; look for unilateral facial drooping.)
  - Arm weakness (Ask client to raise both arms; look for downward drift.)
  - Speech impairment or difficulty speaking (Ask client to repeat simple phrases; listen for unexpected findings such as slurred speech.)
  - Time to call 911. (If any of the above findings present, call 911 immediately.)

Ⓝ *NCLEX® Connection: Health Promotion and Maintenance, Health Promotion and Disease Prevention*

Application Exercises Key

1. A, 5; B, 4; C, 3; D, 2; E, 1
   When taking actions, the nurse should identify that agnosia is the inability to recognize familiar objects by touch, sight, or hearing. Aphasia is the inability to speak or understand language. Agraphia is difficulty writing. Ataxia is the loss of balance or coordination. Apraxia is the inability to perform simple commands.
   Ⓝ *NCLEX® Connection: Physiological Adaptation, Basic Pathophysiology*

2. A, B, E. **CORRECT:** When taking actions, the nurse should identify that clients who have global aphasia have difficulty with speaking and understanding speech. The nurse should implement actions, such as speaking at slower rate, and use alternate forms of communication, such as cards with pictures, a communication board, or a computer, and give instructions one step at a time.
   Ⓝ *NCLEX® Connections: Physiological Adaptation, Alterations in Body Systems*

3. A, B, C, E. **CORRECT:** When generating solutions, the nurse should identify a client who has dysphagia is at risk for aspiration. Therefore, it is important for the nurse to keep the client NPO until a swallowing evaluation has been performed by SLP. When planning care, the nurse should have suction equipment available, eliminate distractions during mealtime, place food on the unaffected side of mouth, and inform the client to swallow with their neck flexed forward. These measures will reduce the risk for aspiration and decrease the risk of choking.
   Ⓝ *NCLEX® Connection: Reduction of Risk Potential, Potential for Alterations in Body Systems*

4. B. **CORRECT:** When taking actions, the nurse should identify that a client who has left homonymous hemianopsia has lost the left visual field of both eyes, which causes vision impairment on their left side. Therefore, the nurse should place the bedside table and wheelchair on the client's right side of the bed for visualization of the items on the table and instruct the client to turn their head to the left to visualize the entire field of vision.
   Ⓝ *NCLEX® Connection: Physiological Adaptation, Alterations in Body Systems*

5. B. **CORRECT:** When taking actions, the nurse should identify that alteplase is a thrombolytic agent that is administered IV for a client who is suspected of having an ischemic stroke. The nurse should monitor for adverse effects of bleeding (GI bleeding, epistaxis, hemoptysis, and intracranial hemorrhage).
   Ⓝ *NCLEX® Connections: Adverse Effects/Contraindications/Side Effects/Interactions*

When reviewing the following chapters, keep in mind the relevant topics and tasks of the NCLEX outline.

Basic Care and Comfort

NUTRITION AND ORAL HYDRATION: Monitor impact of disease/illness on client nutritional status.

Physiological Adaptation

ALTERATIONS IN BODY SYSTEMS
Provide care to correct client alteration in body system.

Notify primary health care provider of a change in client status.

Pharmacological Therapies

ADVERSE EFFECTS/CONTRAINDICATIONS/SIDE EFFECTS/INTERACTIONS
Monitor client for actual and potential adverse effects of medications.

Monitor and document client response to management of medication side effects including prescribed, over-the-counter and herbal supplement.

Reinforce client teaching on possible effects of medications.

EXPECTED ACTIONS/OUTCOMES: Monitor client use of medications over time.

CHAPTER 14 *Disorders of the Eye*

Disorders of the eye can be caused by injury, disease processes, and the aging process.

Disorders of the eye that nurses should be knowledgeable about include macular degeneration, cataracts, and glaucoma.

Macular degeneration

Macular degeneration, often called age-related macular degeneration (AMD), is the central loss of vision that affects the macula of the eye.
- There is no cure for macular degeneration.
- AMD is a common cause of vision loss in older adults. ⓖ

Two types of macular degeneration

Dry macular degeneration is the most common and is caused by a gradual blockage in retinal capillary arteries, which results in the macula becoming ischemic and necrotic due to the lack of retinal cells.

Wet macular degeneration is a less common form and is caused by the new growth of blood vessels that have thin walls that leak blood and fluid.

DATA COLLECTION

RISK FACTORS

Dry macular degeneration
- Smoking
- Hypertension
- Female sex
- Short body stature
- Family history
- Diet lacking carotene and vitamin E
- Age greater than 60
- Caucasian race

Wet macular degeneration can occur at any age.

EXPECTED FINDINGS

- Lack of depth perception
- Objects appear distorted
- Blurred vision
- Loss of central vision
- Blindness

DIAGNOSTIC PROCEDURES

Ophthalmoscopy: An ophthalmoscope is used to examine the back part of the eyeball (fundus), including the retina, optic disc, macula, and blood vessels.

Visual acuity tests: Snellen and Rosenbaum eye charts

PATIENT-CENTERED CARE

Wet macular degeneration

- Laser therapy to seal leaking blood vessels
- Ocular injections to inhibit blood vessel growth
  - Ocular injections include an endothelial growth factor inhibitor, bevacizumab, or ranibizumab.

CLIENT EDUCATION

- Encourage clients to consume foods high in antioxidants, carotene, and vitamins E and B_{12}. The provider may prescribe a daily supplement high in carotene and vitamin E. Ⓠ**PCC**
- As loss of vision progresses, clients may be challenged with the inability to eat, drive, write, and read, as well as other activities of daily living.

Refer clients to community organizations that can assist with transportation, reading devices, and large-print books.

Cataracts

A cataract is an opacity in the lens of an eye that impairs vision.

Common causes of cataracts

Age-related: Drying of lens due to water loss; increase in lens density due to lens fiber compaction

Traumatic: Blunt or penetrating injury or foreign body in the eye, exposure to radiation or ultraviolet light

Toxic: Long-term use of corticosteroids, phenothiazine derivatives, beta blockers, or miotic medications

Associated: Diabetes mellitus, hypoparathyroidism, Down syndrome, chronic sunlight exposure

Complicated: Intraocular disease (retinitis pigmentosa, glaucoma, retinal detachment)

HEALTH PROMOTION AND DISEASE PREVENTION

- Teach clients to wear sunglasses while outside.
- Educate clients to wear protective eyewear while playing sports and performing hazardous activities, such as welding and yard work. Ⓠ**s**
- Encourage annual eye examinations and good eye health, especially in adults over the age of 40. ⓖ

DATA COLLECTION

RISK FACTORS

- Advanced age Ⓖ
- Diabetes
- Heredity
- Smoking
- Eye trauma
- Excessive exposure to the sun
- Chronic use of corticosteroids, phenothiazine derivatives, beta blockers, or miotic medications

EXPECTED FINDINGS

- Decreased visual acuity (prescription changes, reduced night vision, decreased color perception)
- Blurred vision
- Diplopia (double vision)

PHYSICAL FINDINGS
- Progressive and painless loss of vision
- Visible opacity
- Absent red reflex

DIAGNOSTIC PROCEDURES

Cataracts can be determined upon examination of the lens using an ophthalmoscope.

PATIENT-CENTERED CARE

NURSING CARE

- Check visual acuity using the Snellen chart.
- Examine external and internal eye structures using an ophthalmoscope.
- Determine the client's functional capacity due to decreased vision.
- Increase the amount of light in a room. Ⓠs
- Provide adaptive devices that accommodate for reduced vision.
  - Magnifying lens and large-print books/newspapers
  - Talking devices, such as clocks

MEDICATIONS

Anticholinergic agents (atropine 1% ophthalmic solution): This medication prevents pupil constriction for prolonged periods of time (mydriasis) and relaxes muscles in the eye (cycloplegia). It is used to dilate the eye preoperatively and for visualization of the eye's internal structures.

NURSING ACTIONS: The medication has a long duration but a fast onset.

CLIENT EDUCATION
- Remind the client that the effects of the medication can last 7 to 12 days.
- The medication can cause photosensitivity, so remind the client to wear sunglasses to protect the eyes. Ⓠpcc

INTERPROFESSIONAL CARE

Consult with an ophthalmologist (eye surgeon) for cataract surgery.

THERAPEUTIC PROCEDURES

Surgical removal of the lens

A small incision is made, and the lens is either removed in one piece or in several pieces, after being broken up using sound waves. The posterior capsule is retained. A replacement or intraocular lens is inserted. Replacement lenses can correct refractive errors, resulting in improved vision.

NURSING ACTIONS: Postoperative care should focus on the following.
- Preventing an increase in intraocular pressure
- Preventing infection
- Administering ophthalmic medications
- Providing pain relief
- Teaching the client about self-care at home and fall prevention Ⓠs

CLIENT EDUCATION
- Wear sunglasses while outside or in brightly lit areas.
- Report manifestations of infection, such as yellow or green drainage.
- Avoid activities that increase IOP.
  - Bending over at the waist
  - Sneezing
  - Blowing nose
  - Coughing
  - Straining
  - Head hyperflexion
  - Restrictive clothing, such as tight shirt collars
  - Sexual intercourse

14.1 Normal and cataract-clouded lenses

normal lense

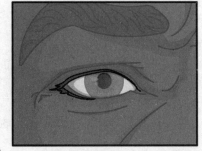

cataract-clouded lense

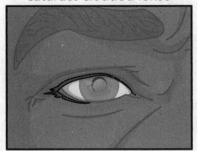

- Limit activities.
  - Tilting the head back to wash hair
  - Cooking and housekeeping
  - Rapid, jerky movements, such as vacuuming
  - Driving and operating machinery
  - Playing sports
- Report pain with nausea/vomiting (indications of increased IOP or hemorrhage).
- Best vision is not expected until 4 to 6 weeks following the surgery.
- Report if any changes occur, such as lid swelling, decreased vision, bleeding or discharge, sharp sudden eye pain, flashes of light, or floating shapes.

COMPLICATIONS

Infection

Infection can occur after surgery.

CLIENT EDUCATION: Manifestations of infection that should be reported include yellow or green drainage, increased redness or pain, reduction in visual acuity, increased tear production, and photophobia. Q_{PCC}

Bleeding

Bleeding is a potential risk several days following surgery.

CLIENT EDUCATION: Immediately report any sudden change in visual acuity or an increase in pain. Q_{PCC}

Glaucoma

Glaucoma is a disturbance of the functional or structural integrity of the optic nerve. Decreased fluid drainage or increased fluid secretion increases intraocular pressure (IOP) and can cause atrophic changes of the optic nerve and visual defects. The expected reference range for IOP is 10 to 20 mm/Hg.
- There are two primary types of glaucoma.
  - **Primary open-angle glaucoma (POAG):** This is the more common form. Open-angle refers to the angle between the iris and sclera. The aqueous humor outflow is decreased due to blockages in the eye's drainage system (Canal of Schlemm and trabecular meshwork), causing a gradual rise in IOP.
  - **Primary angle-closure glaucoma:** IOP rises suddenly. The angle between the iris and the sclera suddenly closes, causing a corresponding increase in IOP. The onset is sudden and requires immediate treatment.
- Glaucoma is a frequent cause of blindness. Early diagnosis and treatment are essential in preventing vision loss from glaucoma.
- Secondary glaucoma can result from trauma, eye surgery, tumors of the eye, uveitis, iritis, neovascular disorders, degenerative disease, or central retinal vein occlusion.

HEALTH PROMOTION AND DISEASE PREVENTION

- Encourage annual eye examinations and good eye health, especially adults over the age of 40. Ⓖ
- Educate clients about the disease process and early indications of glaucoma, such as reduced vision and mild eye pain.

DATA COLLECTION

RISK FACTORS

- Age
- Infection
- Tumors
- Diabetes mellitus
- Genetic predisposition
- Hypertension
- Eye trauma
- Severe myopia
- Retinal detachment

EXPECTED FINDINGS

Primary open-angle glaucoma

- Headache
- Mild eye pain
- Loss of peripheral vision
- Decreased accommodation
- Halos seen around lights
- Elevated IOP (greater than 20 mm Hg: usually 22 to 32)

Primary angle-closure glaucoma

- Rapid onset of elevated IOP (30 mm Hg or higher)
- Decreased or blurred vision
- Colored halos seen around lights
- Pupils nonreactive to light
- Severe pain and nausea
- Photophobia

DIAGNOSTIC PROCEDURES

Visual assessments: Measures decrease in visual acuity and peripheral vision

Tonometry: Measures IOP (expected reference range is 10 to 20 mm Hg). IOP is elevated with glaucoma, especially angle-closure.

Gonioscopy: Used to determine the drainage angle of the anterior chamber of the eyes

PATIENT-CENTERED CARE

NURSING CARE

- Monitor for increased IOP (greater than 20 mm Hg).
- Monitor for decreased vision and light sensitivity.
- Assess for aching or discomfort around the eye.
- Explain the disease process and allow clients to express their feelings.
- Treat severe pain and nausea that accompanies angle-closure glaucoma with analgesics and antiemetics.

MEDICATIONS

The priority intervention for treating glaucoma is medication therapy.

CLIENT EDUCATION
- Prescribed eye medication is beneficial if used every 12 hr.
- Instill one drop in each eye twice daily.
- Wait 5 to 10 min between eye drops if more than one is prescribed to prevent one medication from diluting another.
- Avoid touching the tip of the application bottle to the eye.
- Always wash hands before and after use.
- Once an eye drop is instilled, apply pressure using the punctal occlusion technique (placing pressure on the inner corner of the eye).

Cholinergic agents (carbachol, echothiophate, pilocarpine)

These are miotic medications, which constrict the pupil and allow for improved circulation and outflow of the aqueous humor. Miotics can cause blurred vision. Pilocarpine is considered a second-line drug for POAG.

CLIENT EDUCATION: Use good lighting to avoid falls.

Adrenergic agonists (apraclonidine, brimonidine tartrate, dipivefrin hydrochloride)

These medications reduce intraocular pressure by limiting production of aqueous humor and dilate the pupils to improve the fluid flow to the site of absorption.

CLIENT EDUCATION: Wear sunglasses in bright light because of pupil dilation.

Beta blockers (timolol)

Beta blockers are first-line drug therapy for glaucoma and decrease IOP by reducing aqueous humor production.

NURSING CONSIDERATIONS: Can be absorbed systemically and cause bronchoconstriction and hypoglycemia. Use with caution in clients who have asthma, COPD, and diabetes mellitus. Can potentiate systemic effects of oral beta-blockers and cause bradycardia and hypotension

Carbonic anhydrase inhibitors (acetazolamide, dorzolamide, and brinzolamide)

Decrease IOP by reducing aqueous humor production

NURSING ACTIONS: Ask clients whether they are allergic to sulfa. Carbonic anhydrase inhibitors are sulfa-based.

Prostaglandin analogs

Prostaglandin analogs, such as bimatoprost and latanoprost, increase outflow of the uveosclera by dilating blood vessels in the trabecular mesh where aqueous humor is collected and then drain the humor at a more rapid rate.

CLIENT EDUCATION
- Check for corneal abrasions and do not instill this medication if the corneal is not intact.
- Can cause the iris to change color by darkening with long-term use

Systemic osmotics (IV mannitol, oral glycerin)

IV mannitol is an osmotic diuretic used in the emergency treatment for primary angle-closure glaucoma to quickly decrease IOP.

THERAPEUTIC PROCEDURES

Glaucoma surgery

Laser trabeculectomy, iridotomy, or the placement of a shunt are procedures used to improve the flow of the aqueous humor by opening a channel out of the anterior chamber of the eye.

NURSING ACTIONS: Educate clients about the disease and importance of adhering to the medication schedule to treat IOP.

CLIENT EDUCATION
- Wear sunglasses while outside or in brightly lit areas.
- Report manifestations of infection, such as yellow or green drainage.
- Avoid activities that increase IOP.
  - Bending over at the waist
  - Sneezing
  - Coughing
  - Straining
  - Head hyperflexion
  - Restrictive clothing, such as tight shirt collars
  - Sexual intercourse
- Do not lie on the operative side, and report severe pain or nausea (possible hemorrhage).
- Report if any changes occur (lid swelling, decreased vision, bleeding, discharge, a sharp, sudden pain in the eye, flashes of light, floating shapes).

- Limit activities.
  - Tilting head back to wash hair
  - Cooking and housekeeping
  - Rapid, jerky movements, such as vacuuming
  - Driving and operating machinery
  - Playing sports
- Report pain with nausea/vomiting (indications of increased IOP or hemorrhage).
- Final best vision is not expected until 4 to 6 weeks after surgery.

INTERPROFESSIONAL CARE

Refer to an ophthalmologist if surgery is necessary.

CLIENT EDUCATION

Set up services such as community outreach programs, meals on wheels, and services for the blind. Qs

COMPLICATIONS

Blindness

Blindness is a potential consequence of untreated glaucoma.

CLIENT EDUCATION: Have regular glaucoma checks. Ⓖ
- Before age 40: every 2 to 4 years
- Ages 40 to 54: every 1 to 3 years
- Ages 55 to 64: every 1 to 2 years
- Ages 65 and over: every 6 to 12 months

Active Learning Scenario

A nurse is reviewing discharge instructions for a client who has a new diagnosis of primary open-angle glaucoma and a new prescription for timolol 0.25% eye drops. Use the ATI Active Learning Template: Medication and the ATI Pharmacology Review Module to complete this item.

COMPLICATIONS: List at least three adverse effects that should be included in the teaching.

Application Exercises

1. A nurse is reinforcing teaching for a client who has a new diagnosis of dry macular degeneration. Which of the following instructions should the nurse include in the teaching?
   - A. Increase intake of deep yellow and orange vegetables.
   - B. Administer eye drops twice daily.
   - C. Avoid bending at the waist.
   - D. Wear an eye patch at night.

2. A nurse is caring for a client who has a new diagnosis of cataracts. Which of the following manifestations should the nurse expect? (Select all that apply.)
   - A. Eye pain
   - B. Floating spots
   - C. Blurred vision
   - D. White pupils
   - E. Bilateral red reflexes

3. A nurse is providing postoperative teaching to a client following cataract surgery. Which of the following statements should the nurse include in the teaching?
   - A. "You can resume playing golf in 2 days."
   - B. "You need to tilt your head back when washing your hair."
   - C. "You can get water in your eyes in 1 day."
   - D. "You need to limit your housekeeping activities."

4. A nurse is caring for a client who has diabetes mellitus and reports a gradual loss of peripheral vision. The nurse should recognize this as a manifestation of which of the following diseases?
   - A. Cataracts
   - B. Open-angle glaucoma
   - C. Macular degeneration
   - D. Angle-closure glaucoma

Active Learning Scenario Key

Using the ATI Active Learning Template: Medication and the ATI Pharmacology Review Module

COMPLICATIONS
- CNS: Lethargy, fatigue, anxiety, headache, somnolence, depression
- CV: Bradycardia, palpitations, syncope, hypotension, AV conduction disturbances, CHF
- Specific senses: Eye stinging, tearing, photophobia, eye irritation
- GI: Nausea, dry mouth
- Respiratory: Difficulty breathing, bronchospasm
- Metabolic: Hypoglycemia

Ⓝ *NCLEX® Connection: Pharmacological Therapies, Medication Administration*

Application Exercises Key

1. A. **CORRECT:** When taking action, the nurse should instruct the client to increase dietary intake of carotenoids and antioxidants to slow the progression of the macular degeneration. A client who has primary open-angle glaucoma should administer eye drops twice daily. A client who is at risk for increased intraocular pressure, such as following cataract surgery, should avoid bending at the waist. A client who has had eye surgery, such as cataract surgery, should wear an eye patch at night to protect the eye from injury.

   Ⓝ *NCLEX® Connection: Physiological Adaptation, Basic Pathophysiology*

2. C, D. **CORRECT:** The nurse recognizes blurred vision and white pupils are both manifestations associated with cataracts. Eye pain is associated with primary angle-closure glaucoma, and floating spots are a manifestation associated with retinal detachment. Bilateral red reflexes are absent in a client who has cataracts.

   Ⓝ *NCLEX® Connection: Physiological Adaptation, Basic Pathophysiology*

3. D. **CORRECT:** Instruct the client to limit housekeeping activities following cataract surgery. This activity could cause a rise in IOP or injury to the eye. Do not instruct the client to resume playing golf for several weeks. This could cause a rise in intraocular pressure (IOP) or possible injury to the eye. Do not instruct the client to tilt the head back when washing their hair. This could cause a rise in IOP or possible injury to the eye. The client should not get water in their eyes for 3 to 7 days following cataract surgery to reduce the risk for infection and promote healing.

   Ⓝ *NCLEX® Connection: Reduction of Risk Potential, Therapeutic Procedures*

4. B. **CORRECT:** This is a manifestation of open-angle glaucoma. A gradual loss of peripheral vision is a manifestation associated with this diagnosis. A client who has cataracts experiences a decrease in peripheral and central vision due to opacity of the lens. A client who has macular degeneration experiences a loss of central vision. A client who has angle-closure glaucoma experiences sudden nausea, severe pain, and halos around lights.

   Ⓝ *NCLEX® Connection: Physiological Adaptation, Basic Pathophysiology*

CHAPTER 15 # Middle and Inner Ear Disorders

The ear is a sensory organ with two functions: hearing and balance.

The middle ear consists of the tympanic membrane (eardrum) and the three smallest bones (ossicles) of the body (malleus, incus, and stapes) and connects to the nasopharynx via the Eustachian tube.

The inner ear is located deep within the temporal bone, separated from the middle ear by the oval window. It consists of the cochlea (hearing organ) and semicircular canals (responsible for balance). Cranial nerves VII (facial nerve) and VIII (vestibulocochlear nerve) are part of the inner ear anatomy.

Visual, vestibular, and proprioceptive systems provide the brain with input regarding balance. Problems within any of these systems pose a risk for loss of balance. Qs

Nurses should be knowledgeable about the types of middle and inner ear disorders, including infection, tumors, and issues with balance and coordination.

TYPES OF EAR DISORDERS

Hearing loss

- Environmental or workplace exposure to noise can lead to hearing loss.
- Conductive hearing loss is caused by factors such as otitis media, otosclerosis, and presence of a foreign body (such as impacted cerumen).
- Color of cerumen and external ear canal varies depending on client's race and skin tone. Normal variations should be recognized during assessment. Qpcc

- Sensorineural hearing loss is caused by damage to cranial nerve VIII.
- Combined hearing loss is caused by a mixture of conductive and sensorineural problems.
- Changes in the middle and inner ear related to aging include thickening of the tympanic membrane (loss of elasticity), loss of sensory hair cells in the organ of Corti, and limitations to movement of the ossicles. Ⓖ

Conditions of the middle ear

- Conditions of the middle ear can be caused by injury, disease, and the aging process.
- Acute otitis media is a viral or bacterial infection of the middle ear.
- Manifestations include ear pain, pressure, fever, headache, conductive hearing loss, and purulent or bloody drainage if perforation of the eardrum occurs.
- An otoscopic exam can show redness, bulging tympanic membrane, and inability to visualize usual landmarks.
- Medical management includes systemic antibiotic therapy, analgesics, and application of heat for pain, and decongestants.
- Surgical management includes myringotomy (opening of the eardrum made surgically) and placement of a grommet to equalize pressure.
- Refer to **RN PEDIATRIC NURSING CHAPTER 36: ACUTE OTITIS MEDIA.**

Conditions of the inner ear

- Vertigo occurs when the client has the sensation that they or their surroundings are in motion.
- Benign paroxysmal positional vertigo occurs in response to a change in position. It is thought to be caused by the disruption of the debris located within the semicircular canal (small crystals of calcium carbonate). Onset is sudden and can last for a few weeks or years. Bed rest is prescribed along with short course of meclizine.
- Ménière's disease is characterized by episodic vertigo, tinnitus (ringing in the ears), and fluctuating sensorineural hearing loss.
- Labyrinthitis is an inflammation of the labyrinth in the inner ear, often secondary to otitis media. It is characterized by the sudden onset of severe vertigo, nausea, vomiting, and possible hearing loss and tinnitus. Manifestations are treated with bed rest in a darkened environment. Meclizine or dimenhydrinate is prescribed for nausea and vertigo. Systemic antibiotic therapy can also be prescribed.

DATA COLLECTION

RISK FACTORS

Middle ear disorders
- Recurrent colds and otitis media
- Enlarged adenoids
- Trauma
- Changes in air pressure (scuba diving, flying)

Inner ear disorders
- Viral or bacterial infection
- Damage due to ototoxic medications

EXPECTED FINDINGS

Middle ear disorders
- Hearing loss
- Feeling of fullness and/or pain in the ear
- Red, inflamed ear canal and tympanic membrane (TM)
- Bulging TM
- Fluid and/or bubbles behind TM
- Diffuse appearance of or inability to visualize normal light reflex
- Fever

Inner ear disorders
- Hearing loss
- Tinnitus
- Dizziness or vertigo
- Vomiting
- Nystagmus
- Alterations in balance

DIAGNOSTIC PROCEDURES

Audiometry

Audiometry is a noninvasive test of hearing ability, including frequency, pitch, and intensity. The client indicates when a tone is heard through earphones. Nurses might collaborate with an audiologist for this and other diagnostic procedures. Qᴛᴄ

Tympanogram

Tympanogram measures the mobility of the TM and middle ear structures relative to sound (effective in diagnosing middle ear disease).

Weber and Rinne tests

Weber and Rinne tests use tuning forks to determine whether hearing loss is present.

Otoscopy

An otoscope is used to examine the external auditory canal, TM, and malleus bone visible through the TM.

NURSING ACTIONS
- Otoscopic examination is done if audiometry results indicate possible impairment or if a client reports ear pain.
- After selection of a properly sized speculum, an otoscope is introduced into the external ear.
- If the ear canal curves, pull up and back on the auricle of adults, and down and back on the auricle of children, to straighten out the canal and enhance visualization.
- The TM should be a pearly gray color and intact. It should provide complete structural separation of the outer and middle ear structures.
- The light reflex should be visible from the center of the TM anteriorly (5 o'clock right ear; 7 o'clock left ear). **(15.1)**
- In the presence of fluid or infection in the middle ear, the TM becomes inflamed and can bulge from the pressure of the exudate. This also displaces the light reflex, causing it to look diffuse or completely obscured, a significant diagnostic finding.
- Avoid touching the lining of the ear canal, which causes pain due to sensitivity.

CLIENT EDUCATION: To see the TM clearly, the auricle might need to be firmly pulled.

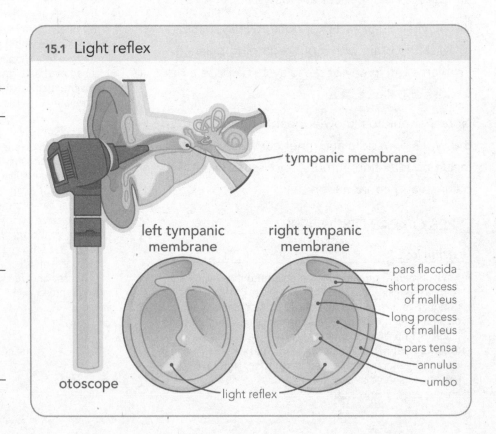

15.1 Light reflex

tympanic membrane

left tympanic membrane

right tympanic membrane

pars flaccida

short process of malleus

long process of malleus

pars tensa

annulus

umbo

otoscope

light reflex

Electronystagmography (ENG)

ENG detects involuntary eye movements (nystagmus) in order to assess for disease of the vestibular system of the ear. Electrodes are taped near the eyes, and movements of the eyes are recorded when the ear canal is stimulated with cold water instillation or injection of air. Recording of eye movements can be interpreted by a specialist as either normal or abnormal.

NURSING ACTIONS

- Intraprocedure, the nurse should ask simple questions (name recall, math problems) to ensure the client remains alert.
- The client should be maintained on bed rest and NPO postprocedure until vertigo subsides. Qs

CLIENT EDUCATION

- Fast immediately before the procedure, and restrict caffeine, alcohol, sedatives, and antihistamines for several days prior to the test.
- This test is not performed on clients who have a pacemaker. (Pacemaker signals inhibit sensitivity of ENG.)

Caloric testing

- Caloric testing can be done concurrently with ENG.
- Water (warmer or cooler than body temperature) is instilled in the ear in an effort to induce nystagmus.
- The eyes' response to the instillation of cold and warm water is diagnostic of vestibular disorders.

NURSING ACTIONS: The client should follow the same restrictions as those for an ENG.

CLIENT EDUCATION: Be aware of the above restrictions.

PATIENT-CENTERED CARE

NURSING CARE

- Monitor functional ability and balance. Take fall risk precautions as necessary. Qs
- Evaluate the client's home situation. Collaborate with home health to assess home safety and fall risks, as needed.
- Encourage a client who has balance or functional limitations to rise slowly and use assistance and assistive devices as needed.
- Monitor blood levels of ototoxic medication and teach clients about adverse effects. Routine audiometry is indicated with use of ototoxic IV antibiotics. Ototoxic medications include the following.
  - Antibiotics: gentamicin, erythromycin
  - Diuretics: furosemide, ethacrynic acid
  - NSAIDs: aspirin, ibuprofen
  - Chemotherapeutic agents: cisplatin
- Assist with ENG and caloric testing as needed.
- Administer antivertigo and antiemetic medications as needed.

MEDICATIONS

Meclizine

Meclizine has antihistamine and anticholinergic effects and is used to treat the vertigo that accompanies inner ear problems.

NURSING ACTIONS: Observe for sedation and take appropriate precautions to ensure safe ambulation. Qs

CLIENT EDUCATION: Be aware of the sedative effects of meclizine. (Avoid driving or operating heavy machinery.)

Antiemetics

Ondansetron is one of several antiemetics used to treat nausea and vomiting associated with vertigo.

NURSING ACTIONS: Contraindicated for clients who have certain cardiac rhythm disorders Qs

CLIENT EDUCATION: Report dizziness or rash.

Diphenhydramine and dimenhydrinate

Antihistamines are effective in the treatment of vertigo and nausea that accompany inner ear problems.

NURSING ACTIONS

- Observe for urinary retention.
- Observe for sedation and take appropriate precautions to ensure safe ambulation. Qs

CLIENT EDUCATION

- Be aware of the sedative effects. (Avoid driving or operating heavy machinery.)
- Dry mouth is expected.

Scopolamine

- Anticholinergics, such as scopolamine, are effective in the treatment of nausea that accompanies inner ear problems.
- It is available transdermally and is used for motion sickness.

NURSING ACTIONS

- Observe for urinary retention.
- Observe for sedation and take appropriate precautions to ensure safe ambulation. Qs
- Monitor clients who have open-angle glaucoma for increasing eye pressure. Contraindicated in clients who have angle-closure glaucoma

CLIENT EDUCATION

- Be aware of the sedative effects. (Avoid driving or operating heavy machinery.)
- Dry mouth is expected.

Diazepam

Diazepam is a benzodiazepine that has a sedative effect that decreases stimuli to the cerebellum and has off-label use for acute vertigo.

NURSING ACTIONS

- Observe for sedation and take appropriate precautions to ensure safe ambulation. Qs
- Restrict use in clients who have closed-angle glaucoma.
- For older adult clients, use the smallest effective dose (prevent oversedation, ataxia). Ⓖ

CLIENT EDUCATION

- Be aware of the sedative effects of diazepam. (Avoid driving or operating heavy machinery.)
- Be aware of diazepam's addictive properties and appropriate use of the medication.

INTERPROFESSIONAL CARE

Vestibular rehabilitation is an option for clients who experience frequent episodes of vertigo or are incapacitated due to vertigo. A team of providers treats the cause and teaches the client exercises that can help them adapt to and minimize the effects of vertigo. A combination of biofeedback, physical therapy, and stress management can be used. Postural education can teach the client positions to avoid and positional exercises that can terminate an attack of vertigo. Qᴛᴄ

THERAPEUTIC PROCEDURES

Vertigo-reducing activities

CLIENT EDUCATION

- Prevent stimulation/exacerbation of vertigo.
- Restrict movement of the head and change positions slowly.
- Avoid caffeine and alcohol.
- Rest in a quiet, darkened environment when vertigo is severe.
- Use assistive devices (cane, walker) as needed for safe ambulation to assist with balance. Qs
- Maintain a safe environment free of clutter.

- Take a diuretic, if prescribed, to decrease the amount of fluid in semicircular canals.
- Space intake of fluids evenly throughout the day.
- Decrease intake of salt and sodium-containing foods (processed meats, MSG).
- Resume these precautions if vertigo returns.

Cochlear implant for sensorineural hearing loss

- Cochlear implants consist of a microphone that picks up sound, a speech processor, a transmitter and receiver that convert sounds into electric impulses, and electrodes that are attached to the auditory nerve.
- The implant's transmitter is located outside the head behind the ear and connects via a magnet to the receiver located immediately below it, under the skin.
- Intensive and prolonged language training is necessary for individuals who did not develop speech.

NURSING ACTIONS: Follow preoperative, intraoperative, and postoperative outpatient surgery guidelines.

CLIENT EDUCATION

- Immediately after surgery, the unit is not turned on.
- The external unit is applied, and the speech processor is programmed 2 to 6 weeks after surgery.
- Be aware of precautions to prevent infection.
- Avoid MRIs.

CLIENT EDUCATION FOLLOWING MIDDLE EAR SURGERY

- Avoid air travel for 2 to 3 weeks.
- Avoid straining or coughing, and blow nose gently with the mouth open for 2 to 3 weeks following surgery.
- Keep ear canal clean and dry. Avoid washing hair or showering for several days to 1 week.
- When able to shower, loosely place a cotton ball with petroleum jelly into the ear canal to prevent water from entering.
- Expect some temporary hearing loss in the affected ear due to presence of fluid or packing.
- Drainage from the ear canal should be reported to the provider.

15.2 Cochlear implant

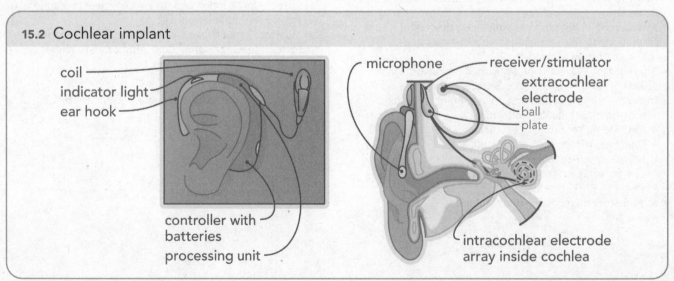

coil
indicator light
ear hook
controller with batteries
processing unit

microphone
receiver/stimulator
extracochlear electrode
ball
plate
intracochlear electrode array inside cochlea

Application Exercises

1. A nurse is caring for a client who has suspected Ménière's disease. Which of the following is an expected finding?

   A. Presence of a purulent lesion in the external ear canal

   B. Feeling of pressure in the ear

   C. Bulging, red bilateral tympanic membranes

   D. Unilateral hearing loss

2. A nurse is reviewing the health record of a client who has severe otitis media. Which of the following are expected findings? (Select all that apply.)

   A. Enlarged adenoids

   B. Report of recent colds

   C. Client prescription for daily furosemide

   D. Light reflex visible on otoscopic exam in the affected ear

   E. Ear pain relieved by meclizine

3. A nurse is performing an otoscopic examination of a client. Which of the following is an unexpected finding?

   A. Pearly gray tympanic membrane (TM)

   B. Malleus visible behind the TM

   C. Presence of soft cerumen in the external canal

   D. Fluid or bubbles seen behind the TM

4. A nurse in a clinic is caring for a client who has been experiencing mild to moderate vertigo due to benign paroxysmal vertigo for several weeks. Which of the following actions should the nurse recommend to help control the vertigo? (Select all that apply.)

   A. Reduce exposure to bright lighting.

   B. Move head slowly when changing positions.

   C. Do not eat fruit high in potassium.

   D. Plan evenly spaced daily fluid intake.

   E. Avoid fluids containing caffeine.

5. A nurse is completing discharge teaching with a client following middle ear surgery. Which of the following statements by the client indicates understanding of the teaching?

   A. "I should restrict rapid movements and avoid bending from the waist for several weeks."

   B. "I should wait until the day after surgery to wash my hair."

   C. "I will remove the dressing behind my ear in 7 days."

   D. "My hearing should be back to normal right after my surgery."

Active Learning Scenario

A nurse in a clinic is reinforcing preoperative teaching for a client who will receive a cochlear implant. What should the nurse include in the teaching? Use the ATI Active Learning Template: Therapeutic Procedure to complete this item.

DESCRIPTION OF PROCEDURE: Describe a cochlear implant.

INDICATIONS: Describe the indication for a cochlear implant.

NURSING INTERVENTIONS: List at least four.

Active Learning Scenario Key

Using the ATI Active Learning Template: Therapeutic Procedure

DESCRIPTION OF PROCEDURE: A cochlear implant consists of a microphone to pick up sound, a speech processor, a transmitter and receiver to convert sounds into electrical impulses, and electrodes that are attached to the auditory nerve. The implant's transmitter is placed outside the head, behind the ear, via a magnet that attaches to the receiver located under the skin below it.

INDICATIONS: A cochlear implant is performed for sensorineural hearing loss.

NURSING INTERVENTIONS
- Pre- and postoperative teaching is completed.
- Intraoperative care is provided in an outpatient setting.
- Client education includes:
  - The unit is not turned on immediately after surgery.
  - The external unit is applied and the speech processor is programmed 2 to 6 weeks after surgery.
  - Prevent infection.
  - MRIs should be avoided.

Ⓝ *NCLEX® Connection: Reduction of Risk Potential, Therapeutic Procedures*

Application Exercises Key

1. D. **CORRECT:** Unilateral sensorineural hearing loss is an expected finding in Ménière's disease. Ménière's disease is an inner ear disorder. A purulent lesion in the external ear canal is not an expected finding. A feeling of pressure in the ear can occur with otitis media but is not an expected finding in Ménière's. Ménière's disease is an inner ear disorder. Bulging, red bilateral tympanic membranes is a finding associated with a middle ear infection.

Ⓝ *NCLEX® Connection: Physiological Adaptation, Basic Pathophysiology*

2. A, B. **CORRECT:** The nurse understands enlarged tonsils and adenoids are a finding associated with a middle ear infection. Frequent colds are also findings associated with a middle ear infection. Furosemide is an ototoxic medication and can cause sensorineural hearing loss, but taking furosemide does not cause a middle ear disorder. Light reflexes are absent or in altered positions in a client who has a middle ear disorder. Meclizine is prescribed to relieve vertigo for inner ear disorders but does not relieve the pain of a middle ear infection.

Ⓝ *NCLEX® Connection: Physiological Adaptation, Basic Pathophysiology*

3. D. **CORRECT:** The nurse should recognize fluid behind the TM indicates the possibility of otitis media and is not an expected finding. A pearly gray TM is an expected finding during an otoscopic examination as is visualization of the malleus behind the TM. Cerumen of various colors, depending on the client's skin color or ethnic background, is also an expected finding in the external ear canal.

Ⓝ *NCLEX® Connection: Reduction of Risk Potential, Potential for Alterations in Body Systems*

4. A, B, D. **CORRECT:** Remaining in a darkened, quiet environment can reduce vertigo, particularly when it is severe. Moving slowly when standing or changing positions can reduce vertigo. Additionally, fluid intake should be planned so that it is evenly spaced throughout the day to prevent excess fluid accumulation in the semicircular canals. The client who has vertigo should be instructed to avoid foods containing high levels of sodium to reduce fluid retention, which can cause vertigo. The client should avoid fluids containing caffeine or alcohol to minimize vertigo.

Ⓝ *NCLEX® Connection: Physiological Adaptation, Alterations in Body Systems*

5. A. **CORRECT:** The client should understand rapid movements and bending from the waist should be avoided for 3 weeks following ear surgery. Avoid showering and washing hair for at least several days up to 1 week following ear surgery. The ear must remain dry during this time. Middle ear surgery is performed through the tympanic membrane, and the client will have a dry dressing within the ear canal. There is no external excision. Decreased hearing is expected following middle ear surgery due to presence of a dressing within the ear canal and possible drainage.

Ⓝ *NCLEX® Connection: Physiological Adaptation, Alterations in Body Systems*

When reviewing the following chapters, keep in mind the relevant topics and tasks of the NCLEX outline.

Pharmacological Therapies

ADVERSE EFFECTS/CONTRAINDICATIONS/SIDE EFFECTS/ INTERACTIONS: Monitor client for actual and potential adverse effects of medications.

EXPECTED ACTIONS/OUTCOMES
Evaluate client response to medication.

Apply knowledge of pathophysiology when addressing client pharmacological agents.

MEDICATION ADMINISTRATION
Reinforce client teaching on client self administration of medications.

Collect required data prior to medication administration.

Reduction of Risk Potential

LABORATORY VALUES: Identify laboratory values for ABGs (pH, PO_2, PCO_2, SaO_2, HCO_3), BUN, cholesterol (total), creatinine, glucose, glycosylated hemoglobin (HgbA1C), hematocrit, hemoglobin, INR, platelets, potassium, PT, PTT & APTT, sodium, WBC.

POTENTIAL FOR COMPLICATIONS OF DIAGNOSTIC TESTS/ TREATMENTS/PROCEDURES: Maintain client tube patency.

POTENTIAL FOR ALTERATION IN BODY SYSTEMS: Perform focused data collection based on client condition (e.g., neurological checks, circulatory checks).

THERAPEUTIC PROCEDURES
Reinforce client teaching on treatments and procedures.

Assist with the performance of a diagnostic or invasive procedure.

CHAPTER 16 # Respiratory Diagnostic and Therapeutic Procedures

Respiratory diagnostic procedures are used to evaluate a client's respiratory status by checking indicators such as the oxygenation of the blood, lung functioning, and the integrity of the airway.

Respiratory diagnostic procedures nurses should be knowledgeable about include pulmonary function tests, arterial blood gases, bronchoscopy, and thoracentesis. The nurse should ensure that the client has signed an informed consent form prior to diagnostic procedures and tests.

Pulmonary function tests

Pulmonary function tests (PFTs) determine lung function and breathing difficulties.
- PFTs measure lung volumes and capacities, diffusion capacity, gas exchange, flow rates, and airway resistance, along with distribution of ventilation.
- Helpful in identifying clients who have lung disease
- Commonly performed for clients who have dyspnea
- Can be performed before surgical procedures to identify clients who have respiratory risks
- If client is a smoker, instruct client not to smoke 6 to 8 hr prior to testing.
- If a client uses inhalers, withhold 4 to 6 hr prior to testing. (This can vary according to facility policy.)

Arterial blood gases

An arterial blood gas (ABG) sample reports the status of oxygenation and acid–base balance of the blood.
- An ABG measures the following.
  - **pH:** amount of free hydrogen ions in the arterial blood (H^+)
  - **PaO_2:** partial pressure of oxygen
  - **$PaCO_2$:** partial pressure of carbon dioxide
  - **HCO_3:** concentration of bicarbonate in arterial blood
  - **SaO_2:** percentage of oxygen bound to Hgb as compared with the total amount that can be possibly carried
- ABGs can be obtained by an arterial puncture or through an arterial line.

INDICATIONS

POTENTIAL DIAGNOSES
- Blood pH levels can be affected by several conditions (respiratory, renal, malnutrition, electrolyte imbalance, endocrine, or neurologic).
- These assessments are helpful in monitoring the effectiveness of various treatments (such as acidosis interventions), in guiding oxygen therapy, and in evaluating client responses to weaning from mechanical ventilation.

INTERPRETATION OF FINDINGS

Blood pH levels less than 7.35 reflect acidosis, and levels greater than 7.45 reflect alkalosis.

COMPLICATIONS

Hematoma, arterial occlusion

A hematoma occurs when blood accumulates under the skin at the puncture site.

NURSING ACTIONS
- Observe for changes in temperature, swelling, color, loss of pulse, or pain.
- Notify the RN or provider immediately if manifestations persist. Qᴛᴄ
- Apply pressure to the hematoma site.

Bronchoscopy

Bronchoscopy permits visualization of the larynx, trachea, and bronchi through either a flexible fiber-optic or rigid bronchoscope.
- Bronchoscopy can be performed as an outpatient procedure, in a surgical suite under general anesthesia, or at the bedside under local anesthesia and moderate (conscious) sedation.
- Bronchoscopy can also be performed on clients who are receiving mechanical ventilation by inserting the scope through the client's endotracheal tube.

16.1 ABG measures and expected reference ranges

ABG MEASURE	EXPECTED REFERENCE RANGE
pH	7.35 to 7.45
PAO_2	80 to 100 mm Hg
$PACO_2$	35 to 45 mm Hg
HCO_3^-	21 to 28 mEq/L
SAO_2	95% to 100%

INDICATIONS

POTENTIAL DIAGNOSES

- Visualization of abnormalities (tumors, inflammation, strictures)
- Biopsy of suspicious tissue (lung cancer)
  - Clients undergoing a bronchoscopy with biopsy have additional risks for bleeding and/or perforation.
- Aspiration of deep sputum or lung abscesses for culture and sensitivity or cytology (pneumonia)

  ! Bronchoscopy is also performed for therapeutic reasons, such as removal of foreign bodies and secretions from the tracheobronchial tree, treating postoperative atelectasis, and to destroy and excise lesions.

CONSIDERATIONS

PREPROCEDURE

NURSING ACTIONS

- Check for allergies to anesthetic agents or routine use of anticoagulants.
- Ensure that a consent form is signed by the client prior to the procedure.
- Remove the client's dentures, if applicable, prior to the procedure.
- Maintain the client on NPO status prior to the procedure, usually 4 to 8 hr, to reduce the risk of aspiration when the cough reflex is blocked by anesthesia.
- Ensure that preprocedure medications are administered (anxiolytic, atropine, viscous lidocaine, local anesthetic throat spray).

INTRAPROCEDURE

NURSING ACTIONS

- Position the client in a sitting or supine position.
- Assist in collecting and labeling specimens. Ensure prompt delivery of specimens to the laboratory.
- Monitor vital signs, respiratory pattern, and oxygenation status throughout the procedure.
- Sedation given to older adult clients who have respiratory insufficiency can precipitate respiratory arrest. Ⓖ

POSTPROCEDURE

NURSING ACTIONS

- Closely monitor respirations, blood pressure, pulse oximetry, heart rate, and level of consciousness during the recovery period.
  - Observe level of consciousness while recognizing that older adult clients can develop confusion or lethargy due to the effects of medications given during the bronchoscopy.
- Observe level of consciousness, presence of gag reflex, and ability to swallow prior to resuming oral intake.
  - Allow adequate time for the cough and gag reflex to return prior to resuming oral intake. The gag reflex can be slower to return in older adult clients receiving local anesthesia due to impaired laryngeal reflex.
  - Once the gag reflex returns, the nurse can offer ice chips to the client and eventually fluids.
- Monitor for development of significant fever (mild fever for less than 24 hr is expected), productive cough, significant hemoptysis indicative of hemorrhage (a small amount of blood-tinged sputum is expected), and hypoxemia.
- Be prepared to intervene for unexpected responses, aspiration, and laryngospasm.
- Provide oral hygiene.
- For older adult clients, encourage coughing and deep breathing every 2 hr. There is an increased risk of respiratory infection and pneumonia in older adult clients due to decreased cough effectiveness and decreased secretion clearance. Respiratory infections can be more severe and last longer in older adult clients. Ⓖ
- The client is not discharged from the recovery room until adequate cough reflex and respiratory effort are present.

CLIENT EDUCATION: Gargling with salt water or using throat lozenges can provide comfort for throat soreness.

COMPLICATIONS

Laryngospasm

Laryngospasm is uncontrolled muscle contractions of the laryngeal cords (vocal cords) that impede the ability to inhale.

NURSING ACTIONS: Continuously monitor for manifestations of respiratory distress. Have resuscitation equipment available.

Pneumothorax

Pneumothorax can occur following a rigid bronchoscopy.

NURSING ACTIONS: Check for diminished or absent breath sounds, changes in oxygen saturation, or sudden onset of chest pain or tightness, and obtain a follow-up chest x-ray.

Aspiration

Aspiration can occur if the client chokes on oral or gastric secretions.

NURSING ACTIONS

- Prevent aspiration by withholding oral fluids or food until the gag reflex returns (usually 2 hr). Ⓠs
- Perform suctioning of airway as needed.

Thoracentesis

Thoracentesis is the surgical perforation of the chest wall and pleural space with a large-bore needle. It is performed to obtain specimens for diagnostic evaluation, instill medication into the pleural space, and remove fluid (effusion) or air from the pleural space for therapeutic relief of pleural pressure.

- Thoracentesis is performed under local anesthesia by a provider at the client's bedside, in a procedure room, or in a provider's office.
- Use of an ultrasound for guidance decreases the risk of complications.

INDICATIONS

POTENTIAL DIAGNOSES

Determine the cause of pleural effusion.

- Transudates (heart failure, cirrhosis, nephrotic syndrome, hypoproteinemia)
- Exudates (inflammatory, infectious, neoplastic conditions)
- Empyema
- Pneumonia
- Blunt, crushing, or penetrating chest injuries/trauma, or invasive thoracic procedures, such as lung or cardiac surgery

CLIENT PRESENTATION

- Large amounts of fluid in the pleural space compress lung tissue and can cause pain, shortness of breath, cough, and other manifestations of pleural pressure.
- Assessment of the effusion area can reveal abnormal breath sounds, dull percussion sounds, and decreased chest wall expansion. Pain can occur due to inflammatory process.

INTERPRETATION OF FINDINGS

Aspirated fluid is analyzed for general appearance, cell counts, protein and glucose content, the presence of enzymes such as lactate dehydrogenase (LDH) and amylase, abnormal cells, and culture.

CONSIDERATIONS

PREPROCEDURE

Percussion, auscultation, radiography, or sonography is used to locate the effusion and needle insertion site. It can be necessary for the nurse to assist the older adult client to maintain an appropriate position for the thoracentesis. Arthritis, tremors, or weakness can make it difficult for the client to remain still in the required position for the procedure. Ⓖ

NURSING ACTIONS

- Ensure that the client has signed the informed consent form.
- Gather all needed supplies.
- Obtain preprocedure x-ray to locate pleural effusion and to determine needle insertion site.
- Position the client sitting upright with arms and shoulders raised and supported on pillows and/or on an overbed table and with feet and legs well-supported.

CLIENT EDUCATION: Remain absolutely still (risk of accidental needle damage) during the procedure and do not cough or talk unless instructed by the provider.

INTRAPROCEDURE

NURSING ACTIONS

- Assist the provider with the procedure (strict surgical aseptic technique). Qᴛᴄ
- Prepare the client for a feeling of pressure with needle insertion and fluid removal.
- Monitor vital signs, skin color, and oxygen saturation throughout the procedure.
- Measure and record the amount of fluid removed from the chest.
- Label specimens at the bedside, and promptly send them to the laboratory.

POSTPROCEDURE

NURSING ACTIONS

- Apply a dressing over the puncture site and assess the dressing for bleeding or drainage.
- Monitor vital signs and respiratory status (respiratory rate and rhythm, breath sounds, oxygenation status) hourly for the first several hours after the thoracentesis.
- Auscultate lungs for reduced breath sounds on side of thoracentesis.
- Encourage the client to deeply breathe to assist with lung expansion.
- Obtain a postprocedure chest x-ray (check resolution of effusions, rule out pneumothorax).

COMPLICATIONS

Pneumothorax

Pneumothorax is a collapsed lung. It can occur due to injury to the lung during the procedure.

NURSING ACTIONS

- Monitor for manifestations of pneumothorax (diminished breath sounds, distended neck veins, asymmetry of the chest wall, respiratory distress, cyanosis).
- Monitor postprocedure chest x-ray results.

CLIENT EDUCATION: A pneumothorax can develop during the first 24 hr following a thoracentesis. Indications include deviated trachea, pain on the affected side that worsens at the end of inhalation and exhalation, affected side not moving in and out upon inhalation and exhalation, increased heart rate, rapid shallow respirations, nagging cough, or feeling of air hunger.

Bleeding

Bleeding can occur if the client is moved during the procedure or is at an increased risk for bleeding.

NURSING ACTIONS
- Monitor for coughing and hemoptysis.
- Monitor vital signs and laboratory results for evidence of bleeding (hypotension, reduced Hgb level).
- Assess thoracentesis site for bleeding.

Infection

Infection can occur due to the introduction of bacteria with the needle puncture.

NURSING ACTIONS
- Ensure that sterile technique is maintained.
- Monitor the client's temperature following the procedure.

Chest tube systems

A disposable three-chamber drainage system is most often used.
- First chamber: drainage collection
- Second chamber: water seal
- Third chamber: suction control (can be wet or dry)

Water seals are created by adding sterile fluid to a chamber up to the 2 cm line. While this is the minimum amount required for functioning, recommended amounts can vary by manufacturer. The water seal chamber allows air to exit from the pleural space on exhalation and stops air from entering the lungs with inhalation.
- To maintain the water seal, keep the chamber upright and below the chest tube insertion site at all times. Routinely monitor the water level due to the possibility of evaporation. Add fluid as needed to maintain the manufacturer's recommended water seal level.
- Wet suction: The height of the sterile fluid in the suction control chamber determines the amount of suction transmitted to the pleural space. A suction pressure of –20 cm H_2O is commonly prescribed. The level of water in the suction control chamber determines the suction pressure. The system is attached to a suction source, and suction is initiated until gentle bubbling begins in the suction chamber.
- Dry suction: When a dry suction control device is used, the provider prescribes a level of suction for the device, typically –20 cm H_2O. When connected to wall suction, the regulator on the chest tube drainage system is set to the manufacturer's recommendation.
- Tidaling (movement of the fluid level with respiration) is expected in the water seal chamber. With spontaneous respirations, the fluid level will rise with inspiration (increase in negative pressure in lung) and will fall with expiration. With positive-pressure mechanical ventilation, the fluid level will rise with expiration and fall with inspiration.

- Cessation of tidaling in the water seal chamber signals lung re-expansion or an obstruction within the system.
- Continuous bubbling in the water seal chamber indicates an air leak in the system. When the tubes are inserted to remove air from the pleural space, intermittent bubbling is expected; it is common to see bubbling during exhalation, sneezing, or coughing. In this case, when bubbling is no longer seen, it indicates that all of the air has been removed.
- When tubes are in the mediastinal space (such as following open heart surgery), bubbling and tidaling are not expected; pulsations in the fluid level might be seen.

Chest tube insertion

INDICATIONS

POTENTIAL DIAGNOSES

Pneumothorax: partial to complete collapse of the lung due to accumulation of air in the pleural space

Hemothorax: partial to complete collapse of the lung due to accumulation of blood in the pleural space

Postoperative chest drainage: thoracotomy or open-heart surgery

Pleural effusion: abnormal accumulation of fluid in the pleural space

Pulmonary empyema: accumulation of pus in the pleural space due to pulmonary infection, lung abscess, or infected pleural effusion

CLIENT PRESENTATION

- Dyspnea
- Distended neck veins
- Hemodynamic instability
- Pleuritic chest pain
- Cough
- Absent or reduced breath sounds on the affected side
- Hyperresonance on percussion of affected side (pneumothorax)
- Dullness or flatness on percussion of the affected side (hemothorax, pleural effusion)
- Asymmetrical chest wall motion

CONSIDERATIONS

PREPROCEDURE

- Verify that the consent form is signed.
- Reinforce with the client that breathing will improve when the chest tube is in place. Qᴘᴄᴄ
- Check for allergies to local anesthetics.
- Assist the client into the desired position (supine or semi-Fowler's).
- Prepare the chest drainage system per the facility's protocol. (Fill the water seal chamber.)
- Administer pain and sedation medications as prescribed.

INTRAPROCEDURE

- When the chest tube is inserted to drain fluid from the lung, the tip of the tube is inserted near the base of the lung on the side. When the chest tube is inserted to remove air from the pleural space, the tip of the tube will be near the apex of the lung.
- Assist the provider with insertion of the chest tube, application of a dressing to the insertion site, and setup of the drainage system. QⓉ🆒
  - Place the chest tube drainage system below the client's chest level with the tubing coiled on the bed. Ensure that the tubing from the bed to the drainage system is straight to promote drainage via gravity.
- Continually monitor vital signs and response to the procedure.

POSTPROCEDURE

- Check vital signs, breath sounds, SaO_2, color, and respiratory effort as indicated by the status of the client and at least every 4 hr.
- Encourage coughing and deep breathing every 2 hr.
- Keep the drainage system below the client's chest level, including during ambulation.
- Monitor chest tube placement and function.
  - Check the water seal level every 2 hr, and add fluid as needed. The fluid level should fluctuate with respiratory effort.
  - Document the amount and color of drainage hourly for the first 24 hr and then at least every 8 hr. Mark the date, hour, and drainage level on the container at the end of each shift. Report excessive drainage (greater than 70 mL/hr) or drainage that is cloudy or red to the provider. Drainage often increases with position changes or coughing.
  - Monitor the fluid in the suction control chamber, and maintain the prescribed fluid level.
  - Ensure the regulator dial on the dry suction device is at the prescribed level.
  - Check for expected findings of tidaling in the water seal chamber and continuous bubbling only in the suction chamber.
- Routinely monitor tubing for kinks, occlusions, or loose connections.
- Monitor the chest tube insertion site for redness, pain, infection, and crepitus (air leakage in subcutaneous tissue).
- Tape all connections between the chest tube and chest tube drainage system.
- Position the client in the semi-to high-Fowler's position to promote optimal lung expansion and drainage of fluid from the lungs.
- Administer pain medications as prescribed. Q🆔🆒🆒
- Keep two enclosed hemostats, sterile water, and an occlusive dressing located at the bedside at all times.

- Due to the risk of causing a tension pneumothorax, chest tubes are clamped only when prescribed in specific circumstances, such as in the case of an air leak, during drainage system change, accidental disconnection of tubing, or damage to the drainage system.
- Do not clamp, strip, or milk tubing; only perform this action when prescribed. Stripping creates a high negative pressure and can damage lung tissue.
- Notify the provider immediately if the client's SaO_2 is less than 90%, if the eyelets of the chest tube become visible, if drainage is above the prescribed amount or stops in the first 24 hr, or complications occur.

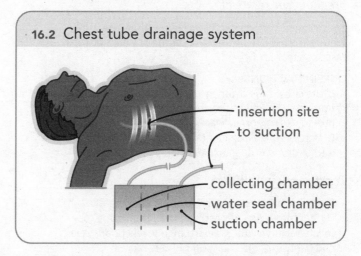

16.2 Chest tube drainage system

- insertion site
- to suction
- collecting chamber
- water seal chamber
- suction chamber

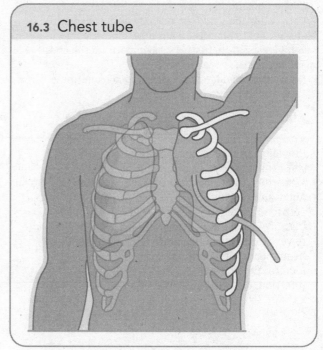

16.3 Chest tube

COMPLICATIONS

Air leaks

Air leaks can result if a connection is not taped securely.

NURSING ACTIONS

- Monitor the water seal chamber for continuous bubbling (air leak finding). If observed, locate the source of the air leak, and intervene accordingly (tighten the connection, replace drainage system).
- Check all connections.
- Notify the charge nurse if an air leak is noted. Q︎TC

Accidental disconnection, system breakage, or removal

These complications can occur at any time and require immediate notification of the provider or rapid response team.

NURSING ACTIONS

- If the chest tube drainage system is compromised, immerse the end of the chest tube in sterile water to provide a temporary water seal.
- If a chest tube is accidentally removed, dress the area with a dry, sterile gauze or occlusive dressing.

Tension pneumothorax

- Sucking chest wounds, prolonged clamping of the tubing, kinks or obstruction in the tubing, or mechanical ventilation with high levels of positive end expiratory pressure (PEEP) can cause a tension pneumothorax.
- Data collection findings include tracheal deviation, absent breath sounds on one side, distended neck veins, respiratory distress, asymmetry of the chest, and cyanosis.
- Notify the provider or rapid response team immediately.

Chest tube removal

- Provide pain medication 30 min before removing chest tubes. Q︎EBP
- Assist the provider with sutures and chest tube removal.
- Apply airtight sterile petroleum jelly gauze dressing. Secure in place with a heavyweight stretch tape.
- Obtain chest x-rays as prescribed. This is performed to verify continued resolution of the pneumothorax, hemothorax, or pleural effusion.
- Monitor for excessive wound drainage, findings of infection, or recurrent pneumothorax.

Application Exercises

1. A nurse is assessing a client following a bronchoscopy. Which of the following findings should the nurse report to the provider?

   A. Blood-tinged sputum

   B. Dry, nonproductive cough

   C. Sore throat

   D. Bronchospasms

2. A nurse is assessing a client following a thoracentesis. Which of the following findings should the nurse report? (Select all that apply.)

   A. Dyspnea

   B. Localized bloody drainage on the dressing

   C. Fever

   D. Hypotension

   E. Report of pain at the puncture site

3. A nurse is assisting with the care of a client who has a chest tube and drainage system in place. The nurse observes that the chest tube was accidentally removed. Which of the following actions should the nurse take first?

   A. Obtain a chest x-ray.

   B. Apply sterile gauze or occlusive dressing to the insertion site.

   C. Check the client's ABGs.

   D. Monitor the client's blood pressure.

4. A nurse is collecting data from a client who has a chest tube and drainage system in place. Which of the following are expected findings? (Select all that apply.)

   A. Continuous bubbling in the water seal chamber

   B. Gentle, constant bubbling in the suction control chamber

   C. Rise and fall in the level of water in the water seal chamber with inspiration and expiration

   D. Exposed sutures without dressing

   E. Drainage system upright at chest level

5. A nurse is assisting a provider with the removal of a chest tube. Which of the following actions should the nurse take?

   A. Instruct the client to lie prone with arms by the sides.

   B. Complete a surgical checklist on the client.

   C. Remind the client that there is minimal discomfort during the removal process.

   D. Place an occlusive dressing over the site once the tube is removed.

Application Exercises Key

1. D. **CORRECT:** When recognizing cues, the nurse should identify that bronchospasms can indicate the client is having difficulty maintaining a patent airway. The nurse should notify the provider immediately. Blood-tinged sputum; a dry, nonproductive cough; and a sore throat are expected findings following a bronchoscopy.

   Ⓝ *NCLEX® Connection: Reduction of Risk Potential, Diagnostic Tests*

2. A, C, D. **CORRECT:** When recognizing cues, the nurse should recognize that dyspnea can indicate a pneumothorax or a re-accumulation of fluid, fever can indicate an infection, and hypotension can indicate intrathoracic bleeding. The nurse should report these findings to the provider immediately.

   Ⓝ *NCLEX® Connection: Reduction of Risk Potential, Potential for Complications of Diagnostic Tests/Treatments/Procedures*

3. B. **CORRECT:** When prioritizing hypotheses, using the airway, breathing, and circulation approach to client care, the nurse should first apply sterile gauze to the site. This prevents air from entering the pleural space and reduces the risk for development of a tension pneumothorax.

   Ⓝ *NCLEX® Connection: Physiological Adaptation, Medical Emergencies*

4. B, C **CORRECT:** When recognizing cues, the nurse should identify that gentle bubbling in the suction control chamber is an expected finding. A rise and fall of the fluid level in the water seal chamber upon inspiration and expiration indicates that the drainage system is functioning properly.

   Ⓝ *NCLEX® Connection: Reduction of Risk Potential, Potential for Complications of Diagnostic Tests/Treatments/Procedures*

5. D. **CORRECT:** When taking actions, the nurse should place an occlusive dressing over the site once the tube is removed and observe the site for drainage.

   Ⓝ *NCLEX® Connection: Reduction of Risk Potential, Therapeutic Procedures*

Active Learning Scenario

A nurse is assessing a client following a thoracentesis. Use the ATI Active Learning Template: Therapeutic Procedure to complete this item.

NURSING INTERVENTIONS (PRE, INTRA, POST):
List three postprocedure nursing actions the nurse should take while caring for this client.

Active Learning Scenario Key

Using the ATI Active Learning Template: Therapeutic Procedure
NURSING INTERVENTIONS (PRE, INTRA, POST)
- Apply a dressing over the puncture site, and check the dressing for bleeding or drainage.
- Monitor vital signs and respiratory status (respiratory rate and rhythm, breath sounds, oxygenation status) every 15 min for the first hour and then hourly for the first several hours after the thoracentesis.
- Auscultate lungs for diminished or absent breath sounds on side of thoracentesis.
- Encourage the client to deeply breathe to assist with lung expansion.
- Ensure that a postprocedure chest x-ray is obtained (check resolution of effusions, and rule out pneumothorax.

Ⓝ *NCLEX® Connection: Reduction of Risk Potential, Potential for Complications From Surgical Procedures and Health Alterations*

UNIT 3   RESPIRATORY DISORDERS
SECTION: DIAGNOSTIC AND THERAPEUTIC PROCEDURES

CHAPTER 17 # Respiratory Management and Mechanical Ventilation

Oxygen is a tasteless and colorless gas that accounts for 21% of atmospheric air.

Oxygen is used to maintain adequate cellular oxygenation. It is used in the treatment of many acute and chronic respiratory problems.

Oxygen is administered in an attempt to maintain an SaO_2 of 95% to 100% by using the lowest amount of oxygen to avoid placing the client at risk for complications.

Clients who cannot spontaneously breathe on their own require mechanical ventilation. This can include clients who need respiratory assistance due to severe respiratory disease, general anesthesia, trauma, and or other illnesses.

Oxygen delivery devices

Supplemental oxygen can be delivered by a variety of methods, based on the client's particular circumstances. The percentage of oxygen delivered is expressed as the fraction of inspired oxygen (FiO_2). While the client is receiving oxygen, the nurse should continue to monitor vital signs, including SaO_2 for changes, and intervene as needed.

LOW-FLOW OXYGEN DELIVERY SYSTEMS

These deliver varying amounts of oxygen based on the method and the client's breathing pattern.

Nasal cannula

- A length of tubing with two small prongs for insertion into the nares
- FiO_2 24% to 44% at flow rates of 1 to 6 L/min

ADVANTAGES
- Safe, easy to apply, comfortable, and well-tolerated
- The client can eat, talk, and ambulate.

DISADVANTAGES
- FiO_2 varies with the flow rate and the client's rate and depth of breathing.
- Extended use can lead to skin breakdown and drying of the mucous membranes.
- Tubing is easily dislodged.

NURSING ACTIONS
- Assess patency of the nares.
- Ensure that the prongs fit in the nares properly.
- Use water-soluble gel to prevent dry nares.
- Provide humidification for flow rates of 4 L/min and greater.

Simple face mask

- Covers the client's nose and mouth
- FiO_2 40% to 60% at flow rates of 5 to 8 L/min (The minimum flow rate is 5 L/min to ensure flushing of CO_2 from the mask.)

ADVANTAGES: A face mask is easy to apply and can be more comfortable than a nasal cannula.

DISADVANTAGES
- Flow rates of less than 5 L/min can result in rebreathing of CO_2.
- Device is poorly tolerated by clients who have anxiety or claustrophobia.
- Eating, drinking, and talking are impaired.
- Use caution with clients who have a high risk of aspiration or airway obstruction. Qs
- Moisture and pressure can collect under the mask and cause skin breakdown.

NURSING ACTIONS: Check for a proper fit to ensure a secure seal over the nose and mouth.

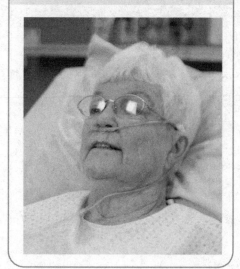

17.1 Nasal cannula

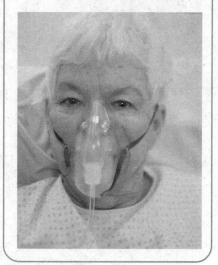

17.2 Simple face mask

Partial rebreather mask

- Covers the client's nose and mouth
- FiO_2 40% to 60% at flow rates of 6 to 11 L/min

ADVANTAGES: The mask has a reservoir bag attached with no valve, which allows the client to rebreathe up to one-third of exhaled air together with room air.

DISADVANTAGES
- Complete deflation of the reservoir bag during inspiration causes CO_2 buildup.
- FiO_2 varies with the client's breathing pattern.
- Mask is poorly tolerated by clients who have anxiety or claustrophobia.
- Eating, drinking, and talking are impaired.
- Use with caution for clients who have a high risk of aspiration or airway obstruction. Qs

NURSING ACTIONS
- Keep the reservoir bag from deflating by adjusting the oxygen flow rate to keep it inflated.
- Monitor for proper fit to ensure a secure seal over the nose and mouth.
- Monitor for skin breakdown beneath the edges of the mask and bridge of nose.

Nonrebreather mask

- Covers the client's nose and mouth
- FiO_2 80% to 95% at flow rates of 10 to 15 L/min to keep the reservoir bag two-thirds full during inspiration and expiration

ADVANTAGES
- Delivers the highest O_2 concentration possible (except for intubation)
- A one-way valve situated between the mask and reservoir allows the client to inhale maximum O_2 from the reservoir bag. The two exhalation ports have flaps covering them that prevent room air from entering the mask.

DISADVANTAGES
- The valve and flap on the mask must be intact and functional during each breath.
- Poorly tolerated by clients who have anxiety or claustrophobia
- Eating, drinking, and talking are impaired.
- Use with caution for clients who have a high risk of aspiration or airway obstruction. Qs

NURSING ACTIONS
- Monitor the valve and flap hourly to ensure patency, proper function, and flaps are not stuck.
- Monitor for proper fit to ensure a secure seal over the nose and mouth.
- Monitor for skin breakdown beneath the edges of the mask and bridge of nose.

HIGH-FLOW OXYGEN DELIVERY SYSTEMS

These deliver precise amounts of oxygen when properly fitted.

Venturi mask

- Covers the client's nose and mouth
- FiO_2 24% to 50% at flow rates of 4 to 10 L/min via different sizes of adapters, which allow specific amounts of air to mix with oxygen

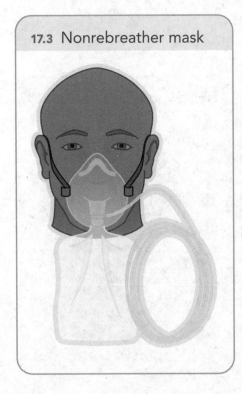

17.3 Nonrebreather mask

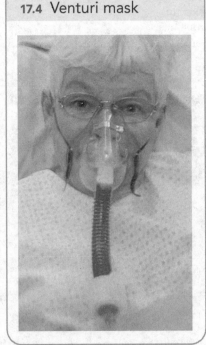

17.4 Venturi mask

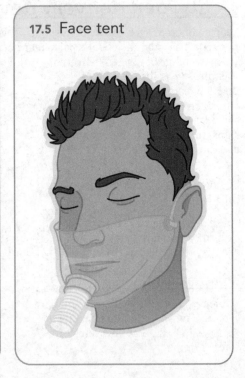

17.5 Face tent

ADVANTAGES

- Delivers the most precise oxygen concentration without intubation
- Humidification is not required.
- Best suited for clients who have chronic lung disease

DISADVANTAGES

- Poorly tolerated by clients who have anxiety or claustrophobia
- Eating, drinking, and talking are impaired.

NURSING ACTIONS

- Assess frequently to ensure an accurate flow rate.
- Make sure the tubing is free of kinks. Qs
- Assess for skin breakdown beneath the edges of the mask, particularly on the nares.
- Ensure that the client wears a nasal cannula during meals.

Aerosol mask, face tent, and tracheostomy collar

- Face tent fits loosely around the face and neck.
- Tracheostomy collar is a small mask that covers a surgically created opening in the trachea.
- FiO_2 24% to 100% at flow rates of at least 10 L/min (Provide high humidification with oxygen delivery.)

ADVANTAGES

- Good for clients who do not tolerate masks well
- Useful for clients who have facial trauma, burns, or thick secretions

DISADVANTAGES: High humidification requires frequent monitoring.

NURSING ACTIONS

- Empty condensation from the tubing often.
- Ensure that there is adequate water in the humidification canister.
- Ensure that the aerosol mist leaves from the vents during inspiration and expiration.
- Make sure the tubing does not pull on the tracheostomy.

T-piece

FiO_2 24% to 100% at flow rates of at least 10 L/min

ADVANTAGES: Can be used for clients who have tracheostomies, laryngectomies, or endotracheal tubes (ET)

DISADVANTAGES: High humidification requires frequent monitoring.

NURSING ACTIONS

- Ensure that the exhalation port is open and uncovered.
- Ensure that the T-piece does not pull on the tracheostomy or ET tube.
- Ensure that the mist is evident during inspiration and expiration.

Oxygen therapy

INDICATIONS

POTENTIAL DIAGNOSES

Hypoxemia and hypoxia

- Hypoxemia is an inadequate level of oxygen in the blood. Hypovolemia, hypoventilation, and interruption of arterial flow can lead to hypoxemia.
- Hypoxia is a decrease in tissue oxygenation.

CLIENT PRESENTATION

Early findings

- Tachypnea
- Tachycardia
- Restlessness
- Pale skin and mucous membranes
- Elevated blood pressure
- Findings of respiratory distress (use of accessory muscles, nasal flaring, tracheal tugging, and adventitious lung sounds)

LATE FINDINGS

- Confusion and stupor
- Cyanotic skin and mucous membranes
- Bradypnea
- Bradycardia
- Hypotension
- Cardiac dysrhythmias

CONSIDERATIONS

PREPARATION OF THE CLIENT

- Explain all procedures to the client.
- Place the client in semi-Fowler's or Fowler's position to facilitate breathing and promote chest expansion.
- Ensure that all equipment is working properly.

ONGOING CARE

- Provide oxygen therapy at the lowest flow that will correct hypoxemia.
- Assess/monitor respiratory rate, rhythm and effort, lung sounds, and SaO_2 to determine the client's need for supplemental oxygen.
  - Manifestations of hypoxemia are shortness of breath, anxiety, tachypnea, tachycardia, restlessness, pallor or cyanosis of the skin or mucous membranes, adventitious breath sounds, and confusion.
  - Manifestations of hypercarbia (elevated levels of CO_2) are restlessness, hypertension, and headache.
- Monitor diagnostic reports that show information related to oxygenation, including ABGs.

- Promote good oral hygiene and provide as needed.
- Promote turning, coughing, deep breathing, use of incentive spirometer, and suctioning.
- Promote rest, and decrease environmental stimuli. Qpcc
- Provide emotional support for clients who appear anxious.
- Assess nutritional status. Provide supplements as prescribed.
- Assess/monitor skin integrity. Provide moisture and pressure-relief devices as indicated.
- Assess/monitor and document the client's response to oxygen therapy.
- Titrate oxygen to maintain prescribed oxygen saturation.
- Discontinue supplemental oxygen gradually.

INTERVENTIONS

Monitor for manifestations of respiratory depression, such as decreased respiratory rate and decreased level of consciousness. Notify the provider if findings are present.

Respiratory distress

- Position the client for maximum ventilation (Fowler's or semi-Fowler's position).
- Complete a focused respiratory assessment.
- Promote deep breathing.
- Use supplemental oxygen as prescribed.
- Stay with the client and provide emotional support to decrease anxiety.
- Promote airway clearance by encouraging coughing and oral/oropharyngeal suctioning if necessary.

COMPLICATIONS

Oxygen toxicity

- Oxygen toxicity can result from high concentrations of oxygen (typically above 50%), long durations of oxygen therapy (typically more than 24 to 48 hr), and the client's degree of lung disease.
- Manifestations include a nonproductive cough, substernal pain, nasal stuffiness, nausea, vomiting, fatigue, headache, sore throat, and hypoventilation.

NURSING ACTIONS
- Use the lowest level of oxygen necessary to maintain the prescribed SaO_2.
- Monitor ABGs. Notify the provider if results are outside the expected or prescribed ranges.
- Use an oxygen mask with continuous positive airway pressure (CPAP) or bi-level positive airway pressure (BiPAP) if prescribed to help decrease the amount of oxygen needed.
- Use positive end expiratory pressure (PEEP) as prescribed while the client is receiving mechanical ventilation to help decrease the amount of needed oxygen.

Oxygen-induced hypoventilation

Oxygen-induced hypoventilation can develop in clients who have COPD and chronic hypoxemia with hypercarbia.

NURSING ACTIONS
- Monitor respiratory rate and pattern, level of consciousness, and SaO_2.
- Provide oxygen therapy at the lowest flow rate that manages hypoxemia.
- If the client tolerates it, use a Venturi mask to deliver precise oxygen levels.
- Notify the provider of findings of respiratory depression, such as a decreased respiratory rate or a decreased level of consciousness.

Combustion

Oxygen is combustible.

NURSING ACTIONS
- Post "No Smoking" or "Oxygen in Use" signs to alert others of a fire hazard. Qs
- Know where the closest fire extinguisher is located.
- Educate the client and others about the fire hazard of smoking during oxygen use.
- Have the client wear a cotton gown because synthetic or wool fabrics can generate static electricity.
- Ensure that all electric devices (razors, hearing aids, radios) are working well.
- Ensure electric machinery (monitors, suction machines) are well-grounded.
- Do not use volatile, flammable materials (alcohol or acetone) near clients who are receiving oxygen.

Noninvasive positive pressure ventilation

Continuous positive airway pressure (CPAP)

Provides positive pressure using a leak-proof mask via noninvasive positive-pressure ventilation device
- The device is to keep the airways throughout the respiratory cycle open and improve gas exchange in the alveoli.
- Most effective treatment for sleep apnea because the positive pressure acts as a splint to keep the upper airway and trachea open during sleep

Bi-level positive airway pressure (BiPAP)

Machine cycles to provide a set positive inspiratory pressure when inspiration takes place and then during expiration to deliver a lower set end expiratory pressure
- Requires wearing a leak-proof mask
- Most often used for clients who have COPD and who require ventilatory assistance.

NURSING ACTIONS
- Monitor the skin around the masks for breakdown as a tight seal is required.
- Check the percentage of oxygen on the machine (both) for both the inspiratory pressure and expiratory pressure when the client is receiving BiPAP.

Transstracheal oxygen therapy

Delivers oxygen directly into the lungs per a small, flexible catheter that is passed through the trachea via a small incision

The catheter is less visible and avoids irritation that occurs from the use of nasal prongs.

Endotracheal tube and endotracheal intubation

INDICATIONS

- A tube is inserted through the client's nose or mouth into the trachea. This allows for emergency airway management of the client.
- Oral intubation is the easiest and quickest form of intubation and is often performed in the emergency department.
- Nasal intubation is performed when the client has facial or oral trauma. This route is not used if the client has a clotting problem.

PLACEMENT

- Intubation is typically performed by a nurse anesthetist, anesthesiologist, critical care or emergency physician, or pulmonologist.
- A chest x-ray verifies correct placement of the endotracheal (ET) tube.
- ET tubes can be cuffed or uncuffed. The cuff on the tracheal end of an ET tube is inflated to ensure proper placement and the formation of a seal between the cuff and the tracheal wall. This prevents air from leaking around the ET tube.
- The seal ensures that an adequate amount of tidal volume is delivered by the mechanical ventilator when attached to the external end of the ET tube.
- The client is unable to talk when the cuff is inflated.

Mechanical ventilation

Mechanical ventilation provides breathing support until lung function is restored, delivering 100% oxygen that is warmed (body temperature 37° C [98.6° F]) and humidified at FiO2 levels between 21% to 100%.

The prevalence of clients who require mechanical ventilation ranges from 6.6 to 23 per 100,000.

The COVID-19 pandemic led to a rise in the number of clients requiring mechanical ventilation, especially among older adults who had multiple comorbidities. Ⓖ

During the COVID-19 pandemic, reported mortality rates for clients receiving mechanical ventilation ranged broadly in care areas: 13.7 to 77.8% in ICU settings; 7.8 to 50% in acute, non-ICU settings; and 12 to 91.8% in nursing home and home health settings.

- Positive-pressure ventilators deliver air to the lungs under pressure throughout inspiration to keep the alveoli open and to prevent alveolar collapse during expiration. Benefits include the following.
  - Forced/enhanced lung expansion
  - Improved gas exchange (oxygenation)
  - Decreased work of breathing
- Mechanical ventilation can be delivered via:
  - ET tube
  - Tracheostomy tube
- Mechanical ventilators can be cycled based on pressure, volume, time, and/or flow.

INDICATIONS

To maintain a patent airway and adequate oxygen saturation of 95% or greater

POTENTIAL DIAGNOSES

- Hypoxemia, hypoventilation with respiratory acidosis
  - Airway trauma
  - Exacerbation of COPD
  - Acute pulmonary edema due to myocardial infarction or heart failure
  - Asthma attack
  - Head injuries, cerebrovascular accident, or coma
  - Neurological disorders (multiple sclerosis, myasthenia gravis, Guillain-Barré)
  - Obstructive sleep apnea
- Respiratory support following surgery (decrease workload)
- Respiratory support while under general anesthesia or heavy sedation

CONSIDERATIONS

PREPARATION OF THE CLIENT

- Explain the procedure to the client.
- Establish a method for the client to communicate, such as asking yes/no questions, providing writing materials, using a dry-erase and/or picture communication board, or lip reading. Ⓠpcc

ONGOING CARE

- Maintain a patent airway.
  - Monitor the position and placement of tube.
  - Keep tubing clear of pooled water and empty as needed.
  - Document tube placement in centimeters at the client's teeth or lips.
  - Use caution when moving the client. Qs
  - Suction oral and tracheal secretions to maintain tube/airway patency.
  - Support ventilator tubing to prevent mucosal erosion and displacement.
  - Have a resuscitation bag with a face mask available at the bedside at all times in case of ventilator malfunction or accidental extubation.
- Check the provider's prescription each shift. Monitor and document ventilator settings hourly.
  - Rate, FiO₂, and tidal volume
  - Mode of ventilation
  - Use of adjuncts (PEEP, CPAP)
  - Plateau or peak inspiratory pressure (PIP)
  - Alarm settings
- Monitor ventilator alarms, which signal if the client is not receiving the correct ventilation.
  - Never turn off ventilator alarms.
- Monitor for skin breakdown.
  - Older adult clients have fragile skin and are more prone to skin and mucous membrane breakdown. Older adult clients have decreased oral secretions. They require frequent, gentle skin and oral care. Ⓖ
- Provide adequate nutrition.
  - Monitor bowel habits.
  - Maintain enteral or parenteral feedings as prescribed.
- Continually monitor the client during the weaning process: vital signs, respiratory rate, ease of breathing, and oxygen saturation.
- Have a manual resuscitation bag with a face mask and oxygen readily available at the client's bedside.
- Have reintubation equipment at bedside.
- Suction the oropharynx and trachea.
- Following extubation, monitor for signs of respiratory distress or airway obstruction (ineffective cough, dyspnea, stridor).
- Encourage coughing, deep breathing, and use of the incentive spirometer.
- Reposition the client to promote mobility of secretions.
- Older adult clients have decreased respiratory muscle strength and chest wall compliance, which makes them more susceptible to aspiration, atelectasis, and pulmonary infections. Older adult clients require more frequent position changes to promote mobility of secretions. Ⓖ

17.4 Common modes of ventilation, adjunctive therapy, and weaning modalities

Mode of ventilation

ASSIST-CONTROL (AC)

- Preset rate and tidal volume. Client initiates breath, and ventilator takes over for the intubated client.
- Hyperventilation can result in respiratory alkalosis.
- Client can require sedation to decrease respiratory rate.

SYNCHRONIZED INTERMITTENT MANDATORY VENTILATION (SIMV)

- Preset rate and tidal volume for machine breaths
- Client initiates breath, and tidal volume will depend upon client's effort.
- Ventilator-initiated breaths are synchronized to reduce competition between ventilator and client.
- Used as a regular mode of ventilation or a weaning mode (rate decreased to allow more spontaneous ventilation) for the intubated client
- Can increase work of breathing, causing respiratory muscle fatigue

INVERSE RATIO VENTILATION (IRV)

- Lengthens inspiratory phase to maximize oxygenation in the intubated client.
- Used for hypoxemia refractory to PEEP
- Uncomfortable for clients and requires sedation and/or neuromuscular blocking agents
- High risk of volutrauma and decreased cardiac output due to air trapping

AIRWAY PRESSURE RELEASE VENTILATION (APRV)

- Allows alveolar gas to be expelled by the lungs, own natural recoil
- Time-triggered and pressure-limited
- Breaths can be initiated spontaneously or by the ventilator.
- Causes less ventilator-induced lung injury and fewer adverse effects on the cardiovascular system

INDEPENDENT LUNG VENTILATION (ILV)

- Double-lumen ET tube allows ventilation of each lung separately.
- Used for clients who have unilateral lung disease
- Requires two ventilators, sedation, and/or use of neuromuscular blocking agents

HIGH-FREQUENCY VENTILATION

- Delivers small amount of gas at rates of 60 to 3,000 cycles/min
- High frequency ventilation often used in children
- Client must be sedated and/or receiving neuromuscular blocking agents.
- Breath sounds difficult to assess

Adjunctive therapy

POSITIVE END EXPIRATORY PRESSURE (PEEP)

- Preset pressure delivered during expiration
- Added to prescribed ventilator settings to treat persistent hypoxemia
- Improves oxygenation by enhancing gas exchanges and preventing atelectasis
- Amount of PEEP added is typically 5 to 15 cm H₂O.

Weaning modality

PRESSURE SUPPORT VENTILATION (PSV)

- Works to keep the alveoli from collapsing during expiration
- Allows for greater oxygenation and makes the work of breathing easier
- Allows for lower levels of FiO₂ to be used
- Can be used with IMV or AC modes to treat or prevent atelectasis.
- Settings 5 to 20 cm H₂O (greater than 20 cm H₂O can cause lung damage)

CONTINUOUS POSITIVE AIRWAY PRESSURE (CPAP)

- Positive pressure supplied during spontaneous breathing. No ventilator breaths delivered unless in conjunction with SIMV
- Risks include volutrauma, decreased cardiac output, and ICP.

COMPLICATIONS

Trauma

Barotrauma (damage to the lungs by positive pressure) can occur due to a pneumothorax, subcutaneous emphysema, or pneumomediastinum.

Volutrauma (damage to the lungs by volume delivered from one lung to the other)

Fluid retention

Fluid retention in clients who are receiving mechanical ventilation is due to decreased cardiac output, activation of renin–angiotensin–aldosterone system, and/or ventilator humidification.

NURSING ACTIONS: Monitor intake and output, weight, breath sounds, and endotracheal secretions.

Oxygen toxicity

Oxygen toxicity can result from high concentrations of oxygen (typically greater than 50%), long durations of oxygen therapy (typically more than 24 to 48 hr), and/or the client's degree of lung disease.

NURSING ACTIONS: Monitor for fatigue, restlessness, severe dyspnea, tachycardia, tachypnea, crackles, and cyanosis.

Gastrointestinal ulceration (stress ulcer)

Gastric ulcers can be evident in clients receiving mechanical ventilation.

NURSING ACTIONS: Monitor gastrointestinal drainage and stools for occult blood.

Infection

Can be related to ventilator intubation or suctioning

NURSING ACTIONS
- Monitor client for fever, changes in sputum color, consistency, quantity, crackles, and rhonchi.
- Monitor WBCs.
- Use aseptic technique during suctioning.

Application Exercises

1. A nurse is caring for a client who has dyspnea and will receive oxygen continuously. Which of the following oxygen devices should the nurse use to deliver a precise amount of oxygen to the client?
   - A. Nonrebreather mask
   - B. Nasal cannula
   - C. Venturi mask
   - D. Tracheostomy collar

2. A nurse is caring for a client who is experiencing respiratory distress. Sort the following manifestations of hypoxemia by whether they are early or late manifestations of hypoxemia.
   - A. Cyanosis
   - B. Tachycardia
   - C. Tachypnea
   - D. Anxiety and restlessness
   - E. Bradycardia

3. A nurse is caring for a group of clients who require mechanical ventilation. Match each type of support with its description.

A. High-frequency ventilation	1. Ventilator only delivers breaths when used with SIMV.
B. Positive end expiratory pressure	2. Ventilator rate and tidal volume are preset, and the rate and volume of client-initiated breaths are controlled by the client.
C. Synchronized intermittent mandatory ventilation (SIMV)	3. Added to ventilator settings to treat persistent hypoxemia
D. Continuous positive airway pressure (CPAP)	4. Delivers a small amount of gas

4. A nurse is caring for a group of clients who are receiving mechanical ventilation. Explain how synchronized intermittent mandatory ventilation (SIMV) and continuous positive airway pressure (CPAP) can increase the work of breathing for the clients.

Active Learning Scenario

A nurse is planning care for a client who is receiving mechanical ventilation. Use the ATI Active Learning Template: Therapeutic Procedure to complete this item.

NURSING INTERVENTIONS: Describe three nursing actions to maintain the client's airway.

Active Learning Scenario Key

Using ATI Active Learning Template: Therapeutic Procedure

NURSING INTERVENTIONS
- Observe the position and placement of the tube.
- Apply protective barriers (soft wrist restraints) according to hospital protocol to prevent self-extubation.
- Use caution when moving the client.
- Suction oral and tracheal secretions to maintain tube patency.
- Support ventilator tubing to prevent mucosal erosion and displacement.
- Have a resuscitation bag with a face mask available at the bedside at all times in case of ventilator malfunction or accidental extubation.

Ⓝ *NCLEX® Connection: Physiological Adaptation, Alterations in Body Systems*

Application Exercises Key

1. C. **CORRECT:** When generating solutions to deliver a precise amount of oxygen to the client, the nurse should suggest that the Venturi mask is the most accurate device to use to deliver a precise, consistent concentration of oxygen because it has an adapter that allows specific amounts of air to mix with oxygen.

Ⓝ *NCLEX® Connection: Physiological Adaptation, Alterations in Body Systems*

2. **EARLY:** B, C, D; **LATE:** A, E

When recognizing cues for a client who is experiencing respiratory distress, the nurse should identify tachycardia, tachypnea, and anxiety and restlessness as early manifestations of altered gas exchange related to hypoxemia. The nurse should identify cyanosis and bradycardia as late manifestations of altered gas exchange related to hypoxemia.

Ⓝ *NCLEX® Connection: Physiological Adaptation, Basic Pathophysiology*

3. A, 4; B, 3; C, 2; D, 1

When taking actions for clients who require ventilatory support, the nurse should recognize that ILV is delivered through a double-lumen ET tube that allows each lung to be separately ventilated. The nurse should recognize that PEEP is a preset pressure delivered during expiration to enhance gas exchange and prevent atelectasis. The nurse should recognize that SIMV synchronizes breaths between the ventilator and client-initiated breaths. The nurse should recognize that APRV in which the pressure is set but the client is allowed unrestricted spontaneous breathing. The nurse should recognize that CPAP applies positive pressure during spontaneous breathing for a client who is ventilated.

Ⓝ *NCLEX® Connection: Physiological Adaptation, Basic Pathophysiology*

4. When recognizing cues in caring for clients who are receiving mechanical ventilation, the nurse identifies that SIMV and CPAP require the client to generate force to take spontaneous breaths.

Ⓝ *NCLEX® Connection: Physiological Adaptation, Basic Pathophysiology*

When reviewing the following chapters, keep in mind the relevant topics and tasks of the NCLEX outline.

Pharmacological Therapies

EXPECTED ACTIONS/OUTCOMES
Evaluate client response to medication.

Apply knowledge of pathophysiology when addressing client pharmacological agents.

MEDICATION ADMINISTRATION
Reinforce client teaching on client self administration of medications.

Collect required data prior to medication administration.

Reduction of Risk Potential

POTENTIAL FOR ALTERATIONS IN BODY SYSTEMS: Perform focused data collection based on client condition (e.g., neurological checks, circulatory checks).

Physiological Adaptation

BASIC PATHOPHYSIOLOGY
Identify signs and symptoms related to an acute or chronic illness.

Consider general principles of client disease process when providing care.

CHAPTER 18 *Acute Respiratory Disorders*

The airway structures permit air to enter and provide for adequate oxygenation and tissue perfusion. Common acute and chronic disorders affect these airway structures. A nursing priority for clients who have acute respiratory disorders is to maintain a patent airway to promote oxygenation. Older adult clients are more susceptible to infections and have decreased pulmonary reserves due to age-related lung changes, including decreased lung elasticity and thickening alveoli.

Acute respiratory disorders include rhinitis, sinusitis, influenza, COVID-19, and pneumonia.

HEALTH PROMOTION AND DISEASE PREVENTION

- Perform hand hygiene to prevent the spread of infection by bacteria and viruses.
- Encourage immunizations that prevent respiratory disorders, especially immunizations for influenza and pneumonia to younger children and older adults, and people who have chronic illnesses or who are immunocompromised. Ⓖ
- Limit exposure to airborne allergens, which trigger a hypersensitivity reaction.
- Promote smoking cessation.

RISK FACTORS

- Extremely young or advanced age Ⓖ
- Recent exposure to viral, bacterial, or influenza infections
- Lack of current immunization status (pneumonia, influenza)
- Exposure to plant pollen, molds, animal dander, foods, medications, and environmental contaminants
- Tobacco smoke
- Substance use (alcohol, cocaine)
- Chronic lung disease (asthma, emphysema)
- Immunocompromised status
- Presence of a foreign body
- Conditions that increase the risk of aspiration (dysphagia)

- Impaired ability to mobilize secretions (decreased level of consciousness, immobility, recent abdominal or thoracic surgery)
- Inactivity and immobility
- Mechanical ventilation (ventilator-acquired pneumonia)

Rhinitis

Rhinitis is an inflammation of the nasal mucosa and often the mucosa in the sinuses that can be caused by infection (viral or bacterial) or allergens. Annually, rhinitis affects approximately 10%–30% of the world population. This condition often coexists with other disorders, such as asthma and allergies. Rhinitis is classified as acute, chronic, nonallergic, and allergic (seasonal or perennial).
- **Viral:** The common cold (coryza) is caused by viruses spread from person to person in droplets from sneezing and coughing or by direct contact.
- **Allergic:** The presence of an allergen causes histamine release and other mediators from WBCs in the nasal mucosa. The mediators bind to blood vessel receptors causing capillary leakage, which leads to local edema and swelling.

DATA COLLECTION

EXPECTED FINDINGS

- Excessive nasal drainage, runny nose (rhinorrhea), and nasal congestion
- Purulent nasal discharge
- Sneezing and pruritus of the nose, throat, and ears
- Itchy, watery eyes
- Sore, dry throat
- Red, inflamed, swollen nasal mucosa
- Low-grade fever, fatigue, cough (viral)
- Diagnostic testing can include allergy tests to identify possible allergens.

PATIENT-CENTERED CARE

NURSING CARE

- Encourage rest (8 to 10 hr/day) and increased fluid intake (at least 2,000 mL/day).
- Encourage the use of a home humidifier or breathing steamy air after running hot shower water.
- Promote proper disposal of tissues and use of cough etiquette (sneeze or cough into tissue, elbow, or shoulder and not the hands).
- Encourage use of saline nasal spray to sooth nasal passages and soften secretions and warm water mouth gargles to alleviate sore throat.
- Promote proper hand hygiene to reduce the risk of spreading the infection to others.

THERAPEUTIC MANAGEMENT

Varies depending on the cause

MEDICATIONS

Medications that are used to block the release of chemicals from WBCs that bind with receptors in nasal tissues, which prevent edema and itching:

- **Antihistamines**, such as brompheniramine/pseudoephedrine
- **Leukotriene inhibitors**, such as montelukast M
- **Mast cell stabilizers**, such as cromolyn
  - Older adults should be aware of adverse effects (vertigo, hypertension, urinary retention). Ⓖ

Decongestants, such as phenylephrine, constrict blood vessels and decrease edema.

Client education: Use as prescribed for 3 to 4 days to avoid rebound nasal congestion.

Expectorants: guaifenesin, promotes the expectoration of mucus

Intranasal glucocorticoid sprays are the most effective for prevention and treatment of seasonal and perennial rhinitis.

Antipyretics are used if fever is present.

Antibiotics/antimicrobials are given if a bacterial infection can be identified.

CLIENT EDUCATION

- Hand hygiene is a measure to prevent transmission.
- Complementary therapies such as echinacea, vitamin C, and zinc preparations can be used to decrease the intensity and duration of rhinitis. Ⓠ EBP
- Limiting exposure to others will prevent and reduce transmission. This is especially important for vulnerable populations such as the very young, older adults, and people who are immunosuppressed. Ⓖ
- Avoid allergens such as foods, medication, environmental (allergic).

Sinusitis

Sinusitis, often called rhinosinusitis, is an inflammation of the mucous membranes of one or more of the sinuses, usually the maxillary or frontal sinus. Swelling of the mucosa can block the drainage of secretions, which can cause a sinus infection.

- Sinusitis often occurs after rhinitis and can be associated with a deviated nasal septum, nasal polyps, inhaled air pollutants or cocaine, facial trauma, dental infections, or loss of immune function.
- The infection is often caused by a virus, *Streptococcus pneumoniae*, *Haemophilus influenzae*, diplococcus, and bacteroides.

DATA COLLECTION

EXPECTED FINDINGS

- Nasal congestion
- Headache
- Facial pressure or pain (worse when head is tilted forward)
- Cough
- Bloody or purulent nasal drainage
- Tenderness to palpation of forehead, orbital, and facial areas
- Low-grade fever (viral); high-grade fever (bacterial)

DIAGNOSTIC PROCEDURES

- CT scan or sinus x-rays confirm the diagnosis, which is typically based upon findings and physical assessment.
- Endoscopic sinus cavity lavage or surgery to relieve the obstruction and promote drainage of secretions may be done.

PATIENT-CENTERED CARE

NURSING CARE

- Encourage the use of steam humidification, sinus irrigation, saline nasal sprays, and hot and wet packs to relieve sinus congestion and pain.
- Teach the client to increase fluid intake and rest.
- Discourage air travel, swimming, and diving.
- Encourage cessation of tobacco use in any form.
- Instruct the client on correct technique for sinus irrigation and self-administration of nasal sprays.

MEDICATIONS

Nasal decongestants, such as phenylephrine, are used to reduce swelling of the mucosa.

CLIENT EDUCATION
- Begin over-the-counter decongestant use at the first manifestation of sinusitis.
- Manifestations of rebound nasal congestion can occur if decongestants are used for more than 3 to 4 days.

Broad-spectrum antibiotics, such as amoxicillin, are used on a limited basis for a confirmed causative bacterial pathogen.

Pain relief medications include NSAIDs, acetaminophen, and aspirin.

THERAPEUTIC PROCEDURES

- Deviated septum repair
- Surgical excision of nasal polyps

CLIENT EDUCATION

- Sinus irrigation and saline nasal sprays are an effective alternative to antibiotics for relieving nasal congestion.
- Contact the provider for manifestations of a severe headache, neck stiffness (nuchal rigidity), and high fever, which can indicate possible complications.

COMPLICATIONS

Meningitis and encephalitis can occur if pathogens enter the bloodstream from the sinus cavity.

Mucocele: cyst formation in the paranasal sinus

Influenza

Seasonal influenza, or "flu," occurs as an epidemic, usually in the fall and winter months.
- It is a highly contagious, acute viral infection that occurs in children and adults of all ages.
- Influenza can be caused by one of several virus families, and this can vary yearly. Adults are contagious from 24 hr before manifestations develop and up to 5 days after they begin.

Pandemic influenza refers to a viral infection among animals or birds that has mutated and is becoming highly infectious to humans. The resulting viral infection has the potential to spread globally, such as H1N1 ("swine flu") and H5N1 ("avian flu").

DATA COLLECTION

EXPECTED FINDINGS

- Severe headache and muscle aches
- Chills
- Fatigue, weakness
- Severe diarrhea and cough (avian flu)
- Fever
- Hypoxia (avian flu)

DIAGNOSTIC PROCEDURES

Although viral culture and other laboratory tests are available to confirm the diagnosis, the CDC recommends testing only if the results will be used to make treatment decisions.

PATIENT-CENTERED CARE

NURSING CARE

- Maintain droplet and contact precautions for hospitalized clients who have pandemic influenza.
- Provide saline gargles.
- Monitor hydration status, intake, and output.
- Administer fluid therapy as prescribed.
- Monitor respiratory status.

MEDICATIONS

Antivirals

- Amantadine, rimantadine, ribavirin oseltamivir, zanamivira, and peramivir can be prescribed for treatment of influenza.
- Duration of the influenza infection can be shortened by antivirals such as the oral inhalant zanamivir and the oral tablet oseltamivir. In cases of pandemic influenza, these medications may be distributed widely among the population.

CLIENT EDUCATION: Begin antiviral medications within 24 to 48 hr after the onset of manifestations.

Influenza vaccines

- Quadrivalent and trivalent vaccines are prepared yearly depending upon the suspected strain of influenza expected to appear.
  ○ Yearly vaccination is encouraged for everyone older than 6 months of age.
  ○ Clients who have a history of pneumonia, clients who have chronic medical conditions, those who are over age 65, pregnant women, and health care providers are at higher risk and require vaccination.
- H1N1 vaccine is available for the general population.
- H5N1 vaccine is stockpiled for distribution if a pandemic occurs.

INTERPROFESSIONAL CARE

- Respiratory services should be consulted for respiratory support.
- Community health officials are notified of influenza outbreaks.
- State and federal public health officials are consulted for containment and prevention directives during pandemic influenza.

CLIENT EDUCATION

- Obtain an annual influenza immunization when vaccines become available.
- Reduce the risk for spreading viruses by thoroughly washing hands and following cough etiquette.
- Avoid places where people gather. Avoid close personal contact (handshaking, kissing, and hugging).
- If flu manifestations develop, increase fluid intake, rest, and stay home from work or school.
- Avoid travel to areas where pandemic influenza is identified.
- Be aware of public health announcements and activation of the early warning system by public health officials in case of pandemic influenza.

COMPLICATIONS

Pneumonia is a complication of influenza and affects older adults and clients who are debilitated or immunocompromised. Ⓖ

Pneumonia

Pneumonia is an inflammatory process in the lungs that produces excess fluid. Pneumonia is triggered by infectious organisms or by the aspiration of an irritant (fluid or a foreign object). The inflammatory process in the lung parenchyma results in edema and exudate that fills the alveoli. Pneumonia can be a primary disease or a complication of another disease or condition. It affects people of all ages, but young clients, older adult clients, and clients who are immunocompromised are more susceptible. Immobility is a contributing factor in the development of pneumonia. ⓖ

The types of pneumonia include community-acquired pneumonia (CAP), healthcare-associated pneumonia (HCAP), hospital-acquired pneumonia (HAP), and ventilator-associated pneumonia (VAP).

- CAP is the most common type and often occurs as a complication of influenza.
- HCAP has a higher mortality rate and is more likely to be resistant to antibiotics. It usually takes 24 to 48 hr from the time the client is exposed to acquire HCAP. It is related to nonhospital admission and contact with health care personnel.
- HAP is when the condition manifests greater than 48 hours after a hospital admission.
- VAP is when the condition manifests greater than 48 hours after client is intubated.

DATA COLLECTION

EXPECTED FINDINGS

- Anxiety
- Fatigue
- Weakness
- Chest discomfort due to coughing
- Confusion from hypoxia is the most common manifestation of pneumonia in older adult clients. ⓖ

PHYSICAL FINDINGS
- Fever
- Chills
- Flushed face
- Diaphoresis
- Shortness of breath or difficulty breathing
- Tachypnea
- Pleuritic chest pain (sharp)
- Sputum production (yellow-tinged)
- Crackles and wheezes
- Coughing
- Dull chest percussion over areas of consolidation
- Decreased oxygen saturation levels (expected reference range is 95% to 100%)
- Purulent, blood-tinged or rust-colored sputum, which may not always be present

LABORATORY TESTS

Sputum culture and sensitivity
- Obtain specimen before starting antibiotic therapy.
- Obtain specimen by suctioning if the client is unable to cough.
- Older adult clients might have a weak cough reflex and decreased muscle strength. Therefore, older adult clients can have trouble expectorating, which can lead to difficulty in breathing and make specimen retrieval more difficult. ⓖ

CBC: Elevated WBC count (might not be present in older adult clients)

ABGs: Hypoxemia (decreased PaO_2 less than 80 mm Hg)

Blood culture: To rule out organisms in the blood

Electrolytes: To identify manifestations of dehydration (elevated BUN, hypernatremia)

DIAGNOSTIC PROCEDURES

Chest x-ray

- A chest x-ray will show consolidation (solidification, density) of lung tissue. **(18.1)**
- Chest x-ray might not indicate pneumonia for a few days after manifestations.
- A chest x-ray is an important diagnostic tool because the early manifestations of pneumonia are often vague in older adult clients. ⓖ

Pulse oximetry

Clients who have pneumonia usually have oximetry levels less than the expected reference range of 95% to 100%.

PATIENT-CENTERED CARE

NURSING CARE

- Position the client to maximize ventilation (high-Fowler's = 90%) unless contraindicated.
- Encourage coughing or suction to remove secretions.
- Administer breathing treatments and medications.
- Administer oxygen therapy.
- Monitor for skin breakdown around the nose and mouth from the oxygen device.
- Encourage deep breathing with an incentive spirometer to prevent alveolar collapse.
- Determine the client's physical limitations and structure activity to include periods of rest. Ⓠᴘᴄᴄ

- Promote adequate nutrition and fluid intake.
  - The increased work of breathing requires additional calories.
  - Proper nutrition aids in the prevention of secondary respiratory infections.
  - Encourage fluid intake of 2 to 3 L/day to promote hydration and thinning of secretions, unless contraindicated due to another condition.
- Provide rest periods for clients who have dyspnea.
- Reassure the client who is experiencing respiratory distress.

MEDICATIONS

Antibiotics

- Antibiotics are given to destroy infectious pathogens. Commonly used antibiotics include penicillins and cephalosporins.
- Antibiotics are often initially given via IV and then switched to an oral form as the condition improves.
- It is important to obtain any culture specimens prior to giving the first dose of an antibiotic. Once the specimen has been obtained, the antibiotics can be given while waiting for the results of the prescribed culture.

NURSING ACTIONS
- Observe clients for frequent stools.
- Monitor kidney function, especially for older adults who are taking penicillins and cephalosporins. Ⓖ

CLIENT EDUCATION: Take penicillins and cephalosporins with food. Some penicillins should be taken 1 hr before meals or 2 hr after.

Bronchodilators

- Bronchodilators are given to reduce bronchospasms and reduce irritation.
- Short-acting beta₂ agonists, such as albuterol, provide rapid relief.
- Cholinergic antagonists (anticholinergic medications), such as ipratropium, block the parasympathetic nervous system, allowing for increased bronchodilation and decreased pulmonary secretions.
- Methylxanthines, such as theophylline, require close monitoring of blood medication levels due to the narrow therapeutic range.

NURSING ACTIONS
- Monitor blood medication levels for toxicity for clients taking theophylline. Adverse effects will include tachycardia, nausea, and diarrhea.
- Watch for tremors and tachycardia for clients taking albuterol.
- Observe for dry mouth in clients taking ipratropium and monitor heart rate. Adverse effects can include headache, blurred vision, and palpitations, which can indicate toxicity.

CLIENT EDUCATION
- Suck on hard candies to moisten dry mouth while taking ipratropium. Ⓠᴱᴮᴾ
- Increase fluid intake unless contraindicated.

Anti-inflammatories

- Anti-inflammatories decrease airway inflammation.
- Glucocorticosteroids, such as fluticasone and prednisone, are prescribed to reduce inflammation. Monitor for immunosuppression, fluid retention, hyperglycemia, hypokalemia, and poor wound healing.

NURSING ACTIONS
- Monitor for decreased immunity function.
- Monitor for hyperglycemia.
- Observe for fluid retention and weight gain. This can be common.
- Monitor the throat and mouth for aphthous lesions (canker sores).

CLIENT EDUCATION
- Report black, tarry stools.
- Drink plenty of fluids to promote hydration.
- Take glucocorticosteroids with food.
- Avoid discontinuing glucocorticosteroids without consulting the provider.

INTERPROFESSIONAL CARE

- Respiratory services should be consulted for inhalers, breathing treatments, and suctioning for airway management.
- Nutritional services can be contacted for weight loss or gain related to medications or diagnosis.
- Rehabilitation care can be consulted if the client has prolonged weakness and needs assistance with increasing level of activity.

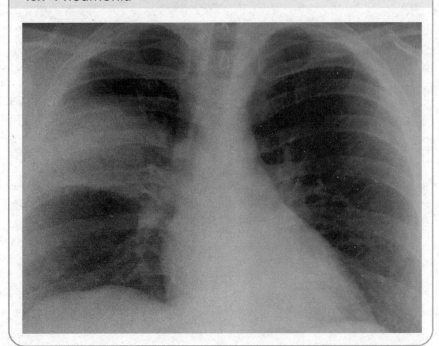

18.1 Pneumonia

CLIENT EDUCATION

- It is important to continue medications for treatment of pneumonia. ⓆPCC
- Rest as needed.
- Maintain hand hygiene to prevent infection.
- Avoid crowded areas to reduce the risk of infection. ⓆEBP
- Treatment and recovery from pneumonia can take time.
- Obtain immunizations for influenza and pneumonia.
- Discontinue tobacco use if needed.

COMPLICATIONS

ATELECTASIS

- Airway inflammation and edema lead to alveolar collapse and increase the risk of hypoxemia.
- The client reports shortness of breath and exhibits findings of hypoxemia.
- The client has diminished or absent breath sounds over the affected area.
- A chest x-ray shows an area of density.

Bacteremia (sepsis): This occurs if pathogens enter the bloodstream from the infection in the lungs.

ACUTE RESPIRATORY DISTRESS SYNDROME

- Hypoxemia persists despite oxygen therapy.
- Lung volume capacity and elasticity is reduced.
- Dyspnea worsens as bilateral pulmonary edema develops that is noncardiac-related.
- A chest x-ray shows an area of density with a ground-glass appearance.
- Blood gas findings demonstrate high arterial blood levels of carbon dioxide (hypercarbia) even though pulse oximetry shows decreased saturation.

Active Learning Scenario

A nurse in a clinic is discussing health promotion and disease management with a client who has rhinitis. What should the nurse include in this discussion? Use the ATI Active Learning Template: System Disorder to complete this item.

RISK FACTORS: Identify three risk factors for rhinitis.

EXPECTED FINDINGS: Describe at least four.

CLIENT EDUCATION: Describe two client self-care activities.

MEDICATIONS: Identify two over-the-counter medications the client can use.

Application Exercises

1. A nurse in a clinic is collecting data from a client who has sinusitis. Which of the following techniques should the nurse use to identify manifestations of this disorder?

   A. Percussion of posterior lobes of lungs

   B. Auscultation of the trachea

   C. Inspection of the conjunctiva

   D. Palpation of the orbital areas

2. A nurse is reinforcing teaching with a group of clients about influenza. Which of the following client statements indicates an understanding of the teaching?

   A. "I should wash my hands after blowing my nose to prevent spreading the virus."

   B. "I need to avoid drinking fluids if I develop symptoms."

   C. "I need a flu shot every 2 years because of the different flu strains."

   D. "I should cover my mouth with my hand when I sneeze."

3. A nurse is monitoring a group of clients for increased risk for developing pneumonia. Which of the following clients should the nurse expect to be at risk? (Select all that apply.)

   A. Client who has dysphagia

   B. Client who has AIDS

   C. Client who was vaccinated for pneumococcus and influenza 6 months ago

   D. Client who is postoperative and has received local anesthesia

   E. Client who has a closed head injury and is receiving mechanical ventilation

   F. Client who has myasthenia gravis

4. A nurse is assessing a client who, upon awakening, was disoriented to person, place, and time. The client reports chills and chest pain that is worse upon inspiration. Which of the following actions is the nursing priority?

   A. Obtain baseline vital signs and oxygen saturation.

   B. Obtain a sputum culture.

   C. Obtain a complete history from the client.

   D. Inform client about recommended pneumococcal vaccine.

5. A nurse is caring for a client who has pneumonia. Assessment findings include temperature 37.8° C (100° F), respirations 30/min, blood pressure 130/76, heart rate 100/min, and SpO2 91% on room air. Sort the following nursing interventions by priority.

   A. Administer antibiotics.

   B. Administer oxygen therapy.

   C. Instruct the client to obtain a yearly influenza vaccination.

   D. Perform a sputum culture.

Application Exercises Key

1. D. **CORRECT:** A client who has sinusitis may report tenderness when the orbital, frontal, and facial areas are palpated. Lung percussion is an advanced technique that can be used to check for pulmonary conditions. Auscultation of the trachea is used to check for respiratory conditions. Inspection of the conjunctiva is used to check for eye conditions.

   Ⓝ *NCLEX® Connection: Health Promotion and Maintenance, Data Collection Techniques*

2. A. **CORRECT:** Hand hygiene decreases the risk of the client spreading influenza viruses. The client should increase fluid intake to loosen mucous, promote expectoration, and maintain hydration. The client should receive an influenza vaccination yearly to reduce the risk for acquiring influenza. The client should sneeze into the shoulder or elbow, rather than the hands, to reduce the risk of spreading the influenza virus.

   Ⓝ *NCLEX® Connection: Health Promotion and Maintenance, Health Promotion and Disease Prevention*

3. A, B, E, F. **CORRECT:** The client who has difficulty swallowing is at increased risk for pneumonia due to aspiration. The client who has AIDS is immunocompromised, which increases the risk of opportunistic infections, such as pneumonia. Mechanical ventilation is invasive and places the client at risk for ventilator-associated pneumonia. A client who has myasthenia gravis has generalized weakness and can have difficulty clearing airway secretions, which increases the risk of pneumonia. The client who has recently been vaccinated in the past few months has a decreased risk of acquiring pneumonia. A client who is postoperative and has received local anesthesia has a decreased risk of acquiring pneumonia.

   Ⓝ *NCLEX® Connection: Health Promotion and Maintenance, Health Promotion and Disease Prevention*

4. A. **CORRECT:** The first action the nurse should take using the nursing process is to assess the client in order to determine the next nursing intervention and provide safe and effective client care. The nurse should obtain a sputum culture to determine sensitivity for antibiotic therapy. However, there is another action the nurse should take first. The nurse should obtain a complete history from the client to determine the plan of care. However, there is another action the nurse should take first. The nurse should provide information for a pneumococcal vaccination to decrease the risk of pneumonia in the future. However, there is another action the nurse should take first.

   Ⓝ *NCLEX® Connection: Physiological Adaptation, Alterations in Body Systems*

5. B, D, A, C

   The client's respiratory and heart rates are elevated, and their oxygen saturation is 91% on room air. Using the ABC priority framework, the nurse should identify that providing oxygen is the first intervention. Obtaining a sputum culture is the second nursing intervention. It should be done prior to administering oral medications to obtain an accurate specimen. Administration of antibiotics is the third action the nurse should take. The sputum culture should be obtained prior to antibiotic administration. The last action the nurse should take is to instruct the client to receive yearly influenza vaccinations to reduce the risk of acquiring influenza that can lead to pneumonia.

   Ⓝ *NCLEX® Connection: Pharmacological Therapies, Expected Actions/Outcomes*

Active Learning Scenario Key

Using the ATI Active Learning Template: System Disorder

RISK FACTORS
- Recent exposure to viral, bacterial or influenza infections
- Lack of current immunization status (pneumonia, influenza)
- Exposure to plant pollen, molds, animal dander, foods, medications, and environmental contaminants
- Tobacco smoke
- Substance use (alcohol, cocaine)
- Presence of a foreign body
- Inactivity and immobility

EXPECTED FINDINGS
- Excessive nasal drainage, runny nose (rhinorrhea), nasal congestion
- Purulent nasal drainage
- Sneezing and pruritus of the nose, throat, and ears
- Itchy, watery eyes
- Sore, dry throat
- Red, inflamed, swollen nasal mucosa
- Low-grade fever

CLIENT EDUCATION
- Rest (8 to 10 hr/day), increased fluid intake (at least 2,000 mL/day)
- Use of a home humidifier or breathing steamy air after running hot shower water
- Proper disposal of tissues and use of cough etiquette

MEDICATIONS: Brompheniramine/pseudoephedrine, cromolyn sodium, phenylephrine, antipyretics

Ⓝ *NCLEX® Connection: Health Promotion and Maintenance, Health Promotion/Disease Prevention*

CHAPTER 19 *Asthma*

Asthma is a chronic disorder of the airways that results in intermittent and reversible airflow obstruction of the bronchioles. The obstruction occurs either by inflammation or airway hyperresponsiveness. Approximately 8.4% of the population in the U.S. has asthma. Asthma can occur at any age. The cause is unknown. Manifestations of asthma include mucosal edema, bronchoconstriction, and excessive mucus production. The goals for Healthy People 2030 includes reducing asthma deaths, attacks, and ED visits.

HEALTH PROMOTION AND DISEASE PREVENTION

- If the client smokes, promote smoking cessation.
- Advise the client to use protective equipment (mask) and ensure proper ventilation while working in environments that contain carcinogens or particles in the air. Qs
- Encourage influenza and pneumonia vaccinations for older adults and all clients who have asthma. Qs
- Instruct the client how to recognize and avoid triggering agents.
  - Environmental factors, such as changes in temperature (especially warm to cold) and humidity
  - Air pollutants
  - Strong odors (perfume)
  - Seasonal allergens (grass, tree, and weed pollens) and perennial allergens (mold, feathers, dust, roaches, animal dander, foods treated with sulfites)
  - Stress and emotional distress
  - Medications (aspirin, NSAIDs, beta blockers, cholinergics)
  - Enzymes, including those in laundry detergents
  - Chemicals (household cleaners)
  - Sinusitis with postnasal drip
  - Viral respiratory tract infection
- Reinforce with the client how to self-administer medications (nebulizers and inhalers).
- Reinforce teachings with the client regarding infection prevention techniques.
- Encourage regular exercise as part of asthma therapy.
  - Promotes ventilation and perfusion
  - Maintains cardiac health
  - Enhances skeletal muscle strength
  - Clients can require premedication
- Instruct the client to use hot water to eliminate dust mites in bed linens.

DATA COLLECTION

Diagnosis is based on findings and classified into one of the following four categories.
- **Mild intermittent**: Symptoms occur less than once a week.
- **Mild persistent**: Symptoms arise more than twice a week but not daily.
- **Moderate persistent**: Daily symptoms occur in conjunction with exacerbations twice a week.
- **Severe persistent:** Symptoms occur continually, along with frequent exacerbations that limit physical activity and quality of life.

RISK FACTORS

- Older adult clients have decreased pulmonary reserves due to physiologic lung changes that occur with the aging process. Ⓖ
  - Older adult clients are more susceptible to infections.
  - The sensitivity of beta-adrenergic receptors decreases with age. As the beta receptors age and lose sensitivity, they are less able to respond to agonists, which relax smooth muscle and can result in bronchospasms.
- Family history of asthma
- Smoking
- Secondhand smoke exposure
- Environmental allergies
- Exposure to chemical irritants or dust
- Gastroesophageal reflux disease (GERD)

EXPECTED FINDINGS

- Dyspnea
- Chest tightness
- Anxiety or stress

PHYSICAL FINDINGS
- Coughing
- Wheezing
- Mucus production
- Use of accessory muscles
- Prolonged exhalation
- Poor oxygen saturation (low SaO_2)

Obtain history regarding current and previous asthma exacerbations. Qpcc
- Onset and duration
- Precipitating factors (stress, exercise, exposure to irritant)
- Changes in medication regimen
- Medications that provide relief
- Other medications taken
- Self-care methods used to promote relief

LABORATORY TESTS

Arterial blood gases

Evaluates oxygenation status during acute attacks.

Sputum cultures

Bacteria can indicate infection. Ⓖ

DIAGNOSTIC PROCEDURES

Pulmonary function tests (PFTs) are the most accurate tests for diagnosing asthma and its severity.
- Forced vital capacity (FVC) is the volume of air exhaled from full inhalation to full exhalation.
- Forced expiratory volume in the first second (FEV1) is the volume of air blown out as hard and fast as possible during the first second of the most forceful exhalation after the greatest full inhalation.
- Peak expiratory flow rate (PEFR) is the fastest airflow rate reached during exhalation.
- A decrease in FEV1 by 15% to 20% below the expected value is common in clients who have asthma.

PATIENT-CENTERED CARE

NURSING CARE

- Position the client to maximize ventilation (high-Fowler's). Ⓠ**EBP**
- Administer oxygen therapy as prescribed.
- Monitor cardiac rate and rhythm for changes during an acute attack (can be irregular, tachycardic, or with PVCs).
- Monitor respiratory rate and rhythm for changes in effort, symmetry, SaO_2; auscultate lung sounds.
- Maintain IV access.
- Remain calm and reassuring.
- Provide rest periods for older adult clients who have dyspnea. Design room and walkways with opportunities for rest. Incorporate rest into ADLs. Ⓖ

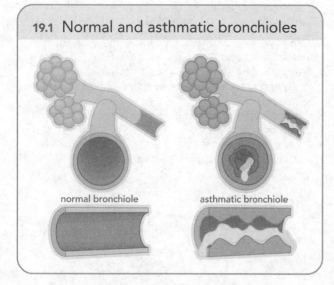

19.1 Normal and asthmatic bronchioles

normal bronchiole   asthmatic bronchiole

- Encourage prompt medical attention for infections and appropriate immunizations.
- Administer medications as prescribed.
- Reinforce with the client to perform daily peak flow meter testing. If only able to achieve a reading in the red zone, immediately use the reliever medications and seek emergency care.

MEDICATIONS

Bronchodilators (inhalers)

- **Short-acting beta₂ agonists**, such as albuterol, provide rapid relief of acute manifestations and prevent exercise-induced asthma.
- **Anticholinergic medications**, such as ipratropium, block the parasympathetic nervous system. This allows for the sympathetic nervous system effects of increased bronchodilation and decreased pulmonary secretions. These medications are long-acting and used to prevent bronchospasms.
- **Methylxanthines**, such as theophylline, require close monitoring of blood medication levels due to a narrow therapeutic range. Use only when other treatments are ineffective.
- **Long-acting beta₂ agonists**, such as salmeterol, primarily are used for asthma attack prevention.

NURSING ACTIONS
- Albuterol: Watch for tremors and tachycardia.
- Ipratropium: Observe for dry mouth.
- Theophylline: Monitor blood levels for toxicity. Adverse effects include tachycardia, nausea, and diarrhea.

CLIENT EDUCATION
- Ipratropium: Suck on hard candies to help relieve dry mouth; increase fluid intake; and report headache, blurred vision, or palpitations, which can indicate toxicity of ipratropium. Monitor heart rate.
- Salmeterol: Use to prevent an asthma attack and not at the onset of an attack. Do not use during acute exacerbations.

Anti-inflammatory agents

These medications are for prophylaxis and are used to decrease airway inflammation.
- **Corticosteroids**, such as fluticasone and prednisone
- **Leukotriene antagonists**, such as montelukast
- **Mast cell stabilizers**, such as cromolyn
- **Monoclonal antibodies**, such as omalizumab

NURSING ACTIONS
- Watch for decreased immunity function and wound healing.
- Monitor for hyperglycemia.
- Observe for fluid retention and weight gain. This can be common.
- Monitor the throat and mouth for aphthous lesions (canker sores).
- Omalizumab can cause anaphylaxis.

CLIENT EDUCATION

- Report black, tarry stools.
- Drink plenty of fluids to promote hydration.
- Take prednisone with food.
- Use these medications to prevent asthma, not for the onset of an attack.
- Avoid people who have respiratory infections.
- Use good mouth care and hand washing regimen.
- Do not discontinue medication suddenly.
- Rinse mouth and gargle after inhaled glucocorticoids to minimize dysphonia and candidiasis.

Combination agents (bronchodilator and anti-inflammatory)

If prescribed separately for inhalation administration at the same time, administer the bronchodilator first in order to increase the absorption of the anti-inflammatory agent.

- Ipratropium and albuterol
- Fluticasone and salmeterol

INTERPROFESSIONAL CARE

- Respiratory services should be consulted for inhalers and breathing treatments for airway management.
- Nutritional services can be contacted for weight loss or gain related to medications or diagnosis.
- Rehabilitation care can be consulted if the client has prolonged weakness and needs assistance with increasing level of activity.

COMPLICATIONS

Respiratory failure

Persistent hypoxemia related to asthma can lead to respiratory failure.

NURSING ACTIONS

- Monitor oxygenation levels and acid-base balance.
- Prepare for intubation and mechanical ventilation.
- Monitor and report inaudible breath sounds, wheezing, retractions, and ineffective cough.

Status asthmaticus

This is a life-threatening episode of airway obstruction that is often unresponsive to common treatment. It involves extreme wheezing, labored breathing, use of accessory muscles, distended neck veins, and creates a risk for cardiac and/or respiratory arrest.

NURSING ACTIONS

- Prepare for emergency intubation.
- Assist with preparing to administer IV fluids, oxygen, bronchodilators, and epinephrine. Assist with initiating systemic steroid therapy.

Application Exercises

1. A nurse is collecting data from a client who has a history of asthma. Which of the following factors should the nurse identify as a risk for asthma?

   A. Sex

   B. Environmental allergies

   C. Alcohol use

   D. History of diabetes

2. A nurse is collecting data from a client who is experiencing an acute asthma attack. Which of the following findings indicates that the client's respiratory status is declining? (Select all that apply.)

   A. SaO$_2$ 95%

   B. Wheezing

   C. Retraction of sternal muscles

   D. Pink mucous membranes

   E. Tachycardia

3. A nurse collecting data from a client who has an SaO$_2$ of 91%, audible wheezing and is using accessory muscles when breathing. Which of the following classes of medications should the nurse anticipate a provider prescription?

   A. Third-generation cephalosporin

   B. Beta-blocker

   C. Nonsteroidal anti-inflammatory

   D. Short-acting beta$_2$ agonist

4. A nurse is reinforcing discharge teaching with a client who has a new prescription for prednisone for asthma. Which of the following client statements indicates understanding?

   A. "I will decrease my fluid intake while taking this medication."

   B. "I will expect to have black, tarry stools."

   C. "I will take my medication with meals."

   D. "I will monitor for weight loss while on this medication."

5. A nurse is reinforcing teaching with a client on the purpose of taking a bronchodilator. Which of the following client statements indicates understanding?

   A. "This medication can decrease my immune response."

   B. "I take this medication to prevent asthma attacks."

   C. "I need to take this medication with food."

   D. "This medication has a slow onset to treat my symptoms."

Active Learning Scenario

A nurse is caring for a client who has asthma and a prescription for prednisone. Use the ATI Active Learning Template: Medication to complete this item.

NURSING INTERVENTIONS: Include at least three.

Active Learning Scenario Key

Using the ATI Active Learning Template: Medication
NURSING INTERVENTIONS
- Watch for decreased immune function.
- Monitor for hyperglycemia.
- Advise the client to report black, tarry stools.
- Observe for fluid retention and weight gain.
- Monitor the throat and mouth for aphthous lesions (canker sores).

Ⓝ *NCLEX® Connection: Pharmacological Therapies, Medication Administration*

Application Exercises Key

1. B. **CORRECT:** Environmental allergies are a risk factor associated with asthma. A client who has environmental allergies typically has other allergic problems, such as rhinitis or a skin rash. Sex, alcohol use, and history of diabetes are not risk factors associated with asthma.

Ⓝ *NCLEX® Connection: Health Promotion and Maintenance, Health Promotion and Disease Prevention*

2. B, C, E. **CORRECT:** Wheezing indicates narrowing of the airway and is a finding that could indicate that the client's respiratory status is declining. Tachycardia is a finding that caused by decreased oxygenation and is a finding that could indicate that the client's respiratory status is declining. Retraction of sternal muscles is associated with increased work of breathing and is a finding that could indicate that the client's respiratory status is declining. An oxygen saturation of 95% and pink mucous membranes are expected findings and do not indicate the client's condition is declining.

Ⓝ *NCLEX® Connection: Physiological Adaptation, Basic Pathophysiology*

3. D. **CORRECT:** The nurse should anticipate a provider prescription for a short-acting beta$_2$ agonist, which is administered to cause dilation of the bronchioles, opening of airways which reduces wheezing. An anticipation of a provider prescription for a third-generation cephalosporin, beta-blocker, and non-steroidal anti-inflammatory medication is not indicated because the client is having an acute respiratory condition. A third-generation cephalosporin is an anti-infective such as that is used to manage infections. A beta blocker is used to manage cardiac conditions such as dysrhythmias heart disease, or hypertension. A non-steroidal anti-inflammatory is used to manage pain and fever.

Ⓝ *NCLEX® Connection: Pharmacological Therapies, Expected Actions/Outcomes*

4. C. **CORRECT:** Prednisone is a corticosteroid that is used to manage inflammation for a client who has asthma. The client should be informed to take prednisone with food because taking it on an empty stomach can cause gastrointestinal distress. The client should drink plenty of fluids while taking prednisone because it can cause the client to have a dry mouth or to become thirsty. The client should inform the provider of any black, tarry stools because this medication can increase bleeding tendency and black stools can be an indication of blood in the stool. The client should monitor the mouth for canker sores because medication can cause bleeding of the gums and soreness in the mouth. It also decreases immune function.

Ⓝ *NCLEX® Connection: Pharmacological Therapies, Medication Administrations*

5. B. **CORRECT:** A long-acting bronchodilator is used to prevent asthma attacks from occurring. A long-acting bronchodilator does not decrease the body's immune response. However, an anti-inflammatory medication can cause this effect. A long-acting bronchodilator does not need to be taken with food. However, an anti-inflammatory medication can cause gastrointestinal distress and needs to be to be given with food. A long-acting bronchodilator has a faster onset of action.

Ⓝ *NCLEX® Connection: Pharmacological Therapies, Expected Actions/Outcomes*

UNIT 3   RESPIRATORY DISORDERS
SECTION: RESPIRATORY SYSTEM DISORDERS

CHAPTER 20 ## Chronic Obstructive Pulmonary Disease

Chronic obstructive pulmonary disease (COPD) encompasses two diseases: emphysema and chronic bronchitis. Most clients who have emphysema also have chronic bronchitis. More than 4% of the population has received a diagnosis of COPD, and it is the 6th leading cause of death in the United States. COPD is irreversible.

Emphysema is characterized by the loss of lung elasticity and hyperinflation of lung tissue. Emphysema causes destruction of the alveoli, leading to a decreased surface area for gas exchange, carbon dioxide retention, and respiratory acidosis.

Chronic bronchitis is an inflammation of the bronchi and bronchioles due to chronic exposure to irritants.

COPD typically affects middle-age to older adults. ⓒ

HEALTH PROMOTION AND DISEASE PREVENTION

- Promote smoking cessation.
- Avoid exposure to secondhand smoke.
- Use protective equipment (a mask) and ensure proper ventilation while working in environments that contain carcinogens or particles in the air.
- Influenza and pneumonia immunizations are important for all clients who have COPD, but especially for older adults. ⓒ

DATA COLLECTION

RISK FACTORS

- Advanced age: Older adult clients have a decreased pulmonary reserve due to age-related lung changes.
- Cigarette smoking is the primary risk factor for the development of COPD.
- Alpha$_1$-antitrypsin (AAT) deficiency.
- Exposure to environmental factors (air pollution).

EXPECTED FINDINGS

Chronic dyspnea. The respiratory rate can reach 40 to 50/min during acute exacerbations.

PHYSICAL FINDINGS

- Dyspnea upon exertion
- Productive cough that is most severe upon rising in the morning
- Hypoxemia
- Crackles and wheezes
- Rapid and shallow respirations
- Use of accessory muscles
- Barrel chest or increased chest diameter (with emphysema)
- Hyperresonance on percussion due to "trapped air" (with emphysema)
- Irregular breathing pattern
- Thin extremities and enlarged neck muscles
- Dependent edema secondary to right-sided heart failure
- Clubbing of fingers and toes (late stages of the disease)
- Pallor and cyanosis of nail beds and mucous membranes (late stages of the disease)
- Decreased oxygen saturation levels (expected reference range is 95% to 100%)
- In older adults or clients who have dark-colored skin, oxygen saturation levels can be slightly lower. ⓒ

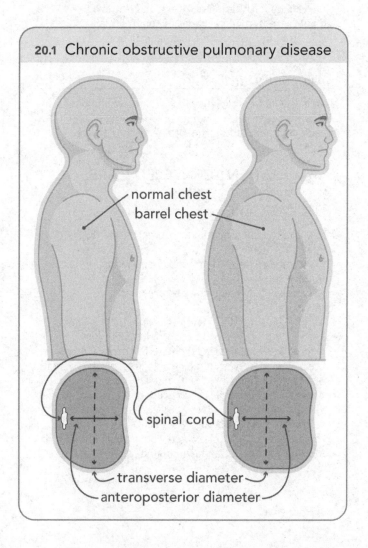

20.1 Chronic obstructive pulmonary disease

normal chest
barrel chest

spinal cord

transverse diameter
anteroposterior diameter

LABORATORY TESTS

- Increased hematocrit level is due to low oxygenation levels.
- Use sputum cultures and WBC counts to diagnose acute respiratory infections.
- Arterial blood gases (ABGs).
  - Hypoxemia (decreased PaO_2 less than 80 mm Hg)
  - Hypercarbia (increased $PaCO_2$ greater than 45 mm Hg)
- Blood electrolytes.

DIAGNOSTIC PROCEDURES

Pulmonary function tests

These tests are used for diagnosis, as well as determining the effectiveness of therapy.

- Comparisons of forced expiratory volume (FEV) to forced vital capacity (FVC) are used to classify COPD as mild to very severe.
- As COPD advances, the FEV-to-FVC ratio decreases. The expected reference range is 100%. For mild COPD, the FEV/FVC ratio is decreased to less than 70%. As the disease progresses to moderate and severe, the ratio decreases to less than 50%.

Chest x-ray

- Reveals hyperinflation of alveoli and flattened diaphragm in the late stages of emphysema.
- It is often not useful for the diagnosis of early or moderate disease.

Alpha₁ antitrypsin levels

Used to check for deficiency in AAT, an enzyme produced by the liver that helps regulate other enzymes (which help break down pollutants) from attacking lung tissue.

PATIENT-CENTERED CARE

NURSING CARE

- Position the client to maximize ventilation (high-Fowler's). Q EBP
- Encourage effective coughing, or suction to remove secretions.
- Encourage deep breathing and use of an incentive spirometer.
- Administer breathing treatments and medications.
- Administer oxygen as prescribed. In COPD, low arterial levels of oxygen serve as the primary drive for breathing. However, in most cases, oxygen levels should be maintained between 88% and 92%.
- Clients who have COPD can need 2 to 4 L/min of oxygen via nasal cannula or up to 40% via Venturi mask. Clients who have chronically increased $PaCO_2$ levels usually require 1 to 2 L/min of oxygen via nasal cannula.
- Monitor for skin breakdown around the nose and mouth from the oxygen device.

- Promote adequate nutrition.
  - Increased work of breathing increases caloric demands.
  - Proper nutrition aids in the prevention of infection.
  - Encourage fluids to promote adequate hydration.
  - Dyspnea decreases energy available for eating, so soft, high-calorie foods should be encouraged.
  - Provide fluids between and at the end of meals to prevent early satiety.
- Monitor weight and note any changes.
- Instruct the client to practice breathing techniques to control dyspneic episodes. Q EBP
  - For diaphragmatic (abdominal) breathing, instruct the client to:
    - Take breaths deep from the diaphragm.
    - Lie on back with knees bent.
    - Rest a hand over the abdomen to create resistance.
    - If the client's hand rises and lowers upon inhalation and exhalation, the breathing is being performed correctly.
  - For pursed-lip breathing, instruct the client to:
    - Form the mouth as if preparing to whistle.
    - Take a breath in through the nose and out through the lips/mouth.
    - Not puff the cheeks.
    - Take breaths deep and slow.
- **Positive expiratory pressure device**
  - Assists client to remove airway secretions.
  - Client inhales deeply and exhales through device.
  - While exhaling, a ball inside the device moves, causing a vibration that results in loosening secretions.
- **Exercise conditioning**
  - Includes improving pulmonary status by strengthening the condition of the lungs by exercise.
  - The client walks daily at a self-paced rate until dyspnea occurs, then stops to rest. Once dyspnea resolves, the client resumes.
  - The client walks 20 min daily 2 to 3 times weekly.
  - Determine the client's physical limitations, and structure activity to include periods of rest.
  - Provide rest periods for older adult clients who have dyspnea. Design the room and walkways with opportunities for relaxation. Ⓒ
- Provide support to the client and family. Talk about disease and lifestyle changes, including home care services such as portable oxygen. Q PCC
- Increase fluid intake. Encourage the client to drink 2 to 3 L/day to liquefy mucus.

Incentive spirometry

Incentive spirometry is used to monitor optimal lung expansion.

NURSING ACTIONS: Show the client how to use the incentive spirometry machine.

CLIENT EDUCATION: Keep a tight mouth seal around the mouthpiece and inhale and hold breath for 3 to 5 seconds. During inhalation, the needle of the spirometry machine will rise. This promotes lung expansion.

MEDICATIONS

Bronchodilators (inhalers)

Short-acting beta₂ agonists, such as albuterol, provide rapid relief.

Cholinergic antagonists (anticholinergic medications), such as ipratropium, block the parasympathetic nervous system. This allows for the sympathetic nervous system effects of increased bronchodilation and decreased pulmonary secretions. These medications are long-acting and are used to prevent bronchospasms.

NURSING ACTIONS
- Watch for tremors and palpations when taking albuterol.
- Observe for dry mouth when taking ipratropium.

CLIENT EDUCATION
- Suck on hard candies to help moisten dry mouth while taking ipratropium.
- Increase fluid intake, report headaches, or blurred vision.
- Monitor heart rate. Palpitations can occur, which can indicate toxicity of ipratropium.

Anti-inflammatory agents

These medications decrease airway inflammation.
- If **corticosteroids**, such as fluticasone and prednisone, are given systemically, monitor for serious adverse effects (immunosuppression, fluid retention, hyperglycemia, hypokalemia, poor wound healing).
- **Leukotriene antagonists,** such as montelukast; mast cell stabilizers, such as cromolyn; and monoclonal antibodies, such as omalizumab, can be used.

NURSING ACTIONS
- Watch for a decrease in immunity function.
- Monitor for delayed wound healing.
- Monitor for hyperglycemia.
- Observe for fluid retention and weight gain. This is common.
- Check the throat and mouth for aphthous lesions (canker sores).
- Omalizumab can cause anaphylaxis.

CLIENT EDUCATION
- Drink plenty of fluids to promote hydration.
- Report black, tarry stools.
- Take glucocorticoids with food.
- Use medication to prevent and control bronchospasms.
- Avoid people who have respiratory infections.
- Use good mouth care.
- Use medication as a prophylactic prevention of COPD manifestations.
- Do not discontinue medication suddenly.

Mucolytic agents

These agents help thin secretions, making them easier for the client to expel.
- Nebulizer treatments include acetylcysteine and dornase alfa.
- Guaifenesin is an oral agent that can be taken.
- A combination of guaifenesin and dextromethorphan also can be taken orally to loosen secretions.

THERAPEUTIC PROCEDURES

- Chest physiotherapy uses percussion and vibration to mobilize secretions.
- Raising the foot of the bed slightly higher than the head can facilitate optimal drainage and removal of secretions by gravity.
- Humidifiers can be useful for who live in a dry climate or who use dry heat during the winter.

INTERPROFESSIONAL CARE

- Consult respiratory services for inhalers, breathing treatments, and suctioning for airway management.
- Contact nutritional services for weight loss or gain related to medications or diagnosis.
- Consult rehabilitative care if the client has prolonged weakness and needs assistance with increasing activity level.
- COPD is debilitating for older adult clients. Management of the disease is continuous. Referrals to assistance programs, such as food delivery services, can be indicated. Ⓖ
- Assist with setting up referral services, including home care services such as portable oxygen.
- Provide support to the client and family.

CLIENT EDUCATION

- Eat high-calorie foods to promote energy. Ⓠᴘᴄᴄ
- Rest as needed.
- Practice hand hygiene to prevent infection.
- Take medications (inhalers, oral medications) as prescribed.
- Stop smoking if needed.
- Obtain immunizations, such as influenza and pneumonia, to decrease the risk of infection.
- Use oxygen as prescribed. Inform other caregivers not to smoke around the oxygen due to flammability.
- Acute infections and other complications often require hospital stays. Report unusual findings or concerns to the provider.
- Ensure fluid intake of at least 2 L (68 oz) daily to thin secretions, unless the provider recommends otherwise.

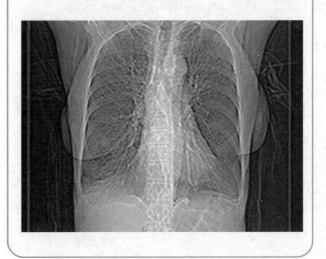

20.2 X-ray of lungs with emphysema

COMPLICATIONS

Respiratory infection

Respiratory infections result from increased mucus production and poor oxygenation levels.

NURSING ACTIONS
- Administer oxygen therapy.
- Monitor oxygenation levels.
- Monitor for indications of infection (increased WBC, CRP, decreased SaO_2, change in temperature).
- Administer antibiotics and other medications.

CLIENT EDUCATION
- Avoid crowds and people who have respiratory infections.
- Obtain pneumonia and influenza immunizations.

Right-sided heart failure (cor pulmonale)

- Air trapping, airway collapse, and stiff alveoli lead to increased pulmonary pressures.
- Blood flow through the lung tissue is difficult. This increased workload leads to enlargement and thickening of the right atrium and ventricle.

MANIFESTATIONS
- Low oxygenation levels
- Cyanosis
- Enlarged and tender liver
- Distended neck veins
- Dependent edema

NURSING ACTIONS
- Monitor respiratory status and administer oxygen therapy.
- Monitor for GI disturbances (nausea, anorexia).
- Monitor heart rate and rhythm.
- Administer medications as prescribed.
- Administer IV fluids and diuretics to maintain fluid balance.

Active Learning Scenario

A nurse is reinforcing discharge instructions to a client who has a new prescription for ipratropium. Use the ATI Active Learning Template: Medication to complete this item.

NURSING INTERVENTIONS: List at least three.

Application Exercises

1. A nurse is reinforcing teaching to a client on how to perform pursed-lip breathing. Which of the following statements should the nurse include?
   - A. "Take quick breaths upon inhalation."
   - B. "Place your hand over your stomach."
   - C. "Take a deep breath in through your nose."
   - D. "Puff your cheeks upon exhalation."

2. A nurse is reinforcing teaching to a client on the use of an incentive spirometer. Which of the following statements by the client indicates an understanding of the teaching?
   - A. "I will place the adapter on my finger to read my blood oxygen saturation level."
   - B. "I will lie on my back with my knees bent."
   - C. "I will rest my hand over my abdomen to create resistance."
   - D. "I will take in a deep breath and hold it before exhaling."

3. A nurse is reinforcing discharge teaching to a client who has COPD and a new prescription for albuterol. Which of the following statements by the client indicates an understanding of the teaching?
   - A. "This medication can increase my blood sugar levels."
   - B. "This medication can decrease my immune response."
   - C. "I can have an increase in my heart rate while taking this medication."
   - D. "I can have mouth sores while taking this medication."

4. A nurse is preparing to administer an initial dose of prednisone to a client who has COPD. The nurse should monitor for which of the following adverse effects of this medication? (Select all that apply.)
   - A. Hypokalemia
   - B. Tachycardia
   - C. Fluid retention
   - D. Nausea
   - E. Black, tarry stools

5. A nurse is assisting with the discharge of a client who has COPD. The client is concerned about not being able to leave the house due to the need for staying on continuous oxygen. Which of the following responses should the nurse make?
   - A. "There are portable oxygen delivery systems that you can take with you."
   - B. "When you go out, you can remove the oxygen and then reapply it when you get home."
   - C. "You probably will not be able to go out as much as you used to."
   - D. "Home health services will come to you so you will not need to get out."

Application Exercises Key

1. A. The client should take a slow deep breath upon inhalation. This improves breathing and allows oxygen into lungs.
   B. The client should place a hand on the stomach while performing diaphragmatic or abdominal breathing. This allows resistance to be met and serves as a guide that the client is inhaling and exhaling correctly.
   C. **CORRECT:** When taking actions, the nurse should identify that the client should take a deep breath in through the nose while performing pursed-lip breathing. This controls the client's breathing.
   D. The client should not puff their cheeks upon exhalation. This does not allow the client to optimally exhale the carbon dioxide from the lungs.

   Ⓝ NCLEX® Connection: Physiological Adaptation, Alterations in Body Systems

2. A. The client should place an adapter on a finger to read the blood oxygen saturation level while performing a pulse oximetry reading.
   B. The client who practices diaphragmatic or abdominal breathing should lie supine with knees bent.
   C. The client who practices diaphragmatic or abdominal breathing should rest a hand over the abdomen to determine if the breathing is done correctly.
   D. **CORRECT:** When evaluating outcomes, the nurse should identify that the client who is using the spirometer should take in as deep a breath as possible before exhaling. As the client inhales, the needle of the spirometer rises. This promotes lung expansion.

   Ⓝ NCLEX® Connection: Reduction of Risk Potential, Diagnostic Tests

3. C. **CORRECT:** When evaluating outcomes, the nurse should identify that bronchodilators, such as albuterol, can cause tachycardia.
   A, B, D. Anti-inflammatory agents, such as corticosteroids, can cause hyperglycemia, a decreased immune response, and mouth sores.

   Ⓝ NCLEX® Connection: Pharmacological Therapies, Medication Administration

4. A, C, E. **CORRECT:** When generating solutions, the nurse should observe for hypokalemia, fluid retention, and black, tarry stools. These are adverse effects of prednisone.
   B. Tachycardia is an adverse effect of a bronchodilator.
   D. Nausea is an adverse effect of a bronchodilator.

   Ⓝ NCLEX® Connection: Physiological Adaptation, Alterations in Body Systems

5. A. **CORRECT:** When taking actions, the nurse should inform the client that there are portable oxygen systems that can be used when leaving the house. This should alleviate the client's anxiety.
   B, C, D. When assisting with discharge teaching, the nurse should tell the client to use oxygen at all times to prevent becoming hypoxic, encourage the client to return to a daily routine, but include periods of rest, and home health services promote a client's independence.

   Ⓝ NCLEX® Connection: Physiological Adaptation, Alterations in Body Systems

Active Learning Scenario Key

Using ATI Active Learning Template: Medication

NURSING INTERVENTIONS

- Observe the client for dry mouth when taking this medication.
- Encourage the client to suck on hard candies to help moisten dry mouth while taking ipratropium.
- Encourage the client to increase fluid intake, and to report headaches or blurred vision.
- Monitor heart rate. Palpitations can occur, which can indicate toxicity of ipratropium.

Ⓝ NCLEX® Connection: Pharmacological Therapies, Medication Administration

CHAPTER 21 *Tuberculosis*

Tuberculosis (TB) is an infectious disease caused by Mycobacterium tuberculosis. TB is transmitted through aerosolization (airborne route). Once inside the lung, the body encases the TB bacillus with collagen and other cells. This can appear as a round nodule or tubercle on a chest x-ray. The infection rate of TB in the United States (US) is 2.2/100,000. There is approximately 13 million people living in the US with latent tuberculosis.

Only a small percentage of people infected with TB develop an active form of the infection. The TB bacillus can lie dormant for many years before producing the disease. TB primarily affects the lungs but can spread to any organ in the blood. The risk of transmission decreases after 2 to 3 weeks of antituberculin therapy.

HEALTH PROMOTION AND DISEASE PREVENTION

- Clients who live in high-risk areas for tuberculosis should be screened on a yearly basis.
- Family members of clients who have tuberculosis should be screened.
- Screening is particularly important for people born outside the U.S. and migrant workers.
- Early detection and treatment are vital. TB has a slow onset, and the client might not be aware until the disease is advanced. TB diagnosis should be considered for any client who has a persistent cough, chest pain, weakness, weight loss, anorexia, hemoptysis, dyspnea, fever, night sweats, or chills.
- National and global health goals for tuberculosis include increasing the percentage of clients who complete treatment for TB.
- Individuals who have been exposed to TB but have not developed the disease can have latent TB. This means that Mycobacterium tuberculosis is in the body, but the body has been able to fight off the infection. If not treated, it can lie dormant for several years and then become active as the individual becomes older or immunocompromised. Ⓖ

DATA COLLECTION

RISK FACTORS

- Frequent and close contact with an untreated individual
- Lower socioeconomic status and without housing
- Immunocompromised status (HIV, chemotherapy, kidney disease, diabetes mellitus, Crohn's disease, selected malignancies such as head and neck cancers, organ transplants)
- Poorly ventilated, crowded environments (correctional or long-term care facilities)
- Advanced age
- Recent travel outside of the United States to areas where TB is endemic
- Immigration (from high prevalence rate areas such as Southeastern Asia, Africa, the Caribbean and Latin America)
- Substance use
- Health care occupation that involves performance of high-risk activities (respiratory treatments, suctioning, coughing procedures)

EXPECTED FINDINGS

- Persistent cough lasting longer than 3 weeks
- Purulent sputum, possibly blood-streaked
- Fatigue and lethargy
- Weight loss and anorexia
- Night sweats and low-grade fever in the afternoon

PHYSICAL FINDINGS: Older adult clients often present with atypical findings of the disease (altered mentation or unusual behavior, fever, anorexia, weight loss). Ⓖ

LABORATORY TESTS

Nucleic acid amplification testing

- Detects the presence of M. tuberculosis in respiratory secretions and can check for rifampin resistance. Results are available in less than 2 hr.
- The most rapid and accurate screening test for TB.

QuantiFERON-TB Gold and T-SPOT (interferon-gamma release assays or IGRAS)

Blood test that detects release of interferon-gamma (IFN-g) in fresh heparinized whole blood from sensitized people.
- Diagnostic for infection, whether active or latent.
- Results are available within 24 to 36 hrs.
- Preferred diagnostic for those who have received the bacille Calmette-Guerin (BCG) vaccine.

Acid-fast bacilli smear and culture

- A positive acid-fast test suggests an active infection.
- The diagnosis is confirmed by a positive culture for Mycobacterium tuberculosis.

NURSING ACTIONS

- Obtain three early-morning sputum samples.
- Wear personal protective equipment when obtaining specimens.
- Samples should also be obtained in a negative airflow room.

DIAGNOSTIC PROCEDURES

Mantoux test

- A client will have a positive intradermal TB test within 2 to 10 weeks of exposure to the infection.
- An intradermal injection of an extract of the tubercle bacillus is made. It should be read in 48 to 72 hr.
- An induration (palpable, raised, hardened area) of 5 mm is considered a positive test for clients who are at high risk (have HIV, had recent contact with someone who has TB, have positive chest x-ray, or immunosuppressed).
- An induration of 10 mm or greater in diameter indicates a positive test for clients who are at moderate risk (born in a country where TB is common, have a substance use disorder, work in a high-risk area such as a laboratory of congregate setting, have medical conditions which place them at high risk, or are younger than 5 years old).
- An induration of 15mm or more indicates a positive test for clients who have known risk factors for TB.
- A positive Mantoux test can indicate that the client has developed an immune response to TB. It does not confirm that active disease is present.
- Clients who have had a positive Mantoux test or have received a Bacillus Calmette-Guerin vaccine within the past 10 years can have a false-positive Mantoux test. These clients need a chest x-ray or QuantiFERON-TB Gold test to evaluate the presence of active TB infection. Ⓠ EBP

- Clients experiencing immunocompromise can demonstrate anergy, or lack of response to Mantoux testing, even if M. tuberculosis is present in the body. In this case, other diagnostic testing is indicated to rule out infection.
- Individuals who have latent TB can have a positive Mantoux test and can receive treatment to prevent development of an active form of the disease.
- Clients who are immunocompromised (such as those who have HIV) and older adult clients should be tested for TB. Clients starting immunosuppressive therapy (such as tumor necrosis factor antagonists) should be tested for TB prior to starting treatment.

CLIENT EDUCATION: Return for a reading of the injection site by a health care personnel between 48 and 72 hr.

Chest x-ray

Can be prescribed to detect active lesions in the lungs.

PATIENT-CENTERED CARE

NURSING CARE

- Administer humidified oxygen therapy as prescribed.
- Prevent infection transmission.
  - Wear a N95 HEPA filter or powered air purifying respirator when caring for clients who are hospitalized with TB.
  - Place the client in a negative-airflow room, and implement airborne precautions.
  - Use barrier protection when the risk of hand or clothing contamination exists.
  - Have the client wear a surgical mask if transportation to another department is necessary. The client should be transported using the shortest and least busy route.
  - Instruct the client to cough and expectorate sputum into tissues that are disposed of by the client into provided plastic bags or no-touch receptacles.

21.1 Mantoux test

21.2 N95 mask

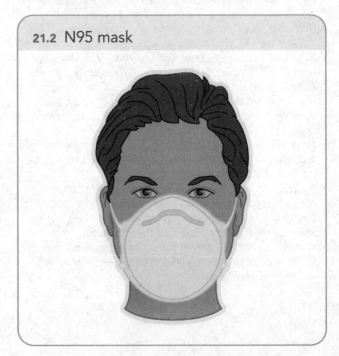

- Administer prescribed medications.
- Promote adequate nutrition.
  - Encourage fluid intake and a well-balanced diet for adequate caloric intake.
  - Encourage foods that are rich in protein, iron, and vitamins C and B.
- Provide emotional support.
- Test exposed family members for TB

MEDICATIONS

Due to the resistance that is developing against the antituberculin medications, combination therapy of two or more medications at a time is recommended.

- Because these medications must be taken for 6 to 12 months, medication noncompliance is a significant contributing factor in the development of resistant strains of TB.
- The typical four-medication regimen includes isoniazid, rifampin, pyrazinamide, and ethambutol.

CLIENT EDUCATION: Complete the series of prescribed medication to ensure all bacteria are eliminated and to decrease the chance of resistance.

Isoniazid

Isoniazid, commonly referred to as INH, is bactericidal and inhibits growth of mycobacteria by preventing synthesis of mycolic acid in the cell wall.

NURSING ACTIONS
- This medication should be taken on an empty stomach.
- Monitor for hepatotoxicity (jaundice, anorexia, malaise, fatigue, and nausea) and neurotoxicity (such as tingling of the hands and feet).
- Vitamin B6 (pyridoxine) is often prescribed concurrently to prevent neurotoxicity from isoniazid.
- Liver function testing should be completed prior to and monthly after starting INH.

CLIENT EDUCATION
- Do not drink alcohol while taking isoniazid, because it can increase the risk for hepatotoxicity. Qs
- Report any manifestations of hepatotoxicity.

Rifampin

Rifampin, commonly referred to as RIF, is a bacteriostatic and bactericidal antibiotic that inhibits DNA-dependent RNA polymerase activity in susceptible cells.

NURSING ACTIONS
- Observe for hepatotoxicity.
- Liver function testing should be completed prior to and at least monthly after starting RIF.

CLIENT EDUCATION
- Urine and other secretions will be orange.
- Discoloration of contact lenses can occur.
- Immediately report pain or swelling of joints, loss of appetite, jaundice, or malaise.
- This medication can interfere with the efficacy of oral contraceptives.

Pyrazinamide

Pyrazinamide, commonly referred to as PZA, is a bacteriostatic and bactericidal. Its exact mechanism of action is unknown.

NURSING ACTIONS
- Observe for hepatotoxicity.
- Check for history of gout, as the medication will cause an adverse effect of non-gouty polyarthralgia.
- Liver enzymes should be completed baseline and every 2 weeks after starting PZA.

CLIENT EDUCATION
- Drink a glass of water with each dose and increase fluids during the day to help prevent gout and kidney problems.
- Immediately report yellowing of the skin or eyes, pain or swelling of joints, loss of appetite, or malaise.
- Avoid using alcohol while taking pyrazinamide.

Ethambutol

- Ethambutol, commonly referred to as EMB, is a bacteriostatic and works by suppressing RNA synthesis, subsequently inhibiting protein synthesis.
- This medication should not be given to children younger than 8 years of age.

NURSING ACTIONS
- Obtain baseline visual acuity tests, and complete monthly after starting treatment.
- Determine color discrimination ability before starting treatment, and periodically.
- Stop medication immediately if ocular toxicity occurs.

CLIENT EDUCATION: Report changes in vision immediately. QEBP

Streptomycin sulfate

Streptomycin sulfate is an aminoglycoside antibiotic. It potentiates the efficacy of macrophages during phagocytosis.

NURSING ACTIONS
- Due to its high level of toxicity, this medication should be used only in clients who have multidrug-resistant TB (MDR-TB).
- Streptomycin can cause ototoxicity, so monitor hearing function and tolerance often.
- Report significant changes in urine output and renal function studies.

CLIENT EDUCATION
- Drink at least 2 L of fluid daily.
- Notify the provider if hearing declines.

INTERPROFESSIONAL CARE

- Contact social services if the client will need assistance in obtaining prescribed medications.
- Assist with referring the client to a community clinic as needed for follow-up appointments to monitor medication regimen and status of disease.

CLIENT EDUCATION

- TB is often treated in the home setting. Q_{PCC}
- Airborne precautions are not needed in the home setting because family members have already been exposed.
- Exposed family members should be tested for TB.
- Continue medication therapy for its full duration of 6 to 12 months, even up to 2 years for multidrug-resistant TB. Failure to take the medications can lead to a resistant strain of TB.
- Continue with follow-up care for 1 full year.
- Sputum samples are needed every 2 to 4 weeks to monitor therapy effectiveness. Clients are no longer considered infectious after three consecutive negative sputum cultures and can resume work and social interactions.
- Practice proper hand hygiene.
- Cover mouth and nose when coughing or sneezing.
- Contaminated tissues should be disposed of in plastic bags.
- While TB is active, wear a mask when in public places or in contact with crowds.

COMPLICATIONS

Miliary TB

The organism invades the bloodstream and can spread to multiple body organs with complications including the following.

- Headaches, neck stiffness, and drowsiness (can be life-threatening)
- Pericarditis: Dyspnea, swollen neck veins, pleuritic pain, and hypotension due to an accumulation of fluid in pericardial sac that inhibits the heart's ability to pump effectively

NURSING ACTIONS: Treatment is the same as for pulmonary TB.

Active Learning Scenario

A nurse is caring for a client who has tuberculosis. Use the ATI Active Learning Template: System Disorder to complete this item.

PATHOPHYSIOLOGY RELATED TO CLIENT PROBLEM

NURSING CARE: Include three nursing interventions.

COMPLICATIONS: Identify one potential complication.

Application Exercises

1. A nurse is providing information about tuberculosis to a group of clients at a local community center. Which of the following manifestations should the nurse include? (Select all that apply.)

   A. Persistent cough

   B. Weight gain

   C. Fatigue

   D. Night sweats

   E. Purulent sputum

2. A nurse in an outpatient facility is caring for a client who has HIV and is desiring to have a reading of their Mantoux test 48 hours following administration. What amount of Mantoux test induration (in mm) is considered a positive for this client?

3. A nurse is caring for a client who has a new diagnosis of tuberculosis and has been placed on a multi-medication regimen. Which of the following instructions should the nurse give the client related to ethambutol?

   A. "Your urine can turn a dark orange."

   B. "Watch for a change in the sclera of your eyes."

   C. "Watch for any changes in vision."

   D. "Take vitamin B_6 daily."

4. A nurse is assisting in the care of a client who has a new prescription for isoniazid (INH) and is providing education about the adverse effects. Which of the following statements should the nurse make? (Select all that apply.)

   A. "You might notice yellowing of your skin."

   B. "You might experience pain in your joints."

   C. "You might develop ringing in your ears."

   D. "You might notice tingling of your hands."

   E. "You might experience a loss of appetite."

5. Monitor client for actual and potential adverse effects of medications (e.g., prescribed, over-the-counter and/or herbal supplements)

A. Ethambutol	1. Color discrimination testing needs to be done prior to starting treatment and then periodically
B. Rifampin	2. Advise clients who wear contact lenses to wear eyeglasses while under treatment.
C. Isoniazid	3. Report client complaints of tinnitus
D. Streptomycin	4. Check client for complaints of paresthesia

Application Exercises Key

1. A, C, D, E. **CORRECT:** A persistent cough, fatigue, night sweats and purulent sputum are manifestations of tuberculosis
   B. Weight loss is a manifestation of tuberculosis.

   Ⓝ *NCLEX® Connection: Physiological Adaptation, Basic Pathophysiology*

2. The size of induration is significant in determining reaction. A reaction of 5 mm or greater is considered positive for a client who has HIV. An induration of 10 mm or greater is considered positive in a client with expected immunity.

   Ⓝ *NCLEX Connection: Health Promotion and Maintenance, Health Promotion/Disease Prevention*

3. A. The client who is taking rifampin should expect to see the urine turn a dark orange
   B. Ethambutol does not have an adverse effect resulting in changes to the sclera of the eyes.
   C. **CORRECT:** The client who is receiving ethambutol will need to watch for visual changes due to optic neuritis, which can result from taking this medication.
   D. The client taking isoniazid should take vitamin B$_6$ daily and observe for signs of hepatotoxicity.

   Ⓝ *NCLEX® Connection: Pharmacological Therapies, Expected Actions/Outcomes*

4. A. **CORRECT:** Yellowing of the skin can be an adverse effect of isoniazid, rifampin or pyrazinamide as a result of hepatotoxicity in a client who has light skin.
   B. Pain in the joints and loss of appetite can be adverse effects of rifampin.
   C. Streptomycin can cause ototoxicity, so monitor hearing function and often.
   D. **CORRECT:** Tingling of the hands can be an adverse effect of isoniazid.
   E. Pain in the joints and loss of appetite can be adverse effects of rifampin.

   Ⓝ *NCLEX Connection: Pharmacological Therapies, Adverse Effects/ Contraindications/Side Effects/Interaction*

5. A, 4; B, 3; C. 2; D, 1;

   Streptomycin - Report client complaints of tinnitus. Streptomycin can cause ototoxicity. Isoniazid – Check client for complaints of paresthesia. Isoniazid can cause neurotoxicity. Rifampin – Advise clients who wear contact lenses to wear eyeglasses while under treatment. Rifampin discolors bodily fluids such as tears and can discolor contact lenses. Ethambutol – Color discrimination needs to be done prior to starting treatment and then periodically. Ethambutol can cause ocular toxicity.

   Ⓝ *NCLEX Connection: Pharmacological Therapies, Adverse Effects/ Contraindications/Side Effects/Interaction*

Active Learning Scenario Key

Using the ATI Active Learning Template: System Disorder

PATHOPHYSIOLOGY RELATED TO CLIENT PROBLEM: Tuberculosis (TB) is an infectious disease caused by *Mycobacterium tuberculosis*. TB is transmitted through aerosolization (airborne route). Once inside the lung, the body encases the TB bacillus with collagen and other cells. This can appear as a Ghon tubercle on a chest x-ray. Only a small percentage of people infected with TB actually develop an active form of the infection. The TB bacillus can lie dormant for many years before producing the disease. TB primarily affects the lungs but can spread to any organ in the blood.

NURSING CARE

Nursing Interventions
- Administer humidified oxygen therapy as prescribed.
- Prevent infection transmission.
- Wear an N95 or HEPA respirator when caring for clients who are hospitalized with TB.
- Place the client in a negative airflow room, and implement airborne precautions.
- Use barrier protection when the risk of hand or clothing contamination exists.
- Have the client wear a surgical mask if transportation to another department is necessary.
- Transport the client using the shortest and least busy route.
- Instruct the client to cough and expectorate sputum into tissues that are disposed of by the client into provided sacks.
- Administer medications as prescribed.
- Promote adequate nutrition.
- Encourage fluid intake and a well-balanced diet for adequate caloric intake.

COMPLICATIONS

Miliary TB: The organism invades the bloodstream and can spread to multiple body organs with complications including the following:
- Headaches, neck stiffness, and drowsiness (can be life-threatening)
- Pericarditis: dyspnea, swollen neck veins, pleuritic pain, and hypotension due to an accumulation of fluid in the pericardial sac that inhibits the heart's ability to pump effectively
- Nursing Actions: Treatment is the same as for pulmonary TB.

Ⓝ *NCLEX® Connection: Physiological Adaptation, Alterations in Body Systems*

When reviewing the following chapters, keep in mind the relevant topics and tasks of the NCLEX outline.

Pharmacological Therapies

EXPECTED ACTIONS/OUTCOMES
Evaluate client response to medication.

Apply knowledge of pathophysiology when addressing client pharmacological agents.

MEDICATION ADMINISTRATION
Reinforce client teaching on client self administration of medications.

Collect required data prior to medication administration.

Reduction of Risk Potential

POTENTIAL FOR COMPLICATIONS OF DIAGNOSTIC TESTS/TREATMENTS/PROCEDURES: Maintain client tube patency.

POTENTIAL FOR ALTERATIONS IN BODY SYSTEMS: Perform focused data collection based on client condition (e.g., neurological checks, circulatory checks).

Physiological Adaptation

ALTERATIONS IN BODY SYSTEMS
Provide care to client on ventilator.

Intervene to improve client respiratory status.

MEDICAL EMERGENCIES: Respond and intervene to a client life-threatening situation.

CHAPTER 22 *Pulmonary Embolism*

A pulmonary embolism (PE) occurs when a substance (solid, gaseous, or liquid) enters venous circulation and forms a blockage in the pulmonary vasculature.

Emboli originating from venous thromboembolism (VTE) are the most common cause. Other types of emboli include fat, air, septic (due to bacterial invasion of a thrombus), and amniotic fluid.

Increased hypoxia to pulmonary tissue and impaired blood flow can result from a large embolus. A PE is a medical emergency.

Mortality from PE is greater in older adults while young females assigned at birth are more prone to die from PE than males assigned at birth within the same age group. A recent study indicated PE occurred more frequently in clients with COVID-19 versus those with influenza, and mortality was significantly higher in those clients as compared to the general client population. Prevention, rapid recognition, and treatment of a PE are essential for a positive outcome.

HEALTH PROMOTION AND DISEASE PREVENTION

- Promote smoking cessation.
- Encourage maintenance of appropriate weight for height and body frame.
- Encourage a healthy diet and physical activity.
- Prevent DVT by encouraging clients to do leg exercises, wear compression stockings, and avoid sitting for long periods of time.

DATA COLLECTION

RISK FACTORS

- Long-term immobility
- Oral contraceptive use and estrogen therapy
- Pregnancy
- Tobacco use
- Hypercoagulability (elevated platelet count)
- Obesity
- Surgery (especially orthopedic surgery of the lower extremities or pelvis)
- Central venous catheters
- Heart failure or chronic atrial fibrillation
- Autoimmune hemolytic anemia (sickle cell)
- Long bone fractures
- Cancer
- Trauma
- Septicemia
- Advanced age ⑥
  - Older adult clients have decreased pulmonary reserves due to normal lung changes, including decreased lung elasticity and thickening alveoli. Older adult clients can decompensate more quickly.
  - Certain pathological conditions and procedures that predispose clients to DVT formation (peripheral vascular disease, hypertension, hip and knee arthroplasty) are more prevalent in older adults.
  - Many older adult clients experience decreased physical activity levels, thus predisposing them to DVT formation and pulmonary emboli.

EXPECTED FINDINGS

- Anxiety
- Feelings of impending doom
- Sudden onset of chest pressure
- Pain upon inspiration and chest wall tenderness
- Dyspnea and air hunger
- Cough
- Hemoptysis

PHYSICAL FINDINGS

- Pleurisy
- Pleural friction rub
- Tachycardia
- Hypotension
- Tachypnea
- Adventitious breath sounds (crackles) and cough
- Heart murmur in S3 and S4
- Diaphoresis
- Low-grade fever
- Decreased oxygen saturation levels (expected reference range is 95% to 100%), low SaO2, cyanosis
- Petechiae (red dots under the skin) over chest and axillae
- Distended neck veins
- Syncope
- Cyanosis

LABORATORY TESTS

ABG analysis

- PaCO2 levels are low (expected reference range is 35 to 45 mm Hg) due to initial hyperventilation (respiratory alkalosis).
- As hypoxemia progresses, respiratory acidosis occurs.
- Further progression leads to metabolic acidosis due to buildup of lactic acid from tissue hypoxia.

D-dimer

Elevated above expected reference range in response to clot formation and release of fibrin degradation products (expected reference range is less than 0.4 mcg/mL).

DIAGNOSTIC PROCEDURES

Computed tomography scan

The multidetector-row computed tomography angiography (MDCTA) is the criterion standard for detecting PE when available, as it provides high-quality visualization of the lung parenchyma.

Ventilation-perfusion scan

Ventilation-perfusion (V/Q) scan images show circulation of air and blood in the lungs and can detect a PE. Useful when client allergy to contrast media is a contraindication to other types of imaging.

Chest x-ray

The chest x-ray can provide data to support the occurrence of pulmonary embolism (elevation of the diaphragm on the affected side or pleural effusion).

PATIENT-CENTERED CARE

NURSING CARE

- Administer oxygen therapy to relieve hypoxemia and dyspnea. Position the client to maximize ventilation (high-Fowler's = 90°).
- Initiate and maintain IV access.
- Administer medications as prescribed.
- Check respiratory status at least every 30 min. Q PCC
  - Auscultate lung sounds.
  - Measure rate, rhythm, and ease of respirations.
  - Inspect skin color and capillary refill.
  - Examine for position of trachea.
- Monitor cardiac status. Q PCC
  - Check for dysrhythmias on cardiac monitor.
- Provide emotional support and comfort to control client anxiety.
- Monitor changes in level of consciousness and mental status.

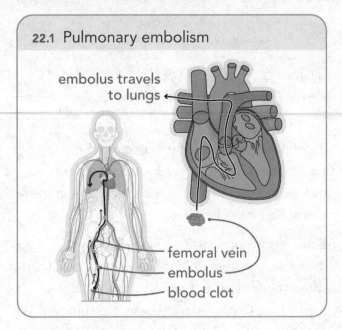

22.1 Pulmonary embolism

embolus travels to lungs ←

femoral vein
embolus
blood clot

MEDICATIONS

Anticoagulants

Unfractionated and low molecular weight heparin, enoxaparin, and warfarin are used to prevent clots from getting larger or additional clots from forming.

NURSING ACTIONS
- Check for contraindications (active bleeding, peptic ulcer disease, history of stroke, recent trauma).
- Monitor bleeding times: Prothrombin time (PT) and international normalized ratio (INR) for warfarin, partial thromboplastin time (aPTT) for heparin, and complete blood count (CBC). Q EBP
- Monitor for adverse effects of anticoagulants (thrombocytopenia, anemia, hemorrhage).

Direct factor Xa inhibitor

Rivaroxaban, apixaban, and fondaparinux bind directly with the active center of factor Xa, which inhibits the production of thrombin.

NURSING ACTIONS
- Check for bleeding from any site. (Clients have experienced epidural hematomas, as well as intracranial, retinal, adrenal, and GI bleeds.)
- Hold medication for 18 hr prior to and 6 hr after removal of an epidural catheter.

Direct thrombin inhibitor

Dabigatran acts as a direct inhibitor of thrombin.

NURSING ACTIONS: Check for bleeding and manifestations of blood loss.

Thrombolytic therapy

- Alteplase, reteplase, and tenecteplase are used to dissolve blood clots and restore pulmonary blood flow.
- Similar adverse effects and contraindications as anticoagulants.

NURSING ACTIONS

- Check for contraindications (known bleeding disorders, uncontrolled hypertension, active bleeding, peptic ulcer disease, history of stroke, recent trauma or surgery, pregnancy).
- Monitor for evidence of bleeding, thrombocytopenia, and anemia.
- Monitor blood pressure, heart rate, respirations, and oxygen saturation per facility protocol before, during, and after administration of medication. Qs

INTERPROFESSIONAL CARE

- Cardiology and pulmonary services should be consulted to manage a PE and treatment.
- Respiratory services should be consulted for oxygen therapy, breathing treatments, and ABGs.
- Radiology should be consulted for diagnostic studies to determine PE.

THERAPEUTIC PROCEDURES

Embolectomy

Surgical removal of embolus

NURSING ACTIONS

- Prepare the client for the procedure (NPO status, informed consent).
- Monitor postoperatively (vital signs, SaO2, incision drainage, pain management).

Inferior vena cava filter (ICVF)

Typically used for clients in which anticoagulation therapy is contraindicated, a filter is inserted in the vena cava to prevent emboli from reaching the pulmonary vasculature

NURSING ACTIONS

- Prepare the client for the procedure (NPO status, informed consent).
- Monitor postoperatively (vital signs, SaO2, incision drainage, pain management).

CLIENT EDUCATION

- If homebound, set up home care services to perform weekly blood draws.
- For severe dyspnea, set up referral services to supply portable oxygen.
- Follow recommendations for prevention of a PE. Qpcc
- If smoking, consider smoking cessation.
  - Avoid long periods of immobility.
  - Perform physical activity, such as walking.
  - Wear compression stockings to promote circulation.
  - Avoid crossing the legs.
- If taking warfarin, do not increase or decrease the amount of vitamin K foods consumed (green, leafy vegetables). Vitamin K can reduce the anticoagulant effects of warfarin.

- Adhere to a schedule for monitoring PT and INR, and follow instructions regarding medication dosage adjustments (if on warfarin) and regular blood draws.
- There is an increased risk for bruising and bleeding.
  - Avoid taking aspirin products, unless specified by the provider.
  - Check the mouth and skin daily for bleeding and bruising.
  - Use electric shavers and soft-bristled toothbrushes.
  - Avoid blowing the nose hard, and gently apply pressure if nose bleeds occur.
- If traveling, take measures to prevent PE.
  - Arise from a sitting position for 5 min out of every hour.
  - Wear support stockings.
  - Remain hydrated by drinking plenty of water.
  - Perform active ROM exercises when sitting (ankle pump exercises).

COMPLICATIONS

Decreased cardiac output

Blood volume is decreased.

NURSING ACTIONS

- Monitor for hypotension, tachycardia, cyanosis, jugular venous distention, and syncope.
- Check for the presence of S3 or S4 heart sounds.
- Initiate and maintain IV access.
- Monitor urinary output (should be 30 mL/hr or more).
- Administer IV fluids (crystalloids) to replace vascular volume.
- Continuously monitor the ECG.
- Monitor pulmonary pressures. IV fluids can contribute to pulmonary hypertension for clients who have right-sided heart failure (cor pulmonale).
- Administer inotropic agents (milrinone, dobutamine) to increase myocardial contractility.
- Vasodilators can be needed if pulmonary artery pressure is high enough to interfere with cardiac contractility.

Hemorrhage

Risk for bleeding increases due to anticoagulant therapy.

NURSING ACTIONS

- Check for bleeding from or bruising around injection and surgical sites at least every 2 hr.
- Monitor cardiovascular status (blood pressure, heart rate and rhythm).
- Monitor CBC (hemoglobin, hematocrit, platelets) and bleeding times (PT, aPTT, INR).
- Administer IV fluids and blood products as required.
- Test stool, urine, and emesis for occult blood.
- Monitor for internal bleeding (measure abdominal girth and check for abdominal or flank pain) at least every 8 hr.
- Have antidote available for use if necessary.

Active Learning Scenario

A nurse is caring for a client who has a pulmonary embolism. Use the ATI Active Learning Template: System Disorder to complete this item.

PATHOPHYSIOLOGY RELATED TO CLIENT PROBLEM

NURSING CARE: Describe three nursing interventions.

MEDICATIONS: Identify two.

Application Exercises

1. A nurse is caring for a group of clients. Which of the following clients are at risk for a pulmonary embolism? (Select all that apply.)
   A. A client who has a BMI of 30
   B. A female client who is postmenopausal
   C. A client who has a fractured femur
   D. A client who is a marathon runner
   E. A client who has chronic atrial fibrillation

2. A nurse is collecting data on a client who has a pulmonary embolism. Which of the following manifestations should the nurse expect? (Select all that apply.)
   A. Bradypnea
   B. Cough
   C. Hypertension
   D. Chest pain
   E. Tachycardia

3. A nurse is reviewing prescriptions for a client who has acute dyspnea and diaphoresis. The client states, "I am anxious and unable to get enough air." Vital signs are heart rate 117/min, respirations 38/min, temperature 38.4° C (101.2° F), and blood pressure 100/54 mm Hg. Which of the following nursing actions is the priority?
   A. Notify the provider.
   B. Assist with administering heparin via IV infusion.
   C. Administer oxygen therapy.
   D. Obtain a CT scan..

4. A nurse is caring for a client who has a new prescription for heparin therapy. Which of the following statements by the client should indicate an immediate concern for the nurse?
   A. "I am allergic to morphine."
   B. "I take antacids several times a day for my ulcer."
   C. "I had a blood clot in my leg several years ago."
   D. "It hurts to take a deep breath."

5. A nurse is caring for a client who is to receive thrombolytic therapy. Which of the following factors should the nurse recognize as a contraindication to the therapy?
   A. Hip arthroplasty 2 weeks ago
   B. Elevated sedimentation rate
   C. Incident of exercise-induced asthma 1 week ago
   D. Elevated platelet count

Application Exercises Key

1. **A, C, E. CORRECT:** When analyzing cues, the nurse should recognize a client who has a BMI of 30 is considered obese and is at risk for a blood clot which can lead to a pulmonary embolism. The nurse should also recognize a client who has turbulent blood flow of the heart such as with atrial fibrillation is at risk for a blood clot, which can lead to a pulmonary embolism.

Ⓝ *NCLEX® Connection: Health Promotion and Maintenance, Health Promotion/Disease Prevention*

2. **B, D, E. CORRECT:** When recognizing cues, the nurse should identify a cough, chest pain and tachycardia are manifestations of a pulmonary embolism.

Ⓝ *NCLEX Connection: Physiological Adaptation, Basic Pathophysiology*

3. A. The nurse should notify the provider about the condition to obtain guidance on treatment. However, another action is the priority.
   B. The nurse should assist with administering IV heparin as a treatment to prevent growth of the existing clot and to prevent additional clots from forming. However, another action is the priority.
   C. **CORRECT:** When using the airway, breathing, circulation (ABC) approach to client care, the nurse determines that the priority finding is to address the client's respiratory status; therefore the nurse should administer oxygen therapy to relieve the client's dyspnea, diaphoresis and tachypnea.
   D. The nurse should request to obtain a CT scan to detect the presence and location of the blood clot. However, another action is the priority.

Ⓝ *NCLEX® Connection: Physiological Adaptation, Basic Pathophysiology*

4. A. The nurse should document the client's allergy to morphine to manage the client's discomfort due to a blood clot. However, another action is the priority.
   B. **CORRECT:** The greatest risk to the client is the possibility of bleeding from a peptic ulcer; therefore, the priority intervention is to notify the provider of the finding.
   C. The nurse should document the client's history of a blood clot to provide preventative measures. However, another action is the priority.
   D. The nurse should expect the client to report pain with breathing. However, another action is the priority.

Ⓝ *NCLEX® Connection: Pharmacological Therapies, Expected Actions/Outcomes*

5. A. **CORRECT:** When analyzing cues, the nurse should recognize a contraindication to the client receiving thrombolytic therapy is undergoing major surgery within the last three weeks due to the risk of bleeding from the surgical site.

Ⓝ *NCLEX® Connection: Pharmacological Therapies, Expected Actions/Outcomes*

Active Learning Scenario Key

Using the ATI Active Learning Template: System Disorder

PATHOPHYSIOLOGY RELATED TO CLIENT PROBLEM: A pulmonary embolism (PE) occurs when a substance (solid, gaseous, or liquid) enters venous circulation and forms a blockage in the pulmonary vasculature. Emboli originating from deep-vein thrombosis (DVT) are the most common cause. Tumors, bone marrow, amniotic fluid, and foreign matter can also become emboli.

NURSING CARE
- Administer oxygen therapy as prescribed to relieve hypoxemia and dyspnea.
- Position the client to maximize ventilation (high-Fowler's = 90%).
- Initiate and maintain IV access.
- Administer medications as prescribed.
- Provide emotional support and comfort to control client anxiety.
- Monitor changes in level of consciousness and mental status.

MEDICATIONS
- Anticoagulants: enoxaparin, heparin, and warfarin
- Thrombolytic therapy: alteplase, reteplase, and tenecteplase

Ⓝ *NCLEX® Connection: Physiological Adaptation, Alterations in Body Systems*

CHAPTER 23

CHAPTER 23
Pneumothorax, Hemothorax, and Flail Chest

A pneumothorax is the presence of air or gas in the pleural space that causes lung collapse.

A tension pneumothorax occurs when air enters the pleural space during inspiration through a one-way valve and is not able to exit upon expiration. The trapped air causes pressure on the heart and the lung. As a result, the increase in pressure compresses blood vessels and limits venous return, leading to a decrease in cardiac output. Death can result if not treated immediately. As a result of a tension pneumothorax, air and pressure continue to rise in the pleural cavity, which causes a mediastinal shift.

A hemothorax is an accumulation of blood in the pleural space.

A spontaneous pneumothorax can occur when there has been no trauma. A small bleb on the lung ruptures and air enters the pleural space.

A flail chest occurs when at least two neighboring ribs, usually on one side of the chest, sustain multiple fractures, causing instability of the chest wall and paradoxical chest wall movement. This results in significant limitation in chest wall expansion.

Pneumothorax and hemothorax

DATA COLLECTION

RISK FACTORS
- Blunt chest trauma
- Penetrating chest wounds
- Closed/occluded chest tube
- Chronic obstructive pulmonary disease (COPD)

EXPECTED FINDINGS
- Anxiety
- Pleuritic pain

PHYSICAL FINDINGS
- Manifestations of respiratory distress (tachypnea, tachycardia, hypoxia, cyanosis, dyspnea, and use of accessory muscles)
- Tracheal deviation to the unaffected side (tension pneumothorax)
- Reduced or absent breath sounds on the affected side
- Asymmetrical chest wall movement
- Hyperresonance on percussion due to trapped air (pneumothorax)
- Subcutaneous emphysema (air accumulating in subcutaneous tissue)

23.1 Pneumothorax

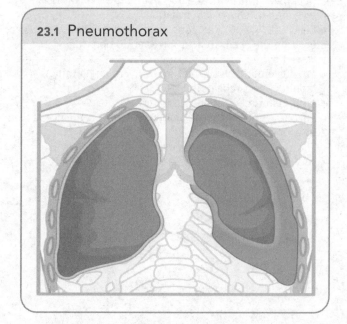

DIAGNOSTIC PROCEDURES

Chest x-ray

Used to confirm pneumothorax or hemothorax

Thoracentesis

Thoracentesis is the surgical perforation of the chest wall and pleural space with a large-bore needle.

NURSING ACTIONS
- Ensure that informed consent has been obtained.
- Assist with client positioning and specimen transport.
- Monitor status (vital signs, SaO_2, injection site).
- Assist the client to the edge of the bed and to lean over a bedside table.

CLIENT EDUCATION
- Remain still during the procedure (no moving, coughing, or deep breathing).
- Discomfort will be felt when the local anesthetic solution is injected. When the needle is inserted into the pleural space, some pressure can be felt, but no pain.

PATIENT-CENTERED CARE

NURSING CARE

- Administer oxygen therapy.
- Auscultate heart and lung sounds and monitor vital signs every 4 hr.
- Document ventilator settings hourly if the client is receiving mechanical ventilation.
- Check ABGs, SaO_2, CBC, and chest x-ray results.
- Position the client to maximize ventilation (high-Fowler's = 90°).
- Provide emotional support to the client and family.
- Monitor chest tube drainage. ⓠEBP
- Administer medications as prescribed.
- Encourage prompt medical attention when evidence of infection occurs.
- Set up referral services (home health, respiratory services) to provide portable oxygen if needed. ⓠTC

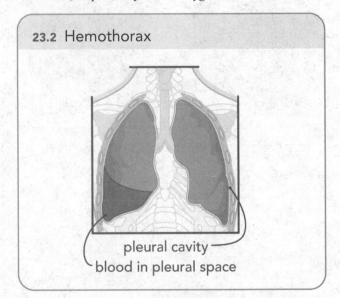

23.2 Hemothorax

pleural cavity
blood in pleural space

MEDICATIONS

Benzodiazepines (sedatives)

Lorazepam or diazepam can be used to decrease anxiety.

NURSING ACTIONS
- Monitor vital signs. (Benzodiazepines can cause hypotension and respiratory distress.)
- Remember that the medications have amnesiac effects.
- Monitor for paradoxical effects (euphoria, rage).

CLIENT EDUCATION: Medications have amnesic effects and cause drowsiness.

Opioid agonists (pain medications)

- Morphine sulfate and fentanyl are opioid agents used to treat moderate to severe pain. These medications act on the mu and kappa receptors that help alleviate pain.
- Activation of these receptors produces analgesia (pain relief), respiratory depression, euphoria, sedation, and decrease in gastrointestinal motility.

NURSING ACTIONS
- Use cautiously for clients who have asthma or emphysema, due to the risk of respiratory depression.
- Check pain every 4 hr.
- Monitor clients, especially older adults, for manifestations of respiratory depression. If respirations are 12/min or less, stop the medication and notify provider immediately.
- Monitor vital signs for hypotension and bradypnea.
- Monitor for nausea and vomiting.
- Monitor level of sedation (drowsiness, level of consciousness).
- Monitor for constipation.
- Encourage fluid intake and activity related to a decrease in gastric motility.
- Monitor intake and output. Report fluid retention as an adverse effect of opioid medications.

CLIENT EDUCATION
- If receiving a fentanyl patch, the initial patch takes several hours to take effect. A short-acting pain medication is administered for breakthrough pain.
- If there are no fluid restrictions due to other conditions, drink plenty of fluids to prevent constipation.
- Follow instructions on how to use a patient-controlled analgesia (PCA) pump if applicable. The client is the only person who should push the medication administration button. The safety lockout mechanism on the PCA prevents the client from using too much medication.

INTERPROFESSIONAL CARE

Respiratory services should be consulted for ABGs, breathing treatments, and suctioning for airway management.

Pain management services can be consulted if pain persists or is uncontrolled.

Rehabilitation care can be consulted if the client has prolonged weakness and needs assistance with an increasing level of activity.

THERAPEUTIC PROCEDURES

Chest tube insertion

Chest tubes are inserted in the pleural space to drain fluid, blood, or air; re-establish a negative pressure; facilitate lung expansion; and restore normal intrapleural pressure.

NURSING ACTIONS

- Assist with obtaining informed consent, gather supplies, monitor the client's status (vital signs, SaO₂, chest tube drainage), report abnormalities to the provider, and administer pain medications.
- Continually monitor vital signs and the client's response to the procedure.
- Monitor chest tube placement, function of chest drainage system, and dressing.

CLIENT EDUCATION

- Take deep breaths to promote lung expansion.
- Take rest periods as needed.
- Use proper hand hygiene to prevent infection.
- Participate in coughing, deep breathing, and use of incentive spirometry.
- Obtain immunizations for influenza and pneumonia.
- Recovery from a pneumothorax/hemothorax can be lengthy.
- Talk with family or other support people to express feelings about the condition and recovery.
- If applicable, consider smoking cessation.
- Follow up with the provider as instructed, and report the following to the provider.
  - Upper respiratory infection
  - Fever
  - Cough
  - Difficulty breathing
  - Sharp chest pain

COMPLICATIONS

Decreased cardiac output

- The amount of blood pumped by the heart decreases as intrathoracic pressure rises.
- Hypotension develops.

NURSING ACTIONS

- Administer IV fluids and blood products as prescribed.
- Monitor heart rate and rhythm.
- Monitor intake and output (chest tube drainage).

Respiratory failure

Inadequate gas exchange due to lung collapse

NURSING ACTIONS

- Prepare for mechanical ventilation.
- Continue respiratory data collection.

Flail chest

As a result of the free-floating rib segments, the lung below the flail segment caves in on inhalation and balloons out on exhalation. The portion of the lung below the flail segment cannot participate in gas exchange, so oxygenation is compromised.

DATA COLLECTION

RISK FACTORS

Multiple rib fractures from blunt chest trauma

EXPECTED FINDINGS

- Unequal chest expansion (the unaffected side of the chest will expand, while the affected side can appear to diminish in size or remain stationary)
- Paradoxical chest wall movement (inward movement of segment during inspiration, outward movement of segment during expiration)
- Tachycardia
- Hypotension
- Dyspnea
- Cyanosis
- Anxiety
- Chest pain

PATIENT-CENTERED CARE

NURSING CARE

- Administer humidified oxygen.
- Monitor vital signs and SaO₂.
- Review findings of pulmonary function tests, periodic chest x-rays, and ABGs.
- Monitor lung sounds, color, and capillary refill.
- Promote lung expansion by encouraging deep breathing and proper positioning.
- Maintain mechanical ventilation in the event of severe injury to establish adequate gas exchange and stabilize the injury. (Flail chest is usually stabilized by positive-pressure ventilation.)
- Suction trachea and endotracheal tube as needed.
- Administer pain medication. Patient-controlled analgesia or an epidural block commonly is used.
- Administer IV fluids as prescribed.
- Monitor intake and output.
- Offer support and reassurance by explaining all procedures.

Active Learning Scenario

A nurse is reinforcing teaching to a newly licensed nurse regarding care for a client who has a hemothorax. What should be included in this review? Use the ATI Active Learning Template: System Disorder to complete this item.

DESCRIPTION OF DISORDER/DISEASE PROCESS

NURSING CARE: Describe three nursing interventions.

MEDICATIONS: Describe two medications used for hemothorax.

Application Exercises

1. A nurse is collecting data from a client following a gunshot wound to the chest. For which of the following findings should the nurse monitor to detect a pneumothorax? (Select all that apply.)
   A. Tachypnea
   B. Deviation of the trachea
   C. Bradycardia
   D. Decreased use of accessory muscles
   E. Pleuritic pain

2. A nurse is assisting the provider with care for a client who has developed a spontaneous pneumothorax. Which of the following actions should the nurse perform first?
   A. Collect data regarding the client's pain.
   B. Obtain a large-bore IV needle for decompression.
   C. Administer lorazepam.
   D. Prepare for chest tube insertion.

3. A nurse is reinforcing discharge instructions with a client who has COPD and experienced a pneumothorax. Which of the following statements should the nurse include?
   A. "Notify your provider if you experience weakness."
   B. "You should be able to return to work in 1 week."
   C. "You need to wear a mask when in crowded areas."
   D. "Notify your provider if you experience a productive cough."

4. A nurse in the emergency department is collecting data from a client who has sustained multiple rib fractures and has a flail chest. Which of the following findings should the nurse expect? (Select all that apply.)
   A. Bradycardia
   B. Cyanosis
   C. Hypotension
   D. Dyspnea
   E. Paradoxical chest movement

Application Exercises Key

1. A. **CORRECT:** The client who has a pneumothorax can experience tachypnea related to respiratory distress caused by the injury.
   B. **CORRECT:** The client who has a pneumothorax can experience deviation of the trachea as tension increases within the chest.
   C. The client who has a pneumothorax can experience tachycardia related to respiratory distress and pain.
   D. The client who has a pneumothorax can experience an increase in the use of accessory muscles as respiratory distress occurs.
   E. **CORRECT:** The client who has a pneumothorax can experience pleuritic pain related to the inflammation of the pleura of the lung caused by the injury.

   Ⓝ *NCLEX® Connection: Physiological Adaptation, Basic Pathophysiology*

2. A. Assessing the client's pain and administer pain medication is important. However, another action is the priority.
   B. **CORRECT:** The priority action when using the airway, breathing, circulation (ABC) approach to client care is to establish and maintain the client's respiratory function. Obtaining a large-bore IV needle for decompression is the priority action by the nurse.
   C. Administering a benzodiazepine will treat the client's anxiety. However, another action is the priority.
   D. Gathering supplies to prepare for chest tube insertion is important. However, another action is the priority.

   Ⓝ *NCLEX® Connection: Physiological Adaptation, Alterations in Body Systems*

3. A. Weakness is an expected finding following recovery from a pneumothorax.
   B. The client should expect a lengthy recovery following a pneumothorax.
   C. It is not necessary to wear a mask following a pneumothorax, unless the client has another condition, such as immunosuppression.
   D. **CORRECT:** The client should notify the provider of a productive or persistent cough. This can indicate that the client might need treatment of a respiratory infection.

   Ⓝ *NCLEX® Connection: Physiological Adaptation, Alterations in Body Systems*

4. A. The client can have tachycardia as a manifestation when experiencing a flail chest due to inadequate oxygenation.
   B. **CORRECT:** The client can have cyanosis as a manifestation when experiencing a flail chest due to inadequate oxygenation.
   C. **CORRECT:** The client can have hypotension as a manifestation when experiencing a flail chest.
   D. **CORRECT:** The client can have dyspnea as a manifestation when experiencing a flail chest due to injury and the client's inability to effectively inhale and exhale.
   E. **CORRECT:** The client can have paradoxical chest movement as a manifestation when experiencing a flail chest due to injury to the chest and the inability to inhale and exhale.

   Ⓝ *NCLEX® Connection: Physiological Adaptation, Basic Pathophysiology*

Active Learning Scenario Key

Using the ATI Active Learning Template: System Disorder

ALTERATION IN HEALTH (DIAGNOSIS): Hemothorax is an accumulation of blood in the pleural space.

NURSING CARE
- Administer oxygen therapy.
- Document ventilator settings hourly if the client is receiving ventilation.
- Monitor ABGs, SaO_2, CBC, and chest x-ray findings.
- Position the client to maximize ventilation (high-Fowler's = 90°).
- Provide emotional support to the client and family.
- Monitor chest tube drainage.
- Administer medications as prescribed.
- Encourage prompt medical attention when manifestations of infection occur.
- Auscultate heart and lung sounds and monitor vital signs every 4 hr.

MEDICATIONS
- Benzodiazepines (sedatives): Lorazepam or midazolam can be used to decrease anxiety.
- Opioid agonists (pain medications): Morphine sulfate and fentanyl are opioid agents used to treat moderate to severe pain. These medications act on the mu and kappa receptors that help alleviate pain.

Ⓝ *NCLEX® Connection: Physiological Adaptation, Medical Emergencies*

CHAPTER 24 *Respiratory Failure*

Respiratory failure includes acute respiratory failure (ARF), acute respiratory distress syndrome (ARDS), and severe acute respiratory syndrome (SARS). Because older adult clients have decreased pulmonary reserves due to expected lung changes associated with aging, including decreased lung elasticity and thickening alveoli, they can decompensate more quickly. ©

Acute respiratory failure

ARF is caused by failure to adequately ventilate and/or oxygenate that causes a ventilation-perfusion mismatch.

- Ventilatory failure is due to a mechanical abnormality of the lungs or chest wall, impaired function of the respiratory muscles (especially the diaphragm), or a malfunction in the respiratory control center of the brain.
- Oxygenation failure can result from a lack of perfusion to the pulmonary capillary bed (pulmonary embolism) or a condition that alters the gas exchange medium (pulmonary edema, pneumonia).
- Both inadequate ventilation and oxygenation can occur in clients who have diseased lungs (asthma, emphysema, or cystic fibrosis). Diseased lung tissue can cause oxygenation failure and increased work of breathing, eventually resulting in respiratory muscle fatigue and ventilatory failure. Combined failure leads to more profound hypoxemia than either ventilatory failure or oxygenation failure alone.
- Criteria for acute respiratory failure are based on ABG values.

Acute respiratory distress syndrome

ARDS is caused by trauma to the lungs (caused by burns, sepsis, physical trauma, aspiration, and transfusions) resulting in fluid accumulation in the alveoli preventing adequate gas exchange.

- A systemic inflammatory response injures the alveolar-capillary membrane and pulmonary vasculature. It becomes permeable to large molecules, and the lung space is filled with fluid and proteins inhibiting gas exchange.
- A reduction in surfactant weakens the alveoli, which causes collapse or filling of fluid, leading to worsening edema. Edema compresses terminal airways, closing and eventually destroying them.

Severe acute respiratory syndrome

SARS is the result of a viral infection from a mutated strain of the coronaviruses (e.g., SARS–CoV–2), a group of viruses that also cause the common cold.

- The virus invades the pulmonary tissue, which leads to an inflammatory response.
- The virus is spread easily through airborne droplets from sneezing, coughing, or talking.

DATA COLLECTION

EXPECTED FINDINGS

Acute respiratory failure

- Dyspnea
- Orthopnea
- Cyanosis
- Hypoxemia
- Tachycardia
- Confusion
- Irritability or agitation
- Restlessness
- Hypercarbia (high levels of carbon dioxide in the blood)

Acute respiratory distress syndrome

- Dyspnea
- Bilateral noncardiogenic pulmonary edema R
- Reduced lung compliance
- Dense patchy bilateral pulmonary infiltrates on x-ray
- Severe hypoxemia despite administration of 100% oxygen
- Cyanosis
- Pallor
- Intercostal and substernal retractions

Severe Acute Respiratory Syndrome (SARS–CoV–2)

- **Mild to moderate**
  - Dyspnea
  - Sore throat
  - Loss of ability to taste and smell
  - Cough
  - Fatigue
  - Myalgia
  - Headache
- **Severe**
  - Unrelenting pressure and pain in the chest
  - Cyanosis
  - Altered level of consciousness
  - ARDS
  - Sepsis (may progress to septic shock)
  - Kidney damage
  - Cardiomyopathy
  - Pneumonia
  - Irregular heartbeat

LABORATORY TESTS

ABGs to confirm and monitor ARF, ARDS, and SARS
- PaO_2 less 60 mm Hg and oxygen saturation less than 90% on room air (hypoxemia)
- $PaCO_2$ greater than 50 mm Hg and pH less than 7.35 (hypoxemia, hypercarbia)
- SaO_2 less than 90%

Acute respiratory failure

ABGs to confirm and monitor combined ventilatory and oxygenation failure
- Room air, PaO_2 less than 60 mm Hg (hypoxemic/oxygenation failure), OR $PaCO_2$ greater than 50 mm Hg in conjunction with a pH less than 7.35 (hypercapnic/ventilatory failure)
- AND SaO_2 less than 90% in both cases

DIAGNOSTIC PROCEDURES

Chest X-ray ⓠEBP

Results can include:
- Pulmonary edema (ARF, ARDS)
- Cardiomegaly (ARF)
- Diffuse infiltrates and white-out or ground-glass appearance (ARDS, SARS)
- Infiltrates (SARS)

CT Scan

Results can include: scattered ground glass opacities (SARS)

NURSING ACTIONS
- Assist with client positioning before and after the x-ray.
- Communicate the results to the appropriate personnel in a timely manner.

Electrocardiogram (ECG)

To rule out cardiac involvement.

PATIENT-CENTERED CARE

NURSING CARE

- Maintain a patent airway and monitor respiratory status every hour and more often as needed.
- Mechanical ventilation is often required with positive-end expiratory pressure (PEEP) or continuous positive airway pressure (CPAP) to prevent alveolar collapse during expiration. Follow facility protocol for monitoring and documenting ventilator settings.
- Oxygenate before suctioning secretions to prevent further hypoxemia.
- Suction the client as needed (most common indicator for need to suction is coarse crackles over the trachea).
- Assess and document sputum color, amount, and consistency.

24.1 Risk factors for acute respiratory failure and distress syndrome

Acute respiratory failure

VENTILATORY FAILURE
- COPD
- Pulmonary embolism
- Pneumothorax
- Flail chest
- ARDS
- Asthma ⓠEBP
- Pulmonary edema
- Fibrosis of lung tissue
- Neuromuscular disorders (multiple sclerosis, Guillain-Barré; syndrome), spinal cord injuries, and cerebrovascular accidents that impair the client's rate and depth of respiration
- Elevated intracranial pressure (closed-head injuries, cerebral edema, hemorrhagic stroke)

OXYGENATION FAILURE
- Pneumonia
- Hypoventilation
- Hypovolemic shock
- Pulmonary edema
- Pulmonary embolism
- ARDS
- Low hemoglobin
- Low concentrations of oxygen in the blood (carbon monoxide poisoning, high altitude, smoke inhalation)

COMBINED VENTILATORY AND OXYGENATION FAILURE

Decreased gas exchange results in poor diffusion of oxygen into arterial blood with carbon dioxide retention
- Hypoventilation (poor respiratory movement)
- Chronic bronchitis
- Asthma attack
- Emphysema
- Cardiac failure

Acute respiratory distress syndrome

- Can result from localized lung damage or from the effects of other systemic problems
- Shock
- Disseminated intravascular coagulopathy (DIC)
- Aspiration
- Pulmonary emboli (fat, amniotic fluid)
- Pneumonia and other pulmonary infections
- Sepsis
- Near-drowning
- Trauma
- Multiple blood transfusions
- Damage to the central nervous system
- Smoke or toxic gas inhalation
- Drug ingestion/toxicity (heroin, opioids, salicylates)
- SARS-COV-2

Severe acute respiratory syndrome

- Exposure to an individual infected with a coronavirus
- Immunocompromised individuals (chemotherapy, AIDS)
- Clients 65 years of age and older
- Chronic kidney, liver, and lung disease
- History of smoking or substance use disorder
- Obesity
- Cardiovascular disease
- Diabetes mellitus type 1 & 2
- Pregnancy
- Vitamin D deficiency

- Assess vital signs, breathing patterns, and lung sounds per facility protocol.
- Monitor for pneumothorax (a high PEEP can cause the lungs to collapse).
- Obtain ABGs as prescribed and following each ventilator setting adjustment.
- Maintain continuous ECG monitoring for changes that can indicate increased hypoxemia, especially when repositioning and applying suction.
- Continually monitor vital signs, including SaO_2. Assess pain level.
- Position the client to facilitate ventilation and perfusion.
  - Prone position as prescribed (ARDS/SARS)
- Prevent infection.
  - Perform frequent hand hygiene.
  - Use appropriate suctioning technique.
  - Provide oral care every 2 hr and as needed.
  - Wear protective clothing (gown, gloves, mask) when appropriate.
    - Maintain droplet and contact precautions for the client who has SARS-CoV-2 infection
    - Airborne precautions apply if the client is receiving a procedure that generates aerosols
- Promote nutrition.
  - Assess bowel sounds.
  - Monitor elimination patterns.
  - Obtain daily weights. Qs
  - Monitor intake and output.
  - Administer enteral and/or parenteral feedings as prescribed.
  - Prevent aspiration with enteral feedings (elevate the head of the bed 30° to 45°).
  - Confirm nasogastric (NG) tube placement prior to feeding.
- Provide emotional support to the client and family.
  - Encourage verbalization of feelings.
  - Provide alternative communication means (dry erase board, pen and paper).

MEDICATIONS

Benzodiazepines

EXAMPLES
- Lorazepam
- Midazolam

ACTIONS: Reduces anxiety and resistance to ventilation and decreases oxygen consumption

Corticosteroids

EXAMPLES
- Cortisone acetate
- Methylprednisolone sodium succinate
- Dexamethasone sodium phosphate
- Recommended for hospitalized clients who have the SARS-CoV-2 virus and require supplemental oxygenation

ACTIONS: Reduces WBC migration and decreases inflammation

NURSING ACTIONS
- Discontinue medication gradually.
- Administer with an antiulcer medication to prevent peptic ulcer formation.
- Monitor weight and blood pressure.
- Monitor glucose and electrolytes. QEBP

CLIENT EDUCATION: Take oral doses with food and avoid stopping the medication suddenly.

Opioid analgesics

EXAMPLES
- Morphine sulfate
- Fentanyl

ACTIONS: Provides pain management

NURSING ACTIONS
- Monitor respirations for clients who are not receiving mechanical ventilation.
- Monitor blood pressure, heart rate, and SaO_2.
- Monitor ABGs. (Hypercapnia can result from depressed respirations.)
- Use cautiously in conjunction with hypnotic sedatives.
- Assess pain level and response to medication.
- Have naloxone and resuscitation equipment available for severe respiratory depression in clients who are not receiving mechanical ventilation.

Antibiotics sensitive to cultured organism(s)

EXAMPLES: Vancomycin

ACTIONS: Treats identified organisms

NURSING ACTIONS
- Culture sputum prior to administration of first dose.
- Monitor for a hypersensitivity reaction.
- Give IV doses slowly (over at least 60 min) to avoid red man syndrome.
- Monitor the IV site for infiltration.
- Do not give with other medications.
- Monitor coagulopathy and renal function.

CLIENT EDUCATION: Take oral doses with food and finish the prescribed dose.

Antivirals: (SARS-CoV-2)

EXAMPLES: Remdesivir
Remdesivir is the only antiviral medication currently approved by the FDA for treatment of the SARS-CoV-19 infection

ACTIONS: Slows replication of the virus

NURSING ACTIONS
- Obtain glomerular filtration rate (GFR), liver enzymes, prothrombin time (PT), and INR before initiating and throughout therapy.
- Monitor for a hypersensitivity reaction.
- Monitor the IV site for infiltration.
- Monitor coagulopathy and renal function.
- Monitor for adverse gastrointestinal effects.

Antirheumatics (SARS-CoV-2)

EXAMPLES: Baricitinib and tocilizumab

ACTIONS: Inhibit inflammatory processes associated with SARS-CoV-2 infection

NURSING ACTIONS
- Monitor for a hypersensitivity reaction.
- Monitor for manifestations of arterial and deep vein thrombosis.
- Monitor liver and kidney function.
- Obtain CBC with differential and absolute neutrophil count before initiating and throughout therapy.

Anticoagulants (SARS-CoV-2)

EXAMPLES: Dalteparin and enoxaparin

ACTIONS: Inhibit blood coagulation

NURSING ACTIONS
- Monitor for a hypersensitivity reaction.
- Assess injection site for bruising and inflammation.
- Monitor for manifestations of bleeding.
- Obtain CBC with differential and absolute neutrophil count before initiating and throughout therapy.

Immunizations: (SARS-CoV-2)

Refer to CDC guidelines for various age groups.

INTERPROFESSIONAL CARE

Respiratory therapy
- The respiratory therapist typically manages the ventilator, adjusts the settings, and provides chest physiotherapy to improve ventilation and chest expansion.
- The respiratory therapist also can suction the endotracheal tube and administer inhalation medications, such as bronchodilators.

Nutritional therapy
- Enteral or parenteral feeding
- Nutritional support following extubation

THERAPEUTIC PROCEDURES

Intubation and mechanical ventilation

Artificial airway insertion with mechanical ventilation

NURSING ACTIONS
- Monitor ECG, SaO2, lung sounds, and color.
- Sedate as needed.
- Explain the procedure and Provide reassurance to calm the client.
- Have suction equipment, manual resuscitation bag, and face mask available at all times.
- Suction secretions as needed.
- **Preintubation**
  - Oxygenate with 100% oxygen.
  - Assist ventilation with manual resuscitation bag and face mask.
  - Have emergency resuscitation equipment readily available.

- **Postintubation**
  - Assess end-tidal carbon dioxide levels, bilateral lung sounds, symmetrical chest movement, and chest x-ray findings to confirm placement of the endotracheal tube. Q$_{PCC}$
  - Secure the endotracheal tube per facility guidelines.
  - Assess the balloon cuff for air leaks periodically Monitor cuff pressure to maintain between 20 to 30 cm. H_2O to stabilize the tube without causing tracheal injury.
- **PEEP**
  - Positive pressure is applied during expiration to keep the alveoli expanded.
  - PEEP is added to the ventilator setting to enhance gas exchange and improve lung expansion, thus preventing atelectasis.

CLIENT EDUCATION: Alternate methods of communication will be provided because speaking is not possible while the endotracheal tube is in place.

Kinetic therapy

A kinetic bed that rotates laterally alters client positioning to reduce atelectasis and improve ventilation.

NURSING ACTIONS
- Begin slowly and gradually to increase the degree of rotation as tolerated.
- Monitor ECG, SaO2, breath sounds, and blood pressure.
- Stop rotation if the client becomes distressed.
- Provide routine skin care to prevent breakdown.
- Sedate as needed.

COMPLICATIONS

ENDOTRACHEAL TUBE

Trauma

- Trauma during intubation or long-term intubation can cause damage to trachea and vocal cords.
- A tracheostomy might be required for long-term ventilation.

Altered position of endotracheal tube

NURSING ACTIONS
- Check tube positioning every 1 to 2 hr and as needed Monitor cuff pressure to maintain between 20 to 30 cm H_2O.
- Assess lung sounds, SaO2, and chest movement each time the client is moved, transferred, or turned.
- Secure endotracheal tube per facility guidelines to maintain tube placement and document level of tube.

Aspiration pneumonia

NURSING ACTIONS
- Check the cuff on the endotracheal tube for leaks.
- Assess suction contents for gastric secretions.
- Verify NG tube placement.

Infection

NURSING ACTIONS
- Prevent infection by using proper hand hygiene, suctioning technique, and meticulous oral care.
- Assess color, amount, and consistency of secretions.

Blocked endotracheal tube

Indicated by high-pressure alarm on ventilator

NURSING ACTIONS: Suction secretions to relieve a mucous plug or insert an oral airway to prevent biting on the tube.

MECHANICAL VENTILATION

Increased intrathoracic pressure

- PEEP increases intrathoracic pressure, which can cause a decreased blood return to the heart, decreased cardiac output, and/or hypotension.
- Decreased cardiac output can activate the renin-angiotensin-aldosterone system, leading to fluid retention and/or decreased urine output.

NURSING ACTIONS: Monitor input and output, weight, and hydration status.

CLIENT EDUCATION: Avoid using the Valsalva maneuver (straining with bowel movement), because it can further increase intrathoracic pressure.

Barotrauma

Ventilation with positive pressure causes damage to the lungs (pneumothorax, subcutaneous emphysema).

NURSING ACTIONS
- Monitor oxygenation status, blood gases, electrolytes, and chest x-ray.
- Assess for subcutaneous emphysema (crackles and/or air movement felt under skin).
- Monitor for a high-pressure ventilator alarm, which can indicate pneumothorax.

Immobilization

Can result in muscle atrophy, pneumonia, and pressure injury

NURSING ACTIONS
- Reposition and suction every 2 hr and as needed.
- Provide routine skin care.
- Implement range-of-motion exercises to prevent muscle atrophy.

SARS-COV-2 Infection

Post-Acute Coronavirus Syndrome
Continued manifestations of SARS-CoV-2 infection occurring 4-weeks or more after onset of initial manifestations

NURSING ACTIONS
- Educate client about manifestations of Post-Acute Coronavirus Syndrome
- Dizziness, myalgia, continues loss of taste or smell, brain fog, depression, shortness of breath, headache, fatigue
- Assess clients for manifestations of Post-Acute Coronavirus Syndrome with each follow-up visit and make referrals as necessary

PATIENT EDUCATION (SARS-COV-2)

Instruct caregivers about prevention of SARS-CoV-2 (infection).
- Frequent hand hygiene
- Maintain distance of at least 6 ft from others when indicated
- Wear face mask when indicated
- Avoid touching face, mouth, and eyes
- Obtain COVID-19 vaccination according to current CDC guidelines

Active Learning Scenario

A nurse is reviewing the plan of care for a client who has acute respiratory distress syndrome (ARDS). What should be included in the plan of care? Use the ATI Active Learning Template: System Disorder to complete this item.

RISK FACTORS: Describe three conditions related to ARDS.

NURSING CARE: Describe three nursing actions to maintain oxygenation.

COMPLICATIONS: Identify two complications of ARDS.

Application Exercises

1. A nurse is reviewing the health records of five clients. Which of the following clients should the nurse identify as being at risk for developing acute respiratory distress syndrome? (Select all that apply.)
   A. A client who experienced a near-drowning incident
   B. A client following coronary artery bypass graft surgery
   C. A client who has a hemoglobin of 15.1 g/dL (14 to 18 g/dL)
   D. A client who has sepsis
   E. A client who experienced acute drug toxicity

2. A nurse is contributing the to the plan of care for a client who is receiving mechanical ventilation with positive end expiratory pressure (PEEP) for acute respiratory distress syndrome. Which of the following interventions should the nurse recommend be included in the plan?
   A. Use clean technique when performing endotracheal suctioning
   B. Maintain the client in a supine position
   C. Monitor for pneumothorax
   D. Place the client in protective isolation

3. A nurse is orienting a newly licensed nurse on the purpose of administering vecuronium to a client who has acute respiratory distress syndrome (ARDS). Which of the following statements by the newly licensed nurse indicates understanding of the teaching?
   A. "This medication is given to treat infection."
   B. "This medication is given to relieve pain."
   C. "This medication is given to decrease inflammation."
   D. "This medication is given to reduce anxiety."

4. A nurse is discussing intubation with a newly licensed nurse. Which of the following complications associated with intubation should the nurse identify?
   A. Changes in the client's voice
   B. Mucositis
   C. Inflammation of the Eustachian tube
   D. Development of rhinorrhea

Active Learning Scenario Key

Using the ATI Active Learning Template: System Disorder

RISK FACTORS

- Can result from localized lung damage or from the effects of other systemic problems
- Aspiration
- Pulmonary emboli (fat, amniotic fluid)
- Pneumonia and other pulmonary infections
- Sepsis
- Near-drowning accident
- Trauma
- Damage to the central nervous system
- Smoke or toxic gas inhalation
- Drug ingestion/toxicity (heroin, opioids, salicylates)

NURSING CARE

- Maintain a patent airway and monitor respiratory status every hour as needed.
- Suction the client as needed.
- Monitor lung sounds.
- Monitor and document sputum color, amount, and consistency.
- Oxygenate before suctioning secretions to prevent further hypoxemia.
- Mechanical ventilation often is required. PEEP often is used to prevent alveolar collapse during expiration.
- Monitor for pneumothorax. (A high PEEP can cause the lungs to collapse.)
- Maintain continuous ECG monitoring for changes that can indicate increased hypoxemia, especially when repositioning and applying suction.
- Continually monitor vital signs, including SaO_2.
- Position the client to facilitate ventilation and perfusion.

COMPLICATIONS

- Endotracheal tube
  - Trauma during intubation or long-term intubation
  - Can cause damage to trachea and vocal cords
  - Nursing Actions: Consider a tracheostomy for long-term ventilation.
- Aspiration pneumonia nursing actions
  - Check the cuff on the endotracheal tube for leaks.
  - Monitor suction contents for gastric secretions.
  - Verify NG tube placement.
- Infection nursing actions
  - Prevent infection by using proper hand hygiene and suctioning technique.
  - Monitor color, amount, and consistency of secretions.
- Blocked endotracheal tube
  - The high-pressure alarm on the ventilator can indicate a blocked endotracheal tube.
  - Nursing Actions: Suction secretions to relieve a mucous plug or insert an oral airway to prevent biting on the tube.
- Altered position of endotracheal tube nursing actions
  - Check tube positioning every 1 to 2 hr and as needed.
  - Monitor breath sounds, SaO_2, and chest movement.
  - Secure endotracheal tube per institution's guidelines to maintain tube placement.
- Mechanical ventilation
  - Increased intrathoracic pressure.
  - PEEP increases intrathoracic pressure, which can cause a decreased blood return to the heart, decreased cardiac output and/or hypotension.
  - Decreased cardiac output can activate the renin-angiotensin-aldosterone system, leading to fluid retention and/or decreased urine output.
  - Nursing Actions: Monitor input and output, weight, and hydration status.
  - Client Education: Avoid using the Valsalva maneuver (straining with bowel movement), because it can further increase intrathoracic pressure.
- Barotrauma: Ventilation with positive pressure causes damage to the lungs (pneumothorax, subcutaneous emphysema).

Ⓝ *NCLEX® Connection: Physiological Adaptation, Alterations in Body Systems*

Application Exercises Key

1. A, B, D, E. **CORRECT:** When reviewing the health records of five clients for the risk for developing acute respiratory distress syndrome (ARDS), the nurse should identify the client who has experienced a near drowning accident, the client who has had a coronary artery bypass graft surgery, the client who has dysphagia, and the client who has experienced acute drug toxicity as at risk for developing ARDS. ARDS develops after a client experiences an acute lung injury that stimulates the inflammatory process within the lungs.
   C. Hemoglobin of 15.1 mg/dL is within the expected reference range. A client who has a low hemoglobin is at risk for developing ARDS.

Ⓝ *NCLEX® Connection: Health Promotion and Maintenance, Health Promotion and Disease Prevention*

2. A. Use sterile technique when providing endotracheal suctioning because of the risk of ventilator associated pneumonia.
   B. Elevate the heat of the bed to improve ventilation and decrease the risk of ventilator associated pneumonia.
   C. **CORRECT:** When generating solutions while contributing to the plan of care for a client who is receiving mechanical ventilation with PEEP, the nurse should include to monitor for a pneumothorax. Tension pneumothorax is a complication associated with PEEP.
   D. A client who has neutropenia should be placed in protective isolation

Ⓝ *NCLEX® Connection: Physiological Adaptation, Alterations in Body Systems*

3. A. Antibiotics are given to treat infection.
   B. Opioid analgesics are given to relieve pain.
   C. Corticosteroids are given to treat inflammation.
   D. **CORRECT:** When evaluating the teaching to a newly license nurse about the purpose of administering lorazepam to a client who has acute respiratory distress syndrome (ARDS), the nurse should identify that the statement, "This medication is given to reduce anxiety," indicates understanding of the teaching. Lorazepam is a benzodiazepine given to treat anxiety.

Ⓝ *NCLEX Connection: Pharmacological Therapies, Expected Actions/Outcomes*

4. A. **CORRECT:** When discussing complications of intubation with a newly license nurse, the nurse should identify a change in the client's voice as a complication. Trauma during intubation can cause damage to the vocal cords, changing the client's voice.
   B. Mucositis is an inflammation and irritation of the mouth resulting from chemotherapy.
   C. Inflammation of the Eustachian tube is not associated with intubation.
   D. Rhinorrhea is not associated with intubation.

Ⓝ *NCLEX® Connection: Physiological Adaptation, Alterations in Body Systems*

When reviewing the following chapters, keep in mind the relevant topics and tasks of the NCLEX outline.

Pharmacological Therapies

ADVERSE EFFECTS/CONTRAINDICATIONS/SIDE EFFECTS/ INTERACTIONS
Identify a contraindication to the administration of a prescribed or over-the-counter medication to the client.

Withhold medication dose if client experiences adverse effect to medication.

PHARMACOLOGICAL PAIN MANAGEMENT: Identify client need for pain medication.

MEDICATION ADMINISTRATION
Collect required data prior to medication administration.

Assist in preparing the client for insertion of a central line.

Administer intravenous piggyback (secondary) medications.

Reduction of Risk Potential

CHANGES/ABNORMALITIES IN VITAL SIGNS: Compare vital signs to client baseline vital signs.

DIAGNOSTIC TESTS
Reinforce client teaching about diagnostic test.

Perform diagnostic testing.

POTENTIAL FOR COMPLICATIONS OF DIAGNOSTIC TESTS/ TREATMENTS/PROCEDURES: Reinforce teaching to prevent complications due to client diagnostic tests/treatments/procedures.

POTENTIAL FOR ALTERATIONS IN BODY SYSTEMS: Perform focused data collection based on client condition.

Physiological Adaptation

ALTERATIONS IN BODY SYSTEMS
Recognize and report basic abnormalities on a client cardiac monitor strip.

Assist in the care of a client with a pacing device.

Reinforce education to client regarding care and condition.

UNEXPECTED RESPONSES TO THERAPIES: Intervene in response to client unexpected negative response to therapy.

CHAPTER 25

Cardiovascular Diagnostic and Therapeutic Procedures

Cardiovascular diagnostic procedures evaluate the functioning of the heart by monitoring for enzymes in the blood; using ultrasound to visualize the heart; determining the heart's response to exercise; and using catheters to determine blood volume, perfusion, fluid status, how the heart is pumping, and degree of artery blockage.

Cardiovascular diagnostic procedures that nurses should be familiar with include cardiac enzymes and lipid profile, echocardiogram, stress testing, hemodynamic monitoring, and angiography. Cardiovascular therapeutic procedures include central vascular IV access placement and percutaneous coronary interventions.

Cardiac enzymes and lipid profile

Cardiac enzymes are released into the bloodstream when the heart muscle is injured.

A lipid profile provides information regarding cholesterol levels and is used for early detection of heart disease. Cardiac enzymes are specific markers in diagnosing a myocardial infarction (MI).

INDICATIONS

- Angina
- MI
- Heart disease
- Hyperlipidemia

CONSIDERATIONS

PREPROCEDURE: Fasting for 12 to 14 hr is recommended prior to lipid profile sampling.

INTERPRETATION OF FINDINGS

25.1 Cardiac enzymes

EXPECTED REFERENCE RANGE	ELEVATED LEVELS FIRST DETECTABLE FOLLOWING MYOCARDIAL INJURY	EXPECTED DURATION OF ELEVATED LEVELS
Creatine kinase MB isoenzyme more sensitive to myocardium		
0% of total CK (30 to 170 units/L)	3 to 6 hr	2 to 3 days
Troponin T		
Less than 0.1 ng/mL	2 to 3 hr	10 to 14 days
Troponin I		
Less than 0.03 ng/mL	2 to 3 hr	7 to 10 days
Myoglobin		
Less than 90 mcg/L	2 to 3 hr	24 hr

25.2 Cardiac tests

EXPECTED REFERENCE RANGE	PURPOSE
Cholesterol (total)	
Less than 200 mg/dL	Screening for heart disease
LDL	
Less than 130 mg/dL	"Bad" cholesterol Transports cholesterol to the body's cells from the liver
Triglycerides	
MALES: 40 to 160 mg/dL FEMALES: 35 to 135 mg/dL	Evaluates the client's risk for heart disease
HDL	
FEMALES: greater than 55 mg/dL MALES: greater than 45 mg/dL	"Good" cholesterol Protects coronary arteries from heart disease by transporting cholesterol from the body's cells to the liver

Transthoracic echocardiography

A transthoracic echocardiogram is used to diagnose valve disorders and cardiomyopathy; evaluate the size, shape, and motion of the structure of the heart; and measure the ejection fraction.

INDICATIONS

- Cardiomyopathy
- Heart failure
- Angina
- MI

CONSIDERATIONS

PREPROCEDURE: Explain that this is a noninvasive test and takes up to 1 hr.

INTRAPROCEDURE: Instruct the client to lie on the left side and remain still.

POSTPROCEDURE: Provider reviews test results and a plan for follow-up care with the client.

Transesophageal Echocardiography

Transesophageal echocardiography provides clearer ultrasonic images than a transthoracic echocardiogram, because the waves pass through less tissue. A small transducer is passed through the mouth and into the esophagus to provide images of the heart.

INDICATIONS

- Heart failure
- Valvular heart disease
- Atrial or ventricular thrombi
- Monitoring during valve replacement and coronary artery bypass surgeries

CONSIDERATIONS

PREPROCEDURE: Ensure that informed consent has been signed. Instruct the client to be NPO for 4 to 6 hr prior to the procedure. Insert an IV access.

INTRAPROCEDURE: Monitor the client's level of consciousness, ECG, blood pressure, heart rate, respiratory rate, and oxygenation status, as moderate sedation is needed for the procedure.

POSTPROCEDURE: Monitor the client's vital signs, oxygenation status, level of consciousness, and return of gag reflex (topical anesthetics are used in the throat). Maintain the head of the bed at 45°.

Stress testing

The client exercises the cardiac muscle by walking on a treadmill, which is called exercise stress testing. This provides information regarding the workload of the heart. The test is discontinued once the heart rate reaches a certain rate.

Fatigue or disability can prevent traditional exercise testing or test completion. The provider can prescribe the test to be done as a pharmacological (chemical) stress test.

INDICATIONS

- Angina
- Heart failure
- MI
- Dysrhythmia

CONSIDERATIONS

PREPROCEDURE

- Assist the provider in obtaining a signed informed consent form.
- Explain to the client that they will be walking on a treadmill, and comfortable athletic shoes and clothing are recommended.
  - If pharmacological stress testing is prescribed, a medication (dipyridamole, adenosine, regadenoson, dobutamine) is given to stress the heart instead of walking on the treadmill.
- Instruct the client to fast 2 to 4 hr before the procedure according to facility policy and to avoid tobacco, alcohol, and caffeine before the test. Qs
- Instruct the client to get adequate rest the night before the procedure.

INTRAPROCEDURE

- Apply a 12-lead ECG to monitor heart rate during the test. Monitor for dysrhythmias throughout the procedure.
- Instruct the client to report any chest pain, shortness of breath, or dizziness during the procedure.

POSTPROCEDURE

- Monitor the client by 12-lead ECG.
- Check blood pressure frequently until the client is stable.
- The provider reviews findings with the client.

Hemodynamic monitoring

Hemodynamic monitoring involves special indwelling catheters, which provide information about blood volume and perfusion, fluid status, and how well the heart is pumping.

- Hemodynamic status is assessed with several parameters.
  - Central venous pressure (CVP)
  - Pulmonary artery pressure (PAP)
  - Pulmonary artery wedge pressure (PAWP)
  - Cardiac output (CO)
  - Intra-arterial blood pressure
- Mixed venous oxygen saturation (SvO_2) indicates the balance between oxygen supply and demand. It is measured by a pulmonary artery catheter with fiber optics.

- A hemodynamic monitoring system is used to display a client's hemodynamic data.
  - Pressure transducer
  - Pressure tubing
  - Monitor
  - Pressure bag and flush device
- Arterial lines are placed in the radial (most common), brachial, or femoral artery.
  - Arterial lines provide continuous information about changes in blood pressure and permit the withdrawal of samples of arterial blood. Intra-arterial pressures can differ from cuff pressures.
  - The integrity of the arterial waveform should be assessed to verify the accuracy of blood pressure readings.
  - Monitor circulation in the limb with the arterial line (capillary refill, temperature, color).
  - Monitor for bleeding around the insertion site. Maintain secure connections.
  - Arterial lines are not used for IV fluid administration.

Pulmonary artery (PA) catheters

The PA catheter is inserted into a large vein (internal jugular, femoral, subclavian, brachial) and threaded through the right atria and ventricle into a branch of the PA.
- PA catheters have multiple lumens, ports, and components that allow for various hemodynamic measurements, blood sampling, and infusion of IV fluids.
  - The proximal lumen can be used to measure right atrial pressure (CVP), infuse IV fluids, and obtain venous blood samples.
  - The distal lumen can be used to measure PAPs (PA systolic, PA diastolic, mean PA pressure, and PA wedge pressure). This lumen is not used for IV fluid administration.
  - The balloon inflation port is intermittently used for PAWP measurements. When not in use, it should be left deflated and in the locked position.
  - The thermistor measures the temperature differences between the right atrium and the PA in order to determine CO.
  - Additional infusion ports can be available, depending on the brand.

INDICATIONS

- Serious or critical illness
- Heart failure
- Post coronary artery bypass graft (CABG) clients
- ARDS
- Acute kidney injury
- Burn injury
- Trauma injury

INTERPRETATION OF FINDINGS

The intravascular volume in older adult clients is often reduced. The nurse should anticipate lower hemodynamic values, particularly if dehydration is a complication. ©

25.3 Hemodynamic monitoring

	EXPECTED REFERENCE RANGES
CVP	2 to 6 mm Hg
Pulmonary Artery Systolic	15 to 28 mm Hg
Pulmonary Artery Diastolic	5 to 16 mm Hg
PAWP	6 to 15 mm Hg
CO	3 to 6 L/min
SVO$_2$	60% to 80%

COMPLICATIONS

Infection/Sepsis

Infection at insertion site can occur if aseptic technique is not used.

Embolism

Plaque or a clot can become dislodged during the procedure.

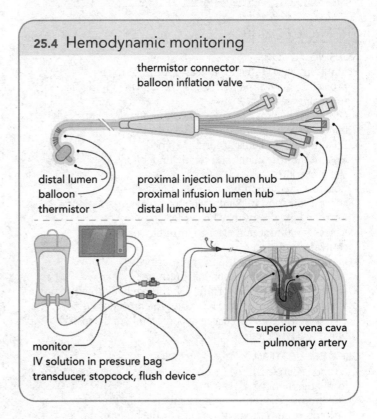

25.4 Hemodynamic monitoring

thermistor connector
balloon inflation valve

distal lumen
balloon
thermistor

proximal injection lumen hub
proximal infusion lumen hub
distal lumen hub

superior vena cava
pulmonary artery

monitor
IV solution in pressure bag
transducer, stopcock, flush device

Angiography

Coronary angiography, also called a cardiac catheterization, is an invasive diagnostic procedure used to evaluate the presence and degree of coronary artery blockage.

- A renal or liver angiogram, cerebral angiogram, or upper and lower extremity angiogram can be done to determine blood flow and areas of possible blockage of a vessel. Procedural care is the same for any type of angiography or according to facility protocol.
- Coronary angiography involves the insertion of a catheter into a femoral, brachial, or radial vessel and threading it into the right or left side of the heart. Coronary artery narrowings and/or occlusions are identified by the injection of contrast media under fluoroscopy.

INDICATIONS

- Unstable angina and ECG changes (T wave inversion, ST segment elevation, depression).
- Confirm and determine location and extent of heart disease.

CONSIDERATIONS

PREPROCEDURE

NURSING ACTIONS

- Maintain NPO status for at least 4 hr prior to the procedure due to the risk for aspiration when lying flat for the procedure.
- Obtain vital signs, auscultate heart and lung sounds, and assess peripheral pulses.
- Ensure that the consent form is signed.
- Ensure that the client and family understand the procedure.
- Contrast media (iodine) may not always be a contraindication in clients who have a shellfish allergy. Further assessment may be needed.
- Assess renal function prior to introduction of contrast media.
- Administer premedications as prescribed (methylprednisolone, diphenhydramine).
- If the client takes metformin, ask the provider about withholding prior to and following the procedure (up to 48 hr). Metformin can cause hypoglycemia or acidosis when receiving iodine media.

CLIENT EDUCATION

- A mild sedative will be given to promote relaxation, and local anesthetic.
- The groin is the most common site used for the procedure; sensations of warmth or flushing might be felt when the dye is injected.
- After the procedure, pressure will be held on the access site. If a vascular closure device is not used, the extremity must be kept straight for a prescribed amount of time to prevent bleeding. Qᴾᶜᶜ

POSTPROCEDURE

NURSING ACTIONS

- Obtain vital signs every 15 min × 4; every 30 min × 2; every hour × 4; and then every 4 hr. (Follow facility protocol.)
- Inspect the affected extremity at the same intervals for:
  - Bleeding and hematoma formation at the insertion site.
  - Thrombosis. (Document pedal pulse, extremity color, and temperature.)
- Maintain bed rest in supine position with extremity straight for prescribed time.
  - A vascular closure device can be used to hasten hemostasis following catheter removal.
  - Older adult clients can have arthritis, which can make lying in bed for 4 to 6 hr after the procedure painful. The provider can prescribe medication. Ⓖ
- Administer antiplatelet as prescribed to prevent clot formation and restenosis.
  - Aspirin
  - Clopidogrel (if having percutaneous coronary intervention [PCI], other antiplatelet medication—such as ticagrelor, prasugrel, or cangrelor—can be administered)
  - Heparin
  - Low molecular weight heparin (enoxaparin)
  - GP IIb/IIIa inhibitors, such as eptifibatide
- Administer anxiolytics and analgesics as needed.
- Monitor urine output and administer IV fluids for hydration.
  - Contrast media acts as an osmotic diuretic.

CLIENT EDUCATION

- Leave the dressing in place for the first 24 hr following discharge. Qᴱᴮᴾ
- Avoid strenuous exercise for the prescribed period of time.
- Immediately report bleeding from the insertion site, chest pain, shortness of breath, and changes in the color or temperature of the extremity.
- Restrict lifting to less than 10 lb (4.5 kg), bending at the waist, or straining for at least 24 hr or for the prescribed period of time if the groin was used for access. Restrict lifting to 5 lb or less if a vessel in the arm or wrist was used for at least 48 hr or for the prescribed period of time.
- Resume metformin as prescribed.

If a having a stent placement

- Take antiplatelet therapy as prescribed, which can be for up to 12 months.
  - Take the medication at the same time each day.
  - Have regular laboratory tests to determine therapeutic levels.
  - Avoid activities that could cause bleeding. (Use soft toothbrush. Wear shoes when out of bed.)
- Follow lifestyle guidelines. (Manage weight. Consume a low-fat/low-sodium diet. Exercise regularly. Stop smoking. Decrease alcohol intake.)

COMPLICATIONS

Artery dissection

- Perforation of an artery by the catheter can cause cardiac tamponade or require emergency coronary artery bypass surgery.
- Findings include severe hypotension and tachycardia, and might require extended occlusion or perforation with a balloon catheter and reversal of anticoagulants.

Cardiac tamponade

Cardiac tamponade can result from fluid accumulation in the pericardial sac.

- Manifestations include hypotension, jugular venous distention, muffled heart sounds, and paradoxical pulse (variance of 10 mm Hg or more in systolic blood pressure between expiration and inspiration).
- Hemodynamic monitoring reveals intracardiac and PAPs are similar and elevated (plateau pressures).

NURSING ACTIONS

- Notify the provider immediately.
- Administer IV fluids to combat hypotension.
- Obtain a chest x-ray or echocardiogram to confirm diagnosis.
- Prepare the client for pericardiocentesis. (Verify informed consent. Gather materials. Administer medications as appropriate.)
- Monitor hemodynamic pressures.
- Monitor heart rhythm. Changes indicate improper positioning of the needle.
- Monitor for reoccurrence of manifestations after the procedure.
- Monitor for dyspnea, and provide oxygen as indicated.

Hematoma formation

Blood clots can form near the insertion site.

NURSING ACTIONS

- Monitor for sensation, color, capillary refill, and peripheral pulses in the extremity distal to the insertion site.
- Collect data regarding the groin at prescribed intervals and as needed.
- Hold pressure for uncontrolled oozing/bleeding.
- Monitor peripheral circulation.
- Notify the provider.

Allergic reaction related to the contrast media

Manifestations can include chills, fever, rash, wheezing, tachycardia, and bradycardia.

NURSING ACTIONS

- Monitor for an allergic reaction.
- Have resuscitation equipment readily available.
- Administer diphenhydramine or epinephrine if prescribed.

External bleeding at the insertion site

NURSING ACTIONS

- Monitor insertion site for bleeding or swelling.
- Apply pressure to site.
- Keep client's leg or arm straight.

Embolism

Plaque or a clot can become dislodged.

NURSING ACTIONS

- Monitor for chest pain during and after the procedure.
- Monitor vital signs and SaO_2.

Restenosis of treated vessel

Clot reformation in the coronary artery can occur immediately or several weeks after procedure.

NURSING ACTIONS

- Assess ECG patterns and for occurrence of chest pain.
- Notify the provider immediately.
- Prepare the client for return to the cardiac catheterization laboratory.

CLIENT EDUCATION: Notify the provider of cardiac manifestations, and take medications as prescribed.

Retroperitoneal bleeding

Bleeding into retroperitoneal space (abdominal cavity behind the peritoneum) can occur due to femoral artery puncture.

NURSING ACTIONS

- Monitor for flank pain and hypotension.
- Notify the provider immediately and hold firm pressure at the puncture site.

CLIENT EDUCATION

- Keep the leg straight.
- Report chest pain, shortness of breath, and cardiac manifestations.

Acute kidney injury

Damage to the kidney can result from use of contrast agent, which is nephrotoxic.

NURSING ACTIONS

- Monitor urine output, BUN, and blood creatinine and electrolyte levels.
- Promote adequate hydration (oral, IV).

Vascular access

The site and type of vascular access device (VAD) is determined by the characteristics of the prescribed therapy (medication type, pH and osmolality, length of time for therapy). The goal is to minimize the number of catheter insertions and the risk for adverse reactions.

Central intravenous therapy

- Central IV catheters are used to infuse any fluids due to rapid hemodilution in the superior vena cava (SVC).
- Ensure x-ray verification of tip placement prior to use.
- Central IV catheters are inserted using sterile technique by a provider, physician assistant, or specifically trained nurses. Insertion occurs in the OR, the client's room, or in an outpatient facility.
- Tunneled and implanted catheters require surgical removal.
- Central IV catheter types include nontunneled percutaneous central venous catheters, peripherally inserted central catheters, tunneled central venous catheters (Hickman, Groshong), and implanted ports.

Nontunneled percutaneous central venous catheter (CVC)

- Description: 18 to 25 cm (7 to 10 in) in length with one to five lumens
- Length of use: short-term use only (less than 6 weeks)
- Insertion location: subclavian vein, jugular vein; tip in the distal third of the superior vena cava
- Indications: Emergent or trauma use, administration of blood, administration of chemotherapeutic agents, antibiotics, and total parenteral nutrition

Tunneled percutaneous central venous catheter

- For long-term use.
- Insertion location: A portion of the catheter lies in a subcutaneous tunnel separating the point where the catheter enters the vein from where it enters the skin with a cuff. Tissue granulates into the cuff to provide a mechanical barrier to organisms and an anchoring for the catheter.
- Indications: Frequent and long-term need for vascular access.
- No dressing is needed because entrance into skin and vein are separate and tissue granulates into catheter cuff, providing a barrier. Groshong catheters have pressure-sensitive valves to prevent blood reflux and do not require a clamp.

Peripherally inserted central catheter (PICC)

- Description: 45 to 74 cm (18 to 29 in) with single or multiple lumens
- Length of use: up to 12 months
- Insertion location: basilic or cephalic vein at least one fingerbreadth below or above the antecubital fossa. The catheter should be advanced until the tip is positioned in the lower one-third of the SVC.
- Indications: administration of blood, long-term administration of chemotherapeutic agents, antibiotics, and total parenteral nutrition
- When possible, insert a PICC early in the course of therapy before veins are exposed to repeated venipunctures.

CONSIDERATIONS

PREPROCEDURE

- Ensure informed consent has been signed.
- Cleanse the site with chlorhexidine.
- Ensure sterility of equipment.
- Place a STOP sign on the door to the room to restrict entry during the procedure.

POSTPROCEDURE

- Confirm placement of the PICC with an x-ray.
- Monitor the site for redness, swelling, drainage, tenderness, and condition of the dressing.
- Clean the insertion port with alcohol for 15 seconds and allow it to dry completely prior to accessing it. Valve disinfection caps which contain alcohol are available for single use.
- Use transparent dressing to allow for visualization. Follow facility protocol for dressing changes, usually every 7 days and when indicated (wet, loose, soiled).
- Advise the client not to immerse the arm in water. To shower, cover dressing site to avoid water exposure.
- Reinforce to the client not to have venipuncture or blood pressure taken in arm with PICC line.
- Take preventive measures.
  - Practice hand hygiene before working with a CVC.
  - Observe the site every 2 hr for infection or infiltration.
  - Nontunneled catheters require an intact sterile dressing (tunneled catheters do not).
  - Clean the site with chlorhexidine for 30 seconds and allow to air dry prior to insertion.

Occlusion

Occlusion is a blockage in the central IV catheter that impedes flow. Thrombosis/emboli can coagulate and cause an occlusion.

25.5 Case study

Part 1

Amy is a nurse in a provider's office caring for Joe Smith. Mr. Smith has returned to the provider's office to review laboratory results that were obtained during a routine physical.

Part 2

John is a nurse on a cardiac unit caring for Joe Smith. Mr. Smith is scheduled for a coronary angiography.

Part 3

Ann, a nurse in a cardiac unit, is orienting Steve, a newly licensed nurse. Ann and Steve are caring for Joe Smith who is preoperative for coronary artery bypass graph. Mr. Smith is having a central venous pressure (CVP) catheter inserted prior to the procedure.

1. The nurse at the provider's office is reviewing the laboratory test results for the client. The nurse should identify that which of the following results indicates the client is at risk for heart disease? (Select all that apply.)

   A. Cholesterol (total) 245 mg/dL

   B. HDL 90 mg/dL

   C. LDL 140 mg/dL

   D. Triglycerides 125 mg/dL

   E. Troponin I 0.02 ng/mL

2. A nurse is reinforcing teaching with a client who is scheduled for an echocardiogram. Which of the following statements should the nurse include in the teaching?

   A. "You may experience a warm feeling when the dye is injected."

   B. "The test will require 2 hours to complete."

   C. "You will be placed onto your right side during the procedure."

   D. "The test allows us to see how your heart valves work."

3. The nurse is teaching the client who is scheduled for a coronary angiography. Which of the following statements should the nurse make?

   A. "You should have nothing to eat or drink for 2 hours prior to the procedure."

   B. "You will be given general anesthesia during the procedure."

   C. "You should not have this procedure done if you are allergic to eggs."

   D. "You will need to keep your affected leg straight following the procedure."

4. The nurse is teaching the newly licensed nurse about caring for the client who is to have a CVP line placed. Which of the following statements by the newly licensed nurse indicates an understanding?

   A. "Air should be instilled into the monitoring system prior to the procedure."

   B. "The client should be positioned on the left side during the procedure."

   C. "The transducer should be level with the second intercostal space after the line is placed."

   D. "A chest x-ray is needed to verify placement after the procedure."

5. A nurse is teaching a newly licensed nurse about vascular access devices. Match the following vascular access devices with the associated characteristics.

   A. Implanted port

   B. Percutaneous inserted central catheter (PICC)

   C. Nontunneled percutaneous central venous catheter

   1. Used for short-term access

   2. Inserted above or below the antecubital fossa

   3. Surgically inserted into the chest wall

Active Learning Scenario

A nurse is reviewing the plan of care for a client who is scheduled for a cardiac exercise stress test. What information should the nurse include in the review? Use the ATI Active Learning Template: Diagnostic Procedure to complete this item.

DESCRIPTION OF THE PROCEDURE

INDICATIONS: List at least two.

NURSING INTERVENTIONS (PRE, INTRA, POST)

- Describe at least four preprocedure actions.
- Describe at least two intraprocedure actions.

Active Learning Scenario Key

Using the ATI Active Learning Template: Diagnostic Procedure

DESCRIPTION OF THE PROCEDURE: During a cardiac exercise stress test, the cardiac muscle is exercised by walking on a treadmill. This provides information regarding the workload of the heart.

INDICATIONS
- Angina
- Heart failure
- Myocardial infarction
- Dysrhythmia

NURSING ACTIONS (PRE, INTRA, POST)

Preprocedure
- Ensure that a signed informed consent form is obtained.
- Explain to the client that they will walk on a treadmill. Comfortable athletic shoes and clothing are recommended.
- Explain that a pharmacological stress test can be prescribed if the client cannot walk on the treadmill and complete the test. A medication (dipyridamole, adenosine, dobutamine) is administered to stress the heart instead of walking on the treadmill.
- Instruct the client to fast 2 to 4 hr before the procedure or according to facility policy and to avoid tobacco, alcohol, and caffeine before the test.
- Instruct the client to get adequate rest the night before the test.

Intraprocedure
- Monitor heart rate and rhythm with a 12-lead ECG during the test.
- Instruct the client to report any chest pain, shortness of breath, or dizziness during the test.

Ⓝ *NCLEX® Connection: Reduction of Risk Potential, Therapeutic Procedures*

Application Exercises Key

1. A, C. **CORRECT:** When analyzing cues, the nurse should identify a total cholesterol level greater than 200 mg/dL, and a LDL level greater than 130 mg/dL indicate an increased risk for heart disease.

   Ⓝ *NCLEX® Connection: Reduction of Risk Potential, Laboratory Values*

2. D. **CORRECT:** When taking actions, the nurse should instruct the client that an echocardiogram is an ultrasound test that is used to evaluate the heart's position and the function of the valves.

   Ⓝ *NCLEX® Connection: Reduction of Risk Potential, Diagnostic Tests*

3. D. **CORRECT:** When taking actions, the nurse should instruct the client they will remain on bed rest in the supine position with the affected leg straight for a prescribed amount of time. This positioning decreases the client's risk for bleeding and hematoma formation at the catheter insertion site.

   Ⓝ *NCLEX® Connection: Reduction of Risk Potential, Therapeutic Procedures*

4. D. **CORRECT:** When evaluating outcomes, the statement by the newly licensed nurse to obtain a chest x-ray indicates an understanding of the teaching. A chest x-ray is obtained to confirm proper placement of the lines and evaluate for a pneumothorax.

   Ⓝ *NCLEX® Connection: Reduction of Risk Potential, Potential for Complications of Diagnostic Tests/Treatments/Procedures*

5. A, 3; B, 2; C, 1

   When taking actions, the nurse should instruct that a nontunneled percutaneous central venous catheter is used for short-term treatment. A PICC line is inserted into the basilic or cephalic vein at least one fingerbreadth below or above the antecubital fossa. An implanted port is surgically inserted into the chest wall. (Iggy 2021, 282, 283, 284)

   Ⓝ *NCLEX® Connection: Reduction of Risk Potential, Potential for Complications of Diagnostic Tests/Treatments/Procedures*

UNIT 4   CARDIOVASCULAR DISORDERS

SECTION: DIAGNOSTIC AND THERAPEUTIC PROCEDURES

CHAPTER 26 *Electrocardiography and Dysrhythmia Monitoring*

Cardiac electrical activity can be monitored by using an electrocardiogram (ECG). The heart's electrical activity can be monitored by a standard 12-lead ECG (resting ECG), ambulatory ECG (Holter monitoring), continuous cardiac monitoring, or by telemetry.

Cardiac monitoring is used to diagnose dysrhythmias, chamber enlargement, myocardial ischemia, injury, or infarction and to monitor the effects of electrolyte imbalances or medication administration.

Cardiac dysrhythmias are heartbeat disturbances (beat formation, beat conduction, or myocardial response to beat).

Nurses should be familiar with cardioversion and defibrillation procedures for treating dysrhythmias.

Electrocardiography

Electrocardiography uses an electrocardiograph to record the electrical activity of the heart over time. The electrocardiograph is connected by wires (leads) to skin electrodes placed on the chest and limbs of a client.

- Continuous cardiac monitoring requires the client to be in close proximity to the monitoring system.
- Telemetry allows the client to ambulate while maintaining proximity to the monitoring system.
- Inform clients receiving continuous ECG monitoring that the monitoring will not detect shortness of breath, chest pain, or other manifestations of acute coronary syndrome. The client should be instructed to report new or worsening manifestations. Qs

INDICATIONS

DYSRHYTHMIAS

- Sinus bradycardia and tachycardia
- Atrioventricular (AV) blocks
- Atrial fibrillation
- Premature atrial complexes (PACs) and premature ventricular complexes (PVCs)
- Supraventricular tachycardia
- Ventricular tachycardia
- Ventricular fibrillation

CLIENT PRESENTATION

- Cardiovascular disease
- Myocardial infarction (MI)
- Hypoxia
- Acid–base imbalances
- Electrolyte disturbances
- Pericarditis
- Drug or alcohol use
- Shock

CONSIDERATIONS

PREPROCEDURE

NURSING ACTIONS

Prepare the client for a 12-lead ECG, if prescribed.

- Position the client in a supine position with chest exposed.
- Wash the client's skin to remove oils.
- Attach one electrode to each of the client's extremities by applying electrodes to flat surfaces above the wrists and ankles and the other six electrodes to the chest, avoiding chest hair. (Chest hair can be shaved or clipped if needed.)

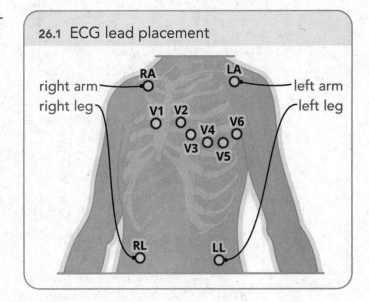

26.1 ECG lead placement

INTRAPROCEDURE

NURSING ACTIONS: Monitor for manifestations of dysrhythmia (chest pain, decreased level of consciousness, shortness of breath) and hypoxia.

CLIENT EDUCATION: Remain still and breathe normally while the 12-lead ECG is performed.

POSTPROCEDURE

NURSING ACTIONS

- Remove leads from the client, print the ECG report, and notify the provider.
- Apply a Holter monitor if the client is on a telemetry unit and/or needs continuous cardiac monitoring.
- Continue to monitor the client for dysrhythmia.
- To conduct a rhythm analysis, perform the following steps:
  - Determine the heart rate.
  - Determine whether the heart rhythm is regular or irregular.
  - Analyze the P waves for regularity and shape.
  - Measure the PR interval for consistency (0.12 to 0.20 seconds).
  - Measure the QRS duration and for consistency in appearance.

Dysrhythmias

- Dysrhythmias are classified by the following:
  - Site of origin: sinoatrial (SA) node, atria, atrioventricular (AV) node, or ventricle
    - Electrophysiological study is performed to determine the area of the heart causing the dysrhythmia. Ablation of the area is possible.
  - Effect on the rate and rhythm of the heart: bradycardia, tachycardia, heart block, premature beat, flutter, fibrillation, or asystole
- Dysrhythmias can be benign or life-threatening.
- The life-threatening effects of dysrhythmias are generally related to decreased cardiac output and ineffective tissue perfusion.
- Cardiac dysrhythmias are a primary cause of death in clients suffering acute MI and other sudden death disorders.
- Rapid recognition and treatment of serious dysrhythmias is essential to preserve life. Treatment is based on the cardiac rhythm, which can require cardioversion, defibrillation or pacemaker insertion, and/or medications. **(26.4)**
- Findings of a dysrhythmia in older adults might be present only with increased activity.
- Risks for heart disease, hypertension, dysrhythmias, and atherosclerosis increase with age.
- Treatment of dysrhythmias follows Advanced Cardiac Life Support (ACLS) evidence-based protocols. (See **CHAPTER 2: EMERGENCY NURSING PRINCIPLES AND MANAGEMENT** for further information).

26.2 ECG strip

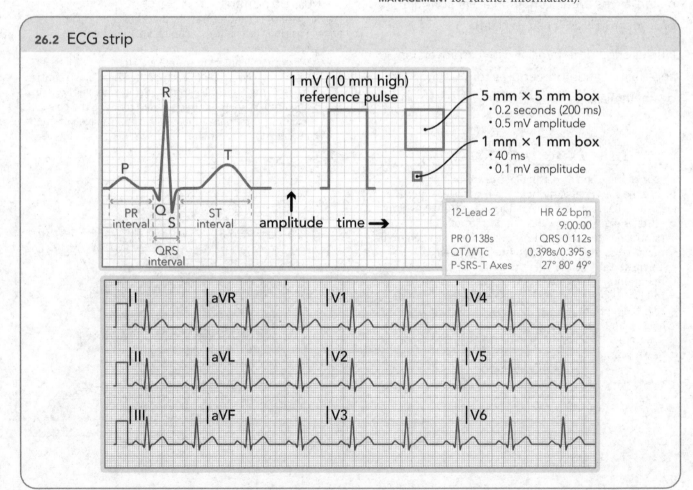

Cardioversion and defibrillation

Cardioversion is the delivery of a direct countershock to the heart synchronized to the QRS complex. Defibrillation is the delivery of an unsynchronized, direct countershock to the heart. Defibrillation stops all electrical activity of the heart, allowing the SA node to take over and reestablish a perfusing rhythm.

INDICATIONS

Cardioversion: Elective treatment of atrial dysrhythmias, supraventricular tachycardia, and ventricular tachycardia with a pulse. Cardioversion is the treatment of choice for clients who are symptomatic.

Defibrillation: Ventricular fibrillation or pulseless ventricular tachycardia.

CONSIDERATIONS

PREPROCEDURE

Clients who have atrial fibrillation of unknown duration must receive adequate anticoagulation for at least 3 weeks prior to cardioversion therapy to prevent dislodgement of thrombi into the bloodstream.

NURSING ACTIONS
- Reinforce teaching about the procedure to the client, and assist with obtaining consent.
- Administer oxygen.
- Document preprocedure l rhythm.
- Have emergency equipment available.

INTRAPROCEDURE

NURSING ACTIONS
- All staff must stand clear of the client, equipment connected to the client, and the bed when a shock is delivered.
- Perform CPR for cardiac asystole or other pulseless rhythms.
- Assist with immediate defibrillation of the client for ventricular fibrillation.

26.3 Dysrhythmias

ATRIAL FIBRILLATION

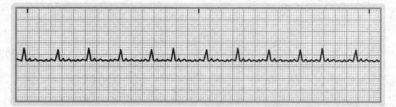

PREMATURE ATRIAL COMPLEXES

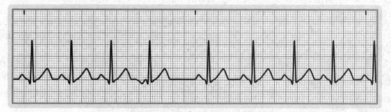

PREMATURE VENTRICULAR COMPLEXES

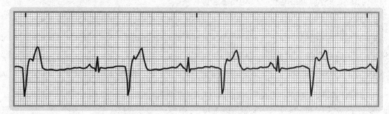

VENTRICULAR TACHYCARDIA

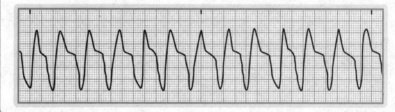

26.4 Dysrhythmia treatments

	MEDICATION	ELECTRICAL MANAGEMENT
Bradycardia (any rhythm less than 60/min) Treat if the client is symptomatic	Atropine; dopamine or epinephrine infusion if unresponsive to atropine	Pacemaker
Atrial fibrillation *Supraventricular tachycardia* *Ventricular tachycardia with pulse*	Amiodarone, adenosine, and verapamil	Synchronized cardioversion
Ventricular tachycardia without pulse or ventricular fibrillation	Amiodarone, lidocaine, and epinephrine	Defibrillation

POSTPROCEDURE

NURSING ACTIONS

- Provide the client/family with reassurance and emotional support.
- Document the following:
  - Postprocedure rhythm
  - Number of defibrillation or cardioversion attempts, energy settings, time, and response
  - The client's condition and state of consciousness following the procedure
  - Skin condition under the electrodes

CLIENT EDUCATION

- Follow instructions on checking your pulse.
- Report palpitations or irregularities.

Active Learning Scenario

A nurse is assisting a nurse educator who is reviewing electrocardiography with a group of nurses. What information should the nurse recommend be included in this discussion? Use the ATI Active Learning Template: Therapeutic Procedure to complete this item.

DESCRIPTION OF PROCEDURE: Describe electrocardiography and describe the difference between continuous cardiac monitoring and telemetry.

INDICATIONS: List four dysrhythmias that can be identified.

NURSING INTERVENTIONS (PRE, INTRA, POST): Identify at least two preprocedure, one intraprocedure, and two postprocedure.

Application Exercises

1. A nurse assisting with the care of a group of clients. The nurse should recognize which of the following clients is at risk for the development of a dysrhythmia? (Select all that apply.)

   A. A client who has metabolic alkalosis

   B. A client who has a blood potassium level of 4.3 mEq/L

   C. A client who has an SaO_2 of 96%

   D. A client who has alcohol use disorder

   E. A client who underwent stent placement in a coronary artery

2. A nurse is assisting with the care of a client who is on telemetry. The nurse recognizes the client's heart rate is 46/min and notifies the provider. Which of the following prescriptions should the nurse anticipate the provider to prescribe?

   A. Defibrillation

   B. Pacemaker insertion

   C. Synchronized cardioversion

   D. Administration of IV Lidocaine

3. A nurse is caring for a client following cardioversion. Which of the following should the nurse include in the documentation of this procedure? (Select all that apply.)

   A. Follow-up ECG

   B. Energy settings used

   C. IV fluid intake

   D. Urinary output

   E. Skin condition under electrodes

4. A nurse is providing teaching to a client who has atrial fibrillation and has a new prescription for an anticoagulant. Which of the following information should the nurse include in the teaching?

   A. The anticoagulant will improve blood pressure.

   B. The anticoagulant can resume the heart to a normal rhythm.

   C. The anticoagulant can prevent infection.

   D. The anticoagulant will decrease the risk of blood clots.

Application Exercises Key

1. A, D, E. **CORRECT:** A client who has an acid-base imbalance (metabolic alkalosis) is at risk for developing a dysrhythmia. A client who has a substance use disorder such as alcohol use disorder is at risk for developing a dysrhythmia. A client who has cardiac disease and underwent stent placement surgery is at risk for developing a dysrhythmia.

   Ⓝ *NCLEX Connection: Physiological Adaptation, Basic Pathophysiology*

2. B. **CORRECT:** When recognizing cues, the nurse should anticipate the provider to prescribe pacemaker insertion for the client. The client who has bradycardia is a candidate for pacemaker insertion which assists with increasing the rate of the heart at a set rate.

   Ⓝ *NCLEX Connection: Physiological Adaptation, Medical Emergencies*

3. A, B, E. **CORRECT:** When taking actions, the nurse should document the client's follow-up ECG results following the procedure. The nurse should also document the energy settings used during the procedure. The nurse should also document the condition of the client's skin where the electrodes were placed for the procedure.

   Ⓝ *NCLEX Nursing Connection: Reduction of Risk Potential, Therapeutic Procedures*

4. D. **CORRECT:** When taking actions, the nurse should inform the client who has atrial fibrillation that they are at risk for clot formation; therefore, the use of an anticoagulant decreases the blood clot formation and the risk of a stroke or pulmonary embolism.

   Ⓝ *NCLEX Connection: Reduction of Risk Potential, Therapeutic Procedures*

Active Learning Scenario Key

Using the ATI Active Learning Template: Therapeutic Procedure

DESCRIPTION OF PROCEDURE
- Electrocardiography is the use of an electrocardiograph to record the electrical activity of the heart over time by connecting wires (leads) to skin electrodes placed on the chest and limbs of the client.
- Continuous monitoring requires the client to be in close proximity to the monitoring system. Telemetry allows the client to ambulate.

INDICATIONS
- Sinus bradycardia and tachycardia
- Atrioventricular (AV) blocks
- Atrial fibrillation
- Supraventricular tachycardia
- Ventricular fibrillation
- Premature ventricular complexes (PVCs)
- Premature atrial complexes (PACs)

NURSING INTERVENTIONS (PRE, INTRA, POST)

Preprocedure
- Position the client in a supine position with chest exposed.
- Wash the skin to remove oils.
- Attach one electrode to each of the client's extremities by applying electrodes to flat surfaces above the wrists and ankles and the other six electrodes to the chest, avoiding chest hair, which can be clipped or shaved.

Intraprocedure
- Instruct the client to remain still and breathe normally.
- Monitor for manifestations of dysrhythmia (chest pain, decreased level of consciousness, shortness of breath) and hypoxia.

Postprocedure
- Remove leads, print ECG report, and notify the provider.
- Apply Holter monitor if the client is on the telemetry unit and/or needs continuous monitoring.
- Continue monitoring for manifestations of dysrhythmia and hypoxia.

Ⓝ *NCLEX® Connection: Reduction of Risk Potential, Potential for Complications of Diagnostic Tests/Treatments/Procedures*

UNIT 4   CARDIOVASCULAR DISORDERS

SECTION: DIAGNOSTIC AND THERAPEUTIC PROCEDURES

CHAPTER 27 *Invasive Cardiovascular Procedures*

Cardiovascular procedures include invasive methods used to improve blood flow for occluded arteries and veins.

Invasive cardiovascular procedures are indicated after noninvasive interventions have been tried, such as diet, exercise, and medications.

Invasive cardiovascular procedures that nurses should be knowledgeable about include percutaneous coronary intervention (PCI), coronary artery bypass grafts (CABG), and peripheral bypass grafts.

Percutaneous coronary intervention

PCI is a nonsurgical procedure performed to open coronary arteries through one of the following means.
- **Atherectomy:** Used to break up and remove plaques within cardiac vessels
- **Stent:** Placement of a mesh-wire device that contains no medication to hold an artery open and prevent restenosis
  - ○ **Bare metal**
  - ○ **Drug-eluting stents (DES)**
- **Percutaneous transluminal coronary angioplasty:** Also referred to simply as angioplasty, this involves inflating a balloon to dilate the arterial lumen and the adhering plaque, thus widening the arterial lumen. This can include stent placement.

INDICATIONS

- Can be performed on an elective basis to treat coronary artery disease when there is occlusion of one to two coronary arteries. The area of occlusion is confined, not scattered, and easy to access (proximal).
- Might reduce ischemia during the occurrence of an acute myocardial infarction (MI) by opening coronary arteries and restoring perfusion. It is usually performed within 4 to 6 hr of the onset of manifestations if having a non-ST-elevation (NSTEMI) or myocardial infarction (MI) or within 60 to 90 min for an ST-elevation myocardial infarction (STEMI).
- Might be used as an alternative to coronary artery bypass graft
- Angioplasty might be used with stent placement to prevent artery reocclusion and to dilate the coronary artery.

CLIENT PRESENTATION

SUBJECTIVE DATA: Chest pain might occur with or without exertion. Pain might radiate to the jaw, left arm, through the back, or to the shoulder. Manifestations might increase in cold weather or with exercise. Other manifestations might include dyspnea, nausea, fatigue, and diaphoresis.

OBJECTIVE DATA: ECG changes might include ST elevation, depression, or nonspecific ST changes. Other findings might include bradycardia, tachycardia, hypotension, elevated blood pressure, vomiting, and mental disorientation.

CONSIDERATIONS

Refer to **PN ADULT MEDICAL SURGICAL NURSING CHAPTER 25: CARDIOVASCULAR DIAGNOSTIC AND THERAPEUTIC PROCEDURES**.

COMPLICATIONS

Artery dissection

- Perforation of an artery by the catheter might cause cardiac tamponade or require emergency bypass surgery.
- Artery dissection findings include severe hypotension and tachycardia and might require extended occlusion of perforation with a balloon catheter and reversal of anticoagulants.

Cardiac tamponade

Cardiac tamponade can result from fluid accumulation in the pericardial sac.
- Findings include hypotension, jugular venous distention, muffled heart sounds, and paradoxical pulse (variance of 10 mm Hg or more in systolic blood pressure between expiration and inspiration).
- Hemodynamic monitoring reveals that intracardiac and pulmonary artery pressures are similar and elevated (plateau pressures) and that cardiac output is decreased.

NURSING ACTIONS

- Notify the provider immediately. ⓠs
- Assist with the administration of IV fluids to manage hypotension.
- Obtain a chest x-ray or echocardiogram to confirm findings.
- Prepare the client for pericardiocentesis or return to surgical suite (informed consent; gather materials; administer medications as appropriate).
  - Monitor hemodynamic pressures and heart rhythm for recurrence of findings after the procedure.

Hematoma formation near insertion site

NURSING ACTIONS

- Monitor for sensation, color, capillary refill, and peripheral pulses in the extremity distal to the insertion site.
- Assess insertion site for development of a hematoma at prescribed intervals and as needed.
- Hold pressure for uncontrolled oozing/bleeding.
- Notify the provider.

Allergic reaction related to the contrast dye

Manifestations can include chills, fever, rash, wheezing, tachycardia, and bradycardia.

NURSING ACTIONS

- Monitor for an allergic reaction.
- Have resuscitation equipment readily available.
- Administer diphenhydramine or epinephrine if prescribed.

External bleeding at the insertion site

NURSING ACTIONS

- Monitor insertion site for bleeding or swelling.
- Apply pressure to site.
- Keep client's leg or arm straight.

Embolism

Plaque or a clot can become dislodged.

NURSING ACTIONS

- Monitor for chest pain during and after the procedure.
- Monitor vital signs and SaO_2.

Retroperitoneal bleeding

Bleeding in the retroperitoneal space (abdominal cavity behind the peritoneum) can occur due to femoral artery puncture.

NURSING ACTIONS

- Monitor for flank pain and hypotension.
- Notify the provider immediately.
- Administer IV fluids and assist with monitoring blood products.

CLIENT EDUCATION

- Pressure will be applied to the insertion site.
- Keep leg straight.
- Report chest pain, shortness of breath, and cardiac manifestations.

Restenosis of treated vessel

Clot formation can occur in the coronary vessel immediately or several days after the procedure.

NURSING ACTIONS

- Monitor ECG patterns and for report of chest pain.
- Notify the provider immediately.
- Prepare the client for return to the cardiac catheterization laboratory.

CLIENT EDUCATION: Notify the provider of cardiac manifestations.

Acute kidney injury

Damage to the kidney can result from use of contrast agent, which is nephrotoxic.

Older adults who have mild renal failure or chronic dehydration are at high risk.

NURSING ACTIONS

- Monitor urine output, BUN, creatinine, and electrolytes.
- Promote adequate hydration (oral and IV).

Coronary artery bypass grafts

- CABG is an invasive surgical procedure that aims to restore vascularization of the myocardium.
  - Performed to bypass an obstruction in one or more of the coronary arteries, CABG does not alter the atherosclerotic process but improves the quality of life for clients restricted by painful coronary artery disease.
  - The procedure is most effective when a client has sufficient ventricular function (ejection fraction greater than 50%).
  - Older adult clients are more likely to experience transient neurologic changes, toxic effects from cardiac medications, and dysrhythmias. ⓖ
- Less invasive revascularization procedures have been developed to reduce risk and improve client outcomes (off-pump coronary artery bypass, robotic heart surgery, minimally invasive direct coronary artery bypass). These procedures have characteristics similar to traditional CABG.

INDICATIONS

POTENTIAL DIAGNOSES

- More than 50% blockage of left main coronary artery with anginal episodes (blockage inaccessible to angioplasty and stenting)
- Significant two-vessel disease with unstable angina
- Triple-vessel disease with or without angina
- Persistent ischemia or likely MI following coronary angiography, PCI, or stent placement

- Heart failure or cardiogenic shock with acute MI or ischemia (might not be reasonable for clients who have poor ejection fractions)
- Coronary arteries that are unable to be accessed or treated by angioplasty and stent placement (narrow or calcified)
- Coronary artery disease nonresponsive to medical management
- Heart valve disease

CLIENT PRESENTATION

SUBJECTIVE DATA: Chest pain can occur with or without exertion. Pain can radiate to jaw, left arm, through the back, or to the shoulder. Effects can increase in cold weather or with exercise. Other findings can include dyspnea, nausea, fatigue, and diaphoresis.

OBJECTIVE DATA: ECG changes can include ST elevation, depression, or nonspecific ST changes. Other findings can include bradycardia, tachycardia, hypotension, elevated blood pressure, vomiting, and mental disorientation.

CONSIDERATIONS

PREPROCEDURE

NURSING ACTIONS

- A CABG can be an elective procedure or done as an emergency. When planned, preparation begins before the client comes to the facility for the procedure.
- Verify that the client has signed the informed consent form.
- Confirm that recent chest x-ray, ECG, and laboratory reports are available if needed.
- Complete a baseline assessment of the client's cognitive status, identify any health issues that can complicate postoperative recovery (diabetes, hypertension, stroke) and the client's support system.
- Administer preoperative medications.
  - Anxiolytics, such as lorazepam and diazepam
  - Prophylactic antibiotics
  - Anticholinergics, such as scopolamine, to reduce secretions
- Provide safe transport of the client to the operating suite. Monitor heart rate and rhythm, oxygenation, and other vital indicators.
- Ensure the client understands the procedure and postsurgical environment.
- Assess client and family anxiety levels surrounding the procedure. Qᴘᴄᴄ

CLIENT EDUCATION

- Understand the importance of coughing and deep breathing after the procedure to prevent complications.
- Splint the incision when coughing and deeply breathing. Provide a return demonstration to the nurse when being instructed.
- Perform arm and leg exercises to prevent complications.
- Report pain to the nursing staff. The majority of pain stems from the harvest site for the vein.
- Expect the following postoperatively.
  - Endotracheal tube and mechanical ventilator for airway management for several hours following surgery
  - Inability to talk while endotracheal tube is in place
  - Sternal incision and possible leg incision
  - Early ambulation to prevent complications
  - Administration of analgesics for pain control
  - One or two mediastinal chest tubes
  - Indwelling urinary catheter
  - Pacemaker wires
  - Hemodynamic monitoring devices (pulmonary artery catheter, arterial line)
- Alter or discontinue regular medications as prescribed.
  - Medications frequently discontinued for CABG
    - Diuretics 2 to 3 days before surgery
    - Aspirin and other anticoagulants 1 week before surgery
  - Medications often continued for CABG
    - Potassium supplements
    - Scheduled antidysrhythmics, such as amiodarone
    - Scheduled antihypertensives (metoprolol, a beta blocker; diltiazem, a calcium-channel blocker)
    - Insulin (clients who have diabetes mellitus and are insulin-dependent usually receive half the regular insulin dose)
  - Verbalize any feelings with family and the nurse.

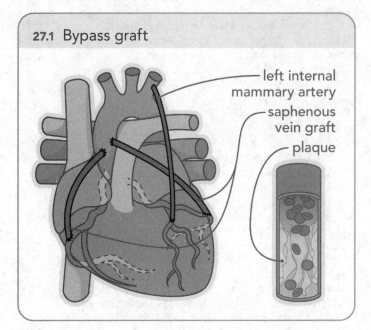

27.1 Bypass graft

left internal mammary artery
saphenous vein graft
plaque

INTRAPROCEDURE

- An extracardiac vein (saphenous vein), artery (usually the radial or mammary artery), or synthetic graft can be used to bypass an obstruction in one or more of the coronary arteries.
- Most often, a median sternotomy incision is made to visualize the heart and the great vessels.
- The client is placed on cardiopulmonary bypass, and the client's core temperature can be lowered to decrease the rate of metabolism and demand for oxygen. A normal core temperature can be maintained during cardiopulmonary bypass to improve postoperative myocardial function and reduce postoperative complications.
- A cardioplegic solution is used to stop the heart. This prevents myocardial ischemia and allows for a motionless operative field.
- The artery or vein to be used is harvested.
- The harvested vessel is anastomosed from the aorta to the affected coronary artery distal to the occlusion. When the mammary artery is used as a graft, the proximal end remains intact, and the distal end is grafted just past the coronary artery occlusion.
- Once the bypass is complete, the hypothermic client is rewarmed by heat exchanges on the bypass machine. Grafts are monitored for patency and leakage as the client is weaned from the bypass machine and blood is redirected through coronary vasculature.
- Lastly, pacemaker wires can be sutured into the myocardium, and chest tubes are placed. The incision is closed with wire sutures, and the client is transported to the intensive care unit.

NURSING ACTIONS

- Provide padding to bony prominences to provide comfort and prevent skin breakdown.
- Communicate surgical progress to family members, if appropriate.
- Assist in monitoring urine output and blood loss.
- Document appropriate surgical events.
- Assist in arranging intensive care unit placement and communicate the client's postoperative needs.

POSTPROCEDURE

NURSING ACTIONS

- Maintain patent airway and adequate ventilation.
  - Monitor respiratory rate and effort.
  - Auscultate breath sounds and verify adventitious sounds with RN. Report crackles.
  - Monitor SaO_2.
  - Document ventilator settings.
  - Suction as needed.
  - Assist with extubation.
- Dangle the client's legs and turn the client from side to side as tolerated within 2 hr following extubation. Assist the client to a chair within 24 hr. Ambulate the client 25 to 100 ft three times a day by first postoperative day.
- Consult respiratory services to aid in recovery and client education.

- Consult case management services to initiate discharge planning: need for home oxygen therapy, transfer to tertiary care facility.
- Continually monitor heart rate and rhythm. Treat dysrhythmias per protocol.
- Maintain an adequate circulating blood volume.
  - Monitor blood pressure.
    - Hypotension can result in graft collapse.
    - Hypertension can result in bleeding from grafts and sutures.
    - Titrate IV drips (dopamine, dobutamine, milrinone, sodium nitroprusside) per protocol to control blood pressure and/or increase cardiac output.
  - Monitor hemodynamic pressures and catheter placement. Observe waveforms and markings on the catheter.
  - Monitor level of consciousness. Assess neurologic status every 30 to 60 min until the client awakens from anesthesia, then every 2 to 4 hr or per facility policy.
  - Notify the surgeon of significant changes in values.
- Monitor chest tube patency and drainage.
  - Measure drainage at least once an hour.
  - Volume exceeding 150 mL/hr could be a manifestation of hemorrhage and should be reported to the surgeon.
  - Avoid dependent loops in tubing to facilitate drainage.
- Assess and control pain.
  - Determine source of pain (angina, incisional pain).
    - Anginal pain often radiates and is unaffected by breathing.
    - Incisional pain is localized, sharp, aching, burning, and often worsens with deep breathing.
- Administer analgesics (morphine, fentanyl).
  - Pain will stimulate the sympathetic nervous system, resulting in increased heart rate and systemic vascular resistance.
  - Provide frequent and adequate doses to control pain. Maintain around-the-clock administration.
- Monitor fluid and electrolyte status.
  - Fluid administration is determined by blood pressure, pulmonary artery wedge pressure, right atrial pressure, cardiac output and index, systemic vascular resistance, blood loss, and urine output.
  - Follow provider or unit-specific orders for fluid administration.
  - Monitor for electrolyte imbalances, especially for hypokalemia and hyperkalemia.
- Prevent and monitor for infection.
  - Practice proper hand hygiene.
  - Use surgical aseptic technique during procedures such as dressing changes and suctioning.
  - Administer antibiotics.
  - Monitor WBC counts, incisional redness and drainage, and fever.
  - Monitor temperature and provide warming measures if indicated.
- Encourage physical activity. Consult the cardiac rehabilitation program or a physical therapist to devise a specific program.
- Discuss home environment and social supports. Consult case management to assist with home planning needs.

CLIENT EDUCATION

- Splint the incision while deeply breathing and coughing.
- Monitor and report manifestations of infection (fever, incisional drainage, redness).
- Treat angina.
  - Maintain a fresh supply of sublingual nitroglycerin.
  - Store nitroglycerin in a light-resistant container.
  - Discontinue activity and rest with the onset of pain. Follow directions for treating anginal pain.
  - Older female clients might show milder manifestations (dyspnea, indigestion). Ⓖ
- Adhere to the pharmacological regimen.
- Those who have diabetes mellitus should closely monitor blood glucose levels.
- Consume a heart-healthy diet (low fat, low cholesterol, high fiber, low salt).
- Quit smoking if applicable. Use resources on smoking cessation provided by nurse.
- Remain home during the first week after surgery and resume normal activities slowly.
  - Week 2: possible return to work part-time, increase in social activities
  - Week 3: lifting of up to 15 lb (Avoid heavier lifting for 6 to 8 weeks.)
- Resume sexual activity based on provider advice.
  - Walking one block or climbing two flights of stairs without shortness of breath or manifestations of angina generally indicates that it is safe for the client to resume normal sexual activity.
- Verbalize feelings.

COMPLICATIONS

Pulmonary complications

These include the primary complication of atelectasis, as well as pneumonia and pulmonary edema.

NURSING ACTIONS

- While the client is intubated, suction every 1 to 2 hr and as needed.
- Turn the client every 2 hr and advance them out of bed as soon as possible.
- Monitor breath sounds, SaO_2, ABGs, pulmonary artery pressures, cardiac output, and urine output, and obtain a chest x-ray as indicated.

CLIENT EDUCATION: Engage in coughing, deep breathing, and use of an incentive spirometer. Increasing activity reduces postoperative complications.

Hypothermia

Hypothermia can cause vasoconstriction, metabolic acidosis, and hypertension.

NURSING ACTIONS

- Monitor temperature and provide warming measures (warm blankets, heat lamps).
- Monitor blood pressure.
- Administer vasodilators if prescribed.

CLIENT EDUCATION: Shivering is common following surgery.

Decreased cardiac output

Decreased cardiac output can result from dysrhythmias, cardiac tamponade, hypovolemia, left ventricular failure, or MI.

Cardiac tamponade results from bleeding while chest tubes are occluded, causing fluid to build up in the pericardium. Increased pericardial fluid compresses heart chambers and inhibits effective pumping.

Indications include a sudden decrease/cessation of chest-tube drainage following heavy drainage, jugular-venous distention with clear lung sounds, and equal pulmonary artery wedge pressure and central venous pressure values.

Hypovolemia can be the result of bleeding, decreased intravascular volume, or vasodilation; hypotension and decreased urine output are the results.

Left ventricular heart failure can occur with an MI or fluid overload.

NURSING ACTIONS

- Monitor ECG, blood pressure, pulmonary artery pressures, cardiac output, urine output, and bleeding through the chest tube.
- Administer inotropic medications and fluid and blood products.
- Treat dysrhythmias.
  - Use pacemaker wires if heart block is present.
- Treatment of cardiac tamponade involves volume expansion (fluid administration) and an emergency sternotomy with drainage. Pericardiocentesis is avoided because blood can have clotted.

Electrolyte disturbances

Potassium and magnesium depletion is common.

NURSING ACTIONS

- Always dilute potassium in adequate fluid (20 to 40 mEq in 100 mL of IV solution).
- Administer via infusion pump to control the rate of delivery. The administration rate is 10 mEq/hr.
- Monitor ECG and electrolytes.

Neurologic deficits

Transient hypertension, hypotension, or a blood clot might cause an intraoperative cerebrovascular accident.

NURSING ACTIONS

- Monitor neurologic status, including pupils, level of consciousness, and sensory and motor function.
- Maintain the client's blood pressure within prescribed parameters.

CLIENT EDUCATION

- Understand the procedures.
- Memory loss and neurologic deficits can be temporary.

Peripheral bypass grafts

Peripheral bypass graft surgery aims to restore adequate blood flow to the areas affected by peripheral artery disease.

- A peripheral bypass graft involves suturing graft material or autogenous saphenous veins proximal and distal to occluded area of an artery. This procedure improves blood supply to the area normally served by the blocked artery.
- Aortoiliac and aortofemoral bypasses are performed for vessel occlusions in the lower extremities.
- If bypass surgery fails to restore circulation, the client might need to undergo amputation of the limb.

INDICATIONS

- Acute circulatory compromise in limb
- Severe pain at rest that interferes with the ability to work

CLIENT PRESENTATION

SUBJECTIVE DATA

- Numbness or burning pain to the lower extremity with exercise; can stop with rest (intermittent claudication)
- Numbness or burning pain to the lower extremity at rest; can wake the client at night; pain can be relieved by lowering the extremity below the level of the heart

OBJECTIVE DATA

- Decreased or absent pulses to feet
- Dry, hairless, shiny skin on calves
- Muscles can atrophy with advanced disease.
- Skin can be cold and darkened.
- Feet and toes can be mottled and dusky, and toenails might be thick.
- Skin can become reddened (rubor) when extremity is dropped to a dependent position.
- Ulcers or lesions can be noted on toes (arterial ulcers) or ankles (venous ulcers).

CONSIDERATIONS

PREPROCEDURE

NURSING ACTIONS

- Assess client and family understanding of the procedure.
- Verify that the client has signed the informed consent form.
- Assess for allergies.
- Document baseline vital signs and peripheral pulses.
- Administer prophylactic antibiotic therapy.
- Understand information about postoperative pain management and deep breathing/incentive spirometer exercises.

CLIENT EDUCATION

- Maintain NPO status for at least 8 hr prior to surgery.
- Do not cross legs.
- An arterial line might be inserted for blood and blood pressure.
- Pedal pulses will be checked frequently.

INTRAPROCEDURE

NURSING ACTIONS

- Provide padding to bony prominences to provide comfort and to prevent skin breakdown.
- Communicate surgical progress to family members, if appropriate.
- Assist in monitoring urine output and blood loss.
- Document appropriate surgical events.
- Communicate the client's postoperative needs to the postanesthesia care unit.

POSTPROCEDURE

NURSING ACTIONS

- Assess vital signs every 15 min for 1 hr and then hourly after the first hour (or per facility policy).
- Follow standing orders to maintain blood pressure within the prescribed range. Hypotension might reduce blood flow to graft, and hypertension might cause bleeding.
- Assess the operative limb every 15 min for 1 hr and then hourly after that, paying particular attention to the following.
  - Incision site for bleeding
  - Peripheral pulses, capillary refill, skin color/temperature, and sensory and motor function for indications of bypass graft occlusion. In clients who have dark skin, assess nail beds and soles of feet to detect early cyanosis.
  - Site is marked with an indelible marker.
- Administer IV fluids.
- Assess the type of pain experienced by the client. **Qs**
  - Throbbing pain is experienced due to an increase in blood flow to extremity.
  - Ischemic pain is often difficult to relieve with opioid administration.
- Assist with administration of analgesics, such as morphine sulfate and fentanyl.
- Administer antibiotics.
- Use surgical aseptic technique for dressing changes.
- Monitor incision sites for evidence of infection (erythema, tenderness, drainage).
- Administer anticoagulant therapy (warfarin, heparin, enoxaparin) to prevent reocclusion.
- Administer antiplatelet therapy (clopidogrel, aspirin). Alternate medications are tirofiban and eptifibatide.
- Help the client turn, cough, and deeply breathe every 2 hr.
- Maintain bed rest for 18 to 24 hr. The leg should be kept straight during this time.
- Assist the client to get out of bed and ambulate. Encourage the use of a walker initially.
- Discourage the client from sitting for long periods of time.
- Apply antiembolic stockings to promote venous return.
- Set up a progressive exercise program that includes walking. Consider a physical therapy consult.

CLIENT EDUCATION

- Completely abstain from smoking. Consider a smoking-cessation program suggested by the nurse.
- Follow activity restrictions.
- Avoid crossing legs.
- Avoid elevating legs above heart level.
- Reduce risk factors for atherosclerosis (smoking, sedentary lifestyle, uncontrolled diabetes mellitus).
- Learn techniques of foot inspection and care from the nurse.
  - Keep feet dry and clean.
  - Avoid extreme temperatures.
  - Use lotion.
  - Avoid socks with tight cuffs.
  - Wear clean, white cotton socks, and always wear shoes.

COMPLICATIONS

Graft occlusion

The graft might occlude due to reduced blood flow and clot formation. Occurs primarily in first 24 hr after the procedure

NURSING ACTIONS

- Notify the provider immediately for changes in pedal pulse, extremity color, or temperature.
- Prepare the client for thrombectomy or thrombolytic therapy.
- Monitor for bleeding with thrombolytics.
- Monitor coagulation studies.
- Monitor for anaphylaxis.

Compartment syndrome

Pressure from tissue swelling or bleeding within a compartment or a restricted space causes reduced blood flow to the area. Untreated, the affected tissue will become necrotic and die.

NURSING ACTIONS

- Monitor for worsening pain, swelling, and tense or taut skin.
- Report unusual findings to the provider immediately.
- Prepare the client for a fasciotomy to relieve compartmental pressure.

Infection

Infection of the surgical site might result in the loss of the graft and increased ischemia.

NURSING ACTIONS

- Assess the wound for increased redness, swelling, and drainage.
- Monitor WBC count and temperature.
- Collect specimens (wound or blood cultures).
- Administer antibiotic therapy.

CLIENT EDUCATION: Notify the provider of decreased sensation, increased ischemic pain, redness, or swelling at the incisional site or in the affected limb.

Active Learning Scenario

A nurse is developing the plan of care for a client who is returning to the unit following angioplasty. What should be included in the plan of care? Use the ATI Active Learning Template: Therapeutic Procedure to complete this item.

NURSING INTERVENTIONS: Describe five postprocedure nursing actions.

POTENTIAL COMPLICATIONS

- Describe at least two.
- Describe at least two actions related to each of these complications.

---

1. A nurse is collecting data from clients who are experiencing complications following angioplasty that was performed by insertion through the femoral artery. Match the findings to the complication the nurse should suspect.

   A. Hemorrhage

   B. Elevated BUN and creatinine

   C. Rash and wheezing

   D. Jugular venous distention (JVD)

   1. Hematoma at the groin

   2. Cardiac tamponade

   3. Allergic reaction to contrast dye

   4. Acute kidney injury (AKI)

2. A nurse is reviewing information with a newly licensed nurse about the use of cardiopulmonary bypass during surgery for coronary artery bypass grafting. Which of the following statements should the nurse include? (Select all that apply.)

   A. "The client's demand for oxygen is lowered."

   B. "Motion of the heart stops."

   C. "Rewarming of the client takes place."

   D. "The client's metabolic rate is increased."

   E. "Blood flow to the heart is stopped."

3. A nurse is assisting with care for a client who is one day postoperative following coronary artery bypass grafting (CABG) surgery. The client declines to perform coughing and deep breathing because they are concerned about causing pain at their incision site. Which action should the nurse take?

   A. Allow the client to rest, and return in 1 hr.

   B. Reinforce teaching with the client to splint their incision with a pillow.

   C. Document that the client is not adhering to the prescribed treatment.

   D. Tell the client they must perform coughing and deep-breathing exercises before discharge.

4. A nurse is reviewing discharge instructions with a client following an femoropopliteal bypass graft. Which of the following instructions should the nurse include? (Select all that apply.)

   A. Elevate legs above the heart whenever sitting.

   B. Keep the temperature of the home cold.

   C. Avoid frequent position changes.

   D. Sit with legs uncrossed.

   E. Walk regularly.

5. A nurse is assisting with collecting data from a client following peripheral bypass graft surgery of the left lower extremity and recognizes unexpected manifestations that should be immediately reported to the provider. Sort the following by whether they are expected or unexpected findings.

   A. Trace of serosanguinous drainage on dressing

   B. Capillary refill of affected limb of 6 seconds

   C. Pallor of the limb

   D. Pulse of 2+ in the affected limb

Application Exercises Key

1. 1, A; 2, D; 3, C; 4, B

   When analyzing cues for clients experiencing complications following angioplasty, the nurse determines that flank pain is a manifestation of blood collecting in the retroperitoneal space. The nurse determines that JVD is a manifestation of fluid collecting in the pericardial cavity from increased venous pressure caused by cardiac tamponade. The nurse determines that rash and wheezing are manifestations of an allergic reaction. The nurse determines that ECG changes and chest pain are manifestations of arterial occlusion in the coronary vessels. The nurse determines that elevated BUN and creatinine are manifestations of nephrotoxic effects to the kidney from the contrast agent.

   Ⓝ *NCLEX® Connection: Reduction of Risk Potential, Potential for Alterations in Body Systems*

2. A, B, C. **CORRECT:** When taking actions to review the use of cardiopulmonary bypass, the nurse should explain to the newly licensed nurse that the use of cardiopulmonary bypass reduces the oxygen demand during surgery, which reduces the risk for inadequate oxygenation of vital organs. The nurse should also include that the motion of the heart also stops during bypass to allow the graft to be placed near the affected coronary artery. Lastly, the nurse should include that the client's core body temperature is lowered during surgery, and rewarming occurs through heat exchanges in the bypass machine.

   Ⓝ *NCLEX® Connection: Reduction of Risk Potential, Therapeutic Procedures*

3. B. **CORRECT:** When taking actions to encourage the client to perform coughing and deep breathing, the nurse should teach them to splint their incision with a pillow to lessen the discomfort associated with coughing.

   Ⓝ *NCLEX® Connection: Reduction of Risk Potential, Therapeutic Procedures*

4. D, E. **CORRECT:** When taking actions, the nurse should instruct the client following a femoropopliteal bypass graft to keep their legs uncrossed to prevent constriction of blood vessels and to walk regularly to stimulate circulation.

   Ⓝ *NCLEX® Connection: Reduction of Risk Potential, Therapeutic Procedures*

5. **EXPECTED FINDINGS:** A, D;
   UNEXPECTED FINDINGS: B, C

   When recognizing cues, the nurse identifies a trace of serosanguinous drainage on the dressing, throbbing pain caused by increased blood flow to the extremity that is relieved by medication administration, and a pulse of 2+ as expected findings for a client following peripheral bypass graft. The nurse identifies that the capillary refill greater than 3 seconds is outside the expected range and should be reported to the provider. The nurse identifies that warmth and redness are expected outcomes and a change in color of the limb such as mottling may indicate graft occlusion and should be reported to the provider.

   Ⓝ *NCLEX® Connection: Reduction of Risk Potential, Therapeutic Procedures*

Active Learning Scenario Key

Using ATI Active Learning Template: Therapeutic Procedure

NURSING INTERVENTIONS
- Assess vital signs every 15 min × 4, every 30 min × 2, every hour × 4, and then every 4 hr (or per facility protocol).
- Assess the groin site with vital signs.
- Maintain bed rest in supine position with leg straight for prescribed time.
- Conduct continuous cardiac monitoring for dysrhythmia.
- Administer antiplatelet or thrombolytic agents.
- Administer anxiolytics and analgesics.
- Monitor urine output and administer IV fluids for hydration.
- Assist with sheath removal from insertion site.

POTENTIAL COMPLICATIONS
- Cardiac tamponade: Notify the provider; administer IV fluids to manage hypotension; obtain chest x-ray or echocardiogram; prepare for pericardiocentesis.
- Hematoma formation: Monitor sensation, color, capillary refill, and pulse in extremity distal to insertion site; hold pressure for uncontrolled oozing/bleeding; notify the provider.
- Allergic reaction: Monitor the client; have resuscitation equipment available; administer diphenhydramine or epinephrine as needed.
- External bleeding: Monitor insertion site for bleeding or swelling; apply pressure to insertion site; keep client's leg straight.
- Embolism: Monitor for chest pain; monitor vital signs and SaO_2.
- Retroperitoneal bleeding: Assess for flank pain and hypotension; notify the provider; administer IV fluids and blood products.
- Restenosis of vessel: Assess ECG pattern and for report of chest pain; notify the provider; prepare for return to cardiac catheterization laboratory.

Ⓝ *NCLEX® Connection: Reduction of Risk Potential, Therapeutic Procedures*

When reviewing the following chapters, keep in mind the relevant topics and tasks of the NCLEX outline.

Pharmacological Therapies

ADVERSE EFFECTS/CONTRAINDICATIONS/SIDE EFFECTS/INTERACTIONS

Identify a contraindication to the administration of a prescribed or over-the-counter medication to the client.

Withhold medication dose if client experiences adverse effect to medication.

MEDICATION ADMINISTRATION

Collect required data prior to medication administration.

Assist in preparing the client for insertion of a central line.

Administer intravenous piggyback (secondary) medications.

Reduction of Risk Potential

POTENTIAL FOR ALTERATIONS IN BODY SYSTEMS

Perform focused data collection based on client condition.

Reinforce client teaching on methods to prevent complications associated with activity level/diagnosed illness/disease.

Physiological Adaptation

ALTERATIONS IN BODY SYSTEMS

Assist in the care of a client with a pacing device.

Reinforce education to client regarding care and condition.

BASIC PATHOPHYSIOLOGY: Identify signs and symptoms related to an acute or chronic illness.

CHAPTER 28   Angina and Myocardial Infarction

Angina pectoris is a term used to describe chest pain and often occurs when the heart has decreased perfusion that can be caused by narrowing of the blood vessels (atherosclerosis). When blood flow to the heart is compromised, ischemia causes chest pain. The types of anginas include:

- **Stable (exertional) angina** occurs with exercise or emotional stress and is relieved by rest or nitroglycerin.

- **Unstable (preinfarction/crescendo) angina** occurs with exercise or at rest but increases in occurrence, severity, and duration over time.

- **Variant (Prinzmetal/vasoplastic) angina** is due to a coronary artery spasm, often occurring during periods of rest.

Acute coronary syndrome (ACS) is an acute onset of ischemia to myocardium that can result in myocardial death. It's an emergent situation that encompasses unstable angina and non-ST-elevation and ST-elevation myocardial infarction (NSTEMI, STEMI). Annually, approximately 800,000 individuals experience a myocardial infarction (MI) and 365,000 individuals experience death from an MI. Manifestations of ACS are due to an imbalance between myocardial oxygen supply and demand. The area of infarction in clients experiencing an MI develops over minutes to hours.

Early recognition and treatment of an acute MI is essential to prevent death. Research shows improved outcomes following an MI in clients treated with aspirin, beta blockers, and angiotensin-converting enzyme inhibitors or angiotensin receptor blockers. Pain unrelieved by rest or nitroglycerin and lasting for more than 15 min differentiates an MI from angina. Females (sex assigned at birth) and older adults do not always experience manifestations typically associated with angina or MI. Ⓖ

An abrupt interruption of oxygen to the heart muscle produces myocardial ischemia. Ischemia can lead to tissue necrosis (infarction) if blood supply and oxygen are not restored. Ischemia is reversible. An infarction results in permanent damage. When the cardiac muscle suffers ischemic injury, cardiac enzymes are released into the bloodstream, providing specific markers of MI.

MIs are classified based on:

- Affected area of the heart: anterior, lateral, inferior, or posterior

- ECG changes produced: ST elevation myocardial infarction (STEMI) vs. non-ST elevation myocardial infarction (NSTEMI)

The time frame within the progression of the infarction: acute, evolving, old

HEALTH PROMOTION AND DISEASE PREVENTION

- Maintain an exercise routine to remain physically active. Consult with a provider before starting any exercise regimen.
- Have cholesterol level and blood pressure checked regularly.
- Consume a diet low in saturated fats and sodium. Consult with a provider regarding diet restrictions.
- Promote smoking cessation.

28.1 Myocardial infarction

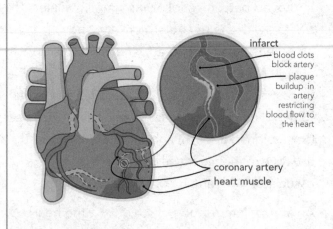

infarct
- blood clots block artery
- plaque buildup in artery restricting blood flow to the heart

coronary artery
heart muscle

28.2 Anginal pain

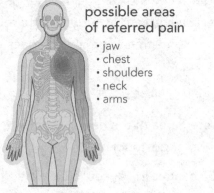

possible areas of referred pain
- jaw
- chest
- shoulders
- neck
- arms

28.3 Distinguishing characteristics

Stable angina

Precipitated by exertion or stress

Relieved by rest or nitroglycerin

Manifestations last less than 15 min.

Not associated with nausea, epigastric distress, dyspnea, anxiety, diaphoresis

Myocardial infarction

Can occur without cause, often in the morning after rest

Relieved only by opioids

Manifestations last more than 30 min.

Associated with nausea, epigastric distress, dyspnea, anxiety, diaphoresis

DATA COLLECTION

RISK FACTORS

- Male sex assigned at birth or postmenopausal clients
- Ethnic background
- Sedentary lifestyle
- Hypertension
- Tobacco use
- Hyperlipidemia
- BMI greater than 30
- Excessive alcohol consumption
- Metabolic disorders (diabetes mellitus, metabolic syndrome, hyperthyroidism)
- Methamphetamine or cocaine use
- Stress (with ineffective coping skills)
- An increased risk of coronary artery disease exists for older adult clients who are physically inactive, have one or more chronic diseases (hypertension, heart failure, and diabetes mellitus), or have lifestyle habits (smoking and diet) that contribute to atherosclerosis. Atherosclerotic changes related to aging predispose the heart to poor blood perfusion and oxygen delivery. Ⓖ
- Incidence of cardiac disease increases with age, especially in the presence of hypertension, diabetes mellitus, hypercholesterolemia, elevated homocysteine, and highly sensitive C-reactive protein (hs-CRP).

EXPECTED FINDINGS

The findings for angina and MI can vary. It's important to know the distinguishing characteristics for both. With stable angina, the pain is generally relieved with rest or the administration of nitroglycerin.
- Anxiety, feeling of impending doom
- Anginal pain: substernal or precordial
  - Reports of tight squeezing, crushing, heavy/aching pressure, or constricting feeling in the chest
  - Can radiate to neck, shoulder, or arm, or present as jaw pain (MI)
  - Weakness or numbness in arms
- Indigestion, nausea
- Dizziness
- Females (sex assigned at birth) and older adult clients can experience atypical angina, which is characterized by pain between the shoulders, ache in the jaw, or sensation of choking with exertion.

PHYSICAL FINDINGS
- Pallor and cool, clammy skin
- Tachycardia and heart palpitations
- Tachypnea and shortness of breath
- Diaphoresis
- Vomiting
- Decreased level of consciousness

LABORATORY TESTS

Cardiac enzymes released with cardiac muscle injury:
- **Myoglobin:** Earliest marker of injury to cardiac or skeletal muscle. Levels no longer evident after 24 hr
- **Creatine kinase–MB:** Peaks around 24 hr after onset of chest pain. Levels no longer evident after 3 days
- **Troponin I or T:** Any positive value indicates damage to cardiac tissue and should be reported.
  - **Troponin I and troponin T:** Levels no longer evident approximately after 10 days

DIAGNOSTIC PROCEDURES

Refer to **PN ADULT MEDICAL NURSING CHAPTER 25: CARDIOVASCULAR DIAGNOSTIC AND THERAPEUTIC PROCEDURES.**

Electrocardiogram (ECG)

Recording of electrical activity of the heart over time

NURSING ACTIONS
- Monitor for changes on serial ECGs.
- Angina: ST depression and/or T-wave inversion indicates presence of ischemia.
- MI: T-wave inversion indicates ischemia; ST-segment elevation indicates injury; abnormal Q-wave indicates necrosis.
  - NSTEMI: no significant ECG changes or persistent ST elevations
  - STEMI: ST segment elevations in 2 separate leads

Stress test

Also known as exercise electrocardiography. Client tolerance of activity is tested using a treadmill, bicycle, or medication to evaluate response to increased heart rate.

Thallium scan

Check for ischemia or necrosis. Radioisotopes cannot reach areas with decreased or absent perfusion, and the areas appear as "cold spots."

CLIENT EDUCATION: Avoid smoking and consuming caffeinated beverages prior to the procedure. These can affect the test.

Cardiac catheterization

- A coronary angiogram, also called a cardiac catheterization, is an invasive diagnostic procedure used to evaluate the presence and degree of coronary artery blockage.
- Angiography involves the insertion of a catheter into a femoral (sometimes a brachial) vessel and threading it into the right or left side of the heart. Coronary artery narrowing and occlusions are identified by the injection of contrast media under fluoroscopy.

NURSING ACTIONS
- Ensure the client understands the procedure prior to signing informed consent. Qᴘᴄᴄ
- Ensure that the client remains NPO 4 to 8 hr prior to procedure.
- Monitor for iodine/shellfish allergy (contrast media).

PATIENT-CENTERED CARE

NURSING CARE

- Monitor the following.
  - Vital signs every 5 min until stable, then every hour
  - Serial ECG, continuous cardiac monitoring
  - Location, precipitating factors, severity, quality, and duration of pain
  - Hourly urine output: greater than 30 mL/hr indicates expected kidney perfusion
  - Laboratory data: cardiac enzymes, electrolytes, ABGs
- Administer oxygen via cannula or face mask.
- Assist with obtaining and maintaining IV access.
- Promote energy conservation. Cluster nursing interventions.

THERAPEUTIC MANAGEMENT

A client who is experiencing symptoms of angina or an MI requires prompt therapeutic interventions to prevent further complications. The initial management includes the administration of **M**orphine, **O**xygen, **N**itrate, **A**spirin. The Joint Commission has established Core Measures to ensure effective client outcomes. The Core Measures for a client who is admitted with an MI include the following.
- The administration of aspirin upon arrival, beta blocker within 24 hours, and thrombolytic within 30 minutes
- Prescription for aspirin/antiplatelet and beta blocker at discharge if indicated

MEDICATIONS

Vasodilators

Nitroglycerin prevents coronary artery vasospasm and reduces preload and afterload, decreasing myocardial oxygen demand.

NURSING ACTIONS
- Use to treat angina and help control blood pressure.
- Use cautiously with other antihypertensive medications.
- Monitor for orthostatic hypotension.
- Ensure the client has not taken a phosphodiesterase inhibitor for erectile dysfunction within 24 to 48 hr, as severe hypotension can result.

CLIENT EDUCATION FOR CHEST PAIN
- Stop activity and rest.
- Place a nitroglycerin tablet under the tongue to dissolve (quick absorption).
- If pain is unrelieved in 5 min, call 911 or be driven to an emergency department.
- Up to two more doses of nitroglycerin can be taken at 5-min intervals. Qᴘᴄᴄ
- Headache is a common adverse effect of this medication.
- Change positions slowly.

Analgesics

Morphine sulfate is an opioid analgesic that is recommended to treat moderate to severe pain. Analgesics act on the mu and kappa receptors that help alleviate pain. Activation of these receptors produces analgesia (pain relief), respiratory depression, euphoria, and sedation and decreases in myocardial oxygen consumption and gastrointestinal (GI) motility.

> ! Use cautiously with clients who have asthma or emphysema due to the risk of respiratory depression.

NURSING ACTIONS
- For the client having chest pain, monitor pain every 5 to 15 min.
- Watch for manifestations of respiratory depression, especially in older adults. If respirations are less than 12/min, stop medication, and notify the provider immediately. ©
- Monitor vital signs for hypotension and decreased respirations.
- Monitor for nausea and vomiting.

CLIENT EDUCATION
- If nausea and vomiting persist, notify a nurse.
- If a PCA pump is prescribed, the client is the only person who should push the medication administration button. The safety lockout mechanism on the PCA pump prevents overdosing of the medication.

Beta blockers

- Metoprolol has antidysrhythmic and antihypertensive properties that decrease the imbalance between myocardial oxygen supply and demand by reducing afterload and slowing heart rate.
- In an acute MI, beta blockers decrease infarct size and improve short- and long-term survival rates.

NURSING ACTIONS
- Beta blockers can cause bradycardia and hypotension. Hold the medication if the apical pulse rate is less than 50/min, and notify the provider. Qs
- Avoid giving to clients who have asthma. Cardioselective beta blockers (which affect only beta₁ receptors), such as metoprolol, are preferred because they minimize the effects on the respiratory system.
- Use with caution in clients who have heart failure.
- Monitor for decreased level of consciousness, crackles in the lungs, and chest discomfort.

CLIENT EDUCATION
- Change positions slowly.
- Notify the provider immediately of shortness of breath, edema, weight gain, or cough.

Thrombolytic agents (also called fibrinolytic agents)

- Alteplase and reteplase are used to break up blood clots.
- Thrombolytic agents have similar adverse effects and contraindications as anticoagulants.
- For best results, give within 6 hr of infarction.

NURSING ACTIONS
- Monitor for contraindications (active bleeding, peptic ulcer disease, history of stroke, recent trauma).
- Monitor for effects of bleeding (mental status changes, hematuria).
- Monitor bleeding times: PT, aPTT, INR, fibrinogen levels, and CBC.
- Monitor for the same adverse effects as anticoagulants (thrombocytopenia, anemia, hemorrhage).
- Administer streptokinase slowly to prevent hypotension.

CLIENT EDUCATION: There is a risk for bruising and bleeding while on this medication.

Antiplatelet agents

- Aspirin and clopidogrel prevent platelets from forming together, which can produce arterial clotting.
- Aspirin prevents vasoconstriction. Due to this and antiplatelet effects, it should be administered with nitroglycerin at the onset of chest pain. Qᴇʙᴘ
- Antiplatelet agents can cause GI upset.

NURSING ACTIONS
- Use cautiously with clients who have a history of GI ulcers.
- Tinnitus (ringing in the ears) can be a manifestation of aspirin toxicity.

CLIENT EDUCATION
- There is risk for bruising and bleeding while on this medication.
- If aspirin is prescribed, choose the enteric-coated form and take with food to minimize GI upset.
- Report ringing in the ears.

Anticoagulants

Heparin and enoxaparin are used to prevent clots from becoming larger or other clots from forming.

NURSING ACTIONS
- Monitor for contraindications (active bleeding, peptic ulcer disease, history of stroke, recent trauma).
- Monitor platelet levels and bleeding times: PT, aPTT, INR, and CBC.
- Monitor for adverse effects of anticoagulants (thrombocytopenia, anemia, hemorrhage).

CLIENT EDUCATION: There is risk for bruising and bleeding while on this medication.

Glycoprotein IIB/IIIA inhibitors

Eptifibatide is used to prevent binding of fibrinogen to platelets, in turn blocking platelet aggregation.

• In combination with aspirin therapy, IIB/IIIA inhibitors are standard therapy.
• This medication can cause active bleeding.

NURSING ACTIONS: Monitor platelet levels.

CLIENT EDUCATION: Report evidence of bleeding during medication therapy.

INTERPROFESSIONAL CARE

There are several social determinants of health (SDOH) that could affect the clients who have MI outcomes such as economic stability, education access and quality, health care access and quality, neighborhood and built environment, and social and community context. It's important for the nurse to collaborate with the interprofessional team to ensure the client's needs are being met. (Refer to PN ADULT MEDICAL NURSING CHAPTERS 1 AND 2 for more information about SDOH.)

• Case manager, social worker, pharmacist
• Pain management services can be consulted if pain persists or is uncontrolled.
• Cardiac rehabilitation care can be consulted if the client has prolonged weakness and needs assistance with increasing level of activity.
• Nutritional services can be consulted for diet modification to promote food choices low in sodium and saturated fat.

28.4 Case study

Scenario introduction

A nurse in a primary care clinic is collecting data from a client who reports headaches, blurred vision, and fatigue for the past week. This is the client's first follow-up appointment since being discharged from the hospital 4 months ago following a myocardial infarction.

The client was prescribed daily doses of metoprolol, simvastatin, and aspirin upon discharge from the hospital. The client has told the nurse today that for the past month, they have been taking the prescribed daily medications every other day to save money.

Scene 1

Nurse: "Tell me your concerns about the cost of your medications."

Client: "I don't have very good medical insurance, so I must pay a lot out of pocket for doctor's appointments, prescriptions, and lab work. It's going to take me a long time to pay the hospital bills. That's why I just had the blood work done that I was supposed to get last month. Also, I take the bus everywhere. We don't have any doctors' offices in our neighborhood, and I must take two buses to get to this clinic."

Scene 2

The nurse measures the client's blood pressure and reviews the client's chart.

Nurse: "Your blood pressure is 162/98 mm Hg, which is elevated, and the laboratory results show that your cholesterol and triglyceride levels are out of expected ranges. You mentioned that you are not taking your medications every day. Let's talk about your diet. What do you eat in a typical day?"

Client: "I work at a fast-food restaurant, and I get a free meal with every shift. Sometimes, I work extra shifts. So, most days, I eat fast food once or twice a day. I know that's not the best thing for me, but I like it because I do not have to buy as much food to keep at home."

Nurse: "What kinds of foods do you eat at home?"

Client: "Mostly canned foods or boxed foods that I can get at the dollar store. They are easy to make. I don't buy a lot of fruits and vegetables because I won't eat them all before they go bad. I must take the bus when I go to the big grocery store, and I can walk to the dollar store that is a few blocks away."

Scene 3

Nurse: "What did you find helpful when you were attending the cardiac rehabilitation program after you were discharged from the hospital?"

Client: "Well, I was supposed to go three days a week. I started going once or twice a week, but then I just stopped going. I had to take the bus and turn down extra shifts at work. It just didn't work out. My grandmothers both had heart attacks and said they never needed cardiac rehab. My relatives go to the doctor as little as possible."

Scenario conclusion

The nurse is assisting with the development of a plan of care and collaborating with other members of the interprofessional team to provide the client with care and services.

Case study exercises

1. The nurse recognizes that the client has reported multiple factors that impact their health. Which of the following social determinants of health (SDOH) were mentioned by the client? (Select all that apply.)

   A. Economic stability

   B. Education access and quality

   C. Health care access and quality

   D. Neighborhood and built environment

   E. Social and community context

2. Which of the following statements by the client is most related to the SDOH of social and community context?

   A. "I can walk to the dollar store that is a few blocks away."

   B. "It's going to take me a long time to pay the hospital bills."

   C. "My relatives go to the doctor as little as possible."

   D. "I had to take the bus and had to turn down extra shifts at work."

3. When assisting with developing the plan of care, what types of referrals should the nurse consider making to other members of the interprofessional team?

THERAPEUTIC PROCEDURES

- Percutaneous transluminal coronary angioplasty (PTCA)
- Bypass graft (also known as CABG)

CLIENT EDUCATION

- Cardiac rehabilitation should be consulted for a specific exercise program related to the heart.
- Nutritional services, such as a dietitian, can be consulted for diet modification or weight management.
- Monitor and report findings of infection (fever, incisional drainage, redness).
- Avoid straining, strenuous exercise, or emotional stress when possible.
- Regarding response to chest pain: Follow instructions on use of sublingual nitroglycerin.
- Consider smoking cessation, if applicable.
- Remain active and exercise regularly.

COMPLICATIONS

ACUTE MI

A complication of angina not relieved by rest or nitroglycerin

NURSING ACTIONS

- Administer oxygen to maintain oxygen saturations of 90% or greater.
- Notify the provider immediately. Qs

HEART FAILURE/CARDIOGENIC SHOCK

Injury to the left ventricle can lead to decreased cardiac output and heart failure. Progressive heart failure can lead to cardiogenic shock.

- This is a serious complication of pump failure, commonly following an MI of 40% blockage.
- Manifestations include tachycardia; hypotension; inadequate urinary output; altered level of consciousness; respiratory distress (crackles and tachypnea); cool, clammy skin; decreased peripheral pulses; and chest pain.

NURSING ACTIONS

- Administer oxygen. Intubation and ventilation can be required. QEBP
- Medications that can be administered include morphine, diuretics, and/or nitroglycerin to decrease preload. Vasopressors and/or positive inotropes can be administered to increase cardiac output and maintain organ perfusion.
- Maintain continuous hemodynamic monitoring.

ISCHEMIC MITRAL REGURGITATION

Evidenced by development of a new cardiac murmur

NURSING ACTIONS

- Administer oxygen.
- Notify the provider immediately.

DYSRHYTHMIAS

- An inferior wall MI can lead to an injury to the AV node, resulting in bradycardia and second-degree AV heart block.
- An anterior wall MI can lead to an injury to the ventricle, resulting in premature ventricular contractions, bundle branch block, or complete heart block.

NURSING ACTIONS

- Monitor ECG and vital signs.
- Administer oxygen.
- Administer antidysrhythmic medications.
- Prepare for cardiac pacemaker or implantable cardioverter defibrillator if needed.

1. A nurse is assisting with the admission of a client who has a suspected myocardial infarction (MI) and a history of angina. Which of the following findings will help the nurse distinguish stable angina from an MI?

   A. Stable angina can be relieved with rest and nitroglycerin.

   B. The pain of an MI resolves in less than 15 min.

   C. The type of activity that causes an MI can be identified.

   D. Stable angina can occur for longer than 30 min.

2. A nurse is reviewing the laboratory findings of a client who is being evaluated for a myocardial infarction (MI). Which of the following laboratory studies are likely to show elevations if the MI occurred within the last 6 hours? (Select all that apply.)

   A. CK-MB

   B. Troponin I

   C. Troponin T

   D. Myoglobin

   E. BNP

   F. Cholesterol

   G. High-density lipoproteins

3. A nurse is assisting with the care of clients who have had MI and is reviewing the medications prescribed for them. Match each classification with the name of the medication.

   A. Antiplatelet agent   1. Nitroglycerin

   B. Anticoagulant   2. Metoprolol

   C. Beta blocker   3. Heparin

   D. Vasodilator   4. Clopidogrel

4. A nurse is caring for a client who asks why the provider prescribed a daily aspirin after their MI. How should the nurse respond?

Active Learning Scenario

A nurse is reinforcing teaching with a client who has a new diagnosis of angina about coronary syndrome. What information should the nurse include in the teaching? Use the ATI Active Learning Template: System Disorder to complete this item.

RISK FACTORS: Describe five.

CLIENT EDUCATION: Describe at least two teaching points the nurse can use to help the client decrease risk of having angina or an MI.

EXPECTED FINDINGS

LIST FIVE SUBJECTIVE FINDINGS.

DESCRIBE FOUR PHYSICAL FINDINGS.

Case Study Exercises Key

1. A, C, D, E. **CORRECT:** When recognizing cues, the nurse should recognize that the SDOH mentioned by the client are economic stability, (out-of-pocket health care costs, bus fares, food insecurity), health care access and quality (medical insurance and lack of providers in community), neighborhood and built environment (lack of grocery stores), and social and community context (the way relatives use health care services).

   Ⓝ *NCLEX® Connection: Health Promotion and Maintenance, Community Resources*

2. C. **CORRECT:** When recognizing cues, the nurse should recognize that the statement most related to the SDOH of social and community context is, "My relatives go to the doctor as little as possible." Relatives, friends, and community members can influence an individual's health and well-being.

   Ⓝ *NCLEX® Connection: Health Promotion and Maintenance, Community Resources*

3. When generating solutions, the nurse should suggest referrals to a dietitian for nutrition education and resources. The nurse should suggest referrals to case managers and social workers for identification of community resources and assistance programs for food, transportation, and financial assistance for health care services. The nurse may suggest a referral to a pharmacist for consultation about lower-cost options for medications.

   Ⓝ *NCLEX® Connection: Health Promotion and Maintenance, Community Resources*

Active Learning Scenario Key

Using the ATI Active Learning Template: System Disorder

RISK FACTORS
- Male sex or postmenopausal clients
- Sedentary lifestyle
- Hypertension
- Substance use (tobacco, cocaine, methamphetamine, excessive alcohol)
- Hyperlipidemia
- Metabolic disorders (diabetes mellitus, hyperthyroidism)
- Stress (with ineffective coping skills)

CLIENT EDUCATION
- Have routine cholesterol, blood pressure, and blood sugar screenings.
- Participate in regular physical activity for exercise and stress reduction.

EXPECTED FINDINGS
- Subjective findings: Feeling of impending doom; chest pain, pressure, or crushing radiating to the arm or jaw; nausea; dizziness; anxiety
- Physical findings: Pale, cool, clammy skin; tachycardia; tachypnea; diaphoresis

Ⓝ *NCLEX® Connection: Physiological Adaptation, Alterations in Body Systems*

Application Exercises Key

1. A. **CORRECT:** When recognizing cues, the nurse should recognize that stable angina can be relieved by rest and nitroglycerin. Chest pain from an MI is not relieved by nitrates or rest.

Ⓝ *NCLEX® Connection: Physiological Adaptation, Alterations in Body Systems*

2. A, B, C, D. **CORRECT:** When analyzing cues, the nurse determines that CK-MB, Troponin I, Troponin T, CPK, and myoglobin are likely to start elevating within a few hours after an MI. CK-MB begins to increase within a few hours after an MI. Troponin I and Troponin T are specific to cardiac muscle tissue and increase within 4 to 6 hours after an MI. The presence of myoglobin indicates muscle damage and starts to increase within 1 to 3 hours of damage to the myocardium.

Ⓝ *NCLEX® Connection: Reduction of Risk Potential, Laboratory Values*

3. A, 4; B, 3; C, 2; D, 1

When recognizing cues, the nurse should identify nitroglycerin as a vasodilator that dilates the coronary arteries. The nurse should identify metoprolol as a beta blocker that slows the heart rate and decreases the force of cardiac contraction. The nurse should identify heparin as an anticoagulant that prevents further clot formation. The nurse should identify clopidogrel as an antiplatelet agent that prevents platelet aggregation.

Ⓝ *NCLEX® Connection: Pharmacological Therapies, Expected Actions/Outcomes*

4. When taking actions to reinforce education with the client about a daily dose of aspirin, the nurse should respond by explaining to the client that aspirin reduces the formation of blood clots that could cause a heart attack. Aspirin decreases platelet aggregation that can cause a myocardial infarction.

Ⓝ *NCLEX® Connection: Pharmacological Therapies, Expected Actions/Outcomes*

UNIT 4   CARDIOVASCULAR DISORDERS
SECTION: CARDIAC DISORDERS

CHAPTER 29 *Heart Failure and Pulmonary Edema*

Heart failure occurs when the heart muscle is unable to pump effectively, resulting in inadequate cardiac output, myocardial hypertrophy, and pulmonary/systemic congestion. The heart is unable to maintain adequate circulation to meet tissue needs.

Heart failure is the result of an acute or chronic cardiopulmonary problem, such as systemic hypertension, myocardial infarction (MI), pulmonary hypertension, dysrhythmias, valvular heart disease, pericarditis, or cardiomyopathy. (29.1)

Pulmonary edema is a severe, life-threatening accumulation of fluid in the alveoli and interstitial spaces of the lung that can result from severe heart failure.

Heart failure

New York Heart Association's functional classification scale

The severity of heart failure is graded on the New York Heart Association's (NYHA) functional classification scale indicating the level of activity it takes to induce manifestations of impaired function (chest pain, shortness of breath).

CLASS I: Client exhibits no manifestations with activity.

CLASS II: Client has manifestations with ordinary exertion (everyday ADLs).

CLASS III: Client displays manifestations with minimal exertion.

CLASS IV: Client has manifestations at rest.

American College of Cardiology and American Heart Association staging heart failure

The American College of Cardiology and American Heart Association developed evidence-based guidelines for staging and managing heart failure in comparison with the NYHA system.
- **A:** High risk for developing heart failure
- **B:** Cardiac structural abnormalities or remodeling but no manifestations of heart failure
- **C:** Current or prior manifestations of heart failure
- **D:** Refractory end-stage heart failure

Low-output heart failure

Low-output heart failure can initially occur on either the left or right side of the heart.
- Left-sided heart (ventricular) failure results in inadequate left ventricle (cardiac) output and consequently in inadequate tissue perfusion.
  - Systolic heart (ventricular) failure (ejection fraction below 40%, pulmonary and systemic congestion)
  - Diastolic heart (ventricular) failure (inadequate relaxation or "stiffening" prevents ventricular filling)
- Right-sided heart (ventricular) failure results in inadequate right ventricle output and systemic venous congestion (peripheral edema).

High-output heart failure

A less common form of heart failure is high-output failure, in which cardiac output is within the expected reference range or greater than the expected reference range. Caused by an elevated metabolic demand, such as in septicemia, hyperthyroidism, fever, and anemia.

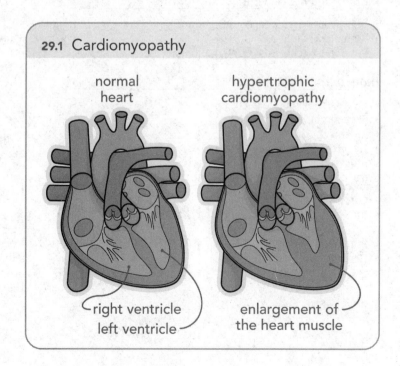

29.1 Cardiomyopathy

normal heart

hypertrophic cardiomyopathy

right ventricle
left ventricle

enlargement of the heart muscle

HEALTH PROMOTION AND DISEASE PREVENTION

- Maintain an exercise routine to remain physically active, and consult with the provider before starting any exercise regimen.
- Consume a diet low in sodium, along with fluid restrictions, and consult with the provider regarding diet specifications.
- Refrain from smoking.
- Follow medication regimen, and follow up with the provider as needed.

DATA COLLECTION

RISK FACTORS

Older adults have an increased risk for heart failure and can have worse manifestations due to increased systolic blood pressure and some medications.

SOCIAL DETERMINANTS OF HEALTH FACTORS:
- Less access to health care in vulnerable populations
- Cost of health care and medications compete with the need of food and housing
- Unemployment is associated with alcohol use disorders, smoking, and depression
- Food insecurity can lead to undernutrition and lack of access to fresh fruits and vegetables

Left-sided heart (ventricular) failure

- Hypertension
- Coronary artery disease, angina, MI
- Valvular disease (mitral and aortic)
- Smoking

Right-sided heart (ventricular) failure

- Left-sided heart (ventricular) failure
- Right ventricular MI
- Pulmonary problems (COPD, pulmonary fibrosis)

High-output heart failure

- Increased metabolic needs
- Septicemia (fever)
- Anemia
- Hyperthyroidism

Cardiomyopathy (leading to heart failure)

- Coronary artery disease
- Infection or inflammation of the heart muscle
- Various cancer treatments
- Prolonged alcohol use
- Heredity

EXPECTED FINDINGS

The presence of other chronic illnesses (lung disease, kidney failure) can mask the presence of heart failure in older adult clients. Ⓒ

Left-sided failure

- Dyspnea, orthopnea (shortness of breath while lying down), nocturnal dyspnea
- Fatigue
- Displaced apical pulse (hypertrophy)
- S_3 heart sound (gallop)
- Pulmonary congestion (dyspnea, cough, bibasilar crackles)
- Frothy sputum (can be blood-tinged)
- Altered mental status
- Manifestations of organ failure, such as oliguria (decrease in urine output)
- Nocturia

Right-sided failure

- Jugular vein distention
- Ascending dependent edema (legs, ankles, sacrum)
- Abdominal distention, ascites
- Fatigue, weakness
- Nausea and anorexia
- Polyuria at rest (nocturnal)
- Liver enlargement (hepatomegaly) and tenderness
- Weight gain

Cardiomyopathy (leading to heart failure)

Blood circulation to the lungs is impaired when the cardiac pump is compromised. (29.1)

TYPES
- Dilated (most common)
- Hypertrophic
- Restrictive

MANIFESTATIONS
- Fatigue, weakness
- Heart failure (left with dilated type, right with restrictive type)
- Dysrhythmias (heart block)
- S_3 gallop
- Cardiomegaly (enlarged heart), more severe with dilated type
- Angina (hypertrophic type)

LABORATORY TESTS

B-type natriuretic peptides (BNP)

In clients who have dyspnea, elevated BNP confirms a diagnosis of heart failure rather than a problem originating in the respiratory system. BNP levels direct the aggressiveness of treatment interventions.
- Less than 100 pg/mL indicates no heart failure.
- Greater than 400 pg/mL indicates heart failure.
- BNP increases with the severity of the heart failure.

DIAGNOSTIC PROCEDURES

Hemodynamic monitoring

Used to identify the client's cardiac function and response to treatment. A catheter is inserted into a central vein into the right side of the heart and pulmonary artery. This can measure the client's central venous pressure, pulmonary artery pressures, and cardiac output.

Ultrasound

Two-dimensional or three-dimensional ultrasound (also called cardiac ultrasound or echocardiogram) is used to measure the systolic and diastolic functioning of the heart.

Left ventricular ejection fraction: The volume of blood pumped from the left ventricle into the arteries upon each beat. Expected reference range is 55% to 70%.

Right ventricular ejection fraction: The volume of blood pumped from the right ventricle to the lungs upon each beat. Expected reference range is 45% to 60%.

Transesophageal echocardiography (TEE)

Uses a transducer placed in the esophagus behind the heart to obtain a detailed view of cardiac structures. The nurse prepares the client for a TEE in the same manner as for an upper endoscopy.

Chest x-ray

A chest x-ray can reveal cardiomegaly and pleural effusions.

ECG, cardiac enzymes, electrolytes, and ABGs

Used to identify factors contributing to heart failure and/or the impact of heart failure. Monitor potassium level closely if the client is taking diuretics.

PATIENT-CENTERED CARE

NURSING CARE

- Monitor daily weight and I&O.
- Monitor for shortness of breath and dyspnea on exertion.
- Administer oxygen as prescribed.
- Monitor vital signs and hemodynamic pressures.
- Position the client to maximize ventilation (high-Fowler's).
- Monitor diagnostic results to track progress.
- Monitor for manifestations of medication toxicity (digoxin toxicity).
- Encourage bed rest until the client is stable.
- Encourage energy conservation by assisting with care and ADLs.
- Maintain dietary restrictions as prescribed (restricted fluid intake, restricted sodium intake).
- Provide emotional support to the client and family.

MEDICATIONS

Herbal medications and supplements can interact with medications taken for disorders of the cardiovascular system. Obtain a list of herbal supplements the client takes, and advise the client of potential contraindications. Q_{EBP}

Diuretics

Diuretics are used to decrease preload.

Loop diuretics, such as furosemide and bumetanide

Thiazide diuretics, such as hydrochlorothiazide

Potassium-sparing diuretics, such as spironolactone

NURSING ACTIONS
- Ensure that furosemide IV is administered IV no faster than 20 mg/min.
- Loop and thiazide diuretics can cause hypokalemia, and potassium supplementation can be required.

CLIENT EDUCATION: If taking loop or thiazide diuretics, ingest foods and beverages that are high in potassium to counter the effects of hypokalemia. If taking potassium-sparing diuretics, watch for hidden sources of potassium, such as salt substitutes. Q_s

Afterload-reducing agents

Afterload-reducing agents help the heart pump more easily by altering the resistance to contraction. These are contraindicated for clients who have renal deficiency.

Angiotensin-converting enzyme (ACE) inhibitors, such as enalapril and captopril

Angiotensin receptor II blockers, such as losartan

Calcium channel blockers, such as diltiazem and nifedipine

Phosphodiesterase-3 inhibitors, such as milrinone

NURSING ACTIONS
- Monitor clients taking ACE inhibitors for hypotension following the initial dose.
- ACE inhibitors can cause angioedema (swelling of the tongue and throat), decreased sense of taste, or skin rash.
- Monitor for increased levels of potassium.

CLIENT EDUCATION: ACE INHIBITORS
- This medication can cause a dry cough.
- Notify the provider if a rash or decreased sense of taste occurs.
- Notify the provider if swelling of the face or extremities occurs.
- Blood pressure should be monitored for 2 hr after the initial dose to detect hypotension.

Inotropic agents

Inotropic agents (digoxin, dopamine, dobutamine, milrinone) are used to increase contractility and thereby improve cardiac output.

NURSING ACTIONS

- For a client taking digoxin, take the apical heart rate for 1 min. Hold the medication if apical pulse is less than 60/min, and notify the provider. For some clients, the provider might allow the heart rate to be as low as 50/min.
- Observe the client for nausea and vomiting.

CLIENT EDUCATION

If self-administering digoxin, be sure to:

- Count pulse for 1 min before taking the medication. If the pulse rate is irregular or the pulse rate is outside of the limitations set by the provider (usually less than 60/min or greater than 100/min), hold the dose and contact the provider. Qs
- Take the digoxin dose at the same time each day.
- Do not take digoxin at the same time as antacids. Separate the two medications by at least 2 hr.
- Report manifestations of toxicity, including nausea, fatigue, muscle weakness, confusion, and loss of appetite.
- Have blood digoxin and potassium levels checked regularly.

Beta adrenergic blockers (beta blockers)

Medications such as carvedilol and metoprolol can be used to improve the condition of the client who has sustained increased levels of sympathetic stimulation and catecholamines. This includes clients who have chronic heart failure.

NURSING ACTIONS

- Monitor blood pressure, pulse, activity tolerance, and orthopnea.
- Check orthostatic blood pressure readings.

CLIENT EDUCATION

- Weigh daily.
- Check blood pressure daily.
- Follow the provider's instructions for increasing medication dosage.

Vasodilators

Nitroglycerin and isosorbide mononitrate prevent coronary artery vasospasm and reduce preload and afterload, decreasing myocardial oxygen demand.

NURSING ACTIONS

- Vasodilators are given to treat angina and help control blood pressure.
- Use cautiously with other antihypertensive mediations.
- Vasodilators can cause orthostatic hypotension.

CLIENT EDUCATION

- A headache is a common adverse effect of this medication.
- Change positions down slowly.

Hyperpolarization-activated cyclic nucleotide-gated channel blocker (HCN channel blocker: Ivabradine

- Slows heart rate by inhibiting sinus node channel
- Used for clients who can not take beta blockers or are receiving the maximum dose

NURSING ACTIONS

Monitor for bradycardia and dizziness

Anticoagulants

Anticoagulants, such as warfarin, can be prescribed if the client has a history of thrombus formation.

NURSING ACTIONS

- Check for contraindications: active bleeding, peptic ulcer disease, history of cerebrovascular accident, and recent trauma.
- Monitor bleeding times: PT, aPTT, INR, and CBC.

CLIENT EDUCATION

- Remember the risk for bruising and bleeding while on this medication.
- Have blood monitored routinely to check bleeding times.

INTERPROFESSIONAL CARE

Cardiology and pulmonary services should be consulted to manage heart failure.

Respiratory services should be consulted for inhalers, breathing treatments, and suctioning for airway management.

Cardiac rehabilitation services can be consulted if the client has prolonged weakness and needs assistance with increasing level of activity.

Nutritional services can be consulted for diet modification to promote low-sodium and low-saturated fat food choices.

THERAPEUTIC PROCEDURES

Ventricular assist device (VAD)

A VAD is a mechanical pump that assists a heart that is too weak to pump blood through the body. It is used in clients who are awaiting heart transplants or who have severe end-stage heart failure and are not candidates for heart transplants.

- Heart transplantation is the treatment of choice for clients who have severe dilated cardiomyopathy.
- Contraindications to VAD surgery include severe chronic lung disease, end-stage kidney disease, clotting disorders, and infections unresponsive to antibiotic therapy.

NURSING ACTIONS

- Assist with preparing the client for the procedure (NPO status and informed consent).
- Monitor postoperatively: vital signs, SaO$_2$, incision drainage, and pain management.

Heart transplantation

- Heart transplantation is a possible option for clients who have end-stage heart failure. Immunosuppressant therapy is required post-transplantation to reduce the risk for rejection.
- Eligibility for transplantation depends on several factors, including life expectancy, age, psychosocial status, and absence of substance use disorders.

NURSING ACTIONS
- Assist with preparing the client for the procedure (NPO status and informed consent).
- Monitor postoperatively: vital signs, SaO₂, incision drainage, and pain management.
- Monitor for complications. Organ transplant recipients are at risk for infection, thrombosis, and rejection.

CLIENT EDUCATION
- Take diuretics in the early morning and early afternoon.
- Restrict fluid and sodium as instructed. Regulate potassium intake as instructed to prevent high or low potassium levels. A dietitian can help with menu planning.
- Check weight daily at the same time and notify the provider for a weight gain of 0.9 kg (2 lb) in 24 hr or 2.3 kg (5 lb) in 1 week.
- Schedule regular follow-up visits with the provider.
- Obtain the pneumococcal and yearly influenza vaccines.
- Initiate regular exercise as tolerated and prescribed.
- Participate in cardiac rehabilitation program.

COMPLICATIONS

Acute pulmonary edema

Acute pulmonary edema is a life-threatening medical emergency. Effective intervention should result in diuresis (carefully monitor output), reduction in respiratory distress, improved lung sounds, and adequate oxygenation.

EXPECTED FINDINGS: Anxiety, tachycardia, acute respiratory distress, dyspnea at rest, change in level of consciousness, and an ascending fluid level within the lungs (crackles, cough productive of frothy, blood-tinged sputum).

NURSING ACTIONS
- Prompt response to this emergency includes assisting with the following.
  - Positioning the client in high-Fowler's position
  - Administration of oxygen, positive airway pressure, intubation and mechanical ventilation
  - IV morphine (to decrease anxiety, respiratory distress, and decrease venous return)
- IV administration of rapid-acting loop diuretics, such as furosemide. Administer prescribed medications to improve cardiac output.
- Reinforce teaching with the client about measures to improve tolerance to activity, such as alternating periods of activity with periods of rest.

Cardiogenic shock

This is a serious complication of pump failure that occurs commonly following an MI with injury to greater than 40% of the left ventricle.

EXPECTED FINDINGS: Tachycardia, hypotension, inadequate urinary output, altered level of consciousness, respiratory distress (crackles, tachypnea), cool, clammy skin, decreased peripheral pulses, chest pain

NURSING ACTIONS
- Monitor breath sounds. Check for crackles or wheezing.
- Monitor heart sounds.
- Assist with administering oxygen and preparing the client for intubation and ventilation, if required.
- The RN can administer IV morphine, diuretics, and/or nitroglycerin to decrease preload. The RN can administer IV vasopressors and/or positive inotropes are used to increase cardiac output and maintain organ perfusion.
- Ensure continuous hemodynamic monitoring.

Cardiac tamponade

Cardiac tamponade can result from fluid accumulation in the pericardial sac.

EXPECTED FINDINGS: Hypotension, jugular venous distention, muffled heart sounds, and paradoxical pulse (variance of 10 mm Hg or more in systolic blood pressure between expiration and inspiration)

DIAGNOSTIC PROCEDURES: Hemodynamic monitoring will reveal intracardiac and pulmonary artery pressures similar and elevated (plateau pressures).

NURSING ACTIONS
- Notify the provider immediately.
- Assist with administering IV fluids to combat hypotension while monitoring for fluid overload.
- Ensure that a chest x-ray or echocardiogram is obtained to confirm diagnosis.
- Assist with preparing the client for pericardiocentesis (informed consent, gather materials, administer medications as prescribed).
- Monitor heart rhythm; changes can indicate improper positioning of the needle.
- Monitor for recurrence of findings after the procedure.

Pulmonary edema

Cardiogenic factors are the most common cause of pulmonary edema. It is a complication of various heart and lung diseases and usually occurs from increased pulmonary vascular pressure secondary to severe cardiac dysfunction.

Noncardiac pulmonary edema can occur due to barbiturate or opiate toxicity, inhalation of irritating gases, rapid administration of IV fluids, and after a pneumonectomy evacuation of pleural effusion.

Neurogenic pulmonary edema develops following a head injury.

OLDER ADULTS: Increased risk for pulmonary edema related to decreased cardiac output and heart failure Ⓖ

- Increased risk for fluid and electrolyte imbalances occurs when the older adult client receives treatment with diuretics.
- IV infusions must be administered at a slower rate to prevent circulatory overload.

HEALTH PROMOTION AND DISEASE PREVENTION

- Remain physically active, but consult with the provider before starting any exercise regimen.
- Consume a diet low in sodium; some clients require fluid restrictions. (Consult with the provider regarding diet specifications.)
- Refrain from tobacco use.

DATA COLLECTION

RISK FACTORS

- Acute MI ⓆEBP
- Fluid volume overload
- Hypertension
- Valvular heart disease
- Postpneumonectomy
- Postevacuation of pleural effusion
- Acute respiratory failure
- Left-sided heart failure
- High altitude exposure or deep-sea diving
- Trauma
- Sepsis
- Medication toxicity

EXPECTED FINDINGS

- Anxiety
- Inability to sleep
- Persistent cough with pink, frothy sputum (key finding)
- Tachypnea, dyspnea, and orthopnea
- Hypoxemia
- Cyanosis (later stage)
- Crackles
- Tachycardia
- Reduced urine output
- Confusion, stupor
- S_3 heart sound (gallop)
- Increased pulmonary artery occlusion pressure

PATIENT-CENTERED CARE

NURSING CARE

- Position the client in high-Fowler's position with feet and legs dependent or sitting on the side of the bed to decrease preload.
- Administer high-flow oxygen using a face mask or nonrebreather mask. Bilevel positive airway pressure or intubation/ventilation can become necessary. Be prepared to intervene quickly.
- Monitor vital signs every 15 min until stable.
- Monitor intake and output.
- Check ABGs, electrolytes (especially potassium if on diuretics), SaO2, and chest x-ray findings.
- Maintain a patent airway. Suction as needed.
- Ensure the restriction of fluid intake (slow or discontinue infusing IV fluids).
- Monitor hourly urine output. Watch for intake greater than output or hourly urine less than 30 mL/hr.
- Provide emotional support for the client and family.

MEDICATIONS

Rapid-acting diuretics, such as furosemide and bumetanide, promote fluid excretion.

Morphine decreases sympathetic nervous system response and anxiety and promotes mild vasodilation.

Vasodilators (nitroglycerin, sodium nitroprusside) decrease preload and afterload.

Inotropic agents, such as digoxin and dobutamine, improve cardiac output.

Antihypertensives, such as ACE inhibitors and beta-blockers, decrease afterload.

CLIENT EDUCATION

- Use techniques to promote effective breathing techniques.
- Understand prescribed medications and how to administer them.
- Continue to take medications even if feeling better.
- Follow instructions for reasons to contact the provider.
- Remain on a low-sodium diet and restrict fluids as prescribed.
- Measure weight daily at the same time. Notify the provider of a gain of more than 0.9 kg (2 lb) in 24 hr or 2.3 kg (5 lb) in 1 week.
- Report swelling of feet or ankles or any shortness of breath or angina.

Application Exercises

1. A nurse on a cardiac unit is collecting data on a group of clients who have heart failure. Sort the following findings into manifestations of left-sided heart failure and manifestations of right-sided heart failure.

   A. Crackles in lungs

   B. Jugular vein distention

   C. Pink frothy sputum

   D. Dependent edema

   E. S₃ heart sound (gallop)

   F. Abdomen distention

2. A nurse is assisting with the care of a client who has heart failure. What actions should the nurse take?

3. A nurse is reinforcing teaching with a client who has heart failure and new prescriptions for furosemide and digoxin. Which of the following instructions should the nurse include? (Select all that apply.)

   A. Monitor daily weight.

   B. Decrease intake of potassium.

   C. Expect to experience muscle weakness.

   D. Hold digoxin if heart rate is less than 60/min.

   E. Decrease sodium intake.

4. A nurse is assisting with teaching a class about medications used to treat heart failure. Match the medication class with the associated adverse effect.

A. Anticoagulants	1. Hypokalemia
B. ACE inhibitors	2. Dry cough
C. Loop diuretics	3. Bruising

5. A nurse is collecting data on a client who has pulmonary edema. Which of the following findings should the nurse expect? (Select all that apply.)

   A. Tachypnea

   B. Persistent cough

   C. Increased urinary output

   D. Thick, yellow sputum

   E. Orthopnea

Active Learning Scenario

A nurse is assisting with a presentation on heart failure to a group of clients. What should the nurse include in this presentation? Use the ATI Active Learning Template: System Disorder to complete this item.

ALTERATION IN HEALTH (DIAGNOSIS): Describe the difference between left- and right-sided heart failure.

LABORATORY TESTS: Describe one and its importance.

DIAGNOSTIC PROCEDURES: Describe two.

MEDICATIONS: Describe two groups of medications and an example of one medication for each group.

Active Learning Scenario Key

Using the ATI Active Learning Template: System Disorder

ALTERATION IN HEALTH (DIAGNOSIS): Left-sided heart failure results in inadequate output from the left ventricle, leading to poor tissue perfusion. Systolic failure includes an ejection fraction below 40% with pulmonary and systemic congestion. Diastolic failure includes stiffening or inadequate relaxation of the ventricle. Right-sided heart failure results in inadequate output from the right ventricle, leading to systemic venous congestion and peripheral edema.

LABORATORY TESTS: B-type natriuretic peptides (BNP) confirms a diagnosis of heart failure, and findings direct the aggressiveness of the treatment.

DIAGNOSTIC PROCEDURES
- Hemodynamic monitoring
- Ultrasound
- Chest x-ray
- Electrocardiogram

MEDICATIONS
- Diuretics: furosemide, bumetanide, hydrochlorothiazide, spironolactone
- Afterload-reducing agents: enalapril, captopril, losartan, diltiazem, nifedipine, milrinone

(N) *NCLEX® Connection: Health Promotion and Maintenance, Health Promotion/Disease Prevention*

Application Exercises Key

1. **LEFT-SIDED FAILURE:** A, C, E;
   RIGHT-SIDED FAILURE: B, D, F

   When recognizing cues, the nurse should identify crackles in lungs, pink, frothy sputum, and an S_3 heart sound (gallop), are manifestations of left-sided heart failure due to decreased cardiac output and increased pulmonary congestion. The nurse should identify that jugular vein distention, dependent edema, and abdominal distention, are manifestations of right-sided heart failure due to systemic congestion.

   (N) *NCLEX® Connection: Physiological Adaptation, Medical Emergencies*

2. When taking actions, the nurse should place the client upright in high-Fowler's position to maximize ventilation, administer oxygen as prescribed, and monitor the client's vital signs and hemodynamic pressures. The nurse should monitor the client's daily weight and I&O, check for shortness of breath and dyspnea on exertion, monitor diagnostic results to track progress, and check the client for manifestations of medication toxicity. The nurse should encourage bed rest and energy conservation until the client is stable, and maintain dietary restrictions as prescribed, such as restricted fluid and sodium intake.

   (N) *NCLEX® Connection: Physiological Adaptation, Medical Emergencies*

3. A. **CORRECT:** When taking actions, the nurse should instruct the client to weigh themselves daily when first getting out of bed to monitor fluid loss or gain.
   D. **CORRECT:** The client should hold digoxin if heart rate is less than 50 to 60/min as prescribed by the provider to reduce the risk of bradycardia.
   E. **CORRECT:** The client should reduce sodium intake to decrease fluid retention and heart failure.

   (N) *NCLEX® Connection: Pharmacological Therapies, Expected Actions/Outcomes*

4. A, 3; B, 2; C, 1

   When taking actions, the nurse should instruct that loop diuretics can cause hypokalemia, ACE inhibitors can cause a dry cough, and anticoagulants can cause bleeding and bruising.

   (N) *NCLEX® Connection: Pharmacological Therapies, Expected Actions/Outcomes*

5. A, B, E. **CORRECT:** When recognizing cues, the nurse should identify that tachypnea, a persistent, productive cough with pink, frothy sputum, and orthopnea are expected findings in a client who has pulmonary edema.

   (N) *NCLEX® Connection: Physiological Adaptation, Basic Pathophysiology*

CHAPTER 30 *Valvular Heart Disease and Inflammatory Disorders*

Valvular heart disease describes an abnormality or dysfunction of any of the heart's four valves: the mitral and aortic valves (left side), the tricuspid, and pulmonic valves (right side). Tricuspid valve dysfunction occurs secondary to endocarditis or IV illicit drug use ands is rare.

Valve dysfunction reduces the efficiency of the heart as a pump and reduces stroke volume. Over time, there might be remodeling of the heart itself (hypertrophy) and heart failure.

With age, fibrotic thickening occurs in the mitral and aortic valves. The aorta is stiffer in older adult clients, increasing systolic blood pressure and stress on the mitral valve. (30.1) Ⓒ

HEALTH PROMOTION AND DISEASE PREVENTION

- Prevent and treat bacterial infections.
- Encourage clients to consume a diet low in sodium and to follow fluid restrictions prescribed by the provider to prevent heart failure.
- Control chronic illnesses (diabetes mellitus, hypertension, hypercholesterolemia).
- Encourage increased activity and exercise to boost high-density lipoprotein (HDL) levels.

DATA COLLECTION

- Valvular heart disease is classified as:
  - **Stenosis:** Narrowed opening impedes blood moving forward.
  - **Insufficiency/Improper closure:** Some blood flows backward (regurgitation) as a result of valves not closing completely.

- Valvular heart disease can have congenital or acquired causes.
  - **Congenital** valvular heart disease can affect all four valves and cause either stenosis or insufficiency.
  - **Acquired** valvular heart disease is classified as one of three types.
    - **Degenerative disease:** Due to damage over time from mechanical stress, atherosclerosis, and hypertension. Most common in developed countries.
    - **Rheumatic disease:** Gradual fibrotic changes, calcification of valve cusps. Most common in developing countries. Streptococcal infections are a common cause.

RISK FACTORS

- Hypertension
- Rheumatic fever (mitral stenosis and insufficiency)
- Infective endocarditis
- Congenital malformations
- Marfan syndrome (connective tissue disorder that affects the heart and other areas of the body)
- In older adult clients, the predominant causes of valvular heart disease are degenerative calcification and atherosclerosis, and papillary muscle dysfunction

EXPECTED FINDINGS

- Clients who have valvular heart disease often do not have manifestations until late in the progression of the disease.
- A murmur is heard with turbulent blood flow. The location of the murmur and timing (diastolic versus systolic) help determine the valve involved. Murmurs are graded on a scale of I (very faint) to VI (extremely loud).
- Left-sided valve damage causes increased pulmonary artery pressure, left ventricular hypertrophy, and decreased cardiac output, resulting in orthopnea, paroxysmal nocturnal dyspnea (PND), and fatigue.

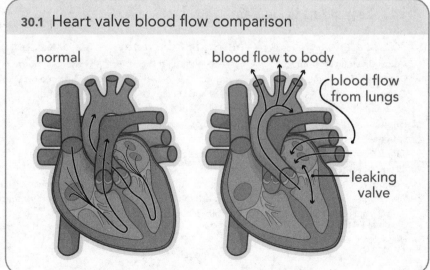

30.1 Heart valve blood flow comparison

normal

blood flow to body

blood flow from lungs

leaking valve

DIAGNOSTIC PROCEDURES

Chest x-ray shows chamber enlargement (with stenosis and insufficiencies) and pulmonary congestion (with aortic stenosis).

12-lead electrocardiogram (ECG) shows chamber hypertrophy.

Echocardiogram shows chamber size, hypertrophy, specific valve dysfunction, ejection function, and amount of regurgitant flow.

Transesophageal echocardiography (TEE) provides visualization of the mitral and aortic valves; TEE can be used intraoperatively during valve replacement and repair.

Exercise tolerance testing/stress echocardiography is used to monitor the impact of the valve problem on cardiac functioning during stress.

Radionuclide studies determine ejection fraction during activity and rest.

Angiography is used to evaluate the coronary arteries and the degree of atherosclerosis. Cardiac catheterization might be used as a diagnostic tool in valvular disease.

PATIENT-CENTERED CARE

NURSING CARE

- Check daily weight to monitor for heart failure.
- Monitor heart rhythm (can be irregular or bradycardic, monitor for murmur).
- Administer oxygen and medications.
- Check hemodynamic monitoring.
- Maintain fluid and sodium restrictions.
- Assist the client to conserve energy.
- Monitor for bleeding.

Oxygen therapy

NURSING ACTIONS
- Monitor oxygen saturation levels.
- Monitor ABGs.
- Monitor client's response to therapy.

MEDICATIONS

Diuretics

Diuretics are used to treat heart failure by removing excessive extracellular fluid.
- Loop diuretics, such as furosemide
- Thiazide diuretics, such as hydrochlorothiazide
- Potassium-sparing diuretics, such as spironolactone

NURSING ACTIONS: Monitor for hypokalemia with loop and thiazide diuretics, and administer potassium supplements as indicated.

CLIENT EDUCATION: If taking loop or thiazide diuretics, ingest foods (dried fruits, nuts, spinach, citrus fruits, bananas and potatoes) and beverages that are high in potassium to decrease the risk of developing hypokalemia. Q EBP

Afterload-reducing agents

Afterload-reducing agents help the heart pump more easily by altering the resistance to contraction.
- Angiotensin-converting enzyme (ACE) inhibitors (enalapril, captopril, lisinopril)
- Angiotensin-receptor blockers (losartan, valsartan)
- Beta blockers, metoprolol, carvedilol
- Calcium-channel blockers (diltiazem, nifedipine, amlodipine)
- Vasodilators, such as hydralazine or nitroglycerin

NURSING ACTIONS: Monitor clients taking ACE inhibitors for initial dose hypotension.

30.2 Left-sided valve damage

Mitral stenosis	Mitral insufficiency	Aortic stenosis	Aortic insufficiency
Apical diastolic murmur	Systolic murmur at the apex	Systolic murmur	Diastolic murmur
Dyspnea on exertion	S_3 sounds	Dyspnea on exertion	Sinus tachycardia
Orthopnea	Fatigue and weakness	S_4 sounds	Exertional dyspnea
Atrial fibrillation	Atrial fibrillation	Angina	Orthopnea
Palpitations	Dyspnea on exertion	Syncope on exertion	Palpitations
Fatigue	Orthopnea	Fatigue	Fatigue
Jugular venous distention	Atypical chest pain	Orthopnea	Nocturnal angina with diaphoresis
Pitting peripheral edema	Palpitations	PND	Widened pulse pressure
Hemoptysis	Jugular venous distention	Narrowed pulse pressure	Bounding arterial pulse on palpation (Corrigan's pulse)
Dry cough	Pitting edema	Peripheral cyanosis	Elevated systolic and diminished diastolic pressures
Paroxysmal nocturnal dyspnea (PND)	Possible diminished lung sounds		PND
Hepatomegaly	PND		
	Hepatomegaly		

Inotropic agents

Inotropic agents, such as digoxin, are used to increase contractility and thereby improve cardiac output. If toxicity develops from digoxin, the antidote is digoxin immune Fab.

CLIENT EDUCATION
If self-administering digoxin:
- Count pulse for 1 min before taking the medication. If the pulse rate is irregular or the pulse rate is outside of the limitations set by the provider (usually less than 60/min or greater than 100/min), the hold the dose and contact the provider.
- Take the dose of digoxin at the same time every day.
- Do not take digoxin at the same time as antacids. Separate the two medications by at least 2 hr.
- Report manifestations of toxicity, including fatigue, muscle weakness, confusion, nausea, diarrhea, visual changes (halos around lights), and loss of appetite.

Anticoagulants

Anticoagulation therapy is used for clients who have a mechanical valve replacement, atrial fibrillation, or severe left ventricle dysfunction to reduce the risk of thrombus.
- Monitor for manifestations of a stroke, such as neurological changes.
- Monitor PT and INR.
- Monitor for manifestations of bleeding, such as bruising.

THERAPEUTIC PROCEDURES

NURSING ACTIONS: Postsurgery care is similar to coronary artery bypass surgery (care for sternal incision, activity limited for 6 weeks, report fever).

Percutaneous balloon valvuloplasty

This procedure can open aortic or mitral valves affected by stenosis. A catheter is inserted through the femoral artery and advanced to the heart. A balloon is inflated at the stenotic lesion to open the fused commissures and improve leaflet mobility. There is an increased chance of recurrence within 6 months.

Valve replacement

This procedure replaces damaged heart valves with mechanical, xenografts (from other species), allografts (from cadavers), or autografts (formed from the client's pulmonic valve and a portion of the pulmonary artery). It is often done with an open-heart approach, although minimally invasive surgery is also performed in some instances.
- Mechanical valves require lifelong anticoagulant therapy.
- Tissue valves need to be replaced every 7 to 10 years.

NURSING ACTIONS
- Monitor insertion site for bleeding.
- Monitor for manifestations of emboli.

Miscellaneous surgical management

- Other surgeries used in the treatment of valvular disorders include chordae tendineae reconstruction, commissurotomy (relieve stenosis on leaflets), annuloplasty ring insertion (correct dilatation of valve annulus by narrowing the opening), and leaflet repair.
- Medical management is appropriate for many older adult clients; surgery is indicated when manifestations interfere with daily activities. The goal of surgery can be to improve the quality of life rather than to prolong life. Ⓖ

INTERPROFESSIONAL CARE

- Respiratory services should be consulted for inhalers, breathing treatments, and suctioning for airway management.
- Cardiology can be consulted for cardiac management.
- Nutritional services can be contacted for weight loss or gain related to medications or diagnosis.
- Rehabilitative care might need to be consulted if the client has prolonged weakness and needs assistance with increasing level of activity. Qтc

CLIENT EDUCATION

- Prophylactic antibiotic use is important before any invasive dental or respiratory procedure that might cause infection. Qs
- Weigh daily and notify the provider of 3 lb (1.4 kg) gain in 1 day or 5 lb (2.3 kg) gain in 1 week.
- Coordinate activities with planned rest periods.
- Follow the prescribed exercise program.
- Adhere to dietary restrictions, including avoidance of caffeine and alcohol; consider nutritional consultation.
- Maintain heart healthy diet, increase fiber, decrease sodium and no trans fat.
- Perform energy conservation.
- Open wounds need to be cleaned carefully and antibiotic ointment should be used.
- Read labels of over-the-counter medication to avoid those which include alcohol, ephedrine, or epinephrine (might cause dysrhythmias).
- Report heart failure manifestations to the provider immediately.
- If smoke or use smokeless tobacco, consider smoking cessation program.

COMPLICATIONS

Heart failure

Heart failure is the inability of the heart to maintain adequate circulation to meet tissue needs for oxygen and nutrients. Ineffective valves result in heart failure.

NURSING ACTIONS: Monitoring the client's heart failure class (I to IV) is often the gauge for surgical intervention for valvular problems.

Inflammatory disorders

Inflammation related to the heart is an extended inflammatory response that often leads to the destruction of healthy tissue. This primarily includes the layers of the heart (epicardium, myocardium, and endocardium).

Inflammatory disorders related to the cardiovascular system that nurses should be familiar with include pericarditis, myocarditis, rheumatic heart disease.

HEALTH PROMOTION AND DISEASE PREVENTION

- Early treatment of streptococcal infections can prevent rheumatic fever.
- Prophylactic treatments (including antibiotics for clients who have cardiac defects) can reduce the risk of infective endocarditis. Take all antibiotics as prescribed.
- Influenza, pneumonia, and COVID-19 immunizations are important for all clients (especially older adults) in order to decrease the incidence of myocarditis. Ⓖ

DATA COLLECTION

RISK FACTORS

- Congenital heart defect/cardiac anomalies
- Intravenous substance use
- Heart valve replacement
- Immunosuppression
- Rheumatic fever and other infections
- School-age children who have a long duration of streptococcus infection
- Malnutrition
- Overcrowding
- Lower socioeconomic status

EXPECTED FINDINGS

Pericarditis: Inflammation of the pericardium
- Commonly follows a viral infection.
- Can be due to a myocardial infarction.
- Can be due to acute exacerbation of a systemic connective tissue disease such as systemic lupus erythematosus, and rheumatoid arthritis.
- Findings include chest pressure/pain aggravated by breathing (mainly inspiration), coughing, and swallowing; pericardial friction rub auscultated at left lower sternal border; shortness of breath; and relief of pain when sitting and leaning forward.

Myocarditis: Inflammation of the myocardium
- Can be due to a viral, fungal, or bacterial infection, or a systemic inflammatory disease (Crohn's disease). COVID-19 might increase the risk for myocarditis.
- Findings include tachycardia, murmur, friction rub auscultated in the lungs, cardiomegaly, chest pain, and dysrhythmias.

Rheumatic heart disease: An infection of the endocardium due to a complication of rheumatic fever. Higher incidence in children.
- Preceded by group A beta-hemolytic streptococcal pharyngitis
- Produces lesions in the heart
- Findings include fever, chest pain, joint pain, tachycardia, shortness of breath, rash on trunk and extremities, friction rub, murmur, muscle spasms

LABORATORY TESTS Q︎EBP

- Blood cultures can detect a bacterial infection.
- An elevated WBC count can be indicative of a bacterial infection.
- Cardiac enzymes can be elevated with pericarditis and endocarditis.
- Elevated ESR and CRP indicate inflammation in the body.
- Throat cultures can detect a streptococcal infection, which can lead to rheumatic fever.

DIAGNOSTIC PROCEDURES

Electrocardiography (ECG)

Can detect a heart block, which is associated with rheumatic fever or demonstrate ST segment elevation in almost all leads in the case of pericarditis

Echocardiography

Can evaluate the structure and function of the heart and reveal inflamed heart layers or pericardial effusion

PATIENT-CENTERED CARE

NURSING CARE

- Auscultate heart sounds. (Listen for murmur or friction rub.)
- Review ABGs, SaO$_2$, and chest x-ray results.
- Administer oxygen.
- Monitor vital signs. (Watch for fever.)
- Monitor ECG, and notify the provider of changes.
- Monitor for cardiac tamponade and heart failure.
- Obtain throat cultures to identify bacteria to be treated by antibiotic therapy.
- Administer antibiotics.
- Administer antipyretics.
- Determine onset, quality, duration, and severity of pain.
- Administer pain medication.
- Encourage bed rest.
- Provide emotional support to the client and family and encourage verbalization of feelings regarding the illness.

MEDICATIONS

Penicillin

Antibiotic given to treat infection

NURSING ACTIONS
- Monitor for skin rash and hives.
- Monitor electrolyte and kidney levels.

CLIENT EDUCATION
- Report skin rash or hives.
- The medication can cause gastrointestinal (GI) distress.

Ibuprofen

NSAIDs are given to treat fever and inflammation associated with pericarditis and infective endocarditis. No longer used for treatment of pain and inflammation with myocarditis.

NURSING ACTIONS
- Do not use with clients who have peptic ulcer disease.
- Watch for indications of GI distress.
- Monitor platelets as well as liver and kidney function levels.

CLIENT EDUCATION
- The medication can cause GI distress. Taking with food reduces the risk.
- Avoid alcohol consumption while taking the medication.

Prednisone

Glucocorticosteroid given to treat inflammation

NURSING ACTIONS
- Use in low doses.
- Monitor blood pressure.
- Monitor electrolytes and blood glucose levels.
- Monitor for impaired healing in clients taking this medication.

CLIENT EDUCATION
- Take the medication with food.
- Avoid stopping the medication abruptly.
- Report unexpected weight gain.

Amphotericin B

Antifungal given to treat fungal infection

NURSING ACTIONS: Monitor liver and kidney function levels.

CLIENT EDUCATION: The medication can cause GI distress.

INTERPROFESSIONAL CARE

- Cardiology services are consulted to manage cardiac dysfunction.
- Infectious disease services can be consulted to manage infection.
- Physical therapy can be consulted to increase the client's level of activity once prescribed.

THERAPEUTIC PROCEDURES

Pericarditis

Pericardiocentesis is the insertion of a needle into the pericardium to aspirate pericardial fluid. This can be done in the emergency department or a procedure room.

NURSING ACTIONS
- Pericardial fluid can be sent to the laboratory for culture and sensitivity.
- Monitor for recurrence of cardiac tamponade.

CLIENT EDUCATION

- Take rest periods as needed.
- Wash hands to prevent infection.
- Report fever.
- Avoid crowded areas to reduce the risk of infection.
- Good oral hygiene and the prevention of infection is important.
- Taking medications as prescribed is important.
- Demonstrate the administration of intravenous antibiotics and management before discharge.
- Participate in cessation of tobacco use if applicable.
- Understand the illness, and express any feelings.
- Advise all providers, including dentists, of history of endocarditis so that antibiotic prophylaxis is prescribed if needed. Qs

CARE AFTER DISCHARGE
- Home health services can be indicated if the client had surgery. Qtc
- Intravenous antibiotic therapy can be given by the home health service.
- Pharmaceutical services can be indicated for IV supplies and medications.
- Rehabilitation services can be indicated to help the client increase the level of activity.

COMPLICATIONS

Cardiac tamponade

Cardiac tamponade, considered a medical emergency, can result from fluid accumulation in the pericardial sac.
- Manifestations include dyspnea, dizziness, report of "tightness" in the chest, increasing restlessness, pulsus paradoxus (a decrease of 10 mm Hg or more in systolic blood pressure during inspiration), tachycardia, muffled heart sounds, and jugular venous distention.
- Hemodynamic monitoring reveals intracardiac and pulmonary artery pressures similar and elevated (plateau pressures).

NURSING ACTIONS: Notify the provider immediately.

Active Learning Scenario

A nurse educator is preparing a poster on valvular heart disease to be displayed at a health fair. What content should be included on the poster? Use the ATI Active Learning Template: System Disorder to complete this item.

ALTERATION IN HEALTH (DIAGNOSIS)

- Describe the difference between valve stenosis and insufficiency.
- Describe the difference between acquired and congenital valvular heart disease.

CLIENT EDUCATION: Describe two actions to prevent valvular disease.

Application Exercises

1. A nurse is reviewing the medical records of several clients to identify risk factors for valvular heart disease. What are the risk factors for valvular heart disease?

2. A nurse is assisting with teaching a class about valvular heart disease. Match the valvular dysfunction with the associated manifestations.

   A. Aortic insufficiency   1. Apical diastolic murmur

   B. Aortic stenosis   2. S_3 heart sound

   C. Mitral insufficiency   3. Narrowed pulse pressure

   D. Mitral stenosis   4. Bounding pulse

3. A nurse is collecting data on a client who has mitral valve insufficiency. Which of the following findings should the nurse expect?

   A. S_4 heart sound

   B. Petechiae

   C. Neck vein distention

   D. Splenomegaly

4. A nurse is assisting with the care of a client who has pericarditis. Which of the following findings should the nurse expect? (Select all that apply.)

   A. Petechiae

   B. Friction rub

   C. Splinter hemorrhages under the nails

   D. Cough

   E. Chest pain

5. A nurse is assisting with teaching a class about risk factors for inflammatory heart disease. The nurse should instruct that which of the following conditions is a risk factor for rheumatic heart disease?

   A. COPD

   B. Streptococcal pharyngitis

   C. Lupus erythematosus

   D. A new tattoo

Application Exercises Key

1. When analyzing cues, the nurse should identify that a history of hypertension, rheumatic fever, infective endocarditis, congenital malformations, Marfan syndrome (connective tissue disorder that affects the heart and other areas of the body) are risk factors for valvular heart disease. Older adult clients are at risk for valvular heart disease due to degenerative calcification and atherosclerosis.

Ⓝ *NCLEX® Connection: Health Promotion and Maintenance, Health Promotion/Disease Prevention*

2. A, 4; B, 3; C, 2; D, 1

When taking actions, the nurse should instruct an apical diastolic murmur is a manifestation of mitral stenosis. An S3 heart sound is a manifestation of mitral insufficiency. Narrowed pulse pressure is a manifestation of aortic stenosis. A bounding pulse is a manifestation of aortic insufficiency.

Ⓝ *NCLEX® Connection: Physiological Adaptation, Basic Pathophysiology*

3. C. **CORRECT:** When analyzing cues, the nurse should identify that neck vein distention is an expected finding in a client who has pulmonary congestion due to mitral valve insufficiency.

Ⓝ *NCLEX® Connection: Physiological Adaptation, Basic Pathophysiology*

4. B, D, E. **CORRECT:** When recognizing cues, the nurse should identify manifestations of pericarditis include a pericardial friction rub, chest pain, and a cough.

Ⓝ *NCLEX® Connection: Physiological Adaptation, Basic Pathophysiology*

5. B. **CORRECT:** When taking actions, the nurse should instruct that streptococcal pharyngitis is a risk factor for developing rheumatic fever, which can result in rheumatic endocarditis.

Ⓝ *NCLEX® Connection: Health Promotion and Maintenance, Health Promotion/Disease Prevention*

Active Learning Scenario Key

Using the ATI Active Learning Template: System Disorder

ALTERATION IN HEALTH (DIAGNOSIS)

- Stenosis is the narrowed opening of a heart valve, which prevents blood from moving forward. Insufficiency is the improper closure of a valve resulting in blood flowing backward (regurgitation) through the valve.
- Congenital valvular heart disease can affect all four valves and can cause either stenosis or insufficiency. Acquired valvular heart disease occurs due to degenerative changes from mechanical stress over time; rheumatic disease, which causes calcifications and fibrotic changes, often to the mitral valve; and infective endocarditis, in which infectious organisms destroy the valve.

CLIENT EDUCATION

- Prevent and manage hypertension.
- Prevent and seek early treatment of bacterial infections.
- Consume a low-sodium diet.

Ⓝ *NCLEX® Connection: Health Promotion and Maintenance, Health Promotion/Disease Prevention*

When reviewing the following chapters, keep in mind the relevant topics and tasks of the NCLEX outline.

Pharmacological Therapies

ADVERSE EFFECTS/CONTRAINDICATIONS/SIDE EFFECTS/INTERACTIONS
Identify a contraindication to the administration of a prescribed or over-the-counter medication to the client.

Withhold medication dose if client experiences adverse effect to medication.

MEDICATION ADMINISTRATION
Collect required data prior to medication administration.

Assist in preparing the client for insertion of a central line.

Administer intravenous piggyback (secondary) medications.

Reduction of Risk Potential

POTENTIAL FOR ALTERATIONS IN BODY SYSTEMS
Perform focused data collection based on client condition.

Reinforce client teaching on methods to prevent complications associated with activity level/diagnosed illness/disease.

Physiological Adaptation

ALTERATIONS IN BODY SYSTEMS: Reinforce education to client regarding care and condition.

BASIC PATHOPHYSIOLOGY: Identify signs and symptoms related to an acute or chronic illness.

UNIT 4 CARDIOVASCULAR DISORDERS

SECTION: VASCULAR DISORDERS

CHAPTER 31 *Peripheral Vascular Diseases*

Peripheral vascular diseases include peripheral arterial disease (PAD) and peripheral venous disorders, both of which interfere with normal blood flow. PAD affects arteries (blood vessels that carry blood away from the heart), and peripheral venous disease affects veins (blood vessels that carry blood toward the heart).

Peripheral arterial disease

- PAD results from atherosclerosis that usually occurs in the arteries of the lower extremities and is characterized by inadequate flow of blood.
- Atherosclerosis is caused by a gradual thickening of the intima and media of the arteries, ultimately resulting in the progressive narrowing of the vessel lumen. Plaques can form on the walls of the arteries, making them rough and fragile.
- Progressive stiffening of the arteries and narrowing of the lumen decreases the blood supply to affected tissues and increases resistance to blood flow.
- Atherosclerosis is a type of arteriosclerosis, which means "hardening of the arteries" and alludes to the loss of elasticity of arteries over time due to thickening of their walls.
- Buerger's disease, subclavian steal syndrome, thoracic outlet syndrome, Raynaud's disease, and popliteal entrapment are examples of PAD.

DATA COLLECTION

RISK FACTORS

- Hypertension
- Hyperlipidemia
- Diabetes mellitus
- Cigarette smoking
- Obesity
- Sedentary lifestyle
- Familial predisposition
- Advanced age
- Elevated C-reactive protein
- Hyperhomocysteinemia

EXPECTED FINDINGS

- Burning, cramping, and pain in the legs during exercise (intermittent claudication)
- Numbness or burning pain primarily in the feet when in bed
- Pain that is relieved by placing legs at rest in a dependent position

PHYSICAL FINDINGS

- Decreased capillary refill of toes (greater than 3 seconds)
- Decreased or nonpalpable pulses
- Loss of hair on lower calf, ankle, and foot
- Dry, shiny, mottled skin
- Thick toenails
- Cold and cyanotic extremity
- Pallor of extremity with elevation
- Dependent rubor (redness) of the extremity
- Muscle atrophy
- Ulcers and possible gangrene of toes

DIAGNOSTIC PROCEDURES

Arteriography

- Arteriography of the lower extremities involves arterial injection of contrast medium to visualize areas of decreased arterial flow on an x-ray. Q**EBP**
- It is usually done only to determine isolated areas of occlusion that can be treated during the procedure with percutaneous transluminal angioplasty and possible stent placement.

NURSING ACTIONS

- Observe for bleeding and hemorrhage.
- Palpate pedal pulses to identify possible occlusions.

Exercise tolerance testing

A stress test is done with or without the use of a treadmill (medications such as dipyridamole and adenosine can be given to mimic the effects of exercise in clients who cannot tolerate a treadmill) with measurement of pulse volumes and blood pressures prior to and following the onset of manifestations or 5 min of exercise. Delays in return to normal pressures and pulse waveforms indicate arterial disease. It is used to evaluate claudication during exercise.

Plethysmography

- Plethysmography is used to determine the variations of blood passing through an artery, thus identifying abnormal arterial flow in the affected limb.
- Blood pressure cuffs are attached to the client's upper extremities, a lower extremity, and the plethysmograph machine. Variations in peripheral pulses between the upper and lower extremity are recorded.
- A decrease in pulse pressure of the lower extremity indicates a possible blockage in the leg.

Segmental systolic blood pressure measurements

- A Doppler probe is used to take various blood pressure measurements (thigh, calf, ankle, brachial) for comparison. In the absence of PAD, pressures in the lower extremities are higher than those of the upper extremities.
- With arterial disease, the pressures in the thigh, calf, and ankle are lower.

Magnetic resonance angiography

A contrast medium, such as gadolinium, is injected to help visualize blood flow through peripheral arteries.

Ankle-brachial index (ABI)

The ankle pressure is compared to the brachial pressure. The expected finding for ABI is 0.9 to 1.3. ABI less than 0.9 in either leg is diagnostic for PAD.

Doppler-derived maximal systolic acceleration

A technique that is especially helpful for evaluating PAD in clients who have diabetes mellitus.

PATIENT-CENTERED CARE

NURSING CARE

- Encourage the client to exercise to build up collateral circulation.
  - Initiate exercise gradually and increase slowly.
  - Instruct the client to walk until the point of pain, stop and rest, and then walk a little farther.
- Promote vasodilation and avoid vasoconstriction.
  - Provide a warm environment for the client.
  - Have the client wear insulated socks.
  - Tell the client to never apply direct heat, such as a heating pad, to the affected extremity because sensitivity is decreased, and this can cause a burn.
  - Instruct the client to avoid exposure to cold (causes vasoconstriction and decreased arterial flow).
  - Instruct the client to avoid stress, caffeine, and nicotine, which also cause vasoconstriction.
    - Vasoconstriction is avoided when the client completely abstains from smoking or chewing tobacco. Qᴱᴮᴾ
    - Vasoconstriction of vessels lasts up to 1 hr after smoking or chewing tobacco.

POSITIONING

- Instruct the client to avoid crossing the legs.
- Tell the client to refrain from wearing restrictive garments.
- Tell the client to elevate the legs to reduce swelling, but not to elevate them above the level of the heart because extreme elevation slows arterial blood flow to the feet.

MEDICATIONS

Antiplatelet medications

Aspirin, clopidogrel, pentoxifylline
Antiplatelet medications reduce blood viscosity by decreasing blood fibrinogen levels, enhancing erythrocyte flexibility, and increasing blood flow in the extremities. Medications, such as aspirin and clopidogrel, can be prescribed. Pentoxifylline, sometimes referred to as a hemorheologic medication, was one of the first to be used and is still used, but less commonly than other medications. It can be given to specifically treat intermittent claudication in clients who have PAD.

CLIENT EDUCATION

- The medication's effects might not be apparent for several weeks.
- Monitor for evidence of bleeding (abdominal pain; coffee-ground emesis; black, tarry stools).
- Avoid taking herbal supplements with clopidogrel because they can increase the risk of bleeding.

Statins

Simvastatin, atorvastatin: Can relieve manifestations associated with PAD (intermittent claudication)

THERAPEUTIC PROCEDURES

Percutaneous transluminal angioplasty and laser-assisted angioplasty

- Percutaneous transluminal angioplasty is an invasive intra-arterial procedure using a balloon and stent to open and help maintain the patency of the vessel.
- Laser-assisted angioplasty is an invasive procedure in which a laser probe is advanced through a cannula to the site of stenosis.
  - The laser is used to vaporize atherosclerotic plaque and open the artery.

NURSING ACTIONS

- The priority action is to observe for bleeding at the puncture site. Qs
- Monitor vital signs, peripheral pulses, and capillary refill.
- Keep the client on bed rest with their limb straight for 2 to 6 hr before ambulation.
- Anticoagulant therapy is used during the procedure, followed by antiplatelet therapy for 1 to 3 months.

Mechanical rotational abrasive atherectomy

Uses a rotational device to scrape plaque from the inside of the client's peripheral artery. The device is designed to cause minimal damage to the surface of the artery.

NURSING ACTIONS

- The priority action is to observe for bleeding at the puncture site. Qs
- Monitor vital signs, peripheral pulses, and capillary refill.
- Keep the client on bed rest with their limb straight for 2 to 6 hr before ambulation.
- Anticoagulant therapy is used during the procedure, followed by antiplatelet therapy for 1 to 3 months.

Arterial revascularization surgery

Used with clients who have severe claudication and/or limb pain at rest, or with clients who are at risk for losing a limb due to poor arterial circulation.

- Bypass grafts are used to reroute the circulation around the arterial occlusion.
- Grafts can be harvested from the client (autologous) or made from synthetic materials.

NURSING ACTIONS

- The priority action is to maintain adequate circulation in the repaired artery. The location of the pedal or dorsalis pulse should be marked, and its pulsatile strength compared with the contralateral leg on a scheduled basis using a Doppler. Qs
- Color, temperature, sensation, and capillary refill should be compared with the contralateral extremity on a scheduled basis.
- Monitor for warmth, redness, and possibly edema of the affected limb as a result of increased blood flow.
- Monitor for pain. Pain can be severe due to the reestablishment of blood flow to the extremity.
- Monitor blood pressure. Hypotension can result in an increased risk of clotting or graft collapse, while hypertension increases the risk for bleeding from sutures.

CLIENT EDUCATION

- Limit bending of the hip and knee to decrease the risk of clot formation.
- Avoid crossing or raising legs above the level of the heart.
- Wear loose clothing.
- Perform wound care if revascularization surgery was done.
- Avoid smoking and cold temperatures.
- Perform foot care (keep feet clean and dry, wear good-fitting shoes, never go barefoot, cut toenails straight across or have the podiatrist cut nails).

COMPLICATIONS

Graft occlusion

Graft occlusion is a serious complication of arterial revascularization and often occurs within the first 24 hr following surgery.

NURSING ACTIONS

- Promptly notify the surgeon of manifestations of occlusion (absent or reduced pedal pulses, increased pain, change in extremity color or temperature). Qs
- Prepare to assist with treatment, which can include an emergency thrombectomy (removal of a clot), local intra-arterial thrombolytic therapy with an agent such as tissue plasminogen activator, infusion of a platelet inhibitor, or a combination of these. With these treatments, monitor for indications of bleeding.

Wound or graft infection

An infection of the surgical wound or graft is a potentially life-threatening complication.

NURSING ACTIONS

- Use sterile technique when changing the surgical dressing or providing wound care.
- Indications of infection include localized induration, warmth, tenderness, erythema, edema, purulent drainage, and an elevated WBC. Promptly report findings to the provider.

Compartment syndrome

Compartment syndrome is considered a medical emergency. Tissue pressure within a confined body space can restrict blood flow, and the resulting ischemia can lead to irreversible tissue damage.

NURSING ACTIONS

- Manifestations of compartment syndrome include tingling, numbness, worsening pain, edema, pain on passive movement, and unequal pulses. Immediately report findings to the provider.
- Loosen dressings.
- Prepare to assist with fasciotomy (surgical opening into the tissues), which can be necessary to prevent further injury and to save the limb.
- Monitor for comfort, impaired mobility, and decreased sensory perception of the affected extremity by following the data collection of the "6 P's" (pain, pressure, paralysis, paresthesia, pallor, pulselessness). Paresthesia (numbness, tingling) is often the first manifestation of compartment syndrome. Then the distal area becomes pale and cool, with pulselessness, pain, and inability to move the distal area (hand, foot).

Peripheral venous disorders

Peripheral venous disorders are problems with the veins that interfere with adequate return of blood flow from the extremities, and can result in blood stasis.

- There are superficial and deep veins in the lower extremities that have valves that prevent backflow of blood as it returns to the heart. The action of the skeletal muscles of the lower extremities during walking and other activities also promotes venous return.
- Three peripheral venous disorders that nurses should be familiar with are venous thromboembolism (VTE), venous insufficiency, and varicose veins.

VTE is a blood clot believed to form as a result of venous stasis, endothelial injury, or hypercoagulability. Thrombus formation can lead to a pulmonary embolism, a life-threatening complication. Thrombophlebitis refers to a thrombus that is associated with inflammation.

Venous insufficiency occurs secondary to incompetent valves in the deeper veins of the lower extremities, which allows pooling of blood and dilation of the veins. The veins' inability to carry fluid and wastes from the lower extremities precipitates the development of swelling, venous stasis ulcers, and in advanced cases, cellulitis.

Varicose veins are enlarged, twisted, and superficial veins that can occur in any part of the body; however, they are commonly observed in the lower extremities and in the esophagus.

DATA COLLECTION

RISK FACTORS

Venous thromboembolism: Associated with Virchow's triad (hypercoagulability, impaired blood flow, damage to blood vessels)
- Hip surgery, total-knee replacement, open prostate surgery
- Heart failure
- Immobility
- Pregnancy
- Oral contraceptives
- Active cancer
- Central venous and dialysis access catheters
- Factor V Leiden defect
- Severe COVID-19 with an elevated D-dimer assay indicating a high risk of thrombosis

Venous insufficiency: Results from periods of prolonged venous hypertension that results in damage to the valve, causing backup of blood, edema, and damage to the deep tissue
- Sitting or standing in one position for a long period of time
- Obesity
- Pregnancy
- Thrombophlebitis

Varicose veins
- Assigned female gender at birth
- Working in an occupation requiring prolonged standing
- Pregnancy
- Obesity
- Systemic diseases (heart disease)
- Family history

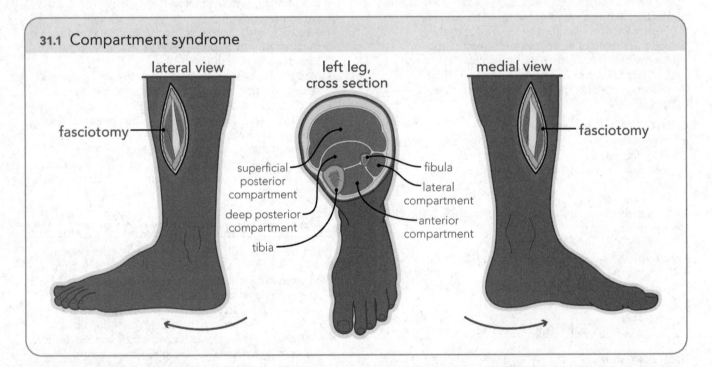

31.1 Compartment syndrome

lateral view

left leg, cross section

medial view

fasciotomy

fasciotomy

superficial posterior compartment

deep posterior compartment

tibia

fibula

lateral compartment

anterior compartment

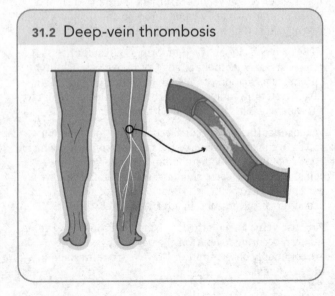

31.2 Deep-vein thrombosis

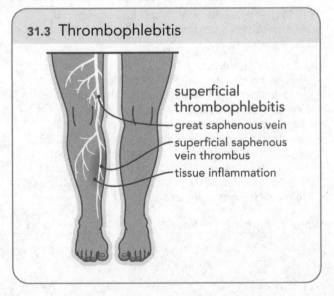

31.3 Thrombophlebitis

superficial thrombophlebitis

great saphenous vein

superficial saphenous vein thrombus

tissue inflammation

EXPECTED FINDINGS

Limb pain: Aching pain and feeling of fullness or heaviness in the legs after standing

PHYSICAL FINDINGS

- **Deep vein thrombosis (DVT) and thrombophlebitis**
  - Client can be asymptomatic.
  - Calf or groin pain, tenderness, and a sudden onset of edema of the extremity. ○EBP
  - Warmth, edema, and induration and hardness over the involved blood vessel.
  - Changes in circumferences of right and left calf and thigh over time; localized edema over the affected area.

  ! Shortness of breath and chest pain can indicate that the embolus has moved to the lungs (pulmonary embolism).

- **Venous insufficiency**
  - Stasis dermatitis is a brown discoloration along the ankles that extends up the calf relative to the level of insufficiency.
  - Edema
  - Stasis ulcers (typically found around ankles)
- **Varicose veins**
  - Distended, superficial veins can be visible just below the skin and are tortuous in nature.
  - Clients often report muscle cramping and aches, pain after sitting, and pruritus.

LABORATORY TESTS

D-dimer test measures fibrin degradation products present in the blood produced from fibrinolysis. A positive test indicates that thrombus formation has possibly occurred.

DIAGNOSTIC PROCEDURES

DVT and thrombophlebitis

- Venous duplex ultrasonography uses high-frequency sound waves to provide a real-time picture of the blood flow through a blood vessel.
- Doppler flow study produces an audible sound when venous circulation is normal and little or no sound when veins are thrombosed.
- Impedance plethysmography can be used to determine the variations of blood passing through a vein, thus identifying abnormal venous flow in the affected limb.
- If the above tests are negative for a DVT, but one is still suspected, a venogram, which uses contrast material, or magnetic resonance imaging might be needed for accurate diagnosis.

Varicose veins: Trendelenburg test

NURSING ACTIONS

- Place the client in a supine position with legs elevated.
- A tourniquet is applied.
- When the client stands, if the veins remain flat the cause is the valves of the deep veins. If the veins distend rapidly, the valves of the superficial veins are affected.

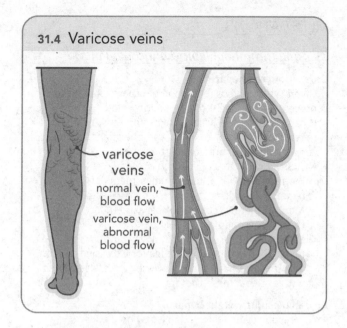

31.4 Varicose veins

varicose veins

normal vein, blood flow

varicose vein, abnormal blood flow

PATIENT-CENTERED CARE

NURSING CARE

DVT and thrombophlebitis

- Encourage ambulation following initiation of anticoagulant therapy.
  - Encourage dorsiflexion/plantar flexion exercises of the foot when in bed.
  - Occasionally elevate the legs above the level of the heart while the client is in bed. (Avoid using a knee gatch or pillow under the knees.)
- Administer intermittent or continuous warm moist compresses as prescribed.
- Do not massage the affected limb. ○s
- Provide thigh-high compression or anti-embolism stockings.
- Prepare the client for an inferior vena cava interruption surgery (a filter traps emboli and prevents them from reaching the heart) as indicated.

Venous insufficiency

- Elevate legs for at least 20 min, four to five times a day.
- Elevate the legs above the heart when in bed.

CLIENT EDUCATION

- Avoid crossing legs and wearing constrictive clothing or stockings.
- Wear elastic compression stockings. Apply them after the legs have been elevated and when swelling is at a minimum. ○EBP

MEDICATIONS

DVT and thrombophlebitis: anticoagulants

Unfractionated heparin

- Given IV to prevent formation of other clots and to prevent enlargement of the existing clot.
- It has significant adverse effects and must be given in the facility. Prior to discharge, the client will be converted to oral anticoagulation therapy with warfarin.
- NURSING ACTIONS
  - Monitor aPTT to allow for adjustments of heparin dosage.
  - Monitor platelet counts for heparin-induced thrombocytopenia. Qs
  - Ensure that protamine sulfate, the antidote for heparin, is available if needed for excessive bleeding.
  - Monitor for hazards and adverse effects associated with anticoagulant therapy.

Low-molecular weight heparin

- Given subcutaneously and is based on a client's weight.
- Enoxaparin is used for the prevention and treatment of DVT. It is usually given in the facility, but the twice-daily injections can be given in the home setting.
- CLIENT EDUCATION
  - Observe for evidence of bleeding.
  - Take bleeding precautions (use electric instead of bladed razor, brush teeth with a soft toothbrush). Qs

Warfarin

- Inhibits synthesis of the four vitamin K–dependent clotting factors.
- The therapeutic effect takes 3 to 4 days to develop, so administration of the medication is begun while the client is still on heparin.
- NURSING ACTIONS
  - Monitor for bleeding.
  - Monitor PT and INR.
  - Ensure that vitamin K (the antidote for warfarin) is available in case of excessive bleeding.
- CLIENT EDUCATION
  - Be aware of food sources of vitamin K (green leafy vegetables) and avoid fluctuations in the amount and frequency of consumption.
  - Observe for evidence of bleeding.
  - Take bleeding precautions (use electric instead of bladed razor, and brush teeth with soft toothbrush).

Factor Xa inhibitors:
Inhibit Factor Xa in prevention of development of thromboses (fondaparinux [subcutaneous administration], rivaroxaban and apixaban [oral administration])

Direct thrombin inhibitor

- Acts as a direct inhibitor of thrombin to prevent thrombus formation (dabigatran).
- Idarucizumab is the antidote to reverse dabigatran in life-threatening events by preventing dabigatran from inhibiting thrombin.
- Initial lab values are PT and aPTT. Recurrent laboratory monitoring is not necessary.
- Not recommended if the client has renal insufficiency.

DVT and thrombophlebitis: thrombolytic therapy

Thrombolytic therapy dissolves clots that have already developed. Therapy must be started within 5 days after the development of the clot for the therapy to be effective. Tissue plasminogen activator, a thrombolytic agent, and platelet inhibitors (such as abciximab and eptifibatide) can be effective in dissolving a clot or preventing new clots during the first 24 hr. Administering the medication in a manner that provides direct contact with the thrombus can be more effective and lessen the chance of bleeding.

NURSING ACTIONS: Monitor for bleeding (intracerebral bleeding).

CLIENT EDUCATION: Take bleeding precautions (use electric instead of bladed razor and brush teeth with a soft toothbrush).

THERAPEUTIC PROCEDURES

DVT

An **inferior vena cava filter** can be inserted when a client is unresponsive to medical therapy or when anticoagulation is contraindicated. It is inserted via the femoral vein and passed into the inferior vena cava where it traps emboli before they progress to the lungs.

Varicose veins

Sclerotherapy

- A sclerosing irritating chemical solution is injected into the varicose vein to produce localized inflammation, which will close the lumen of the vessel over time.
- For larger vessels, an incision and drainage of the trapped blood in a sclerosed vein might need to be performed 2 to 3 weeks after the injection.
- Pressure dressings are applied for approximately 1 week after each procedure to keep the vessel free of blood.
- CLIENT EDUCATION
  - Wear elastic stockings for the prescribed time.
  - Mild analgesics, such as acetaminophen, can be taken for discomfort.

Vein stripping

Vein stripping is the removal of large varicose veins that cannot be treated with less-invasive procedures.

- PREOPERATIVE NURSING ACTIONS
  - Assist the provider with vein marking.
  - Assist with evaluating pulses as a baseline for postoperative comparison.
- POSTOPERATIVE NURSING ACTIONS
- Maintain elastic bandages on the legs.
  - Monitor groin and leg for bleeding through the elastic bandages.
  - Monitor extremity for edema, warmth, color, and pulses.
  - Assist with the evaluation of legs above the level of the heart.
- CLIENT EDUCATION
  - Understand the importance of wearing elastic stockings after bandage removal.
  - Elevate the legs when sitting and avoid dangling them over the side of the bed.
  - Engage in range-of-motion exercises of the legs.

Endovenous laser treatment: This type of treatment uses a laser fiber that is inserted into the vessel proximal to the area to be treated and then threaded to the involved area, where heat from the laser is used to close the dilated vein.

Application of radio frequency energy: This type of treatment uses a small catheter with a radio frequency electrode, instead of a laser, that is inserted into the vessel proximal to the area to be treated that scars and closes a dilated vein.

INTERPROFESSIONAL CARE

Venous insufficiency

- Care of venous stasis ulcers requires long-term management.
- Recommend a consultation with a dietitian and wound care specialist to facilitate the healing process. Qᴛᴄ

COMPLICATIONS

Ulcer formation

- Venous stasis ulcers often form over the medial malleolus. Venous ulcers are chronic, hard to heal, and often recur. They can lead to amputation or death.
- Clients who have neuropathy might not feel as much discomfort from the ulcer as its appearance can warrant.

NURSING ACTIONS

- Administer and assist with treatments to improve circulation (wound vacuum, hyperbaric chamber).
- Monitor and assist with treatment of pain as prescribed.
- Apply oxygen-permeable polyethylene films to superficial ulcers.
- Apply occlusive hydrocolloid dressings on deeper ulcers to promote granulation tissue and reepithelialization. Qᴇʙᴘ
- Leave a dressing on for 3 to 7 days.
- If a wound needs chemical debridement, assist with the application of prescribed topical enzymatic agents to debride the ulcer, eliminate necrotic tissue, and promote healing.
- Assist with the administration of systemic antibiotics as prescribed.
- Prepare for oxygen therapy and blood gas analysis while continuing to monitor the client for other manifestations.
- If the wound has a large amount of drainage, a vacuum assisted drainage device can be prescribed.

CLIENT EDUCATION

- Adhere to a diet high in zinc, protein, iron, and vitamins A and C.
- Understand the use of compression stockings.
- Prepare to administer prescribed anticoagulation.

Pulmonary embolism

A pulmonary embolism occurs when a thrombus is dislodged, becomes an embolus, and lodges in a pulmonary vessel. This can lead to obstruction of pulmonary blood flow, decreased systemic oxygenation, pulmonary tissue hypoxia, and possible death.

NURSING ACTIONS

- Manifestations include sudden onset dyspnea, pleuritic chest pain, restlessness, apprehension, feelings of impending doom, cough, and hemoptysis.
- Findings include tachypnea, crackles, pleural friction rub, tachycardia, S_3 or S_4 heart sounds, diaphoresis, low-grade fever, petechiae over chest and axillae, and decreased arterial oxygen saturation.
- Notify the provider immediately. Reassure the client. Assist the client to a position of comfort with the head of the bed elevated. Qꜱ
- Prepare for oxygen therapy and blood gas analysis while continuing to monitor the client for other manifestations.
- Prepare to administer prescribed anticoagulation.

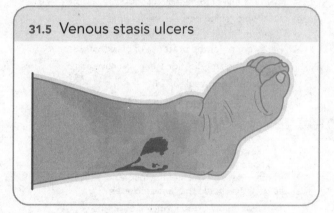

31.5 Venous stasis ulcers

Active Learning Scenario

A nurse is assisting with a poster presentation on peripheral arterial disease (PAD) for a community health fair. What content should the nurse recommend to include on the poster? Use the ATI Active Learning Template: System Disorder to complete this item.

ALTERATION IN HEALTH (DIAGNOSIS)

RISK FACTORS: Describe at least six.

EXPECTED FINDINGS: Describe at least six findings.

CLIENT EDUCATION: Describe at least two actions by the client related to proper positioning and two actions related to promoting vasodilation.

1. A nurse is collecting data from a client who has chronic peripheral arterial disease (PAD). Which of the following findings should the nurse expect?

   A. Edema around the ankles and feet

   B. Ulceration around the medial malleoli

   C. Scaling eczema of the lower legs with stasis dermatitis

   D. Pallor on elevation of the limbs, and rubor when the limbs are dependent

2. A nurse is reviewing the results of client's ankle-brachial index report in the medical record. The nurse notes the results are consistent with presence of peripheral arterial disease (PAD) indicating need for client education if what value is noted?

3. A nurse is reinforcing teaching with client who has a new prescription for clopidogrel. Which of the following statements should the nurse make? (Select all that apply.)

   A. "Avoid taking herbal supplements while taking this medication."

   B. "Monitor for the presence of black, tarry stools."

   C. "Take this medication when you have pain."

   D. "Schedule a weekly PT test."

   E. "Limit food sources containing vitamin K while taking this medication."

4. A nurse is reinforcing teaching with a client who has a new diagnosis of severe peripheral arterial disease. Which of the following instructions should the nurse include?

   A. Wear tightly-fitted insulated socks with shoes when going outside.

   B. Elevate both legs above the heart when resting.

   C. Apply a heating pad to both legs for comfort.

   D. Place both legs in a dependent position while sleeping.

5. A nurse is caring for a client who has chronic venous insufficiency and a prescription for thigh-high compression stockings. Which of the following actions should the nurse take?

   A. Elevate the client's legs for 10 min, two to three times daily while wearing stockings.

   B. Apply the stockings to the client in the morning upon awakening and before getting out of bed.

   C. Roll the stockings down to the client's knees to relieve discomfort on the legs.

   D. Remove the stockings while out of bed for 1 hr, four times a day, to allow the client's legs to rest.

6. A nurse is caring for a client who has a deep-vein thrombosis (DVT) and has been taking unfractionated heparin for 1 week. Two days ago, the provider also prescribed warfarin. The client asks the nurse about receiving both heparin and warfarin at the same time. Which of the following statements should the nurse make?

   A. "I will remind your provider that you are already receiving heparin."

   B. "Your laboratory findings indicated that two anticoagulants were needed."

   C. "It takes 3 to 4 days before the therapeutic effects of warfarin are achieved, and then the heparin can be discontinued."

   D. "Only one of these medications is being given to treat your deep-vein thrombosis."

1. A. The nurse should also expect findings of edema around the ankles and feet, ulceration around the medial malleoli, and scaling eczema of the lower legs with stasis dermatitis in a client who has venous stasis.
   B. The nurse should also expect findings of edema around the ankles and feet, ulceration around the medial malleoli, and scaling eczema of the lower legs with stasis dermatitis in a client who has venous stasis.
   C. The nurse should also expect findings of edema around the ankles and feet, ulceration around the medial malleoli, and scaling eczema of the lower legs with stasis dermatitis in a client who has venous stasis.
   D. **CORRECT:** When recognizing cues in a client who has chronic PAD, the nurse should expect pallor to be seen in the extremities when the limbs are elevated, and rubor to occur when they are lowered.

   Ⓝ *NCLEX® Connection: Physiological Adaptation, Basic Pathophysiology*

2. When analyzing cues, the nurse should identify an ankle brachial index (ABI) less than 0.9 in either leg is diagnostic for PAD. The expected finding for ABI is 0.9 to 1.3.

   Ⓝ *NCLEX® Connection: Reduction of Risk Potential, Laboratory Tests*

3. A. **CORRECT:** When taking actions, the nurse should reinforce to the client to avoid herbal supplements while taking clopidogrel. Herbal supplements (garlic, ginger, ginkgo, ginseng) can increase the risk of bleeding.
   B. **CORRECT:** The client should also be reminded to monitor for evidence of GI bleeding (abdominal pain; coffee-ground emesis; black, tarry stools). If this occurs, the client should report this to the provider.
   C. The client should take clopidogrel routinely as prescribed because it can take several weeks to be effective.
   D. The PT and INR levels are monitored regularly in a client taking warfarin.
   E. A client who is taking warfarin should be advised about food sources containing vitamin K.

   Ⓝ *NCLEX® Connection: Pharmacological Therapies, Adverse Effects/Contraindications/Side Effects/Interactions*

4. A. While insulated socks can promote warmth, they should be loose-fitting to promote circulation.
   B. The client should avoid elevating the legs above the heart while resting as this can cause a restriction in arterial blood flow to the feet.
   C. The client should not apply a heating pad to the legs due to the loss in sensation as a result of the disease. Applying direct heat to the legs can burn the client.
   D. **CORRECT:** When taking actions, the nurse should instruct the client to place their legs in a dependent position, such as hanging off the edge of the bed, while sleeping. This can alleviate swelling and discomfort of the legs.

   Ⓝ *NCLEX® Connection: Physiological Adaptation, Alterations in Body Systems*

5. A. The client who has venous insufficiency should sit with their legs elevated for at least 20 min, four to five times daily.
   B. **CORRECT:** When taking actions, the nurse should apply the stockings to the client in the morning upon awakening and before getting out of bed reduces venous stasis and assists in the venous return of blood to the heart. Legs are also less edematous at this time making the stockings easier to apply.
   C. Rolling stockings down can restrict circulation and cause edema.
   D. Stockings should remain in place throughout the day and are removed before going to bed to provide continuous venous support. If the stockings are removed, such as for a bath or shower, then the legs should be elevated before the stockings are reapplied.

   Ⓝ *NCLEX® Connection: Reduction of Risk Potential, Potential for Alterations In Body Systems*

6. C. **CORRECT:** When taking actions, the nurse should identify that warfarin depresses synthesis of clotting factors but does not have an effect on clotting factors that are present. It takes 3 to 4 days for the clotting factors that are present to decay and for the therapeutic effects of warfarin to occur. For this reason warfarin is prescribed for 3 to 4 days before discontinuing IV heparin. In order to determine if the IV heparin can be discontinued the PT must be 1.5 to 2 times normal with a goal INR of 2.0 to 3.0 to determine if warfarin has achieved the therapeutic effect. The nurse should explain to the client there can be an overlap of intravenous heparin and oral warfarin until the desired anticoagulation has been achieved.

   Ⓝ *NCLEX® Connection: Pharmacological Therapies, Expected Actions/Outcomes*

Active Learning Scenario Key

Using the ATI Active Learning Template: System Disorder

ALTERATION IN HEALTH (DIAGNOSIS): PAD is inadequate blood flow of the lower extremities due to atherosclerosis. The intima and media of the arteries become thickened, and plaque can form on the walls of the arteries, making them rough and fragile. The arteries progressively stiffen and the lumen narrows, decreasing blood supply to tissues and increasing resistance to blood flow. It is classified as either an inflow or outflow type of PAD.

RISK FACTORS

- Hypertension
- Hyperlipidemia
- Diabetes mellitus
- Cigarette smoking
- Obesity
- Sedentary lifestyle
- Familial predisposition
- Age: older adult clients

EXPECTED FINDINGS

- Decreased capillary refill of toes (greater than 3 seconds)
- Decreased or nonpalpable pulses
- Loss of hair on the lower extremities
- Dry, shiny, mottled skin
- Thick toenails
- Cold, cyanotic extremity
- Pallor of extremity with elevation
- Dependent rubor
- Muscle atrophy
- Ulcers and possible gangrene of toes

CLIENT EDUCATION

- Adhere to the following positions.
  - Avoid crossing the legs.
  - Avoid wearing restrictive garments.
  - Keep legs elevated to reduce swelling, but not above the level of the heart.
- Promote vasodilation.
  - Maintain a warm environment.
  - Wear insulated socks.
  - Avoid applying direct heat to the extremity.
  - Avoid exposure to cold.
  - Avoid stress, caffeine, and nicotine.

Ⓝ *NCLEX® Connection: Health Promotion and Maintenance, Health Promotion/Disease Prevention*

UNIT 4   CARDIOVASCULAR DISORDERS
SECTION: VASCULAR DISORDERS

CHAPTER 32 *Hypertension*

For an adult client, hypertension occurs when systolic blood pressure is at or greater than 130 mm Hg or diastolic blood pressure is at or greater than 80 mm Hg for two or more data collections of blood pressure at least 2 weeks apart. More than 40% of adults over the age of 20 in the United States are treated for hypertension. Hypertension and related diseases account for more than 40,000 deaths yearly. Lifestyle changes are necessary for these clients to help prevent cardiovascular disease.

Essential hypertension, also called primary hypertension, accounts for most cases of hypertension. There is no known cause. **Secondary hypertension** can be caused by disease states (kidney disease) or as an adverse effect of some medications. Treatment for secondary hypertension occurs by removing the cause (adrenal tumor, medication).

Prolonged, untreated, or poorly-controlled hypertension can cause peripheral vascular disease that primarily affects the heart, brain, eyes, and kidneys. The risk of developing complications increases as blood pressure increases. Hypertrophy of the left ventricle can develop as the heart pumps against resistance caused by the hypertension.

There are four bodily mechanisms that regulate blood pressure:

- **Arterial baroreceptors** are located in the carotid sinus, aorta, and left ventricle. They control blood pressure by altering the heart rate. They also cause vasoconstriction or vasodilation.

- **Regulation of body-fluid volume:** Properly functioning kidneys retain fluid when a client is hypotensive and excrete fluid when a client is hypertensive.

- **Renin-angiotensin-aldosterone system:** Renin is converted into angiotensin II, which causes vasoconstriction and controls aldosterone release, causing the kidneys to reabsorb sodium and inhibit fluid loss.

- **Vascular autoregulation:** This maintains consistent levels of tissue perfusion.

HEALTH PROMOTION AND DISEASE PREVENTION

- Maintain body mass index of less than 25.
- Clients who have diabetes mellitus should keep blood glucose within a recommended reference range.
- Limit caffeine and alcohol intake.
- Use stress-management techniques during times of stress.
- Stop smoking. Nicotine patches or engaging in a smoking cessation class are potential strategies.
- Engage in exercise that provides aerobic benefits at least 3 times a week.
- Follow recommended dietary guidelines (Heart healthy diet, DASH diet).
- Limit sodium and fat intake.

DATA COLLECTION

RISK FACTORS

Essential hypertension
- Positive genetic history
- Excessive sodium intake
- Physical inactivity
- BMI greater than 25
- High alcohol consumption
- African American ethnicity
- Smoking
- Diabetes mellitus
- Hyperlipidemia
- Stress
- Age greater than 60 or postmenopausal

Secondary hypertension
- Kidney disease
- Cushing's disease (excessive glucocorticoid secretion)
- Primary aldosteronism (causes hypertension and hypokalemia)
- Pheochromocytoma (excessive catecholamine release)
- Brain tumors, encephalitis
- Medications (estrogen, steroids, sympathomimetics)
- Pregnancy

EXPECTED FINDINGS

Clients who have hypertension can experience few or no manifestations. Monitor for the following.
- Headache
- Facial flushing
- Dizziness
- Fainting
- Retinal changes, visual disturbances

PHYSICAL FINDINGS: When a blood pressure reading is elevated, take it in both arms and with the client sitting and standing. Ensure that proper cuff size is used. Refer to image (32.1) for the classifications of hypertension according to the American Heart Association.

LABORATORY TESTS

No laboratory tests exist to diagnose hypertension. However, several laboratory tests can identify the causes of secondary hypertension and target organ damage.
- BUN, creatinine elevation is indicative of kidney disease.
- Elevated blood corticoids can indicate Cushing's disease.
- Blood glucose and cholesterol studies can identify contributing factors related to blood vessel changes.

DIAGNOSTIC PROCEDURES

ECG evaluates cardiac function. Tall R-waves are often seen with left-ventricular hypertrophy.
Chest x-ray can show cardiomegaly.

PATIENT-CENTERED CARE

NURSING CARE

- Reinforce with client about factors that increase the risk of hypertension and how to manage them.
- Monitor blood pressure and labs frequently.

32.1 Classifications of blood pressure

	SYSTOLIC BP (mm HG)	DIASTOLIC BP (mm HG)
EXPECTED	Less than 120	Less than 80
ELEVATED	120 to 139	Less than 80
STAGE 1 HYPERTENSION	130 to 139	80 to 89
STAGE 2 HYPERTENSION	Equal to or greater than 140	Equal to or greater than 90
HYPERTENSIVE CRISIS	Greater than 180	Equal to or greater than 120

Source: American Heart Association, 2022

MEDICATIONS

REFER TO THE PHARMACOLOGY REVIEW MODULE FOR ADDITIONAL MEDICATIONS.

Medications are added to treat hypertension that is not responsive to lifestyle changes alone. Diuretics are often first-line medications. However, clients can require a combination of medications to control hypertension.

CLIENT EDUCATION: If taking antihypertensives, change positions slowly, and be careful when getting out of bed, driving, and climbing stairs until the medication's effects are fully known. Qs

Diuretics

- Thiazide diuretics (hydrochlorothiazide) inhibit water and sodium reabsorption and increase potassium excretion.
- Other diuretics can treat hypertension that is not responsive to thiazide diuretics.
  - Loop diuretics (furosemide) decrease sodium reabsorption and increase potassium excretion.
  - Potassium-sparing diuretics (spironolactone) affect the distal tubule and prevent reabsorption of sodium in exchange for potassium.

NURSING ACTIONS: Monitor potassium levels and watch for muscle weakness, irregular pulse, and dehydration. Thiazide and loop diuretics can cause hypokalemia, and potassium-sparing diuretics can cause hyperkalemia.

CLIENT EDUCATION
- Keep all appointments with the provider to monitor efficacy of pharmacological treatment and possible electrolyte imbalance (hyponatremia, hyperkalemia).
- If taking multiple doses of a diuretic daily, take last dose prior to 6PM.
- If taking a potassium-depleting diuretic, increase consumption of potassium-rich foods (bananas).

Calcium-channel blockers

Verapamil, amlodipine, and diltiazem alter the movement of calcium ions through the cell membrane, causing vasodilation and lowering blood pressure.

NURSING ACTIONS
- Monitor blood pressure and pulse. Change the client's position slowly. Hypotension is a common adverse effect.
- Use calcium-channel blockers cautiously with clients who have heart failure.

CLIENT EDUCATION
- Constipation can occur with verapamil, so intake foods that are high in fiber.
- A decrease or increase in heart rate and atrioventricular (AV) block can occur. Take pulse and call the provider if it is irregular or lower than the established rate.
- Avoid grapefruit juice, which potentiates the medication's effects, increases hypotensive effects, and increases the risk of medication toxicity.

Angiotensin-converting enzyme (ACE) inhibitors

ACE inhibitors (lisinopril, enalapril) prevent the conversion of angiotensin I to angiotensin II, which prevents vasoconstriction.

NURSING ACTIONS
- Monitor blood pressure and pulse. Hypotension is a common adverse effect.
- Monitor for evidence of heart failure (edema). ACE inhibitors can cause heart and kidney complications.

CLIENT EDUCATION
- Report a cough, which is an adverse effect of ACE inhibitors. Notify the provider of this adverse effect, as the medication can be discontinued due to its persistent nature and occasional relationship to angioedema (swelling of the tissues under the skin) that affects the lips, tongue and glottis, and can progress to a life-threatening obstruction). Qs
- Report manifestations of heart failure (edema).

Angiotensin-receptor blockers (ARBs)

ARBs such as valsartan, losartan are a good option for clients taking ACE inhibitors who report a cough or have hyperkalemia. ARBs block the effects of angiotensin II at the receptor and decrease peripheral resistance. ARBs do not require a dosage adjustment for older adult clients.

NURSING ACTIONS: Monitor for manifestations of angioedema or heart failure. Angioedema is a serious, but uncommon, adverse effect, and heart failure can result from taking this medication.

CLIENT EDUCATION
- Change positions slowly.
- Report findings of angioedema (swollen lips or face) or heart failure (edema).
- Avoid foods that are high in potassium and have potassium levels monitored because ARBs can cause hyperkalemia.

Aldosterone-receptor antagonists

Aldosterone-receptor antagonists (eplerenone, spironolactone) block aldosterone action. The blocking effect of eplerenone on aldosterone receptors promotes the retention of potassium and excretion of sodium and water.

NURSING ACTIONS
- Monitor kidney function, triglycerides, sodium, and potassium levels. The risk of adverse effects increases with deteriorating kidney function. Hypertriglyceridemia, hyponatremia, and hyperkalemia can occur as the dose increases.
- Monitor potassium levels every 2 weeks for the first few months and every 2 months thereafter. The client should avoid taking potassium supplements or potassium-sparing diuretics.

CLIENT EDUCATION
- Be aware of potential food, medication, and herbal interactions. Grapefruit juice and St. John's wort can increase adverse effects.
- Do not take salt substitutes with potassium or other foods that are rich in potassium.

Beta blockers

Beta blockers (metoprolol, atenolol) block the sympathetic nervous system (beta adrenergic receptors) and produce a slower heart rate and lowered blood pressure.

NURSING ACTIONS: Monitor blood pressure and pulse.

CLIENT EDUCATION
- These medications can cause fatigue, weakness, depression, and sexual dysfunction.
- If heart rate is less than 50/min, withhold medication and notify provider.
- Do not suddenly stop taking the medication without consulting with the provider. Stopping suddenly can cause rebound hypertension.
- Beta blockers can reduce some manifestations of hypoglycemia (tachycardia). Monitor for other indicators.

Central-alpha$_2$ agonists

Central-alpha$_2$ agonists (clonidine) reduce peripheral vascular resistance and decrease blood pressure by inhibiting the reuptake of norepinephrine.

NURSING ACTIONS: Monitor blood pressure and pulse.

CLIENT EDUCATION
- Adverse effects include sedation, orthostatic hypotension, and impotence.
- This medication is not for first-line management of hypertension.

Alpha-adrenergic antagonists

Alpha-adrenergic antagonists (prazosin, doxazosin) reduce blood pressure by causing vasodilation.

NURSING ACTIONS
- Start treatment with a low dose of the medication, usually given at night.
- Monitor blood pressure for 2 hr after initiation of treatment.

CLIENT EDUCATION: Rise slowly to prevent postural hypotension. Use caution when driving until the effects of the medication are known. Qs

CLIENT EDUCATION

- Report manifestations of electrolyte imbalance (hyperkalemia, hypokalemia, hyponatremia).
- Understand the importance of adhering to the medication regimen, even if there are no manifestations of hypertension.
- Understand the prescribed medications and their adverse effects.
- Have the resources necessary to pay for and obtain prescribed antihypertensive medication.
- Schedule regular provider appointments to monitor hypertension and cardiovascular status.
- Monitor blood pressure at home.
- Report findings and adverse effects, as they can be indicative of additional problems. Medications can often be changed to alleviate adverse effects.
- Older adult clients are more likely to experience medication interactions and orthostatic hypotension. ©
- Treatment involves making lifestyle changes.

NUTRITION

- Monitor for hyperkalemia with salt substitute use.
- Consume less than 2.3 g/day of sodium.
- Consume a diet low in fat, saturated fat, and cholesterol.
- Limit alcohol intake to 2 servings per day for males and 1 serving per day for females. A serving of alcohol is equivalent to 1.5 oz liquor, 5 oz wine, or 12 oz beer.
- Dietary approaches to stop hypertension (DASH) are effective in the prevention and treatment of hypertension. Qᴇʙᴘ
- The DASH diet is high in fruits, vegetables, and low-fat dairy foods.
- Avoid foods high in sodium and fat (trans and saturated fat).
- Consume foods rich in calcium and magnesium.
- Increase potassium consumption if not contraindicated by medications (potassium sparing diuretics, ARBs).

WEIGHT REDUCTION AND MAINTENANCE

- Begin slowly and gradually advance the program with the guidance of the provider and physical therapist.
- Exercise at least three times a week in a manner that provides aerobic benefits.

Smoking cessation: Explore smoking cessation options such as nicotine replacement therapy, medications (bupropion, varenicline), and support groups. Qᴘᴄᴄ

Stress reduction: Try yoga, massage, hypnosis, or other forms of relaxation.

COMPLICATIONS

HYPERTENSIVE CRISIS

Hypertensive crisis often occurs when clients do not follow the medication therapy regimen.

NURSING ACTIONS
- Recognize manifestations:
  - Severe headache
  - Extremely high blood pressure (generally, systolic blood pressure greater than 180 mm Hg, diastolic greater than 120 mm Hg)
  - Blurred vision, dizziness, and disorientation
  - Epistaxis
- The RN will administer IV antihypertensive therapies (nitroprusside, nicardipine, labetalol).
- The goal is to lower the blood pressure by 20% to 25% the first hour but not to drop the blood pressure to less than 140/90 mm Hg.
- Before, during, and after administration of an IV antihypertensive, monitor blood pressure every 5 to 15 min.
- Assist with monitoring neurologic status (pupils, level of consciousness, muscle strength) to monitor for cerebrovascular change.
- Monitor the ECG to check cardiac status.

Application Exercises

1. A nurse is screening a client for hypertension. Which of the following statements by the clients increases their risk for developing hypertension? (Select all that apply.)

    A. "I drink 8 oz nonfat milk daily."

    B. "Buttered popcorn is one of my favorite daily snacks."

    C. "I walk at least one mile per day."

    D. "I drink at least 2-3 beers a day."

    E. "A weekly massage is good for me."

2. A nurse is reinforcing teaching with a client who has hypertension and received a new prescription for spironolactone. Which of the following statements by the client indicates an understanding of the teaching?

    A. "I should eat foods that are high potassium."

    B. "I should monitor rhythm of my heart rate."

    C. "I should season my food with a salt substitute."

    D. "I should decrease the dose of this medication after 2 weeks."

3. A nurse in an outpatient clinic is assisting with collecting data from a client who has type 2 diabetes mellitus and hypertension who has recently received a new prescription for metoprolol. Which of the following client data should the nurse report to the provider?

    A. The client takes psyllium daily.

    B. The client drinks 8 oz of skim milk at bedtime.

    C. The client has a heart rate of 50/min.

    D. The client takes metoprolol with grapefruit juice.

4. A nurse is reinforcing discharge teaching for a client who has a new prescription for furosemide 20 mg PO twice daily. What information should the nurse include about the timing of the administration of furosemide when providing discharge teaching?

5. A nurse in the emergency department is assisting with admitting a client who has a blood pressure of 266/147 mm Hg and reports severe headache and blurred vision. Which of the following actions should the nurse suggest taking first?

    A. Administer an analgesic.

    B. Check the client's neurovascular status.

    C. Assist with obtaining IV access.

    D. Check the client's cardiac status.

Active Learning Scenario

A nurse is helping prepare a community education presentation on hypertension. What information should the nurse recommend for inclusion in the presentation? Use the ATI Active Learning Template: System Disorder to complete this item.

ALTERATION IN HEALTH (DIAGNOSIS):
Describe hypertension to include essential, secondary, and prehypertension.

RISK FACTORS: Describe at least four risk factors each for essential and secondary hypertension.

EXPECTED FINDINGS

- Describe at least three expected subjective data findings for hypertension.

- Describe the objective data stages of hypertension.

Active Learning Scenario Key

Using the ATI Active Learning Template: System Disorder

ALTERATION IN HEALTH (DIAGNOSIS)

- Hypertension is when systolic blood pressure is at or above 130 mm Hg or diastolic blood pressure is at or greater than 80 mm Hg for an adult client or greater than 150/90 mm Hg for a client older than 60.
- Essential (primary) hypertension has no known cause.
- Secondary hypertension is caused by diseases such as kidney disorders, or as an adverse effect of a medication. Treatment occurs by removing the cause.
- Elevated blood pressure is when a client has a systolic blood pressure of 120 to 129 mm Hg and a diastolic blood pressure of less than 80 mm Hg.

RISK FACTORS

- Primary hypertension: Positive family history, excessive sodium intake, physical inactivity, obesity, high alcohol consumption, African-American, nicotine use, hyperlipidemia, stress, age greater than 60, postmenopausal
- Secondary hypertension: Kidney disease, Cushing's disease, primary aldosteronism (caused by hypertension and hypokalemia), pheochromocytoma (excessive catecholamine release), brain tumors, encephalitis, and medications (estrogen, steroids, sympathomimetics)

EXPECTED FINDINGS

Subjective data: Few or no manifestations
- Can include headaches, particularly in the morning
- Dizziness, fainting, retinal changes, visual disturbances, nocturia, facial flushing

Objective data stages: Obtain blood pressure readings in both arms with the client sitting and standing:
- Elevated: systolic 120 to 129 mm Hg, diastolic less than 80 mm Hg
- Stage I: systolic 130 to 139 mm Hg, diastolic 80 to 89 mm Hg
- Stage II: systolic greater than or equal to 140 mm Hg, diastolic greater than or equal to 90 mm Hg

ⓝ *NCLEX® Connection: Health Promotion and Maintenance, Health Promotion/Disease Prevention*

Application Exercises Key

1. A. Consuming low-fat beverages and foods lowers the risk for developing hypertension.
   B. **CORRECT:** The nurse should identify that eating buttered popcorn daily increases the client's risk for developing hypertension because of the high sodium and fat content of this snack.
   C. Engaging in regular exercise (walking) lowers the risk of developing hypertension.
   D. **CORRECT:** Consuming more than 12-24 oz beer (varies depending on gender) increases the client's risk for developing hypertension.
   E. Stress management activities (a massage) lower the risk of hypertension.

ⓝ *NCLEX® Connection: Health Promotion and Maintenance, Health Promotion/Disease Prevention*

2. A. The nurse should inform the client to limit consumption of foods that are high in potassium.
   B. **CORRECT:** Spironolactone is a potassium sparing diuretic that is used to manage hypertension and has adverse effects of hyperkalemia, which can cause an irregular heart rate. The nurse should reinforce with the client to monitor their heart rate and report any changes to the provider.
   C. The client should be informed that salt substitutes are commonly high in potassium and can lead to hyperkalemia when taken with a potassium-sparing diuretic such as spironolactone.
   D. The client should continue taking their medication as prescribed even if they do not have any manifestations of hypertension.

ⓝ *NCLEX® Connection: Pharmacological Therapies, Medication Administration*

3. A. Adverse effects of psyllium do not include hypoglycemia.
   B. Skim milk increases blood glucose levels and lowers cholesterol.
   C. **CORRECT:** Metoprolol is a beta blocker that decreases heart rate and blood pressure by blocking the sympathetic nervous system. It has adverse effects of fatigue, weakness, depression and sexual dysfunction, and can mask the effects of hypoglycemia in clients who have diabetes mellitus.
   D. Grapefruit juice increases blood glucose levels and is not a contraindication while taking metoprolol.

ⓝ *NCLEX® Connection: Pharmacological Therapies, Adverse Effects/Contraindications/Side Effects/Interactions*

4. The nurse should include in the discharge education that the client should take the second dose of this medication no later than 5:00 pm to prevent a disruption in their sleep cycle.

ⓝ *NCLEX® Connection: Pharmacological Therapies, Medication Administration*

5. A. Administering an analgesic is a non-priority action the nurse should suggest taking.
   B. Checking the client's neurovascular status is a non-priority action the nurse should suggest taking.
   C. **CORRECT:** The nurse should identify that the greatest risk to the client is injury due to a blood pressure of 266/147 mm Hg, which can be life-threatening and should be lowered as soon as possible. Therefore, the client is experiencing a hypertensive crisis and the nurse should first assist with obtaining an IV access to allow for the administration of an IV antihypertensive, which would decrease the client's blood pressure quickly.
   D. Checking the client's cardiac status is a non-priority action the nurse should suggest taking.

ⓝ *NCLEX® Connection: Pharmacological Therapies, Medication Administration*

UNIT 4   CARDIOVASCULAR DISORDERS
SECTION: VASCULAR DISORDERS

CHAPTER 33   *Shock*

Shock is a state of inadequate tissue perfusion that impairs cellular function and can lead to organ failure. Any condition that compromises oxygen delivery to organs and tissues can lead to shock. Shock is a rapidly progressing, life-threatening process. Early detection with rapid response is necessary to improve client outcome.

Older adult clients can have reduced compensatory mechanisms and rapidly progress through the stages of shock. Decreased ability to compensate due to decreased vascular tone, impaired cardiac function, and impaired vasoconstriction of vessels from antihypertensive medications can cause sustained low cardiac output and blood pressure. Ⓖ

The type and stage of shock guide treatment.

TYPES OF SHOCK

The type of shock is identified by its underlying cause.

Cardiogenic: Failure of the heart to pump effectively due to a cardiac factor

Hypovolemic: A decrease in intravascular volume of at least 15% to 30%

Obstructive: Impairment of the heart to pump effectively because of a noncardiac factor

Distributive: Widespread vasodilation and increased capillary permeability, including neurogenic, septic, and anaphylactic shock

STAGES

All types of shock progress through the same stages and produce similar effects on body systems

Initial: Minimal changes in client parameters; only changes on the cellular level

Compensatory (non-progressive): Measures to increase cardiac output to restore tissue perfusion and oxygenation Progressive: Compensatory mechanisms beginning to fail

Refractory: Irreversible shock and total body failure

STAGES OF SHOCK

Initial

The mean arterial pressure (MAP) decreases 5 to 10 mm Hg from the client's baseline, mild vasoconstriction occurs, and the heart rate increases to maintain cardiac output

Compensatory

Vasoconstriction increases, the heart rate increases, the MAP decreases 10 to 15 mm Hg from baseline, and the client experiences mild acidosis and mild hyperkalemia.

Progressive

The MAP decreases more than 20 mm Hg from baseline, the vital organs experience hypoxia, and the client experiences moderate acidosis and moderate hyperkalemia.

Refractory

The client experiences severe tissue hypoxia, multiple organ dysfunction syndrome (MODS), and possibly death.

HEALTH PROMOTION AND DISEASE PREVENTION

CARDIOGENIC SHOCK

Reinforce education to the client about ways to reduce the risk of a myocardial infarction (MI), such as exercise, diet, stress reduction, and smoking cessation.

HYPOVOLEMIC SHOCK

Reinforce education to the client to drink plenty of fluids when exercising or when in hot weather and to recognize manifestations of dehydration, including thirst, decreased urine output, and dizziness.

OBSTRUCTIVE/NEUROGENIC/ HYPOVOLEMIC SHOCK

Educate the client about wearing seat belts and helmets, and the use of caution with dangerous equipment, machinery, or activities.

SEPTIC SHOCK

- Reinforce education to the client to obtain early medical attention with evidence of an infection (localized redness, swelling, drainage, fever, urinary frequency and burning).
- Reinforce instruction to the client to complete the entire course of antibiotics as directed.
- Sequential Organ Failure Assessment (SOFA), also called Sepsis-Related Organ Failure Assessment Score: recommended tool for all hospitalized clients who have infections
  - Parameters related to cardiovascular status, respiration, liver function, renal function, coagulation, and central nervous system function.
  - Sepsis and risk for septic shock are suspected if score indicates organ dysfunction.

Anaphylactic shock

Reinforce instructions to the client to wear a medical identification wristband, avoid allergens, and to have an epinephrine pen available at all times. Qs

DATA COLLECTION

RISK FACTORS

Cardiogenic shock

- Cardiac pump failure occurs due to a direct cardiac cause, such as MI (especially anterior wall infarction), heart failure, cardiomyopathy, dysrhythmias, and valvular rupture or stenosis.
- Older adult clients are at increased risk for MI and cardiomyopathy.

Hypovolemic shock

- Excessive fluid loss from diuresis, vomiting, or diarrhea; or blood loss secondary to surgery, trauma, gynecologic/obstetric causes, burns, and diabetic ketoacidosis.
- Older adult clients are more prone to dehydration due to decreased fluid and protein intake and the use of medications, such as diuretics. Minimal amounts of fluid loss (vomiting, diarrhea) can cause the older adult client to become dehydrated. ⓖ

Obstructive shock

Cardiac pump failure occurs due to an indirect cardiac factor (blockage of great vessels, pulmonary artery stenosis, pulmonary embolism, cardiac tamponade, tension pneumothorax, aortic dissection).

Distributive shock

Divided into three types:

Neurogenic: Loss of sympathetic tone causing massive vasodilation. Head trauma, spinal cord injury, and epidural anesthesia are among the causes.

Septic: Infection from elsewhere in body enters blood stream, causing massive vasodilation. Most common cause is gram-negative bacteria.
- Sepsis affects 1.7 million adults annually in the United States with more than 250,000 deaths.
- Studies indicate that sepsis occurs in 30 to 50 percent of hospitalizations culminating in death.
- Urosepsis is more frequent in older adult clients due to increased use of catheters in long-term care facilities and late detection of urinary tract infection (decreased sensation of burning, urgency). ⓖ

Anaphylactic: Allergen exposure results in an antigen-antibody reaction causing massive vasodilation. Common causes include antibiotics, foods (such as peanuts), latex, and bee stings.

EXPECTED FINDINGS

Manifestations can include chest pain, lethargy, somnolence, restlessness, anxiousness, dyspnea, diaphoresis, thirst, muscle weakness, nausea, and constipation.

DATA COLLECTION FINDINGS

- Hypoxia, tachypnea progressing to greater than 40/min, hypocarbia
- Skin moist and cool or cold. Pallor and cyanosis (first in mucous membranes, then extremities the trunk). Skin mottling (clients who have dark skin tones appear darker and lack reddish undertones; clients who have light skin tones appear grayish-blue). Skin can be flushed initially with anaphylactic and septic shock.
- Angioedema (anaphylactic shock)
- Wheezing
- Decreased blood pressure with narrowed pulse pressure.
- Postural hypotension
- Tachycardia
- Pulse that is weak, thready
- Decreased cardiac output
- Central venous pressure decreased (hypovolemic shock)
- Central venous pressure increased with increased systemic vascular resistance (cardiogenic shock)
- Decreased urine output
- Seizures

LABORATORY TESTS

ABGs: Decreased tissue oxygenation (decreased pH, decreased PaO2, increased PaCO2)

Blood lactic acid: Increases due to anaerobic metabolism

Blood glucose and electrolytes: Blood glucose can increase during shock due to hypermetabolism; electrolyte balance can be altered depending on cause (dehydration).

Cardiogenic shock

Cardiac enzymes: elevation can indicate cardiac ischemia or infarction.

B-type natriuretic peptide: elevated in response to increased left ventricular pressures.

Hypovolemic shock

Hgb and Hct: Decreased with hemorrhage, increased with dehydration

Septic shock

Cultures: Blood, urine, wound

Coagulation tests: PT, INR, aPTT

DIAGNOSTIC PROCEDURES

Hemodynamic monitoring

- Continuous monitoring of blood pressure and ECG
- Monitor ABGs
- Have resuscitation medications and equipment ready
- Reinforce explanations of procedures to the client. The client can be anxious and scared.

Cardiogenic and obstructive shock

ECG: Used to monitor ECG changes associated with MI and dysrhythmias. Q**EBP**

Echocardiogram: Used for cardiomegaly, cardiomyopathy, evaluation of cardiac contractility and function, ejection fraction, and valve function

Computerized tomography (CT): Used for cardiomegaly, cardiac tamponade, pulmonary emboli, cardiomyopathy, aortic dissection or aneurysm, and pericardial effusion

Cardiac catheterization: Used to identify coronary artery blockage

Chest x-ray: Used to diagnose cardiomegaly and pneumothorax, and to evaluate lungs

Hypovolemic shock: miscellaneous diagnostic procedures

Investigate possible sources of bleeding.
- Blood in nasogastric drainage or stools
- Esophagogastroduodenoscopy
- CT scan of abdomen

NURSING ACTIONS
- Continuously monitor airway and vital signs.
- Assist with administration of fluids and medications because a client who has suspected shock can be hemodynamically unstable.
- Have resuscitation equipment available when transporting the client to and from procedures.
- Reinforce explanations of procedures to the client.

PATIENT-CENTERED CARE

NURSING CARE

- Monitor the following.
  - Oxygenation status (priority)
  - Vital signs
  - Cardiac rhythm with continuous cardiac monitoring
  - Urine output: hourly, report if less than 30 mL/hr
  - Level of consciousness
  - Skin color, temperature, moisture, capillary refill, turgor
  - Assist with hemodynamic monitoring—central venous pressure, pulmonary artery pressures, cardiac output, pulse pressure.

- Reinforce teaching about procedures and findings to the client and family while providing reassurance.
- Prepare to place the client on high-flow oxygen, such as a 100% non-rebreather face mask. If the client has COPD, prepare to insert a 2 L/min nasal cannula and increase the oxygen flow as needed.
- Be prepared to assist with intubation of the client. Have emergency resuscitation equipment ready. Q**s**
- Insert indwelling urinary catheter.
- Monitor patent IV access.
- For hypotension, place the client flat with both legs elevated to increase venous return.
- If change in status occurs, notify the rapid response team and provider of the findings.
- Assist with client care during transfer to the intensive care unit, surgery, other specialty unit, or diagnostic area.

MEDICATIONS

Inotropic agents

Milrinone lactate, dobutamine

ACTIONS: Strengthens cardiac contraction and increases cardiac output

NURSING ACTIONS
- Monitor continuous IV infusion via central line
- Constant hemodynamic monitoring.

Vasopressors

Dopamine hydrochloride, norepinephrine

ACTIONS
- Strengthens cardiac contraction and increases cardiac output
- Increases kidney perfusion at low doses
- Decreases kidney perfusion at high doses

NURSING ACTIONS
- Monitor administration by continuous IV infusion.
- Constant hemodynamic monitoring.
- Monitor urine output.

Pituitary hormone: Vasopressin

ACTIONS: Causes vasoconstriction, increases systemic vascular resistance, increases blood pressure

NURSING ACTIONS
- Monitor continuous IV infusion
- Constant hemodynamic monitoring.
- Monitor urine output.

Sympathomimetics: Epinephrine

ACTIONS
- Rapid-acting bronchodilator
- Increases heart rate and cardiac output

NURSING ACTIONS
- Monitor blood pressure, pulse, and cardiac output.
- Epinephrine can cause sloughing if it infiltrates tissue.

Opioid analgesics: Morphine sulfate

ACTIONS: Pain management

NURSING ACTIONS
- Monitor respirations of clients who are nonventilated.
- Monitor blood pressure, heart rate, and SaO2.
- Monitor ABGs.
- Use opioid analgesics cautiously in conjunction with hypnotic sedatives.
- Use cautiously due to risk of increased vasodilation and hypotension.
- Have naloxone and resuscitation equipment available for severe respiratory depression in a client who is nonventilated. Qs

Proton-pump inhibitors: Pantoprazole

ACTIONS: Protects against stress ulcer development

NURSING ACTIONS: Do not mix with other medications.

Anticoagulants

Low-molecular weight heparin, enoxaparin sodium

ACTIONS: Deep-vein thrombosis prophylaxis

NURSING ACTIONS
- Administer subcutaneously, usually in abdomen.
- Do not rub injection site.

Isotonic crystalloids or colloids (including blood products)

0.9% sodium chloride or lactated Ringer's

ACTIONS: Hypovolemic shock: volume replacement

NURSING ACTIONS: Assist with fluid volume replacement before vasopressor medications are used and only if blood pressure remains low after volume is replaced.

> ! During hypovolemic shock, replace volume first.

Antihistamines: Diphenhydramine

ACTIONS
- Used as a secondary medication to treat angioedema and urticaria associated with anaphylactic shock
- Blocks histamine at receptor sites

NURSING ACTIONS: Can cause drowsiness, hypotension, and tachycardia.

Vasodilator: Sodium nitroprusside

ACTIONS
- Used to treat cardiogenic shock
- Reduces afterload and preload
- Causes vasodilation
- Decreases cardiac output and afterload

NURSING ACTIONS
- Continuous arterial blood pressure monitoring is recommended.
- Protect the solution from light.

Corticosteroids: Hydrocortisone, methylprednisolone

ACTIONS: Reduces WBC migration and decreases inflammation

NURSING ACTIONS
- Hydrocortisone can cause hypertension.
- Discontinue medication gradually.
- Hydrocortisone is administered with an antiulcer medication to prevent peptic ulcer formation.
- Monitor weight and blood pressure.
- Monitor blood glucose and electrolytes.

Antibiotics sensitive to cultured organism(s)

Because septic shock is most commonly caused by gram-negative bacteria, the Joint Commission's National Patient Safety Goals recommends the administration of IV antibiotics that are effective against gram-negative bacteria within 1 hr of a septic shock diagnosis. Qs

Vancomycin: Antibiotics sensitive to the cultured organism, such as vancomycin, can then be prescribed once the causative organism is identified.
- ACTIONS
  - Used to treat septic shock
  - Inhibits cell growth or reproduction of causative organism
- NURSING ACTIONS
  - Monitor for hypersensitivity reaction.
  - Administered slowly and separately from other IV medications.
  - Culture infected area prior to administration of the first dose of vancomycin.
  - Monitor the IV site for infiltration.
  - Monitor coagulopathy and kidney function.

THERAPEUTIC PROCEDURES

Needle decompression and chest tube insertion

This procedure is used to relieve pressure from a tension pneumothorax that can be causing obstructive shock.

NURSING ACTIONS
- Monitor ECG, SaO₂, breath sounds, and color.
- Assist with sedation as needed.
- Assist with the set up a water seal chest-drainage system and attach it to suction.
- Apply a dressing.
- Observe the chest tube for air leaks.
- Monitor and document the drainage.
- Obtain a chest x-ray postprocedural.

CLIENT EDUCATION: Needle decompression provides temporary relief while chest tube insertion allows for lung reinflation.

Pericardiocentesis

Pericardial fluid that is causing cardiac tamponade and obstructive shock is drained.

NURSING ACTIONS
- Monitor postprocedural vital signs ECG, SaO₂, breath sounds, and color.
- Monitor the dressing.
- Obtain a postprocedural chest x-ray.

CLIENT EDUCATION: Additional procedures are often necessary to resolve acute tamponade (pericardial window, pericardiectomy).

Surgical interventions

Surgery might be needed to correct the cause of shock (hemorrhaging ulcer, wound, artery, vein).

PREPROCEDURE NURSING ACTIONS
- Monitor the airway and provide supplemental oxygen if needed.
- Assist with hemodynamic support with fluids and medications to stabilize the client prior to surgical intervention, if possible.

POSTPROCEDURE NURSING ACTIONS
- Continue to assist with monitoring—blood pressure, ECG, pulmonary artery pressures, cardiac output, central venous pressure, and urine output.
- Assist with administrations of medications as prescribed.
- Monitor the surgical site for bleeding.
- Monitor airway, breath sounds, and ABGs.
- Monitor CBC.
- Reinforce explanations of procedures to the client.

INTERPROFESSIONAL CARE

Respiratory therapy: For a client who is being mechanically ventilated, the respiratory therapist typically manages the ventilator, adjusts the settings, and provides chest physical therapy to improve ventilation and chest expansion. The respiratory therapist can also suction the endotracheal tube and administer inhalation medications, such as bronchodilators. Qᴛᴄ

COMPLICATIONS

Multiple organ dysfunction syndrome (MODS)

MODS occurs from the release of toxic metabolites and destructive enzymes in response to inadequate oxygenation.
- MODS can develop from inadequate tissue perfusion (severe hypotension) and reperfusion of ischemic cells, causing further tissue injury. Organ failure usually first occurs in the lungs (adult respiratory distress syndrome), but can occur in the kidneys, heart (decreased coronary artery perfusion, decreased cardiac contractility), and the gastrointestinal tract (necrosis).
- MODS is most commonly associated with sepsis. Other risk factors include malnutrition, coexisting disease, and advanced age.

NURSING ACTIONS
- Monitor vital signs and peripheral pulses.
- Monitor urine output.

Disseminated intravascular coagulation (DIC)

DIC is a complication of septic shock. Thousands of small clots form within organ capillaries (liver, kidney, heart, brain), creating hypoxia and anaerobic metabolism. As a result of massive, multiple clot formation, platelets and other clotting factors such as fibrinogen are depleted, and the client is at increased risk for hemorrhage. The client can develop diffuse petechiae and ecchymoses, and blood can leak from membranes and puncture sites.

NURSING ACTIONS
- Note client preference related to transfusion of blood products. Some clients might not accept this treatment for various reasons (religion, fear of contamination). Qᴘᴄᴄ
- Assist with the administration of platelets, clotting factors, and other blood products as prescribed.
- Monitor hemodynamic levels.
- Monitor results of laboratory tests (PT, PTT, blood fibrinogen, fibrin degradation products).
- Monitor for bleeding from mucous membranes, venipuncture sites, gums, and around IV catheters.
- Apply pressure to leaking IV/central line/arterial line sites.
- Reinforce explanations about procedures and care to the client and family.

Active Learning Scenario

A nurse is reviewing care of a client who is in shock with a newly hired nurse. What should the nurse include in this discussion? Use the ATI Active Learning Template: System Disorder to complete this item.

RISK FACTORS: List each type of shock and at least one risk factor for each.

EXPECTED FINDINGS: Describe expected findings related to blood pressure, pulse, respirations, and urine output.

Application Exercises

1. A nurse is assisting with the care of a client who has a possible dissecting abdominal aortic aneurysm. Which of the following actions is the priority for the nurse to take?

   A. Septic

   B. Distributive

   C. Obstructive

   D. Hypovolemic

   E. Cardiogenic

   1. Failure of the heart to pump effectively due to a cardiac cause

   2. Significant loss of fluid volume

   3. Failure of the heart to pump effectively due to a non-cardiac cause

   4. Widespread vasodilation and increased capillary permeability

   5. Type of distributive shock, caused by infection elsewhere in the body entering bloodstream

2. A nurse in the emergency department is collecting data from a client who is being treated for shock. Which of the following manifestations should the nurse expect to find? (Select all that apply.)

   A. Increased urinary output

   B. Bounding pulse

   C. Slow capillary refill

   D. Hypotension

   E. Tachypnea

3. A nurse is reinforcing teaching about diagnostic procedures with the family of a client who is experiencing cardiogenic shock. Match each procedure with its description.

   A. Chest x-ray

   B. Cardiac catheterization

   C. Computerized tomography (CT)

   D. Echocardiogram

   E. ECG

   1. Used to monitor ECG changes

   2. Used to detect cardiomegaly and cardiomyopathy; evaluate of cardiac contractility and function, ejection fraction, and valve function

   3. Used to detect structural changes of the heart, including cardiomegaly, cardiac tamponade, cardiomyopathy, aortic dissection or aneurysm, and pericardial effusion

   4. Used to identify coronary artery blockage

   5. Used to diagnose cardiomegaly and pneumothorax, and to evaluate lungs

4. A nurse is preparing to assist with the administration of medications to a client who is experiencing septic shock. Why should the nurse expect the RN to administer IV antibiotics within 1 hr of diagnosis?

Application Exercises Key

1. A, 5; B, 4; C, 3; D, 2; E, 1

   When recognizing cues, the nurse should identify that cardiogenic shock occurs because the heart is unable to pump effectively to provide adequate oxygenation to the body. Hypovolemic shock occurs when external or internal fluid losses cause a decrease in intravascular volume of 15 to 30% (750 to 1000 mL). Obstructive shock occurs when a non-cardiac factor (such as tension pneumothorax or cardiac tamponade) decreases the pumping ability of the heart. Distributive shock occurs when widespread vasodilation shifts fluid into interstitial spaces and away from intravascular volume. Septic shock, a type of distributive shock, occurs when the inflammatory responses associated with widespread infections cause poor tissue perfusion.

   Ⓝ *NCLEX® Connection: Physiological Adaptation, Basic Pathophysiology*

2. C, D, E. **CORRECT:** When evaluating outcomes for a client who is being treated for shock, the nurse should identify that capillary refill greater than 3 seconds, systolic blood pressure less than 100 mm Hg or MAP less than 65 mm Hg, and respiratory rate of greater than 22 breaths per minute are manifestations of a client is experiencing shock.

   Ⓝ *NCLEX® Connection: Physiological Adaptation, Alterations in Body Systems*

3. A, 5; B, 4; C, 3; D, 2; E; 1

   Ⓝ *NCLEX® Connection: Physiological Adaptation, Alterations in Body Systems*

4. When generating solutions for a client who is experiencing septic shock, commonly caused by gram-negative bacteria, the nurse should expect the RN to administer IV antibiotics per the Joint Commission's National Patient Safety Goals recommendation that IV antibiotics effective against gram-negative bacteria are administered within 1 hr of a septic shock diagnosis.

   Ⓝ *NCLEX® Connection: Pharmacological Therapies, Expected Actions/Outcomes*

Active Learning Scenario Key

Using the ATI Active Learning Template: System Disorder

RISK FACTORS
- Cardiogenic: Pump failure due to myocardial infarction, heart failure, cardiomyopathy, dysrhythmia, and valvular rupture or stenosis
- Hypovolemic: Excessive fluid loss from diuresis, vomiting, diarrhea, blood loss
- Obstructive: Blockage of great vessels, pulmonary artery stenosis, pulmonary embolism, cardiac tamponade, tension pneumothorax, and aortic dissection
- Septic: Endotoxins (gram-negative bacteria) and mediators causing massive vasodilation
- Neurogenic: Loss of sympathetic tone causing massive vasodilation due to trauma, spinal shock, epidural anesthesia
- Anaphylactic: Antigen-antibody reaction causing massive vasodilation due to allergens (inhaled, swallowed, contacted, or introduced IV)

EXPECTED FINDINGS
- Blood pressure: Decreased blood pressure with narrowed pulse pressure, postural hypotension
- Pulse: Tachycardia, can be weak or thready, bounding with distributive shock
- Respirations: Tachypnea progressing to greater than 40/min, hypocarbia, hypoxia
- Urine output: Decreased

Ⓝ *NCLEX® Connection: Physiological Adaptation, Medical Emergencies*

CHAPTER 34 *Aneurysms*

A weakness in a section of a dilated artery that causes a widening or ballooning in the arterial wall is called an aneurysm. Aneurysms can occur in two forms. They can be saccular (only affecting one side of the artery), or fusiform (involving the complete circumference of the artery). Aneurysms mostly develop in the abdomen or thoracic area; however, other areas include the peripheral vasculature.

Aortic dissection (also known as a dissecting aneurysm) can occur when blood accumulates within the artery wall (hematoma) following a tear in the lining of the artery (usually due to hypertension). This is a life-threatening condition because of the increased risk of rupture.

HEALTH PROMOTION AND DISEASE PREVENTION

- Promote smoking cessation.
- Maintain appropriate weight for height and body frame.
- Encourage a healthy diet and physical activity.
- Control blood pressure with regular monitoring and medication if needed.

34.1 Common aneurysm sites

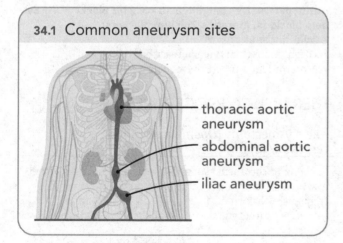

thoracic aortic aneurysm

abdominal aortic aneurysm

iliac aneurysm

DATA COLLECTION

RISK FACTORS

- Atherosclerosis (most common cause)
- Males (sex assigned at birth)
- Uncontrolled hypertension
- Tobacco use
- Hyperlipidemia
- Genetic predisposition
- Blunt force trauma
- Older adults: with age, arterial stiffening caused by loss of elastin in arterial walls, thickening of intima of arteries, and progressive fibrosis of media occurs. Older adult clients are more prone to aneurysms and have a higher mortality rate from aneurysms than younger individuals. Ⓒ

EXPECTED FINDINGS

Initially, clients are often asymptomatic.

Abdominal aortic aneurysm (AAA)

Most common, related to atherosclerosis
- Constant gnawing feeling in abdomen
- Low back pain (due to pressure on lumbar nerves by aneurysm)
- Pulsating abdominal mass (do not palpate; can cause rupture Qs)
- Bruit over the area of the aneurysm
- Elevated blood pressure (unless in cardiac tamponade or rupture of aneurysm)

34.2 Aneurysm types

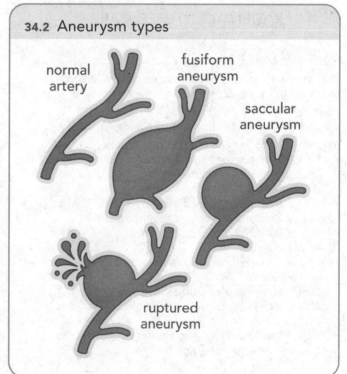

normal artery

fusiform aneurysm

saccular aneurysm

ruptured aneurysm

Thoracic aortic aneurysm

- Severe back pain (most common)
- Hoarseness, cough, shortness of breath, and difficulty swallowing
- Decrease in urinary output (secondary to hypovolemic shock)
- Nodule above suprasternal area
- Report of pressure in substernal/tracheal area

Aortic dissections

Often associated with Marfan syndrome
- Sudden onset of "tearing," "ripping," and "stabbing" abdominal or back pain
- Hypovolemic shock
  - Diaphoresis, nausea, vomiting, faintness, apprehension
  - Decreased or absent peripheral pulses
  - Neurologic deficits
  - Hypotension and tachycardia (initial)
  - Oliguria

DIAGNOSTIC PROCEDURES

X-ray: Can be used to detect the presence of an aneurysm.

Computed tomography (CT) and ultrasonography: Used to monitor the size and location of aneurysms. Often repeated at periodic intervals to monitor the progression of an aneurysm.

Transesophageal echocardiography (TEE): Useful in identifying aortic dissections.

PATIENT-CENTERED CARE

NURSING CARE

The priority intervention is to maintain client's blood pressure within the expected range. Elevated blood pressure can result in rupture. Qs

Nursing care for aortic dissection consist of emergent interventions to prevent severe complications.
- Assist with obtaining and monitoring vital signs every 15 min until stable, then every hour. Monitor for an increase in blood pressure.
- Assist with administering antihypertensives, analgesics as prescribed (may require IV administration).
- Monitor the onset, quality, duration, and severity of pain.
- Monitor temperature, circulation, and range of motion of extremities.
- Assist with monitoring cardiac rhythm.
- Assist with monitoring ABGs, SaO₂, electrolytes, and CBC findings.
- Monitor hourly urine output. Greater than 30 mL/hr indicates adequate kidney perfusion.

- Insert indwelling urinary catheter if prescribed.
- Administer oxygen as prescribed.
- Assist with maintaining IV access. (May require two IV sites).
- Assist with preparing the client for surgery and reinforcing teaching.

> ! All aneurysms can be life-threatening and require medical attention.

THERAPEUTIC MANAGEMENT

Nonsurgical

- Varies and depends on the size of the aneurysm and client findings
- Noninvasive approach can be used if the aneurysm is small. This includes monitoring for enlargement by having frequent ultrasounds/CT scans and blood pressure control.

CLIENT EDUCATION

- Review manifestations of aneurysm rupture (abdominal fullness or pain, chest or back pain, shortness of breath, cough, difficulty swallowing, hoarseness). Report these immediately.
- Avoid strenuous activity and restrict heavy lifting.
- Monitor and maintain blood pressure. Stay within parameters set by the provider. Taking medications as prescribed prevents complications (rupture). Qs
- Follow up on scheduled CT scans or ultrasounds to monitor aneurysm size (nonsurgical client). Collaborate with case management services to assist with transportation needs.
- Consider smoking cessation if the client smokes. Qpcc
- Adhere to a proper diet (low-fat, high-protein).

MEDICATIONS

Antihypertensives (angiotensin receptor blockers (ARBs), beta blockers, diuretics, calcium blockers)
- Administer as prescribed.
- Often, more than one is prescribed
- Monitor blood pressure frequently

THERAPEUTIC PROCEDURES

Aneurysmectomy (Open-aneurysm resection/ repair)

Excision of the aneurysm and the placement of a synthetic graft (elective or emergency). This procedure is not frequently performed.
- Elective surgery is used to manage large AAA or thoracic aneurysms
- Emergency surgery is indicated for a rupturing aneurysm.
- Risks include significant blood loss and the consequences of reduced cardiac output and tissue ischemia (myocardial infarction, acute kidney injury, respiratory distress, and paralytic ileus).

- Thoracic repair procedure is like thoracic surgery (open heart) in which a cardiopulmonary bypass can be used. Nursing care following procedure is like coronary artery bypass graft surgery. (Monitor respiratory status. Respiratory distress is common after this type of procedure.)
- Client may require monitor in intensive care unit following procedure.

POSTPROCEDURE NURSING ACTIONS
- Assist with monitoring for evidence of graft occlusion or rupture postoperatively.
- Assist with obtaining and monitoring vital signs and circulation (pulses distal to graft) every 15 min.
- Report evidence of graft occlusion or rupture immediately (changes in pulses, coolness of extremity below graft, white or blue extremities or flanks, severe pain, abdominal distention, decreased urine output). Qs
- Maintain a warm environment to prevent temperature-induced vasoconstriction.
- Monitor administration of IV fluids at prescribed rates to ensure adequate hydration and kidney perfusion.
- Monitor for altered kidney perfusion and acute kidney injury caused by clamping aorta during surgery (urine output less than 30 mL/hr, weight gain, elevated BUN or blood creatinine).
- Monitor drainage tubes (chest tubes for thoracic repair), NG tube (abdominal repair)
- Encourage incentive spirometry every hour. Coughing is discouraged but if it occurs, encourage splinting.
- Monitor onset, quality, duration, and severity of pain. Administer pain medication as prescribed.
- Monitor bowel sounds, and observe for abdominal distention. Maintain nasogastric suction as prescribed.
- Prevent thromboembolism. Maintain sequential compression devices. Encourage early ambulation.
- Monitor for infection. Administer antibiotics as prescribed.
- Nursing care after thoracic aneurysm repair is similar to care following coronary artery bypass graft surgery.

CLIENT EDUCATION

- Prevent infection (good hand hygiene, wound care management). Report evidence of infection following surgical intervention (wound redness, edema, drainage; elevated temperature).
- Adhere to a proper diet (low-fat, high-protein, vitamins A and C, zinc to promote wound healing).
- Encourage smoking cessation if the client smokes. Qpcc
- Avoid strenuous activity and restrict heavy lifting to less than 15 lbs.

Endovascular repair/stent grafts

Procedure is more commonly performed to repair aneurysms. During the procedure involves the percutaneous insertion of endothelial stent grafts for aneurysm repair which avoids abdominal/thoracic incision and shortens the postoperative period.
- Nursing care after the procedure is like the care following an arteriogram or cardiac catheterization (monitor pedal pulse).
- Client may require care on medical-surgical unit or telemetry unit following procedure; however, most clients are discharged home following procedure.

POST PROCEDURE NURSING ACTIONS: REFER TO CHAPTER 26: INVASIVE CARDIOVASCULAR PROCEDURES.
- Monitor pulses distal to stent graft (may need Doppler for auscultation).
- Check site for hematoma, bleeding (femoral site common).
- Monitor vital signs frequently and urine output.
- Monitor for complications (infection, embolism, bleeding).
- Monitor for graft occlusion or rupture.

CLIENT EDUCATION
- Adhere to prescribed activity level and restrictions (avoid climbing large number of stairs, avoid heavy lifting, driving)
- Monitor procedure site and provide incisional care as prescribed
- Take prescribed analgesics as indicated

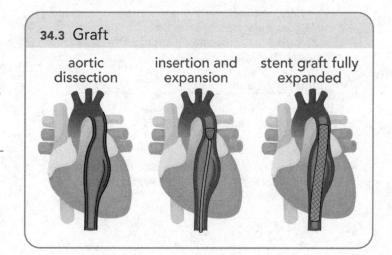

34.3 Graft

aortic dissection   insertion and expansion   stent graft fully expanded

INTERPROFESSIONAL CARE

- Cardiology services can assist in managing and treating hypertension.
- Radiology should be consulted for diagnostic studies to diagnose and monitor an aneurysm.
- Vascular services may be consulted for surgical intervention.
- Social worker, case manager (assist client with managing their identified needs).
- Home health care (assist client with ADLs) temporarily if indicated.
- Cardiac rehabilitation services are often consulted for prolonged weakness and assistance in increasing the client's level of activity.
- Nutritional services can be consulted for food choices that are low in fat and cholesterol.

COMPLICATIONS

Rupture

- Aneurysm rupture is a life-threatening emergency, often resulting in massive hemorrhage, shock, and death. A priority action is to control and prevent bleeding.
- Treatment requires simultaneous resuscitation and immediate surgical repair.
- Monitor and report client findings of a sudden unexpected increase in pain intensity, apprehension or client report of lightheadedness which could indicate a rupture.
- Older adult clients who have an aneurysm greater than 6 cm (2.4 in) along with hypertension are at greater risk of death due to spontaneous rupture than of dying during surgical repair.

Thrombus formation

- A thrombus can form inside the aneurysm. Emboli can be dislodged, blocking arteries distal to the aneurysm, which causes ischemia and shuts down other body systems.
- Monitor circulation distal to aneurysm, including pulses and color and temperature of the lower extremities. Monitor urine output.

Active Learning Scenario

A nurse is assisting the nurse manager with a presentation to a group of nurses about care of the client who has an aneurysm. What information should the nurse recommend be included in the presentation? Use the ATI Active Learning Template: System Disorder to complete this item.

RISK FACTORS: Describe three.

DIAGNOSTIC PROCEDURES: Describe two.

NURSING CARE: Describe at least four nursing actions.

Application Exercises

1. A nurse is reinforcing teaching to a client who has a new diagnosis of an aneurysm. The client asks the nurse to explain what causes an aneurysm to rupture. Which of the following statements should the nurse give?

   A. "This can occur when the wall of an artery becomes thin and flexible."

   B. "This can occur when there is turbulence in blood flow in the artery."

   C. "It is due to abdominal enlargement."

   D. "It is due to hypertension."

2. A nurse is collecting data on a client who has a new diagnosis of a thoracic aortic aneurysm. Which of the following findings should the nurse expect? (Select all that apply.)

   A. Cough

   B. Shortness of breath

   C. Upper chest pain

   D. Diaphoresis

   E. Altered swallowing

3. A nurse in the emergency department (ED) is assisting with the care of a client who has a possible dissecting abdominal aortic aneurysm. Which of the following actions is the priority for the nurse to take?

   A. Provide comfort measures.

   B. Provide a warm environment.

   C. Ensure the client has IV access.

   D. Assist with preparing the client for a 12-lead ECG.

4. A nurse is collecting data from a client who has a suspected occlusion of a graft of the abdominal aorta. Which of the following manifestations should the nurse expect?

   A. Increase in urine output

   B. Bounding pedal pulse

   C. Report of headache

   D. Coolness of inferior graft extremity

5. A nurse is contributing to the plan of care for a client following a surgical placement of an endovascular stent graft to repair an aneurysm. Which of the following interventions should the nurse recommend for inclusion in the plan of care? (Select all that apply.)

   A. Monitor pulses distal from procedure site.

   B. Monitor for an increase in pain below the graft site.

   C. Monitor procedure site for bleeding.

   D. Report hourly urine output of 60 mL.

   E. Monitor vital signs frequently

Application Exercises Key

1. D. **CORRECT:** When taking actions, the nurse should instruct the client that an aneurysm ruptures because of thickening in the intima of the artery and a lack of elasticity in the vessel wall, which is typically under pressure due to hypertension.

   Ⓝ *NCLEX® Connection: Physiological Adaptation, Alterations in Body Systems*

2. A, B, E. **CORRECT:** When recognizing cues, the nurse should recognize a client who has a thoracic aneurysm can experience cough, shortness of breath, and altered swallowing because of the aneurysm's location and potential pressure exerted in the thoracic cavity.

   Ⓝ *NCLEX® Connection: Physiological Adaptation, Basic Pathophysiology*

3. C. **CORRECT:** The nurse should analyze the findings of a client who has an aortic dissecting aneurysm is a medical emergency and determine that the priority hypothesis is that the client is at greatest risk for rupture; therefore, when breathing, circulation approach to client care, the priority action for the nurse to take is to ensure the client has IV access which may be required for medication and IV fluid administration, and possible surgery.

   Ⓝ *NCLEX® Connection: Physiological Adaptation, Basic Pathophysiology*

4. D. **CORRECT:** When recognizing cues, the nurse should identify coolness of extremity below graft a can be indication of graft occlusion/rupture which is an emergent condition that should be reported immediately to the provider.

   Ⓝ *NCLEX® Connection: Physiological Adaptation, Basic Pathophysiology*

5. A, B, C, E. **CORRECT:** When generating solutions following endovascular stent graft procedure, the nurse should recommend including in the client's plan of care to monitor distal pulses, increased pain below graft site, monitor bleeding and monitor vital signs frequently. These actions allow the nurse to identify complications such as graft occlusion and intervene promptly.

   Ⓝ *NCLEX® Connection: Physiological Adaptation, Reduction of Risk Potential*

Active Learning Scenario Key

Using the ATI Active Learning Template: System Disorder

RISK FACTORS
- Atherosclerosis (most common cause)
- Males (sex assigned at birth)
- Uncontrolled hypertension
- Tobacco use
- Hyperlipidemia
- Genetic predisposition
- Blunt force trauma
- Older adults

DIAGNOSTIC PROCEDURES
- X-rays
- CT scans
- Ultrasonography
- Transesophageal echocardiography (TEE)

NURSING CARE
- Assist with obtaining and monitoring vital signs every 15 min until stable, then every hour. Monitor for an increase in blood pressure.
- Assist with administering antihypertensives, analgesics as prescribed (may require IV administration).
- Monitor the onset, quality, duration, and severity of pain.
- Monitor temperature, circulation, and range of motion of extremities.
- Assist with monitoring cardiac rhythm.
- Assist with monitoring ABGs, SaO_2, electrolytes, and CBC findings.
- Monitor hourly urine output.
- Insert indwelling urinary catheter if prescribed.
- Administer oxygen as prescribed.
- Assist with maintaining IV access.
- Assist with preparing the client for surgery and reinforcing teaching.

Ⓝ *NCLEX® Connection: Coordinated Care, Collaboration with Multidisciplinary Team*

When reviewing the following chapters, keep in mind the relevant topics and tasks of the NCLEX outline.

Pharmacological Therapies

MEDICATION ADMINISTRATION: Monitor transfusion of blood product.

Reduction of Risk Potential

LABORATORY VALUES
Identify laboratory values for ABGs (pH, PO2, PCO2, SaO2, HCO3), BUN, cholesterol (total), creatinine, glucose, glycosylated hemoglobin (HgbA1C), hematocrit, hemoglobin, INR, platelets, potassium, PT, PTT & APTT, sodium, WBC.

Compare client laboratory values to normal laboratory values.

Reinforce client teaching on purposes of laboratory tests.

POTENTIAL FOR COMPLICATIONS OF DIAGNOSTIC TESTS/ TREATMENTS/PROCEDURES: Notify primary health care provider if client has signs of potential complications.

Physiological Adaptation

UNEXPECTED RESPONSE TO THERAPIES: Intervene in response to client unexpected negative response to therapy.

CHAPTER 35 *Hematologic Diagnostic Procedures*

Hematologic assessment and diagnostic procedures evaluate blood function by testing indicators such as erythrocytes (RBCs), leukocytes (WBCs), platelets, and coagulation times. By testing the blood, diagnosis of a disease and efficacy of treatment can be determined.

Bone marrow is responsible for the production of many blood cells including RBCs, WBCs, and platelets. A bone marrow biopsy provides diagnostic information about how the bone marrow is functioning.

Blood collection/testing

- Hematologic diagnostic procedures of blood components that nurses should be knowledgeable about include the following.
  - RBC count
  - WBC count
  - Mean corpuscular volume (MCV)
  - Mean corpuscular Hgb (MCH)
  - Total iron-binding count (TIBC)
  - Iron
  - Platelets
  - Hemoglobin (Hgb)
  - Hematocrit (Hct)
  - Coagulation studies
    - Prothrombin time (PT)
    - Partial thromboplastin time (aPTT)
    - International normalized ratio (INR)
    - D-dimer
    - Fibrinogen levels
    - Fibrin degradation products
- CBC is a series of tests that includes RBC, WBC, MCV, MCH, Hgb, and Hct.

CONSIDERATIONS

PREPROCEDURE

NURSING ACTIONS: Use standard precautions in collecting and handling blood for specimen collection.

INTRAPROCEDURE

NURSING ACTIONS: For coagulation studies, draw blood at specific times and immediately send to the laboratory.

POSTPROCEDURE

NURSING ACTIONS
- Results of hematologic tests are usually available preliminarily within 24 to 48 hr, with final results in 72 hr.
- If results are out of the expected reference range, it is the nurse's responsibility to report the results to the provider for further intervention.
- Adjust the dose of anticoagulant therapy based on the results and prescription.

Bone marrow aspiration/biopsy

- A biopsy is the extraction of a very small amount of tissue, such as bone marrow, to definitively diagnose cell type and to confirm or rule out malignancy. A bone marrow tissue sample is removed by needle aspiration for cytological (histological) examination.
- Biopsies are commonly performed with local anesthesia or conscious sedation in an ambulatory setting, intraoperatively, or during endoscopic procedures.

INDICATIONS

A bone marrow biopsy is commonly performed to diagnose causes of blood disorders, such as anemia or thrombocytopenia; to diagnose diseases of the bone marrow, such as leukemia, and infection; or to stage lymphoma or other forms of cancer.

CONSIDERATIONS

PREPROCEDURE

NURSING ACTIONS
- Ensure that the client has provided informed consent.
- Place the client in a prone or side-lying position to expose the iliac crest for the procedure.
- Reinforce teaching about the procedure.

CLIENT EDUCATION
- The biopsy site will be anesthetized with a local anesthetic, and there can be a feeling of pressure and brief pain during the aspiration.
- There will be a sensation of pressure as the biopsy needle is inserted, and a crunching sound might be heard when the needle enters the bone.

35.1 Expected reference ranges for blood diagnostic procedures

	EXPECTED REFERENCE RANGE	INTERPRETATION OF FINDINGS
RBC	Females: 4.2 to 5.4 million/uL Males: 4.7 to 6.1 million/uL	Elevated level: Erythrocytosis, polycythemia vera, severe dehydration Decreased level: Anemia, hemorrhage, kidney disease
WBC	5,000 to 10,000/mm³	Elevated level: Infection, inflammation. Decreased level: Immunosuppression, autoimmune disease
MCV	80 to 95 fL	Elevated level: Macrocytic (large) RBCs, megaloblastic anemia. Decreased level: Microcytic (small) RBCs, iron deficiency anemia.
MCH	27 to 31 pg/cell	Elevated/decreased level: Same as above for MCV
TIBC	250 to 460 mcg/dL	Elevated level: Iron deficiency anemia, polycythemia vera Decreased level: Malnutrition, cirrhosis, pernicious anemia
Iron	Females: 60 to 160 mcg/dL Males: 80 to 180 mcg/dL	Elevated level: Hemochromatosis, iron excess, liver disorder, or lead toxicity. Decreased level: Iron deficiency anemia, chronic blood loss, inadequate dietary intake of iron.
Platelets	150,000 to 400,000 mm³	Increased level: Malignancy, polycythemia vera, rheumatoid arthritis. Decreased level: Enlarged spleen, hemorrhage, leukemia
Hgb	Females: 12 to 16 g/dL Males: 14 to 18 g/dL	Elevated level: Erythrocytosis, COPD, severe dehydration Decreased level: Anemia, hemorrhage, kidney disease
Hct	Females: 37% to 47% Males: 42% to 52%	Elevated /decreased level: Same as above for Hgb
aPTT	30 to 40 seconds (1.5 to 2.5 times the control value if receiving heparin therapy)	Increased time: Vitamin K deficiency, disseminated intravascular coagulation (DIC), liver disease, heparin administration Decreased time: Extensive cancer
PT	11 to 12.5 seconds, 85% to 100%, or 1:1.1 client-control ratio	Increased time: Clotting factors II, V, VII, or X, liver disease, warfarin therapy, disseminated intravascular coagulation Decreased time: Vitamin K excess, pulmonary embolus, thrombophlebitis
INR	0.8 to 1.1 (desired goal of 2 to 3 on warfarin therapy)	Measures the mean of PT to provide a universally recognized value. Elevated level: Warfarin therapy Decreased level: Cancer disorders
D-dimer	Less than 0.4 mcg/mL	Positive result: Disseminated intravascular coagulation, malignancy Negative result: Can rule out pulmonary embolus or deep vein thrombosis
Fibrinogen levels	200 to 400 mg/dL	Elevated level: Acute inflammation, acute infection, heart disease Decreased levels: Liver disease, advanced cancer, malnutrition
Fibrin degradation products	Less than 10 mcg/mL	Elevated level: Disseminated intravascular coagulation, massive trauma resulting in fibrinolysis Decreased level: Anticoagulation therapy

35.2 Bone marrow biopsy

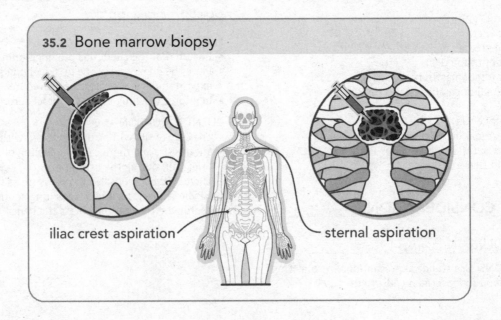

iliac crest aspiration — sternal aspiration

INTRAPROCEDURE

NURSING ACTIONS

- Administer a sedative if prescribed.
  - Older adult clients are at greater risk for complications associated with sedation for biopsy procedures due to chronic illnesses.
  - The nurse should take an older adult's kidney function into consideration when using analgesics for sedation.
- Cleanse the site with an antiseptic solution.
- Maintain sterility of equipment and supplies.
- Assist the provider with the procedure as needed.

CLIENT EDUCATION: The test will last about 20 min.

POSTPROCEDURE

NURSING ACTIONS

- Apply pressure to the biopsy site to control bleeding and prevent hematoma formation.
- Place a sterile dressing over the biopsy site.
- Maintain the client on bed rest for 30 to 60 min.
- Monitor for manifestations of infection (fever, increased WBCs, pain, and swelling at the site) and bleeding.
- Apply ice to the biopsy site to minimize bleeding and bruising.
- Postprocedure discomfort is usually relieved by mild analgesics.
- Avoid aspirin and other medications that affect clotting.

CLIENT EDUCATION

- Report excessive bleeding and evidence of infection to the provider.
- Check the biopsy site daily. Keep the dressing clean, dry, and intact.
- If sutures are in place, return in 7 to 10 days to have them removed.

INTERPRETATION OF FINDINGS

After a procedure is completed, the tissue sample is sent to pathology for interpretation.

COMPLICATIONS

Infection

Infection can occur at the aspiration site.

NURSING ACTIONS: Monitor the site, and keep the dressing clean and dry.

Bleeding

Bleeding can occur from the site.

NURSING ACTIONS

- Report bleeding to the provider immediately.
- Apply a pressure dressing over the site.

Application Exercises

1. A nurse in a clinic is caring for a client who has suspected anemia. Which of the following laboratory test results should the nurse review?
   A. Iron 90 mcg/dL
   B. RBC 6.5 mm³
   C. WBC 4,800 mm³
   D. Hgb 10 g/dL

2. A nurse is caring for a client who is receiving warfarin for anticoagulation therapy. Which of the following laboratory test results indicates to the nurse that the client needs an increase in the dosage?
   A. aPTT 38 seconds
   B. INR 1.1
   C. PT 22 seconds
   D. D-dimer negative

3. A nurse is reinforcing teaching for a client who is scheduled for a bone marrow biopsy of the iliac crest. Which of the following statements made by the client indicates an understanding of the teaching?
   A. "This test will be performed while I am lying flat on my back."
   B. "I will need to stay in bed for about an hour after the test."
   C. "This test will determine which antibiotic I should take for treatment."
   D. "I will receive general anesthesia for the test."

4. A nurse is caring for a client who has disseminated intravascular coagulation (DIC). Which of the following laboratory values is most useful to evaluate the intrinsic clotting cascade?
   A. INR
   B. MCV
   C. PTT
   D. Iron

5. A nurse caring for a client who has bone marrow suppression. The nurse should identify which of the following lab values as consistent with this diagnosis? (Select all that apply.)
   A. WBC 2,100 mm³
   B. Iron 220 mc/dL
   C. Platelet count 75,000 mm³
   D. PT 30 seconds

Application Exercises Key

1. D. **CORRECT:** The nurse should analyze the cues from the client's laboratory findings, and determine that the Hgb is the result to review for a client who has suspected anemia A Hgb of 10 g/dL is below the expected reference range and is an expected finding of anemia.

   (N) *NCLEX® Connection: Reduction of Risk Potential, Laboratory Values*

2. B. **CORRECT:** The nurse should analyze the cues from the client's laboratory findings and determine that reviewing the INR can indicate a need for a change in dosage of warfarin. An INR of 1.1 is within the expected reference range for a client who is not receiving warfarin. However, this value is subtherapeutic for anticoagulation therapy. Expect the client to receive an increased dosage of warfarin until the INR is 2 to 3.

   (N) *NCLEX® Connection: Reduction of Risk Potential, Laboratory Values*

3. B. **CORRECT:** When evaluating outcomes of client education, the nurse should identify client understanding when the client states that they will need to stay on bed rest for 30 to 60 min following the test to reduce the risk for bleeding.

   (N) *NCLEX® Connection: Reduction of Risk Potential, Diagnostic Tests*

4. C. **CORRECT:** The nurse should analyze cues from the client's laboratory values and determine that the PTT evaluates the action of clotting factors and the clotting cascade. This value may be prolonged in the client experiencing disseminated intravascular coagulation.

   (N) *NCLEX® Connection: Reduction of Risk Potential, Laboratory Values*

5. A, C. **CORRECT:** The nurse should analyze the cues from the client's laboratory findings and determine that the client with bone marrow suppression can have alterations in the RBCs, WBCs, and platelets. The WBC count of 2,100 and the platelet count of 75,000 are both indicative of bone marrow suppression.

   (N) *NCLEX® Connection: Reduction of Risk Potential, Laboratory Values*

Active Learning Scenario

A nurse is caring for a client who is having a bone marrow biopsy. What actions should the nurse take? Use the ATI Active Learning Template: Diagnostic Procedure to complete this item.

NURSING INTERVENTIONS (PRE, INTRA, POST): Describe two for each of the pre-, intra-, and postprocedure periods.

POTENTIAL COMPLICATIONS: Identify two.

CLIENT EDUCATION: Describe two discharge teaching points.

Active Learning Scenario Key

Using the ATI Active Learning Template: Diagnostic Procedure
NURSING INTERVENTIONS (PRE, INTRA, POST)

Preprocedure
- Ensure that the client has signed the informed consent form.
- Position the client in a prone or side-lying position.
- Reinforce teaching about the procedure to the client. Inform the client that they might feel pressure and brief pain during the bone marrow aspiration.

Intraprocedure
- Administer sedative medication.
- Assist with the procedure.
- Inform the client that the procedure lasts about 20 min.
- Cleanse the site with an antiseptic solution.
- Maintain sterility of equipment and supplies.

Postprocedure
- Apply pressure to the biopsy site.
- Place a sterile dressing over the biopsy site.
- Monitor for evidence of infection and bleeding.
- Apply ice to the biopsy site.
- Administer mild analgesics. Avoid aspirin or medications that affect clotting.

POTENTIAL COMPLICATIONS
- Bleeding and infection
- Older adults at greater risk for complications associated with anesthesia

CLIENT EDUCATION
- Report excessive bleeding and evidence of infection to the provider.
- Check the biopsy site daily. Keep the dressing clean, dry and intact.
- If there are sutures, return in 7 to 10 days for removal.

   (N) *NCLEX® Connection: Reduction of Risk Potential, Potential for Complications from Surgical Procedures and Health Alterations*

CHAPTER 36 Blood and Blood Product Transfusions

Clients can receive transfusions of whole blood or components of whole blood for replacement due to blood loss or blood disease.

Blood components include packed RBCs, washed red blood cells (WBC-poor RBCs), white blood cells (WBCs), fresh frozen plasma, albumin, clotting factors, cryoprecipitate, and platelets.

TRANSFUSION TYPES

Standard donation: Transfusion from compatible donor blood.

Autologous transfusions: The client's blood is collected in anticipation of future transfusions (elective surgery). This blood is designated for and used only by the client. Clients can donate up to 6 weeks prior to the scheduled surgery. If the client's hemoglobin and hematocrit remain stable, donation can occur weekly until the desired amount of blood for the anticipated transfusion is collected.

Intraoperative blood salvage: Sterile blood lost during a procedure is saved or retrieved into a device that filters and drains the blood into a bag for transfusion intraoperatively or postoperatively. Reinfusion must occur within 6 hr of salvaged blood collection.

INDICATIONS

POTENTIAL DIAGNOSES

Excessive blood loss: packed RBCs

Anemia (Hgb less than 6, or 6 to 10 g/dL, depending on findings): packed RBCs

Kidney failure: packed RBCs

Coagulation factor deficiencies such as hemophilia: fresh frozen plasma

Thrombocytopenia/platelet dysfunction: platelets

Hemophilia A: cryoprecipitate

Burns, hypoproteinemia: albumin

CONSIDERATIONS

Platelet transfusion

Platelets do not need to match the client blood type. Platelet infusion bags contain 200 to 300 mL.

NURSING ACTIONS
- Platelets are fragile and must be immediately infused once brought to the client's room, and given over 15 to 30 min using a special transfusion set with a small filter and short tubing.
- Vital signs are taken before the infusion, 15 min after the infusion starts, and upon completion.

Plasma transfusion

- Plasma is frozen immediately following donation and is then in the form of fresh frozen plasma (FFP).
- FFP is transfused as soon as the unit is thawed while clotting factors are still active.
- The client can react to the FFP transfusion if the ABO compatibility is not matched.

NURSING ACTIONS: A unit of 200 mL of FFP should be infused rapidly over 30 to 60 min through a regular Y-set or straight filtered tubing.

White blood cell transfusion (granulocyte)

- Immunocompromised clients rarely receive WBC transfusions because of the risk for severe reaction.
- If the client is receiving amphotericin B antibiotics, 4 to 6 hr should be between the administration of the antibiotic and the WBC transfusion because amphotericin B can hemolyze the WBCs.

NURSING ACTIONS: WBCs suspended in 400 mL plasma should be infused over 45 to 60 min and vital signs are taken every 15 min. The presence of the provider may be required according to agency policy.

Washed RBCs (WBC-poor packed RBCs)

NURSING ACTIONS
- Should be transfused a unit of 200 mL over 2 to 4 hr.
- Administer to a client who has a history of transfusion reactions or to a client who has had a hematopoietic stem cell transplant.

PREPROCEDURE

- Incompatibility is a major concern when administering blood or blood products. Preventing incompatibility requires strict adherence to blood transfusion protocols.
- Type and cross match is necessary for packed red blood cells. Blood products containing RBCs are typed and cross-matched for antigens.
- Plasma products are typed for ABO compatibility but not cross-matched for antigens. The other cells (WBCs, platelets) in the plasma products can carry ABO antigens.
- Blood is typed based on the presence of antigens.
- Another consideration is the Rh factor. Clients who are Rh-negative are born without the Rh antigen in their RBCs. As a result, they do not develop antibodies unless sensitization occurs. Once this occurs, any transfusion with Rh-positive blood will cause a reaction.

NURSING ACTIONS

- Ensure the procedure has been explained to the client.
- Check vital signs and the client's temperature prior to transfusion.
- Remain with the client during the initial 15 to 30 min of the transfusion. Most severe reactions occur within this time frame.
- Review laboratory values to ensure the client requires transfusion and to compare to post-transfusion values.
- Verify the prescription for a specific blood product.
- Ensure that the client has given consent for procedure if required.
- Ensure that blood samples have been obtained for compatibility determination, such as type and cross-match.
- Check for a history of blood-transfusion reactions.
- Ensure that the client has a large-bore IV access. An 18- or 20-gauge needle is standard for administering blood products.
- Assist with obtaining blood products from the blood bank. Inspect the blood for discoloration, excessive bubbles, or cloudiness.
- Prior to transfusion, two RNs (or an RN and a PN, depending on facility policy) must identify the correct blood product and client by looking at the hospital identification number (noted on the blood product) and the number identified on the client's identification band to make sure the numbers match.
- The nurse completing the blood product verification must be one of the nurses who administers the blood product.
- Ensure that the blood administration set has been primed with 0.9% sodium chloride only. Never add medications to blood products. Y-tubing with a filter is used to transfuse blood.
- Use a blood warmer if indicated.
- The transfusion should be started by the RN within 30 min of obtaining the blood product to reduce the risk of bacterial growth.
- **OLDER ADULT CLIENTS** ©
  - No larger than a 19-gauge needle is used.
  - Monitor kidney function, fluid status, and circulation prior to blood product administration. Older adult clients are at an increased risk for fluid overload.
  - Use blood products that are less than 1 week old.
  - Ensure the client understands the reason for the blood transfusion.

36.1 Blood type compatibility

BLOOD TYPE	ANTIGEN	ANTIBODIES AGAINST	COMPATIBLE WITH
A	A	B	A, O
B	B	A	B, O
AB	AB	None	A, B, AB, O
O	None	A, B	O

INTRAPROCEDURE

NURSING ACTIONS

- Remain with the client for the first 15 to 30 min of the infusion (reactions occur most often during the first 15 min) and monitor vital signs and rate of infusion per facility policy. **Qs**
- **OLDER ADULT CLIENTS:** Check vital signs every 15 min throughout the transfusion because changes in pulse, blood pressure, and respiratory rate can indicate fluid overload, or can be the sole indicators of a transfusion reaction. Older adult clients who have cardiac or kidney dysfunction are at an increased risk for heart failure and fluid-volume excess when receiving a blood transfusion. The blood transfusion should be administered over 2 to 4 hr for older adult clients. Withhold administration of other IV fluids during blood product administration to prevent fluid overload. ©
- Notify the provider immediately if indications of a reaction occur.

POSTPROCEDURE

NURSING ACTIONS

- Obtain vital signs upon completion of the transfusion.
- Dispose of the blood-administration set according to facility policy.
- Complete paperwork, and file in the appropriate places.
- Document the client's response.

COMPLICATIONS

Acute hemolytic transfusion reaction

ONSET: Immediate or can manifest during subsequent transfusions

FINDINGS

- Results from a transfusion of blood products that are incompatible with the client's blood type or Rh factor. Can occur following the transfusion of as few as 10 mL of a blood product.
- Can be mild or life-threatening, resulting in disseminated intravascular coagulation (DIC) or circulatory collapse.
- Include chills, fever, low-back pain, tachycardia, flushing, hypotension, chest tightening or pain, tachypnea, nausea, anxiety, hemoglobinuria, and an impending sense of doom.

NURSING ACTIONS

- Stop the transfusion.
- Assist with removing the blood tubing from the IV access. Avoid infusing further blood products into the circulatory system.
- Ensure that an infusion of 0.9% sodium chloride using new tubing is initiated.
- Monitor vital signs and fluid status.
- Send the blood bag and administration set to the lab for testing.

Febrile transfusion reaction

ONSET: Commonly occurs within 2 hr of starting the transfusion

FINDINGS
- Results from the development of anti-WBC antibodies. Can be seen when the client has received multiple transfusions.
- Findings include chills, increase of 1° C (2° F) or greater from the pretransfusion temperature, flushing, hypotension, and tachycardia.

NURSING ACTIONS
- Use WBC filter for administration to catch the WBCs and prevent the reaction from occurring.
- Stop the transfusion and administer antipyretics.
- Ensure an infusion of 0.9% sodium chloride using new tubing is initiated.

Allergic transfusion reaction

ONSET: During or up to 24 hr after transfusion

FINDINGS
- Results from a sensitivity reaction to a component of the transfused blood products.
- Findings are usually mild and include itching, urticaria, and flushing.
- The client can develop an anaphylactic transfusion reaction resulting in bronchospasm, laryngeal edema, hypotension, and shock.

NURSING ACTIONS

Mild reaction
- Stop the transfusion.
- Ensure that an infusion of 0.9% sodium chloride using new tubing has been initiated.
- Administer an antihistamine, such as diphenhydramine.
- If the provider prescribes to restart the transfusion, ensure it is administered slowly.

Anaphylactic reaction
- Stop the transfusion.
- Assist with the administration of epinephrine, corticosteroids, vasopressors, oxygen, or CPR if indicated.
- Remove the blood tubing from the client's IV access.
- Ensure an infusion of 0.9% sodium chloride is initiated using new tubing.

Bacterial transfusion reaction

ONSET: During or up to several hours after transfusion

FINDINGS
- Results from a transfusion of contaminated blood products.
- Include wheezing, dyspnea, chest tightness, cyanosis, hypotension, and shock.

NURSING ACTIONS
- Stop the transfusion.
- Ensure that antibiotics and an IV infusion of 0.9% sodium chloride using new tubing is administered.
- Send a blood culture specimen to the lab for analysis.

Circulatory overload

ONSET: Can occur any time during the transfusion

FINDINGS
- Results from a transfusion rate that is too rapid for the client. Older adult clients or those who have a preexisting increased circulatory volume are at an increased risk.
- Include crackles, dyspnea, cough, anxiety, jugular vein distention, and tachycardia. Manifestations can progress to pulmonary edema.

NURSING ACTIONS
- Slow or stop the transfusion depending on the severity of manifestations.
- Position the client upright with feet lower than the level of the heart.
- Assist with the administration of oxygen, diuretics, and morphine as prescribed.

Active Learning Scenario

A nurse is caring for a client who is receiving a blood transfusion. What nursing actions should the nurse plan to take if a transfusion reaction is suspected? Use the ATI Active Learning Template: Nursing Skill to complete this item.

INDICATIONS
- Describe the types of reactions and the time of onset.
- Describe three medications that can be administered and for which reaction.

NURSING INTERVENTIONS: Describe actions for each type of reaction.

1. A nurse is reinforcing preoperative teaching for a client who requests autologous donation in preparation for a scheduled orthopedic surgical procedure. Which of the following statements should the nurse include while reinforcing the teaching?

   A. "You should make an appointment to donate blood 10 weeks prior to the surgery."

   B. "If you need an autologous transfusion, the blood a sibling donates can be used."

   C. "You can donate blood during the weeks prior to surgery."

   D. "Any unused blood that is donated can be used for other clients."

2. A nurse is assisting the charge nurse with the administration of a blood transfusion to an older adult client. Which of the following actions by the newly licensed nurse indicates an understanding of the procedure?

   A. Inserts an 18-gauge IV catheter in the client

   B. Verifies blood compatibility and expiration date of the blood with an assistive personnel (AP)

   C. Administers dextrose 5% in 0.9% sodium chloride IV with the transfusion

   D. Obtains vital signs frequently throughout the procedure.

3. A nurse is assisting with the administration of packed RBCs to a client who has a Hgb of 6 g/dL. Which of the following actions should the nurse plan to take during the first 15 min of the transfusion?

   A. Obtain consent from the client for the transfusion.

   B. Monitor the client for an acute hemolytic reaction.

   C. Explain the transfusion procedure to the client.

   D. Obtain blood culture specimens to send to the lab.

4. A nurse is monitoring a client who began receiving a unit of packed RBCs 10 min ago. Which of the following findings should the nurse identify as an indication of a febrile transfusion reaction? (Select all that apply.)

   A. Temperature change from 37° C (98.6° F) pretransfusion to 37.2° C (99.0° F)

   B. Current blood pressure 178/90 mm Hg

   C. Heart rate change from 88/min pretransfusion to 120/min

   D. Client report of itching

   E. Client appears flushed

5. A nurse is assisting with the care of a client who is receiving a blood transfusion. Which of the following actions should the nurse take if the client develops manifestations of an allergic transfusion reaction? (Select all that apply.)

   A. Stop the transfusion.

   B. Monitor for hypertension.

   C. Maintain an IV infusion with 0.9% sodium chloride.

   D. Position the client in an upright position with the feet lower than the heart.

   E. Administer diphenhydramine.

Active Learning Scenario Key

Using the ATI Active Learning Template: Nursing Skill

INDICATIONS

Types of reactions and onset
- Acute hemolytic: immediate or during subsequent transfusions
- Febrile: within 2 hr of starting the transfusion
- Allergic: during or up to 24 hr after transfusion
- Bacterial: during or up to several hours after the transfusion
- Circulatory overload: any time during the transfusion

Medications
- Antipyretics (acetaminophen): febrile
- Antihistamines (diphenhydramine): mild allergic
- Antihistamines, corticosteroids, vasopressors, epinephrine: anaphylactic
- Antibiotics: bacterial
- Diuretics, morphine: circulatory overload

NURSING ACTIONS

Acute hemolytic
- Stop the transfusion.
- Remove the blood tubing.
- Ensure the initiation of an infusion of 0.9% sodium chloride.
- Monitor vital signs and fluid status.
- Send the blood bag and administration set to the lab for testing.

Febrile
- Use a WBC filter to help prevent a febrile reaction.
- Stop the transfusion.
- Administer antipyretics.
- Ensure the initiation of an infusion of 0.9% sodium chloride.

Mild allergic reaction
- Stop the transfusion.
- Ensure the initiation of an infusion of 0.9% sodium chloride.
- Administer an antihistamine.
- If prescribed, ensure the RN restarts the transfusion slowly to continue.

Anaphylactic reaction
- Stop the transfusion.
- Assist with the administration of epinephrine, corticosteroids, vasopressors, and oxygen.
- Administer CPR if indicated.
- Remove the blood tubing from the client's IV access.
- Ensure the initiation of an infusion of 0.9% sodium chloride.

Circulatory overload
- Slow or stop the transfusion depending on the severity.
- Position the client upright with feet lower than the level of the heart.
- Assist with the administration of oxygen, diuretics, and morphine.

Bacterial
- Stop the transfusion.
- Administer antibiotics as prescribed.
- Ensure the initiation of an infusion of 0.9% sodium chloride.
- Ensure blood samples are obtained for culture.

(N) *NCLEX® Connection: Physiological Adaptation, Unexpected Response to Therapies*

Application Exercises Key

1. C. **CORRECT:** When taking actions and reinforcing teaching a client about autologous blood donations, the nurse should teach the client that beginning 6 weeks prior to surgery, the client can donate blood each week for autologous transfusion if their Hgb and Hct remain stable.

(N) *NCLEX® Connection: Reduction of Risk Potential, Potential for Complications from Surgical Procedures and Health Alterations*

2. D. **CORRECT:** The nurse should plan to generate solutions to address the older adult's increased risk of fluid overload which include checking the client's vital signs every 15 min throughout the transfusion to allow for early detection of fluid overload or other transfusion reaction.

(N) *NCLEX® Connection: Pharmacological Therapies, Medication Administration*

3. B. **CORRECT:** The nurse should plan to generate solutions to address the potential for blood transfusion reactions while receiving packed RBCs. The nurse should plan to monitor the client for an acute hemolytic reaction during the first 15 min of the transfusion. This form of a reaction can occur following the transfusion of as little as 10 mL of blood product.

(N) *NCLEX® Connection: Pharmacological Therapies, Medication Administration*

4. C, E. **CORRECT:** The nurse should analyze cues from the client's manifestations and determine that tachycardia and a flushed appearance can be indications of a febrile transfusion reaction.

(N) *NCLEX® Connection: Pharmacological Therapies, Medication Administration*

5. A, C, E. **CORRECT:** When taking actions for a client who is developing manifestations of an allergic blood transfusion reaction, the nurse should stop the infusion and administer an antihistamine, such as diphenhydramine Maintain an IV infusion of 0.9% sodium chloride solution through new IV tubing.

(N) *NCLEX® Connection: Physiological Adaptation, Unexpected Response to Therapies*

ⓝ NCLEX® Connections

When reviewing the following chapters, keep in mind the relevant topics and tasks of the NCLEX outline.

Basic Care and Comfort

NUTRITION AND ORAL HYDRATION: Monitor impact of disease/illness on client nutritional status.

Pharmacological Therapies

MEDICATION ADMINISTRATION
Collect required data prior to medication administration.

Reinforce client teaching on client self administration of medications.

Reduction of Risk Potential

POTENTIAL FOR ALTERATIONS IN BODY SYSTEMS: Identify client with increased risk for insufficient blood circulation.

POTENTIAL FOR COMPLICATIONS OF DIAGNOSTIC TESTS/TREATMENTS/PROCEDURES: Notify primary health care provider if client has signs of potential complications.

Physiological Adaptation

ALTERATIONS IN BODY SYSTEMS: Provide care to correct client alteration in body system.

FLUID AND ELECTROLYTE IMBALANCES: Provide care for a client with a fluid and electrolyte imbalance.

CHAPTER 37 *Anemias*

Anemia is an abnormally low number of circulating RBCs, Hgb concentration, or both is an indicator of an underlying disease or disorder. Anemia results in diminished oxygen-carrying capacity and delivery to tissues and organs. The goal of treatment is to restore and maintain adequate tissue oxygenation.

Iron-deficiency anemia, due to an inadequate intake of iron in the diet, is the most common type of anemia. Iron-deficiency anemia due to blood loss (such as from a gastrointestinal ulcer) is the most common cause of anemia in adult clients. Clients who are menstruating can develop anemia secondary to menorrhagia.

CAUSES OF ANEMIA

- Blood loss
- Inadequate RBC production (hypoproliferative)
- Increased RBC destruction (hemolytic)
- Deficiency of necessary components (folic acid, iron, erythropoietin, vitamin B_{12})

HEALTH PROMOTION AND DISEASE PREVENTION

- Clients who are pregnant or menstruating should ensure that their diet contains adequate amounts of iron-rich foods. Otherwise, they should take an iron supplement.
- Individuals who are iron-deficient and have elevated cholesterol levels should integrate iron-rich foods that are not red or organ meats into their diets (iron-fortified cereal and breads, fish, poultry, and dried peas and beans).
- Clients should regularly consume foods high in folate (spinach, lentils, bananas) and folic acid fortified grains and juices.

DATA COLLECTION

RISK FACTORS

Acute or chronic blood loss
- Trauma
- Menorrhagia
- Gastrointestinal bleed (ulcers, tumor)
- Intra or postsurgical blood loss or hemorrhage
- Cancer
- Hemorrhoids

Rapid metabolic activity
- Pregnancy
- Adolescence
- Infection

Increased hemolysis
- Defective Hgb (sickle-cell disease): RBCs become malformed during periods of hypoxia and obstruct capillaries in joints and organs
- Impaired glycolysis: glucose-6-phosphate-dehydrogenase (G6PD) deficiency anemia
- Immune disorder or destruction (transfusion reactions, autoimmune diseases)
- Mechanical trauma to RBCs (mechanical heart valve, cardiopulmonary bypass)

Inadequate dietary intake or malabsorption
- Iron deficiency
- Vitamin B_{12} deficiency: pernicious anemia due to deficiency of intrinsic factor produced by gastric mucosa, which is necessary for absorption of vitamin B_{12}
- Folic acid deficiency
- Pica, or a persistent eating of substances not normally considered food (nonnutritive substances), such as soil or chalk, for at least 1 month, which can limit the amount of healthy food choices a client makes

Bone-marrow suppression
- Exposure to radiation or chemicals (such as insecticides or solvents)
- Aplastic anemia, which results in a decreased number of RBCs as well as decreased platelets and WBCs
- Viral infections such as HIV or mononucleosis

Age
- Older adult clients are at risk for nutrition-deficient anemias (iron, vitamin B_{12}, folate). Ⓖ
- Anemia can be misdiagnosed as depression or debilitation in older adult clients.
- Gastrointestinal bleeding is a common cause of anemia in older adult clients. Check stools for occult blood.

EXPECTED FINDINGS

- Little to no manifestations in mild cases
- Pallor
- Fatigue, somnolence, and headache
- Irritability
- Numbness and tingling of extremities
- Dyspnea on exertion
- Sensitivity to cold
- Pain and hypoxia with sickle-cell crisis

PHYSICAL FINDINGS

- Shortness of breath/fatigue, especially upon exertion
- Tachycardia, palpitations, and angina
- Dizziness or syncope upon standing or with exertion
- Pallor of the nail beds and mucous membranes
- Nail bed deformities (spoon-shaped nails)
- Smooth, sore, bright-red tongue (vitamin B_{12} deficiency)
- Paresthesia in hands and feet with possible loss of balance (vitamin B_{12} deficiency)

LABORATORY TESTS

CBC count

- RBCs are the major carriers of hemoglobin in the blood.
- Hgb transports oxygen and carbon dioxide to and from the cells and can be used as an index of the oxygen-carrying capacity of the blood.
- Hct is the percentage of RBCs in relation to the total blood volume.

RBC indices

Used to determine the type and cause of most anemias

Mean corpuscular volume (MCV): Size of red blood cells
- Normocytic: Normal size
- Microcytic: Small cells
- Macrocytic: Large cells

Mean corpuscular Hgb (MCH): Determines the amount of Hgb per RBC
- Normochromic: Normal amount of Hgb per cell
- Hypochromic: Decreased Hgb per cell

Mean corpuscular Hgb concentration (MCHC): Indicates Hgb amount relative to the size of the cell

Iron studies

- Total iron-binding capacity (TIBC) reflects an indirect measurement of all proteins that bind with iron and transports it for storage. Transferring represents the largest amount of iron-binding proteins.
- Ferritin is an indicator of total iron stores in the body.
- Low blood iron levels and elevated TIBC indicate iron-deficiency anemia.

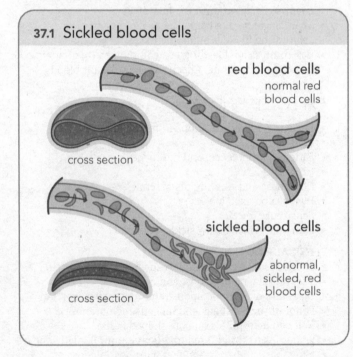

37.1 Sickled blood cells

red blood cells

normal red blood cells

cross section

sickled blood cells

abnormal, sickled, red blood cells

cross section

Hgb electrophoresis

Separates normal Hgb from abnormal. It is used to detect thalassemia and sickle-cell disease.

Sickle-cell test

Evaluates the sickling of RBCs in the presence of decreased oxygen tension

Schilling test

Measures vitamin B_{12} absorption with and without intrinsic factor. It is used to differentiate between malabsorption and pernicious anemia.

DIAGNOSTIC PROCEDURES

Bone-marrow aspiration/biopsy is used to diagnose aplastic anemia (failure of bone marrow to produce RBCs as well as platelets and WBCs).

PATIENT-CENTERED CARE

NURSING CARE

- Encourage increased dietary intake of the deficient nutrient (iron, vitamin B_{12}, folic acid). Supply clients with a list of foods high in these nutrients.
- Monitor oxygen saturation to determine a need for oxygen therapy.
- Administer medications, as prescribed, at the proper time for optimal absorption, and using an appropriate technique.
- Reinforce teaching with the client and family about energy conservation and the risk of the client experiencing dizziness upon standing.
- Reinforce teaching with the client about the time frame for resolution.

MEDICATIONS

Iron supplements

Ferrous sulfate, ferrous fumarate, ferrous gluconate
- Oral iron supplements are used to replenish iron in the blood and iron stores. Iron is an essential component of Hgb, and subsequently, oxygen transport.
- Parenteral iron supplements (iron dextran) are only given for severe anemia.

NURSING ACTIONS: Administer parenteral iron using the Z-track method.

CLIENT EDUCATION
- Have hemoglobin checked in 4 to 6 weeks to determine efficacy.
- Vitamin C can increase oral iron absorption.
- Take iron supplements between meals to increase absorption, if tolerated.
- Stools can appear green to black in color while taking iron.

37.2 RBC indices

	NORMAL MCV, MCH, MCHC	DECREASED MCV, MCH, MCHC	INCREASED MCV
Classification	Normocytic, normochromic anemia	Microcytic, hypochromic anemia	Macrocytic anemia, normochromic anemia
Possible causes	Acute blood loss Chronic illness (kidney disease, sepsis, tumor) Aplastic anemia Iron deficiency anemia (early detection)	Iron-deficiency anemia (late detection) Thalassemia Chronic blood loss	Vitamin B$_{12}$ deficiency Folic acid deficiency Chemotherapy Dysfunction of the thyroid gland

Erythropoietin: epoetin alfa

A hematopoietic growth factor used to increase production of RBCs

NURSING ACTIONS
- Monitor for an increase in blood pressure.
- Monitor Hgb and Hct twice per week.
- Monitor for a cardiovascular event if Hgb increases too rapidly (greater than 1 g/dL in 2 weeks).

CLIENT EDUCATION: Have Hgb and Hct evaluated on a twice-per-week basis until targeted levels are reached.

Vitamin B$_{12}$ supplementation (cyanocobalamin)

- Vitamin B$_{12}$ is necessary to convert folic acid from its inactive form to its active form. All cells rely on folic acid for DNA production.
- Vitamin B$_{12}$ supplementation can be given orally if the deficit is due to inadequate dietary intake. However, if deficiency is due to lack of intrinsic factor being produced by the parietal cells of the stomach or malabsorption syndrome, it must be administered parenterally or intranasally to be absorbed.

NURSING ACTIONS
- Administer vitamin B$_{12}$ according to appropriate route related to cause of vitamin B$_{12}$ anemia (parenteral vs. oral).
- Administer parenteral forms of vitamin B$_{12}$ IM or deep subcutaneous to decrease irritation. Do not mix other medications in the syringe.

CLIENT EDUCATION
- If lacking intrinsic factor or have an irreversible malabsorption syndrome, this therapy must be continued for the rest of life.
- Receive vitamin B$_{12}$ injections on a monthly basis.

Folic acid supplements

Folic acid is a water-soluble, B-complex vitamin. It is necessary for the production of new RBCs.

NURSING ACTIONS: Folic acid can be given orally or parenterally.

CLIENT EDUCATION
- Large doses of folic acid can mask vitamin B$_{12}$ deficiency.
- Large doses of folic acid will turn urine dark yellow.

Hydroxyurea

Hydroxyurea is used for clients who have sickle cell disease. It reduces sickling and episodes by promoting hemoglobin production.

THERAPEUTIC PROCEDURES

Blood transfusions

- Blood transfusions lead to an immediate improvement in blood-cell counts and manifestations of anemia.
- Typically only used when the client has significant manifestations of anemia, because of the risk of blood-borne infections.

COMPLICATIONS

Heart failure

Heart failure can develop due to the increased demand on the heart to provide oxygen to tissues. A low Hct decreases the amount of oxygen carried to tissues in the body, which makes the heart work harder and beat faster (tachycardia, palpitations).

NURSING ACTIONS
- Administer oxygen and monitor oxygen saturation.
- Monitor cardiac rhythm.
- Obtain daily weight.
- Monitor the client during a blood transfusion.
- Administer cardiac medications as prescribed (diuretics, antidysrhythmics).
- Administer anti-anemia medications as prescribed.

Active Learning Scenario

A nurse is assisting with preparing a community education program on anemia. What should be included in this presentation? Use the *ATI Active Learning Template: System Disorder* to complete this item.

PATHOPHYSIOLOGY RELATED TO CLIENT PROBLEM: Describe at least three causes of the disorder.

EXPECTED FINDINGS: Identify at least six.

LABORATORY TESTS: Describe the importance of the total iron-binding capacity (TIBC) test.

Application Exercises

1. A nurse is collecting data from a client who has anemia. Which of the following findings should the nurse expect?
   - A. Absent turgor
   - B. Spoon-shaped nails
   - C. Shiny, hairless legs
   - D. Yellow mucous membranes

2. A nurse is contributing to the plan of care for a client who has Hgb 7.5 g/dL and Hct 21.5%. Which of the following actions should the nurse include in the plan of care? (Select all that apply.)
   - A. Provide assistance with ambulation.
   - B. Monitor oxygen saturation.
   - C. Weigh the client weekly.
   - D. Obtain stool specimen for occult blood.
   - E. Schedule daily rest periods.

3. A nurse is reinforcing teaching with a client who has a new prescription for ferrous sulfate. Which of the following information should the nurse include?
   - A. Stools will be dark red.
   - B. Take with a glass of milk if gastrointestinal distress occurs.
   - C. Foods high in vitamin C will promote absorption.
   - D. Take for 14 days.

4. A nurse in a clinic receives a phone call from a client seeking information about a new prescription for erythropoietin. Which of the following information should the nurse review with the client?
   - A. The client needs an erythrocyte sedimentation rate (ESR) test weekly.
   - B. The client should have their hemoglobin checked weekly until stable.
   - C. Oxygen saturation levels should be monitored.
   - D. Folic acid production will increase

5. Match each client statement to the correct category of either Understanding Teaching or Needs Further Teaching regarding reinforcing discharge teaching for a client who had a gastrectomy for stomach cancer.
   - A. "I will need a monthly injection of vitamin B_{12} for the rest of my life."
   - B. "An oral supplement of vitamin B_{12} taken on a daily basis can meet my B_{12} needs."
   - C. "Using the nasal spray form of vitamin B_{12} on a weekly basis can be an option."
   - D. "I should increase my intake of animal proteins, and legumes to increase vitamin B_{12} in my diet."
   - E. "I can add soy milk fortified with vitamin B_{12} to my diet to decrease the risk of pernicious anemia."

Application Exercises Key

1. B. **CORRECT:** When recognizing cues, the nurse should identify those deformities of the nails (such as being spoon-shaped) can be a finding in a client who has anemia.

   Ⓝ *NCLEX® Connection: Physiological Adaptation, Basic Pathophysiology*

2. A, B, D, E. **CORRECT:** The nurse should also plan to obtain the client's stool to test for occult blood, which can identify a possible cause of anemia caused from gastrointestinal bleeding and schedule rest periods throughout the day for the client to rest to decrease fatigue. Rest periods should be planned to conserve energy.

   Ⓝ *NCLEX® Connection: Physiological Adaptation, Basic Pathophysiology*

3. C. **CORRECT:** When taking action and reinforcing teaching a client about a new prescription for ferrous sulfate, the nurse should reinforce with the client that vitamin C enhances the absorption of iron by the intestinal tract.

   Ⓝ *NCLEX® Connection: Pharmacological Therapies, Expected Actions/Outcomes*

4. B. **CORRECT:** When taking action and reviewing information about erythropoietin with a client, the nurse should include that a hemoglobin and hematocrit levels should be monitored weekly until the targeted levels are reached and then continue monthly checks or after a dose adjustment.

   Ⓝ *NCLEX® Connection: Pharmacological Therapies, Medication Administration*

5. **UNDERSTANDS TEACHING:** A, C
   NEEDS FURTHER TEACHING: B, D, E

   Ⓝ *NCLEX® Connection: Pharmacological Therapies, Medication Administration*

Active Learning Scenario Key

Using the ATI Active Learning Template: System Disorder

PATHOPHYSIOLOGY RELATED TO CLIENT PROBLEM: Anemia is an abnormally low amount of circulating red blood cells, hemoglobin concentration, or both. It can be due to blood loss, inadequate production or increased destruction of red blood cells, and dietary deficiencies of folic acid, iron, erythropoietin, and/or vitamin B_{12}.

EXPECTED FINDINGS
- Shortness of breath and fatigue with exertion
- Tachycardia, palpitations, dizziness, or syncope upon standing or with exertion
- Pallor of the nail beds and mucous membranes, nail bed deformities
- Smooth, sore, bright-red tongue
- Irritability, numbness and tingling of extremities, dyspnea on exertion, sensitivity to cold, pain, and hypoxia with sickle-cell crisis

LABORATORY TESTS: A total iron-binding capacity (TIBC) test is an indirect measurement of transferrin, a protein that binds with iron and transports it for storage. Transferrin is an indicator of the total iron stores in the body.

Ⓝ *NCLEX® Connection: Health Promotion and Maintenance, Health Promotion/Disease Prevention*

When reviewing the following chapters, keep in mind the relevant topics and tasks of the NCLEX outline.

Physiological Adaptation

FLUID AND ELECTROLYTE IMBALANCES

Identify signs and symptoms of client fluid and/or electrolyte imbalances.

Provide care for a client with a fluid and electrolyte imbalance.

MEDICAL EMERGENCIES

Review and document client response to emergency interventions.

Reinforce teaching of emergency intervention explanations to client.

BASIC PATHOPHYSIOLOGY: Consider general principles of client disease process when providing care.

UNIT 6   FLUID/ELECTROLYTE/ACID-BASE IMBALANCES

CHAPTER 38 *Fluid Imbalances*

The body maintains homeostasis when the characteristics of body fluid remain in balance: volume, concentration (osmolality), composition (electrolyte concentration), and acidity (pH). In the healthy adult client, 55% to 60% of body weight is comprised of body fluid. This decreases to about 50% to 55% in a healthy older adult client.

Fluid moves between compartments through selectively permeable membranes by a variety of methods (diffusion, active transport, filtration, osmosis) to maintain homeostasis.

Balance is maintained through input and output. Thirst sensation, social factors, and personal habits can impact fluid intakes. Fluid output occurs in all of the following organs, the kidneys, skin, lungs, and GI tract. The kidneys are the major regulator of fluid output.

Volume imbalances occur when too little or too much isotonic fluid is present. Osmolality imbalances occur when body fluid becomes either hypertonic or hypotonic. Hypernatremia (water deficit) and hyponatremia (water excess or intoxication) are good examples of this type of imbalance.

BODY FLUIDS

Body fluids are distributed between two compartments.

Intracellular fluid (ICF)
• Two thirds of body water
• Body fluids within the cell

Extracellular fluid (ECF)
• One third of body water
• Body fluids outside of the cell membrane
• Further divided into parts
  ○ **Intravascular fluid:** The liquid part of blood or the plasma
  ○ **Interstitial fluid:** Located between the cells and outside of the blood vessels
  ○ **Transcellular body fluids:** Secreted by epithelial cells (cerebrospinal, pleural, peritoneal, synovial fluids)

38.1 Intracellular/Extracellular/Plasma

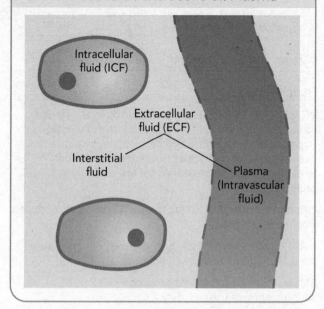

Dehydration

A lack of fluid in the body, from insufficient intake or excessive loss
• Actual dehydration is a lack of fluid in the body; relative dehydration involves a shift of water from the plasma (blood) to the interstitial space.
• Hypovolemia, or isotonic dehydration, is a lack of both water and electrolytes, causing a decrease in circulating blood volume. This is also called fluid volume deficit.

DATA COLLECTION

RISK FACTORS

Causes of isotonic fluid volume deficit (hypovolemia)

• Excessive gastrointestinal (GI) loss: vomiting, nasogastric suctioning, diarrhea
• Excessive skin loss: diaphoresis without sodium and water replacement
• Excessive renal system losses: diuretic therapy, kidney disease, adrenal insufficiency
• Third spacing: burns
• Hemorrhage or plasma loss
• Altered intake: anorexia, nausea, impaired swallowing, confusion, nothing by mouth (NPO) (decreased intake of water and sodium)

Causes of dehydration

• Hyperventilation or excessive perspiration without water treatment
• Prolonged fever
• Diabetic ketoacidosis
• Insufficient water intake (enteral feeding without water administration, decreased thirst sensation, aphasia)

- Diabetes insipidus
- Osmotic diuresis
- Excessive intake of salt, salt tablets, or hypertonic IV fluids

EXPECTED FINDINGS

Hypovolemia

VITAL SIGNS: Hypothermia, tachycardia (in an attempt to maintain a normal blood pressure), thready pulse, hypotension, orthostatic hypotension, decreased central venous pressure, tachypnea (increased respirations to compensate for lack of fluid volume within the body), hypoxia

NEUROMUSCULOSKELETAL: Dizziness, syncope, confusion, weakness, fatigue Qs

GASTROINTESTINAL: Thirst, dry furrowed tongue, nausea, vomiting, anorexia, acute weight loss

RENAL: Oliguria (decreased production and concentration of urine)

OTHER FINDINGS
- Diminished capillary refill, cool clammy skin, diaphoresis, sunken eyeballs, flattened neck veins, poor skin turgor and tenting, weight loss, low central venous pressure
- The effect of fluid imbalance in older adults is greater due to the loss of elasticity of the skin, decrease in glomerular filtration and concentrating ability of the kidneys, loss of muscle mass (muscle tissue holds more body water), and diminished thirst reflex. Ⓒ
- In dehydration, the client can have an elevated temperature (cause or finding). Rapid/severe dehydration can induce seizures.

LABORATORY TESTS

With fluid loss due to hemorrhage, hemoconcentration does not occur.

Hematocrit (Hct): Increased in hypovolemia

BUN: Increased (greater 25 mg/dL) due to hemoconcentration

Urine specific gravity: Greater than 1.030

Blood sodium: Greater than 145 mEq/L with dehydration

Blood osmolality: Greater than 295 mOsm/kg with dehydration/hypernatremia

38.3 Case study

Scenario introduction

1200: Amy is a nurse assisting in an urgent care center caring for Joseph Smith. Mr. Smith presents to the urgent care center with a 2-day history of nausea, diarrhea, anorexia, headache, and abdominal pain.

Scene 1

Amy: "Hello, Mr. Smith. My name is Amy. What brings you to the urgent care center?

Ms. Smith: "I have had a headache for the past 2 days. I have been vomiting and I have diarrhea."

Amy: "Have you been able to eat or drink fluids?"

Mr. Smith: "I'm feeling weak, and I haven't felt like eating."

Scene 2

Amy: "When was the last time you had anything to eat or drink?"

Mr. Smith: "I had a little broth yesterday and some sips of water today."

Scene 3

Amy: "I would like to collect some data, check your vital signs, and obtain some blood work, if that is okay with you."

Mr. Smith: "That's fine, thank you."

Scenario conclusion

Amy documents the following information.

1215
- T 38.6° C (101.5)°F
- BP 108/60 mm Hg
- P 118/min
- R 22/min
- Pulse oximetry 95% on room air
- Bilateral breath sounds are clear and present throughout.
- Neck veins flat
- Skin is warm and dry with poor skin turgor.
- Abdomen is soft, non-distended, hyperactive bowel sounds are present in 4 quadrants.
- Lab work reviewed and charge nurse notified of results:
- Hct 58% (42% to 52%)
- Hgb 20 g/dL (14 g/dL to 18 g/dL)
- Potassium 3.5 mEq/L (3.5 mEq/L to 5 mEq/L)
- Urine specific gravity 1.032 (1.005 to 1.03)

Case study exercises

1. The nurse is collecting data on the client who reports nausea, vomiting, and weakness. Which of the following findings should the nurse recognize are manifestations of fluid volume deficit? (Select all that apply.)

   A. Potassium level

   B. Urine specific gravity

   C. Heart rate

   D. Temperature

   E. Oxygen saturation

2. The nurse is assisting with the plan of care for the client who has fluid volume deficit. What interventions should the nurse include in the plan of care?

PATIENT-CENTERED CARE

NURSING CARE

- Provide oral or IV rehydration therapy.
- Monitor I&O.
- Monitor vital signs. Check orthostatic measurements, as a client is at increased risk of falls when orthostatic hypotension present.
- Monitor for changes in mentation and confusion (an indication of worsening fluid imbalance).
- Monitor weight while fluid replacement is in progress.
- Monitor level of gait stability. Encourage the client to use call light and ask for assistance because of the increased risk for falls. Qs
- Encourage the client to change positions, rolling from side to side or standing up slowly.

INTERPROFESSIONAL CARE

Collaborate with other members of the health care team to determine appropriate fluid volume replacement and oxygen management.

CLIENT EDUCATION

- Drink plenty of liquids to promote hydration.
- Causes of dehydration include vomiting; large, draining wounds; and diarrhea or excessive ostomy losses.

COMPLICATIONS

Hypovolemic shock

- Occurs with significant loss of body fluid.
- The client's mean arterial pressure decreases (which slows blood flow and perfusion to tissues of the body) and the cells are no longer able to carry oxygen to the blood adequately (due to the loss of red blood cells).

NURSING ACTIONS
- Volume replacement is essential.
- Administer oxygen, and monitor oxygen saturation. Oxygen saturation less than 70% is a medical emergency.
- Stay with an unstable client suffering from hypovolemic shock.
- Monitor vital signs at least every 15 min.
- Provide fluid replacement with the following.
  - **Colloids:** whole blood, packed RBCs, plasma, synthetic plasma expanders
  - **Crystalloids:** lactated Ringer's, normal saline
- Assist with administering vasoconstrictors (dopamine, norepinephrine, phenylephrine), agents to improve myocardial perfusion (sodium nitroprusside), and/or positive inotropic medications (dobutamine, milrinone).
- Maintain hemodynamic monitoring.

Overhydration

Too much fluid in the body from excessive intake or ineffective removal from the body
- Fluid overload is an excess of fluid or water, such as with water intoxication. This includes hemodilution, which makes the amount of blood components (blood cells, electrolytes) seem lower.
- Hypervolemia, or fluid volume excess, involves an excess of water and electrolytes, so that the two are still in the right proportions. For example, excessive sodium intake causes the body to retain water, so that there is too much of both.
- Clients who have fluid overload are at risk for developing pulmonary edema or congestive heart failure.
- In older adult clients, the risk of fluid imbalance is greater due to changes in the body with age (such as reduced kidney function). ©

HEALTH PROMOTION AND DISEASE PREVENTION

When clients have known heart disease and impairment of kidney function, it important to instruct the client regarding the following.
- Consume a diet low in sodium. Consult with the provider regarding diet restrictions.
- Restrict fluid intake. Consult with provider regarding prescribed restrictions.

DATA COLLECTION

RISK FACTORS

Causes of hypervolemia

- Compromised regulatory systems (heart failure, kidney disease, cirrhosis)
- Overdose of fluids (oral, enteral, IV)
- Fluid shifts that occur following burns
- Prolonged use of corticosteroids
- Severe stress
- Hyperaldosteronism

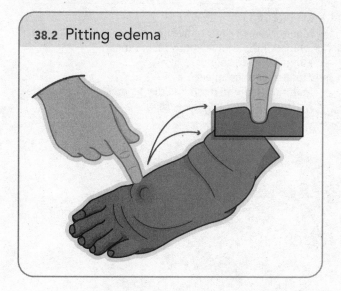

38.2 Pitting edema

Causes of overhydration

- Water replacement without electrolyte replacement, excessive water intake (forced or psychogenic polydipsia)
- Syndrome of inappropriate antidiuretic hormone (SIADH)
- Excessive administration of IV D5W; use of hypotonic solutions for irrigations

EXPECTED FINDINGS

Fluid volume overload

VITAL SIGNS: Tachycardia, bounding pulse, hypertension, tachypnea, increased central venous pressure

NEUROMUSCULAR: Weakness, visual changes, paresthesias, altered level of consciousness, seizures (if severe, sudden hyponatremia/water excess)

GASTROINTESTINAL: Ascites, increased motility, liver enlargement

RESPIRATORY: Crackles, cough, dyspnea

OTHER SIGNS: Peripheral edema due to an excess of fluids within the body and lungs, resulting in weight gain, distended neck veins, and increased urine output, skin cool to touch with pallor

LABORATORY TESTS

- Decreased Hct and Hgb
- Decreased blood osmolarity with water/fluid excess
- Decreased urine sodium and specific gravity
- Decreased BUN due to plasma dilution

DIAGNOSTIC PROCEDURES

Chest x-ray: Reveals possible pulmonary congestion

PATIENT-CENTERED CARE

NURSING CARE

- Monitor I&O.
- Monitor daily weight. A weight gain or loss of 1 kg (2.2 lb) in 24 hr is equivalent to 1 L of fluid.
- Monitor breath sounds.
- Monitor peripheral edema.
- Maintain sodium-restricted diet as prescribed (indicated for isotonic/fluid volume excess).

- Maintain fluid restrictions if prescribed.
- Encourage rest.
- Monitor clients receiving diuretics.
- Encourage the client to discuss use of over-the-counter medications with the provider, as some of these contain sodium.
- Position the client in the semi-Fowler's or Fowler's position and reposition to prevent tissue breakdown in edematous skin.
- Use a pressure-reducing mattress and monitor bony prominence on a regular basis.
- Monitor blood sodium and potassium levels.

INTERPROFESSIONAL CARE

- Respiratory services can be consulted for oxygen management.
- Pulmonology can be consulted if fluid moves into lungs.

CLIENT EDUCATION

- Weigh daily. Notify the provider if there is a 1- to 2-lb gain in 24 hr, or a 3-lb gain in 1 week.
- If excessive sodium intake is the cause of fluid volume excess, consume a low-sodium diet, read food labels to check sodium content, and keep a record of daily sodium intake. Q_{EBP}
- Adhere to fluid restriction. Consult with the provider regarding prescribed restrictions, and divide the 24-hr fluid allotment to allow for fluid intake throughout the day.

COMPLICATIONS

Pulmonary edema

- Pulmonary edema can be caused by severe fluid overload.
- Manifestations include anxiety, tachycardia, increased vein distention, premature ventricular contractions, dyspnea at rest, change in level of consciousness, restlessness, lethargy, ascending crackles (fluid level within lungs), and cough productive of frothy pink-tinged sputum.

NURSING ACTIONS

- Position the client in high-Fowler's to maximize ventilation. Q_{EBP}
- Administer oxygen, positive airway pressure, and/or possible intubation and mechanical ventilation.
- Assist with the administration of morphine, nitrates, and diuretic as prescribed if blood pressure is adequate.

Application Exercises

1. A nurse is assisting with the plan of care for a client who has fluid volume excess. Which of the following interventions should the nurse include in the plan? (Select all that apply.)

   A. Check the client's weight 2 times per week

   B. Place the client in a semi-Fowler's position

   C. Monitor the client's breath sounds

   D. Change the client's position every 4 hrs

   E. Check the client for peripheral edema

2. A nurse is collecting data on two clients. Sort the findings into manifestations associated with either fluid volume deficit or fluid volume excess.

   A. Bounding pulse

   B. Sunken eyeballs

   C. Crackles heard in lung fields

   D. Poor skin turgor

   E. Fever

   F. Distended neck veins

Active Learning Scenario

A nurse is planning care for a client who is experiencing fluid volume excess. What nursing actions should the nurse include in the plan of care? Use the ATI Active Learning Template: System Disorder to complete this item.

NURSING CARE: Describe three interventions the nurse should take.

Active Learning Scenario Key

Using the ATI Active Learning Template: System Disorder

NURSING CARE

- Check CBC and chest x-ray results.
- Position the client in semi-Fowler's to Fowler's position as tolerated.
- Obtain daily weight.
- Monitor intake and output.
- Administer supplemental oxygen as prescribed.
- Ensure that IV flow rates are reduced.
- Administer diuretics (osmotic, loop) as prescribed.
- Limit fluid and sodium intake as prescribed.
- Monitor and document presence of edema (pretibial, sacral, periorbital).
- Reposition the client at least every 2 hr.
- Support arms and legs to decrease dependent edema as appropriate.
- Monitor vital signs and heart rhythm.
- Auscultate lung sounds for crackles.

Ⓝ *NCLEX® Connection: Physiological Adaptation, Fluid and Electrolyte Imbalances*

Case Study Exercises Key

1. B, C, D. **CORRECT:** When recognizing cues, the nurse should identify that concentrated urine, tachycardia, and elevated temperature are manifestations of fluid volume deficit.

Ⓝ *NCLEX® Connection: Physiological Adaptation, Fluid and Electrolyte Imbalances*

2. When generating solutions, the nurse should plan to provide oral or IV rehydration therapy, monitor the client's intake and output, monitor the client's vital signs, monitor for orthostatic hypotension, and encourage the client to change positions slowly. The nurse should plan to monitor the client for changes in mentation and confusion and monitor the client's weight every 8 hr while fluid replacement is in progress. Check the client for gait stability and encourage the client to ask for assistance ambulating to reduce the risk for falls.

Ⓝ *NCLEX® Connection: Physiological Adaptation, Fluid and Electrolyte Imbalances*

Application Exercises Key

1. B, C, E. **CORRECT:** When generating solutions, the nurse should place the client in semi-Fowler's or Fowler's position, and reposition every 2 hrs to reduce the risk for tissue breakdown. The nurse should monitor the client's breath sounds, because the client is at risk for pulmonary edema. The nurse should check the client for peripheral edema.

Ⓝ *NCLEX® Connection: Physiological Adaptation, Fluid and Electrolyte Imbalances*

2. **FLUID VOLUME DEFICIT:** B, D, E;
   FLUID VOLUME EXCESS: A, C, F

   When recognizing cues, the nurse should identify that bounding pulse, crackles heard in lung fields, and distended neck veins are manifestations of fluid volume excess. Sunken eyeballs, poor skin turgor, and fever are manifestations of fluid volume deficit.

Ⓝ *NCLEX® Connection: Physiological Adaptation, Fluid and Electrolyte Imbalances*

CHAPTER 39 ## Electrolyte Imbalances

Electrolytes are charged ions dissolved in body fluids. Cations are positively charged, and anions are negatively charged. Electrolytes are distributed between intracellular (ICF) and extracellular (ECF) fluid compartments. The distributions of ions differs in ICF and ECF. The difference in the concentration of electrolytes in the ICF and ECF maintains cell excitability and allows for the transmission of nerve impulses.

Body fluids should be electrically neutral; the negative and positive ions in the body fluids are equal in number. Electrolytes conduct either a positive (cations: magnesium, potassium, sodium, calcium, and hydrogen ions) or negative (anions: phosphate, sulfate, chloride, bicarbonate, and proteinate ions) electrical current.

Clients can develop an imbalance of electrolytes from an imbalance of intake and output. Clients who are ill and older adult clients are at higher risk of electrolyte imbalance. Although laboratory tests can accurately reflect the electrolyte concentrations in plasma, it is not possible to directly measure electrolyte concentrations within cells.

EXPECTED REFERENCE RANGES

Sodium: 136 to 145 mEq/L

Calcium: 9.0 to 10.5 mg/dL

Potassium: 3.5 to 5.0 mEq/L

Magnesium: 1.3 to 2.1 mEq/L

Chloride: 98 to 106 mEq/L

Phosphorus: 3.0 to 4.5 mg/dL

Sodium imbalances

- Sodium (Na^+) is the major electrolyte (cation) found in ECF, and maintains ECF osmolarity.
- Sodium within ICF is low (14 mEq/L). The difference in ICF and ECF sodium levels is very important in maintaining skeletal muscle contraction, cardiac contraction, and nerve impulse transmission.
- Water flows in the direction of sodium concentration. The ECF sodium level influences fluid retention, excretion, and movement of fluid from one body space to another.
- The kidneys regulate sodium levels with the assistance of aldosterone, antidiuretic hormone (ADH), and natriuretic peptide.

Hyponatremia

Hyponatremia is a net gain of water or loss of sodium-rich fluids that results in sodium levels less than 136 mEq/L.
- Hyponatremia delays and slows the depolarization of membranes.
- Water moves from the ECF into the ICF, causing cells to swell (cellular edema).
- Urine sodium levels helps to differentiate between non-kidney fluid loss (vomiting, diarrhea, and sweating) and kidney salt wasting, which can occur with diuretic use.
- Hyponatremia generally is caused by fluid imbalance, which results in sodium loss.
- Compensatory mechanisms include the kidney excretion of sodium-free water.

DATA COLLECTION

RISK FACTORS

Actual sodium deficits
- Excessive sweating
- Diuretics
- Wound drainage (especially gastrointestinal)
- Nasogastric tube suction of isotonic gastric contents
- Decreased secretion of aldosterone
- Kidney disease
- Inadequate sodium intake (nothing by mouth [NPO] status)
- Liver disease with ascites

Relative sodium deficits due to dilution
- Hypotonic fluid excess (forced oral intake, psychogenic polydipsia, irrigation with hypotonic solutions)
- Kidney failure (nephrotic syndrome)
- Heart failure
- Syndrome of inappropriate ADH secretion
- Older adult clients at a greater risk due to increased incidence of chronic illnesses, use of diuretic medications, and risk for insufficient sodium intake Ⓖ

EXPECTED FINDINGS

- Clinical indicators depend on whether the ECF volume is normal (euvolemic), decreased (hypovolemic), or increased (hypervolemic).
- If the client is hypervolemic with hyponatremia, the pulse quality is usually bounding. The client's blood pressure can be within or above the expected reference range.

VITAL SIGNS (WITH HYPOVOLEMIA): Hypothermia, tachycardia, rapid thready pulse, hypotension, orthostatic hypotension, diminished peripheral pulses

NEUROMUSCULOSKELETAL: Headache, confusion, lethargy, muscle weakness to the point of possible respiratory compromise, fatigue, decreased deep-tendon reflexes (DTRs), seizures, lightheadedness, dizziness

GASTROINTESTINAL: Increased motility, hyperactive bowel sounds, abdominal cramping, nausea, vomiting

LABORATORY TESTS

Blood sodium: Decreased, less than 136 mEq/L

Blood osmolarity: Decreased (except in azotemia with toxin accumulation)

Urine sodium: Less than 20 mEq/L (in sodium loss); greater than 20 mEq/L (in SIADH)

Urine specific gravity: Decreased (1.002 to 1.004 in sodium loss; increased in SIADH)

PATIENT-CENTERED CARE

NURSING CARE

- If the client can tolerate PO fluids, sodium can be easily replaced by intake of foods and fluids. Encourage foods and fluids high in sodium (beef broth, tomato juice).
- Administer IV fluids (lactated Ringer's, 0.9% isotonic saline).
- Replacement of sodium should not exceed 12 mEq/L in a 24-hr period because rapid rise in sodium level risks development of neurologic damage due to demyelination. Qs
- For fluid overload, restrict water intake as prescribed.
- Monitor I&O and daily weight.
- Monitor vital signs and level of consciousness. Report abnormal findings to the provider.

INTERPROFESSIONAL CARE

- Nephrology can be consulted for electrolyte and fluid replacement.
- Respiratory services can be consulted for oxygen management.
- Nutritional services can be consulted for high-sodium food choices and restricting fluid intake. Qtc

CLIENT EDUCATION

- Weigh daily and notify the provider of a 1- to 2-lb gain in 24 hr, or 3-lb (1.4 kg) gain in 1 week.
- Consume a high-sodium diet, including reading food labels to check sodium content and keeping a daily record of sodium intake.

COMPLICATIONS

Severe hyponatremia

Complications (coma, seizures, respiratory arrest) can result from acute hyponatremia if not treated immediately.

NURSING ACTIONS

- The goal is to elevate the blood sodium level enough to decrease neurologic manifestations associated with hyponatremia (lethargy, confusion, seizures).
- Maintain an open airway, and monitor vital signs.
- Maintain seizure precautions, and take appropriate action if seizures occur.
- Monitor level of consciousness.
- Assist with administering hypertonic oral and IV fluids as prescribed.
- Ensure the administration of 3% sodium chloride slowly, and monitor sodium levels frequently.
- Administer medications as prescribed (such as conivaptan or tolvaptan, which promote excretion of excess fluid).

Hypernatremia

Increased sodium causes hypertonicity of the blood. This causes a shift of water out of the cells, resulting in dehydrated cells.

- Hypernatremia is a blood sodium level greater than 145 mEq/L.
- Hypernatremia is a serious electrolyte imbalance. It can cause significant neurologic, endocrine, and cardiac disturbances.

DATA COLLECTION

RISK FACTORS

Actual sodium excess

- Kidney failure
- Cushing's syndrome
- Aldosteronism
- Excessive intake of oral sodium

Relative sodium excess due to decreased fluid volume

- Water deprivation (NPO)
- Hypertonic enteral feedings without adequate water supplement
- Diabetes insipidus
- Heatstroke

- Hyperventilation
- Watery stools
- Burns
- Excessive sweating
- High sodium dietary intake

EXPECTED FINDINGS

- Thirst
- Dry, sticky mucous membranes
- Red, swollen tongue
- Hot, dry skin
- Flushing
- Oliguria
- Decrease in sweating

VITAL SIGNS: Hyperthermia, tachycardia, orthostatic hypotension

NEUROMUSCULOSKELETAL: Restlessness, irritability, muscle twitching to the point of muscle weakness, decreased or absent DTRs, seizures, coma

GASTROINTESTINAL: Nausea, vomiting, anorexia, occasional diarrhea

LABORATORY TESTS

Blood sodium: Increased to greater than 145 mEq/L

Blood osmolarity: Increased to greater than 300 mOsm/L

Urine specific gravity and osmolarity: Increased

PATIENT-CENTERED CARE

NURSING CARE

- Monitor level of consciousness, and ensure safety.
- Monitor vital signs and heart rhythm.
- Auscultate lung sounds.
- Provide oral hygiene and other comfort measures to decrease thirst, and encourage fluid intake.
- Monitor I&O, and alert the provider of inadequate urinary output.
- Monitor potassium level if diuretics are administered.

Fluid loss

Based on blood osmolarity and hemodynamic stability
- Dextrose 5% in 0.45% sodium chloride is a hypertonic solution prior to infusion. However, once infused, the glucose rapidly metabolizes and it becomes a hypotonic solution.
- 0.3% sodium chloride can be prescribed as a hypotonic solution, which provides a more gradual reduction in blood sodium levels and reduces the risk of cerebral edema. This is the preferred IV solution if the client also has severe hyperglycemia.
- Dextrose 5% in water and 0.9% sodium chloride are isotonic solutions.

Excess sodium

- Encourage water intake, and discourage sodium intake.
- Administer diuretics (loop diuretics) for clients who have poor kidney excretion.

INTERPROFESSIONAL CARE

Nutritional services can be consulted for low-sodium food choices and to restrict fluid intake. Q℠

CLIENT EDUCATION

- Weigh daily. Notify the provider of a 1- to 2-lb gain in 24 hr, or 3-lb (1.4 kg) gain in 1 week.
- Consume a low-sodium diet, read food labels for sodium content, and keep a record of daily sodium intake.
- Adhere to fluid intake as prescribed.
- Over-the-counter medications that contain sodium bicarbonate can increase sodium levels.

COMPLICATIONS

Severe hypernatremia

Seizures, convulsion, and death can result from severe hypernatremia if not treated immediately.

NURSING ACTIONS
- Maintain open airway, and monitor vital signs.
- Maintain seizure precautions, and take appropriate action if seizures occur.
- Monitor level of consciousness.

Potassium imbalances

- Potassium (K^+) is the major cation in ICF. 98% of the body's potassium is within the cells.
- Potassium plays a vital role in cell metabolism; transmission of nerve impulses; functioning of cardiac, lung, and muscle tissues; and acid–base balance.
- Potassium has a reciprocal action with sodium.
- Minor variations in the level of potassium in the body is a significant finding.

Hypokalemia

Hypokalemia is the result of an increased loss of potassium from the body or movement of potassium into the cells, resulting in a blood potassium less than 3.5 mEq/L.

DATA COLLECTION

RISK FACTORS

Actual potassium deficits
- Overuse of diuretics, digitalis, corticosteroids
- Increased secretion of aldosterone
- Cushing's syndrome
- Loss via GI tract: vomiting, diarrhea, prolonged nasogastric suctioning, and excessive use of laxatives or tap water enema administered repeatedly because tap water is hypotonic, and gastrointestinal losses are isotonic
- NPO status
- Kidney disease, which impairs the reabsorption of potassium

Relative potassium deficit
- Alkalosis
- Hyperinsulinism
- Hyperalimentation
- Total parenteral nutrition
- Water intoxication
- Older adult clients due to increased use of diuretics and laxatives ©

EXPECTED FINDINGS

VITAL SIGNS: Decreased blood pressure; weak, irregular pulse; orthostatic hypotension

NEUROLOGIC: Altered mental status, anxiety, and lethargy that progresses to acute confusion and coma

CARDIOVASCULAR: Dysrhythmias

GASTROINTESTINAL: Hypoactive bowel sounds, nausea, vomiting, constipation, abdominal pain and distention. Paralytic ileus can develop.

MUSCULAR: Weakness, leg cramps. Deep-tendon reflexes can be reduced.

RESPIRATORY: Shallow breathing

LABORATORY TESTS

Blood potassium: Decreased to less than 3.5 mEq/L

ABGs: Evaluate acid-base status (alkalosis)

DIAGNOSTIC PROCEDURES

Electrocardiogram (ECG): Inverted/flat T waves, ST depression. An elevated U wave is a finding specific to hypokalemia. Other dysrhythmias possible.

PATIENT-CENTERED CARE

NURSING CARE

- Administer prescribed potassium replacement. Never give potassium via IM or subcutaneous route, which can cause necrosis of the tissues.
- Monitor and maintain adequate urine output.
- Observe for shallow ineffective respirations and diminished breath sounds.
- Monitor cardiac rhythm, and report unexpected findings.
- Monitor clients receiving digoxin. Hypokalemia increases the risk for digoxin toxicity.
- Monitor level of consciousness, and maintain client safety.
- Monitor bowel sounds and abdominal distention, and intervene as needed.
- Monitor oxygen saturation levels, which should remain greater than 95%.
- Check hand grasps for muscle weakness.
- Check DTRs.
- Implement fall precautions due to muscle weakness.

Oral replacement of potassium

- Encourage foods high in potassium: avocados, broccoli, dairy products, dried fruit, cantaloupe, bananas, juices, melon, lean meats, milk, whole grains, and citrus fruits. Salt substitutes are high in potassium and can facilitate increased oral potassium intake.
- Provide oral potassium medications.

IV potassium supplementation

- Never administer by IV bolus (high risk of cardiac arrest).
- Do not give IV potassium unless urine output is at least 30 mL/hr.
- Monitor IV site for phlebitis (tissue irritant).

INTERPROFESSIONAL CARE

- Nephrology can be consulted for electrolyte and fluid management.
- Respiratory services can be consulted for oxygen management.
- Nutritional services can be consulted for food choices and potassium-rich foods.
- Cardiology can be consulted for dysrhythmias.

CLIENT EDUCATION

- Understand which potassium-rich foods to consume.
- Prevent a decrease in potassium by avoiding excessive use of diuretics and laxatives.

COMPLICATIONS

Respiratory failure

NURSING ACTIONS
- Maintain an open airway, and monitor vital signs.
- Monitor level of consciousness.
- Monitor for hypoxemia and hypercapnia.
- Assist with intubation and mechanical ventilation if indicated.

Cardiac arrest

NURSING ACTIONS
- Assist with maintaining continuous cardiac monitoring.
- Report dysrhythmias promptly.

Hyperkalemia

Hyperkalemia is the result of an increased intake of potassium, movement of potassium out of the cells, or inadequate kidney excretion resulting in a blood potassium level greater than 5.0 mEq/L.

Increased risk of cardiac arrest

DATA COLLECTION

RISK FACTORS

Clients who are chronically ill

Actual potassium excess
- Older adult clients due to decreases in renin and aldosterone, and increased use of salt substitutes, ACE inhibitors, and potassium-sparing diuretics Ⓖ
- Overconsumption of high-potassium foods or salt substitutes
- Excessive or rapid potassium replacement (oral or IV)
- RBC transfusions
- Adrenal insufficiency
- ACE inhibitors or potassium-sparing diuretics
- Kidney failure
- Digitalis toxicity

Relative potassium excess
- Extracellular shift caused from decreased insulin production
- Acidosis (diabetic ketoacidosis)
- Tissue damage (sepsis, trauma, burns surgery, fever, myocardial infarction)
- Intestinal obstruction

EXPECTED FINDINGS

Vital signs: Slow irregular pulse, hypotension

Neuromusculoskeletal: Restlessness, irritability, weakness to the point of ascending flaccid paralysis, paresthesia

Cardiovascular: Dysrhythmias

Gastrointestinal: Increased motility, diarrhea, hyperactive bowel sounds, nausea, abdominal cramping

LABORATORY TESTS

Blood potassium: Increased to greater than 5.0 mEq/L

Hemoglobin and hematocrit
- Increased with dehydration
- Decreased with kidney failure

BUN and creatinine: Increased with kidney failure

Arterial blood gases: Metabolic acidosis (pH less than 7.35) with kidney failure

DIAGNOSTIC PROCEDURES

Electrocardiogram: Peaked T waves, prolonged PR and wide QRS, possible dysrhythmias (heart block)

PATIENT-CENTERED CARE

NURSING CARE

Priority nursing care is to prevent falls, collect data for cardiac complications, and reinforce health teaching.
- Monitor cardiac rhythm, and report unexpected findings.
- Monitor I&O.
- Check for muscle weakness.
- Observe for GI manifestations, such as nausea and intestinal colic.
- For clients who have elevated potassium levels, report and stop IV infusion of potassium, maintain IV access, stop all potassium supplements, and promote a potassium-restricted diet.
- Monitor for manifestations of hypokalemia while receiving medications to reduce the potassium level.
- Monitor blood potassium levels.
- Severe hyperkalemia can require administration of calcium gluconate. Chronic or severe hyperkalemia can require dialysis.
- Promote movement of potassium from ECF to ICF. The nurse should monitor the administration of:
  - IV fluids with dextrose and regular insulin.
  - Sodium bicarbonate to reverse acidosis.

Prevention of hyperkalemia
- Encourage the client to avoid foods high in potassium (citrus fruits, legumes, whole-grain foods, lean meat, milk, eggs, cocoa, some cola beverages). Encourage the client to read food labels for potassium content.
- Fruits and juices low in potassium include raw apples, cranberries, grapes, canned peaches, and cranberry and grape juice. Vegetables low in potassium include lettuce, cabbage, cucumbers, green peppers, sweet onions, green peas, and green beans. It is possible to reduce the content of most vegetables by leaching them (slice, peel, soak overnight, drain water, and boil). Refined grains have less potassium than whole grains and cereals. Beverages low in potassium include brewed tea and coffee, ginger ale, and root beer. Other food items with low potassium content include applesauce, angel food cake, butter, margarine, hard candy, sugar, and honey.
- Clients who have impaired kidney function and are taking potassium-conserving diuretics should not receive potassium replacement or salt substitutes.

MEDICATIONS

To increase potassium excretion

Loop diuretics (furosemide)

- Administer if kidney function is adequate.
- Loop diuretics increase the depletion of potassium from the renal system.

NURSING ACTIONS
- Monitor intake and output.
- Ensure IV access.
  - Monitor weight daily.
  - Observe for edema.
- Check for fluid depletion dizziness, tachycardia, and orthostatic hypotension.

Cation exchange resins

Sodium polystyrene sulfonate works in the intestine and excretes excess potassium from the body through the feces.

NURSING ACTIONS: If potassium levels are extremely high, dialysis can be required.

CLIENT EDUCATION
- Adhere to a potassium-restricted diet.
- Hold oral potassium supplements until advised by the provider.

IV insulin and glucose

Lowers blood potassium by causing potassium to shift into intracellular space.

INTERPROFESSIONAL CARE

- Nephrology can be consulted if dialysis is needed and for electrolyte and fluid management.
- Nutritional services can be consulted for food choices containing potassium-restricted foods.
- Cardiology can be consulted for dysrhythmias.

CLIENT EDUCATION

- Remember which potassium-restricted foods to consume.
- Prevent an increase in potassium by reading food labels and avoiding salt substitutes containing potassium. Qᴘᴄᴄ

COMPLICATIONS

Cardiac arrest

NURSING ACTIONS
- Monitor for dysrhythmias.
- Perform continuous cardiac monitoring.

Other electrolyte imbalances

CALCIUM: Hypocalcemia, hypercalcemia

CHLORIDE: Hypochloremia, hyperchloremia

MAGNESIUM: Hypomagnesemia, hypermagnesemia

PHOSPHORUS: Hypophosphatemia, hyperphosphatemia

In particular, nurses should be aware of the implications of hypocalcemia and hypomagnesemia.

Hypocalcemia

Hypocalcemia is a total blood calcium less than 9.0 mg/dL.

DATA COLLECTION Qᴘᴄᴄ

RISK FACTORS

Actual calcium deficit

- Inadequate intake of calcium, including lactose intolerance, malabsorption issues
- Diarrhea or steatorrhea
- Inadequate vitamin D intake
- End-stage kidney disease
- Metastatic cancer
- Abuse of phosphate laxatives and enemas
- Bariatric surgery

Relative calcium deficit

- Conditions: alkalosis, acute pancreatitis, hypomagnesemia, hyperphosphatemia, immobility
- Treatments: calcium chelators, citrate
- Immobility
- Parathyroid removal or damage, causing hyposecretion of parathyroid hormone, necessary for calcium regulation.

EXPECTED FINDINGS

Tetany is the most common manifestation seen in clients in a hypocalcemic state. It is caused by neural excitability-spontaneous discharges from both the sensory and motor fibers (peripheral nerves).
- Paresthesia of the fingers and lips (early manifestation)
- Muscle twitches as hypocalcemia progresses
- Seizure due to irritability of the central nervous system
- Frequent, painful muscle spasms at rest in the foot or calf (Charley horses)
- Hyperactive DTRs
- Positive Chvostek's sign (tapping on the facial nerve triggering facial twitching)
- Positive Trousseau's sign (hand/finger spasms with sustained blood pressure cuff inflation)
- History of thyroid surgery or irradiation of the upper chest or neck, which places a client at risk for developing hypocalcemia
- Laryngospasm if severe

CARDIOVASCULAR: Decreased heart rate and hypotension when hypocalcemia is severe

GASTROINTESTINAL: Hyperactive bowel sounds, diarrhea, and abdominal cramps

OTHER MANIFESTATIONS: Anxiety, confusion

LABORATORY TESTS

- Calcium level less than 9.0 mg/dL.
- Decreased blood albumin level can make the total blood calcium level falsely low.
- The ionized calcium level should give the true calcium level when the client appears to have hypocalcemia with hypoalbuminemia.

DIAGNOSTIC PROCEDURES

Electrocardiogram changes: Prolonged QT and ST interval, dysrhythmias, bradycardia, ventricular tachycardia

PATIENT-CENTERED CARE

NURSING CARE

- Ensure the administration of oral or IV calcium supplements. Vitamin D supplements enhance the absorption of calcium.
- Implement seizure and fall precautions.
- Avoid overstimulation. Keep the client's room quiet, limit visitors, and use soft lighting in the room.
- Have emergency equipment on standby.
- Encourage foods high in calcium, including dairy products, canned salmon, sardines, fresh oysters, and dark leafy green vegetables.
- A client exhibiting life-threatening manifestations of hypocalcemia will require rapid treatment with calcium gluconate or calcium chloride (not used as often due to risk of tissue damage if infiltrated). IV administration should be diluted in dextrose 5% and water and given as a bolus infusion (using an infusion pump) by an RN. If administered too quickly, cardiac arrest could occur.

INTERPROFESSIONAL CARE

- Endocrinology can be consulted for electrolyte and fluid management.
- Respiratory services can be consulted for oxygen management.
- Nutritional services can be consulted for food choices high in calcium. Qᴛᴄ
- Cardiology can be consulted for dysrhythmias.

CLIENT EDUCATION

- Consume foods high in calcium (yogurt, milk).
- Increase calcium in diet by reading food labels.

39.1 Case study

Scenario introduction

0800: John is a nurse on a medical-surgical unit assisting with the care of Joseph Smith. Mr. Smith has been admitted following a 2-day history of nausea, diarrhea, anorexia, headache, and abdominal pain.

Scene 1

John: "Hello, Mr. Smith. My name is John. How are you feeling?
Mr. Smith: "I still have abdominal cramps and I have numbness and tingling in my hands and feet."

Scene 2

John: "I would like to collect some data, check your vital signs, and review your laboratory results."
Mr. Smith: "That's fine, thank you."

Scenario conclusion

John documents the following information.

0815
- T 38.6° C (101.5)°F)
- BP 106/58 mm Hg
- P 106/min
- R 18/min
- Pulse oximetry 96% on room air
- Bilateral breath sounds are clear and present throughout.
- Neck veins flat
- Skin is warm and dry with poor skin turgor.
- Fine muscle twitching noted in fingers
- Abdomen is non-distended, hyperactive bowel sounds are present in 4 quadrants
- Positive Chvostek's and Trousseau's signs noted.
- Lab work reviewed and provider notified of results:
- Potassium 3.4 mEq/L (3.5 mEq/L to 5 mEq/L)
- Calcium 7.8 mg/dL (9 to 10.5 mg/dL)
- Magnesium 1.3 mEq/L (1.3 to 2.1 mEq/L)

Case study exercises

1. The nurse is checking the client for the Chvostek's sign. Which of the following actions should the nurse take?

   A. Apply a blood pressure cuff to the client's arm.

   B. Place a stethoscope bell over the client's carotid artery.

   C. Ask the client to lower their chin to their chest.

   D. Tap lightly on the client's cheek.

2. The nurse is collecting data on the client who reports nausea, vomiting, and weakness. Which of the following findings are manifestations of hypocalcemia? (Select all that apply.)

   A. Tingling in fingers

   B. Poor skin turgor

   C. Abdominal pain

   D. Elevated temperature

   E. Muscle twitching

Hypomagnesemia

Hypomagnesemia is a blood magnesium level less than 1.3 mg/dL.

DATA COLLECTION

RISK FACTORS

- Celiac disease, Crohn's disease, acute pancreatitis
- Malnutrition (insufficient magnesium intake)
- Ethanol ingestion (magnesium excretion)
- Diarrhea, steatorrhea, or chronic laxative use
- Steatorrhea
- Myocardial infarction or heart failure
- Concurrent hypokalemia and hypocalcemia
- Medication therapy (aminoglycoside antibiotics, amphotericin B, loop diuretics)
- Pancreatitis, chronic alcoholism

EXPECTED FINDINGS

Cardiovascular: Risk for increased blood pressure and dysrhythmias

Neuromuscular: Increased nerve impulse transmission (hyperactive DTRs, paresthesias, muscle tetany, seizures), positive Chvostek's and Trousseau's signs

Gastrointestinal: Hypoactive bowel sounds, constipation, abdominal distention, paralytic ileus

Other: Possible depressed mood, apathy, seizures, or agitation

DIAGNOSTIC PROCEDURES

Electrocardiogram changes: Prolonged QT intervals

PATIENT-CENTERED CARE

NURSING CARE

- Correct concurrent imbalance of other electrolytes to prevent worsening of either condition.
- Encourage foods high in magnesium (dark green vegetables, nuts, whole grains, seafood, peanut butter, cocoa). If there is mild hypomagnesemia, dietary changes can be used to correct it.
- Discontinue magnesium-depleting medications (loop diuretics, osmotic diuretics, medications that contain phosphorus).
- Administer oral magnesium sulfate for mild hypomagnesemia. Oral magnesium can cause diarrhea and increase magnesium depletion.
- IV magnesium sulfate is prescribed if hypomagnesemia is severe. Monitor DTRs hourly during administration.
- Monitor clients taking digitalis closely if magnesium is low because it predisposes the client to digitalis toxicity.
- Have calcium gluconate readily available to reverse hypermagnesemia.

INTERPROFESSIONAL CARE

- Endocrinology can be consulted for electrolyte and fluid management.
- Respiratory services can be consulted for oxygen management.
- Nutritional services can be consulted for food choices high in magnesium.
- Cardiology can be consulted for dysrhythmias.

CLIENT EDUCATION

- Intake foods that are high in magnesium.
- Increase magnesium in diet by reading food labels.

Application Exercises

1. A nurse is assisting with the care of a client who has a nasogastric tube attached to low intermittent suctioning. The nurse should monitor the client for which electrolyte imbalances?

2. A nurse is assisting with teaching a class about electrolyte imbalances. The nurse should include that which of the following conditions places a client at risk for hyperkalemia?
   - A. Diabetic ketoacidosis
   - B. Heart failure
   - C. Cushing's syndrome
   - D. Thyroidectomy

Active Learning Scenario

A nurse is caring for a client who has hypokalemia. Use the ATI Active Learning Template: System Disorder to complete this item.

ALTERATION IN HEALTH (DIAGNOSIS)

NURSING CARE: Describe at least six actions.

INTERPROFESSIONAL CARE: Describe one action.

CLIENT EDUCATION: Describe one teaching point.

COMPLICATIONS: Describe one.

Active Learning Scenario Key

Using the ATI Active Learning Template: System Disorder

ALTERATION IN HEALTH (DIAGNOSIS): Hypokalemia is the result of an increased loss of potassium from the body or movement of potassium into the cells, resulting in a blood potassium less than 3.5 mEq/L.

NURSING CARE

- Report abnormal findings to the provider.
- Replacement of potassium
  - Encourage foods high in potassium (avocados, broccoli, dairy products, dried fruit, cantaloupe, bananas, juices, melon, lean meats, milk, whole grains, and citrus fruits).
  - Provide oral potassium supplementation.
- Assist with providing IV potassium supplementation.
  - Never administer by IV bolus (high risk of cardiac arrest).
  - Check IV site for phlebitis (tissue irritant).
- Potassium must never be given by IM or subcutaneous route, which can cause necrosis of the tissues.
- Monitor and maintain adequate urine output.
- Observe for shallow ineffective respirations and diminished breath sounds.
- Monitor cardiac rhythm, and report unexpected findings.
- Monitor clients receiving digoxin. Hypokalemia increases the risk for digoxin toxicity.
- Monitor level of consciousness, and maintain client safety.
- Monitor bowel sounds and abdominal distention, and intervene as needed.
- Monitor oxygen saturation levels, which should remain greater than 95%.
- Check hand grasps for muscle weakness.
- Check deep-tendon reflexes.

INTERPROFESSIONAL CARE

- Nephrology can be consulted for electrolyte and fluid management.
- Respiratory services can be consulted for oxygen management.
- Nutritional services can be consulted for food choices and potassium-rich foods.
- Cardiology can be consulted for dysrhythmias.

CLIENT EDUCATION

- Understand which potassium-rich foods to consume.
- Prevent a decrease in potassium by avoiding excessive use of diuretics and laxatives.

COMPLICATIONS

- Respiratory failure
- Cardiac arrest

Ⓝ *NCLEX® Connection: Physiological Adaptation, Fluid and Electrolyte Imbalances*

Case Study Exercises Key

1. D. **CORRECT:** When taking actions, the nurse should tap the client's cheek over the facial nerve just below and anterior to the ear to elicit Chvostek's sign. A positive response is indicated when the client exhibits facial twitching on this side of the face.

   Ⓝ *NCLEX® Connection: Physiological Adaptation, Fluid and Electrolyte Imbalances*

2. A, C, E. **CORRECT:** When analyzing cues, the nurse should identify that numbness and tingling in fingers and toes, abdominal cramps and diarrhea, and muscle twitching are manifestations of hypocalcemia.

   Ⓝ *NCLEX® Connection: Physiological Adaptation, Fluid and Electrolyte Imbalances*

Application Exercises Key

1. When taking actions, the nurse should monitor the client who has a nasogastric tube for hyponatremia and hypokalemia due to loss of these electrolytes through gastric drainage.

   Ⓝ *NCLEX® Connection: Physiological Adaptation, Fluid and Electrolyte Imbalances*

2. A. **CORRECT:** When taking actions, the nurse should instruct that diabetic ketoacidosis places a client at risk for hyperkalemia. During acidosis, hydrogen enters cells and potassium is pushed out of cells, causing blood potassium levels to rise.

   Ⓝ *NCLEX® Connection: Physiological Adaptation, Fluid and Electrolyte Imbalances*

UNIT 6   FLUID/ELECTROLYTE/ACID-BASE IMBALANCES

CHAPTER 40 *Acid-Base Imbalances*

For cells to function optimally, metabolic processes must maintain a steady balance between the acids and bases found in the body. Acid-base balance represents homeostasis of hydrogen (H^+) ion concentration in body fluids. Hydrogen shifts between the extracellular and intracellular compartments to compensate for acid-base imbalances. Minor changes in hydrogen concentration have major effects on normal cellular function.

Arterial pH is an indirect measurement of hydrogen ion concentration and is a result of respiratory and kidney compensation function. Arterial blood gases (ABGs) are most commonly used to evaluate acid-base balance. The pH is the expression of the balance between carbon dioxide (CO_2), which is regulated by the lungs, and bicarbonate (HCO_3^-), a base regulated by the kidneys. The greater the concentration of hydrogen, the more acidic the body fluids and the lower the pH. The lower the concentration of hydrogen, the more alkaline the body fluids and the higher the pH.

MAINTENANCE OF ACID-BASE BALANCE

Acid-base balance is maintained by chemical, respiratory, and kidney function.

Chemical (bicarbonate and intracellular fluid) and protein buffers (albumin and globulins)
- First line of defense
- Either bind or release hydrogen ions as needed
- Respond quickly to changes in pH QEBP

Respiratory buffers
- Second line of defense
- Control the level of hydrogen ions in the blood through the control of CO_2 levels
- When a chemoreceptor senses a change in the level of CO_2, a signal is sent to the brain to alter the rate and depth of respirations.
  - **Hyperventilation:** Triggered by an increase in CO_2. Results in a decrease in hydrogen ions (exhalation of excess hydrogen ions)
  - **Hypoventilation:** Triggered by a decrease in CO_2. Results in an increase in hydrogen ions (retaining hydrogen ions)

Kidney buffers
- Kidneys are the third line of defense.
- This buffering system is much slower to respond, but it is the most effective buffering system with the longest duration.
- Kidneys control the movement of bicarbonate in the urine. Bicarbonate can be reabsorbed into the bloodstream or excreted in the urine in response to blood levels of hydrogen.
- Kidneys can also produce more bicarbonate when needed.
  - High hydrogen ions: (pH less than 7.35): Bicarbonate reabsorption and production
  - Low hydrogen ions: (pH greater than 7.45): Bicarbonate excretion

COMPENSATION

Compensation refers to the process by which the body attempts to correct changes and imbalances in pH levels.
- Full compensation occurs when the pH level of the blood returns to normal (7.35 to 7.45).
- If the pH level is not able to normalize, it is referred to as partial compensation.

40.1 Compensation

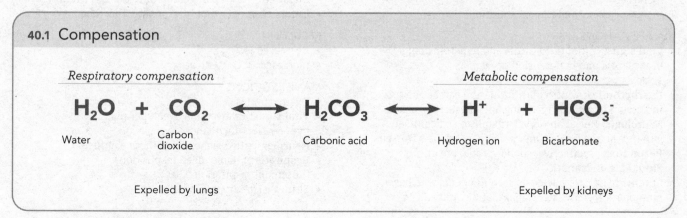

Respiratory compensation   *Metabolic compensation*

$$H_2O + CO_2 \longleftrightarrow H_2CO_3 \longleftrightarrow H^+ + HCO_3^-$$

Water   Carbon dioxide   Carbonic acid   Hydrogen ion   Bicarbonate

Expelled by lungs   Expelled by kidneys

EXAMPLES

- Metabolic alkalosis, metabolic acidosis, respiratory alkalosis, and respiratory acidosis are examples of acid-base imbalances.
- Acid-base imbalances are a result of insufficient compensation. Respiratory and kidney function play a large role in the body's ability to effectively compensate for acid-base alterations. Organ dysfunction negatively affects acid-base compensation. (40.1) Q EBP

HEALTH PROMOTION AND DISEASE PREVENTION

- Encourage a healthy diet and physical activity.
- Limit the consumption of alcohol.
- Encourage drinking six to eight cups of water daily.
- Maintain an appropriate weight for height and body frame.
- Promote smoking cessation.

DATA COLLECTION

RISK FACTORS

Respiratory acidosis: Hypoventilation

RESULTS FROM

- Respiratory depression from opioids, poisons, anesthetics
- Clients who have brain tumors, cerebral aneurysm, stroke or overhydration, trauma, or neurologic diseases (myasthenia gravis, Guillain-Barré when respiratory effort is affected)
- Inadequate chest expansion due to muscle weakness, pneumothorax/hemothorax, flail chest, obesity, sleep apnea, tumors, or deformities
- Airway obstruction that occurs from neck edema, or localized lymph node enlargement, foreign bodies or mucus
- Alveolar-capillary blockage secondary to a pulmonary embolus, thrombus, acute respiratory distress syndrome, chest trauma, drowning, or pulmonary edema
- Inadequate mechanical ventilation

RESULTS IN

- Increased CO_2
- Increased or normal H^+ concentration

MANIFESTATIONS

- **Vital signs:** Initial tachycardia and hypertension; bradycardia and hypotension develop as acidosis worsens
- **Dysrhythmias:** Ventricular fibrillation can be the first indication in a client receiving anesthesia.
- **Neurologic:** Initial anxiety, irritability, and confusion; lethargy and possibly coma develop as acidosis worsens
- **Respiratory:** Ineffective, shallow, rapid breathing
- **Skin:** Pale or cyanotic
- Chronic respiratory acidosis seen in clients who have pulmonary disease, sleep apnea, and obesity

NURSING CARE: Oxygen therapy, maintain patent airway, and enhance gas exchange (positioning and breathing techniques, ventilatory support, bronchodilators, mucolytics). Q s

Respiratory alkalosis: Hyperventilation

RESULTS FROM

- Hyperventilation due to fear, anxiety, intracerebral trauma, salicylate toxicity, or excessive mechanical ventilation
- Hypoxemia from asphyxiation, high altitudes, shock, or early-stage asthma or pneumonia

RESULTS IN

- Decreased CO_2
- Decreased or normal H^+ concentration

MANIFESTATIONS

- **Vital signs:** Tachypnea
- **Neurologic:** Inability to concentrate, numbness, tingling, tinnitus, and possible loss of consciousness
- **Cardiovascular:** Tachycardia, ventricular, and atrial dysrhythmias
- **Respiratory:** Rapid, deep respirations

NURSING CARE: Oxygen therapy, anxiety reduction interventions, and rebreathing techniques

Metabolic acidosis

RESULTS FROM

- Excess production of hydrogen ions
- Diabetic ketoacidosis (DKA)
- Starvation
- Lactic acidosis can result from:
  - Heavy exercise
  - Seizure activity
  - Hypoxia
- Excessive intake of acids
  - Ethyl alcohol
  - Methyl alcohol
  - Acetylsalicylic acid (aspirin)
- Inadequate elimination of hydrogen ions
  - Kidney failure
  - Severe lung problems
- Inadequate production of bicarbonate
  - Kidney failure
  - Pancreatitis
- Impaired liver or pancreatic function: Liver failure
- Excess elimination of bicarbonate: Diarrhea

RESULTS IN

- Decreased HCO_3^-
- Increased H^+ concentration

MANIFESTATIONS

- Dysrhythmias
- **Vital signs:** Bradycardia, weak peripheral pulses, hypotension, tachypnea
- **Neurologic:** Headache, drowsiness, confusion
- **Respiratory:** Rapid, deep respirations (Kussmaul respirations)
- **Skin:** Warm, dry, pink

NURSING CARE: Varies with causes. If DKA, administer insulin. If related to GI losses, administer antidiarrheals and provide rehydration. If blood bicarbonate is low, administer sodium bicarbonate 1 mEq/kg.

Metabolic alkalosis

RESULTS FROM

- Base excess
- Oral ingestion of excess amount of bases (antacids)
- Venous administration of bases (blood transfusions, total parenteral nutrition, or sodium bicarbonate)
- Acid deficit
  ○ Loss of gastric secretions (through prolonged vomiting, nasogastric suction)
  ○ Potassium depletion (due to thiazide diuretics, laxative overuse, Cushing's syndrome, hyperaldosteronism)
- Increased digitalis toxicity

RESULTS IN

- Increased HCO_3^-
- Decreased H^+ concentration

MANIFESTATIONS

- **Vital signs:** Tachycardia, normotensive or hypotensive
- **Dysrhythmias:** Atrial tachycardia, ventricular issues when pH increases
- **Neurologic:** Numbness, tingling, tetany, muscle weakness, hyperreflexia, confusion, convulsion
- **Respiratory:** Depressed skeletal muscles resulting in ineffective breathing

NURSING CARE: Varies with causes (GI losses: administer antiemetics, fluids, and electrolyte replacements). If related to potassium depletion, discontinue causative agent.

DIAGNOSTIC PROCEDURES

To determine the type of imbalance, follow these steps. (40.2)

STEP 1: **Look at pH.**
- If less than 7.35, identify as acidosis.
- If greater than 7.45, identify as alkalosis. Q**EBP**

STEP 2: **Look at $PaCO_2$ and HCO_3^- simultaneously.**
- Determine which is in the expected reference range.
- Conclude that the other is the indicator of imbalance.
- Identify $PaCO_2$ less than 35 or greater than 45 mm Hg as respiratory in origin.
- Identify HCO_3^- less than 21 or greater than 28 mEq/L as metabolic in origin.

STEP 3: **Combine diagnoses of Steps 1 and 2 to name the type of imbalance.**

STEP 4: **Evaluate the PaO_2 and SaO_2.** If the results are less than the expected reference range, the client is hypoxic.

STEP 5: **Determine compensation as follows.**
- **Uncompensated:** The pH is outside the expected reference range, and either the HCO_3^- or the $PaCO_2$ is outside the expected reference range.
- **Partially compensated:** The pH, HCO_3^-, and $PaCO_2$ are outside the expected reference range.
- **Fully compensated:** The pH is within the expected reference range, but the $PaCO_2$ and HCO_3^- are both outside the expected reference range. Looking at the pH will provide a clue as to which system initiated the problem, respiratory or metabolic. If the pH is less than 7.40, think "acidosis," and determine which system has the acidosis value. If the pH is greater than 7.40, think "alkalosis," and determine which system has the alkalosis value.

PATIENT-CENTERED CARE

NURSING CARE

- For all acid-base imbalances, it is imperative to treat the underlying cause.
- Education can vary in relation to the client's condition.

INTERPROFESSIONAL CARE

- Respiratory services can be consulted for oxygen therapy, breathing treatments, and ABGs.
- Pulmonology services can be consulted for respiratory management. Q**TC**

CLIENT EDUCATION

- Adhere to the prescribed diet and dialysis regimen, if with kidney dysfunction.
- Weigh daily and notify the provider if there is a 1- to 2-lb (0.5 to 0.9 kg) gain in 24 hr or a 3-lb (1.4 kg) gain in 1 week.
- Consider smoking cessation if a smoker.
- Take medication as prescribed. Adhere to the medication regimen if with COPD.
- Set up referral services (home oxygen). Q**PCC**

40.2 Types of results

The following are the five classic types of ABG results demonstrating balance and imbalance.

Step 1: Look at pH	Step 2: Determine which is in the normal range		Step 3: Combine names
pH	$PaCO_2$	HCO_3^-	DIAGNOSIS
7.35 to 7.45	35 to 45	21 to 28	Homeostasis
Less than 7.35	Greater than 45	21 to 28	Respiratory acidosis
Less than 7.35	35 to 45	Less than 21	Metabolic acidosis
Greater than 7.45	Less than 35	21 to 28	Respiratory alkalosis
Greater than 7.45	35 to 45	Greater than 28	Metabolic alkalosis

COMPLICATIONS

Convulsions, coma, and respiratory arrest

NURSING ACTIONS

- Implement seizure precautions, and perform management interventions if necessary.
- Provide life–support interventions if necessary.

Active Learning Scenario

A nurse is caring for a client who has liver cancer. The client's arterial blood gases reveal metabolic acidosis. Use the ATI Active Learning Template: System Disorder to complete this item.

RISK FACTORS: Include three conditions related to metabolic acidosis.

NURSING CARE: Include two nursing actions.

COMPLICATIONS: Identify one.

Application Exercises

1. A nurse is assisting with teaching a group of nurses about conditions that can cause metabolic acidosis. Which of the following conditions should the nurse include?

   A. Diabetic ketoacidosis

   B. Myasthenia gravis

   C. Asthma

   D. Laxative overuse

2. A nurse is collecting data on a client who has pancreatitis. The client's arterial blood gases reveal metabolic acidosis. What findings should the nurse expect?

3. A nurse is reviewing ABG results for a client who has vomited for 24 hr. Which of the following acid-base imbalances should the nurse expect?

   A. Respiratory acidosis

   B. Respiratory alkalosis

   C. Metabolic acidosis

   D. Metabolic alkalosis

4. A nurse is reviewing information about acid-base imbalances. Match the acid-base imbalance with the ABG result.

A. Metabolic alkalosis	1. pH 7.30 $PaCO_2$ 48 mm Hg HCO_3^- 26 mEq/L
B. Metabolic acidosis	2. pH 7.50 $PaCO_2$ 28 mm Hg HCO_3^- 24 mEq/L
C. Respiratory alkalosis	3. pH 7.32 $PaCO_2$ 35 mm Hg HCO_3^- 18 mEq/L
D. Respiratory acidosis	4. pH 7.50 $PaCO_2$ 38 mm Hg HCO_3^- 30 mEq/L

5. A nurse is caring for assisting with the care of a client who was in a motor-vehicle accident and reports chest pain and difficulty breathing. A chest x-ray reveals the client has a pneumothorax. Which of the following ABG results should the nurse expect?

   A. pH 7.25 $PaCO_2$ 52 mm Hg HCO_3^- 24 mEq/L

   B. pH 7.42 $PaCO_2$ 38 mm Hg HCO_3^- 23 mEq/L

   C. pH 7.30 $PaCO_2$ 36mm Hg HCO_3^- 18mEq/L

   D. pH 7.50 $PaCO_2$ 29 mm Hg HCO_3^- 26 mEq/L

Application Exercises Key

1. A. **CORRECT:** When analyzing cues, the nurse should identify that metabolic acidosis results from an excess production of hydrogen ions, which occurs in diabetic ketoacidosis.

Ⓝ *NCLEX® Connection: Physiological Adaptation, Fluid and Electrolyte Imbalances*

2. When recognizing cues, the nurse should expect the client who has metabolic acidosis to have dysrhythmias, bradycardia, weak peripheral pulses, hypotension, tachypnea, headache, drowsiness, confusion, rapid, deep respirations, and warm, dry, pink skin.

Ⓝ *NCLEX® Connection: Physiological Adaptation, Fluid and Electrolyte Imbalances*

3. D. **CORRECT:** When analyzing cues, the nurse should expect the client who has vomited for 24 hrs to have metabolic alkalosis. Excessive vomiting causes a loss of gastric acids and an accumulation of bicarbonate in the blood, resulting in metabolic alkalosis.

Ⓝ *NCLEX® Connection: Physiological Adaptation, Fluid and Electrolyte Imbalances*

4. A, 4; B, 3; C, 2; D, 1

When taking actions, the nurse should instruct that in respiratory acidosis, the pH is less than 7.35, the $PaCO_2$ is greater than 45 mm Hg, and the HCO_3^- is 22 to 26 mEq/L. The nurse should instruct that in respiratory alkalosis, the pH is greater than 7.45, the $PaCO_2$ is less than 35 mm Hg, and the HCO_3^- is 22 to 26 mEq/L. The nurse should instruct that in metabolic acidosis, the pH is less than 7.35, the $PaCO_2$ is 35 to 45 mm Hg, and the HCO_3^- is less than 22 mEq/L. The nurse should instruct that in metabolic alkalosis, the pH is greater than 7.45, the $PaCO_2$ is 35 to 45 mm Hg, and the HCO_3^- is greater than 26 mEq/L.

Ⓝ *NCLEX® Connection: Physiological Adaptation, Fluid and Electrolyte Imbalances*

5. A. **CORRECT:** When analyzing cues, the nurse should expect the client who has a pneumothorax to have respiratory acidosis. A pneumothorax can cause alveolar hypoventilation and increased carbon dioxide levels, resulting in a state of respiratory acidosis.

Ⓝ *NCLEX® Connection: Reduction of Risk Potential, Laboratory Values*

Active Learning Scenario Key

Using the ATI Active Learning Template: System Disorder

RISK FACTORS

Metabolic acidosis results from:
- Excess production of hydrogen ions.
- Diabetic ketoacidosis (DKA).
- Starvation.

Lactic acidosis can result from:
- Heavy exercise.
- Seizure activity.
- Hypoxia.
- Excessive intake of acids such as the following.
  ○ Ethyl alcohol
  ○ Methyl alcohol
  ○ Acetylsalicylic acid (aspirin)
- Inadequate elimination of hydrogen ions.
  ○ Kidney failure
  ○ Severe lung problems
- Inadequate production of bicarbonate.
  ○ Kidney failure
  ○ Pancreatitis
  ○ Impaired liver or pancreatic function
  ○ Liver failure
- Excess elimination of bicarbonate (diarrhea).

Metabolic acidosis results in:
- Decreased HCO_3^-.
- Increased H^+ concentration.

NURSING CARE: Varies with causes. If DKA, administer insulin. If related to GI losses, administer antidiarrheals and provide rehydration. If blood bicarbonate is low, administer sodium bicarbonate 1 mEq/kg.

COMPLICATIONS: Convulsions, coma, and respiratory arrest

NURSING ACTIONS
- Implement seizure precautions, and perform management interventions if necessary.
- Provide life-support interventions if necessary.

Ⓝ *NCLEX® Connection: Physiological Adaptation, Basic Pathophysiology*

When reviewing the following chapters, keep in mind the relevant topics and tasks of the NCLEX outline.

Pharmacological Therapies

MEDICATION ADMINISTRATION: Administer medication by gastrointestinal tube.

PHARMACOLOGICAL PAIN MANAGEMENT: Identify client need for pain medication.

Reduction of Risk Potential

DIAGNOSTIC TESTS: Perform diagnostic testing.

LABORATORY VALUES: Monitor diagnostic or laboratory test results.

POTENTIAL FOR COMPLICATIONS OF DIAGNOSTIC TESTS/ TREATMENTS/PROCEDURES: Maintain client tube patency.

THERAPEUTIC PROCEDURES: Assist with the performance of a diagnostic or invasive procedure.

Physiological Adaptation

ALTERATIONS IN BODY SYSTEMS: Reinforce education to client regarding care and condition.

CHAPTER 41 *Gastrointestinal Diagnostic Procedures*

Gastrointestinal diagnostic procedures often involve endoscopes and x-rays to visualize parts of the gastrointestinal system and to evaluate gastrointestinal contents. Procedures include liver function tests, other blood tests, urobilinogen, fecal occult blood test (FOBT), stool samples, endoscopy, and gastrointestinal (GI) series.

Liver function tests and other blood tests

- Liver function tests are aspartate aminotransferase (AST), alanine aminotransferase (ALT), alkaline phosphatase (ALP), bilirubin, and albumin.
- Other blood tests that provide information on the functioning of the GI system include amylase, lipase, alpha–fetoprotein, and ammonia.

41.1 Blood tests: Interpretation of findings

BLOOD TEST	EXPECTED REFERENCE RANGE	INTERPRETATION OF FINDINGS
Aspartate aminotransferase	0 to 35 units/L	Elevation occurs with hepatitis or cirrhosis.
Alanine aminotransferase	4 to 36 units/L	
Alkaline phosphatase	30 to 120 units/L	Elevation indicates liver damage.
Amylase	30 to 220 units/L	Elevation occurs with pancreatitis.
Lipase	0 to 160 units/L	
Total bilirubin	0.3 to 1 mg/dL	Elevations indicate altered liver function, bile duct obstruction, or other hepatobiliary disorder.
Direct (conjugated) bilirubin	0.1 to 0.3 mg/dL	
Indirect (unconjugated) bilirubin	0.2 to 0.8 mg/dL	
Albumin	3.5 to 5 g/dL	Decrease can indicate hepatic disease.
Alpha-fetoprotein	Less than 40 mcg/L	Elevated in liver cancer, cirrhosis, hepatitis.
Ammonia	10 to 80 mcg/dL	Elevated in liver disease.

INDICATIONS

Suspected liver, pancreatic, or biliary tract disorder

CONSIDERATIONS

PREPROCEDURE: Explain to the client how blood is obtained and what information this will provide.

Urine bilirubin

Also known as urobilinogen, this is a urine test to determine the presence of bilirubin in the urine.

INDICATIONS

Suspected liver or biliary tract disorder

CONSIDERATIONS

PREPROCEDURE

NURSING ACTIONS: The test can be performed by using a dipstick (urine bilirubin) or a 24-hr urine collection (urobilinogen).

CLIENT EDUCATION: Collect urine using the provided proper collection container.

POSTPROCEDURE

NURSING ACTIONS: Inform the client when and how results are provided.

INTERPRETATION OF FINDINGS

A positive or elevated finding indicates possible liver disorder (cirrhosis, hepatitis), biliary obstruction, hemolytic anemia, or pernicious anemia.

Fecal occult blood test and stool samples

A stool sample is collected and can be tested for blood, ova and parasites (*Giardia lamblia*), and bacteria (*Clostridium difficile*).

INDICATIONS

CLIENT PRESENTATION
- GI bleeding
- Unexplained diarrhea

CONSIDERATIONS

PREPROCEDURE

NURSING ACTIONS
- **Occult blood:** Provide the client with cards impregnated with guaiac that can be mailed to provider or with a specimen collection cup. If the cards are used, three samples are usually required.
- **Stool for ova and parasites and bacteria:** Provide the client with a specimen collection cup.

CLIENT EDUCATION
- **Occult blood:** Adhere to the proper collection technique. Be aware of any dietary restrictions to follow (avoid vitamin C rich foods, red meat, poultry, fish for 3 days prior to the test) prior to obtaining samples. **Qpcc**
- **Stool for ova and parasites and bacteria:** Adhere to the proper collection technique (time frame for submission to laboratory, need for refrigeration).

POSTPROCEDURE

NURSING ACTIONS: Inform the client when and how the results are provided.

INTERPRETATION OF FINDINGS

- At least three stool specimens on three separate days are needed for accurate results.
- A positive finding for blood is indicative of GI bleeding (ulcer, colitis, cancer).

Stool samples
- A positive finding for ova and parasites is indicative of a GI parasitic infection.
- A positive finding for Clostridium difficile is indicative of this opportunistic infection, which becomes established secondary to use of broad-spectrum antibiotics, immunosuppression, or excessive evacuation of the bowels.

Endoscopy

- Endoscopic procedures allow direct visualization of body cavities, tissues, and organs through the use of a flexible, lighted tube (endoscope). They are performed for diagnostic and therapeutic purposes.
- Endoscopic procedures are performed in a variety of facilities. The provider can perform biopsies, remove abnormal tissue, and perform minor surgery, such as cauterizing a bleeding ulcer.

GASTROINTESTINAL SCOPE PROCEDURES
- Colonoscopy
- Esophagogastroduodenoscopy (EGD)
- Endoscopic retrograde cholangiopancreatography (ERCP)
- Small bowel capsule endoscopy (M2A)
- Sigmoidoscopy

INDICATIONS

POTENTIAL DIAGNOSES: GI bleeding, ulcerations, inflammation, polyps, malignant tumors

CLIENT PRESENTATION
- Anemia (secondary to bleeding)
- Abdominal discomfort
- Abdominal distention or mass

41.2 Case study

Part 1: Scenario introduction
Kennedy is a nurse who is caring for a client, Marquis, in a gastroenterology clinic. They report a two-month history of anorexia, weight loss, abdominal pain, nausea, vomiting, and diarrhea. They also report a family history of colon cancer.

Scene 1
Kennedy: "The provider has ordered liver function tests, a CBC, and electrolytes. I'd like to draw your blood now if that's okay. We're also going to ask you to give us a urine specimen."

Marquis: "What does all that mean?"

Part 2
Kennedy: "Marquis, we're also going to send you home with a test for fecal occult blood."

Marquis: "What does that mean?"

Kennedy: "Fecal occult blood is blood that can't be seen in your stool."

Marquis: "Do I have to do that test myself?"

Kennedy: "We'll give you the specimen cards with instructions, and you'll bring them back or mail them to us."

Part 3
Marquis has returned to the clinic for a follow up appointment after learning about the positive result of the fecal occult blood test.

Scene 3
Kennedy: "Because you had a positive result on the fecal occult blood test, your provider would like to schedule a colonoscopy for you."

Marquis: "I thought that might happen. Don't I have to eat a lot of gelatin and take a bunch of laxatives?"

Scenario conclusion
Kennedy reinforces instructions to Marquis about the pre-procedure diet and bowel prep. She also reinforces education about what to expect before, during, and after the procedure.

CONSIDERATIONS

General endoscopic procedures

Preprocedure
- NURSING ACTIONS
- Verify that a consent form has been signed.
  - Obtain vital signs, and verify the client's allergies.
  - Assist in the evaluation of baseline laboratory tests and report unexpected findings to the provider (can include CBC, electrolyte panel, BUN, creatinine, PT, aPTT, and liver function studies). Report unexpected findings in reports for chest x-ray, ECG, and ABGs, as indicated.
  - Review the client's medical history for increased risk of complications.
  - **Age** can influence the client's ability to understand the procedures, tolerance of the required positioning, and compliance with pretest preparation. Ⓖ
  - **Current health status:** Consider conditions and medications that can affect the client's tolerance of and recovery from the procedure.
  - **Cognitive status:** Determine the client's understanding of the procedure and baseline mental status.
  - **Support system:** Determine whether a support person will assist the client after the procedure.
  - **Recent food or fluid intake:** Can affect the provider's ability to visualize key structures and increase the risk for complications (aspiration). Notify the provider if dietary restrictions were not followed.
  - **Medications:** Some medications (NSAIDs, warfarin, aspirin) place the client at risk for complications. Notify the provider if medication restrictions were not followed.
  - **Previous radiographic examinations:** Any recent radiographic examinations using barium can affect the provider's ability to view key structures. Endoscopic procedures should take place prior to barium contrast studies.
  - **Electrolyte and fluid status:** Imbalances secondary to repeated enemas can affect bowel preparation tolerance, especially in older adult clients.
  - Ensure that the client followed proper bowel preparation (laxatives, enemas). Inadequate bowel preparation can result in cancellation and delays the examination. This can also lead to the client experiencing extended periods of being NPO or on a liquid diet.
  - Ensure that the client is NPO for the prescribed period prior to the examination.
- CLIENT EDUCATION
  - Understand the given instructions regarding medication and food restrictions.
  - Receive prescriptions for medications used for the bowel prep.
  - Remember the number and type of enemas, if prescribed.

Postprocedure
- NURSING ACTIONS
  - Monitor vital signs.
  - Collect data regarding complications.
- CLIENT EDUCATION: If a biopsy was performed, food restrictions can be prescribed. Ⓠpcc

Colonoscopy

Use of a flexible fiber optic colonoscope, which enters through the anus, to visualize the rectum and the sigmoid, descending, transverse, and ascending colon

ANESTHESIA: **Moderate sedation:** Midazolam and an opiate such as fentanyl are commonly used medications.

POSITIONING: Left side with knees to chest

Preparation
- Bowel prep
- Prep can include laxatives, such as bisacodyl and polyethylene glycol.
- Polyethylene glycol is not recommended for older adult clients because it can cause fluid and electrolyte imbalances. Ⓖ
- Polyethylene glycol can inhibit the absorption of some medications. Review the client's medications and consult with the provider.
- Clear liquid diet (avoid red, purple, orange fluids) 1 to 2 days prior to the test. NPO 8 hr prior to the test.
- The client must avoid medications indicated by the provider (aspirin, anticoagulants, antiplatelet).

Postprocedure
- Notify the provider of severe pain (possible perforation) or indication of hemorrhage.
- Monitor for rectal bleeding.
- Monitor vital signs and respiratory status. Maintain an open airway until the client is awake. Ⓠpcc
- Resume normal diet as prescribed.
- Encourage increased fluid intake.
- Instruct the client that there can be increased flatulence due to air instillation during the procedure.
- Instruct the client not to drive or use equipment for 12 to 18 hr after the procedure.

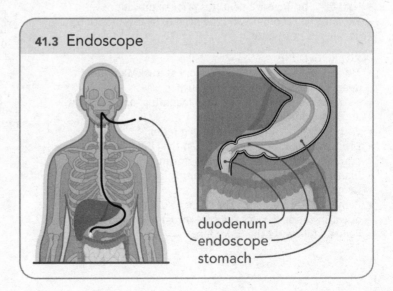

41.3 Endoscope

duodenum
endoscope
stomach

Esophagogastroduodenoscopy (EGD)

Insertion of endoscope through the mouth into the esophagus, stomach, and duodenum to identify or treat areas of bleeding, dilate an esophageal stricture, and diagnose gastric lesions.

ANESTHESIA: Moderate sedation per IV access:
Topical anesthetic to depress the gag reflex, atropine to decrease secretions

POSITIONING: Left side-lying with head of bed elevated

PREPARATION: NPO for 8 hr. Remove dentures prior to procedure.

POSTPROCEDURE
- Monitor vital signs and respiratory status. Maintain an open airway until the client is awake.
- Notify the provider of bleeding, abdominal or chest pain, and any evidence of infection.
- Withhold fluids until return of gag reflex. Qs
- Discontinue IV fluid therapy when the client tolerates oral fluids without nausea and vomiting.
- Instruct the client not to drive or use equipment for 12 to 18 hr after the procedure.
- Reinforce teaching with the client to use throat lozenges if a sore throat or hoarse voice persists following the procedure.

Endoscopic retrograde cholangiopancreatography (ERCP)

Insertion of an endoscope through the mouth into the biliary tree via the duodenum. Allows visualization of the biliary ducts, gall bladder, liver, and pancreas. X-rays are taken after a contrast medium is injected into the common duct.

ANESTHESIA: Moderate sedation per IV access:
Topical anesthetic to depress the gag reflex, atropine to decrease secretions

POSITIONING: Initially semi-prone with repositioning throughout procedure

PREPARATION
- NPO for 8 hr. Remove dentures prior to procedure.
- Explain the procedure and the need to change positions during the procedure.

POSTPROCEDURE
- Monitor vital signs and respiratory status. Maintain an open airway until the client is awake.
- Notify the provider of bleeding, abdominal or chest pain, and any evidence of infection.
- Withhold fluids until return of gag reflex.
- Discontinue IV fluid therapy when the client tolerates oral fluids without nausea and vomiting.
- Instruct the client not to drive or use equipment for 12 to 18 hr after the procedure.
- Reinforce teaching with the client to use throat lozenges or warm saline gargles if a sore throat or hoarse voice persists following the procedure.

Capsule endoscopy

Swallow the capsule with a glass of water for a video enteroscopy to visualize the entire small bowel over an 8-hr period. The capsule is not used to view the colon.

ANESTHESIA: None

POSITIONING: Return to normal activity during the study

PREPARATION
- Fast (water only) for 8 to 10 hr before the test and NPO for first 2 hr of the testing. Normal eating 4 hr after swallowing the capsule.
- The abdomen is marked for the location of the sensor. Eight-lead sensors are placed and connected to a data recorder, which captures images of the small intestines. Qᴸ

POSTPROCEDURE
- After 8 hr, the client returns the recorder for downloading of the images.
- The client will evacuate the capsule in the stool.

Sigmoidoscopy

Scope is shorter than colonoscope, allowing visualization of the anus, rectum, and sigmoid colon to test for colon cancer, investigate for a GI bleed, and diagnose or monitor inflammatory bowel disease.

ANESTHESIA: None required

POSITIONING: On left side

PREPARATION
- Bowel prep, which can include laxatives (such as bisacodyl), cleansing enema, or sodium biphosphate enema
- Clear liquid diet at least 24 hr before the procedure
- NPO after midnight
- The client must avoid medications as indicated by the provider

POSTPROCEDURE
- Monitor vital signs and respiratory status.
- Monitor for rectal bleeding.
- Resume normal diet as prescribed.
- Encourage increased fluid intake.
- Instruct the client that there can be increased flatulence due to air instillation during the procedure.

INTERPRETATION OF FINDINGS

Can indicate a need for medication or surgical removal of a lesion.

COMPLICATIONS

Oversedation

Use of moderate sedation places the client at risk for oversedation. Qs

MANIFESTATIONS: Difficult to arouse, poor respiratory effort, evidence of hypoxemia, tachycardia, and elevated or low blood pressure

NURSING ACTIONS
- Be prepared to assist with the administration of antidotes for sedatives administered prior to and during the procedure.
- Administer oxygen, and monitor vital signs. Maintain an open airway until awake.
- Notify the provider immediately, and call for assistance.

CLIENT EDUCATION: Driving and major decision-making are restricted until the effects of the sedation have worn off. This varies with the type of agent used.

Hemorrhage

MANIFESTATIONS: Bleeding, cool and clammy skin, hypotension, tachycardia, dizziness, and tachypnea

NURSING ACTIONS
- Monitor for hemorrhage from the site. Monitor vital signs.
- Monitor diagnostic test results (particularly Hgb and Hct).
- Notify the provider immediately.

CLIENT EDUCATION: Report fever, pain, and bleeding to the provider.

Aspiration

Using moderate sedation or topical anesthesia can affect the gag reflex.

MANIFESTATIONS: Dyspnea, tachypnea, adventitious breath sounds, tachycardia, and fever

NURSING ACTIONS
- Keep the client NPO until the gag reflex returns. Ensure that the client is awake and alert prior to consuming food or fluid. Encourage the client to deep breathe and cough to promote removal of secretions.
- Notify the provider if there is a delay in gag reflex return.

CLIENT EDUCATION: Report any respiratory congestion or compromise to the provider.

Perforation of the gastrointestinal tract

Manifestations include chest or abdominal pain, fever, nausea, vomiting, and abdominal distention.

NURSING ACTIONS: Monitor diagnostic tests for evidence of infection, including elevated WBC, and notify the provider of unexpected findings.

CLIENT EDUCATION: Report fever, pain, and bleeding to the provider.

Gastrointestinal series

GI studies are done with or without contrast and help define anatomic or functional abnormalities.
- These include radiographic imaging of the esophagus, stomach, and entire intestinal tract.
- Upper GI imaging is done by having the client drink a radiopaque liquid (barium). For small bowel follow-through, barium is traced through the small intestine to the ileocecal junction.
- A barium enema is done by instilling a radiopaque liquid into the rectum and colon.

INDICATIONS

POTENTIAL DIAGNOSES: Gastric ulcers, peristaltic disorders, tumors, varices, and intestinal enlargements or constrictions

CLIENT PRESENTATION: Abdominal pain, altered elimination habits (constipation, diarrhea), or GI bleeding

CONSIDERATIONS

PREPROCEDURE

NURSING CONSIDERATIONS
- Inform the client about medications, food and fluid restrictions (clear liquid and/or low residue diet, NPO after midnight), and avoiding smoking or chewing gum (increases peristalsis).
- Determine the client's understanding of bowel preparation (laxatives, enemas) so the image will not be distorted by feces.
- Barium enema studies must be scheduled prior to upper GI studies. QEBP
- Determine if there are any contraindications to bowel preparation (possible bowel perforation or obstruction, inflammatory disease).

CLIENT EDUCATION
- Restrict food and fluids for bowel preparation.
- If the small intestine is to be visualized, additional radiographs will be done over the next 24 hr.

POSTPROCEDURE

NURSING ACTIONS
- Monitor elimination of contrast material, and administer a laxative if prescribed.
- Increase fluid intake to promote elimination of contrast material.

CLIENT EDUCATION
- Monitor elimination of contrast material and report retention of contrast material (constipation) or diarrhea accompanied by weakness.
- An over-the-counter medication can be needed to prevent constipation resulting from the barium. QPCC
- Stools will be white for 24 to 72 hr until barium clears. Report abdominal fullness, pain, or delay in return to brown stool.

INTERPRETATION OF FINDINGS

Include altered bowel shape and size, increased motility, or obstruction.

Active Learning Scenario

A nurse in a clinic is reinforcing teaching with a client who will undergo a gastrointestinal series of x-rays. What should the nurse include when reinforcing the teaching? Use the ATI Active Learning Template: Diagnostic Procedure to complete this item.

DESCRIPTION OF PROCEDURE: Describe the procedure and technique involved.

INDICATIONS: Identify at least three potential diagnoses and two manifestations.

CLIENT EDUCATION: Describe three teaching points.

Application Exercises

1. Kennedy discusses liver function tests, a complete blood count, electrolytes, and a urinalysis with Marquis. When reinforcing education to the client about the laboratory tests and findings, which tests should the nurse discuss as liver function tests? (Select all that apply.)

   A. Aspartate aminotransferase (AST)

   B. Alanine aminotransferase (ALT)

   C. Urobilinogen

   D. Amylase

   E. Albumin

   F. Lipase

2. Kennedy reinforces instructions with Marquis about the fecal occult blood test, which requires the client to mail multiple specimens collected on consecutive days. Which statement by Marquis indicates understanding of the test?

   A. "I will continue to take my daily aspirin while I complete this test."

   B. "I'm glad I don't have to follow a special diet while I'm collecting these samples."

   C. "This test will determine if I have parasites in my bowels."

   D. "This test is part of the screening for colon cancer."

3. The nurse reinforces instructions about the colonoscopy procedure, including the diet the client should follow during the bowel prep. The client states, "Oh, good. I have a few boxes of cherry gelatin I need to use." How should the nurse respond?

4. A nurse caring for clients in an endoscopy center is preparing to reinforce instructions to clients who are scheduled to undergo colonoscopies, sigmoidoscopies, and ERCPs. Sort the descriptions the nurse will include by the type of procedure the clients are having.

   A. Allows visualization of entire colon

   B. Requires an extensive bowel prep at least 1 day before the procedure

   C. Allows visualization of bile duct and pancreatic duct

   D. Side effects may include sore throat

   E. Prep may include a light breakfast

Application Exercises Key

1. A, B, C, E. **CORRECT:** When taking actions to reinforce education about liver function tests to the client, the nurse should explain that increased levels of liver enzymes, including AST and ALT, and urobilinogen in the urine can indicate liver disease.

   Ⓝ *NCLEX® Connection: Reduction of Risk Potential, Laboratory Values*

2. D. **CORRECT:** When evaluating outcomes of reinforcing instructions about fecal occult blood testing to the client, the nurse should recognize that the statement, "This test is part of the screening for colon cancer" indicates understanding by the client that a tumor in the large intestine may cause occult blood in the stool.

   Ⓝ *NCLEX® Connection: Reduction of Risk Potential, Laboratory Values*

3. When generating solutions with the client for clear liquid intake during the bowel prep, the nurse should reinforce that any foods or liquids that are red, orange, blue, or green in color may interfere with visualization of the colon and interpretation of the results of the test.

   Ⓝ *NCLEX® Connection: Reduction of Risk Potential, Diagnostic Tests*

4. **COLONOSCOPY:** A, B; **SIGMOIDOSCOPY:** E; **ERCP:** C, D

   When generating solutions for reinforcing instructions to clients who are undergoing endoscopic procedures, the nurse will describe a colonoscopy as a procedure that requires an extensive bowel prep at least one day before to ensure the colon is clear of stool to allow the provider to visualize the entire colon through a flexible scope. The nurse will reinforce instruction to clients who are undergoing sigmoidoscopies that they may eat a light breakfast, because digestive contents will not reach the sigmoid colon before the procedure. The nurse will reinforce instructions to clients who are undergoing ERCP that the provider will use an endoscope and radiographic dye to obtain radiographic images of the bile duct and pancreatic duct and that because the endoscope is passed through the pharynx, the client may experience a sore throat for several days.

   Ⓝ *NCLEX® Connection: Reduction of Risk Potential, Diagnostic Tests*

Active Learning Scenario Key

Using the ATI Active Learning Template: Diagnostic Procedure

DESCRIPTION OF PROCEDURE: Radiographic images are used to define anatomic or functional abnormalities of the esophagus, stomach, and intestinal tract. These can include an upper GI image, which includes the client drinking radiopaque barium liquid that is traced through the small intestine. The client can have a barium enema, in which liquid barium is instilled into the rectum and colon.

INDICATIONS

- Diagnoses: Gastric ulcers, peristaltic disorders, tumors, varices, intestinal enlargements or constrictions
- Manifestations: Abdominal pain, altered elimination habits (constipation, diarrhea), gastrointestinal bleeding

CLIENT EDUCATION

- Follow fluid and food restrictions for bowel preparation.
- Additional radiographs can be done over a 24-hr period.
- Monitor elimination of contrast media, and report retention of contrast media (constipation) or diarrhea accompanied by weakness. Over-the-counter medication can be used to prevent constipation.
- Stool can be white for 24 to 72 hr until barium clears the system. Report abdominal fullness, pain, or a delay in a return to brown stool.

Ⓝ *NCLEX® Connection: Reduction of Risk Potential, Diagnostic Tests*

CHAPTER 42 *Gastrointestinal Therapeutic Procedures*

Gastrointestinal therapeutic procedures are performed for maintenance of nutritional intake, and treatment of gastrointestinal obstructions, obesity, and other disorders.

Gastrointestinal therapeutic procedures nurses should be knowledgeable about enteral feedings, total parenteral nutrition (TPN), abdominal paracentesis, nasogastric decompression, bariatric surgeries, and ostomies.

Enteral feedings

Enteral feedings are instituted for a client who has a functioning GI tract but is unable to swallow or take in adequate calories and protein orally. It can be in addition to an oral diet, or it can be the only source of nutrition.

INDICATIONS

POTENTIAL DIAGNOSES

- Inability to eat due to a medical condition (head and neck cancer)
- Pathologies that cause difficulty swallowing or increase risk of aspiration (stroke, advanced Parkinson's disease, multiple sclerosis)
- Inability to maintain adequate oral nutritional intake and need for supplementation due to increased metabolic demands (burns, sepsis)

CLIENT PRESENTATION

- Malnutrition (decreased prealbumin, decreased transferrin or total iron-binding capacity)
- Aspiration pneumonia

COMPLICATIONS

Overfeeding

Overfeeding results from infusion of a greater quantity of feeding than can be readily digested, resulting in abdominal distention, nausea, and vomiting.

NURSING ACTIONS
- Check facility policy regarding residual check, which is usually every 4 to 6 hr, and take corrective actions as prescribed. Some facilities no longer require residual checks.
- Follow protocol for slowing or withholding feedings for excess residual volumes. Many facilities hold for residual volumes of 100 to 200 mL and then restart at a lower rate after a period of rest.
- Check pump for proper operation and ensure feeding infused at correct rate.

Diarrhea

Diarrhea occurs secondary to concentration of feeding or its constituents.

NURSING ACTIONS
- Slow the rate of feeding and notify the provider.
- Confer with a dietitian.
- Provide skin care and protection.
- Recommend evaluation for *Clostridium difficile* if diarrhea continues, especially if it has a very foul odor.

Constipation

Constipation occurs secondary to inactivity, lack of free water, or lack of fiber.

NURSING ACTIONS
- Add water during flushes of the tube.
- Confer with a dietitian to select a formula that contains fiber.
- Collaborate with provider or physical therapist about increased physical activity. Qᴛᴄ

Aspiration pneumonia

Pneumonia can occur secondary to aspiration of feeding, and can be a life-threatening complication. Tube displacement is the primary cause of aspiration of feeding.

NURSING ACTIONS
- For prevention, confirm tube placement before feedings, and elevate the head of the bed at least 30° during feedings, and for at least 1 hr after.
- Stop the feeding. Qs
- Turn the client to one side and suction the airway. Administer oxygen if indicated.
- Monitor vital signs for an elevated temperature.
- Auscultate breath sounds for increased congestion and diminishing breath sounds.
- Notify the provider and obtain a chest x-ray if prescribed.

Refeeding syndrome

Refeeding syndrome is a potentially life-threatening condition that occurs when enteral feeding is started in a client who is in a starvation state and whose body has begun to catabolize protein and fat for energy.

NURSING ACTIONS

- Monitor for new onset of confusion or seizures.
- Monitor for shallow respirations.
- Monitor for increased muscular weakness.
- Notify the provider and obtain blood electrolytes if needed.

Total parenteral nutrition

TPN is a hypertonic IV bolus solution. The purpose of TPN administration is to prevent or correct nutritional deficiencies and minimize the adverse effects of malnourishment.

- TPN administration is usually through a central line (a tunneled triple lumen catheter or a single- or double-lumen peripherally inserted central [PICC] line).
- TPN contains complete nutrition, including calories in a high concentration (10% to 50%) of dextrose, lipids/essential fatty acids, protein, electrolytes, vitamins, and trace elements. Standard IV bolus therapy is typically no more than 700 calories/day.
- Partial parenteral nutrition or peripheral parenteral nutrition (PPN) is less hypertonic, intended for short-term use, and administered in a large peripheral vein. Usual dextrose concentration is 10% or less. Risks include phlebitis.

INDICATIONS

Any condition that
- Affects the ability to absorb nutrition
- Has a prolonged recovery
- Creates a hypermetabolic state
- Creates a chronic malnutrition

POTENTIAL DIAGNOSES

- Chronic pancreatitis
- Diffuse peritonitis
- Short bowel syndrome
- Gastric paresis from diabetes mellitus
- Severe burns

CLIENT PRESENTATION

- Weight loss greater than 10% of body weight and NPO or unable to eat or drink for more than 5 days
- Muscle wasting, poor tissue healing, burns, bowel disease disorders, acute kidney failure

CONSIDERATIONS

PREPARATION OF THE CLIENT

- Determine the client's readiness for TPN. Q PCC
- Obtain daily laboratory values, including electrolytes. Solutions are customized for each client according to daily laboratory results.

ONGOING CARE

- The flow rate is gradually increased or decreased to allow body adjustment (usually no more than a 10% hourly increase in rate).

  > ! Never abruptly stop TPN. Speeding up/slowing down the rate is contraindicated. An abrupt rate change can alter blood glucose levels significantly. Q s

- Obtain vital signs every 4 to 8 hr and weights daily.
- Follow sterile procedures to minimize the risk of sepsis.
  - TPN solution is prepared by the pharmacy using aseptic technique with a laminar flow hood.
  - Change tubing and solution bag every 24 hr (even if not empty).
  - Do not use the line for other IV bolus solutions (prevents contamination and interruption of the flow rate).
  - Do not add anything to the solution due to risks of contamination and incompatibility.
  - Use sterile technique, including a mask, when changing the central line dressing (per facility procedure).

INTERVENTIONS

- Check capillary glucose every 4 to 6 hr for at least the first 24 hr.
- Clients receiving TPN frequently need supplemental regular insulin until the pancreas can increase its endogenous production of insulin.
- Keep dextrose 10% in water at the bedside in case the solution is unexpectedly ruined or the next bag is not available. This will minimize the risk of hypoglycemia with abrupt changes in dextrose concentrations.
- If a bag is unavailable and administered late, do not attempt to catch up by increasing the infusion rate because the client can develop hyperglycemia.
- **OLDER ADULT CLIENTS** have an increased incidence of glucose intolerance. G

COMPLICATIONS

Metabolic complications

Metabolic complications include hyperglycemia, hypoglycemia, and vitamin deficiencies.

NURSING ACTIONS
- Review results of daily laboratory monitoring to ensure that the components prescribed in the client's TPN match the client's needs.
- Fluid needs are typically replaced with a separate IV bolus to prevent fluid volume excess.
- Monitor for hyperglycemia.

Air embolism

A pressure change during tubing changes can lead to an air embolism.

NURSING ACTIONS
- Monitor for manifestations of an air embolism (sudden onset of dyspnea, chest pain, anxiety, hypoxia).
- Clamp the catheter immediately and place the client on their left side in Trendelenburg position to trap air. Administer oxygen and notify the provider so trapped air can be aspirated.

Infection

Concentrated glucose is a medium for bacteria.

NURSING ACTIONS
- Observe the central line insertion site for local infection (erythema, tenderness, exudate).
- Change the sterile dressing on a central line per protocol (typically every 48 to 72 hr).
- Change IV tubing per protocol (typically every 24 hr).
- Monitor the client for manifestations of systemic infection (fever, increased WBC, chills, malaise). Qᴘᴄᴄ

> ! Do not use TPN line for other IV bolus fluids and medications (repeated access increases the risk for infection).

Fluid imbalance

TPN is a hyperosmotic solution (three to six times the osmolarity of blood), which poses a risk for fluid shifts, placing client at increased risk of fluid volume excess.

OLDER ADULT CLIENTS are more vulnerable to fluid and electrolyte imbalances. Ⓖ

NURSING ACTIONS
- Auscultate the lungs for crackles and monitor for respiratory distress.
- Monitor daily weight and I&O.
- Use a controlled infusion pump to administer TPN at the prescribed rate.
- Do not speed up the infusion to catch up.
- Gradually increase the flow rate until the prescribed infusion rate is achieved.

Paracentesis

A paracentesis is performed by inserting a needle or trocar through the abdominal wall into the peritoneal cavity. The therapeutic goal is relief of abdominal ascites pressure.
- A paracentesis can be performed in a provider's office, outpatient center, radiology department, or acute care setting at the bed side.
- Usually performed with ultrasound as a safety precaution.
- Once drained, ascitic fluid can be sent for laboratory culture.

INDICATIONS

POTENTIAL DIAGNOSES

Abdominal ascites

- Ascites is an abnormal accumulation of protein-rich fluid in the abdominal cavity most often caused by cirrhosis of the liver. The result is increased abdominal girth and distention.
- Respiratory distress is the determining factor in the use of a paracentesis to treat ascites, and in the evaluation of treatment effectiveness.

CLIENT PRESENTATION

Compromised lung expansion, increased abdominal girth, rapid weight gain

CONSIDERATIONS

PREPROCEDURE

NURSING ACTIONS
- Determine the client's readiness for the procedure. Variables (the age of the client and chronic and acute diseases) can influence ability to tolerate and recover from this procedure. Ⓖ
- Review pertinent blood testing results (albumin, protein, glucose, amylase, BUN, and creatinine).
- Verify that the client has signed the informed consent form.
- Gather equipment for the procedure.
- Have the client void, or insert an indwelling urinary catheter.
- Position the client in an upright position, either on the edge of the bed with feet supported or a high-Fowler's position in the bed. Clients who have ascites are typically more comfortable sitting up.
- Review baseline vital signs, record weight, and measure abdominal girth.

CLIENT EDUCATION
- Local anesthetics will be used at the insertion site.
- There can be pressure or pain with needle insertion.

INTRAPROCEDURE

NURSING ACTIONS

- Monitor vital signs.
- Label laboratory specimens and send to the laboratory.
- Up to 4 L of fluid is slowly drained from the abdomen by gravity. Monitor the amount of drainage and notify the provider of any evidence of complications.

POSTPROCEDURE

NURSING ACTIONS

- Maintain pressure at the insertion site for several minutes. Apply a dressing to the site.
- If the insertion site continues to leak after holding pressure for several minutes, dry sterile gauze dressings should be applied and changed as often as necessary.
- Check vital signs, record weight, and measure abdominal girth. Document and compare to preprocedure measurements.
- Continue to monitor vital signs and insertion site per facility protocol.
- Monitor temperature every 4 hr for a minimum of 48 hr. Fever can indicate a bowel perforation.
- Measure I&O every 4 hr.
- Administer medication.
  - Diuretics (spironolactone and furosemide) can be prescribed to control fluid volume.
  - Potassium supplements can be necessary when a loop diuretic (furosemide) has been administrated.
- Monitor the infusion of IV bolus fluids or albumin as prescribed.
- Assist the client into a position of comfort with the head of the bed elevated to promote lung expansion.
- Document color, odor, consistency, and amount of fluid removed; location of insertion site; evidence of leakage at the insertion site; manifestations of hypovolemia; and changes in mental status.
- Continue monitoring of blood albumin, protein, glucose, amylase, electrolytes, BUN, and creatinine levels.

CLIENT EDUCATION

- Avoid alcohol, maintain a low-sodium diet, and monitor the puncture site for bleeding or leakage of fluid.
- Report changes in mental and cognitive status due to change in fluid and electrolyte balance.
- Change positions slowly to decrease the risk of falls, which can be related to hypovolemia from the removal of ascites fluid.

COMPLICATIONS

Hypovolemia

Albumin levels can drop dangerously low because the peritoneal fluid removed contains a large amount of protein. The removal of this protein-rich fluid can cause shifting of intravascular volume, resulting in hypovolemia.

NURSING ACTIONS

- Preventive measures include slow drainage of fluid and administration of plasma expanders (albumin) to counter albumin losses.
- Monitor for manifestations of hypovolemia (tachycardia, hypotension, pallor, diaphoresis, dizziness).

Nasogastric decompression

Clients who have an intestinal obstruction require NG decompression. An NG tube is inserted, then suction is applied to relieve abdominal distention. Treatment continues until the obstruction resolves or is removed. The obstruction can be mechanical or functional.

INDICATIONS

POTENTIAL DIAGNOSES

Any disorder that causes a mechanical (tumors, adhesions, impaction) or functional (surgery, trauma, GI tract infections, conditions in which peristalsis is absent) intestinal obstruction

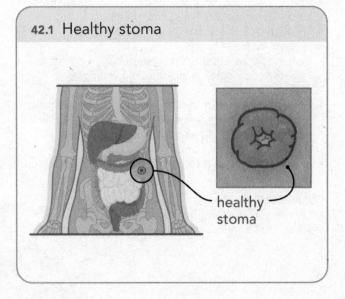

42.1 Healthy stoma

healthy stoma

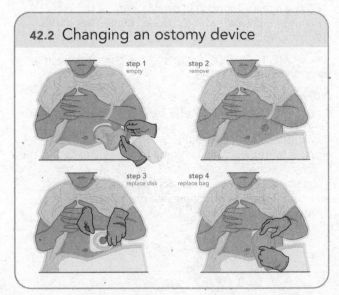

42.2 Changing an ostomy device

step 1
empty

step 2
remove

step 3
replace disk

step 4
replace bag

CLIENT PRESENTATION

- Vomiting (begins with stomach contents and continues until fecal material is also being regurgitated)
- Bowel sounds absent (paralytic ileus) or hyperactive and high-pitched (obstruction)
- Intermittent, colicky abdominal pain and distention
- Hiccups
- Abdominal distention

CONSIDERATIONS

PREPROCEDURE

NURSING ACTIONS: Inform the client of the purpose of the NG tube and the client's role in its placement.

POSTPROCEDURE

NURSING ACTIONS
- Check and maintain proper function of the NG tube and suction equipment.
- Incorporate NG tube flushes and drainage into I&O calculations.
- Monitor bowel sounds and abdominal girth; return of flatus.
- Monitor tube for displacement (decrease in drainage, increased nausea, vomiting, distention).
- Check pertinent lab results (electrolytes, hematocrit).
- Provide frequent oral and nares care.

CLIENT EDUCATION
- Maintain NPO status.
- Reposition frequently when in bed, and get out of the bed as able to promote movement of the intestines.

COMPLICATIONS

Fluid/electrolyte imbalance

NURSING ACTIONS
- Monitor for fluid and electrolyte imbalance (metabolic acidosis: low obstruction; alkalosis: high obstruction).
- Monitor I&O, observing for discrepancies.

Skin breakdown

NURSING ACTIONS: Inspect nasal skin for irritation.

Ostomies

An ostomy is a surgical opening from the inside of the body to the outside and can be located in various areas of the body. Ostomies can be permanent or temporary.
- A stoma is the artificial opening created during the ostomy surgery.
- Main types of ostomies performed in the abdominal area
  - **Ileostomy:** A surgical opening into the ileum to drain stool, which is typically frequent and liquid because large intestine is bypassed
  - **Colostomy:** A surgical opening into the large intestine to drain stool, with the ascending colon producing more liquid stools, the transverse colon producing more formed stools, and the sigmoid colon producing near-normal stool

---

42.3 Expected output for ostomies

ILEOSTOMY	TRANSVERSE COLOSTOMY	SIGMOID COLOSTOMY
Normal postoperative output		
More than 1,000 mL/day Can be bile-colored and liquid	Small semi-liquid with some mucus 2 to 3 days after surgery Blood can be present in the first few days after surgery	Small to moderate amount of mucus with semi-formed stool 4 to 5 days after surgery
Postoperative changes in output		
After several days to weeks, the output decreases to approximately 500 to 1,000 mL/day Becomes more paste-like as the small intestine assumes the absorptive function of the large intestine	After several days to weeks, output becomes more stool-like, semi-formed, or formed	After several days to weeks, output resembles semi-formed stool
Pattern of output		
Continuous output	Unpredictable	Resumes a pattern similar to the preoperative pattern

---

INDICATIONS

POTENTIAL DIAGNOSES

Ileostomy: when the entire colon must be removed due to disease (Crohn's disease, ulcerative colitis).

Colostomy: when a portion of the bowel must be removed (cancer, ischemic injury) or requires rest for healing (diverticulitis, trauma).

CONSIDERATIONS

PREPROCEDURE

NURSING ACTIONS
- Determine the client's readiness for the procedure, including visual acuity, manual dexterity, cognitive status, cultural influences, and support systems. Qpcc
- Recommend referral to the wound ostomy care nurse (WOCN) for ostomy placement marking and client teaching. Qtc
- Work collaboratively with the WOCN to reinforce teaching the client and support person about ostomy care and management.

CLIENT EDUCATION: Perform care and management of an ostomy.

POSTPROCEDURE

NURSING ACTIONS
- Observe the type and fit of the ostomy appliance. Monitor for leakage (risk to skin integrity). The ostomy appliance is based on the following.
  - Type and location of the ostomy
  - Visual acuity and manual dexterity of the client
- Monitor peristomal skin integrity and appearance of the stoma. The stoma should appear pink and moist.
- Apply skin barriers and creams (adhesive paste) to peristomal skin and allow to dry before applying a new appliance.
- Observe stoma output. Output should be more liquid and more acidic the closer the ostomy is to the proximal small intestine.
- Empty the ostomy bag when it is one-third to one-half full of drainage.
- Monitor for fluid and electrolyte imbalances, particularly with a new ileostomy.
- Determine ability of the client or support person to perform ostomy care.

CLIENT EDUCATION
- Follow instructions regarding dietary changes, and use ostomy appliances that can help manage flatus and odor.
  - Foods that can cause odor include fish, eggs, asparagus, garlic, beans, and dark green leafy vegetables. Buttermilk, cranberry juice, parsley, and yogurt help to decrease odor.
  - Foods that can cause gas include dark green leafy vegetables, beer, carbonated beverages, dairy products, and corn. Chewing gum, skipping meals, and smoking can also cause gas. Yogurt, crackers, and toast can be ingested to decrease gas.
  - After an ostomy involving the small intestine is placed, avoid high-fiber foods for the first 2 months after surgery, chew food well, increase fluid intake, and evaluate for evidence of blockage when slowly adding high-fiber foods to the diet.
  - Proper appliance fit and maintenance prevent odor when pouch is not open. Filters, deodorizers, or a breath mint can be placed in the pouch to minimize odor while the pouch is open.
- Discuss feelings about the ostomy and concerns about its effect on life. Look at and touch the stoma. Qpcc
- Consider joining a local ostomy support group. Qtc

COMPLICATIONS

Stomal ischemia/necrosis

Stomal appearance should normally be pink or red and moist.

- Manifestations of stomal ischemia are a pale pink or bluish purple color and dry appearance.
- If the stoma appears black or purple in color, this indicates a serious impairment of blood flow and requires immediate intervention.

NURSING ACTIONS: Obtain vital signs, oxygen saturation, and current laboratory results.

CLIENT EDUCATION: Watch for indications of stomal ischemia/necrosis.

Intestinal obstruction

Intestinal obstruction can occur for a variety of reasons.

NURSING ACTIONS
- Monitor and record output from the stoma.
- Check for manifestations of obstruction, including abdominal pain, hypoactive or absent bowel sounds, distention, nausea, and vomiting.

CLIENT EDUCATION: Note indications of an intestinal obstruction following discharge.

1. A nurse is caring for a group of clients who are experiencing complications from enteral feedings. Match each potential complication with potential cause for that complication.

   A. Refeeding syndrome
   B. Nausea and vomiting
   C. Aspiration pneumonia
   D. Tube occlusion
   E. Constipation
   F. Diarrhea

   1. Bacterial contamination
   2. Lack of free water
   3. Crushed medication
   4. Displaced feeding tube
   5. Rapid increase in volume of formula administered
   6. Metabolic changes related to fluid and electrolyte shifts

2. A nurse is assisting with the care of a client who is receiving TPN. The current bag of solution was hung 24 hours ago, and 400 mL is remaining in the bag. Which action should the nurse take?

   A. Suggest discontinuing the current bag and replacing it with a new bag.
   B. Suggest that the remaining solution be infused and then replaced with a new bag.
   C. Suggest that the infusion rate be increased so the remaining solution is administered within an hour.
   D. Suggest that the current bag be discontinued and replaced with a bag of lactated Ringer's.

3. The nurse is assisting in the care of a client who is receiving intermittent enteral feedings and a client who is receiving TPN. Sort the actions by whether they are appropriate for the client who receives enteral feedings or the client who receives TPN.

   A. Monitor the administration of the solution through a central line.
   B. Assist in the dressing change using sterile technique.
   C. Monitor for manifestations of air embolism.
   D. Check residual volume per facility's policy.
   E. Flush tubing after intermittent feeding.

4. A nurse is preparing to care for a client who has cirrhosis and is undergoing paracentesis for ascites. Match each action the nurse prepares to take with the rationale for the action.

   A. Monitor the infusion of albumin as ordered
   B. Assist client to high-Fowler's position
   C. Obtain abdominal girth after the procedure
   D. Encourage client to urinate or perform catheterization

   1. Prevents inadvertent puncture of bladder
   2. Allows comparison with baseline measurement
   3. Facilitates drainage into the peritoneal cavity
   4. Reduces the risk for reaccumulation of ascites

5. A nurse is caring for clients who have undergone ostomy surgeries. Sort the types of ostomies the clients have by the characteristics of fecal output the nurse observes in their ostomy pouches. (Ileostomy, Transverse colostomy, Sigmoid colostomy)

   A. Output is liquid.
   B. Output is continuous.
   C. Output is a small amount of semi-liquid stool several days after surgery.
   D. Output may contain blood for several days after surgery.
   E. Output is semi-formed 4 to 5 days after surgery.

Active Learning Scenario

A clinical nurse educator is reviewing care of a client who will have an ileostomy with a group of newly hired nurses. What should the nurse include in this discussion? Use the ATI Active Learning Template: Therapeutic Procedure to complete this item.

INDICATIONS FOR AND DESCRIPTION OF PROCEDURE: Describe an ileostomy and the reasons it may be performed.

NURSING INTERVENTIONS: Describe at least five nursing interventions related to the care of a client who is postoperative following an ileostomy.

CLIENT EDUCATION: Describe at least five considerations for home care. .

Active Learning Scenario Key

Using the ATI Active Learning Template: Therapeutic Procedure

DESCRIPTION OF AND INDICATIONS FOR PROCEDURE: A procedure to remove the colon and create a surgical opening into the ileum to drain stool, which is typically frequent and liquid because large intestine is bypassed. Common indications for an ileostomy are complications from Crohn's disease and ulcerative colitis, including intestinal perforation, obstruction, or bleeding. Other indications include tumor and trauma.

NURSING INTERVENTIONS
- Inspect stoma; should be moist and pink or red.
- Observe skin around stoma for irritation.
- Monitor bowel sounds.
- Monitor intake and output.
- Monitor electrolyte levels.
- Encourage client to identify psychosocial concerns related to self-image, intimacy, and ability to care for stoma after discharge.
- Consult with certified wound, ostomy, and continence nurse (WOCN).

CLIENT EDUCATION
- Ensure adequate hydration.
- Identify gas-producing foods - for example, carbonated beverages and cruciferous vegetables (broccoli, cauliflower, brussels sprouts, collard greens) and introduce slowly into diet.
- Identify odor-causing foods - for example, beans, cabbage, and fish - and introduce slowly into diet.
- Clean stoma with warm water and pat dry with a towel.
- Empty pouch when it is one-third to one-half full.
- Step-by-step instructions for changing appliance, including measurement of stoma to ensure appropriate size.
- Contact information for ostomy support groups.

(N) *NCLEX® Connection: Reduction of Risk Potential, Therapeutic Procedures*

Application Exercises Key

1. A, 6; B, 5; C, 4; D, 3; E, 2; F, 1

   When recognizing cues for clients who experience complications during enteral feedings, the nurse should identify bacterial contamination from water or nonadherence to aseptic practices is a potential cause for diarrhea. The nurse should identify lack of free water, which promotes peristalsis and the movement of stool through the large intestine, is a potential cause for constipation. The nurse should identify medication tablets that have not been completely crushed and dissolved as a potential cause of tube occlusion. The nurse should identify displacement of the feeding tube into the lungs as a potential cause of aspiration pneumonia. The nurse should identify a rapid increase in the volume or rate of administration of formula as a potential cause of nausea and vomiting. The nurse should identify fluid and electrolyte shifts as potential causes of refeeding syndrome, which can lead to metabolic changes.

   (N) *NCLEX® Connection: Basic care and Comfort, Nutrition and Oral Hydration*

2. A. **CORRECT:** When taking actions for a client who is receiving TPN, the nurse should suggest replacing the container of TPN that has been hanging for 24 hours with a new bag of TPN to prevent infection.

   (N) *NCLEX® Connection: Safety and Infection Control, Standard Precautions/Transmission–Based Precautions/Surgical Asepsis*

3. **ENTERAL FEEDING:** D, E; **TPN:** A, B, C

   When taking actions for care for the client who is receiving TPN, the nurse should monitor the administration of the calorically dense, parenteral solution through a central line. The nurse should assist in performing central line dressing changes at the TPN infusion site using sterile technique to prevent central line associated bloodstream infections (CLABSI). The nurse should monitor the client who is receiving TPN for air embolism during the insertion of the central line and when changing the IV tubing. When taking actions to care for the client who is receiving enteral feedings, the nurse should check residual volume per facility's policy and hold feedings when indicated. The nurse should flush the feeding tube before and after each feeding for the client who is receiving intermittent tube feedings.

   (N) *NCLEX® Connection: Basic Care and Comfort, Nutrition and Oral Hydration*

4. A, 4; B, 3; C, 2; D, 1

   When generating solutions for a client who is undergoing a paracentesis, the nurse should anticipate encouraging the client to urinate to avoid puncture of a full bladder. The nurse should anticipate measuring the abdominal girth pre- and post-procedure to compare the differences. The nurse should anticipate placing the client in high-Fowler's position to facilitate drainage of fluid into the peritoneal cavity. The nurse should anticipate monitoring an infusion of albumin that is administered to compensate for protein loss that can cause fluid shifts.

   (N) *NCLEX® Connection: Reduction of Risk Potential, Potential for Complications of Diagnostic Tests/Treatments/Procedures*

5. **ILEOSTOMY:** A, B; **TRANSVERSE COLOSTOMY:** C, D; **SIGMOID COLOSTOMY:** E

   When recognizing cues, the nurse identifies continuous, liquid fecal material as output from an ileostomy. The nurse identifies semi-liquid stool containing blood several days after surgery as output from a transverse colostomy. The nurse identifies semi-formed stool 4 to 5 days after surgery as output from a sigmoid colostomy.

   (N) *NCLEX® Connection: Physiological Adaptation, Alterations in Body Systems*

When reviewing the following chapters, keep in mind the relevant topics and tasks of the NCLEX outline.

Basic Care and Comfort

NUTRITION AND ORAL HYDRATION: Reinforce client teaching on special diets based on client diagnosis/nutritional needs and cultural considerations.

Pharmacological Therapies

PHARMACOLOGICAL PAIN MANAGEMENT: Identify client need for pain medication.

EXPECTED ACTIONS/OUTCOMES: Reinforce client teaching on actions and therapeutic effects of medications and pharmacological interactions.

Reduction of Risk Potential

LABORATORY VALUES: Monitor diagnostic or laboratory test results.

Physiological Adaptation

ALTERATIONS IN BODY SYSTEMS: Reinforce education to client regarding care and condition.

CHAPTER 43 ## Esophageal Disorders

The esophagus is a muscular tube that leads from the throat to the stomach. The esophagus is about 25 cm (10 in) long. It extends from the base of the pharynx to the stomach, about 4 cm (1.6 in) below the diaphragm. Esophageal disorders can affect any part of the esophagus.

There are two sphincters: upper esophageal (UES), also referred to as the oropharyngeal sphincter, and the lower esophageal (LES), also referred to as gastroesophageal sphincter. They prevent the reflux of food and fluids into the mouth or esophagus.

Disorders of the esophagus, such as structural defects, inflammation, obstruction, and cancer, can interfere with nutritional intake.

Contractions of the esophagus propel food and fluids toward the stomach, while relaxation of the lower esophageal sphincter allows passage into the stomach. Following this, the LES contracts, preventing reflux of food back up into the esophagus.

Esophageal disorders include gastroesophageal reflux disease (GERD), hiatal hernia, and esophageal varices.

Gastroesophageal reflux disease

GERD is a common condition characterized by gastric content and enzyme backflow into the esophagus. Some backflow of stomach contents into the esophagus is normal. When the reflux is excessive due to any of the following conditions—an incompetent LES, pyloric stenosis, hiatal hernia, excessive intra-abdominal or intragastric pressure, or motility problems—the corrosive fluids irritate the esophageal tissue, causing delay in their clearance. This further exposes esophageal tissue to the acidic fluids, causing more irritation.
- The primary treatment of GERD is diet and lifestyle changes, advancing to medication use (antacids, H_2-receptor antagonists, proton pump inhibitors) and surgery. Qᴘᴄᴄ
- Untreated GERD leads to inflammation, breakdown, and long-term complications, such as Barrett's esophagus or adenocarcinoma of the esophagus.

HEALTH PROMOTION AND DISEASE PREVENTION
- Maintain a weight below BMI of 30.
- Stop smoking.
- Limit or avoid alcohol and tobacco use.
- Eat a low-fat diet.
- Avoid foods that lower the LES pressure such as caffeinated drinks, chocolate, nitrates, citrus fruits, and alcohol.
- Avoid eating or drinking 2 hr before bed.
- Avoid tight-fitting clothes.
- Elevate the head of the bed 6 to 8 inches.

DATA COLLECTION

RISK FACTORS
- Obesity
- Older age (delayed gastric emptying and weakened LES tone) Ⓖ
- Sleep apnea
- Nasogastric tube

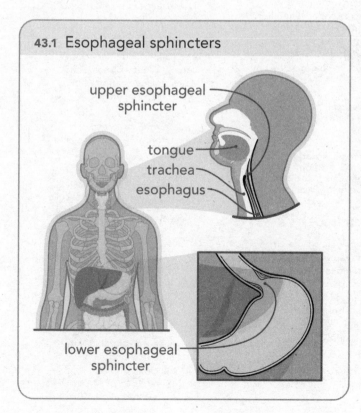

43.1 Esophageal sphincters

upper esophageal sphincter
tongue
trachea
esophagus
lower esophageal sphincter

CONTRIBUTING FACTORS

- Excessive ingestion of foods that relax the LES include fatty and fried foods, chocolate, caffeinated beverages (coffee), peppermint, spicy foods, tomatoes, citrus fruits, and alcohol.
- Prolonged or frequent abdominal distention (from overeating or delayed emptying)
- Increased abdominal pressure from obesity, pregnancy, bending at the waist, ascites, or tight clothing at the waist
- Medications that relax the LES (theophylline, nitrates, calcium channel blockers, anticholinergics, and diazepam)
- Increased gastric acid caused by medications (NSAIDs) or stress (environmental)
- Debilitation resulting in weakened LES tone
- Hiatal hernia (LES displacement into the thorax with delayed esophageal clearance)
- Gastritis due to *Helicobacter pylori* can increase reflux.
- Lying flat

EXPECTED FINDINGS

- Report of dyspepsia (indigestion) after eating an offending food or fluid and regurgitation
- Radiating pain (neck, jaw, or back)
- Report of a feeling of having a heart attack
- Pyrosis (burning sensation in the esophagus)
- Odynophagia (pain on swallowing)
- Pain that worsens with position (bending, straining, lying down)
- Pain that occurs after eating and lasts 20 min to 2 hr
- Throat irritation (chronic cough, laryngitis), hypersalivation, bitter taste in mouth (caused by regurgitation) and dysphagia in chronic GERD
- Increased flatus and eructation (burping)
- Pain relieved (almost immediately) by drinking water, sitting upright, or taking antacids
- Dental caries
- Chest congestion and wheezing due to reflux material entering the tracheobronchial tree
- Manifestations occurring four to five times per week on a consistent basis are considered diagnostic.

43.2 Case study

Part 1

1400: John is a nurse in a provider's office assisting with the care of client Joe Smith. The client reports heartburn that worsens when lying down at night. Client reports a 40-year history of cigarette smoking, drinks 3 cups of coffee daily, and has a BMI of 32.

The client takes magnesium hydroxide as needed for heartburn and has a history of cholelithiasis and a family history of diabetes mellitus.

Part 2

John is a nurse in a provider's office collecting data on Joe Smith.

Scene 1

John: "Hi, I'm John. What brings you to the provider's office?"

Joe Smith: "I'm having heartburn. It's been getting worse, especially at night."

John: "Have you noticed any foods that worsen your heartburn?"

Joe Smith: "Yes, it's worse when I eat spicy foods."

Scene 2

John: "Is there anything that relieves the pain?"

Joe Smith: "Yes, when I take my antacid or sit upright, the pain goes away."

Scene 3

John: "I would like to collect some data, check your vital signs, and obtain some blood work."

Joe Smith: "That is fine, thank you."

Part 2 conclusion

John documents the following information.

1400
- Temp 36° C (96.8° F)
- BP right arm supine: 114/56 mm Hg
- HR 72/min
- Resp 20/min
- Oxygen saturation on room air: 98%
- Abdomen soft, nondistended; audible bowel sounds present in 4 quadrants
- Lab work:
- Hct 37% (37% to 47%)
- Hgb 12 g/dL (12 g/dL to 16 g/dL)

Part 3

John is discussing medication options to treat GERD with a client.

Part 4

Amy is a nurse assisting in a surgery center with the care of client Joe Smith who is postoperative following a laparoscopic Nissen fundoplication for treatment of GERD.

Case study exercises

1. The nurse is collecting data on the client who reports heartburn. The nurse should identify that which of the following findings is a contributing factor for developing gastroesophageal reflux disease (GERD)? (Select all that apply.)
   - A. BMI
   - B. Coffee intake
   - C. Medical history
   - D. Family history
   - E. Smoking history

2. The nurse is collecting data on the client who has GERD. Which of the following findings is a manifestation of GERD?
   - A. Elevated temperature
   - B. Pain relieved by antacids
   - C. Decreased Hct level
   - D. Absence of bowel sounds

3. The nurse is discussing medications and their actions with the client who has GERD. Match the medication with its associated actions.

A. Proton pump inhibitors	1. Neutralize excess gastric acid
B. Prokinetics	2. Inhibits histamine at the gastric parietal cells
C. Histamine₂-receptor antagonists	3. Increases the motility of the esophagus and stomach
D. Antacids	4. Inhibits the cellular pump of the gastric parietal cells

4. The nurse is reinforcing discharge teaching with the client who is postoperative following a Nissen fundoplication. What instructions should the nurse include in the teaching?

DIAGNOSTIC PROCEDURES

Esophagogastroduodenoscopy (EGD)

- EGD is done under moderate sedation to identify tissue damage and to dilate strictures in the esophagus. The esophageal lining should be pink but is often red with persistent GERD. Biopsies can be done to determine if high-grade dysplasia (HGD) is present.
- HGD is evidenced by squamous mucosa of the esophagus replaced by columnar epithelium (cells seen in the stomach or intestines). When HGD is found, there is an increased chance of developing cancer.
- EGD allows visualization of the esophagus, revealing esophagitis or Barrett's epithelium (premalignant cells).

NURSING ACTIONS: Ensure gag response has returned prior to providing oral fluids or food following the procedure to reduce the risk for aspiration. Monitor client for manifestations of esophageal perforation (fever, pain, dyspnea, bleeding). Qs

Esophageal pH monitoring

A small catheter is placed through the nose and into the distal esophagus, or a small capsule is attached to the esophageal wall during endoscopy. pH readings are taken in relation to food, position, and activity for 24 to 48 hr.
- Most accurate method of diagnosing GERD
- Especially helpful in diagnosis for clients who have atypical manifestations

NURSING ACTIONS: Instruct the client to keep a journal of foods and beverages consumed, manifestations, and activity during the 24-hr test period.

Esophageal manometry

Esophageal manometry records lower esophageal sphincter pressure and peristaltic activity of the esophagus. The client swallows three small tubes, and pressure readings and pH levels are tested.

Barium swallow

Barium swallow identifies a hiatal hernia, strictures, or structural abnormalities, which would contribute to or cause GERD.

NURSING ACTIONS: Reinforce with the client to use cathartics to evacuate the barium from the GI tract following the procedure. Failure to eliminate the barium places the client at risk for fecal impaction.

PATIENT-CENTERED CARE

MEDICATIONS

Proton pump inhibitors (PPIs)

Pantoprazole, omeprazole, esomeprazole, rabeprazole, and lansoprazole reduce gastric acid by inhibiting the cellular pump of the gastric parietal cells necessary for gastric acid secretion.

NURSING ACTIONS
- Monitor for electrolyte imbalances such as hypomagnesemia (tremors, muscle cramps).
- Long-term use has been related to the development of community-acquired pneumonia and Clostridium difficile infections.

CLIENT EDUCATION: Long-term use of PPIs increases the risk for fractures, especially in older adults. Ⓖ

Antacids

Aluminum hydroxide, magnesium hydroxide, calcium carbonate, and sodium bicarbonate neutralize excess acid and increase LES pressure.

NURSING ACTIONS: Ensure there are no contraindications with other prescribed medications (levothyroxine). Evaluate kidney function in clients taking magnesium hydroxide.

CLIENT EDUCATION: Take antacids when acid secretion is the highest (1 to 3 hr after eating and at bedtime), and separate from other medications by at least 1 hr.

Histamine₂-receptor antagonists

Famotidine, cimetidine, and nizatidine reduce the secretion of acid by inhibiting histamine at the gastric parietal cells.
The onset is longer than antacids, but the effect has a longer duration.

NURSING ACTIONS: Use cautiously in clients who have kidney disease.

CLIENT EDUCATION
- Take with meals and at bedtime.
- Separate dosages from antacids (1 hr before or after taking antacid).

Prokinetics

Metoclopramide increases the motility of the esophagus and stomach.

NURSING ACTIONS: Monitor the client taking metoclopramide for extrapyramidal adverse effects.

CLIENT EDUCATION: Report abnormal, involuntary movement.

THERAPEUTIC PROCEDURES

Stretta

Uses radiofrequency energy, applied by an endoscope, to decrease vagus nerve activity. This causes the LES muscle tissue to contract and tighten.

Fundoplication

Fundoplication might be indicated for clients who fail to respond to other treatments. The fundus of the stomach is wrapped around and behind the esophagus through a laparoscope to create a physical barrier.

- Complications following fundoplication include temporary dysphagia (monitor for aspiration), gas bloat syndrome (difficulty belching to relieve distention), and atelectasis/pneumonia (monitor respiratory function).
- Monitor for bowel sounds.

CLIENT EDUCATION

- **Diet**
  - Maintain a soft diet for 1 week following procedure.
  - Avoid foods that cause reflux, such as carbonated and caffeinated beverages.
  - Avoid large meals.
  - Avoid carbonated beverages.
  - Remain upright after eating.
  - Avoid eating before bedtime.
  - Consume four to six small meals throughout the day.
- **Lifestyle**
  - Avoid clothing that is tight-fitting around the abdomen.
  - Lose weight, if applicable.
  - Elevate the head of the bed 15.2 to 20.3 cm (6 to 8 in) with blocks.
  - Avoid lifting heavy objects.
  - Walk daily.
  - Stop smoking.
- Report fever, nausea, vomiting, severe pain, dysphagia, or persistent bloating to the surgeon.

COMPLICATIONS

Aspiration of gastric secretion

CAUSES: Reflux of gastric fluids into the esophagus can be aspirated into the trachea.

RISKS ASSOCIATED WITH ASPIRATION
- Asthma exacerbations from inhaled aerosolized acid
- Frequent upper respiratory, sinus, or ear infections
- Aspiration pneumonia

NURSING ACTIONS
- Place the client in a semi-Fowler's position for meals and for 1 to 2 hr after meals.
- Keep oral suction equipment at the client's bedside.

Barrett's epithelium (premalignant) and esophageal adenocarcinoma

CAUSE: Reflux of gastric fluids leads to esophagitis. In chronic esophagitis, the body continuously heals inflamed tissue, eventually replacing normal esophageal epithelium with premalignant tissue (Barrett's epithelium) or malignant adenocarcinoma.

NURSING ACTIONS: Assist with determining the cause of GERD with the client and review lifestyle changes that can decrease gastric reflux. Monitor nutritional status. Qpcc

Hiatal hernia

Hiatal hernia (diaphragmatic hernia) is a protrusion of the stomach (in part or in total) above the diaphragm into the thoracic cavity through the hiatus (the opening in the diaphragm). There are two types of hiatal hernia.

Sliding (more common): A portion of the stomach and gastroesophageal junction move above the diaphragm. This generally occurs with increases in intra-abdominal pressure or while the client is in a supine position.

Paraesophageal (rolling): Part of the fundus of the stomach moves above the diaphragm, although the gastroesophageal junction remains below the diaphragm.

HEALTH PROMOTION AND DISEASE PREVENTION

- Avoid eating immediately prior to going to bed.
- Avoid foods and beverages that decrease LES pressure (fatty and fried foods, chocolate, coffee, peppermint, spicy foods, tomatoes, citrus fruits, and alcohol).
- Exercise regularly.
- Maintain a healthy weight.
- Elevate the head of the bed on 6-inch blocks.
- Avoid straining or excessive vigorous exercise.
- Avoid wearing clothing that is tight around the abdomen.

DATA COLLECTION

EXPECTED FINDINGS

Presenting manifestations depend on the type of hiatal hernia and are typically worse following a meal.

Sliding: heartburn, reflux, chest pain, dysphagia, belching

Paraesophageal: fullness after eating, sense of breathlessness/suffocation, chest pain, worsening of manifestations when reclining

DIAGNOSTIC PROCEDURES

Barium swallow with fluoroscopy

Allows visualization of the esophagus

NURSING ACTIONS: Reinforce with the client to use cathartics to evacuate the barium from the GI tract following the procedure. Failure to eliminate the barium places the client at risk for fecal impaction.

Esophagogastroduodenoscopy (EGD)

Allows visualization of the esophagus and the gastric lining

NURSING ACTIONS: Ensure gag response has returned prior to providing oral fluids or food following the procedure. Qs

CT scan of the chest with contrast

Allows visualization of the esophagus and stomach

NURSING ACTIONS: Check for iodine allergies if IV contrast is to be used. Encourage fluids following procedure to promote dye excretion and minimize risk of renal injury. Monitor BUN/creatinine.

PATIENT-CENTERED CARE

MEDICATIONS

Proton pump inhibitors

Pantoprazole, omeprazole, esomeprazole, rabeprazole, and lansoprazole reduce gastric acid by inhibiting the cellular pump of the gastric parietal cells necessary for gastric acid secretion.

NURSING ACTIONS

- Monitor for electrolyte imbalances and hypoglycemia in clients who have diabetes mellitus.
- Long-term use has been related to the development of community-acquired pneumonia and *Clostridium difficile* infections.

CLIENT EDUCATION: Long-term use of PPIs increases the risk for fractures, especially in older adults. Ⓖ

Antacids

Aluminum hydroxide, magnesium hydroxide, calcium carbonate, and sodium bicarbonate neutralize excess acid and increase LES pressure.

NURSING ACTIONS: Ensure there are no contraindications with other prescribed medications (levothyroxine). Evaluate kidney function in clients taking magnesium hydroxide.

CLIENT EDUCATION: Take antacids when acid secretion is the highest (1 to 3 hr after eating and at bedtime), and separate from other medications by at least 1 hr.

THERAPEUTIC PROCEDURES

Fundoplication: reinforcement of the LES by wrapping a portion of the fundus of the stomach around the distal esophagus

Laparoscopic Nissen fundoplication: minimally invasive with fewer complications

NURSING ACTIONS: Elevate the head of the bed to promote lung expansion. Reinforce with the client to support the incision during movement and coughing to minimize strain on the suture lines.

CLIENT EDUCATION: Consume a soft diet for the first week postoperative. Avoid carbonated beverages. Ambulate, but avoid heavy lifting.

COMPLICATIONS: Temporary dysphagia, gas bloat syndrome (difficulty burping and distention), atelectasis/pneumonia

COMPLICATIONS

Volvulus: twisting of the esophagus and/or stomach

Obstruction (paraesophageal hernia): blockage of food in the herniated portion of the stomach

Strangulation (paraesophageal hernia): compression of the blood vessels to the herniated portion of the stomach

Iron-deficiency anemia (paraesophageal hernia): resulting from bleeding into the gastric mucosa due to obstruction

Esophageal varices

- Esophageal varices are swollen, fragile blood vessels that are generally found in the submucosa of the lower esophagus, but varices can develop higher in the esophagus or extend into the stomach.
- Esophageal varices can occur as a result of portal hypertension, usually due to cirrhosis of the liver.
- When esophageal varices hemorrhage, it is often a medical emergency associated with a high mortality rate. Recurrence of esophageal bleeding is common.

HEALTH PROMOTION AND DISEASE PREVENTION

Avoid alcohol consumption.

DATA COLLECTION

RISK FACTORS

- Portal hypertension (elevated blood pressure in veins that carry blood from the intestines to the liver)
  - Caused by impaired circulation of blood through the liver. Collateral circulation subsequently develops, creating varices in the upper stomach and esophagus. Varices are fragile and can bleed easily.
  - The primary risk factor for development of esophageal varices
- Alcoholic cirrhosis
- Viral hepatitis
- Frequently in older adult clients, depressed immune function, decreased liver function, and cardiac disorders that make them especially vulnerable to bleeding Ⓖ

EXPECTED FINDINGS

- The client can experience no manifestations until the varices begin to bleed. Hematemesis (vomiting blood), melena (black, tarry stools), and a general deterioration of the client's physical and mental status
- Activities that precipitate bleeding are the Valsalva maneuver, lifting heavy objects, coughing, sneezing, and alcohol consumption.

PHYSICAL FINDINGS (BLEEDING ESOPHAGEAL VARICES)
- Shock
- Hypotension
- Tachycardia
- Cool, clammy skin

LABORATORY TESTS

Liver function tests indicate a liver disorder.

Hemoglobin and hematocrit tests can indicate anemia secondary to occult bleeding or overt bleeding.

Elevated blood ammonia level can indicate liver disease. Ammonia is converted to urea in the liver.

DIAGNOSTIC PROCEDURES

Endoscopy

Therapeutic interventions can be performed during the endoscopy.

NURSING ACTIONS: Administer preprocedure sedation. After the procedure, monitor vital signs and take measures to prevent aspiration, such as confirming the gag reflex before offering oral fluids.

PATIENT-CENTERED CARE

NURSING CARE Qs

If bleeding is suspected, establish IV access with a large bore needle, monitor vital signs and hematocrit, type, and cross-match for possible blood transfusions, and monitor for overt and occult bleeding.

MEDICATIONS

Nonselective beta blockers

- Propranolol is prescribed to decrease heart rate and consequently reduce hepatic venous pressure.
- Used prophylactically (not for emergency hemorrhage)

Vasoconstrictors

- Octreotide is a synthetic form of the hormone somatostatin, which decreases the bleeding from the esophageal varices but does not affect the blood pressure.
- Vasopressin causes constriction of the esophageal and proximal gastric veins and reduces portal pressure.

NURSING ACTIONS
- Vasopressin should not be given to clients who have coronary artery disease due to resultant coronary constriction. Potent vasoconstriction can also reduce peripheral and cerebral circulation. If vasopressin is used in combination with nitroglycerin IV in this client population, it can decrease or prevent the vasoconstriction of the coronary arteries.
- Monitor for fluid retention and hyponatremia, as vasopressin has an antidiuretic effect.

THERAPEUTIC PROCEDURES

Endoscopic variceal ligation (EVL)

Endoscopic variceal ligation (esophageal banding therapy) can be used for acute bleeding.
- During endoscopy, the varices are rubber-banded to cut off the circulation to the varices. Necrosis of the tissue occurs with eventual sloughing of the varix.
- There is a significant decrease in rebleeding as well as decreased mortality post procedure.

COMPLICATIONS
- Superficial ulceration
- Dysphagia
- Temporary chest discomfort
- Esophageal strictures (rare)

NURSING ACTIONS: After the procedure, monitor vital signs and take measures to prevent aspiration.

Endoscopic sclerotherapy

During endoscopy, a sclerosing agent is injected into the varices, resulting in thrombosis of the varicosity.

COMPLICATIONS
- Bleeding
- Perforation of the esophagus
- Aspiration pneumonia
- Esophageal stricture

NURSING ACTIONS
- After the procedure, monitor vital signs and take measures to prevent aspiration.
- Antacids, H_2-receptor blockers, or PPIs can be administered after the procedure to protect the esophagus and prevent acid reflux, which is often caused by sclerotherapy.

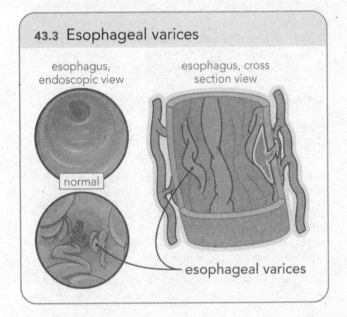

43.3 Esophageal varices

esophagus, endoscopic view

esophagus, cross section view

normal

esophageal varices

Transjugular intrahepatic portal-systemic shunt (TIPS)

- TIPS is used to treat an acute episode of bleeding when EVL and pharmacological measures are not controlling the variceal bleeding. It rapidly lowers the portal pressure. The procedure is costly and therefore is only used when other measures do not work.
- While the client is under sedation or general anesthesia, a catheter is passed into the liver via the jugular vein in the neck. A stent is then placed between the portal and hepatic veins bypassing the liver. Portal hypertension is subsequently relieved.

COMPLICATIONS
- Bleeding
- Sepsis
- Heart failure
- Organ perforation
- Liver failure

NURSING ACTIONS: Monitor vital signs. Keep the head of the bed elevated.

Surgical interventions

- Considered as a last resort. TIPS has replaced many surgical measures. High morbidity and mortality rates continue to be seen with surgical intervention.
- Bypass procedures establish a venous shunt that bypasses the liver, decreasing portal hypertension.
  - Common shunts include **splenorenal** (splenic, left renal veins), **mesocaval** (mesenteric vein, vena cava), and **portacaval** (portal vein, inferior vena cava).
  - Clients commonly have a nasogastric tube inserted during surgery to monitor for hemorrhage.

NURSING ACTIONS (PREPROCEDURE, POSTPROCEDURE)
- Monitor for an increase in liver dysfunction or encephalopathy.
- Monitor nasogastric tube secretions for bleeding.
- Monitor PT, aPTT, platelets, and INR.

INTERPROFESSIONAL CARE

Alcohol recovery program (varices secondary to alcohol use disorder)

COMPLICATIONS

Hypovolemic shock

Due to hemorrhage from varices

NURSING ACTIONS
- Observe for manifestations of hemorrhage and shock (tachycardia, hypotension).
- Monitor vital signs, Hgb, Hct, and coagulation studies.
- Support therapeutic procedures to stop and control bleeding.

Application Exercises

1. A nurse is reinforcing teaching with a client who has a hiatal hernia. Which of the following client statements indicates an understanding of the teaching?
   - A. "I can take my medications with a carbonated drink."
   - B. "Peppermint tea can increase my indigestion."
   - C. "Wearing an abdominal binder will decrease my indigestion."
   - D. "I will drink hot chocolate at bedtime to help me sleep."

2. A nurse is assisting with the plan of care for a client who has bleeding esophageal varices. The nurse should expect a prescription for which of the following medications?
   - A. Propranolol
   - B. Metoclopramide
   - C. Famotidine
   - D. Vasopressin

Active Learning Scenario

A nurse is preparing a poster on GERD to be displayed at a community health fair. What should be included in the poster? Use the ATI Active Learning Template: System Disorder to complete this item.

ALTERATION IN HEALTH (DIAGNOSIS)

RISK FACTORS: Describe at least seven.

EXPECTED FINDINGS: Describe at least seven.

Active Learning Scenario Key

Using the ATI Active Learning Template: System Disorder

ALTERATION IN HEALTH (DIAGNOSIS): Gastroesophageal reflux disease (GERD) is a common condition characterized by gastric content and enzyme backflow into the esophagus. These fluids are corrosive to esophageal tissue, causing a delay in their clearance. This further exposes esophageal tissue to the acidic fluids, increasing tissue irritation.

RISK FACTORS

- Obesity
- Older age
- Sleep apnea
- Excessive ingestion of foods that relax the lower esophageal sphincter (fatty and fried foods, chocolate, caffeinated beverages, peppermint, spicy foods, tomatoes, citrus fruits, and alcohol)
- Pregnancy
- Bending at the waist, wearing tight clothing at the waist
- Medications (theophylline, nitrates, calcium channel blockers, anticholinergics, NSAIDs)
- Stress
- Hiatal hernia
- Lying flat

EXPECTED FINDINGS

- Dyspepsia after eating and regurgitation (classic)
- Throat irritation (chronic cough, laryngitis)
- Hypersalivation
- Bitter taste in mouth
- Chest pain due to esophageal spasm
- Increased flatus and eructation (burping)
- Pain relieved by drinking water, sitting upright, or taking antacids

Ⓝ *NCLEX® Connection: Health Promotion and Maintenance, Health Promotion/Disease Prevention*

Application Exercises Key

1. B. **CORRECT:** When evaluating outcomes, the nurse should identify that the client understands the instructions because peppermint decreases LES pressure and should be avoided by the client who has a hiatal hernia.

Ⓝ *NCLEX® Connection: Physiological Adaptation, Alterations in Body Systems*

2. D. **CORRECT:** When generating solutions, the nurse should plan to administer vasopressin to the client who has bleeding esophageal varices. Vasopressin constricts blood vessels to decrease blood flow and bleeding.

Ⓝ *NCLEX® Connection: Physiological Adaptation, Alterations in Body Systems*

Case Study Exercises Key

1. A, B, E. **CORRECT:** When recognizing cues, the nurse should identify that contributing factors for GERD include obesity, caffeine intake, and cigarette smoking. Obesity can cause an increase in intra-abdominal pressure and gastric reflux. Caffeine intake and cigarette smoking can decrease lower esophageal sphincter pressure, resulting in gastric reflux.

Ⓝ *NCLEX® Connection: Health Promotion and Maintenance, Health Promotion/Disease Prevention*

2. B. **CORRECT:** When recognizing cues, the nurse should identify that pain that is relieved by taking antacids, drinking fluids, and sitting upright is a manifestation of GERD.

Ⓝ *NCLEX® Connection: Physiological Adaptation, Alterations in Body Systems*

3. A, 4; B, 3; C, 2; D, 1

When taking actions, the nurse should instruct the client that antacids reduce GERD by neutralizing gastric acid. Histamine₂receptor antagonists reduce gastric acid secretion by inhibiting histamine at the gastric parietal cells. Prokinetics reduce GERD by increasing the motility of the esophagus and stomach. Proton pump inhibitors reduce gastric acid secretion by inhibiting the cellular pump of the gastric parietal cells. (Burchum, 2022, 952, 953, 956, 980)

Ⓝ *NCLEX® Connection: Physiological Adaptation, Alterations in Body Systems*

4. When taking actions, the nurse should instruct the client to avoid foods that cause reflux, such as carbonated and caffeinated beverages, consume 4 to 6 small meals per day, remain upright after eating and avoid eating, before bedtime. The nurse should instruct the client to avoid clothing that is tight-fitting around the abdomen, reduce weight, if applicable, and elevate the head of the bed 15.2 to 20.3 cm (6 to 8 in) with blocks. The client should avoid lifting heavy objects and walk daily. The client should report fever, nausea, vomiting, severe pain, dysphagia, or persistent bloating to the surgeon.

Ⓝ *NCLEX® Connection: Physiological Adaptation, Alterations in Body Systems*

CHAPTER 44 Peptic Ulcer Disease

A peptic ulcer is an erosion of the mucosal lining of the stomach, esophagus, or duodenum. The most common area for a peptic ulcer is the duodenum. The mucous membranes can become eroded to the point that the epithelium is exposed to gastric acid and pepsin, which can precipitate bleeding and perforation. Perforation that extends through all the layers of the stomach or duodenum can cause peritonitis. An individual who has a peptic ulcer has peptic ulcer disease.

Most peptic ulcers are caused by an infection from gram-negative bacteria *Helicobacter pylori* (*H. pylori*). Contact with the bacteria occurs from food, water, or exposure to body fluids such as saliva. Some people infected with the *H. pylori* bacteria do not develop ulcers. Stress ulcers occur from an acute period of physiological stressful events, such as burns, shock, severe sepsis, or multiple organ trauma. These ulcers are different clinically from a peptic ulcer. They consist of multiple lesions in the stomach and proximal duodenum and can be present in a ventilated client in the intensive care unit. Bleeding is the primary manifestation of the stress ulcer. Clients experiencing trauma often receive proton-pump inhibitor prophylaxis to prevent the development of stress ulcers.

HEALTH PROMOTION AND DISEASE PREVENTION

- Drink alcohol in moderation.
- Stop smoking and use of tobacco products.
- Use stress management techniques.
- Avoid NSAIDs as indicated.
- Limit caffeine-containing beverages.
- Consume a balanced diet.
- Engage regularly in exercise.

DATA COLLECTION

RISK FACTORS

Causes of peptic ulcers
- *Helicobacter pylori* (*H. pylori*) infection
- NSAID and corticosteroid use
- Severe stress
- Familial tendency
- Hypersecretory states
- Excess alcohol consumption
- Zollinger-Ellison syndrome (combination of peptic ulcers, hypersecretion of gastric acid, and gastrin-secreting tumors)
- Pernicious anemia
- Cigarette smoking

EXPECTED FINDINGS

- Dyspepsia: heartburn, bloating, nausea, and vomiting (vomiting is rare but can be caused by a gastric outlet obstruction). Can be perceived as uncomfortable fullness or hunger
- Dull, gnawing pain or burning sensation at the midepigastrium or the back

44.1 Ulcer pain

GASTRIC ULCER	DUODENAL ULCER
• Pain most commonly occurs 30 to 60 min after a meal.	• Pain occurs 1.5 to 3 hr after a meal.
• Less often pain at night (30% to 40% of clients)	• Awakening with pain during the night
• Pain exacerbated by ingestion of food	• Pain relieved by ingestion of food or antacid
• Malnourishment	• Well-nourished
• Hematemesis	• Melena

PHYSICAL FINDINGS
- Pain or epigastric tenderness or abdominal distension
- Bloody emesis (hematemesis) or stools (melena)
- Weight loss

LABORATORY TESTS

H. pylori testing: Gastric samples are collected via an endoscopy to test for *H. pylori*.

Urea breath testing: The client exhales into a collection container (baseline), drinks carbon-enriched urea solution, and is asked to exhale into a collection container. The client should take nothing by mouth (NPO) prior to the test. If *H. pylori* is present, the solution will break down and carbon dioxide will be released. Serologic testing documents the presence of *H. pylori* based on antibody assays.

Stool sample tests for the presence of the *H. pylori* antigen

Hemoglobin and hematocrit (findings below the expected reference range secondary to bleeding)

Stool sample for occult blood

DIAGNOSTIC PROCEDURES

Esophagogastroduodenoscopy (EGD)

Refer to **CHAPTER 41: GASTROINTESTINAL DIAGNOSTIC PROCEDURES**. An EGD provides a definitive diagnosis of peptic ulcers and can be repeated to evaluate the effectiveness of treatment. Gastric samples are obtained to test for *H. pylori*.

NURSING ACTIONS: Monitor vital signs until sedation wears off. Keep client NPO until return of gag reflex. Monitor for manifestations of perforation: pain, bleeding, fever, and vital sign changes.

CLIENT EDUCATION: NPO 6 to 8 hr prior to the exam.

PATIENT-CENTERED CARE

NURSING CARE

- Instruct clients to avoid foods that cause distress (coffee, tea, carbonated beverages).
- Monitor for orthostatic changes in vital signs and tachycardia, as these findings are suggestive of gastrointestinal bleeding or perforation.
- Assist with the administration of saline lavage via nasogastric tube.
- Administer medication as prescribed.
- Decrease environmental stress.
- Encourage rest periods.
- Encourage smoking cessation and avoiding alcohol consumption.
- Monitor laboratory results (hemoglobin, hematocrit, coagulation studies, serum electrolytes, BUN).

MEDICATIONS

Antibiotics

Metronidazole, amoxicillin, clarithromycin, and tetracycline eliminate *H. pylori* infection.

NURSING ACTIONS: A combination of two or three different antibiotics can be administered.

CLIENT EDUCATION: Complete a full course of medication.

Histamine₂-receptor antagonists

Famotidine, cimetidine, and nizatidine suppress the secretion of gastric acid by selectively blocking H_2 receptors in parietal cells lining the stomach.
- Used in conjunction with antibiotics to treat ulcers caused by *H. pylori*
- Used to prevent stress ulcers in clients who are NPO after major surgery; have large areas of burns, multiple trauma, or multisystem disorders, are septic; or have increased intracranial pressure

NURSING ACTIONS
- Famotidine can be administered IV in acute situations.
- Cimetidine and famotidine can be taken with or without food.
- Treatment of peptic ulcer disease is usually started as an oral dose twice a day until the ulcer is healed, followed by a maintenance dose usually taken once a day at bedtime.

CLIENT EDUCATION
- Notify the provider of obvious or occult GI bleeding (coffee-ground emesis).
- Complete the prescribed regimen, even when manifestations subside.

Proton-pump inhibitors

Pantoprazole, esomeprazole, omeprazole, lansoprazole, and rabeprazole suppress gastric acid secretion by irreversibly inhibiting the enzyme that produces gastric acid and inhibit basal and stimulated acid production.

NURSING ACTIONS
- Insignificant adverse effects with short-term treatment
- Long-term use can increase the risk of fractures, pneumonia, acid rebound, and the possibility of developing *Clostridium difficile*.
- Rabeprazole and pantoprazole are enteric-coated tablets and should not be crushed.

CLIENT EDUCATION
- Do not crush, chew, or break sustained-release capsules.
- Take omeprazole and lansoprazole once a day prior to eating the main meal of the day.
- Take rabeprazole with or without food. Q**PCC**
- Avoid alcohol and irritating medications (NSAIDs).
- Complete the prescribed regimen, even when manifestations subside.

Antacids

- Aluminum hydroxide and magnesium hydroxide neutralize acid in the gut. The medication provides manifestation relief but generally does not accelerate healing.
- Antacids can be given 7 times per day, 1 to 3 hr after meals and at bedtime, to neutralize gastric acid, which occurs with food ingestion.

NURSING ACTIONS
- Give 1 to 2 hr apart from other medications to avoid reducing the absorption of other medications.
- Monitor kidney function of clients prescribed aluminum hydroxide and magnesium hydroxide.
- Encourage compliance by reinforcing the intended effect of the antacid (relief of pain; promotes healing of ulcer).
- Aluminum hydroxide can cause constipation.
- Magnesium hydroxide can cause diarrhea.

CLIENT EDUCATION: Take all medications at least 1 to 2 hr before or after taking an antacid.

Mucosal protectants

- Sucralfate coats the ulcer and protects it from the actions of pepsin and acid.
- Bismuth subsalicylate prevents *H. pylori* from binding to the mucosal wall.

NURSING ACTIONS

- Administer on an empty stomach 1 hr before meals and at bedtime.
- Oral suspension is easier for the older adult clients to ingest because the tablet form is large and difficult to swallow.
- Monitor for adverse effect of constipation.

CLIENT EDUCATION

- If taking bismuth subsalicylate, avoid aspirin products to avoid salicylate toxicity.
- If taking bismuth subsalicylate, stools can be black. This is temporary and harmless.

THERAPEUTIC PROCEDURES

Esophagogastroduodenoscopy (EGD)

Areas of bleeding can be treated with epinephrine or laser coagulation.

NURSING ACTIONS

- PREPROCEDURE: Ensure two large-bore IV catheters are in place.
- POSTPROCEDURE
  - Monitor vital signs. Keep client NPO until gag reflex returns.
  - Take vital signs every 15 to 30 min.
  - Observe client for fever, pain, and vital sign changes, which could indicate a perforation.

Surgical interventions

Can be used in clients when ulcers do not heal following 12 to 16 weeks of medical treatment, hemorrhage, perforation, or obstruction

Gastrectomy: All or part of the stomach is removed with laparoscopic or open approach.
- **Antrectomy:** The antrum portion (lower portion of stomach) of the stomach is removed.
- **Gastrojejunostomy (Billroth II procedure):** The lower portion of the stomach is excised, the remaining stomach is anastomosed to the jejunum, and the remaining duodenum is surgically closed.

Vagotomy: The vagus nerve is cut to decrease gastric acid production in the stomach. Often done laparoscopically to reduce postoperative complications

Pyloroplasty: The opening between the stomach and small intestine is enlarged to increase the rate of gastric emptying.

NURSING ACTIONS

- Monitor the incision for evidence of infection.
- Place the client in a semi-Fowler's position to facilitate lung expansion.
- Monitor nasogastric tube drainage. Scant blood can be seen in the first 12 to 24 hr.
- Notify the provider before repositioning or irrigating the nasogastric tube (disruption of sutures). Qs
- Monitor bowel sounds.
- Advance diet as tolerated to avoid undesired effects (abdominal distention, diarrhea).
- Administer medication as prescribed (analgesics, stool softeners).

CLIENT EDUCATION

- Take vitamin and mineral supplements due to decreased absorption after a gastrectomy, including vitamin B_{12}, vitamin D, calcium, iron, and folate.
- Consume small, frequent meals while avoiding large quantities of carbohydrates as directed.
- Notify provider of sudden abdominal or epigastric pain.
- Monitor and report bleeding such as black stools or coffee-ground emesis.

INTERPROFESSIONAL CARE

Nutrition consult: Diet that restricts acid-producing foods: milk products, caffeine, decaffeinated coffee, spicy foods, medications (NSAIDs)

COMPLICATIONS

Perforation/hemorrhage

When peptic ulcers perforate or bleed, it is an emergency situation.
- Perforation presents as severe epigastric pain spreading across the abdomen. The pain can radiate into the shoulders, especially the right shoulder due to irritation of the phrenic nerve. The abdomen can become tender and rigid (boardlike). Hyperactive to diminished bowel sounds can be auscultated, and there is rebound tenderness. The client will display manifestations of shock, hypotension, and tachycardia. Perforation is a surgical emergency.
- Gastrointestinal bleeding in the form of hematemesis or melena can cause manifestations of shock (hypotension, tachycardia, dizziness, confusion), and decreased hemoglobin.

NURSING ACTIONS

- Perform frequent checks of pain and vital signs to detect subtle changes that can indicate perforation or bleeding. Qs
- Provide oxygen and assist with ventilator support as needed.
- Ensure two large-bore IV lines are in place for replacement of blood and fluids.
- Report findings, prepare the client for endoscopic or surgical intervention, assist with blood and fluid replacement to maintain blood pressure, insert nasogastric tube, and assist with saline lavages.

Pernicious anemia

- Occurs due to a deficiency of the intrinsic factor normally secreted by the gastric mucosa
- Manifestations include pallor, glossitis, fatigue, and paresthesias.

CLIENT EDUCATION: Lifelong monthly vitamin B_{12} injections will be necessary.

Dumping syndrome

This can occur following gastrectomy surgery and is a group of manifestations that occur following eating. A shift of fluid to the abdomen is triggered by rapid gastric emptying or high-carbohydrate ingestion. The rapid release of metabolic peptides following ingestion of a food bolus causes dumping syndrome.

- The client can report a full sensation, weakness, diaphoresis, palpitations, dizziness, and diarrhea. Vasomotor manifestations that can occur 5 to 30 min following a meal are pallor, perspiration, palpitations, headache, feeling of warmth, dizziness, and drowsiness.
- Late manifestations of dumping syndrome can be related to the rapid release of blood glucose, followed by an increase in insulin production resulting in hypoglycemia.

NURSING ACTIONS

- Monitor for vasomotor manifestations.
- Assist/instruct the client to lie down when vasomotor manifestations occur.
- Administer medications.
  - Octreotide subcutaneously can be prescribed if manifestations are severe and not effectively controlled with dietary measures. Octreotide blocks gastric and pancreatic hormones, which can lead to findings of dumping syndrome.
  - Acarbose slows the absorption of carbohydrates.
- Malnutrition and fluid electrolyte imbalances can occur due to altered absorption. Monitor I&O, laboratory values, and weight.

44.2 Vasomotor manifestations

	EARLY MANIFESTATIONS	LATE MANIFESTATIONS
Onset	Within 30 min after eating	1.5 to 3 hr after eating
Cause	Rapid emptying	Excessive insulin release
Findings	Nausea, vomiting, sweating, and dizziness	Dizziness and sweating
		Tachycardia and palpitations
	Tachycardia	Shakiness and feelings of anxiety
	Palpitations	Confusion

CLIENT EDUCATION

- Lying down after a meal slows the movement of food within the intestines.
- Limit the amount of fluid ingested at one time.
- Eliminate liquids with meals for 1 hr prior to and following a meal.
- Consume a high-protein, high-fat, low-fiber, and low- to moderate-carbohydrate diet. Qpcc
- Avoid milk and sugars (sweets, fruit juice, sweetened fruit, milk shakes, honey, syrup, jelly).
- Consume small, frequent meals rather than large meals.

Pyloric (gastric outlet) obstruction

- Pyloric obstruction occurs due to scarring, edema, or spasm or loss of muscle tone of the area distal to the pyloric sphincter and prevents emptying of the stomach.
- Manifestations include feeling of fullness, distention, nausea after eating, and emesis consisting of undigested food.

NURSING ACTIONS

- Insert an NG tube for gastric decompression.
- Monitor fluid and electrolyte status.

Application Exercises

1. A nurse is assisting with teaching a class about peptic ulcer disease. Sort the following into features associated with a gastric ulcer and those associated with a duodenal ulcer.

    A. Pain occurs 30 to 60 min after a meal.

    B. Pain occurs 1.5 to 3 hr after a meal.

    C. Hematemesis

    D. Melena

    E. Pain exacerbated by ingestion of food

    F. Pain relieved by ingestion of food

2. A nurse is reinforcing discharge teaching for a client who has an infection due to *Helicobacter pylori* (*H. pylori*). Which of the following statements by the client indicates understanding?

    A. "I will stop taking my medication as soon as I feel better."

    B. "I will take my medications with my morning coffee."

    C. "I will take a combination of medications for treatment."

    D. "I will take an antacid at the same time as my antibiotic medications."

3. A nurse is collecting data on a client who has a peptic ulcer and a suspected stomach perforation. What findings should the nurse expect?

4. Match each type of food listed to the correct answer (foods allowed or encouraged, foods to use with caution, and foods that must be excluded).

    A. Non-spicy soups

    B. Fruit

    C. Sweetened fruit juice

    D. Mayonnaise

    E. Milk products with fat

    F. Whole grain bread

    G. Diet jelly

5. A nurse is reinforcing teaching with a client who has a new diagnosis of dumping syndrome following gastric surgery. Which of the following information should the nurse include?

    A. Eat three moderate-sized meals a day.

    B. Drink at least one glass of water with each meal.

    C. Eat a bedtime snack that contains a milk product.

    D. Increase protein in the diet.

Active Learning Scenario

A nurse is preparing a poster about peptic ulcer disease to be displayed at a community health fair. What information should the nurse include in the poster? Use the ATI Active Learning Template: System Disorder to complete this item.

ALTERATION IN HEALTH (DIAGNOSIS):
Include the types of ulcers.

HEALTH PROMOTION AND DISEASE PREVENTION:
Describe at least three prevention activities.

RISK FACTORS: Describe four risk factors for peptic ulcers.

Active Learning Scenario Key

Using the ATI Active Learning Template: System Disorder

ALTERATION IN HEALTH (DIAGNOSIS): An erosion of the mucosal lining of the stomach or duodenum. Mucous membranes can become eroded to the point that the epithelium is exposed to gastric acid and pepsin, which can precipitate bleeding and perforation. Types of ulcers include gastric, duodenal, and stress ulcers.

HEALTH PROMOTION AND DISEASE PREVENTION
- Drink alcohol in moderation.
- Stop smoking and use of tobacco products.
- Use stress management strategies.
- Avoid NSAIDs.
- Limit caffeine-containing beverages.

RISK FACTORS
- *Helicobacter pylori (H. pylori)*
- NSAID and corticosteroid use
- Severe stress
- Hypersecretory conditions
- Excess alcohol ingestion

Ⓝ *NCLEX® Connection: Health Promotion and Maintenance, Health Promotion/Disease Prevention*

Application Exercises Key

1. **GASTRIC ULCER:** A, C, E; **DUODENAL ULCER:** B, D, F

   When taking actions, the nurse should instruct that manifestations of a gastric ulcer include pain that occurs 30 to 60 min after a meal, hematemesis (bloody emesis), and pain that is exacerbated by ingestion of food. Manifestations of a duodenal ulcer include pain that occurs 1.5 to 3 hr after a meal, melena (blood in stools), and pain that is relieved by ingestion of food.

   Ⓝ *NCLEX® Connection: Physiological Adaptation, Basic Pathophysiology*

2. C. **CORRECT:** When evaluating outcomes, the nurse should identify the client understands to take a combination of medications, such as a proton-pump inhibitor and two antibiotics to treat an infection caused by *H. pylori*.

   Ⓝ *NCLEX® Connection: Pharmacological Therapies, Expected Actions/Outcomes*

3. When recognizing cues, the nurse should check the client for severe epigastric pain that might spread across the abdomen. The pain can radiate into the shoulders, especially the right shoulder due to irritation of the phrenic nerve. The abdomen can become tender and rigid (boardlike). Hyperactive to diminished bowel sounds might be auscultated, and there is rebound tenderness. Gastrointestinal bleeding in the form of hematemesis or melena can cause manifestations of shock (hypotension, tachycardia, dizziness, confusion) and decreased hemoglobin. Stomach or intestinal perforation is a surgical emergency.

   Ⓝ *NCLEX® Connection: Physiological Adaptation, Basic Pathophysiology*

4. **FOODS ALLOWED OR ENCOURAGED:** B, G;
   FOODS TO USE WITH CAUTION: A, D, F;
   FOODS THAT MUST BE EXCLUDED: C, E

   Ⓝ *NCLEX® Connection: Physiological Adaptation, Basic Pathophysiology*

5. D. **CORRECT:** When taking actions, the nurse should instruct the client to eat a high-protein, high-fat, low-fiber, and moderate- to low-carbohydrate diet to slow gastrointestinal transit time.

   Ⓝ *NCLEX® Connection: Physiological Adaptation, Alterations in Body Systems*

CHAPTER 45 *Acute and Chronic Gastritis*

Gastritis is an inflammation in the lining of the stomach, either erosive or nonerosive, and can be acute or chronic.

TYPES OF GASTRITIS

Nonerosive gastritis (acute or chronic) is most often caused by an infection; *Helicobacter pylori*.

Erosive gastritis is likely caused by NSAIDs, alcohol use disorder, or recent radiation treatment.

Acute gastritis has sudden onset, is of short duration, and can result in gastric bleeding if severe. A severe form of acute gastritis is caused by the ingestion of an irritant, (such as a strong acid or alkali) and can result in the development of gangrenous tissue or perforation. Scarring can result, leading to pyloric stenosis.

Chronic gastritis can be related to autoimmune disease, such as pernicious anemia, and *H. pylori*.

Extensive gastric mucosal wall damage can cause **erosive gastritis (peptic ulcers)** and increase the risk of stomach cancer.

HEALTH PROMOTION AND DISEASE PREVENTION

- Assist in the reduction of anxiety related to gastritis.
- Follow a prescribed diet.
- Decrease or eliminate alcohol use.
- Watch for indications of GI bleeding.
- Follow the prescribed medication regimen.
- Eat small, frequent meals, avoiding foods and beverages that cause irritation.
- Report constipation, nausea, vomiting, or bloody stools.
- Stop smoking.

DATA COLLECTION

RISK FACTORS

- Family member who has *H. pylori* infection
- Family history of gastritis
- Prolonged use of NSAIDs, corticosteroids (stops prostaglandin synthesis)
- Excessive alcohol use
- Bile reflux disease
- Advanced age

- Radiation or chemotherapy
- Smoking
- Caffeine
- Excessive stress
- Exposure to contaminated food or water

BACTERIAL INFECTION: *Helicobacter pylori, Salmonella,* staphylococci, or *Escherichia coli*

EXPECTED FINDINGS

PHYSICAL FINDINGS
- Dyspepsia, general abdominal discomfort
- Hiccuping
- Upper abdominal pain or burning, which can increase or decrease after eating
- Nausea and vomiting
- Reduced appetite and weight loss
- Abdominal bloating or distention
- Hematemesis (bloody emesis) and stools that test positive for occult blood
- Gastric hemorrhage
- Anorexia
- Anemia
- Intolerance of spicy and fatty foods

> Manifestations can have rapid onset with acute gastritis.

Erosive gastritis
- Black, tarry stools; coffee-ground emesis
- Acute abdominal pain

LABORATORY TESTS

Noninvasive tests

CBC to check for anemia
- Females assigned at birth: Hgb less than 12 g/dL and RBC less than 4.2 cells/mcL
- Males assigned at birth: Hgb less than 14 g/dL and RBC less than 4.7 cells/mcL

Blood and stool antibody/antigen: test for presence of *H. pylori*

Stool specimen: Test for occult blood

Urea breath test: Used to measure *H. pylori*

DIAGNOSTIC PROCEDURES

Upper endoscopy

A small flexible scope is inserted through the mouth into the esophagus, stomach, and duodenum to visualize the upper digestive tract. This procedure allows for a biopsy, cauterization, removal of polyps, dilation, or diagnosis. (See **CHAPTER 41: GASTROINTESTINAL DIAGNOSTIC PROCEDURES.**)

CLIENT EDUCATION

- Maintain NPO status after midnight the day of the procedure.
- Have a ride home available after the procedure.
- A local anesthetic will be sprayed onto the back of the throat, but the throat can be sore following the procedure. Qs
- Monitor for indications of perforation (chest or abdominal pain, fever, nausea, vomiting, and abdominal distention) and have emergency contact numbers available.

PATIENT-CENTERED CARE

NURSING CARE

- Monitor fluid intake and urine output.
- Assist with the administration of IV fluids as prescribed.
- Monitor electrolytes. (Diarrhea and vomiting can deplete electrolytes and cause dehydration.)
- Assist the client in identifying foods that are triggers.
- Provide small, frequent meals and encourage the client to eat slowly.
- Advise the client to avoid alcohol, caffeine, and foods that can cause gastric irritation.
- Assist the client in identifying ways to reduce stress.
- Monitor for indications of gastric bleeding (coffee-ground emesis; black, tarry stools).
- Monitor for findings of anemia (tachycardia, hypotension, fatigue, shortness of breath, pallor, feelings of lightheadedness or dizziness, chest pain).

MEDICATIONS

Histamine$_2$ antagonists

ACTION: Decreases gastric acid output by blocking gastric histamine$_2$ receptors

MEDICATIONS

- Nizatidine
- Famotidine
- Cimetidine

NURSING INTERVENTIONS

- Allow 1 hr before or after to administer antacid. Antacids can decrease the effectiveness of H$_2$-receptor antagonists. Qpcc
- Monitor for neutropenia.
- Dilute and administer slowly when given IV; rapid administration can cause bradycardia.

CLIENT EDUCATION

- Do not smoke or drink alcohol.
- Take oral dose with meals. Take famotidine 1 hr before meals to decrease heartburn, acid indigestion, and sour stomach.
- Wait 1 hr prior to or following H$_2$-receptor antagonist to take an antacid.
- Monitor for indications of GI bleeding (black stools, coffee-ground emesis).

Antacids

ACTION

- Increases gastric pH and neutralizes pepsin
- Improves mucosal protection

MEDICATIONS

- Aluminum hydroxide
- Magnesium hydroxide with aluminum hydroxide

NURSING INTERVENTIONS

- Do not give to clients who have acute kidney injury or chronic kidney failure.
- Monitor clients taking aluminum antacids for aluminum toxicity and constipation. Monitor magnesium antacids for diarrhea or hypermagnesemia.

CLIENT EDUCATION

- Take antacids on an empty stomach.
- Wait 2 hr to take other medications.

Proton-pump inhibitors

ACTION: Reduces gastric acid by stopping the hydrogen/potassium ATPase enzyme system in parietal cells, blocking acid production

MEDICATIONS

- Omeprazole
- Lansoprazole
- Rabeprazole sodium
- Pantoprazole
- Esomeprazole

NURSING INTERVENTIONS: Can cause nausea, vomiting, and abdominal pain

CLIENT EDUCATION

- Allow 60 min before eating when taking esomeprazole.
- Do not to crush or chew if any of the medications are enteric-coated or sustained-release.
- It can take up to 4 days to see the effects.
- Take medication with or without food according to the instructions.

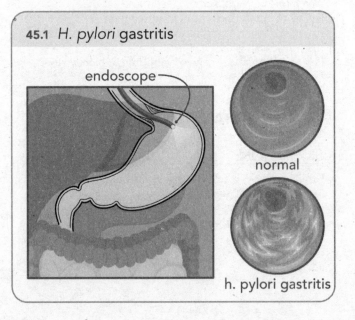

45.1 *H. pylori* gastritis

endoscope

normal

h. pylori gastritis

Anti-ulcer/mucosal barriers

ACTION: Inhibits acid and forms a protective coating over mucosa

MEDICATIONS: Sucralfate

NURSING INTERVENTIONS: Allow 30 min before or after to give antacid.

CLIENT EDUCATION
- Take on an empty stomach.
- Do not smoke or drink alcohol.
- Continue to take medication even if manifestations subside.

Antibiotics

ACTION: Eliminates *H. pylori* infection

MEDICATIONS
- Clarithromycin
- Amoxicillin
- Tetracycline
- Metronidazole

NURSING INTERVENTIONS
- Monitor for increased abdominal pain and diarrhea.
- Monitor electrolytes and hydration if fluid is depleted.
- Use cautiously in clients who have kidney or hepatic impairment. Qpcc

CLIENT EDUCATION
- Complete prescribed dosage.
- Notify the provider of persistent diarrhea, which can indicate superinfection of the bowel.

THERAPEUTIC PROCEDURES

Surgery is prescribed for clients who have ulcerations or significant bleeding or when nonsurgical interventions are ineffective. (See **CHAPTER 44: PEPTIC ULCER DISEASE**.)

Partial gastrectomy: Removal of the involved portion of the stomach

INTERPROFESSIONAL CARE

- A nutritionist can assist in alterations to diet.
- Supportive care might be needed to reduce stress, increase exercise, and stop smoking. Qtc

COMPLICATIONS

Gastric bleeding

CAUSES
- Severe acute gastritis with deep tissue inflammation extending into the stomach muscle
- In chronic erosive gastritis, bleeding can be slow or profuse as in a perforation of the stomach wall.

NURSING ACTIONS
- Monitor vital signs and airway.
- Provide fluid replacement and assist with administration of blood products.
- Monitor CBC and clotting factors.
- Insert a nasogastric (NG) tube for gastric lavage (irrigate with normal saline or water to stop active gastric bleed) as indicated. Obtain an x-ray to confirm placement of NG tube prior to fluid instillation to prevent aspiration. QEBP
- Monitor NG tube for absence or presence of blood, check the amount of bleeding, and prevent gastric dilation.

CLIENT EDUCATION: Monitor for indications of slow gastric bleeding (coffee-ground emesis; black, tarry stools). Seek immediate medical attention with severe abdominal pain or vomiting blood. Take medications as directed.

Gastric outlet obstruction

CAUSE: Severe acute gastritis with deep tissue inflammation extending into the stomach muscle

NURSING ACTIONS
- Monitor fluids and electrolytes because continuous vomiting results in loss of chloride (metabolic alkalosis) and severe fluid and electrolyte depletion.
- Provide fluid and electrolyte replacement. Monitor I&O.
- Prepare to insert an NG tube to empty stomach contents.
- Prepare for a diagnostic endoscopy.

CLIENT EDUCATION: Seek medical attention for continuous vomiting, bloating, and nausea.

Dehydration

CAUSE: Loss of fluid due to vomiting or diarrhea

NURSING ACTIONS
- Monitor fluid intake and urine output.
- Assist with the provision of IV fluids if needed.
- Monitor electrolytes.

CLIENT EDUCATION: Contact a provider for vomiting and diarrhea.

Active Learning Scenario

A nurse is reinforcing teaching about acute and chronic gastritis with a client. What information should the nurse reinforce with the client? Use the ATI Active Learning Template: System Disorder to complete this item.

ALTERATION IN HEALTH (DIAGNOSIS)
- Describe gastritis.
- Compare/contrast acute vs. chronic gastritis.

PATHOPHYSIOLOGY RELATED TO CLIENT PROBLEM: Describe as related to client problem.

RISK FACTORS: Describe six.

Application Exercises

1. A nurse is reinforcing teaching with a client who is scheduled for an upper endoscopy. Which of the following instructions should the nurse include?

    A. You will receive general anesthesia for the procedure.

    B. You should have nothing to eat or drink after midnight the day of the procedure.

    C. You will be intubated during the procedure.

    D. You will be placed on your right side for the procedure.

2. A nurse is collecting data for a client following an upper endoscopy (EGD). Which of the following observations would indicate the development of a complication?

    A. The client is drowsy but responsive.

    B. The client reports a sore throat.

    C. The client's temperature is 100.2° F.

    D. The client eats only 30% of a soft diet.

3. A nurse is reinforcing discharge teaching with a client who has a new prescription for aluminum hydroxide. Which of the following information should the nurse include?

    A. Take the medication with food.

    B. Monitor for diarrhea.

    C. Wait 2 hours before taking other oral medications.

    D. Maintain a low-fiber diet.

4. A nurse is reinforcing teaching for a client who has a new prescription for famotidine. Which of the following statements made by the client indicates an understanding of the teaching?

    A. "This medication coats the lining of my stomach."

    B. "The medication should stop the pain right away."

    C. "I will take this pill at bedtime."

    D. "I will monitor for nosebleeds."

5. A nurse is collecting data from a client with gastritis who reports abdominal pain. Which of the following statements made by the client should the nurse address?

    A. "I have been trying to relax and get more sleep."

    B. "I carry antacids with me in case I get heartburn."

    C. "I gave up drinking coffee and orange juice."

    D. "I use ibuprofen if I get a headache or joint pain."

Application Exercises Key

1. B. **CORRECT:** When taking actions, the nurse should inform the client that they will be NPO after midnight the day of the procedure to prevent vomiting or aspiration.

    Ⓝ NCLEX® Connection: Physiological Adaptation, Alterations in Body Systems

2. C. **CORRECT:** When recognizing cues, the nurse should identify a fever is an indication that perforation or infection has occurred.

    Ⓝ NCLEX® Connection: Reduction of Risk Potential, Potential for Complications of Diagnostic Tests/Treatments/Procedures

3. C. **CORRECT:** When generating solutions, the nurse should inform the client to wait 2 hours before taking other medications as aluminum hydroxide can interfere with the actions and absorption of other medications.

    Ⓝ NCLEX® Connection: Pharmacological Therapies, Adverse Effects/Contraindications/Side Effects/Interactions

4. C. **CORRECT:** When evaluating outcomes, the nurse should identify the client understands the teaching by stating famotidine should be taken at bedtime so that it works by suppressing nocturnal acid production.

    Ⓝ NCLEX® Connection: Pharmacological Therapies, Adverse Effects/Contraindications/Side Effects/Interactions

5. D. **CORRECT:** When generating solutions, the nurse should address the client taking ibuprofen for headaches or joint pain, which can cause GI bleeding.

    Ⓝ NCLEX® Connection: Pharmacological Therapies, Adverse Effects/Contraindications/Side Effects/Interactions

Active Learning Scenario Key

Using the ATI Active Learning Template: System Disorder

ALTERATION IN HEALTH (DIAGNOSIS): Gastritis is an inflammation of the lining of the stomach as a result of irritation to the mucosa.
- Acute: Sudden onset; short duration; can result in gastric bleeding
- Chronic: Slow onset; when profuse, it can damage parietal cells, resulting in pernicious anemia

PATHOPHYSIOLOGY RELATED TO CLIENT PROBLEM: Gastric acid overwhelms the production of COX 1 enzymes, which provide mucosal prostaglandins that line the stomach. This results in an erosion of the mucosa and increases the risk for ulcers and stomach cancer.

RISK FACTORS
- Bacterial infection (*H. pylori*, *Salmonella*, staphylococci, *E. coli*)
- Family history of *H. pylori*
- Prolonged use of NSAIDs or corticosteroids
- Excessive alcohol use
- Bile reflux disease
- Autoimmune diseases
- Advanced age
- Radiation therapy
- Smoking
- Caffeine
- Excessive stress
- Exposure to contaminated food or water

Ⓝ NCLEX® Connection: Physiological Adaptation, Alterations in Body Systems

When reviewing the following chapters, keep in mind the relevant topics and tasks of the NCLEX outline.

Basic Care and Comfort

NUTRITION AND ORAL HYDRATION: Reinforce client teaching on special diets based on client diagnosis/nutritional needs and cultural considerations.

Pharmacological Therapies

PHARMACOLOGICAL PAIN MANAGEMENT: Identify client need for pain medication.

EXPECTED ACTIONS/OUTCOMES: Reinforce client teaching on actions and therapeutic effects of medications and pharmacological interactions.

Reduction of Risk Potential

LABORATORY VALUES: Monitor diagnostic or laboratory test results.

Physiological Adaptation

ALTERATIONS IN BODY SYSTEMS
Reinforce education to client regarding care and condition.

Reinforce client teaching on ostomy care.

CHAPTER 46 # Noninflammatory Bowel Disorders

Noninflammatory bowel disorders can cause pain, changes in bowel pattern, bleeding, and malabsorption. This group of disorders includes hemorrhoids, cancer, hernia, irritable bowel syndrome (IBS), and intestinal obstruction.

Hemorrhoids are distended or edematous intestinal veins resulting from increased intra-abdominal pressure (straining, obesity, prolonged sitting or standing, constipation, weight lifting). Pregnancy increases the risk of hemorrhoids.

Cancer of the small or large intestine can be caused by age-related changes (clients who are 50 years or older have an increased risk), genetic influence, or chronic bowel disease, such as Crohn's disease or ulcerative colitis.

Nurses should be knowledgeable about noninflammatory bowel disorders and treatments. Topics to be reviewed include hernia, irritable bowel syndrome, and intestinal obstruction.

Hernia

Bowel herniation is the displacement of the bowel through a weakness of the abdominal muscle into other areas of the abdominal cavity.

Incisional hernias can occur as a postsurgical complication due to inadequate healing of the incisional site from malnutrition, infection, or obesity.

A hernia that cannot be moved back into place with gentle palpation is considered irreducible and requires immediate surgical evaluation.

In a hernia that is strangulated, blood supply is cut off to a portion of the bowel, increasing the risk for obstruction, necrosis, and perforation. Findings include abdominal distention, tachycardia, vomiting, abdominal pain, and fever. Surgical intervention is necessary.

DATA COLLECTION

RISK FACTORS

- Male sex (indirect inguinal hernia can be large and descend into the scrotum)
- Advanced age (direct hernia) Ⓖ
- Increased intra–abdominal pressure due to pregnancy or obesity (femoral, adult-acquired umbilical hernia)
- Genetics (congenital umbilical hernia)

EXPECTED FINDINGS

Protrusion or lump at involved site (groin area, umbilicus, healed incision)

46.1 Hernia

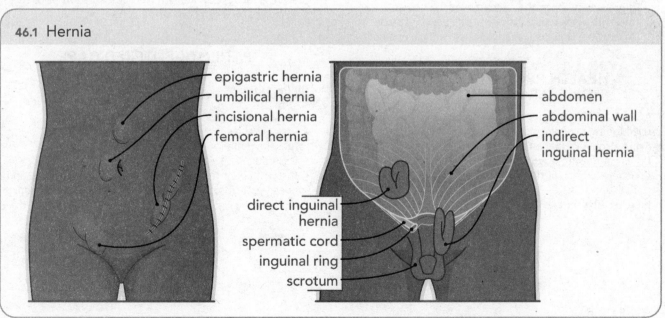

- epigastric hernia
- umbilical hernia
- incisional hernia
- femoral hernia

- direct inguinal hernia
- spermatic cord
- inguinal ring
- scrotum

- abdomen
- abdominal wall
- indirect inguinal hernia

PATIENT-CENTERED CARE

NURSING ACTIONS: If the hernia does not require surgery, instruct the client to wear a truss pad with hernia belt during waking hours to prevent the abdominal contents from bulging into the hernia sac. Inspect skin under the pad daily.

Postoperative client education

- Avoid increased intra-abdominal pressure for 1 to 3 weeks (avoid coughing, straining, and lifting objects greater than 10 lb).
- Apply ice as prescribed and inspect and report redness or swelling at the incisional site.
- Prevent constipation by increasing dietary fiber and fluids.
- Rest for several days and return to work when recommended by the surgeon, usually 1 to 2 weeks postoperatively.

Irritable bowel syndrome

IBS is a disorder of the gastrointestinal system that causes changes in bowel function (chronic diarrhea, constipation, bloating, and/or abdominal pain).

- The etiology of IBS is uncertain, but it is thought that environmental, immunological, genetic, hormonal, and stress -related factors influence the development and course of the disease. Food intolerances worsen the manifestations.
  - **Environmental factors:** Dairy products, caffeinated beverages, infectious agents
  - **Immunological factors:** Cytokine genes (pro-inflammatory interleukins), tumor necrosis factor (TNF) alpha
  - **Stress–related factors:** Anxiety, depression
- IBS is diagnosed primarily based on the presence of manifestations. Criteria can include recurrent abdominal pain for 3 days during a month in the past 3 months and two or more of the following.
  - Improvement when the client moves their bowels
  - Onset when there is a change in frequency of stools
  - Onset when there is a change in appearance of stools

HEALTH PROMOTION AND DISEASE PREVENTION

- Avoid foods that trigger exacerbation (dairy, wheat, corn, fried foods, alcohol, spicy foods, aspartame).
- Avoid alcoholic and caffeinated beverages, and other fluids containing fructose and sorbitol.
- Consume 2 to 3 L of fluid per day from food and fluid sources.
- Increase fiber intake (approximately 30 to 40 g/day).

DATA COLLECTION

RISK FACTORS

- Female sex
- Stress
- Eating large meals containing a large amount of fat
- Caffeine intake
- Alcohol intake

EXPECTED FINDINGS

- Cramping pain in abdomen
- Abdominal pain
- Nausea
- Anorexia
- Abdominal bloating
- Belching
- Diarrhea (diarrhea-predominant IBS)
- Constipation (constipation-predominant IBS)
- Hyperactive or hypoactive bowel sounds
- Sensation of incomplete defecation
- Mucous in stools

LABORATORY TESTS

CBC, blood albumin, erythrocyte sedimentation rate (ESR), and occult stools are all typically within the expected reference range.

DIAGNOSTIC TESTS

Hydrogen breath test

A hydrogen breath test might be performed to identify malabsorption, impaired digestion, or an overgrowth of bacteria. The client is asked to exhale into a hydrogen analyzer before and after ingesting test sugar. Positive test results indicate excess hydrogen in the bloodstream from bacterial overgrowth or malabsorption.

CLIENT EDUCATION: Remain NPO at least 12 hr prior to test, except for sips of water.

PATIENT-CENTERED CARE

NURSING CARE

- Review strategies to reduce stress.
- Instruct the client to limit the intake of irritating agents (gas-forming foods, caffeine, alcohol).
- Encourage a diet high in fiber and fluids.
- Instruct client to keep a food diary to record intake and bowel patterns (to adjust diet to prevent exacerbations).

MEDICATIONS

Diarrhea-predominant IBS (IBS-D)

Loperamide
- Decreases peristalsis and increases bulk
- Can cause drowsiness
- Discontinue if no response after 48 hr.

Psyllium
- Bulk-forming laxative
- Discontinue for abdominal cramping, rectal bleeding, and vomiting.
- Monitor for electrolyte imbalance.

Alosetron
- An IBS-specific medication that selectively blocks $5-HT_3$ receptors that innervate the viscera. The expected result is increased firmness in stools and decreased urgency and frequency of defecation.
- Indicated for IBS-D in females that has lasted more than 6 months and is resistant to conventional management. Use with caution in females and only as a last resort.

NURSING ACTIONS: Contraindicated for clients who have a history of bowel obstruction, Crohn's disease, ulcerative colitis, impaired intestinal circulation, or thrombophlebitis

CLIENT EDUCATION
- Manifestations should resolve within 1 to 4 weeks. Discontinue medication after 4 weeks if manifestations persist.
- Avoid concurrent use of psychoactive drugs and antihistamines.
- Report constipation, fever, increasing abdominal pain, fatigue, dark urine, bloody diarrhea, or rectal bleeding immediately because alosetron can cause ischemic colitis. Discontinue medication if these manifestations occur. Qs

Constipation-predominant IBS (IBS-C)

Lubiprostone: An IBS-specific medication that increases fluid secretion in the intestine to promote intestinal motility. This is indicated for IBS-C in females.
- Contraindicated for clients who have known or possible bowel obstruction
- CLIENT EDUCATION: Take with food and water.

Linaclotide
- Increases fluid and motility in the intestine
- Can relieve pain and cramps
- CLIENT EDUCATION: Take daily about 30 min before breakfast.

Intestinal obstruction

Intestinal obstruction can result from mechanical or nonmechanical causes. Manifestations vary according to type.
- Mechanical obstruction occurs when the bowel is blocked by something outside or inside the intestines (adhesions, fecal impactions). Complete mechanical obstructions should be addressed surgically.
- Nonmechanical obstructions are caused by diminished peristalsis within the bowel (paralytic ileus). This can occur postoperatively due to the handling of the intestines during surgery.
- Treatment focuses on fluid and electrolyte balance, decompressing the bowel, and relief/removal of the obstruction.

DATA COLLECTION

RISK FACTORS

Mechanical obstructions

Result from the following:
- Encirclement or compression of intestine by adhesions, tumors, fibrosis (endometriosis), or strictures (Crohn's disease, radiation)
  - Postsurgical adhesions are often the cause of small bowel obstructions.
  - Carcinomas are often the cause of large intestine obstructions.
  - OLDER ADULT CLIENTS: Diverticulitis, fecal impaction, and tumors are common causes of obstruction. Bowel regimens can be effective in preventing impactions. Ⓖ
- Hernia (bowel becomes trapped in weakened area of abdominal wall)
- Volvulus (twisting) or intussusception (telescoping) of bowel segments

Nonmechanical obstructions

- Nonmechanical obstructions (paralytic ileus) result from decreased peristalsis secondary to the following.
  - Neurogenic disorders (manipulation of the bowel during major surgery and spinal fracture)
  - Vascular disorders (vascular insufficiency and mesenteric emboli)
  - Electrolyte imbalances (hypokalemia)
  - Inflammatory responses (peritonitis or sepsis)
- Manifestations of nonmechanical obstructions include diffuse, constant pain; significant abdominal distention; and frequent vomiting.

EXPECTED FINDINGS

Manifestations vary depending on the location of the obstruction.

Small bowel and large intestine obstructions

- Obstipation: the inability to pass a stool and/or flatus for more than 8 hr despite feeling the urge to defecate
- Abdominal distention
- High-pitched bowel sounds above site of obstruction (borborygmi) with hypoactive bowel sounds below, or overall hypoactive; absent bowel sounds later in process
- Diarrhea or ribbon-like stools around an impaction with large intestine obstruction

Small bowel obstructions

- Severe fluid and electrolyte imbalance
- Metabolic alkalosis
- Visible peristaltic waves (possible)
- Epigastric or upper abdominal distention
- Abdominal pain, discomfort
- Profuse, sudden projectile vomiting with fecal odor

LABORATORY TESTS

- Increased hemoglobin, BUN, creatinine, and hematocrit can indicate dehydration.
- Increased blood amylase and WBC count can occur with strangulating obstructions.
- Arterial blood gases (ABGs) indicate metabolic imbalance, depending on obstruction type.
- Chemistry profiles reveal decreased blood sodium, chloride, and potassium.

DIAGNOSTIC PROCEDURES

X-ray: Flat plate and upright abdominal x-rays evaluate the presence of free air and gas patterns.

Endoscopy determines the cause of obstruction.

CT scan determines the cause and exact location of the obstruction.

PATIENT-CENTERED CARE

NURSING CARE

Nonmechanical cause of obstruction

- Nothing by mouth with bowel rest
- Check bowel sounds.
- Provide oral hygiene.
- Ensure IV fluids and electrolyte replacement (particularly potassium) are administered.
- Manage pain (once diagnosis identified).
- Encourage ambulation.
- Place in semi-Fowler's position.

Mechanical cause of obstruction

- Prepare for surgery and assist with providing preoperative nursing care.
- Withhold intake until peristalsis resumes.

MEDICATIONS

Opioid antagonist (alvimopan) is administered for short-term use to reverse the action of opioids on bowel motility in clients who have a postoperative paralytic ileus. Monitor for myocardial infarction.

THERAPEUTIC PROCEDURES

Nasogastric (NG) tube with a vent (to prevent damage to the stomach mucosa during continuous suctioning) is inserted to decompress the bowel.

NURSING ACTIONS
- Maintain intermittent suction as prescribed.
- Check NG tube patency and placement. Irrigate every 4 hr, or as prescribed.
- Monitor and measure gastric output.
- Monitor nasal area for skin breakdown.
- Provide oral hygiene every 2 hr.
- Monitor vital signs, skin integrity, weight, and I&O.

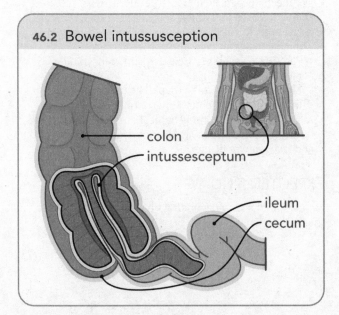

46.2 Bowel intussusception

colon
intussesceptum
ileum
cecum

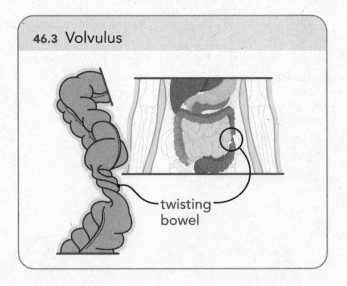

46.3 Volvulus

twisting bowel

Surgical interventions

Procedure varies based on cause of obstruction. These can include lysis of adhesions, colon resection, colostomy creation (temporary or permanent), embolectomy, thrombectomy, resection of gangrenous intestinal tissue, or complete colectomy.

Exploratory laparotomy : To determine and correct the cause of obstruction if possible

NURSING ACTIONS
- Ensure the client understands the type of procedure (open or laparoscopic).
- Monitor vital signs.
- Assist with the administration of IV fluid replacement and maintenance as prescribed.
- Monitor bowel sounds.
- Maintain NG tube patency and measure output.
- Clamp NG tube as prescribed to check the client's tolerance prior to removal.
- Advance diet as tolerated when prescribed, beginning with clear liquids. Clamp tube after eating for 1 to 2 hr.
- Instruct client to report intolerance of intake following NG tube removal (nausea, vomiting, increasing distention).

COMPLICATIONS

Dehydration

CAUSE: Persistent vomiting

NURSING ACTIONS
- Monitor hydration through evaluation of hematocrit, BUN, orthostatic vital signs, skin turgor/mucous membranes, urine output, and specific gravity. Notify the provider of a fluid imbalance.
- Monitor electrolytes, especially potassium levels. Qs
- Notify the provider of an electrolyte imbalance.
- Assist with the administration of IV fluids as prescribed to replace electrolytes.

Active Learning Scenario

A nurse is preparing a poster on caring for a client who has a bowel obstruction. What information should the nurse include on the poster? Use the ATI Active Learning Template: System Disorder to complete this item.

RISK FACTORS: Identify at least two for each form of obstruction.

EXPECTED FINDINGS: Identify at least two expected findings for each type of obstruction.

DIAGNOSTIC PROCEDURES: Identify at least two.

Active Learning Scenario Key

Using the ATI Active Learning Template: System Disorder

RISK FACTORS
- Mechanical
  - Encirclement or compression of intestines by adhesions, tumors, fibrosis, or strictures
  - Volvulus, intussusception
  - Hernia, fecal impaction
- Nonmechanical: decreased peristalsis due to neurogenic or vascular disorders, electrolyte imbalances, and inflammatory responses
  - Small bowel: postsurgical adhesions

EXPECTED FINDINGS
- Mechanical: mild, colicky, intermittent pain
- Nonmechanical: vague, diffuse, constant pain; significant abdominal distention
  - Small bowel obstruction
    - Visible peristaltic waves possible
    - Profuse, sudden projectile vomiting with fecal odor, which relieves pain
    - Severe fluid and electrolyte imbalance, metabolic alkalosis

DIAGNOSTIC PROCEDURES
- X-rays (flat plate, upright abdominal)
- Endoscopy
- CT scan

N *NCLEX® Connection: Physiological Adaptation, Alterations in Body Systems*

Application Exercises

1. A nurse is reinforcing teaching about diet recommendations with a client who has IBS. Which of the following information should the nurse include? (Select all that apply.)

    A. Limit alcohol intake to one drink per day.

    B. Eliminate dairy from diet.

    C. Avoid beverages that contain caffeine.

    D. Limit foods containing fructose.

2. A nurse is reinforcing teaching about diagnostic testing with a client who has manifestations of IBS. The nurse should advise the client that which of the following tests can be used to determine the presence of bacterial overgrowth?

    A. *Helicobacter pylori* breath test

    B. Hydrogen breath test

    C. Glucose tolerance

    D. Pulmonary function test

3. A nurse is collecting data on a client in an extended care facility. The nurse should recognize which of the following findings is a manifestation of an obstruction of the large intestine due to a fecal impaction?

    A. The client reports one bowel movement yesterday morning.

    B. Increased bowel sounds

    C. The client is flatulent.

    D. The client states they vomited once this morning.

4. A nurse is assisting with the care of a client who has a nasogastric tube attached to low suction due to an intestinal obstruction. Which of the following actions should the nurse take?

    A. Maintain in the client in lateral semi-prone recumbent position.

    B. Provide oral hygiene every 12 hr.

    C. Irrigate the NG tube every 4 hr.

    D. Offer ice chips frequently.

5. A nurse is caring for a group of clients who have an intestinal disorder. Match the medication that can be prescribed for the disorder.

    | A. Alosetron | 1. Postoperative paralytic ileus |
    | B. Lubiprostone | 2. Irritable bowel syndrome-constipation |
    | C. Alvimopan | 3. Irritable bowel syndrome-diarrhea |

6. A nurse is reviewing the medical record of a client who has a small bowel obstruction. Which of the following findings should the nurse report to the provider? (Select all that apply.)

    A. Emesis prior to insertion of the nasogastric tube

    B. Urine specific gravity 1.040

    C. Hematocrit 60%

    D. High-pitched bowel sounds

    E. WBC 10,000/ μl

7. A nurse is contributing to the plan of care for a client who has a small bowel obstruction and a nasogastric (NG) tube in place. Which of the following interventions should the nurse include? (Select all that apply.)

    A. Document the NG drainage with the client's output.

    B. Irrigate the NG tube every 8 hr.

    C. Monitor bowel sounds.

    D. Ensure the client is in semi-Fowler's position.

    E. Monitor NG tube for placement.

8. A nurse is caring for a client who has a small bowel obstruction from adhesions. Which of the following findings are consistent with this diagnosis? (Select all that apply.)

    A. Emesis greater than 500 mL with a fecal odor

    B. Report of spasmodic abdominal pain

    C. High-pitched bowel sounds

    D. Abdomen flat with rebound tenderness to palpation

    E. Laboratory findings indicating metabolic acidosis

9. A nurse is caring for a client who has an umbilical hernia. Which of the following should the nurse identify as a risk factor for this type of hernia?

    A. Congenital

    B. Impaired healing

    C. Age

    D. Sex

10. A nurse is reinforcing discharge teaching with a client who has irritable bowel syndrome (IBS). Which of the following instructions should the nurse include?

    A. Keep a food diary to identify triggers to exacerbation.

    B. Consume 15 to 20 g of fiber daily.

    C. Plan three moderate to large meals per day.

    D. Limit fluid intake to 1 L each day.

1. **B, C, D. CORRECT:** When taking actions, the nurse should instruct the client to avoid foods that can initiate manifestations of IBS, such as alcohol, caffeine, fructose, and dairy.

   Ⓝ *NCLEX® Connection: Basic Care and Comfort, Nutrition and Oral Hydration*

2. **B. CORRECT:** When taking action, the nurse should include in the teaching that a hydrogen breath test is used to diagnose the presence of bacterial overgrowth for clients who have IBS.

   Ⓝ *NCLEX® Connection: Reduction of Risk Potential, Laboratory Values*

3. **B. CORRECT:** When recognizing cues, the nurse should identify a client who has a mechanical obstruction due to fecal impaction can have increased bowel sounds of the abdomen above the area of obstruction.

   Ⓝ *NCLEX® Connection: Physiological Adaptation, Basic Pathophysiology*

4. **C. CORRECT:** When taking actions, the nurse should irrigate the NG tube every 4 hr to keep the tube patent.

   Ⓝ *NCLEX® Connection: Reduction of Risk Potential, Potential for Complications of Diagnostic Tests/Treatments/Procedures*

5. A, 3; B, 2; C,1

   Alvimopan is an opioid antagonist that can be used to treat postoperative paralytic ileus. Lubiprostone is an IBS-specific medication that increases fluid secretion in the intestine to promote intestinal motility. This is indicated for IBS-C in females. Alosetron is an IBS-specific medication that is indicated for IBS-D.

   Ⓝ *NCLEX® Connection: Physiological Adaptation, Basic Pathophysiology*

6. A. Profuse emesis is an expected finding for a client who has a small bowel obstruction. Do not report this finding to the provider.
   B. **CORRECT:** This urine specific gravity is greater than the expected reference range of 1.005 to 1.030. An increased urine specific gravity is an indication of dehydration. Report this finding to the provider.
   C. **CORRECT:** The Hct is greater than the expected reference range of 42% to 52% for males and 37% to 47% for females. An elevated HCT indicates hemoconcentration, which is due to dehydration.
   D. **CORRECT:** High-pitched bowel sounds can be heard above the point of the obstruction for a client who has a small bowel obstruction. Report this finding to the provider.
   E. This WBC is within the expected reference range of 5,000 to 10,000/mm³. Do not report this finding to the provider.

   Ⓝ *NCLEX® Connection: Reduction of Risk Potential, Laboratory Values*

7. A. **CORRECT:** Document the NG drainage as output. This helps determine the amount of fluid replacement needed.
   B. The NG tube is irrigated every 4 hr to maintain patency.
   C. **CORRECT:** Bowel sounds should be monitored to evaluate treatment and resolution of the obstruction.
   D. **CORRECT:** The client should be in semi-Fowler's position to prevent aspiration. If the client experiences hypotension, place the client on their left side.
   E. **CORRECT:** Check the placement of the NG tube prior to irrigation to prevent aspiration and periodically to prevent an increase in abdominal distention.

   Ⓝ *NCLEX® Connection: Reduction of Risk Potential, Potential for Complications of Diagnostic Tests/Treatments/Procedures*

8. A. **CORRECT:** Large emesis with a fecal odor is a finding in a client who has a small bowel obstruction.
   B. **CORRECT:** Report of abdominal pain is a finding in a client who has a small bowel obstruction.
   C. **CORRECT:** High-pitched bowel sounds are a manifestation of a small or large bowel obstruction.
   D. Abdominal distention is a finding in a client who has a small bowel obstruction.
   E. Metabolic alkalosis due to the loss of gastric acid is a finding in a client who has a small bowel obstruction.

   Ⓝ *NCLEX® Connection: Physiological Adaptation, Basic Pathophysiology*

9. A. **CORRECT:** Congenital, pregnancy or obesity can be risk factors for umbilical hernias.
   B. Impaired healing of a surgical incision can be a risk factor from a ventral hernia.
   C. Older adults can be a risk factor for inguinal hernias due to weakness of the posterior-inguinal wall.
   D. Being of male sex can be a risk factor for inguinal hernias due to incomplete closure of the tract when the testes descend into the scrotum before birth.

   Ⓝ *NCLEX® Connection: Health Promotion and Maintenance, Health Promotion/Disease Prevention*

10. A. **CORRECT:** The client should keep a food diary to identify foods that trigger exacerbation of manifestations.
    B. The client should increase daily fiber intake to 30 to 40 g.
    C. The client should eat small, frequent meals.
    D. The client should drink 2 to 3 L of fluids per day to promote a consistent bowel pattern.

    Ⓝ *NCLEX® Connection: Basic Care and Comfort, Nutrition and Oral Hydration*

CHAPTER 47 *Inflammatory Bowel Disease*

Inflammatory bowel disease (IBD) can affect structures or segments along the gastrointestinal tract. The term includes both acute and chronic disorders.

Acute and chronic IBD can result in nutritional deficits, altered bowel elimination, infection, pain, and fluid or electrolyte imbalances. The nurse needs to be knowledgeable about acute and chronic IBD in order to collaborate with the client and the interprofessional team in treating and managing these disorders.

ACUTE INFLAMMATORY BOWEL DISEASE

Appendicitis

Inflammation of the appendix
- Caused by an obstruction of the lumen or opening of the appendix
- Fecaliths, or hard pieces of stool, can be the initial cause of the obstruction.
- Adolescents and young adults are at increased risk.
- Refer to the **PEDIATRIC NURSING REVIEW MODULE, CHAPTER 22: GASTROINTESTINAL STRUCTURAL AND INFLAMMATORY DISORDERS.**

Peritonitis

Inflammation of the peritoneum results from infection of the peritoneum due to puncture (surgery or trauma), rupture of part of the gastrointestinal tract (diverticulitis, peptic ulcer disease, appendicitis, bowel obstruction), or infection from continuous ambulatory peritoneal dialysis.

Gastroenteritis

Inflammation of the stomach and small intestine
- Triggered by infection (either bacterial or viral)
- Vomiting and frequent, watery stools place the client at increased risk for fluid and electrolyte imbalance and impaired nutrition.

CHRONIC INFLAMMATORY BOWEL DISEASE

Ulcerative colitis and Crohn's disease are characterized by frequent stools, cramping abdominal pain, exacerbations, and remissions.

Ulcerative colitis

Edema and inflammation primarily in the rectum and rectosigmoid colon
- In severe cases, it can involve the entire length of the colon. Mucosa, submucosa, and the colon will become edematous and reddened and can bleed easily.
- Edema and thickened bowel mucosa can cause partial bowel obstruction. Intestinal mucosal cell changes can lead to colon cancer.

Crohn's disease

Inflammation and ulceration of the gastrointestinal tract, often at the distal ileum
- All bowel layers can become involved; lesions are sporadic. Fistulas and abscesses are common.
- Can involve the entire GI tract from the mouth to the anus.
- Malabsorption and malnutrition can develop when the jejunum and ileum become involved. Requires supplemental vitamins and minerals, possibly including vitamin B_{12} injections

Diverticulitis

Diverticulitis is inflammation and infection of the bowel mucosa caused by bacteria, food, or fecal matter trapped in one or more diverticula (pouch-like herniations in the intestinal wall). Diverticulitis is not to be confused with diverticulosis, which is the presence of many small diverticula in the colon without inflammation.
- Not all clients who have diverticulosis develop diverticulitis.
- Diverticula can perforate and cause peritonitis and/or severe bleeding.

DATA COLLECTION

Etiology of ulcerative colitis and Crohn's disease is unknown but possibly due to a combination of genetic, environmental, and immunological causes.

RISK FACTORS

Genetics: Ulcerative colitis and Crohn's disease

Culture: Non-Hispanic white (ulcerative colitis), Jewish heritage (ulcerative colitis and Crohn's disease), and African Americans (diverticular disease)

Tobacco use: Crohn's disease

EXPECTED FINDINGS

Ulcerative colitis

- Abdominal pain/cramping: often left-lower quadrant pain relieved with defecation
- Anorexia and weight loss

PHYSICAL FINDINGS
- Fever
- Diarrhea: up to 15 to 30 liquid stools/day
- Stools containing mucus or blood
- Abdominal distention, tenderness, and/or firmness upon palpation
- Rectal bleeding

Crohn's disease

- Abdominal pain/cramping: often right-lower quadrant pain that is relieved by defecation
- Anorexia and weight loss

PHYSICAL FINDINGS
- Fever
- Diarrhea: five loose stools/day
- Abdominal distention, tenderness and/or firmness upon palpation
- Anemia
- Malaise

Diverticulitis

- Acute onset of abdominal pain often in left lower quadrant
- Nausea and vomiting

PHYSICAL FINDINGS
- Fever
- Diarrhea or constipation
- Abdominal distention

LABORATORY TESTS

IBD (Ulcerative colitis and Crohn's disease)

- Hematocrit and hemoglobin: Decreased
- Erythrocyte sedimentation rate (ESR): Increased
- WBC: Increased
- Albumin: Decreased
- C-reactive protein: Increased
- Stool for occult blood: Can be positive
- Electrolytes: Decreased

DIAGNOSTIC PROCEDURES

Magnetic resonance enterography: Used with all IBD

CLIENT EDUCATION: Maintain NPO for 4 to 6 hr prior to the exam. Client might be asked to drink a contrast medium prior to the test.

Ulcerative colitis

Sigmoidoscopy or colonoscopy: Intestinal tissue specimens can be collected to differentiate IBD.

Barium enema: Helpful to distinguish ulcerative colitis from other disease processes

CT scan or MRI: Can identify the presence of abscesses

Stool examination: For the presence of parasites or microbes, blood, and mucus

Crohn's disease

Endoscopy
- Newer diagnostic tools used, such as video capsule endoscopy
- **Proctosigmoidoscopy:** Performed to identify inflamed tissue
- **Colonoscopy and sigmoidoscopy:** A lighted, flexible scope inserted into the rectum to visualize the rectum and large intestine and to collect intestinal tissue specimens

Abdominal ultrasound, x-ray, and CT scan: CT scans can show bowel thickening.

Barium enema: Barium is inserted into the rectum as a contrast medium for x-rays. This allows for the rectum and large intestine to be visualized and is used to diagnose ulcerative colitis. A barium enema can show the presence of diverticulosis and is contraindicated in the presence of diverticulitis due to the risk of perforation.

NURSING ACTIONS: Reinforce teachings about the procedure and assist with preparing the bowels prior to the procedure. Qs

FINDINGS
- Small intestine ulcerations and narrowing is consistent with Crohn's disease.
- Ulcerations and inflammation of the sigmoid colon and rectum is significant for ulcerative colitis.

CLIENT EDUCATION
- Remain NPO as required, and perform bowel preparation.
- There can be possible abdominal discomfort and cramping during the barium enema.
- Stools will be white in color after the procedure and return to normal after all of the barium is expelled.

PATIENT-CENTERED CARE

NURSING CARE

Supportive care for a client who has IBD include promoting rest, decreasing stressors, providing nutritional support, and treating symptoms.

Ulcerative colitis and Crohn's disease

- The client should receive instructions regarding the usual course of the disease process.
- The client should receive instructions regarding medication therapy and vitamin supplements.
- Monitor by colonoscopy due to the increased risk of colon cancer.
- Assist the client in identifying foods that trigger manifestations.
- Monitor for electrolyte imbalance, especially potassium. Diarrhea can cause a loss of fluids and electrolytes.
- Monitor I&O, and check for dehydration.

CLIENT EDUCATION

- Seek emergency care for indications of bowel obstruction or perforation (fever, severe abdominal pain, vomiting). Qs
- For extreme or long exacerbations, NPO status and administration of total parenteral nutrition promotes bowel rest while providing adequate nutrition.
- Avoid caffeine, alcohol, and lactose.
- Eat high-protein, high-calorie, low-fiber foods.
- Small, frequent meals can reduce the occurrence of manifestations.
- Dietary supplements that are high in protein and low in fiber (elemental and semi-elemental products, canned nutrition beverages) can be used.
- Weigh 1 or 2 times weekly.
- Use of vitamin supplements and B₁₂ injections, if needed

Diverticulitis

- For severe manifestations (severe pain, high fever), the client is hospitalized; is NPO; and receives nasogastric suctioning, IV fluids, IV antibiotics, and IV opioid analgesics for pain.
- Instruct the client who has mild diverticulitis about self-care at home. The client should take medications as prescribed (antibiotics, analgesics, antispasmodics) and get adequate rest.
- Reinforce instructions to promote normal bowel function and consistency. (Avoid laxatives and the use of enemas. Drink adequate fluids.)

CLIENT EDUCATION

- Consume a clear-liquid diet until manifestations subside.
- Progress to a low-fiber diet once solid foods are tolerated without other manifestations. Slowly advance to a high-fiber diet as tolerated when inflammation resolves.
- Avoid seeds or indigestible material (nuts, popcorn, seeds), which can block diverticulum.
- Avoid foods or drinks that can irritate the bowel. (Avoid alcohol. Limit fat to 30% of daily calorie intake.)

MEDICATIONS FOR ULCERATIVE COLITIS, CROHN'S DISEASE

5-aminosalicylic acid: anti-inflammatory

Reduces inflammation of the intestinal mucosa and inhibits prostaglandins

Sulfonamides: Sulfasalazine
- These medications are contraindicated if the client has a sulfa or salicylate allergy.
- Sulfasalazine is given orally.
- Adverse effects include nausea, fever, and rash.
- NURSING ACTIONS
  ○ Monitor CBC and kidney and hepatic function.
  ○ Monitor for the development of agranulocytosis, hemolytic anemia, and macrocytic anemia.

- CLIENT EDUCATION
  ○ Take the medication with a full glass of water after meals.
  ○ Avoid sun exposure.
  ○ Increase fluid intake to 2 L/day.
  ○ This medication can cause urine, skin, and contact lenses to have a yellow-orange color.
  ○ Notify the provider if nausea, vomiting, anorexia, sore throat, rash, bruising, or fever occur.
  ○ Take medication as directed. The usual maintenance dose of sulfasalazine is 2 to 4 g/day.

Nonsulfonamides
- Mesalamine
- Balsalazide
- The adverse effects are not as serious as sulfasalazine.
- These medications can be contraindicated if the client has a salicylate or sulfa allergy.
- NURSING ACTIONS: Monitor for kidney toxicity.
- CLIENT EDUCATION: Report headache or gastrointestinal problems (abdominal discomfort, diarrhea).

Corticosteroids

Reduce inflammation and pain
- For rectal inflammation, topical steroids can be administered by a retention enema.
- Used to induce remission
- Not for long-term use due to adverse effects
- Prolonged use can lead to adrenal suppression, osteoporosis, risk of infection, and cushingoid syndrome. Use corticosteroids in low doses to minimize adverse effects.
- Can slow healing

MEDICATIONS
- Prednisone
- Prednisolone
- Hydrocortisone
- Budesonide

NURSING ACTIONS
- Monitor blood pressure.
- Reduce systemic dose slowly.
- Monitor electrolytes and glucose.

CLIENT EDUCATION
- Take the oral dose with food.
- Avoid discontinuing dose suddenly.
- Report unexpected increase in weight or other indications of fluid retention.
- Avoid crowds and other exposures to infectious diseases.
- Report evidence of infection (Crohn's disease can mask infection).

Immunosuppressants

Mechanism of action in treatment of IBD is unknown.

MEDICATIONS
- Cyclosporine
- Methotrexate
- Azathioprine
- Mercaptopurine

NURSING ACTIONS
- Monitor for pancreatitis and neutropenia.
- Can take up to 6 months to see therapeutic effects
- Not used as monotherapy
- Reserved for refractory disease due to toxicity

CLIENT EDUCATION
- Avoid crowds and other chances of exposures to infectious diseases, and report evidence of infection.
- Monitor for indications of bleeding, bruising, or infection.

Immunomodulators

- Suppress the immune response
- Inhibit tumor necrosis factor, an antibody found in Crohn's disease

MEDICATIONS
- Infliximab
- Adalimumab (self-administered by subcutaneous injection)
- Natalizumab (can cause progressive multi-focal leukoencephalopathy, a deadly brain infection)
- Certolizumab

NURSING ACTIONS
- Many adverse effects are possible, including chills, fever, hypotension/hypertension, dysrhythmias, and blood dyscrasias.
- Monitor liver enzymes, coagulation studies, and CBC.

CLIENT EDUCATION
- Avoid crowds and other exposures to infectious diseases, and report evidence of infection. There is a risk for development or reactivation of tuberculosis.
- Monitor and report evidence of bleeding, bruising, or infection, and transfusion or allergic reaction.

Antidiarrheals

Suppress the number of stools
- Used to decrease risk of fluid volume deficit and electrolyte imbalance. They also reduce discomfort.
- Use of antidiarrheals can lead to toxic megacolon (massive dilation of the colon with a risk of the development of gangrene and peritonitis). Use cautiously. Qs

MEDICATIONS
- Diphenoxylate and atropine
- Loperamide

NURSING ACTIONS
- Observe for manifestations of toxic megacolon that can result in gangrene and peritonitis (hypotension, fever, abdominal distention, decrease or absence of bowel sounds).
- Observe for indications of respiratory depression, especially in older adult clients.

CLIENT EDUCATION: Due to the central nervous system effects, avoid hazardous activities until the response to the medication is established.

MEDICATION FOR DIVERTICULITIS

Antimicrobials

Treat infection (decrease inflammation in Crohn's disease, used to treat abscesses or fistulas)
- Discontinue ciprofloxacin for tendon pain. Can cause tendon rupture
- Decreased dose should be used for clients who have impaired kidney function.

MEDICATIONS
- Ciprofloxacin
- Metronidazole
- Sulfamethoxazole-trimethoprim

NURSING ACTIONS: Monitor kidney and hepatic studies.

CLIENT EDUCATION
- Can cause a superinfection; observe for manifestations of thrush or vaginal yeast infection
- Urine can darken (expected, harmless effect).
- Monitor for manifestations of CNS effects (numbness of extremities, ataxia, and seizures), and notify the provider immediately.

THERAPEUTIC PROCEDURES

Clients who do not have success with medical treatment or who have complications (bowel perforation, colon cancer) are candidates for surgery.

Ulcerative colitis: Colectomy/proctocolectomy with or without ileostomy

Crohn's disease
- Laparoscopic stricturoplasty to increase the diameter of the bowel for bowel strictures
- Surgical repair of fistulas or in response to other complications related to the disease (perforation)

Diverticulitis (dependent on problem)
- Required for rupture of the diverticulum that results in peritonitis, bowel obstruction, uncontrolled bleeding, or abscess
- Colon resection with or without colostomy

PREOPERATIVE CARE

- Preoperative care is similar to other abdominal surgeries.
- If the creation of a stoma is planned, collaborate with an enterostomal therapy nurse regarding care related to the stoma. Q**TC**
- Administer antibiotic bowel prep, if prescribed.
- Administer cleansing enema or laxatives, if prescribed.

POSTOPERATIVE CARE

- Postoperative care is similar to care for clients who have other types of abdominal surgery.
- The client should be NPO and have a nasogastric tube to suction, unless the surgery was performed laparoscopically.
- Monitor bowel sounds.
- Check for abdominal distension.
- Observe color, amount, and odor of surgical drains or drainage.
- An ileostomy can drain as much as 1,000 mL/day. Prevent fluid volume deficit. Replace fluid loss with IV fluids if the client is NPO. Oral hydration is slowly introduced in 1 to 2 days. Q**S**

CARE AFTER DISCHARGE: Refer the client who has an ostomy to an enterostomal therapist and an ostomy support group.

INTERPROFESSIONAL CARE

- Assist with obtaining a referral for nutritional counseling.
- The client might benefit from complementary therapy (biofeedback, massage, yoga).
- Recommend community support groups or a mental health referral for assistance with coping. Q**PCC**

COMPLICATIONS

Complications of ulcerative colitis, Crohn's disease, and diverticulitis include bleeding and fluid and electrolyte imbalance. Peritonitis can occur due to perforation of the bowel. Abscess formation can occur as a complication of diverticular disease and Crohn's disease.

Peritonitis

- A life-threatening inflammation of the peritoneum and lining of the abdominal cavity
- Often caused by bacteria in the peritoneal cavity

PHYSICAL FINDINGS

- Rigid, board-like abdomen (hallmark indication)
- Abdominal distention
- Nausea, vomiting
- Rebound tenderness
- Tachycardia
- Fever
- Early manifestation in older adult clients: decreased mental status, confusion

NURSING ACTIONS

- Place the client in Fowler's or semi-Fowler's position to promote drainage of peritoneal fluid and improve lung expansion. Q**EBP**
- Monitor respiratory status and administer oxygen as prescribed. Turn, cough, and deeply breathe. Mechanical ventilation can be required.
- Maintain and monitor nasogastric suction.
- Keep the client NPO.
- Monitor fluid and electrolyte status.
- Monitor for hypovolemia.
- Administer analgesics as prescribed.
- Monitor bowel sounds.
- Monitor for reports of passing flatus.
- Monitor for manifestations of paralytic ileus, which include slowing or absence of bowel sounds.
- Assist with the administration of hypertonic IV fluids and broad-spectrum antibiotics as prescribed.
- Collaborate with case management to determine home care and wound management needs. Q**TC**
- If surgery is performed:
  - Closely monitor postoperative vital signs.
  - Monitor I&O every hour immediately after surgery.
  - Monitor surgical dressing for bleeding.
  - If the client requires wound irrigation postoperatively, use sterile technique, and monitor irrigation intake and output to prevent fluid retention.

CLIENT EDUCATION

- Maintain adequate rest and resume home activity slowly, as tolerated. No heavy lifting for at least 6 weeks
- Monitor for evidence of return infection. Notify the provider immediately.

Bleeding due to deterioration of the bowel

NURSING ACTIONS

- Observe for indications of rectal bleeding (black, tarry stools; bright red blood).
- Monitor vital signs.
- Check laboratory values, especially hematocrit, hemoglobin, and coagulation factors.

CLIENT EDUCATION

- Report rectal bleeding.
- Understand the importance of bed rest.

Fluid and electrolyte imbalance

Occurs due to loss of fluid through diarrhea, vomiting, and nasogastric suctioning

NURSING ACTIONS

- Monitor laboratory values, and provide replacement therapy.
- Monitor weight.
- Monitor for indications of fluid volume deficit (loss or absence of skin turgor).

CLIENT EDUCATION

- Record and report the number of loose stools.
- Maintain adequate fluid intake.
- Follow the prescribed diet.

Abscess and fistula formation

Occurs due to the destruction of the bowel wall, leading to an infection

NURSING ACTIONS

- Monitor fluid and electrolytes.
- Observe for manifestations of dehydration (decreased urine output, fever, hypotension, tachycardia, dizziness).
- Provide a diet high in protein and calories (at least 3,000 calories/day) and low in fiber.
- Administer a vitamin supplement.
- Consult with an enterostomal therapist to develop a plan to prevent skin breakdown and promote wound healing. Qтс
- Monitor for evidence of infection, which can indicate abdominal abscesses or sepsis.
- Ensure the function of drainage devices if used.

Toxic megacolon

Occurs due to inactivity of the colon. Massive dilation of the colon occurs, and the client is at risk for perforation.

NURSING ACTIONS

- Maintain nasogastric suction.
- Assist with the administration of IV fluids and electrolytes.
- Administer prescribed medications (antibiotics, corticosteroids).
- Prepare the client for surgery (usually an ileostomy) if the client does not begin to show improvement within 72 hr.

Active Learning Scenario

A nurse is reinforcing teaching with a client who has diverticulitis. What should the nurse include? Use the ATI Active Learning Template: System Disorder to complete this item.

PATHOPHYSIOLOGY RELATED TO CLIENT PROBLEM

EXPECTED FINDINGS: Identify two expected findings.

DIAGNOSTIC PROCEDURES: Identify three.

CLIENT EDUCATION: Describe dietary instruction.

Active Learning Scenario Key

Using the ATI Active Learning Template: System Disorder

PATHOPHYSIOLOGY RELATED TO CLIENT PROBLEM: Inflammation and infection of the bowel mucosa caused by bacteria or fecal matter trapped in one or more diverticula (pouches in the intestine)

EXPECTED FINDINGS

- Hemoglobin and hematocrit are decreased.
- Stool can be positive for occult blood.

DIAGNOSTIC PROCEDURES

- Abdominal x-ray
- CT scan
- Colonoscopy
- Sigmoidoscopy

CLIENT EDUCATION

- Consume clear liquids until manifestations subside. Progress to a low-fiber diet once solid foods are tolerated. Slowly advance to a high-fiber diet.
- Avoid seeds or indigestible material (nuts, popcorn, seeds).
- Avoid alcohol. Limit fat to 30% of daily caloric intake.

Ⓝ *NCLEX® Connection: Physiological Adaptation, Alterations in Body Systems*

1. A nurse is reinforcing teaching about the features of ulcerative colitis and Crohn's disease with a group of nurses on the medical-surgical unit. Sort the features according to ulcerative colitis and Crohn's disease.

   A. Inflammation begins in the rectum.

   B. Primarily affects the terminal ileum

   C. Anemia

   D. B_{12} deficiency

   E. Hemorrhage is a complication.

   F. Fistulas are a complication.

2. A nurse is reviewing the laboratory data for a client who has an acute exacerbation of Crohn's disease. Which of the following serum laboratory results should the nurse expect to be elevated?

   A. Hematocrit

   B. Erythrocyte sedimentation rate (ESR)

   C. B_{12}

   D. Folic acid

   E. Albumin

3. A nurse is assisting with the care of a client who has severe manifestations of diverticulitis. Which of the following prescriptions from the provider should the nurse anticipate?

   A. Liquid diet

   B. Oral antibiotics

   C. Intravenous opioid medication for pain

   D. Seizure precautions

4. A nurse is reinforcing teaching with a client who has a new prescription for sulfadiazine. Which of the following information should the nurse include? (Select all that apply.)

   A. "Notify the provider immediately if you develop a rash."

   B. "Drink 2 liters of water per day."

   C. "Expose skin to sunlight 30 minutes per day to strengthen bones."

   D. "This medication can cause high blood sugar."

   E. "Take the medication with orange juice to increase its absorption."

5. A nurse is collecting data from a client who is experiencing an infection following abdominal surgery. Which of the following findings are manifestations of peritonitis? (Select all that apply.)

   A. Abdominal distention

   B. High fever

   C. Tachycardia

   D. Hypoactive bowel sounds

   E. Vomiting

6. A nurse is reviewing the laboratory data of a client who has an acute exacerbation of Crohn's disease. Which of the following blood laboratory results should the nurse expect to be elevated? (Select all that apply.)

   A. Hematocrit

   B. Erythrocyte sedimentation rate

   C. WBC

   D. Folic acid

   E. Albumin

7. A nurse is collecting data from a client who has been taking prednisone following an exacerbation of inflammatory bowel disease. The nurse should recognize which of the following findings as the priority?

   A. Client reports difficulty sleeping.

   B. The client's urine is positive for glucose.

   C. Client reports having an elevated body temperature.

   D. Client reports gaining 4 lb in the last 6 months.

8. A nurse is reinforcing teaching with a client who has a new prescription for sulfasalazine. Which of the following instructions should the nurse include?

   A. "Take the medication 2 hours after eating."

   B. "Discontinue this medication if your skin turns yellow-orange."

   C. "Notify the provider if you experience a sore throat."

   D. "Expect your stools to turn black."

9. A nurse is reinforcing discharge teaching with a client who has Crohn's disease. Which of the following instructions should the nurse include?

   A. Decrease intake of calorie-dense foods.

   B. Drink canned protein supplements.

   C. Increase intake of high fiber foods.

   D. Eat high-residue foods.

10. A nurse in a clinic is reinforcing teaching with a client who has ulcerative colitis. Which of the following statements by the client indicates understanding of the information provided?

    A. "I will plan to limit lactose in my diet."

    B. "I will restrict fluid intake during meals."

    C. "I will switch to black tea instead of drinking coffee."

    D. "I will try to eat cold foods rather than warm when my stomach feels upset."

1. **ULCERATIVE COLITIS:** A, C, E; **CROHN'S DISEASE:** B, D, F

   Ulcerative colitis and Crohn's disease are inflammatory intestinal disorders that have many similarities. However, some features are different, including the location of the inflammation, anemia, and hemorrhage as a complication.

   Ⓝ *NCLEX® Connection: Physiological Adaptation, Alterations in Body Systems*

2. B. **CORRECT**: When recognizing cues, the nurse should expect the client's ESR to be elevated due to inflammation. Clients who have Crohn's disease are at risk for anemia; therefore, the nurse should expect the client's hematocrit to be decreased. Folic acid, B₁₂, and albumin levels are typically decreased due to malabsorption.

   Ⓝ *NCLEX® Connection: Reduction of Risk Potential, Laboratory Values*

3. C. **CORRECT**: When generating solutions, the nurse should identify acute left lower abdominal pain as a manifestation of diverticulitis; therefore, the client should anticipate a prescription for IV opioid analgesics.

   Ⓝ *NCLEX® Connection: Physiological Adaptation, Alterations in Body Systems*

4. A, B. **CORRECT**: This medication can cause a severe hypersensitivity reaction; therefore, the client should notify the provider immediately at the first sign of sensitivity, such as a rash. Deposit of sulfadiazine in the kidney can cause renal damage; therefore, the nurse should instruct the client to drink 2 liters of water per day to increase urine flow and reduce the risk of renal damage. Sulfadiazine places the client at risk for photosensitivity; therefore, the nurse should instruct the client to avoid sun exposure. Glucocorticoids are often prescribed for clients who have inflammatory bowel disease, and they can cause hyperglycemia; however, hyperglycemia is not an adverse effect of sulfadiazine. Vitamin C, which is found in orange juice, can cause crystalluria when consumed with sulfadiazine, and crystalluria can lead to kidney injury; therefore, the nurse should not include this in the teaching.

   Ⓝ *NCLEX® Connection: Pharmacological Therapies, Adverse Effects/Contraindications/Side Effects/Interactions*

5. A, B, C, E. **CORRECT**: Peritonitis is a life-threating inflammation and infection of the peritoneum. Manifestations include abdominal distension, high fever, tachycardia, and vomiting. Bowel sounds are diminished.

   Ⓝ *NCLEX® Connection: Physiological Adaptation, Alterations in Body Systems*

6. A. Hematocrit is decreased as a result of chronic blood loss.
   B. **CORRECT**: Increased erythrocyte sedimentation rate is a finding in a client who has Crohn's disease as a result of inflammation.
   C. **CORRECT**: Increased WBC is a finding in a client who has Crohn's disease.
   D. A decrease in folic acid level is indicative of malabsorption due to Crohn's disease.
   E. A decrease in sodium is indicative of malabsorption due to Crohn's disease.

   Ⓝ *NCLEX® Connection: Physiological Adaptation, Alterations in Body Systems*

7. A. The client is at risk for sleep deprivation because prednisone can cause anxiety and insomnia. However, another finding is the priority.
   B. The client is at risk for hyperglycemia because prednisone can cause glucose intolerance. However, another finding is the priority.
   C. **CORRECT**: The greatest risk to the client is infection because prednisone can cause immunosuppression. Therefore, identify manifestations of an infection, such as an elevated body temperature, as the priority finding.
   D. The client is at risk for weight gain because prednisone can cause fluid retention. However, another finding is the priority.

   Ⓝ *NCLEX® Connection: Pharmacological Therapies, Adverse Effects/Contraindications/Side Effects/Interactions*

8. A. Sulfasalazine should be taken right after meals and with a full glass of water to reduce gastric upset and prevent crystalluria.
   B. Yellow-orange coloring of the skin and urine is a harmless effect of sulfasalazine.
   C. **CORRECT**: Sulfasalazine can cause blood dyscrasias. The client should monitor and report any manifestations of infection, such as a sore throat.
   D. Sulfasalazine can cause thrombocytopenia and bleeding. Black stools are a manifestation of gastrointestinal bleeding, and the client should report this to the provider.

   Ⓝ *NCLEX® Connection: Pharmacological Therapies, Medication Administration*

9. A. A high-protein diet is recommended for the client who has Crohn's disease.
   B. **CORRECT**: A high-protein diet is recommended for the client who has Crohn's disease. Canned protein supplements are encouraged.
   C. A low-fiber diet is recommended for the client who has Crohn's disease to reduce inflammation.
   D. Instruct the client to eat low-residue foods to reduce inflammation.

   Ⓝ *NCLEX® Connection: Physiological Adaptation, Alterations in Body Systems*

10. A. **CORRECT**: Lactose limitations are recommended for the client who has ulcerative colitis to reduce inflammation.
    B. A client who has dumping syndrome should avoid fluids with meals.
    C. Caffeine can increase diarrhea and cramping. The client should avoid caffeinated beverages, such as black tea.
    D. The client should avoid cold foods because these can increase intestinal motility and cause exacerbation of manifestations.

    Ⓝ *NCLEX® Connection: Basic Care and Comfort, Nutrition and Oral Hydration*

When reviewing the following chapters, keep in mind the relevant topics and tasks of the NCLEX outline.

Basic Care and Comfort

NUTRITION AND ORAL HYDRATION: Reinforce client teaching on special diets based on client diagnosis/nutritional needs and cultural considerations.

Pharmacological Therapies

PHARMACOLOGICAL PAIN MANAGEMENT: Identify client need for pain medication.

EXPECTED ACTIONS/OUTCOMES: Reinforce client teaching on actions and therapeutic effects of medications and pharmacological interactions.

Reduction of Risk Potential

LABORATORY VALUES: Monitor diagnostic or laboratory test results.

Physiological Adaptation

ALTERATIONS IN BODY SYSTEMS: Reinforce education to client regarding care and condition.

CHAPTER 48 *Cholecystitis and Cholelithiasis*

Cholecystitis is an inflammation of the gallbladder. Cholecystitis is most often caused by gallstones (cholelithiasis) obstructing the cystic and/or common bile ducts (bile flows from the gallbladder to the duodenum), causing bile to back up and the gallbladder to become inflamed.

Cholelithiasis is the presence of stones in the gallbladder related to the precipitation of either bile, calcium, or cholesterol into stones. Bile is used for the digestion of fats. It is produced in the liver and stored in the gallbladder. Cholecystitis can be acute or chronic and can obstruct the pancreatic duct, causing pancreatitis. It can also cause the gallbladder to rupture, resulting in secondary peritonitis.

HEALTH PROMOTION AND DISEASE PREVENTION

- Consume a low-fat diet rich in HDL sources (seafood, nuts, olive oil).
- Participate in a regular exercise program.
- Do not smoke.

DATA COLLECTION

RISK FACTORS

- More common in females
- Estrogen therapy and use of some oral contraceptives
- Obesity (impaired fat metabolism, high cholesterol)
- Genetic predisposition
- Older adults (decreased gallbladder contractility, more likely to develop gallstones) Ⓖ
- Type 2 diabetes mellitus (high triglycerides) or Crohn's disease
- Low-calorie diets
- Rapid weight loss (increases cholesterol)
- Native American or Mexican American ethnicity
- Bariatric surgery

EXPECTED FINDINGS

- Sharp pain in the right upper quadrant, often radiating to the right shoulder
- Intense pain with nausea and vomiting after ingestion of high-fat food caused by biliary colic
- Dyspepsia, eructation (belching), and flatulence
- Fever

PHYSICAL FINDINGS

- Jaundice noted in the sclera and skin, clay-colored stools, steatorrhea (fatty stools).
- Older adult clients can have atypical presentation of cholecystitis (absence of pain or fever). Delirium might be the initial manifestation, or the client might have localized tenderness. Ⓖ

LABORATORY TESTS

- Increased WBC indicates inflammation.
- Direct, indirect, and total blood bilirubin can be increased if a bile duct is obstructed.
- Amylase and lipase can be increased with pancreatic involvement.
- Aspartate aminotransferase (AST), alanine aminotransferase (ALT), lactate dehydrogenase (LDH), and alkaline phosphatase (ALP) (increased with liver dysfunction) can indicate the common bile duct is obstructed.

DIAGNOSTIC PROCEDURES

Ultrasound visualizes gallstones and a dilated common bile duct.

Abdominal x-ray or CT scan can visualize calcified gallstones and an enlarged gallbladder.

Hepatobiliary scan (HIDA) determines the patency of the biliary duct system after an IV injection of contrast.

Endoscopic retrograde cholangiopancreatography (ERCP) allows for direct visualization, using an endoscope that is inserted through the esophagus and into the common bile duct via the duodenum which also allows for the removal of gallstones. (Refer to **CHAPTER 41: GASTROINTESTINAL DIAGNOSTIC PROCEDURES.**)

Magnetic resonance cholangiopancreatography combines the use of oral/IV contrast with an MRI. This test assists the provider in determining the cause of cholecystitis or cholelithiasis.

PATIENT-CENTERED CARE

NURSING CARE

- Administer analgesics as needed.
- Place client in Fowler's position to decrease pressure on the abdomen and decrease pain.

MEDICATIONS

Analgesics

Opioid analgesics, such as morphine sulfate or hydromorphone, are preferred for acute biliary pain.

Bile acid

Bile acid (chenodiol, ursodiol) gradually dissolves cholesterol-based gallstones.

NURSING ACTIONS: Use caution in clients who have liver conditions or disorders with varices.

CLIENT EDUCATION: Report abdominal pain, diarrhea, or vomiting. The medication is limited to 2 years of administration and requires a gallbladder ultrasound every 6 months during the first year to determine effectiveness.

THERAPEUTIC PROCEDURES

Extracorporeal shock wave lithotripsy

Shock waves are used to break up stones.

NURSING ACTIONS
- Instruct and assist the client to lay on a fluid-filled pad for delivery of shock waves.
- Administer analgesia.

CLIENT EDUCATION: Several procedures can be required to break up all stones. There can be pain intraprocedural due to gallbladder spasms or movement of the stones.

Cholecystectomy

- Removal of the gallbladder with a laparoscopic, minimally invasive, or open approach
- The client usually is discharged within 24 hr if a laparoscopic approach is used. An open approach can require hospitalization for 2 to 4 days.

NURSING ACTIONS
- **Laparoscopic approach:** Provide immediate postoperative care.
- **Minimally invasive approach:** Natural orifice transluminal endoscopic surgery. Explain to the client that this surgical procedure is performed through entry of the mouth, vagina, or rectum. This approach eliminates visible incisions and decreases the risk of complications for the client.
- **Open approach:** The provider can place a drain in the gallbladder or a T-tube in the common bile duct.
  - Though used less commonly, clients can have a T-tube placed in the common bile duct to drain bile if there were intraoperative complications involving the bile duct.
  - Monitor stools for color (stools clay-colored until biliary flow is reestablished).

- **Care of the drainage tube**
  - Clients can have a drainage tube placed intraoperatively to prevent accumulation of fluid in the gallbladder bed.
  - Monitor and record drainage (initially serosanguineous stained with green-brown bile).
  - Antibiotics are often prescribed to decrease the risk for infection.
- **Care of the T-tube**
  - Instruct client to report an absence of drainage with manifestations of nausea and pain (can indicate obstruction in the T-tube).
  - Inspect the surrounding skin for evidence of infection (redness, swelling, bile leakage, warmth).
  - Keep drainage tube below the level of surgical area.
  - Monitor and record the color and amount of drainage.
  - Clamp the tube per protocol before and after meals.
  - Expect removal of the tube in 1 to 3 weeks.
  - Change wound dressing with caution to prevent accidental removal.

CLIENT EDUCATION
- **Laparoscopic approach**
  - Ambulate frequently to minimize free air pain, which is common following laparoscopic surgery (under the right clavicle, shoulder, scapula).
  - Monitor the incision for evidence of infection.
  - Perform pain control.
  - Report indications of bile leak (pain, vomiting, abdominal distention) to the provider.
  - Resume activity gradually and as tolerated and resume the preoperative diet (low fat).
  - Remove bandages from surgical site the day after surgery, and shower. Do not remove the adhesive surgical strips.
- **Open approach**
  - Resume activity gradually. Avoid heavy lifting or strenuous activities.
  - Begin with clear liquids and advance to solid foods as peristalsis returns.
  - Report sudden increase in drainage, foul odor, pain, fever, or jaundice. Q_s
  - Take showers instead of baths until drainage tube is removed.
  - The color of stools should return to brown in about a week, and diarrhea is common.
  - Inform client to wear loose-fitting clothes.
- **Dietary counseling**
  - Adhere to a low-fat diet (reduce dairy products and avoid fried foods, chocolate, nuts, gravies). The client can have increased tolerance of small, frequent meals.
  - Avoid gas-forming foods (beans, cabbage, cauliflower, broccoli).
  - Consider weight reduction.
  - Take fat-soluble vitamins or bile salts as prescribed to enhance absorption and aid with digestion.

COMPLICATIONS

Obstruction of the bile duct

This can cause ischemia, gangrene, and a rupture of the gallbladder wall. A rupture of the gallbladder wall can cause a local abscess or peritonitis (rigid, board-like abdomen, guarding), which requires a surgical intervention and administration of broad-spectrum antibiotics.

Bile peritonitis

This can occur if adequate amounts of bile are not drained from the surgical site. This is a rare but potentially fatal complication.

Active Learning Scenario

A nurse is assisting with presenting a program on gallbladder disease to a group of clients at a health fair. What information should the nurse include in the program? Use the ATI Active Learning Template: System Disorder to complete this item.

RISK FACTORS: Describe at least four.

EXPECTED FINDINGS: Describe at least eight findings.

CLIENT EDUCATION: Describe three preventative activities.

Application Exercises

1. A nurse is reviewing a client's medical history for risk factors for cholecystitis. The nurse should identify that which of the following findings is a risk factor?
   - A. Obesity
   - B. Rapid weight gain
   - C. Decreased blood triglyceride level
   - D. Male sex

2. A nurse in a clinic is reviewing the laboratory reports of a client who has suspected cholelithiasis. Which of the following is an expected finding?
   - A. Blood amylase 80 units/L
   - B. WBC 9,000/mm3
   - C. Direct bilirubin 2.1 mg/dL
   - D. Alkaline phosphatase 25 units/L

3. A nurse is reinforcing teaching with a client who has cholelithiasis and a new prescription for chenodiol. Which of the following information should the nurse include?
   - A. This medication is used to decrease acute biliary pain.
   - B. This medication requires thyroid function monitoring every 6 months.
   - C. This medication is not recommended for clients who have diabetes mellitus.
   - D. This medication dissolves gallstones gradually over a period of up to 2 years.

4. A nurse is assisting with preparing a presentation for a group of newly licensed nurses on cholecystectomy and extracorporeal shock wave lithotripsy. Sort each finding to the correct procedure.
   - A. Delivery of shock waves to a stone
   - B. Non-invasive procedure
   - C. Minimally invasive procedure
   - D. Removal of the gallbladder
   - E. Usually requires a 24-hr hospital stay
   - F. Removal of stones

5. A nurse is reinforcing discharge teaching with a client who is postoperative following a laparoscopic cholecystectomy. Which of the following instructions should the nurse include in the teaching? (Select all that apply.)
   - A. "Take baths rather than showers."
   - B. "Resume a diet of choice."
   - C. "Cleanse the puncture site using mild soap and water."
   - D. "Remove adhesive strips from the puncture site in 24 hr."
   - E. "Report nausea and vomiting to the surgeon."

6. A nurse is reinforcing preoperative teaching for a client who is scheduled for a laparoscopic cholecystectomy. Which of the following should be included in the teaching?
   - A. "The scope will be passed through your rectum."
   - B. "You might have shoulder pain after surgery."
   - C. "You will have a Jackson-Pratt drain in place after surgery."
   - D. "You should limit how often you walk for 1 to 2 weeks."

Active Learning Scenario Key

Using the ATI Active Learning Template: System Disorder

RISK FACTORS
- Female sex
- Estrogen therapy and some oral contraceptives
- High-fat or low-calorie, liquid protein diets
- Obesity
- Genetic predisposition
- Age over 60 years
- Type 2 diabetes mellitus
- Rapid weight loss
- Native American or Mexican American ethnicity

EXPECTED FINDINGS
- Sharp pain in the right upper quadrant that often radiates to the right shoulder
- Pain upon deep inspiration during right subcostal palpation
- Intense pain with nausea and vomiting after ingestion of high-fat food
- Dyspepsia
- Eructation (belching)
- Flatulence
- Fever
- Jaundice
- Clay-colored stools
- Steatorrhea (fatty stools)
- Dark urine
- Pruritus

CLIENT EDUCATION
- Get regular exercise.
- Stop using tobacco products.
- Consume a low-fat diet rich in HDL sources (seafood, nuts, olive oil).

Ⓝ *NCLEX® Connection: Physiological Adaptation, Alterations in Body Systems*

Application Exercises Key

1. A. **CORRECT:** The nurse should identify that obesity is considered a risk factor for the development of cholecystitis. Rapid weight loss, increased blood cholesterol levels, and female sex are also risk factors for the development of cholecystitis.

Ⓝ *NCLEX® Connection: Health Promotion and Maintenance, Health Promotion/Disease Prevention*

2. C. **CORRECT:** When generating solutions, the nurse should expect the client who has cholelithiasis to have an elevated direct bilirubin level if the bile duct is obstructed. A direct bilirubin level of 2.1 mg/dL is above the expected reference range. The nurse should identify that the client who has cholelithiasis will have an elevated blood amylase level if pancreatic involvement is present. A blood amylase of 80 units/L is within the expected reference range. The nurse should identify that the client who has cholelithiasis will have an elevated WBC level due to inflammation. A WBC of 9,000/mm3 is within the expected reference range. The nurse should identify that the client who has cholelithiasis will have an elevated alkaline phosphatase (ALP) level if the common bile duct is obstructed. An ALP of 25 units/L is less than the expected reference range.

Ⓝ *NCLEX® Connection: Reduction of Risk Potential, Laboratory Values*

3. D. **CORRECT:** When taking action and reinforcing teaching about chenodiol, the nurse should include that chenodiol is a bile acid that gradually dissolves cholesterol-based gallstones. The medication can be taken for up to 2 years. Opioid analgesics are preferred for the treatment of acute biliary pain. The client should have an ultrasound of the gallbladder every 6 months during the first year of treatment to determine effectiveness of the medication. Chenodiol is used cautiously in clients who have hepatic conditions or disorders with varices.

Ⓝ *NCLEX® Connection: Pharmacological Therapies, Medication Administration*

4. **CHOLECYSTECTOMY:** C, D, E, F; **LITHOTRIPSY:** A, B;

When generating solutions, the nurse should identify that clients who undergo a cholecystectomy are having either a laparoscopic, minimally invasive, or open procedure to remove the gallbladder and gallstones. This procedure usually requires the client to stay at least 24 hours following a laparoscopic approach and up to 48 hours for an open procedure. An extracorporeal shock wave lithotripsy is a non-invasive procedure that delivers shock waves to the area that break up cholesterol-based gallstones.

Ⓝ *NCLEX® Connection: Physiological Adaptation, Alterations in Body Systems*

5. B, C, E. **CORRECT:** When taking action, the nurse should instruct the client to resume a regular diet upon discharge. The client should cleanse the puncture site with mild soap and water to decrease the risk of infection. The client should report nausea, vomiting, or abdominal pain to the surgeon. The client should be told to take a bath or shower within 1 to 2 days following surgery and that the adhesive strips covering the puncture site should remain in place until they fall off naturally.

Ⓝ *NCLEX® Connection: Reduction of Risk Potential, Therapeutic Procedures*

6. B. **CORRECT:** When generating solutions, the nurse should include that shoulder pain is expected postoperatively due to free air that is introduced into the abdomen during laparoscopic surgery. Surgery is possibly performed through the rectum during the natural orifice transluminal endoscopic surgery (NOTES) approach. A Jackson-Pratt drain can be placed during the open surgery approach. The client is instructed to ambulate frequently following a laparoscopic surgical approach to minimize the free air that has been introduced.

Ⓝ *NCLEX® Connection: Reduction of Risk Potential, Therapeutic Procedures*

CHAPTER 49 *Pancreatitis*

The islets of Langerhans in the pancreas secrete insulin and glucagon. The pancreatic tissues secrete digestive enzymes that break down carbohydrates, proteins, and fats.

Pancreatitis is an autodigestion of the pancreas by pancreatic digestive enzymes that activate prematurely before reaching the intestines. The estimated number of cases of pancreatitis each year in the United States is 275,000. Pancreatitis has a mortality rate of 1.6/100,000. The mechanism of action is unclear. Inflammation of the pancreatic tissue causes duct obstruction, which can lead to increased pressure and duct rupture, causing the release of pancreatic enzymes into the pancreatic tissue. Pancreatitis can result in pancreatic inflammation, necrosis, and hemorrhage. Classic presentation of an acute attack includes severe, constant, knifelike pain (left upper quadrant, midepigastric, and/or radiating to the back).

- **Acute pancreatitis** is an inflammatory process due to activated pancreatic enzymes autodigesting the pancreas, ranging from mild to necrotizing hemorrhagic pancreatitis (widespread bleeding and necrosis).

- **Chronic pancreatitis** is a progressive, destructive disease of inflammation and fibrosis of the pancreas. Chronic pancreatitis is classified as chronic calcifying pancreatitis (often associated with alcohol use disorder), chronic obstructive pancreatitis (often associated with cholelithiasis), autoimmune pancreatitis, and idiopathic and hereditary pancreatitis.

HEALTH PROMOTION AND DISEASE PREVENTION

- Avoid excessive alcohol consumption.
- Eat a low-fat diet.

DATA COLLECTION

RISK FACTORS

- Biliary tract disease: Gallstones can cause a blockage where the common bile duct and pancreatic duct meet.
- Alcohol use: The primary cause of chronic pancreatitis is alcohol use disorder. Times of increased alcohol consumption, such as vacations or holidays, are associated with acute pancreatitis. Q EBP
- Endoscopic retrograde cholangiopancreatography (ERCP) (postprocedure complication)
- Gastrointestinal surgery
- Metabolic disturbances (hyperlipidemia, hyperparathyroidism, hypercalcemia)
- Kidney failure or transplant
- Genetic predisposition
- Trauma
- Penetrating ulcer (gastric or duodenal)
- Medication toxicity
- Viral infections: coxsackievirus B and human immunodeficiency virus
- Cigarette smoking

EXPECTED FINDINGS

- Sudden onset of severe, boring pain (goes through the body)
  - Epigastric, radiating to back, left flank, or left shoulder
  - Worse when lying down
  - Eating may worsen discomfort (acute).
- Pain relieved somewhat by fetal position or sitting upright, bending forward
- Nausea and vomiting
- Weight loss

PHYSICAL FINDINGS
- Seepage of blood-stained exudates into tissue as a result of pancreatic enzyme actions
  - Ecchymoses on the flanks
  - Bluish-gray periumbilical discoloration: Cullen's sign
- Abdominal distension and rigidity (peritonitis)
- Generalized jaundice
- Absent or decreased bowel sounds (possible paralytic ileus)
- Warm, moist skin; fruity breath (evidence of hyperglycemia)
- Tetany due to hypocalcemia
  - Trousseau's sign: hand spasm when blood pressure cuff is inflated
  - Chvostek's sign: facial twitching when facial nerve is tapped

LABORATORY TESTS

- **Serum amylase** increases within 24 hr and remains increased for 2 to 3 days (continued elevation can indicate pancreatic abscess or pseudocyst). **Blood lipase** increases slowly and can remain increased for days longer than amylase.
  - Urine amylase remains increased for up to 1 week.
  - Increases in enzymes indicate pancreatic cell injury.

> MEMORY AID: In pancreatitis, the "ases" (aces) are high.

- **WBC count:** Increased due to infection and inflammation
- **Platelets:** Decreased
- **Blood calcium and magnesium:** Decreased due to fat necrosis with pancreatitis
- **Blood liver enzymes and bilirubin:** Increased with associated biliary dysfunction
- **Blood glucose:** Increased due to a decrease in insulin production by the pancreas
- **Erythrocyte sedimentation rate:** Elevated

DIAGNOSTIC PROCEDURES

Computed tomography scan with contrast is reliably diagnostic of acute pancreatitis.

PATIENT-CENTERED CARE

NURSING CARE

- Rest the pancreas.
  - NPO: No food until pain-free
  - For severe pancreatitis: Enteral or parenteral nutrition
  - When diet is resumed: Bland, high-protein, low-fat diet with no stimulants (caffeine); small, frequent meals ⓠEBP
  - Antiemetic administered as needed
  - Nasogastric tube: Gastric decompression (for severe vomiting or paralytic ileus)
  - No alcohol consumption
  - No smoking
  - Limit stress
  - Pain management
- Position the client for comfort (fetal, side-lying, head of the bed elevated, sitting up, or leaning forward).
- Administer analgesics and other medications as prescribed.
- Monitor respiratory status and vital signs.
- Monitor blood glucose, and provide insulin as needed (potential for hyperglycemia).
- Monitor hydration status (orthostatic blood pressure, I&O, laboratory values).
- Monitor IV fluids and electrolyte replacements.

49.1 Ecchymoses of the flank

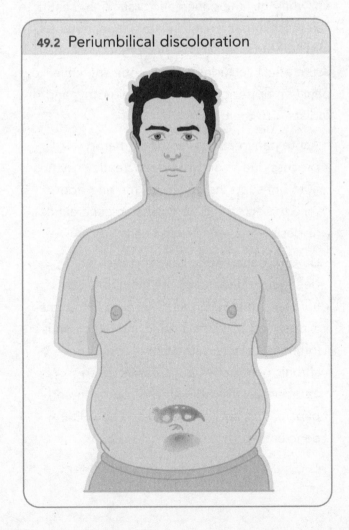

49.2 Periumbilical discoloration

MEDICATIONS

Opioid analgesics

Morphine or hydromorphone for acute pain

Ketorolac, an NSAID, used for mild to moderate pain

NURSING ACTIONS: Meperidine is discouraged due to the risk of seizures, especially in older adult clients.

Histamine-receptor antagonists: cimetidine

Decreases gastric acid secretion.

CLIENT EDUCATION: Take 1 hr before or 1 hr after antacid.

Proton-pump inhibitors: omeprazole

Decreases gastric acid secretion

NURSING CONSIDERATIONS: Monitor for hypomagnesemia.

Pancreatic enzymes: pancrelipase

Aids with digestion of fats and proteins when taken with meals and snacks

CLIENT EDUCATION
- Monitor and report persistent adverse effects such as headache, cough, dizziness, and sore throat.
- Contents of capsules can be sprinkled on nonprotein foods.
- Drink a full glass of water following pancrelipase.
- Wipe lips and rinse mouth after taking medication (to prevent skin breakdown or irritation).
- Take pancrelipase after antacid or histamine-receptor antagonists.
- Take pancrelipase with every meal and snack.

THERAPEUTIC PROCEDURES

ERCP to create an opening in the sphincter of Oddi if pancreatitis is caused by gallstones

INTERPROFESSIONAL CARE

- Dietary referral for postpancreatitis diet and nutritional supplements can be indicated when oral intake is resumed.
- Home health services can be indicated for clients regarding nutritional needs, possible wound care, and assistance with ADLs. Qᴛᴄ
- Substance-related support groups can be indicated for a client or family member who has an alcohol use disorder.

CLIENT EDUCATION

- For pancreatitis induced by alcohol use disorder, abstain from further alcohol intake. Alcohol use support groups can be helpful.
- Avoid high-fat foods or heavy meals to prevent acute pancreatitis. Qᴘᴄᴄ

COMPLICATIONS

Hypovolemia

Up to 6 L of fluid can be third-spaced; caused by retroperitoneal loss of protein-rich fluid from proteolytic digestion. The client can develop hypovolemic shock.

NURSING ACTIONS: Monitor electrolytes and for hypotension and tachycardia. Assist with the provision of IV fluid and electrolyte replacement.

Pancreatic infection

Pseudocyst (outside pancreas); abscess (inside pancreas)

CAUSE: Leakage of fluid out of damaged pancreatic duct

MANIFESTATIONS: Fever, epigastric mass, nausea, vomiting, jaundice

NURSING ACTIONS
- Monitor for rupture and hemorrhage.
- Maintain sump tube if placed for drainage of cyst.
- Monitor skin around tube for breakdown secondary to corrosive enzymes.

Type 1 diabetes mellitus

CAUSE: Lack or absence of insulin (due to destruction of pancreatic beta cells)

NURSING ACTIONS
- Monitor blood glucose.
- Administer insulin as prescribed.

CLIENT EDUCATION: Adhere to long-term diabetes management.

Left lung effusion and atelectasis

Can precipitate pneumonia

CAUSES: Pancreatic ascites

NURSING ACTIONS: Monitor for hypoxia and assist with the provision of ventilatory support.

Coagulation defects

Disseminated intravascular coagulopathy

CAUSES: Release of thromboplastic endotoxins secondary to necrotizing hemorrhagic pancreatitis

NURSING ACTIONS: Monitor coagulation studies and for bleeding.

Multi-system organ failure

Inflammation of pancreas is believed to trigger systemic inflammation.

CAUSE: Necrotizing hemorrhagic pancreatitis

NURSING ACTIONS
- Administer treatments.
- Monitor for evidence of organ failure (respiratory distress, jaundice, oliguria). Qꜱ
- Report unexpected findings to provider.

1. A nurse is collecting data from a client who has pancreatitis. Which of the following findings should the nurse expect?

   A. Pain in right upper quadrant radiating to right shoulder

   B. Report of pain being worse when sitting upright

   C. Pain relieved with defecation

   D. Epigastric pain radiating to the left shoulder

2. A nurse is collecting data from a client who has pancreatitis. Which of the following findings should the nurse identify as a manifestation of pancreatitis?

   A. Generalized cyanosis

   B. Hyperactive bowel sounds

   C. Gray-blue discoloration of the skin around the umbilicus

   D. Wheezing in the lower lung fields

3. A nurse is reviewing the admission laboratory results of a client who has acute pancreatitis. Which of the following findings should the nurse expect?

   A. Decreased blood lipase level

   B. Decreased blood amylase level

   C. Increased blood calcium level

   D. Increased blood glucose level

4. A nurse is preparing to administer pancrelipase to a client who has pancreatitis. Which of the following actions should the nurse take?

   A. Instruct the client to chew the medication before swallowing.

   B. Offer a glass of water following medication administration.

   C. Administer the medication 30 min before meals.

   D. Sprinkle the contents on peanut butter.

5. A nurse is assisting in the plan of care for an older adult client who has pancreatitis. Sort the following actions by whether the nurse should or should not recommend them.

   A. Obtain a prescription for meperidine.

   B. Monitor the client's blood glucose.

   C. Encourage client to decrease alcohol intake.

   D. Ensure the client remains NPO.

   E. Place client in a side-lying or semi-Fowler's position.

6. A nurse is reinforcing nutrition teaching with a client who has pancreatitis. Which of the following statements by the client indicate an understanding of the instruction? (Select all that apply.)

   A. "I plan to eat small, frequent meals."

   B. "I will eat easy-to-digest foods with limited spice."

   C. "I will use skim milk when cooking."

   D. "I plan to drink regular cola."

   E. "I will limit alcohol intake to two drinks per day."

Active Learning Scenario

A nurse is assisting in the plan of care for a client who has pancreatitis. What should the nurse include in the plan? Use the ATI Active Learning Template: System Disorder to complete this item.

ALTERATION IN HEALTH (DIAGNOSIS): Describe the classic presentation of pancreatitis.

LABORATORY TESTS: Describe four tests and expected findings.

NURSING CARE: Describe at least six nursing actions.

Application Exercises Key

1. D. **CORRECT:** When recognizing cues, the nurse should expect that a client who has pancreatitis will report severe, boring epigastric pain that radiates to the back, left flank, or left shoulder. A client who has cholecystitis will report pain in the right upper quadrant radiating to the right shoulder. A client who has pancreatitis will report pain being worse when lying down. A client who has pancreatitis will report that pain is relieved by assuming the fetal position.

Ⓝ *NCLEX® Connection: Physiological Adaptation, Basic Pathophysiology*

2. C. **CORRECT:** When recognizing cues, the nurse should identify that a gray-blue discoloration in the periumbilical area, generalized jaundice, absent or decreased bowel sounds, and diminished breath sounds, as well as dyspnea or orthopnea, are manifestations of pancreatitis.

Ⓝ *NCLEX® Connection: Reduction of Risk Potential, Potential for Alterations in Body Systems*

3. D. **CORRECT:** When analyzing cues, the nurse should expect that the client will experience an increased blood glucose level due to pancreatic cell injury, which results in impaired metabolism of carbohydrates due to a decrease in the release of insulin. The client will experience an elevated blood lipase and amylase level due to pancreatic cell injury and a decreased blood calcium level due to fat necrosis.

Ⓝ *NCLEX® Connection: Physiological Adaptation, Medical Emergencies*

4. B. **CORRECT:** When taking action, the nurse should ensure the client drinks a full glass of water following administration of pancrelipase. Pancrelipase should be swallowed without chewing to reduce irritation and slow the release of the medication. It should be administered with every meal and snack. The contents of the pancrelipase capsule can be sprinkled on nonprotein foods, and peanut butter is a protein food.

Ⓝ *NCLEX® Connection: Pharmacological Therapies, Medication Administration*

5. **SHOULD RECOMMEND:** B, D, E;
   SHOULD NOT RECOMMEND: A, C:

   When generating solutions, the nurse should identify that meperidine is contraindicated in older adult clients due to the risk of seizures. The client should be given an opioid such as morphine or hydromorphone. The nurse should emphasize the importance of abstaining from alcohol. When planning care, the nurse should plan to monitor the client's blood glucose, ensure the client remains NPO to rest the pancreas and decrease secretion of pancreatic enzymes, and place the client in a side-lying or semi-Fowler's position to decrease abdominal pain.

Ⓝ *NCLEX® Connection: Coordinated Care, Collaboration With Multidisciplinary Team*

6. A, B, C. **CORRECT:** When evaluating outcomes, the nurse should identify that the client's statements regarding small, frequent meals; bland, easy-to-digest foods; and low-fat foods indicate an understanding of the instruction about what is recommended for the client who has pancreatitis. Caffeine-free beverages are recommended for the client who has pancreatitis. Regular cola contains caffeine. The client who has pancreatitis should avoid any alcohol intake.

Ⓝ *NCLEX® Connection: Basic Care and Comfort, Nutrition and Oral Hydration*

Active Learning Scenario Key

Using the ATI Active Learning Template: System Disorder

ALTERATION IN HEALTH (DIAGNOSIS): Severe, constant, knifelike pain (left upper quadrant, midepigastric, and/or radiating to the back)

LABORATORY TESTS
- Blood amylase (increases within 12 hr, remains increased for 4 days)
- Blood lipase value (increases slowly and remains increased for up to 2 weeks)
- Urine amylase remains increased for up to 2 weeks.
- Increased WBC count due to inflammation/infection
- Decreased blood calcium and magnesium
- Blood liver enzymes and bilirubin increased with associated biliary dysfunction
- Blood glucose increased

NURSING CARE
- Maintain NPO status until the client is pain-free.
- Assist with the administration of total parenteral nutrition or jejunal feedings (contraindicated if paralytic ileus develops).
- Maintain NG tube (for severe vomiting or paralytic ileus).
- Resume diet, beginning with bland, high-protein, low-fat foods and no caffeine.
- Plan small, frequent meals.
- Administer antiemetics as needed.
- Limit stress.
- Provide pain management.
- Remind the client to not consume alcohol or smoke.

Ⓝ *NCLEX® Connection: Physiological Adaptation, Alterations in Body Systems*

NCLEX® Connections

When reviewing the following chapters, keep in mind the relevant topics and tasks of the NCLEX outline.

Basic Care and Comfort

NUTRITION AND ORAL HYDRATION: Reinforce client teaching on special diets based on client diagnosis/nutritional needs and cultural considerations.

Pharmacological Therapies

PHARMACOLOGICAL PAIN MANAGEMENT: Identify client need for pain medication.

EXPECTED ACTIONS/OUTCOMES: Reinforce client teaching on actions and therapeutic effects of medications and pharmacological interactions.

Reduction of Risk Potential

LABORATORY VALUES: Monitor diagnostic or laboratory test results.

Physiological Adaptation

ALTERATIONS IN BODY SYSTEMS: Reinforce education to client regarding care and condition.

CHAPTER 50 *Hepatitis and Cirrhosis*

Hepatitis is an inflammation of liver cells. Hepatitis can be caused by viral or toxic agents or as a secondary infection in conjunction with another virus. It is classified as acute or chronic.

Cirrhosis is permanent scarring of the liver that is usually caused by chronic inflammation.

Hepatitis

- Viral hepatitis is the most common type of hepatitis.
- Toxic and drug-induced hepatitis occur secondary to an exposure to a chemical or medication agent (alcohol, industrial toxins, acetaminophen).
- After exposure to a virus or toxin, the liver becomes enlarged from the inflammatory process. As the disease progresses, there is an increase in inflammation and necrosis, interfering with blood flow to the liver.
- Individuals can be infected with a hepatitis virus and remain free of manifestations and therefore are unaware that they could be contagious.

Major categories of viral hepatitis
- Hepatitis A virus (HAV)
- Hepatitis B virus (HBV)
- Hepatitis C virus (HCV)
- Hepatitis D virus (HDV)
- Hepatitis E virus (HEV)

HEALTH PROMOTION AND DISEASE PREVENTION

- Follow vaccination recommendations according to the CDC.
- Follow infection control precautions according to the CDC.
- Reinforce and use safe injection practices. Qs
  ○ Aseptic technique for preparation and administration of parenteral medications
  ○ Sterile, single-use, disposable needle and syringe for each injection
  ○ Single-dose vials whenever possible
  ○ Needleless systems or safety caps
- Use proper hand hygiene (before preparing and eating food, after using the toilet or changing a diaper).
- When traveling to underdeveloped countries, drink purified water and avoid sharing eating utensils and bed linens.

DATA COLLECTION

RISK FACTORS

Hepatitis A

ROUTE OF TRANSMISSION: Fecal-oral

RISK FACTORS
- Ingestion of contaminated food or water, especially shellfish
- Contact with infected stool (incontinent individuals, anal sexual activity)

Hepatitis B

ROUTE OF TRANSMISSION: Blood

RISK FACTORS
- Unprotected sex with infected individual
- Infants born to infected mothers
- Contact with infected blood
- Substance use disorder (injectable substances)

Hepatitis C

ROUTE OF TRANSMISSION: Blood

RISK FACTORS
- Substance use disorder (injectable substances)
- Blood, blood products, or organ transplants
- Contaminated needle sticks, unsanitary tattoo equipment
- Sexual contact

Hepatitis D

ROUTE OF TRANSMISSION: Coinfection with HBV

RISK FACTORS
- Substance use disorder (injectable substances)
- Unprotected sex with infected individual

Hepatitis E

ROUTE OF TRANSMISSION: Fecal-oral

RISK FACTORS: Ingestion of food or water contaminated with fecal waste

Additional risk factors

- Unscreened blood transfusions (prior to 1992)
- Hemodialysis
- Percutaneous exposure (dirty needles, sharp instruments, body piercing, tattooing, use of another person's substance use paraphernalia or personal hygiene tools)
- Ingestion of food prepared by a hepatitis-infected person who does not practice proper sanitation precautions
- Travel/residence in underdeveloped country (using tap water to clean food products, drinking contaminated water)
- Eating or living in crowded environments (correctional facilities, dormitories, universities, long-term care facilities, military base housing)

EXPECTED FINDINGS

- History of exposure to infected blood, stool, or body fluid
- Influenza-like manifestations
  - Fatigue
  - Decreased appetite with nausea
  - Abdominal pain
  - Joint pain

PHYSICAL FINDINGS

- Fever
- Vomiting
- Dark-colored urine
- Clay-colored stool
- Jaundice

LABORATORY TESTS QEBP

Alanine aminotransferase (ALT): Elevated; expected reference range is 4 to 36 units/L

Liver function test: Elevated

Prothrombin time: Elevated PT/INR

WBC

Platelets

Bilirubin: Elevated

Aspartate aminotransferase (AST): Elevated; expected reference range is 0 to 35 units/L

Alkaline phosphatase (ALP): Normal or elevated; expected reference range is 30 to 120 units/L

Total bilirubin level: Elevated; expected reference range is 0.3 to 1.0 mg/dL

Hepatitis antibodies: Positive for the specific type of hepatitis (A, B, C, D, E). However, a client who is vaccinated against HBV will have a positive HBsAg, indicating immunity to the disease.

Enzyme immunoassay (EIA): Detects presence of antigens or antibodies to hepatitis

DIAGNOSTIC PROCEDURES

Liver biopsy

This is the most definitive diagnostic approach, and it is used to identify the intensity of the infection and the degree of liver damage.

PREPROCEDURE NURSING ACTIONS

- Reinforce teaching about the procedure.
- Ensure that informed consent has been signed.
- Ensure the client fasts starting at midnight on the day of the procedure in case surgery is needed due to a complication. Qs
- Administer medications as prescribed.

INTRAPROCEDURE NURSING ACTIONS

- Assist the client into the supine position with the upper right quadrant of the abdomen exposed.
- Assist the client with relaxation techniques.
- Instruct the client to exhale and hold for at least 10 seconds while the needle is inserted. Qs
- Instruct the client to resume breathing once the needle is withdrawn.
- Apply pressure to the puncture site.

POSTPROCEDURE NURSING ACTIONS

- Assist the client to a right side-lying position and maintain for several hours.
- Monitor vital signs.
- Monitor for abdominal pain.
- Monitor for bleeding from the puncture site.
- Monitor for manifestations of pneumothorax (dyspnea, cyanosis, restlessness) due to accidental puncture of the pleura or lung.

PATIENT-CENTERED CARE

NURSING CARE

- Most clients will be cared for in the home unless they are acutely ill.
- Always use standard precautions and enforce contact precautions if indicated.
- Provide a high-carbohydrate, high-calorie, moderate-fat, and moderate-protein diet after nausea and anorexia subsides, and provide small, frequent meals to promote nutrition and healing.
- Promote hepatic rest and the regeneration of tissue.
  - Administer only necessary medications, including over-the-counter medications or herbal supplements.
  - Avoid alcohol.
  - Limit physical activity.
- Reinforce teaching with the client and family regarding measures to prevent the transmission of the disease to others at home. QPCC
  - Avoid sexual intercourse until hepatitis antibody testing is negative.
  - Use proper hand hygiene.
  - Avoid sharing household items (towels, toothbrushes).
- Provide culturally sensitive care.
- Discuss use of or interest in complementary and integrative therapies with the client to improve quality of life.

MEDICATIONS

Hepatitis A

- Hepatitis A immunization is recommended for post-exposure protection.
- Immunoglobulin is recommended for post-exposure protection for clients older than 40 years, younger than 12 months, who have chronic liver disease, who are immunosuppressed, or who are allergic to the vaccine.

Hepatitis B

Acute infection: No medications; supportive care

Chronic infection: Antiviral medications: tenofovir, adefovir dipivoxil, interferon alfa-2b, peginterferon alfa-2a, lamivudine, entecavir, and telbivudine

Hepatitis C

Combination therapy with peginterferon alfa-2a and ribavirin is the preferred treatment.

Hepatitis E

No medications; supportive care

INTERPROFESSIONAL CARE

Possible consults with infection control, social worker, primary care provider; connect the client with community resources

COMPLICATIONS

CHRONIC HEPATITIS

- Ongoing inflammation of the liver cells
- Results from hepatitis B, C, or D
- Increases the client's risk for liver cancer

ACUTE LIVER FAILURE

- Extremely severe and potentially fatal form of viral hepatitis
- Clients develop manifestations of viral hepatitis, then within hours or days develop severe liver failure.
- No medications, supportive care
- Irreversible damage to liver cells, with decreased ability to function adequately to meet the body's needs

Cirrhosis of the liver: Permanent scarring of the liver that is usually caused by chronic inflammation

LIVER CANCER

Hepatic encephalopathy: A life-threatening complication of liver failure. Toxic substances, which are normally detoxified by the liver, enter systemic circulation. Ammonia levels rise and enter the brain, causing clients to develop changes in neurologic status.

Cirrhosis

- Cirrhosis is extensive scarring of the liver caused by necrotic injury or a chronic reaction to inflammation over a prolonged period of time. Normal liver tissue is replaced with fibrotic tissue that lacks function.
- Portal and periportal areas of the liver are primarily involved, affecting the liver's ability to handle the flow of bile by nodules blocking the bile ducts and normal blood flow throughout the liver, which can result in portal hypertension.

HEALTH PROMOTION AND DISEASE PREVENTION

- Prevent infection with viral hepatitis (B, C, D).
- Avoid excessive alcohol intake. GPCC

Types of cirrhosis

Postnecrotic: Caused by viral hepatitis, or some medications or toxins

Laennec's: Caused by chronic alcohol use disorder

Biliary: Caused by chronic biliary obstruction or infection

Cardiac: Caused by right-sided heart failure or cor pulmonale

DATA COLLECTION

RISK FACTORS

- Alcohol use disorder
- Chronic viral hepatitis (hepatitis B, C, or D)
- Damage to the liver caused by medications, substances, toxins, infections
- Chronic biliary cirrhosis (bile duct obstruction, bile stasis, hepatic fibrosis)
- Cardiac cirrhosis resulting from severe right heart failure inducing necrosis and fibrosis due to lack of blood flow

EXPECTED FINDINGS

- Fatigue
- Anorexia
- Weakness
- Dyspnea
- Weight loss, abdominal pain, distention
- Pruritus (severe itching of skin)
- Confusion or difficulty thinking (due to the buildup of waste products in the blood and brain that the liver is unable to get rid of)
- Personality and mentation changes, emotional lability, euphoria, depression

PHYSICAL FINDINGS

- Cognitive changes
- Gastroesophageal bleeding (enlarged esophageal veins [varices] develop and burst, causing vomiting and passing of blood in bowel movements) or portal hypertensive gastropathy, which causes bleeding of gastric mucosa
- Splenomegaly caused from backup of blood into the spleen, which can cause thrombocytopenia, leukopenia, and platelet destruction
- Ascites (bloating or swelling due to fluid buildup in abdomen and legs)
- Jaundice (yellowing of skin) and icterus (yellowing of the eyes) from decreased excretion of bilirubin, resulting in an increase of circulating bilirubin levels
- Petechiae (round, pinpoint, red-purple lesions), ecchymoses (large yellow and purple-blue bruises), nosebleeds, hematemesis

- Palmar erythema (redness, warmth of the palms of the hands)
- Spider angiomas (red lesions, vascular in nature with branches radiating on the nose, cheeks, upper thorax, shoulders)
- Dependent peripheral edema of extremities and sacrum
- Asterixis (hand flapping tremor): coarse tremor characterized by rapid, nonrhythmic extension and flexion of the wrists and fingers
- Fetor hepaticus (liver breath): fruity or musty odor
- Urine: dark-colored with a foamy appearance
- Stools: clay-colored

LABORATORY TESTS Q EBP

Blood liver enzymes: elevated initially

Lactate dehydrogenase (LDH), ALT, and AST are elevated due to hepatic inflammation. ALT and AST return to normal when liver cells are no longer able to create an inflammatory response. ALP increases in cirrhosis due to intrahepatic biliary obstruction.

ALT: Expected reference range: 4 to 36 units/L

AST: Expected reference range: 0 to 35 units/L

ALP: Expected reference range: 30 to 120 units/L

Blood bilirubin: elevated

Bilirubin levels are elevated in cirrhosis due to the inability of the liver to excrete bilirubin.

Bilirubin, indirect (unconjugated): Elevated; expected reference range: 0.2 to 0.8 mg/dL

Bilirubin, total: Elevated; expected reference range: 0.3 to 1.0 mg/dL

Blood total protein

- Decreased due to the lack of hepatic synthesis
- Expected reference range: 6.4 to 8.3 g/dL

Blood albumin

- Decreased due to the lack of hepatic synthesis
- Expected reference range: 3.5 to 5 g/dL

Hematological tests

RBC: Decreased

Hemoglobin: Decreased

Hematocrit: Decreased

Platelet count: Decreased

PT/INR

Prolonged due to decreased synthesis of prothrombin

Ammonia levels

- Increase when hepatocellular injury (cirrhosis) prevents the conversion of ammonia to urea for excretion
- Expected reference range: 6 to 47 μmol/L (10 to 80 mcg/dL)

DIAGNOSTIC PROCEDURES

Ultrasound: Used to detect ascites, hepatomegaly, splenomegaly, biliary stones, or biliary obstruction

Abdominal x-rays and CT scan: Used to visualize possible hepatomegaly, ascites, and splenomegaly

MRI: Used to visualize mass lesions and determine whether the liver is malignant or benign

Liver biopsy (most definitive)
- A liver biopsy identifies the progression and extent of the cirrhosis.
- To minimize the risk of hemorrhage, a radiologist can perform the biopsy through the jugular vein, which is threaded to the hepatic vein to obtain tissue for a microscopic evaluation.
- This is done under fluoroscopy for safety because this procedure can be problematic for cirrhosis clients due to an increased risk for bleeding complications. Q s

Esophagogastroduodenoscopy: This is performed under moderate (conscious) sedation to detect the presence of esophageal varices, ulcerations in the stomach, or duodenal ulcers and bleeding.

Magnetic resonance cholangiopancreatography: Used to view the biliary tract

PATIENT-CENTERED CARE

NURSING CARE Q PCC

Respiratory status: Monitor oxygen saturation levels and distress. Provide comfort measures by positioning the client to ease respiratory effort (can be compromised by plasma volume excess and ascites). Have the client sit in a chair or elevate the head of the bed to 30° with feet elevated.

Skin integrity: Monitor closely for skin breakdown. Implement measures to prevent pressure injuries. Pruritus, which is associated with jaundice, will cause the client to scratch. Encourage washing with warm water and applying lotion to decrease the itching.

Fluid balance: Monitor for indications of fluid volume excess. Keep strict I&O, obtain daily weights, and check for ascites and peripheral edema. Restrict fluids and sodium if prescribed. Assist with the administration of blood products such as FFP or albumin.

Vital signs: Monitor vital signs and pain level.

Neurologic status: Monitor for deteriorating mental status and dementia consistent with hepatic encephalopathy. Monitor for asterixis (coarse tremor of wrists and fingers) and fetor hepaticus. Lactulose can be given to aid in excretion of ammonia.

Nutritional status: High-carbohydrate, high-protein, moderate-fat, and low-sodium diet with vitamin supplements, such as thiamine, folate, and multivitamins

Bleeding: Monitor coagulation values and stools. Monitor for mental status changes and restlessness. Do not perform rectal temperatures or administer enemas. Assist with the administration of blood products, such as platelets.

Gastrointestinal status: In the presence of ascites, measure abdominal girth daily over the largest part of the abdomen. Mark the location of tape for consistency. Observe for potential bleeding complications.

Pain status: Collect data about client's pain, and administer analgesics and gastrointestinal antispasmodics as needed.

MEDICATIONS Q EBP

Because the metabolism of most medications is dependent upon a functioning liver, general medications are administered sparingly, especially opioids, sedatives, and barbiturates.

Diuretics: Decrease excessive fluid in the body

Beta-blocking agent: Used for clients who have varices to prevent bleeding and to manage portal hypertension

Lactulose: Used to promote excretion of ammonia from the body through the stool

Oral antibiotics: Antibiotics kill bacteria in the intestine that produce ammonia.

Vitamin K: Promote clotting

Cholesterol binding agents: Decrease pruritus

H₂ antagonist: Decrease gastritis

Oxazepam: Decrease agitation

Vitamin/mineral supplements (thiamine, folate, B₁₂)

THERAPEUTIC PROCEDURES

Paracentesis

Sterile procedure used to relieve ascites

PREPROCEDURE NURSING CARE
- Reinforce information provided about the procedure.
- Ensure that informed consent has been obtained.
- Obtain vital signs and weight.
- Assist the client to void to reduce the risk of injury to the bladder. Q s
- Weigh client.
- Measure abdominal girth.

INTRAPROCEDURE NURSING CARE
- Position the client supine with head of bed elevated.
- Assist the client with relaxation techniques.
- Apply dressing over puncture site.

POSTPROCEDURE NURSING CARE
- Monitor vital signs.
- Maintain bed rest.
- Measure the fluid, and document amount and color.
- Send specimen to the laboratory.
- Monitor puncture site dressing for drainage.
- Weigh client.
- Measure abdominal girth.

Endoscopic variceal ligation/ endoscopic sclerotherapy

- Varices are either sclerosed or banded endoscopically.
- There is a decreased risk of hemorrhage with banding.

Transjugular intrahepatic portosystemic shunt (TIPS)

This is performed in interventional radiology for clients who require further intervention with ascites or hemorrhage. Shunts blood from the portal vein to hepatic vein to bypass the liver

Liver transplantation

- Portions of healthy livers from deceased donors (most commonly trauma victims) or living donors can be used for transplant.
- The transplanted liver portion will regenerate and grow based on the needs of the body.
- The client must meet the transplant criteria to be eligible.
- Clients who have severe cardiac and respiratory disease, metastatic malignant liver cancer, or alcohol/substance use disorder are not candidates for liver transplantation.

INTERPROFESSIONAL CARE

- A dietary consult can assist with specific diet needs.
- Recommend appropriate referrals (social services, Alcoholics Anonymous, Al-Anon).

CLIENT EDUCATION Q PCC

- Abstain from alcohol and engage in an alcohol recovery program if needed.
  - Helps prevent further scarring and fibrosis of liver
  - Allows healing and regeneration of liver tissue
  - Prevents irritation of the stomach and esophagus lining
  - Helps decrease the risk of bleeding
  - Helps prevent other life-threatening complications
- Consult with the provider prior to taking any over-the-counter medications or herbal supplements. Q s

- Follow diet guidelines.
  - High-calorie, moderate-fat diet
  - Low-sodium diet (if the client has excessive fluid in the peritoneal cavity)
  - Low-protein (if encephalopathy, elevated ammonia)
  - Small, frequent, well-balanced nutritional meals
  - Nutritional supplement drinks or shakes and a daily multivitamin
  - Replacement and administration of vitamins due to the inability of the liver to store them
  - Fluid intake restrictions if blood sodium is low

COMPLICATIONS

Hepatic encephalopath /portal systemic encephalopathy

Clients who have a poorly functioning liver are unable to convert ammonia and other waste products to a less toxic form. These products are carried to the brain and cause neurologic manifestations. Reductions in dietary protein are indicated as ammonia is formed when protein is broken down by intestinal flora.

NURSING ACTIONS
- Administer lactulose as prescribed.
- Monitor laboratory findings, including potassium, because clients can become hypokalemic with increased stools from the lactulose therapy.
- Monitor for changes in the level of consciousness and orientation.
- Monitor for fetor hepaticus (sweet, fruity, fecal breath odor).
- Report asterixis (flapping of the hands) and fetor hepaticus immediately to the provider. These are clinical indications that encephalopathy is worsening.

CLIENT EDUCATION: Adhere to the prescribed diet.

Esophageal varices

CAUSES: Portal hypertension (elevated blood pressure in veins that carry blood from the intestines to the liver) is caused by impaired circulation of blood through the liver. Collateral circulation is subsequently developed, creating varices in the upper stomach and esophagus. Varices are fragile and can bleed easily.

NURSING ACTIONS
- Assist with saline lavage (vasoconstriction), esophagogastric balloon tamponade, blood transfusions, ligation and sclerotherapy, and shunts to stop bleeding and reduce the risk for hypovolemic shock.
- Monitor hemoglobin level and vital signs.
- Monitor for any bleeding.

Application Exercises Key

1. A. **CORRECT:** Hepatitis A is transmitted by contaminated food, water, and shellfish.
   B, C. Hepatitis B and C are transmitted by blood.
   D. Hepatitis D coexists with hepatitis B and C and is transmitted in the same way.
   E. **CORRECT:** Hepatitis E is seen in less-developed parts of the world and is transmitted by fecal contamination of water.

   Ⓝ *NCLEX Connection: Safety and Infection Control, Standard Precautions/Transmission-Based Precautions/Surgical Asepsis*

2. A. **CORRECT:** The nurse should have the client lie on their right side for 2 hr after the procedure because this position compresses the liver capsule against the chest wall, therefore decreasing the risk of bleeding.
   B. The nurse should encourage a client who has had testing using radioisotopes to drink large amounts of water to promote the excretion of radioisotopes from the body.
   C. The nurse should place a small dressing over the needle insertion site.
   D. The nurse should inform the client that coughing and straining can cause increased intra-abdominal pressure and cause bleeding.

   Ⓝ *NCLEX® Connection: Reduction of Risk Potential, Potential for Complications of Diagnostic Tests/Treatments/Procedures*

3. A, B, C, E. **CORRECT:** The nurse should monitor the client for fluid volume excess by measuring the client's abdominal girth, daily weights, and intake and output and by checking for peripheral edema.
   D. Reducing fluid intake and sodium intake can be helpful in reducing fluid retention associated with ascites.

   Ⓝ *NCLEX® Connection: Physiological Adaptation, Fluid and Electrolyte Imbalances*

4. A. **CORRECT:** In clients who have hepatic encephalopathy, lactulose enhances the intestinal absorption of ammonia, a substance that accumulates because the liver is unable to detoxify this substance.
   B. Lactulose can cause an increase in sodium.
   C, D. Although bilirubin and AST are elevated in clients who have liver disease, lactulose does not influence bilirubin or AST.

   Ⓝ *NCLEX® Connection: Physiological Adaptation, Alterations in Body Systems*

5. A. **CORRECT:** Fetor hepaticas is breath with a musty, sweet odor that occurs in late liver failure and is a manifestation of hepatic encephalopathy.
   B. **CORRECT:** Asterix, or hand flapping, also occurs in late liver failure and is a manifestation of hepatic encephalopathy.
   C, D, E. Anorexia, ascites, and abdominal pain are manifestations that can occur in the early stages of cirrhosis and are not indications of hepatic encephalopathy.

   Ⓝ *NCLEX® Connection: Physiological Adaptation, Alterations in Body Systems*

Active Learning Scenario

A nurse is caring for a client who has hepatitis C and will undergo liver biopsy. Use the ATI Active Learning Template: Diagnostic Procedure to complete the following.

DESCRIPTION OF PROCEDURE

NURSING INTERVENTIONS (PRE, INTRA, POST): List one preprocedure, one intraprocedure, and one postprocedure.

POTENTIAL COMPLICATIONS: Identify one potential complication of the procedure.

Active Learning Scenario Key

Using the ATI Active Learning Template: Diagnostic Procedure

DESCRIPTION OF PROCEDURE: A liver biopsy is a procedure to collect a sample of liver tissue for diagnostic testing. A needle is inserted in the intercostal space between the two right lower ribs and into the liver. An aspirate of liver tissue is then collected.

NURSING ACTIONS (PRE, INTRA, POST)

Preprocedure
- Reinforce teaching about the procedure to the client/family.
- Ensure that informed consent has been signed.
- Ensure the client has been fasting since midnight.
- Administer medication.

Intraprocedure
- Assist the client into the supine position with the upper right quadrant of the abdomen exposed.
- Assist the client with relaxation techniques.
- Instruct the client to exhale and hold for at least 10 seconds while the needle is inserted.
- Instruct the client to resume breathing once the needle is withdrawn.
- Apply pressure to the puncture site.

Postprocedure
- Assist the client to a right side-lying position and maintain for several hours.
- Monitor vital signs.
- Check for abdominal pain.
- Check for bleeding from puncture site.

Potential Complications
- Bleeding
- Bile peritonitis
- Pneumothorax

Ⓝ *NCLEX® Connection: Reduction of Risk Potential, Diagnostic Tests*

When reviewing the following chapters, keep in mind the relevant topics and tasks of the NCLEX outline.

Basic Care and Comfort

NUTRITION AND ORAL HYDRATION: Reinforce client teaching on special diets based on client diagnosis/nutritional needs and cultural considerations.

Reduction of Risk Potential

LABORATORY VALUES: Monitor diagnostic or laboratory test results.

Physiological Adaptation

ALTERATIONS IN BODY SYSTEMS: Reinforce education to client regarding care and condition.

CHAPTER 51 *Obesity*

Obesity is defined as a BMI greater than 30. Approximately 1/3 of the adult population in the United States are considered obese. It is estimated that 2 in 5 adults and 1 in 5 children in the U.S. will have obesity. Obesity, when combined with chronic conditions, is associated with a reduction in life span. An individual who has an BMI of 25-29.9 is considered overweight. Nurse and health care team members should be aware that complexity of care increases when caring for clients who are overweight or obese. Management and treatment should focus on quality of life and long-term reduction of health risks associated with obesity. For additional information about complications of obesity, see **NUTRITION FOR NURSING: CHAPTER: MALNUTRITION.**

HEALTH PROMOTION AND DISEASE PREVENTION

Lifestyle modifications include establishing a healthy eating pattern, increasing physical activity, and implementing behavior changes, including:
- Reducing calorie intake
- Incorporating cultural preferences
- Increasing aerobic and resistance training exercises
- Avoiding triggers
- Setting goals
- Managing stress
- Using social support
- Identifying emotions related to food intake
- Keeping a food diary

Healthy People 2030

THE OBJECTIVES FOR CLIENTS WHO HAVE OBESITY INCLUDE:
- Reduce proportion of adults who have obesity.
- Increase the proportion of individuals who have obesity to obtain health care visits with the inclusion of counseling on weight loss, physical activity, and dietary recommendations.
- Decrease consumption of added sugars.

DATA COLLECTION

RISK FACTORS

- Lifestyle factors (decreased physical activity)
- Medications (corticosteroids, antidepressants)
- Genetic predisposition
- Cardiovascular disease
- Hypertension
- Stroke
- Stress
- Mood disorders (depression)
- Hyperlipidemia
- Type 2 diabetes mellitus
- Bone/joint conditions
- Gallstones

EXPECTED FINDINGS

BODY MASS INDEX (BMI)
- Overweight: BMI 25 to 29.9
- Class 1 obesity: BMI 30 to 34.9
- Class 2 obesity: BMI 35 to 39.9
- Class 3 obesity: BMI 40 or greater

Waist circumference (central obesity) is a strong predictor of long-term complications related to obesity, such as coronary artery disease.

Central obesity is indicated by a waist circumference of greater than 89 cm (35 inches) for clients who are female (sex assigned at birth) and greater than 102 cm (40 inches) for males (sex assigned at birth).

PATIENT-CENTERED CARE

NURSING INTERVENTIONS

Considerations when caring for a client who has obesity

RISKS DURING HOSPITALIZATION
- Poor wound healing, pressure injury, and infection
  - Fatty tissue has a poor supply of blood, nutrients, and collagen.
  - Mobility limitations
- Pressure injury
- Diminished cardiac function
- Obstructive sleep apnea
  - Enlarged neck circumference
- Reduced lung volume
- Hypoventilation, hypercapnia, and hypoxemia
- Venous thromboembolism (VTE)
- Inadequate pain management
  - Might require larger dosages of medication
- Injury to client or staff members

THERAPEUTIC MANAGEMENT

Weight management involves balancing of the intake of energy with the expenditure of energy. Some of the components of weight loss program include modifications of diet and lifestyle and physical activity.

LIFESTYLE MODIFICATIONS

Client is encouraged to modify their present lifestyle by using strategies such as:
- Setting goals
- Stimulus control
- Cognitive restructuring (correct and address negative thoughts)
- Problem-solving
- Relapse prevention

PHYSICAL ACTIVITY: Moderate exercise at least 30 minutes each day is recommended (walking 1.5 miles per day).

DIETARY MODIFICATIONS

Used in combination with lifestyle changes and physical activity
- Diet is usually individualized and balanced with (protein, carbohydrates, decreased fat, increased fiber).
- Calorie restrictions may be indicated.
- Limit alcohol consumption.
- Limit consumption of refined sugars.

MEDICATIONS

Medication management is indicated for clients who have a BMI greater with increased risk factors for other conditions. It should be used in conjunction with lifestyle modifications, diet modifications, and physical activity. Clients should consider this option before moving to more invasive therapies for weight loss, such as bariatric surgery.
- **Orlistat** inhibits digestion of fats by blocking gastric and pancreatic lipases. Adverse effects include oily rectal discharge and stools, flatulence, and reduced food and vitamin absorption.
  - Psyllium, a bulk-forming laxative, can increase the absorption of dietary fats and decrease the gastrointestinal (GI) adverse effects.
  - Daily supplementation with a multivitamin can prevent vitamin deficiencies.
  - Client should not take orlistat with a meal that does not contain fat.
- **Phentermine-topiramate** suppresses the appetite and induces a feeling of satiety. Adverse effects include headache, dry mouth, constipation, nausea, change in taste, dizziness, insomnia, and paresthesia. Contraindicated if the client has hyperthyroidism, has glaucoma, or is taking an MAO inhibitor
  - Medication may be taken with meals or on an empty stomach.
  - Instruct client to take medication early in the day to prevent insomnia.

- **Naltrexone-bupropion** suppresses the appetite and decreases cravings. Adverse effects include constipation, diarrhea, nausea, vomiting, headache, insomnia, and dry mouth. Contraindicated for clients who have uncontrolled hypertension, eating disorders, seizure disorders, or who are taking MAO inhibitors.
  - Client should not take medication with high-fat meals to avoid increased systemic concentration of naltrexone and bupropion.
  - Bupropion has anti-depressant effect; client should be monitored for suicidal ideation.
- **Liraglutide**: Suppresses appetite and slows gastric emptying to induce satiety. Adverse effects include nausea, vomiting, diarrhea, constipation, increased heart rate, dyspepsia, and hypoglycemia. Also used for management of type 2 diabetes mellitus. Should be used with caution for clients who are taking other medications that lower blood glucose levels
  - Administered by subcutaneous injection.
  - Medication may be taken with meals or on an empty stomach.

CAM THERAPIES Qᴘᴄᴄ

- Acupuncture
- Hypnosis

THERAPEUTIC PROCEDURES

Hydrogel pill: approved by the FDA as an adjunct device to diet and exercise for weight loss for clients who have a BMI 25-40
- Pill is taken with meals.
- Absorbs water to occupy space in the stomach and reduce stomach capacity
- Passes through GI tract and is excreted
- Adverse effects include constipation, obstruction, diarrhea, and dehydration.
- Contraindicated for clients who have Crohn's disease or history of any surgery that altered GI motility

Intragastric balloon therapy: gas-filled or saline-filled balloon placed in stomach during endoscopic procedure
- Weight loss can be related to increased satiety and decreased gastric emptying.
- Adverse effects are nausea and vomiting, potential balloon rupture, and rupture of the stomach or esophagus. Pancreatitis can occur if balloon is in place longer than 6 months. Qₛ

Bariatric surgeries

Bariatric surgeries include open and minimally invasive approaches. These surgeries are performed to assist with weight loss in clients who are obese and have been unable to lose weight through modifications and pharmacological interventions. Bariatric surgeries assist in weight loss through the decrease of the capacity of the stomach causing malabsorption by bypassing part of the small intestine or through a combination of both mechanisms. Some clients undergo plastic surgery, including abdominoplasty and breast reduction, to remove excess skin and tissue following weight loss.

Preoperatively, clients undergo upper endoscopy to rule out GI disease. Postoperatively, clients undergo barium x-ray to evaluate for anastomotic leaks.

Following bariatric surgery, many clients experience decreased complications from previously diagnosed conditions such as hypertension, CAD, hyperlipidemia, asthma, sleep apnea, and diabetes mellitus.

INDICATIONS

Bariatric surgeries are a treatment for obesity when other weight-control methods have failed. Candidates for bariatric surgery are clients who have:
- BMI greater than 40 and no comorbidities
- BMI greater than 35 and at least one complication related to obesity (for example, hypertension, osteoarthritis, type 2 diabetes mellitus)
- BMI 30 to 34.9 and glucose levels inadequately controlled with medications and lifestyle modifications

TYPES OF BARIATRIC SURGERIES

RESTRICTIVE

Create decreased capacity of the stomach; allow for normal digestion. Common types are banding and sleeve gastrectomy.

Gastric banding: Small pouch is created through laparoscopic placement of an adjustable band around the upper part of the stomach that allows only small portions of food to enter the GI tract.
- Performed laparoscopically
- Bladder in subcutaneous reservoir can be inflated or deflated.

Vertical banded gastroplasty: Upper part of stomach is surgically stapled to create a small pouch, and a band is placed to slow the emptying of food from the pouch to the rest of the stomach.

Sleeve gastrectomy: Pouch (sleeve) is created by removal of a large portion of the stomach through open or laparoscopic procedure.

MALABSORPTIVE

Procedures combine decreased capacity with malabsorption created from bypassing part of small intestine.

Gastric bypass

- **Roux-en-Y (RNYGB):** Small pouch is created with the upper part of the stomach. The jejunum is attached to the pouch, causing food to bypass most of the stomach and the duodenum.
- Often performed as a robotic-assisted surgery, open or laparoscopic
- Increased risk of dumping syndrome related to removal of pyloric valve
- **Biliopancreatic diversion with duodenal switch:** Part of the stomach is removed, leaving a pouch that is attached directly to the jejunum.

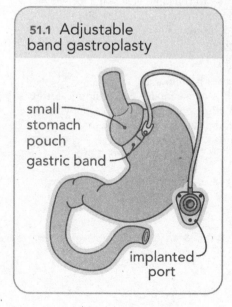

51.1 Adjustable band gastroplasty

small stomach pouch
gastric band
implanted port

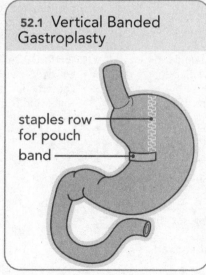

52.1 Vertical Banded Gastroplasty

staples row for pouch
band

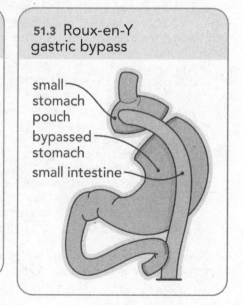

51.3 Roux-en-Y gastric bypass

small stomach pouch
bypassed stomach
small intestine

PATIENT-CENTERED CARE

NURSING ACTIONS

PREPROCEDURE

- To identify psychosocial factors related to obesity, provide the client the opportunity to express emotions about eating behaviors, weight, and weight loss. Qpcc
- Reinforce teaching with the client about necessary diet and lifestyle changes.
- Arrange for availability of a bariatric room, furniture, and other equipment, such as correct size of blood pressure cuff for the client.
- Ensure adequate staff are available for ambulation and transfers.
- Use mechanical lifting devices to prevent client/staff injury. Qs
- Review lab results (CBC, electrolytes, BUN, creatinine, HbA1C, iron, vitamin B_{12}, thiamine, and folate).
- Ensure sequential compression stockings are applied to reduce the risk for deep vein thrombosis.

POSTPROCEDURE

Monitor the airway and oxygen saturation per facility protocol. Maintain client in a semi-Fowler's position to promote lung expansion.

- If the client had an NG tube inserted during surgery, do not reposition it. Repositioning can disrupt the sutures. Postoperatively, an NG tube should not be inserted for a client who has had bariatric surgery.
- Monitor for postoperative complications. Clients who have had bariatric surgery are at a greater risk for developing atelectasis, thromboembolism, skin fold breakdown, incisional hernia, and peritonitis.
- Monitor bowel sounds.
- Apply an abdominal binder as prescribed to prevent dehiscence if there is an abdominal incision.
- Recommend implementation of measures to prevent VTE.
  - Clients who have bariatric surgery are at moderate to high risk for developing VTE.
  - Ambulate the client as soon as possible.
  - Apply pneumatic compression stockings
  - Administer low-molecular-weight heparin as ordered.
- Resume fluids as prescribed. Fluids might be restricted for the first few days and then increased in frequency and volume.
  - Diet progresses from clear liquids to full liquids. Clients usually discharged with full liquid diet
  - Pureed foods one week after surgery
  - Solid foods at six to eight weeks postoperatively
    - Four to six small meals per day
    - Reinforce teaching with client to wait for 30 minutes before drinking liquids following a meal.
    - Reinforce teaching with client to observe for manifestations of dumping syndrome (nausea, weakness, diaphoresis, diarrhea).
      - Empty calories, such as beverages with sugar increase the risk of dumping syndrome for clients who have RYGB)
- Collaborate with interdisciplinary team to assist with long-term behavior modification. Qtc

CLIENT EDUCATION

- Adhere to the limited diet of liquids or pureed foods for the first 6 to 8 weeks, as well as the volume that can be consumed.
- Avoid carbonated beverages.
- Collaborate with physical therapy for exercise instructions. Qtc

COMPLICATIONS

Anastomotic leak

- A frequent, serious complication of gastric bypass surgery
- Life-threatening emergency
- Monitor for manifestations of leak of anastomosis and notify the provider immediately.
  - Increasing abdominal pain
  - Nausea and vomiting
  - Tachycardia
  - Hypotension
  - Fever

Dehydration

- Reinforce with the client that excessive thirst or concentrated urine can be an indication of dehydration and the surgeon should be notified.
- Reinforce goals and schedule for adequate daily fluid intake — at least 1.5 L daily.

Malabsorption/malnutrition

Because bariatric surgeries reduce the size of the stomach or bypass portions of the intestinal tract, fewer nutrients are ingested and absorbed.

NURSING ACTIONS

- Common nutrient deficiencies are vitamin B_{12}, vitamin D, thiamine, calcium, iron, and folate.
- Monitor the client's tolerance of increasing amounts of food and fluids.
- Recommend referral for dietary management. Qtc
- Reinforce teaching to consume meals in a low-Fowler's position and to remain in this position for 30 min after eating to delay stomach emptying and minimize dumping syndrome.

CLIENT EDUCATION

- Eat two servings of protein a day.
- Eat only nutrition-dense foods. Avoid empty calories (colas and fruit juice drinks) and limit carbohydrates.
- Take vitamin and mineral supplements for life.

1. A nurse is reinforcing teaching with a newly licensed nurse about medications used for weight management. The nurse should include that which of the following medications is administered subcutaneously?

   A. Orlistat

   B. Liraglutide

   C. Naltrexone-bupropion

   D. Phentermine-topiramate

2. A nurse is reinforcing teaching about the actions of bariatric medications and devices with a client who is obese and seeking information about weight loss. Match each action to the medication or device it describes.

   A. Suppresses appetite and decreases cravings

   B. Inhibits digestion of fats by blocking lipases

   C. Absorbs water to decrease stomach capacity

   D. Increases satiety with placement of an expandable device filled with saline

   1. Intragastric balloon

   2. Hydrogel pill device

   3. Orlistat

   4. Naltrexone-bupropion

3. A nurse is contributing to planning care for clients who have had bariatric surgery. Sort the procedures by whether they are categorized as restrictive or malabsorptive surgeries.

   A. Gastric banding

   B. Roux-en-Y

   C. Sleeve gastrectomy

   D. Vertical banded gastroplasty

   E. Biliopancreatic diversion with duodenal switch

4. A nurse is reinforcing discharge teaching with a client who had a gastric bypass surgery. Which of the following statements by the client indicates understanding of the instructions? (Select all that apply.)

   A. "I should start to eat solid foods 2 weeks after surgery."

   B. "I should expect very little urine output for the first 2 weeks."

   C. "The most serious complication I can expect is vomiting."

   D. "The amount of refined carbohydrates in my diet should be limited."

   E. "I should drink at least 1.5 liters of water each day."

   F. "After a meal, I should wait for 30 minutes to drink liquids."

A nurse is reinforcing education with a group of newly hired nurses about care of a client who is scheduled to have bariatric surgery. What should the nurse include in this discussion? Use the ATI Active Learning Template: Therapeutic Procedure to complete this item.

DESCRIPTION OF PROCEDURE: Describe three types of surgeries a client can have to assist in weight loss.

NURSING INTERVENTIONS: Provide at least five interventions. Include any equipment that might be required to promote safety of the client and staff.

CLIENT EDUCATION: Discuss postoperative dietary requirements.

Active Learning Scenario Key

Using the ATI Active Learning Template: Therapeutic Procedure

DESCRIPTION OF PROCEDURE

- Vertical banded gastroplasty: Upper part of stomach is surgically stapled to create a small pouch and a band is placed to slow the emptying of food from the pouch to the rest of the stomach.
- Gastric banding – Small pouch is created through laparoscopic placement of an adjustable band around the upper part of the stomach that allows only small portions of food to enter the GI tract.
- Roux-en-Y (RNYGB) – A small pouch is created with the upper part of the stomach. The jejunum is attached to the pouch causing food to bypass most of the stomach and the duodenum.

NURSING INTERVENTIONS

- To identify psychosocial factors related to obesity, provide the client the opportunity to express emotions about eating behaviors, weight, and weight loss
- Reinforce teaching to the client about necessary diet and lifestyle changes.
- Arrange for availability of a bariatric room, furniture, and other equipment, such as an extra-large blood pressure cuff.
- Monitor for leak of anastomosis and notify provider immediately if this occurs.
- Monitor airway and oxygen saturation per facility protocol. Maintain client in a semi-Fowler's position to promote lung expansion and encourage coughing and deep breathing.
- For open surgical procedures, apply an abdominal binder as prescribed to help prevent dehiscence.
- Ambulate client as soon as possible.
- Reinforce teaching with client to observe for manifestations of dumping syndrome (cramps, diarrhea, tachycardia, dizziness, fatigue.
- If NG tube present, monitor placement and function. Do not reposition tube. Repositioning can disrupt the sutures. Postoperatively, an NG tube should not be inserted for a client who has had bariatric surgery.

CLIENT EDUCATION

- Adhere to the limited diet of liquids or pureed foods for the first 6 to 8 weeks.
- Remain in low-Fowler position for 20 to 30 minutes after eating to delay gastric emptying.
- Take vitamin and mineral supplements for life.
- Avoid carbonated beverages.

Application Exercises Key

1. B. **CORRECT:** When taking actions, the nurse should discuss that liraglutide is administered subcutaneously. It should be used with caution for clients who are taking anti-hyperglycemic medications. Liraglutide is also used to lower blood glucose for clients who have diabetes mellitus and can potentiate the effects of other anti-hyperglycemic medications.

   Ⓝ *NCLEX® Connection: Pharmacological Therapies, Expected Actions/Outcomes*

2. A, 4; B, 3; C, 2; D, 1

   When taking actions to reinforce education with the client about bariatric medications and devices, the nurse describes the gas-filled or saline-filled intragastric balloon as a device that is placed during endoscopic surgery to increase satiety and decrease gastric emptying. The nurse describes the hydrogel pill as a device that expands in the stomach to reduce stomach capacity and intake of food. The nurse describes orlistat as a medication that inhibits digestion of fats by blocking gastric and pancreatic lipases. The nurse describes naltrexone-bupropion as a medication that suppresses appetite and decreases cravings.

   Ⓝ *NCLEX® Connection: Pharmacological Therapies, Expected Actions/Outcomes*

3. **RESTRICTIVE:** A, C, D; **MALABSORPTIVE:** B, E

   When generating solutions, the nurse recognizes that gastric banding, sleeve gastrectomy, and vertical banded gastroplasty create decreased stomach capacity while allowing normal digestion of nutrients. The nurse recognizes that although Roux-en-Y and biliopancreatic diversion with duodenal switch are surgeries that also create decreased capacity, they are considered malabsorptive because they bypass part of the small intestine to reduce absorption of nutrients.

   Ⓝ *NCLEX® Connection: Reduction of Risk Potential, Potential for Complications From Surgical Procedures and Health Alterations*

4. D, E, F. **CORRECT:** When participating in the evaluation of outcomes, the nurse recognizes that the client expresses understanding of postoperative instructions by stating they should limit carbohydrates, drink at least 1.5 liters of water per day, and wait for 30 minutes after a meal to drink liquids. Following a gastric bypass surgery, high intake of refined carbohydrates increases the risk for dumping syndrome. Ensuring adequate water intake decreases the risks of dehydration that can be caused by vomiting or diarrhea. Delaying intake of liquids for at least 30 minutes following a meal of solid foods decreases the risk for dumping syndrome.

   Ⓝ *NCLEX® Connection: Reduction of Risk Potential, Potential for Complications From Surgical Procedures and Health Alterations*

When reviewing the following chapters, keep in mind the relevant topics and tasks of the NCLEX outline.

Basic Care and Comfort

NUTRITION AND ORAL HYDRATION: Reinforce client teaching on special diets based on client diagnosis/nutritional needs and cultural considerations.

Pharmacological Therapies

PHARMACOLOGICAL PAIN MANAGEMENT: Monitor and document client response to pharmacological interventions.

ADVERSE EFFECTS/CONTRAINDICATIONS/SIDE EFFECTS/ INTERACTIONS: Identify potential and actual incompatibilities of client medications.

Physiological Adaptation

ALTERATIONS IN BODY SYSTEMS
Provide care to client undergoing peritoneal dialysis.

Provide care to correct client alteration in body system.

FLUID AND ELECTROLYTE IMBALANCES
Provide care for a client with a fluid and electrolyte imbalance.

Monitor client response to interventions to correct fluid and/or electrolyte imbalance.

UNEXPECTED RESPONSE TO THERAPIES: Promote recovery of the client from unexpected negative response to therapy.

CHAPTER 52 # Renal Diagnostic Procedures

Renal diagnostic procedures and laboratory tests are used to evaluate kidney function. By testing kidney function, providers can diagnose disease and evaluate the efficacy of treatment. The nurse should ensure that the client has signed an informed consent for most of the diagnostic procedures and tests.

LABORATORY TESTS

Blood creatinine

Results from protein and muscle breakdown
- Kidney disease is the only condition that increases blood creatinine levels.
- Kidney function loss of at least 50% causes an elevation of blood creatinine values.
- Although muscle mass and amount of creatinine decreases with age, the blood creatinine values remain constant in older adults who do not have kidney disease.

Blood urea nitrogen (BUN)

Results from the breakdown of protein in the liver, creating the byproduct urea nitrogen excreted by the kidneys
- Factors affecting BUN are dehydration, infection, chemotherapy, steroid therapy, and reabsorption of blood in the liver from damaged tissue.
- Elevated BUN suggests kidney disease.
- Because liver failure limits urea production, BUN is decreased when liver and kidney failure occur.

Urinalysis

Evaluates waste products from the kidney and detects urologic disorders
- Collection of an early-morning specimen provides a more concentrated sample.
- Urinalysis identifies color; clarity; concentration or dilution; specific gravity; acidity or alkalinity; and presence of drug metabolites, glucose, ketone bodies, and protein. Glucose, ketone bodies, and protein, including leukocyte esterase and nitrites, are not usually present in urine and can indicate diabetes mellitus; fat metabolism; infection; or, after a cytology analysis, cancer.
- Urine for culture and sensitivity identifies bacteria and determines the type of antibiotic to treat the infection.

- A 24-hr urine collection measures creatinine, urea nitrogen, sodium, chloride, calcium, catecholamines, and proteins.
- A 24-hr collection for creatinine clearance measures the glomerular filtration rate for clients who have impaired kidney function.

GUIDELINES FOR COLLECTING A 24-HR URINE SPECIMEN
- Reinforce client teaching regarding the testing procedure.
  - Void prior to defecating.
  - Avoid placing toilet paper into urine collection container.
- To begin the test, have the client void. The test begins at the time of first void. This first void is discarded. However, all subsequent urine is collected for the next 24 hr.
- Post notices on the client's medical record and over the toilet alerting all personnel of the ongoing test.
- Collect all urine voided over the next 24 hr in an approved container that is kept on ice or refrigerated.
- Collect the last urine sample as close to the end of the 24 hr as possible.
- The test must be restarted if any urine collection sample is missed.

RENAL DIAGNOSTIC PROCEDURES

Radiography (x-ray)

- An x-ray of the kidneys, ureters, and bladder (KUB or a "flat plate") without the use of contrast dye
- Allows for visualization of structures and detects renal calculi, strictures, calcium deposits, or obstructions
- KUB can detect the presence of gas within the GI tract and ascites.

NURSING ACTIONS
- Ask clients if they are pregnant.
- Tell clients to remove clothes over the area and all jewelry and metal objects.

COMPLICATIONS: No known complications

CT scan

- Provides three-dimensional imaging of the renal/urinary system to monitor for kidney size and obstruction, cysts, or masses
- IV contrast media (iodine-based) enhances images.

NURSING ACTIONS
- Ask clients if they are pregnant.
- Check for iodine allergy (the use of contrast media can vary depending on the severity of the client's allergy).
- Tell clients to remove clothes over the area and all jewelry and metal objects.
- Check for metformin use (this medication may need to be withheld prior to procedure because of its adverse effects on the kidneys).
- Monitor for signs of a delayed allergic reaction to dye/contrast media (dyspnea, tachycardia, rash, hives).
- Encourage client to increase fluid intake following procedure.

COMPLICATIONS

- Contrast media can cause acute kidney injury.
- Risk of complications is greater for the following clients.
  - Older adult clients Ⓖ
  - Clients who are dehydrated
  - Clients who have a history of previous renal insufficiency
  - Clients who are taking nephrotoxic drugs

MRI

Useful for staging cancer, similar to CT

NURSING ACTIONS

- Clients lie down and have to remain still for the test.
- Clients who have metal implants are not eligible for an MRI because the magnet can move the metal implant.

COMPLICATIONS: Poor imaging if a client is unable to lie still

Ultrasound

- Evaluates the size of kidneys, and images the ureters, bladder, masses, cysts, calculi, and obstructions of the lower urinary tract
- Good alternative to excretory urography

NURSING ACTIONS: Provide skin care by removing gel after the procedure.

COMPLICATIONS: Minimal risk for the client

Cystography, cystourethrography, voiding cystourethrogram (VCUG)

- VCUG detects urethral or bladder injury after instillation of contrast media through a urinary catheter to provide an image of the bladder (cystography) and the ureters (cystourethrography).
- VCUG detects via an x-ray during urination whether urine refluxes into the ureters.
- Contrast media does not reach the bloodstream or the kidneys and is not nephrotoxic.

NURSING ACTIONS

- Determine for the presence of allergy to contrast media or iodine.
- Monitor for infection for the first 72 hr after the procedure.
- Encourage increased fluid intake to dilute urine and minimize burning on urination.
- Monitor urine output (report less than 30 mL/hr) if suspected pelvic or urethral trauma.
- Reinforce with the client to report bright red bleeding, abdominal or flank pain, chills or fever after the procedure.

COMPLICATIONS: Urinary tract infection (UTI) due to catheter placement

- Cloudy, foul-smelling urine
- Urgency
- Urine positive for leukocyte esterase and nitrites, sediment, and RBCs

Kidney biopsy

Removal of a sample of tissue by excision or needle aspiration for cytological (histological) examination

NURSING ACTIONS: Clients receive sedation and ongoing monitoring.

PREPROCEDURE

- Review coagulation studies.
- Ensure client has been NPO at least 4 hr.
- Position the client prone with a pillow placed under the abdomen.

POSTPROCEDURE

- Monitor vital signs following sedation.
- Check dressings and urinary output (hematuria)
- Review Hgb and Hct values.
- Administer analgesia as needed.
- Ensure that a pressure dressing is on the puncture site.
- Monitor the dressing frequently for signs of infection and hemorrhage.
- Monitor urine for output and gross hematuria. The urine will contain some blood initially but will clear up after 24 hr.
- Reinforce with the client to remain on prescribed bed rest (could be up to 24 hr following procedure).

COMPLICATIONS

- Hemorrhage: Monitor for hypotension, tachycardia, dizziness, or back/flank pain.
- Infection
  - Cloudy, foul-smelling urine
  - Urgency
  - Urine positive for leukocyte esterase and nitrites, sediment, and RBCs
- Urinary retention
- Liver/bowel puncture during kidney biopsy: Monitor abdomen for pain, tenderness, rigidity, and decreased bowel sounds.

Cystoscopy, cystourethroscopy

Used to discover abnormalities of bladder wall (cystoscopy) and/or occlusions of ureter or urethra (cystourethroscopy)

NURSING ACTIONS

- Clients receive anesthesia for the procedure.
- Check for findings of bleeding and infection.

PREPROCEDURE

- NPO after midnight
- Administer laxative or enemas for bowel preparation the night before the procedure.

POSTPROCEDURE

- Monitor vital signs and urine output.
- Document the color of urine (can be pink-tinged).
- Irrigate urinary catheter with 0.9% sodium chloride irrigation if blood clots are present or the urine output is decreased or absent.
- Encourage oral fluids to increase urine output and reduce any burning sensation with urination.
- Reinforce with the client to monitor for urinary retention, hematuria, increased abdominal pain, fever, chills, and dysuria for at least 72 hr following procedure.

COMPLICATIONS

- Bladder or ureter perforation during the procedure
- Sepsis
- Hematuria
- Urinary retention
- UTI
  - Cloudy, foul-smelling urine
  - Urinary urgency
  - Urine positive for leukocytes, nitrates, sediment, and RBCs

Retrograde pyelogram, cystogram, urethrogram

- Identifies obstruction or structural disorders of the ureters and renal pelvis of the kidneys (pyelogram) by instilling contrast media during a cystoscopy
- Identifies fistulas, diverticula, and tumors in the bladder (cystogram) and urethra (urethrogram) by instilling contrast media during a cystoscopy

NURSING ACTIONS: Same as a cystoscopy

COMPLICATIONS: Same as a cystoscopy, in addition to ureter obstruction related to ureteral edema (pyelogram)

Renal scan

Monitors renal blood flow and estimates glomerular filtration rate (GFR) after IV injection of radioactive material to produce a scanned image of the kidneys

NURSING ACTIONS

PREPROCEDURE

- Encourage the client to void prior to the scan.
- Encourage the client to drink fluid as directed prior to scan.
- Reinforce with the client to remain still during the scan.

POSTPROCEDURE

- Monitor blood pressure frequently during and after the procedure if the client receives captopril during the procedure to change the blood flow to the kidneys.
- Alert clients about possible orthostatic hypotension following the procedure if they received captopril.
- Increase fluid intake if hypotension occurs and to promote excretion of the radioisotope.

COMPLICATIONS

- Radioactive material does not cause nephrotoxicity.
- Clients are not at risk from radioactive material they excrete in the urine.

Excretory urography

Detects obstruction and parenchymal masses and observes the size of the kidneys. IV contrast media (iodine-based) enhances the images.

NURSING ACTIONS: Same as KUB

PREPROCEDURE

- Encourage increased fluids the day before procedure.
- Bowel cleansing with a laxative or an enema to remove fecal contents, fluid, and gas from the colon for a clearer visualization
- NPO after midnight
- Determine allergies to iodine, seafood, eggs, milk, or chocolate, or if the client has asthma.
- Check creatinine and BUN levels.
- Withhold metformin for 24 hr before the procedure (risk for lactic acidosis from contrast media with iodine).

POSTPROCEDURE

- Assist with monitoring the administration of parenteral fluid, or encourage oral fluids to flush media through the renal system and prevent complications.
- Diuretics can increase media excretion.
- Monitor creatinine and BUN blood levels before resuming metformin.
- Monitor urine for output and characteristics. Pink tinge is expected. Report hematuria or clots.

COMPLICATIONS

- Media can cause acute kidney injury.
- Allergy to iodine dye
- Hypoglycemia/acidosis (metformin)
- Hemorrhage

GERONTOLOGICAL CONSIDERATIONS ©

- Kidney size and function decrease with aging.
- Blood flow adaptability decreases, especially during a hypotensive or hypertensive crisis.
- GFR decreases by half the rate of a young adult.
- Diabetes mellitus, hypertension, and heart failure can affect GFR.
- Kidney injury can occur more easily from contrast media and medication due to decreased kidney size, blood flow, and GFR.
- Tubular changes can cause urgency and nocturnal polyuria.
- A weak urinary sphincter muscle and a shorter urethra in females can cause incontinence and urinary tract infections.
- An enlarged prostate can cause urinary retention and infection.

Active Learning Scenario

A nurse is assisting with developing a plan of care for a client who will undergo a cystoscopy with retrograde pyelogram. What information should the nurse recommend in the plan of care? Use the ATI Active Learning Template: Diagnostic Procedure to complete this item.

DESCRIPTION OF PROCEDURE: Define the procedure.

INDICATIONS: Identify one indication for cystoscopy and two for retrograde pyelogram.

NURSING INTERVENTIONS (PRE, INTRA, POST): Describe two nursing actions for preprocedure and two for postprocedure.

Application Exercises

1. A nurse is preparing to begin a 24-hr urine collection for a client. Which of the following actions should the nurse take?
   - A. Store collected urine in a designated container at room temperature.
   - B. Discard the first voiding when beginning the test.
   - C. Post a notice on the client's door regarding the testing.
   - D. Document any urine collection that was missed during the 24 hr of the testing.

2. A nurse is reinforcing teaching with a client who is scheduled to have an x-ray of the kidneys, ureters, and bladder (KUB). Which of the following statements should the nurse include?
   - A. "You will receive contrast dye during the procedure."
   - B. "An enema is necessary before the procedure."
   - C. "You will need to lie in a prone position during the procedure."
   - D. "The procedure determines whether you have a kidney stone."

3. A nurse is collecting data from a client who has returned to the medical-surgical unit following a CT scan of the kidneys with IV contrast. Which of the following findings should the nurse identify as an indication the client is experiencing an allergic reaction to the contrast material?
   - A. Bradycardia
   - B. Pink-tinged sputum
   - C. Hyperpyrexia
   - D. Skin hives

4. A nurse is monitoring a client who had a kidney biopsy for postoperative complications. Which of the following complications should the nurse identify as causing the greatest risk to the client?
   - A. Infection
   - B. Hemorrhage
   - C. Hematuria
   - D. Pain

5. A nurse is caring for a client who has type 2 diabetes mellitus and is scheduled for an excretory urography. Prior to the procedure, which of the following actions should the nurse take? (Select all that apply.)
   - A. Identify an allergy to seafood.
   - B. Withhold metformin for 24 hr.
   - C. Administer an enema.
   - D. Obtain a blood coagulation profile.
   - E. Monitor for asthma.

Application Exercises Key

1. B. **CORRECT:** When taking actions for a client who has a 24-hour urine test, the nurse should begin the testing period after discarding the first voiding. This would ensure accuracy of test results.

   Ⓝ *NCLEX® Connection: Reduction of Risk Potential, Diagnostic Tests*

2. A. Contrast dye and bowel prep are not needed for KUB.
   B. Contrast dye and bowel prep are not needed for KUB.
   C. The client can be positioned supine during the procedure.
   D. **CORRECT:** When taking actions, the nurse should inform the client that a KUB can identify renal calculi, strictures, calcium deposits, and obstructions of the urinary system.

   Ⓝ *NCLEX® Connection: Reduction of Risk Potential, Diagnostic Tests*

3. D. **CORRECT:** When analyzing cues, the nurse should identify skin hives is an allergic reaction to contrast media used during a CT of the renal pelvis. Other manifestations that can indicate an allergic reaction to contrast media can include tachycardia, dyspnea, and rash.

   Ⓝ *NCLEX® Connection: Reduction of Risk Potential, Potential for Complications of Diagnostic Tests/Treatments/Procedures*

4. B. **CORRECT:** The nurse should analyze the findings and determine that the priority hypothesis for the client following a kidney biopsy is hemorrhage. The client is at greatest risk for hemorrhage following a kidney biopsy due to a lack of clotting at the puncture site. The nurse should report this finding to the provider immediately.

   Ⓝ *NCLEX® Connection: Reduction of Risk Potential, Potential for Complications of Diagnostic Tests/Treatments/Procedures*

5. A, B, C, E. **CORRECT:** When taking actions, the nurse should identify that clients who have an allergy to seafood are at higher risk for an allergic reaction to the contrast media they will receive during the procedure. Clients who also take metformin are at risk for lactic acidosis from the contrast media with iodine they receive during the procedure. Clients should receive an enema to remove fecal contents, fluid, and gas from the colon for a clear visualization. The nurse should also identify that clients who have asthma have a higher risk of an exacerbation as an allergic response to the contrast media they receive during the procedure.

   Ⓝ *NCLEX® Connection: Reduction of Risk Potential, Potential for Complications of Diagnostic Tests/Treatments/Procedures*

Active Learning Scenario Key

Using the ATI Active Learning Template: Diagnostic Procedure

DESCRIPTION OF PROCEDURE
- Cystoscopy is instrumentation into the urinary tract to inspect the bladder wall.
- Retrograde pyelogram is the injection of media into the ureters to inspect the ureters and pelvis of the kidney.

INDICATIONS
- Cystoscopy discovers abnormalities of the bladder wall (cysts, tumors, stones).
- Retrograde pyelogram discovers obstructions or structural disorders of the ureters and kidney pelvis (strictures, stones, mass).

NURSING INTERVENTIONS (PRE, INTRA, POST)

Preprocedure
- Clients must be NPO after midnight.
- Administer a laxative the night before the procedure.

Postprocedure
- Monitor vital signs.
- Encourage an increase in oral fluid intake to reduce the burning sensation when voiding.
- Document the color of urine.
- For clients who have a urinary catheter, irrigate it with 0.9% sodium chloride irrigation for active bleeding, clots, or decreased or absent urine output.
- Reinforce teaching with the client to monitor for urinary retention, hematuria, increased abdominal pain, fever, chills, and dysuria for at least 72 hr following procedure.

Ⓝ *NCLEX® Connection: Reduction of Risk Potential, Potential for Complications of Diagnostic Tests/Treatments/Procedures*

UNIT 8   RENAL DISORDERS
SECTION: DIAGNOSTIC AND THERAPEUTIC PROCEDURES

CHAPTER 53 *Hemodialysis and Peritoneal Dialysis*

For clients who are experiencing acute kidney injury or chronic kidney disease, dialysis can sustain life (although it does not replace the hormonal function of the kidney). The two types of dialysis are hemodialysis and peritoneal dialysis.

FUNCTIONS OF DIALYSIS

- Rids the body of excess fluid and electrolytes
- Achieves acid–base balance
- Eliminates waste products
- Restores internal homeostasis by osmosis, diffusion, and ultrafiltration

Hemodialysis

Hemodialysis shunts blood from the body through a dialyzer and back into circulation. Hemodialysis requires vascular access. Hemodialysis is started when manifestations of uremia become severe.

INDICATIONS

POTENTIAL DIAGNOSES
- Renal insufficiency
- Acute kidney injury
- Chronic kidney disease
- Medication or illicit drug toxicity
- Persistent hyperkalemia
- Pulmonary edema
- Severe hypertension
- Hypervolemia that does not respond to diuretics

CLIENT PRESENTATION
- Fluid volume changes, electrolyte and pH imbalances, and nitrogenous wastes
- Manifestations include fluid overload, neurologic changes, bleeding, and uremia (cognitive impairment, pruritus, nausea, vomiting).

CONSIDERATIONS

PREPROCEDURE

NURSING ACTIONS
- Check for informed consent.
- Use a temporary hemodialysis dual–lumen catheter or subcutaneous device until the provider inserts a long-term device and it is available for access.
- Monitor the patency of a long-term device: arteriovenous (AV) fistula or AV graft (presence of bruit, palpable thrill, distal pulses, circulation).
- Avoid measuring blood pressure, administering injections, performing venipunctures, or inserting IV catheters on or into an arm with an access site. Elevate the extremity following surgical creation of an AV fistula to reduce swelling.
- Obtain vital signs, laboratory values (BUN, blood creatinine, electrolytes, Hct), and weight.
- Discuss with the provider medications to withhold until after dialysis. Withhold any dialyzable medications and medications that lower blood pressure.

CLIENT EDUCATION: Hemodialysis will be needed three times per week, for 3- to 5-hr sessions. It involves insertion of two needles, one into an artery and the other into a vein.

POSTPROCEDURE

NURSING ACTIONS
- Monitor vital signs and laboratory values (BUN, blood creatinine, electrolytes, Hct). Decreases in blood pressure and changes in laboratory values are common following dialysis.
- Compare the client's preprocedure weight with the postprocedure weight as a way to estimate the amount of fluid the procedure removed. 1 L fluid equals 1 kg (2.2 lb).
- Monitor for the following.
  - Complications (hypotension, clotting of vascular access, headache, muscle cramps, bleeding)
  - Indications of bleeding or infection at the access site
  - Findings of disequilibrium syndrome (nausea, vomiting, headache)
  - Findings of hypovolemia (hypotension, dizziness, tachycardia)
- Avoid invasive procedures for 4 to 6 hr after dialysis due to the risk of bleeding as a result of anticoagulation.
- Monitor access site for bleeding, patency, and infection.
- Reinforce AV fistula or AV graft precautions. Qs

CLIENT EDUCATION

- Alert the nurse of early findings of disequilibrium syndrome, such as nausea and headache.
- Check the access site at intervals following dialysis. Apply light pressure if bleeding.
- Contact the provider if bleeding from the insertion site lasts longer than 30 min following dialysis, for no thrill/ bruit, or for findings of infection.
- Avoid carrying objects that compress or constrict the extremity.
- Avoid sleeping on top of the extremity with the vascular access.

COMPLICATIONS

Clotting/infection of the access site

Anticoagulants prevent blood clots from forming. Monitor for hemorrhage at the insertion site.

- Cannulation can introduce infections at the access site.
- Immunosuppressive disorders increase the risk for infection.
- Advanced age is a risk factor for dialysis–induced hypotension and access site complications due to chronic illnesses or fragile veins. Ⓖ

NURSING ACTIONS

- Avoid compression of the access site.
- Avoid venipuncture or blood pressure measurements on the extremity with the vascular access site.
- Monitor the graft site for a palpable thrill or audible bruit indicating vascular flow.
- Monitor the access site for redness, swelling, or drainage.
- Monitor for fever.

Disequilibrium syndrome

Disequilibrium syndrome results from too rapid a decrease of BUN and circulating fluid volume. It can result in cerebral edema and increased intracranial pressure.

- Early recognition of disequilibrium syndrome is essential. Manifestations include nausea, vomiting, changes in level of consciousness, seizures, and agitation.
- Advanced age is a risk factor for dialysis disequilibrium and hypotension due to rapid changes in fluid and electrolyte status. Ⓖ

NURSING ACTIONS: RN can use a slow dialysis exchange rate, especially for older adult clients and first-time hemodialysis.

Hypotension

Antihypertensive therapy and rapid fluid depletion during dialysis can cause hypotension.

NURSING ACTIONS

- The RN should carefully replace fluid volume by infusing IV fluids or colloid. Slow the dialysis exchange rate.
- Lower the head of the client's bed.

Anemia

Blood loss and removal of folate during dialysis can contribute to the anemia that often accompanies chronic kidney disease (from decreased RBC production due to decreased erythropoietin secretion).

NURSING ACTIONS

- Administer erythropoietin to stimulate the production of RBC.
- Monitor Hgb and RBC level.
- Monitor for hypotension and tachycardia.
- Assist with transfusion of blood products.

Infectious diseases

Blood transfusions and frequent blood access due to hemodialysis pose a risk for transmission of bloodborne infections such as HIV and hepatitis B and C.

NURSING ACTIONS

- Use sterile equipment and skin antisepsis.
- Use standard precautions.

Peritoneal dialysis

- Peritoneal dialysis involves instillation of dialysate solution into the peritoneal cavity, followed by a prescribed dwell time. The peritoneum serves as a semipermeable filtration membrane. Waste products, such as urea and creatinine, and excess fluids and electrolytes are filtered through the peritoneum from an area of high concentration (blood) to an area of low concentration (dialysate). After the prescribed dwell time, the dialysate outflow, or effluent, containing excess fluids, electrolytes, and waste products flows out of the peritoneum into a drainage bag.
- The client should have an intact peritoneal membrane, without adhesions from infection or multiple surgeries.

INDICATIONS

- Peritoneal dialysis is the treatment of choice for the older adults who require dialysis.
- Peritoneal dialysis treats clients requiring dialysis who:
  ○ Are unable to tolerate anticoagulation.
  ○ Have difficulty with vascular access
  ○ Have chronic infections or are unstable
  ○ Have chronic diseases (diabetes mellitus, heart failure, severe hypertension)

CONSIDERATIONS

PREPROCEDURE

NURSING ACTIONS
- Determine dry weight (without dialysate instillation), vital signs, blood electrolytes, blood creatinine, BUN, and blood glucose.
- Determine the client's ability to self-perform peritoneal dialysis and follow sterile technique.
  - Level of alertness
  - Past experience with dialysis
  - Understanding of procedure
- Use standard precautions.
- Use aseptic technique with handling of equipment and during procedure.
- Measure and record abdominal girth.
- Ensure dialysate solution is at room temperature.

CLIENT EDUCATION
- Follow instructions regarding the procedure. Fullness can be felt when the dialysate is dwelling. There can be discomfort initially with dialysate infusion.
- Continuous ambulatory peritoneal dialysis (CAPD) requires 7 days/week for 4 to 8 hr. Clients can continue normal activities during CAPD.
- Continuous-cycle peritoneal dialysis (CCPD) is a 24-hr dialysis. The exchange occurs at night while sleeping. The final exchange is left in to dwell during the day.
- Automated peritoneal dialysis (APD) is regulated by automated machinery in ambulatory settings or the client's home at night.

INTRAPROCEDURE

NURSING ACTIONS
- Monitor vital signs frequently during initial dialysis of clients in a hospital setting.
- Monitor blood glucose level (dialysate contains glucose).
- Record the amount of inflow compared with outflow of dialysate.
- Monitor the color (should be clear, light yellow) and amount (should equal or exceed the amount of dialysate inflow) of outflow.
- Monitor for findings of infection (fever; bloody, cloudy, or frothy dialysate return; drainage at access site) and for complications (respiratory distress, abdominal pain, insufficient outflow, discolored outflow).
- Check the access site dressing for wetness (risk of dialysate leakage) and exit-site infections.
- Adhere to the times for infusion, dwell, and outflow.
- Maintain surgical asepsis of the catheter insertion site and when accessing the catheter.
- Keep the outflow bag lower than the client's abdomen (drain by gravity, prevent reflux).
- Reposition the client if inflow or outflow is inadequate.
- Provide emotional support to the client and family.

POSTPROCEDURE

NURSING ACTIONS: Monitor weight and blood levels of electrolytes, creatinine, glucose, and urea nitrogen (BUN).

CLIENT EDUCATION
- Perform home care of the access site.
- Perform peritoneal dialysis exchanges at home. Support can be provided with home peritoneal dialysis with home visits. Qpcc
- Seek additional information from the National Kidney Foundation for local support groups.

COMPLICATIONS

Peritonitis

Peritoneal dialysis can allow micro-organisms into the peritoneum and cause peritonitis. Cloudy or opaque effluent is the earliest indication of peritonitis.

NURSING ACTIONS
- Maintain surgical asepsis during the procedure.
- Monitor for infection (fever, purulent drainage, redness, swelling, cloudy or discolored drained dialysate).

CLIENT EDUCATION
- Use strict sterile technique during exchanges.
- Notify the provider about any indications of infection.

Infection at the access site

- Infection at the access site can result from leakage of dialysate. Access-site infections can cause peritonitis.
- Advanced age is a risk factor for access-site complications due to chronic illnesses and/or fragile veins. Ⓖ

NURSING ACTIONS
- Maintain surgical asepsis at the access site.
- Monitor for infection (fever, purulent drainage, redness, swelling).

CLIENT EDUCATION
- Use strict sterile technique during exchanges.
- Notify the provider of any indications of infection. Qs
- Monitor the site for leaks, and prevent tugging or twisting of the tubing.

Hyperglycemia and hyperlipidemia

- Hyperglycemia can result from glucose in the dialysate.
- The blood can absorb glucose from the dialysate.
- Hyperlipidemia can also occur from long-term therapy and lead to hypertension.

NURSING ACTIONS: Monitor blood glucose.

Poor dialysate inflow or outflow

Causes include:
- Obstruction or twisting of the tubing
- Constipation
- Client positioning
- Fibrin clot formation
- Catheter displacement

NURSING ACTIONS
- Reposition the client if inflow or outflow is inadequate.
- Check the tubing for kinks or closed clamps.

CLIENT EDUCATION
- Check the tubing for kinks, and follow instructions for how to remove a fibrin clot.
- Monitor the inflow and outflow, and change position or lower or raise the dialysate bag to improve flow.
- Prevent constipation with diet and stool softeners.
- Lie supine with head slightly elevated during CCPD and APD treatment.

Active Learning Scenario

A nurse is reviewing complications that a client can develop when receiving peritoneal dialysis. What complications and nursing actions should the nurse include in the review? Use the ATI Active Learning Template: Diagnostic Procedure to complete this item.

DESCRIPTION OF PROCEDURE: Write out the name, and define the diagnostic test.

POTENTIAL COMPLICATIONS: List three.

NURSING INTERVENTIONS: List two nursing actions for each of the three complications.

Application Exercises

1. A nurse is reinforcing teaching about the function of hemodialysis with a client who has chronic kidney disease. What information should the nurse include?

2. A nurse is assisting with the plan of care of a client who is scheduled for hemodialysis. What actions should the nurse plan to take?

3. A nurse is reinforcing teaching with a client who is scheduled for hemodialysis via an arteriovenous fistula. Which of the following instructions should the nurse include?
   A. Avoid invasive procedures 4 hr after dialysis.
   B. Wear a compression sleeve over the extremity with the vascular access.
   C. Sleep on the side of the extremity with the vascular access.
   D. Expect to experience nausea after dialysis.

4. A nurse assisting with the care of a client who is scheduled for peritoneal dialysis (PD). Which of the following actions should the nurse take?
   A. Monitor the client's blood glucose levels.
   B. Report cloudy dialysate outflow.
   C. Warm the dialysate in a microwave oven.
   D. Watch the client for bleeding.
   E. Check the access site dressing for wetness.
   F. Maintain medical asepsis when accessing the catheter insertion site.

5. A nurse is assisting with teaching a class about dialysis to a group of nurses. Sort the following characteristics into those associated with either hemodialysis or peritoneal dialysis.
   A. Disequilibrium syndrome is a complication.
   B. Peritonitis is a complication.
   C. Accessed through an arteriovenous fistula
   D. Accessed through an intra-abdominal catheter

Application Exercises Key

1. When taking actions, the nurse should instruct the client that hemodialysis is performed to rid the body of excess fluid and electrolytes, achieve acid-base balance, eliminate waste products, and restore internal homeostasis by osmosis, diffusion, and ultrafiltration.

Ⓝ *NCLEX® Connection: Reduction of Risk Potential, Potential for Complications From Surgical Procedures and Health Alterations*

2. When generating solutions, the nurse should plan to check for informed consent. Check the patency of an arteriovenous (AV) fistula or AV graft, such as presence of bruit, palpable thrill, distal pulses, and circulation. Avoid measuring blood pressure, administering injections, performing venipunctures, or inserting IV catheters on or into an arm with a vascular access site. Check vital signs, laboratory values, and weight prior to dialysis. Discuss with the provider medications to withhold until after dialysis. Withhold any dialyzable medications and medications that lower blood pressure.

Ⓝ *NCLEX® Connection: Physiological Adaptation, Alterations in Body Systems*

3. A. **CORRECT:** When taking actions, the nurse should instruct the client to avoid invasive procedures for 4 to 6 hr following dialysis to reduce the risk of bleeding. The client is at risk for bleeding because anticoagulants are administered during dialysis.

Ⓝ *NCLEX® Connection: Physiological Adaptation, Alterations in Body Systems*

4. A, B, D, E. **CORRECT:** When taking actions, the nurse should monitor the client's blood glucose because the client is at risk for hyperglycemia due to glucose in the dialysate. The nurse should monitor the client for manifestations of an infection, such as cloudy effluent, fever, and abdominal pain and monitor the client for bleeding. The client who has a new PD catheter might have blood in effluent for the first week due to trauma during the catheter insertion. Check the access site dressing for wetness and look for kinking, pulling, clamping, or twisting of the tubing, which can increase the risk for exit-site infections.

Ⓝ *NCLEX® Connection: Physiological Adaptation, Alterations in Body Systems*

5. **HEMODIALYSIS:** A, C; **PERITONEAL DIALYSIS:** B, D

When taking actions, the nurse should instruct that disequilibrium syndrome is a complication of hemodialysis. An arteriovenous fistula is accessed in hemodialysis. Peritonitis is a complication of peritoneal dialysis. An intra-abdominal catheter is accessed in peritoneal dialysis.

Ⓝ *NCLEX® Connection: Physiological Adaptation, Alterations in Body Systems*

Active Learning Scenario Key

Using the ATI Active Learning Template: Diagnostic Procedure

DESCRIPTION OF PROCEDURE: Peritoneal dialysis: To instill a hypertonic dialysate solution into the peritoneal cavity, allow the solution to dwell for prescribed amount of time, and drain the solution that includes the waste products.

POTENTIAL COMPLICATIONS
- Peritonitis
- Hyperglycemia
- Poor dialysate inflow or outflow

NURSING INTERVENTIONS

Peritonitis
- Maintain surgical asepsis.
- Monitor color of outflow solution and for pain or fever.

Hyperglycemia: Monitor blood glucose level.

Poor dialysate inflow or outflow
- Reposition the client.
- Check the tubing for kinks or closed clamps.
- Encourage stool softeners and high-fiber diet to prevent constipation.

Ⓝ *NCLEX® Connection: Physiological Adaptation, Alterations in Body Systems*

NCLEX® Connections

When reviewing the following chapters, keep in mind the relevant topics and tasks of the NCLEX outline.

Health Promotion and Maintenance

HEALTH PROMOTION/DISEASE PREVENTION: Assist client in disease prevention activities.

Basic Care and Comfort

NUTRITION AND ORAL HYDRATION: Reinforce client teaching on special diets based on client diagnosis/nutritional needs and cultural considerations.

Pharmacological Therapies

PHARMACOLOGICAL PAIN MANAGEMENT: Monitor and document client response to pharmacological interventions.

ADVERSE EFFECTS/CONTRAINDICATIONS/SIDE EFFECTS/ INTERACTIONS: Identify potential and actual incompatibilities of client medications.

Physiological Adaptation

ALTERATIONS IN BODY SYSTEMS: Reinforce education to client regarding care and condition.

BASIC PATHOPHYSIOLOGY: Identify signs and symptoms related to an acute or chronic illness.

FLUID AND ELECTROLYTE IMBALANCES
Provide care for a client with a fluid and electrolyte imbalance.

Monitor client response to interventions to correct fluid and/or electrolyte imbalance.

UNEXPECTED RESPONSE TO THERAPIES: Promote recovery of the client from unexpected negative response to therapy.

CHAPTER 54
Polycystic Kidney Disease, Acute Kidney Injury, and Chronic Kidney Disease

The kidneys regulate fluid, acid-base, and electrolyte balance and eliminate wastes from the body. Several disorders affect the renal system and its ability to function (acute kidney injury, chronic kidney disease, polycystic kidney disease).

Kidney failure is diagnosed as acute kidney injury or chronic kidney disease. Without aggressive treatment, or when complicating preexisting conditions exist, acute kidney injury can result in chronic kidney disease.

Acute kidney injury

Acute kidney injury (AKI) is the sudden cessation of kidney function that occurs when blood flow to the kidneys is significantly compromised. Manifestations occur abruptly.

PHASES

- **Onset:** Begins with the onset of the event, ends when oliguria develops, and lasts for hours to days
- **Oliguria:** Begins with the kidney insult; urine output is 100 to 400 mL/24 hr with or without diuretics; lasts for 1 to 3 weeks
- **Diuresis:** Begins when the kidneys start to recover; diuresis of a large amount of fluid occurs, 1,000 mL to 2,000 mL per day; can last for 2 to 6 weeks. Death can result from dehydration and imbalances in serum sodium or potassium levels.
- **Recovery:** Continues until kidney function is fully restored and can take up to 12 months

TYPES

- **Prerenal:** Occurs as a result of volume depletion and prolonged reduction of blood flow to the kidneys, which leads to ischemia of the nephrons. Occurs before damage to the kidney. Early intervention restoring fluid volume deficit can reverse AKI and prevent chronic kidney disease (CKD).
- **Intrarenal:** Occurs as a result of direct damage to the kidney from lack of oxygen, indicating damage to the glomeruli, nephrons, or tubules
- **Postrenal:** Occurs as a result of bilateral obstruction of structures leaving the kidney

HEALTH PROMOTION AND DISEASE PREVENTION

- Drink at least 2 L daily. Consult with the provider regarding prescribed fluid restriction if needed.
- Stop smoking.
- Maintain a healthy weight.
- Use NSAIDs and other prescribed medications cautiously.
- Control diabetes and hypertension to prevent complications.
- Take all antibiotics prescribed for infections.

DATA COLLECTION

RISK FACTORS

Prerenal acute kidney injury

- Kidney vascular obstruction
- Shock
- Decreased cardiac output causing decreased kidney profusion
- Sepsis
- Hypovolemia
- Peripheral vascular resistance
- Use of aspirin, ibuprofen, or NSAIDs
- Liver failure

Intrarenal acute kidney injury

- **Physical injury:** trauma
- **Hypoxic injury:** renal artery or vein stenosis or thrombosis
- **Chemical injury:** acute nephrotoxins (antibiotics, contrast dye, heavy metals, blood transfusion reaction, alcohol, cocaine)
- **Immunologic injury:** infection, vasculitis, acute glomerulonephritis

Postrenal acute kidney injury

- Stone, tumor, bladder atony
- Prostate hyperplasia, urethral stricture
- Spinal cord disease or injury

Urinary system

Prerenal
- Blood loss
- Infection
- Dehydration
- Burns
- Myocardial infarction

Intrarenal
- Glomerulonephritis
- Lupus
- Cholesterol deposits that obstruct the blood flow in the kidney
- Medications, such as chemotherapy, antibiotics, and contrast media

Post renal
- Bladder, cervical, colon, or prostate cancer
- Stones
- Enlarged prostate
- Blood clots in the urinary tract

EXPECTED FINDINGS

In most cases, the findings of AKI are related to waste buildup and decreased urine output. However, almost every body system can be affected.

- **CARDIOVASCULAR:** Hypertension, fluid overload (dependent and generalized edema), dysrhythmia (hyperkalemia)
- **RESPIRATORY:** Crackles, decreased oxygenation, shortness of breath
- **RENAL:** Scant to normal or excessive urine output, depending on the phase; possible hematuria
- **NEUROLOGIC:** Lethargy, muscle twitching, seizures
- **INTEGUMENTARY:** Dry skin and mucous membranes

The nurse should also monitor for findings associated with the underlying cause.

LABORATORY TESTS

- Blood creatinine gradually increases 1 to 2 mg/dL every 24 to 48 hr, or 1 to 6 mg/dL in 1 week or less.
- Blood urea nitrogen (BUN) can increase to 80 to 100 mg/dL within 1 week.
- Urine specific gravity varies in postrenal type; can be elevated up to 1.030 in prerenal type or diluted as low as 1.000 in intrarenal type.
- Electrolytes: Sodium can be decreased (prerenal azotemia) or increased (intrarenal azotemia); hyperkalemia, hyperphosphatemia, hypocalcemia.
- Hematocrit: decreased
- Urinalysis: presence of sediment (RBC, casts)
- ABG: metabolic acidosis

DIAGNOSTIC PROCEDURES

Kidney biopsy is performed when the cause of AKI is uncertain, and manifestations continue. This can also be performed to detect immunological disease or determine kidney dysfunction reversibility and need for dialysis therapy.

Imaging procedures
- X-ray of the pelvis, or kidneys, urethra, and bladder (KUB) to detect calculi and hydronephrosis and to determine size of kidneys
- Ultrasound to detect an obstruction in the urinary tract
- CT scan without contrast dye or MRI to detect anatomical changes, tumors, or other obstruction; patency of ureters; kidney perfusion
- Nuclear medicine tests (cystography, retrograde pyelography)

PATIENT-CENTERED CARE

NURSING CARE

- Identify and assist with correcting the underlying cause.
- Monitor central venous pressure (CVP) and for hypotension and tachycardia.
- Monitor fluid intake and output strictly.
- Review laboratory values (BUN, creatinine, electrolytes, hematocrit).
- Avoid using nephrotoxic medications. If necessary, give these medications sparingly and decrease the medication dosage.
- Monitor for edema and manifestations of heart failure or pulmonary edema.
- Restrict fluid intake as prescribed.
- Monitor for flank pain, nausea, and vomiting (nephrolithiasis).
- Monitor for ECG dysrhythmias and changes (tall T waves).
- Monitor daily weights.
- Monitor for changes in urination stream or difficulty starting the stream of urine.
- Monitor the urine for blood or particles.
- Treat fever or infection promptly to prevent increase in the client's metabolic rate.
- Provide skin care to prevent injury (bathe with cool water, reposition frequently, provide adequate moisture).
- Provide psychosocial support to the client and family. Reinforce teaching with the client and family about prescribed treatments.
- Reinforce teaching with the client to perform coughing and deep breathing exercises, if lethargic.

NUTRITION
- Implement potassium, phosphate, sodium, and magnesium restrictions, if prescribed (depending on the stage of injury).
- Restrict fluid intake, if prescribed.
- Protein requirements are individualized based on several factors, including client's nutritional status, catabolic response, and cause of injury. Possible total parenteral nutrition (TPN)

THERAPEUTIC PROCEDURES

Continuous kidney replacement therapy, hemodialysis, peritoneal dialysis

INTERPROFESSIONAL CARE

- Dietitian to calculate protein, calorie, and fluid needs
- Nephrology services to monitor kidney function

Chronic kidney disease

CKD is a progressive, irreversible kidney disease.

- A client who has CKD can be free of manifestations except during periods of stress (infection, surgery, and trauma). As kidney dysfunction progresses, manifestations become apparent.
- Older adult clients are at an increased risk for chronic kidney disease related to the aging process (decreased number of functioning nephrons, decreased GFR). ⓖ
- Older adult clients who are on bed rest, confused, have a lack of thirst, and do not have easy access to water are at a higher risk for dehydration leading to chronic kidney disease.

STAGES

CKD is comprised of five stages.
- **Stage 1:** No manifestations
- **Stage 2:** GFR decreases without manifestations.
- **Stage 3:** Moderate decline in GFR, can advance to end-stage kidney disease (ESKD) with complications such as infection or nephrotoxicity
- **Stage 4:** Chronic manifestations of uremia
- **Stage 5:** End stage: Kidney disease requiring dialysis or kidney transplant

HEALTH PROMOTION AND DISEASE PREVENTION

- Drink at least 2 L water daily. Consult with the provider regarding any restrictions.
- Stop smoking.
- Limit alcohol intake.
- Use diet and exercise to manage weight and prevent or control diabetes and hypertension.
- Adhere to medication prescription guidelines to prevent kidney damage.
- Test for albumin in the urine yearly (clients who have diabetes or hypertension).
- Take all antibiotics until completed.
- Limit over-the-counter NSAIDs. Qs

DATA COLLECTION

- End-stage kidney disease exists when 90% of the functioning nephrons are destroyed and are no longer able to maintain fluid, electrolyte, and acid-base homeostasis.
- Dialysis or kidney transplantation can maintain life, but neither is a cure for CKD.

RISK FACTORS

- Acute kidney injury
- Diabetes mellitus
- Chronic glomerulonephritis
- Nephrotoxic medications (gentamicin, NSAIDs) or chemicals
- Hypertension, especially in African American clients
- Autoimmune disorders (systemic lupus erythematosus)
- Polycystic kidney disease
- Pyelonephrosis
- Renal artery stenosis
- Recurrent, severe infections

EXPECTED FINDINGS

Nausea, fatigue, lethargy, involuntary movement of legs, depression, intractable hiccups

In most cases, findings of chronic kidney disease are related to fluid volume overload and include the following.
- **NEUROLOGIC:** lethargy, decreased attention span, slurred speech, tremors or jerky movements, ataxia, seizures, coma
- **CARDIOVASCULAR:** fluid overload (jugular distention; sacrum, ocular, or peripheral edema), hyperlipidemia, hypertension, dysrhythmias, heart failure, orthostatic hypotension, peaked T wave on ECG (hyperkalemia)
- **RESPIRATORY:** uremic halitosis with deep sighing, yawning, shortness of breath, tachypnea, hyperpnea, Kussmaul respirations, crackles, pleural friction rub, frothy pink sputum
- **HEMATOLOGIC:** anemia (pallor, weakness, dizziness), ecchymoses, petechiae, melena
- **GASTROINTESTINAL:** ulcers in mouth and throat, foul breath, blood in stools, vomiting
- **MUSCULOSKELETAL:** osteodystrophy (thin, fragile bones)
- **RENAL:** Urine contains protein, blood, and particles; change in the amount, color, concentration.
- **SKIN:** decreased skin turgor, yellow cast to skin, dry, pruritus, urea crystal on skin (uremic frost)
- **REPRODUCTIVE:** erectile dysfunction

LABORATORY TESTS

Urinalysis: Hematuria, proteinuria, and decrease in specific gravity

Blood creatinine: Gradual increase over months to years for CKD exceeding 4 mg/dL; can increase to 15 to 30 mg/dL

BUN: Gradual increase with elevated blood creatinine over months to years for CKD; can increase 10 to 20 times the creatinine finding

Blood electrolytes: Decreased sodium (dilutional) and calcium; increased potassium, phosphorus, and magnesium

CBC: Decreased hemoglobin and hematocrit from anemia secondary to the loss of erythropoietin in CKD

DIAGNOSTIC PROCEDURES

- Cystoscopy
- Retrograde pyelography
- Kidney biopsy

Imaging procedures: Radiologic procedures to detect disease processes, obstruction, and arterial defects

- Ultrasound
- Kidneys, ureter, and bladder (KUB)
- Computerized tomography (CT)
- Magnetic resonance imaging (MRI) without contrast dye
- Aortorenal angiography

PATIENT-CENTERED CARE

NURSING CARE

- Report and monitor irregular findings.
  - Urinary elimination patterns: amount, color, odor, and consistency
  - Vital signs: Blood pressure can be increased or decreased.
  - Weight: 1 kg (2.2 lb) of daily weight increase is approximately 1 L of fluid retained.
- Monitor vascular access or peritoneal dialysis insertion site.
- Obtain a detailed medication and herb history to determine the client's risk for continued kidney injury.
- Control protein intake based on the client's stage of CKD and type of dialysis prescribed.
- Restrict dietary sodium, potassium, phosphorous, and magnesium.
- Provide a diet that is high in carbohydrates and moderate in fat.
- Restrict intake of fluids (based on urinary output).
- Monitor for weight-gain trends.
- Adhere to meticulous cleaning of areas on skin not intact and access sites to control infections.
- Balance the client's activity and rest.
- Prepare the client for hemodialysis, peritoneal dialysis, and hemofiltration if indicated.
- Provide skin care in order to increase comfort and prevent breakdown.
- Protect the client from injury. **Qs**
- Provide emotional support to the client and family.
- Encourage the client to ask questions and discuss fears.
- Administer medications as prescribed.

MEDICATIONS

See the **PN PHARMACOLOGY REVIEW MODULE** for detailed information on these medications.

> **!** Avoid administering antimicrobial medications (aminoglycosides and amphotericin B), NSAIDs, angiotensin-converting enzyme inhibitors, angiotensin-receptor blockers, and IV contrast dye, which are nephrotoxic.

Digoxin: a cardiac glycoside that increases contractility of the myocardium and promotes cardiac output

- Monitor digoxin laboratory levels and expect dosages to be reduced due to slow excretion of the medication with CKD.
- Monitor carefully for manifestations of digoxin toxicity (nausea, vomiting, anorexia, visual changes). Monitor potassium level. **Qs**
- Administer digoxin after dialysis.

Sodium polystyrene: increases elimination of potassium Restrict sodium intake. Sodium polystyrene contains sodium and can cause fluid retention and hypertension, a complication of CKD.

Epoetin alfa: stimulates production of red blood cells; given for anemia

Ferrous sulfate: an iron supplement to prevent severe iron deficiency

Calcium carbonate

- Taken with meals to bind phosphate in food and stop phosphate absorption
- Take 2 hr before or after other medications.
- Can cause constipation, so clients can require a stool softener

Furosemide or bumetanide: loop-diuretics administered to excrete excess fluids

- Avoid administering to a client who has end-stage kidney disease.
- Clients can also receive thiazide diuretics, potassium-sparing diuretics, and osmotic diuretics.

THERAPEUTIC PROCEDURES

- Peritoneal dialysis
- Hemodialysis
- Kidney transplantation

INTERPROFESSIONAL CARE

- Nephrology services to manage dialysis or kidney failure
- Nutritional services to manage the nutritional needs

CLIENT EDUCATION **QEBP**

- Monitor the daily intake of carbohydrates, proteins, sodium, and potassium.
- Monitor fluid intake according to prescribed fluid restriction.
- Avoid antacids containing magnesium.
- Take rest periods from activity.
- Follow instructions for home or outpatient peritoneal dialysis or hemodialysis.
- Measure blood pressure and weight at home.
- Ask questions and discuss fears.
- Diet, exercise, and take medication as prescribed.
- Notify the provider of skin breakdown.

CARE AFTER DISCHARGE

- Nephrology services are indicated if receiving outpatient dialysis.
- Consider joining a community support group relating to the disease.
- Consult nutritional services for dietary needs.
- Take part in a smoking-cessation support group and counseling if needed.

COMPLICATIONS

Potential complications include electrolyte imbalance, dysrhythmias, fluid overload, hypertension, metabolic acidosis, secondary infection, and uremia.

Polycystic kidney disease

- Polycystic kidney disease (PKD) is a congenital disorder where clusters of fluid-filled cysts develop in the nephrons. Healthy kidney tissue is replaced by multiple non-functioning cysts.
- PKD is hereditary and is caused by a genetic mutation.
- PKD is more common in Caucasian clients.

DATA COLLECTION

EXPECTED FINDINGS

- Familial history of PKD
- Anxiety, guilt
- Abdominal and/or flank pain
  - Dull pain indicates increased kidney size or possible cyst infection.
  - Sharp pain indicates ruptured cyst or possible renal lithiasis (kidney stone).
- Headaches
- Hypertension caused by kidney ischemia from the enlarging cysts
- Enlarged abdominal girth
- Constipation
- Bloody and/or cloudy urine
- Renal lithiasis
- Hyponatremia
- Nocturia (excessive urination at night)
- Progressive kidney failure

LABORATORY TESTS

- Urinalysis
- Hematuria, proteinuria, and bacteria indicating infection
- Gradual increase of blood creatinine, BUN, creatinine clearance

DIAGNOSTIC PROCEDURES

Imaging procedures: radiologic procedures to detect disease processes and cysts: ultrasound, CT, and MRI

PATIENT-CENTERED CARE

NURSING CARE

HYPERTENSION CONTROL

- Controlling blood pressure is the highest nursing priority for clients who have PKD.
- Manage hypertension with prescribed medication.
- Reinforce teaching with the client and family about how to measure and record blood pressure readings and daily weights.

PAIN MANAGEMENT: Provide prescribed pain medications and nonpharmacological pain methods (relaxation, deep breathing, guided imagery, distraction). Use NSAIDs cautiously in clients who have kidney disease.

INFECTION PREVENTION

- Assist with the administration of antibiotics (ciprofloxacin, trimethoprim–sulfamethoxazole). Monitor for antibiotic-induced nephrotoxicity by evaluating blood creatinine levels and urinary output.
- Monitor urine specific gravity to determine kidney function and hydration status.

CONSTIPATION PREVENTION

- Provide adequate oral fluid intake (as allowed per prescribed fluid restrictions), increase dietary fiber, and encourage client to ambulate.
- Monitor bowel sounds and bowel movements.
- Administer stool softeners as prescribed.

CLIENT EDUCATION

- Monitor blood pressure and weight daily.
- Notify the provider of elevated temperature.
- Adhere to a low-sodium diet.
- Inform the provider if there are any changes in urine or bowel movements.

CARE AFTER DISCHARGE

- Consider joining a community support group related to the disease.
- Consult nutritional services for dietary needs.

Active Learning Scenario

A nurse is preparing to administer medication to a client who has chronic kidney disease (CKD). What information should the nurse consider when administering medication? Use the ATI Active Learning Template: Medication to complete this item.

MEDICATION: Identify two.

THERAPEUTIC USES: Describe how the medication is used to treat CKD.

NURSING INTERVENTIONS: Describe two for each medication.

Application Exercises

1. A nurse is collecting data from a client who has prenatal acute kidney injury (AKI). Which of the following findings should the nurse expect? (Select all that apply.)
   - A. Reduced BUN
   - B. Elevated cardiac enzymes
   - C. Reduced urine output
   - D. Elevated blood creatinine
   - E. Elevated blood calcium

2. A nurse is contributing to the plan of care for a client who has prerenal acute kidney injury (AKI) following an abdominal aortic aneurysm repair. The client's urinary output is 60 mL in the past 2 hr, and blood pressure is 92/58 mm Hg. The nurse should recommend which of the following interventions?
   - A. Prepare the client for a CT scan with contrast dye.
   - B. Plan to administer nitroprusside.
   - C. Prepare to administer a fluid challenge.
   - D. Plan to position the client in Trendelenburg.

3. A nurse is contributing to the plan of care for a client who has postrenal AKI due to metastatic cancer. The client has a blood creatinine of 5 mg/dL. Which of the following interventions should the nurse recommend for the client's plan of care? (Select all that apply.)
   - A. Provide a high-protein diet.
   - B. Monitor the urine for blood.
   - C. Monitor for intermittent anuria.
   - D. Weigh the client once per week.
   - E. Provide NSAIDs for pain.

4. A nurse is reviewing a client's laboratory results. Which of the following findings should the nurse expect for a client who has stage 4 chronic kidney disease?
   - A. Blood urea nitrogen (BUN) 15 mg/dL
   - B. Glomerular filtration rate (GFR) 20 mL/min
   - C. Blood creatinine 1.1 mg/dL
   - D. Blood potassium 5.0 mEq/L

5. A nurse is contributing to the plan of care for a client who has chronic kidney disease. Which of the following actions should the nurse recommend to include in the plan of care? (Select all that apply.)
   - A. Monitor for jugular vein distention.
   - B. Provide frequent mouth rinses.
   - C. Auscultate for a pleural friction rub.
   - D. Provide a high-sodium diet.
   - E. Monitor for dysrhythmias.

Application Exercises Key

1. C, D. **CORRECT:** When recognizing cues, the nurse should expect the client who has prerenal AKI to have reduced urinary output, an elevated blood creatinine, and a reduced calcium level.

   Ⓝ *NCLEX Connection: Physiological Adaptation, Fluid and Electrolyte Imbalances*

2. C. **CORRECT:** When generating solutions, the nurse should recommend a fluid challenge for hypovolemia, which is indicated for the client who has prerenal AKI and has a low urinary output and blood pressure.

   Ⓝ *NCLEX Connection: Physiological Adaptation, Fluid and Electrolyte Imbalances*

3. A, B, C. **CORRECT:** When generating solutions, the nurse should recommend a high-protein diet due to the high rate of protein breakdown that occurs with acute kidney injury. The nurse should monitor the client's urine for blood, stones, and particles, indicating an obstruction of the urinary structures that leave the kidney. The nurse should plan to monitor for intermittent anuria due to obstruction or damage to kidneys or urinary structures.

   Ⓝ *NCLEX® Connection: Physiological Adaptation, Alterations in Body Systems*

4. B. **CORRECT:** When analyzing cues, the nurse should identify that the GFR is decreased to 20 mL/min, which is indicative of stage 4 chronic kidney disease.

   Ⓝ *NCLEX Connection: Reduction of Risk Potential, Laboratory Values*

5. A, B, C. **CORRECT:** When generating solutions, the nurse should plan to monitor for jugular vein distention, which can indicate fluid overload and heart failure. The nurse should provide frequent mouth rinses due to uremic halitosis caused by urea waste in the blood. The nurse should auscultate for a pleural friction rub related to respiratory failure and pulmonary edema caused by acid base imbalances and fluid retention. The nurse should monitor for dysrhythmias related to increased blood potassium caused by stage 4 chronic kidney disease.

   Ⓝ *NCLEX® Connection: Physiological Adaptation, Alterations in Body Systems*

Active Learning Scenario Key

Using the ATI Active Learning Template: Medication

MEDICATION
- Digoxin
- Sodium polystyrene
- Furosemide

THERAPEUTIC USES
- Digoxin: A cardiac glycoside: Increases contractility of the myocardium and promotes cardiac output
- Sodium polystyrene: Increases elimination of potassium
- Calcium carbonate: Binds to phosphate in food and stops phosphate absorption
- Furosemide: A loop diuretic that causes diuresis of excess fluids

NURSING INTERVENTIONS
- Digoxin
  - Monitor blood digoxin and potassium levels.
  - Monitor for manifestations of toxicity (nausea, vomiting, anorexia, visual changes).
- Sodium polystyrene
  - Monitor for hypokalemia.
  - Restrict sodium intake.
- Furosemide
  - Monitor intake and output and blood pressure.
  - Avoid administering to a client who has end-stage kidney disease.

Ⓝ *NCLEX® Connection: Physiological Adaptation, Basic Pathophysiology*

CHAPTER 55 Infections of the Renal and Urinary System

The renal system includes the kidneys and the urinary system.

The function of the renal system includes maintaining fluid volume, removing waste, regulating blood pressure, maintaining acid-base balance, producing erythropoietin, and activating vitamin D.

There are three components to the urinary system: the ureter, bladder, and urethra. The function of the urinary system is to store and remove urine.

Urinary tract infections (UTIs) are infections of the urinary system, and pyelonephritis is an infection of the kidney and renal pelvis. They are the most common outpatient infection in the U.S., with at least 50% of adult females (sex assigned at birth) experiencing a UTI in their lifetime. Acute and chronic glomerulonephritis can develop from a systemic infection and involves the glomeruli of the kidney or the area responsible for filtering particles from the blood to make urine.

Urinary tract infection

- A urinary tract infection (UTI) refers to any portion of the lower urinary tract (ureters, bladder, urethra, prostate). UTIs include the following.
  - Cystitis
  - Urethritis
  - Prostatitis
- An upper UTI refers to conditions such as pyelonephritis (inflammation of the kidney pelvis).
- UTIs are often caused by *Escherichia coli*. Other organisms include Enterobacteriaceae micro-organisms (klebsiella, proteus), pseudomonas, and *Staphylococcus saprophyticus*.
- Untreated UTIs can lead to pyelonephritis and urosepsis, which can result in septic shock and death.

DATA COLLECTION

RISK FACTORS

- Alkaline urine promotes bacterial growth.
- Indwelling urinary catheters (significant source of infection in clients who are hospitalized)
- Stool incontinence
- Bladder distention
- Urinary conditions (anomalies, stasis, calculi, residual urine)
- Possible genetic links
- Disease (diabetes mellitus)

Female (sex assigned at birth)
- Short urethra predisposes females to UTIs.
- Close proximity of the urethra to the rectum
- Decreased estrogen in aging females promotes atrophy of the urethral opening toward the rectum (increases the risk of urosepsis in females). Ⓖ
- Sexual intercourse
- Frequent use of feminine hygiene sprays, tampons, sanitary napkins, and spermicidal jellies
- Pregnancy
- Poorly-fitted diaphragm
- Hormonal influences within the vaginal flora
- Synthetic underwear and pantyhose
- Wet bathing suits
- Frequent submersion into baths or hot tubs

Older adult clients Ⓖ
- Increased risk of bacteremia, sepsis, and shock
- Incomplete bladder emptying caused by an enlarged prostate or prostatitis in males
- Bladder prolapse in females
- Inability to empty bladder (neurogenic bladder) as a result of a stroke or Parkinson's disease
- Fecal incontinence with poor perineal hygiene
- Hypoestrogenism in females affecting the mucosa of the vagina and urethra, causing bacteria to adhere to the mucosal surface
- Renal complications increase due to decreased number of functioning nephrons and fluid intake.

EXPECTED FINDINGS

- Lower back or lower abdominal discomfort and tenderness over the bladder area
- Nausea
- Urinary frequency and urgency
- Dysuria, bladder cramping, spasms
- Feeling of incomplete bladder emptying or retention of urine
- Perineal itching
- Hematuria (red-tinged, smoky, coffee-colored urine)
- Pyuria (WBCs in the urine sample)
- Fever
- Vomiting
- Voiding in small amounts
- Nocturia
- Urethral discharge
- Cloudy or foul-smelling urine

OLDER ADULT MANIFESTATIONS Ⓖ
- Confusion
- Incontinence
- Loss of appetite
- Nocturia and dysuria
- Hypotension, tachycardia, tachypnea, and fever (indications of urosepsis)

LABORATORY TESTS

Urinalysis and urine culture and sensitivity

EXPECTED FINDINGS
- Bacteria, sediment, white blood cells (WBC), and red blood cells (RBC)
- Positive leukocyte esterase and nitrites (68% to 88% of positive results indicates UTI.)

NURSING ACTIONS
- Instruct the client regarding proper technique for the collection of a clean-catch urine specimen.
- Collect catheterized urine specimens using sterile technique.

WBC count and differential
- If urosepsis is suspected
- White blood cell count equal to or greater than 10,000/μL with a shift to the left, indicating an increased number of immature cells (neutrophils) in response to infection

Sexually transmitted infection testing
- STIs can cause manifestations of a UTI.
- *Chlamydia trachomatis*, *Neisseria gonorrhoeae*, and herpes simplex can cause acute urethritis.
- Trichomoniasis or candida can cause acute vaginal infections.

DIAGNOSTIC PROCEDURES

Imaging procedures
- Cystoscopy is used for complicated UTIs.
- Cystourethroscopy detects strictures, calculi, tumors, and cystitis.
- Computed tomography (CT) scan is used to detect pyelonephritis.
- Ultrasonography detects cysts, tumors, calculi, and abscesses.
- Transrectal ultrasonography is used to detect prostate and bladder conditions in males.

PATIENT-CENTERED CARE

NURSING CARE
- Consult with the provider regarding prescribed fluid restrictions if needed.
- Administer antibiotic medications as prescribed.
- Recommend warm sitz bath two or three times a day to provide comfort.
- Avoid the use of indwelling catheters if possible. This reduces the risk for infection.
- Clients who are pregnant require immediate and effective treatment to prevent pyelonephritis that can result in preterm labor. Ⓠs

MEDICATIONS

Fluoroquinolones, nitrofurantoin, trimethoprim, or sulfonamides

Antibiotics used to treat urinary infections by directly killing bacteria and inhibiting bacterial reproduction ⓆEBP
- Penicillins and cephalosporins are administered less frequently because the medication is less effective and tolerated.
- Nitrofurantoin is an antibacterial medication where therapeutic levels are achieved in the urine only.

NURSING ACTIONS
- If a sulfonamide is prescribed, ask the client about allergy to sulfa.
- Advise clients taking fluoroquinolones or sulfonamides that sun-sensitivity is increased and sunburn is a risk for even dark-skinned individuals. These medications can precipitate in the renal tubules, so advise client to take these medications with a full glass of water and to increase fluid intake.

CLIENT EDUCATION
- Understand the need to take all of the prescribed antibiotics even if manifestations subside.
- Take the medication with food.
- Monitor and report watery diarrhea that can indicate pseudomembranous colitis.

Phenazopyridine

Bladder analgesic used to treat UTIs

CLIENT EDUCATION
- The medication will turn urine orange.
- Take the medication with food.
- The medication will not treat the infection, but it will help relieve bladder discomfort, pain, burning, itching, urgency, and frequency.

INTERPROFESSIONAL CARE

Consult with urology services for managing UTIs.

CLIENT EDUCATION

- Drink at least 8 to 10 glasses of fluid daily.
- Bathe daily to promote good body hygiene.
- Empty bladder every 3 to 4 hr instead of waiting until the bladder is completely full.
- Urinate before and after intercourse.
- Drink cranberry juice to decrease the risk of infection. Q EBP
  - The compound in cranberries might stop certain bacteria from adhering to the mucosa of the urinary tract.
  - Clients who have chronic cystitis should avoid cranberry juice, which irritates the bladder.
- Empty the bladder as soon as there is an urgency to void.

Instruct female clients to:
- Wipe the perineal area from front to back.
- Avoid using bubble baths and feminine products and toilet paper containing perfumes.
- Avoid sitting in wet bathing suits.
- Avoid wearing pantyhose with slacks or tight clothing.

CARE AFTER DISCHARGE: Urology services can be consulted for management of long-term antibiotic therapy for chronic UTIs.

COMPLICATIONS

Urethral obstruction, pyelonephritis, chronic kidney disease, urosepsis, septic shock, and death

Pyelonephritis

Pyelonephritis is an infection and inflammation of the kidney pelvis, calyces, and medulla and is classified as acute or chronic. Acute pyelonephritis is the cause of more than 20,000 hospital admissions yearly. The infection usually begins in the lower urinary tract with organisms ascending into the kidney pelvis. *Escherichia coli* organisms are frequently the cause of acute pyelonephritis. Repeated infections can create scarring that changes the blood flow to the kidney, glomerulus, and tubular structure. Filtration, reabsorption, and secretion are impaired, which results in a decrease in kidney function.

Acute pyelonephritis is an active bacterial infection that occurs most frequently in females 20 to 30 years of age and can cause the following.
- Interstitial inflammation
- Tubular cell necrosis
- Abscess formation in the capsule, cortex, or medulla
- Temporarily altered kidney function (This rarely progresses to chronic kidney disease.)

Chronic pyelonephritis is the result of repeated infections that cause progressive inflammation and scarring.
- This can result in the thickening of the calyces and post-inflammatory fibrosis with permanent renal tissue scarring.
- It is more common with obstructions, urinary anomaly, and vesicoureteral urine reflux.
- Reflux of urine occurs at the junction where the ureter connects to the bladder.

DATA COLLECTION

RISK FACTORS

- Young adult females (sex assigned at birth) (acute)
- Pregnancy (acute)
- Neurogenic bladder (chronic)
- Congenital genitourinary malformations (chronic)
- Bladder tumors, chronic urinary stones
- Chronic illness (diabetes mellitus, hypertension, chronic cystitis)
- Alkaline urine which promotes bacterial growth
- Incomplete bladder emptying (prostatitis/BPH)
- Older adult clients can exhibit gastrointestinal or pulmonary manifestations instead of febrile responses because their temperature can vary at a lower-than-normal state. Causes are inadequate diet, loss of adipose tissue, lack of exercise, and reduction in the client's thermoregulator. G

EXPECTED FINDINGS

A client who has chronic pyelonephritis may not experience any manifestations.
- Chills
- Headache
- Nausea and vomiting
- Malaise, fatigue
- Dysuria and urgency, and frequency with urination
- Costovertebral angle tenderness
- Flank and back pain
- Nocturia
- Fever
- Hypertension (chronic)
- Inability to concentrate urine or conserve sodium (chronic)

LABORATORY TESTS

- Urinalysis and urine culture and sensitivity are the same as for a UTI (positive leukocyte esterase and nitrites, WBCs, bacteria, pyuria, hematuria).
- WBC count and differential are the same as for a UTI.
- Blood cultures will be positive for the presence of bacteria if a systemic infection is present.
- Serum creatinine and blood urea nitrogen (BUN) are elevated during acute episodes and consistently elevated with chronic infection.
- C-reactive protein is elevated during exacerbating inflammatory processes of the kidneys. Erythrocyte sedimentation rate (ESR) is elevated during acute or chronic inflammation.

DIAGNOSTIC PROCEDURES

Imaging procedures
- An x-ray of the kidneys, ureters, and bladder (KUB) can demonstrate calculi or structural abnormalities.
- Ultrasonography is used to detect cysts, tumors, calculi, and abscesses.
- Gallium scan is a nuclear medicine test that uses injectable radioactive dye to visualize organs, glands, bones, and blood vessels that have infection and inflammation.
- Intravenous pyelogram can demonstrate calculi, structural, or vascular abnormalities.

PATIENT-CENTERED CARE

NURSING CARE

- Monitor the following.
  - Nutritional status
  - Intake and output
  - Fluid and electrolyte balance
  - Temperature
  - Onset, quality, duration, and severity of pain
- Increase fluid intake to at least 2 L/day unless contraindicated.
- Administer antipyretic, such as acetaminophen, as needed for fever and opioid analgesics for pain associated with pyelonephritis.
- Provide emotional support.
- Assist with personal hygiene.

MEDICATIONS

See the **PHARMACOLOGY REVIEW MODULE** for more detailed information.

Opioid analgesics (opioid agonists), morphine sulfate, and morphine: for moderate to severe pain

Antibiotics Ⓠᴱᴮᴾ
- Mild to moderate pyelonephritis treated at home for 14 days with the following:
  - Anti-infective: trimethoprim, sulfamethoxazole/trimethoprim
  - Quinolone antibiotic: ciprofloxacin, levofloxacin
- Severe pyelonephritis treated in the hospital for 24 to 48 hr with IV medication:
  - Quinolone antibiotics: ciprofloxacin
  - Cephalosporin antibiotics: ceftriaxone, ceftazidime
  - Aminopenicillin antibiotics: ampicillin, ampicillin/sulbactam
  - Aminoglycoside antibiotics: gentamicin, tobramycin

THERAPEUTIC PROCEDURES

Reinforce preoperative/postoperative operative teaching.

Assist with monitoring the administration of intravenous antibiotics and analgesics, which are usually administered for each procedure.

Pyelolithotomy: The removal of a large stone from the kidney that causes infections and blocks the flow of urine from the kidney

Nephrectomy: The removal of the kidney when all procedures to clear the client of infection were unsuccessful

Ureteroplasty: Done to repair or revise the ureter and can involve reimplantation of the ureter in the bladder wall to preserve the function of the kidney and eliminate infection

INTERPROFESSIONAL CARE

- Urology services to manage pyelonephritis
- Nutritional services to promote adequate calories

CLIENT EDUCATION

- Maintain an adequate nutritional status.
- Drink at least 2 L of fluids daily unless otherwise indicated by the provider.
- Notify the provider if acute onset of pain occurs or a fever is present.
- Express any fears and anxiety related to the disease.
- Take rest periods from activity as needed.

CARE AFTER DISCHARGE
- Home care services can be indicated if needing assistance with medications or nutritional therapy.
- Follow up with the provider as directed.

COMPLICATIONS

- Septic shock (hypotension, tachycardia, fever) due to bacterial organism entering the blood stream
- Chronic kidney disease (elevated BUN, creatinine, electrolytes) from inflammation and infection that causes fibrosis of the kidney pelvis and calyx, scarring, and changes in the blood vessels and the glomerular and tubular filtration system
- Hypertension (related to fluid and sodium retention) indicating chronic kidney disease caused by destruction of the filtration system of the kidney due to infection

Glomerulonephritis

Immunologic kidney disorder that can start in the kidneys (genetic basis and immune-inducing inflammation) or be a result of other health disorders (lupus erythematosus, diabetic nephropathy) and results in glomerular injury

- This can lead to end-stage kidney disease (ESKD).
- Acute glomerulonephritis often occurs following an infection.
- Chronic glomerulonephritis develops over a period of 20 to 30 years.

DATA COLLECTION

RISK FACTORS

- Recent infection particularly of the skin or upper respiratory tract
- Recent travel or other possible exposure to bacteria, viruses, fungi or parasites
- Presence of systemic diseases (systemic lupus erythematosus, Goodpasture syndrome)
- Recent surgery or illness

EXPECTED FINDINGS

- Edema (face, hands, eyes, feet)
- Anorexia
- Nausea
- Dysuria, oliguria
- Fatigue
- Hypertension
- Fluid volume excess (difficulty breathing, crackles, weight gain, S3 heart sound)
- Reddish-brown or cola-colored urine
- Older adult clients likely to have the less common manifestations related to circulatory overload, which can be confused with congestive heart failure Ⓒ

LABORATORY TESTS

- Urinalysis shows red blood cells and protein.
- Glomerular filtration rate is decreased.
- Blood, skin, or throat cultures (if indicated)
- 24-hr urine collection for protein assay (increased in acute glomerulonephritis and decreased in chronic glomerulonephritis).
- Blood urea nitrogen and creatinine are increased.
- Antistreptolysin O titers are increased after group A beta hemolytic streptococcus infection.
- C3 complement levels decreased
- Cryoglobulins present
- Anti-nuclear antibody (ANA) presence
- Altered electrolytes: hyperkalemia, hyperphosphatemia, hypocalcemia

DIAGNOSTIC PROCEDURES

Kidney biopsy will diagnose the condition, determine prognosis, and guide treatment.

PATIENT-CENTERED CARE

NURSING CARE

- Coordinate care to conserve client energy.
- Consult with provider to determine if fluid restriction is needed.
- Administer antibiotics as prescribed.
- Reinforce teaching about relaxation exercises to decrease stress.
- Monitor blood pressure.
- Monitor respiratory status.
- Monitor fluid and electrolytes.

MEDICATIONS

Antibiotics: Penicillin, erythromycin, or azithromycin is prescribed for glomerulonephritis infection due to streptococcal infection. ⓆEBP

Antihypertensives: To control hypertension

INTERPROFESSIONAL CARE

- Collaborate with provider and nutritional support regarding any potassium or protein restriction in diet.
- Dialysis or plasmapheresis if necessary

CLIENT EDUCATION

- Complete full course of antibiotics.
- Monitor weight daily and report increases to provider.
- Adhere to dietary and fluid restrictions.
- Perform basic infection control practices, such as hand hygiene.

CARE AFTER DISCHARGE

- Consider home care services for continued dialysis or plasmapheresis if needed.
- Follow up with the provider as directed.

Application Exercises

1. A nurse is reviewing urinalysis results for four clients. Which of the following urinalysis results indicates a urinary tract infection?

   A. Positive for hyaline casts

   B. Positive for leukocyte esterase

   C. Positive for ketones

   D. Positive for crystals

2. A nurse is caring for a client who has a urinary tract infection (UTI). Which of the following is the priority intervention by the nurse?

   A. Offer a warm sitz bath.

   B. Recommend drinking cranberry juice.

   C. Encourage increased fluids.

   D. Administer an antibiotic.

3. A nurse is assisting in the preparation of educational material to present to a female client who has frequent urinary tract infections. Which of the following information should the nurse include? (Select all that apply.)

   A. Avoid sitting in a wet bathing suit.

   B. Wipe the perineal area back to front following elimination.

   C. Empty the bladder when there is an urge to void.

   D. Wear synthetic fabric underwear.

   E. Take a shower daily.

4. A nurse is caring for several clients. Which of the following clients are at risk for developing pyelonephritis? (Select all that apply.)

   A. A client who is at 32 weeks of gestation

   B. A client who has kidney calculi

   C. A client who has a urine pH of 4.2

   D. A client who has a neurogenic bladder

   E. A client who has diabetes mellitus

5. A nurse is contributing to the plan of care for a client who has chronic pyelonephritis. Which of the following actions should the nurse plan to include? (Select all that apply.)

   A. Recommend a referral for nutrition counseling.

   B. Encourage daily fluid intake of 1 L.

   C. Palpate the costovertebral angle.

   D. Monitor urinary output.

   E. Administer antibiotics.

6. A nurse is preparing a presentation about acute pyelonephritis and acute glomerulonephritis for a group of newly licensed nurses. Sort each clinical manifestation to its condition: acute pyelonephritis or acute glomerulonephritis.

   A. Difficulty breathing

   B. Costovertebral angle (CVA) tenderness

   C. Urinary frequency and urgency

   D. Cola-colored urine

   E. Weight gain

   F. Chills

   G. Swelling of face, hands, and extremities

Active Learning Scenario

A nurse is reinforcing teaching with a client who has chronic pyelonephritis. What information should the nurse include? Use the ATI Active Learning Template: System Disorder to complete this item.

ALTERATION IN HEALTH (DIAGNOSIS)

COMPLICATIONS: List three, and explain why these occur.

CLIENT EDUCATION: Include three instructional points.

1. A. Hyaline casts in the urine can indicate proteinuria and can occur following exercise.
   B. **CORRECT:** When analyzing cues, the nurse should identify that a positive leukocyte esterase indicates a urinary tract infection.
   C. Ketones in the urine are a manifestation of poorly-controlled diabetes mellitus or starvation.
   D. Crystals in the urine can indicate a potential for kidney stone formation.

   Ⓝ *NCLEX® Connection: Reduction of Risk Potential, Laboratory Values*

2. A. The nurse should offer a warm sitz bath to provide temporary relief of the manifestations of the UTI. However, another action is the priority.
   B. The nurse should recommend that the client drink cranberry juice to prevent a UTI in the future. However, another action is the priority.
   C. The nurse should encourage the client to increase fluid intake to dilute the urine and flush the kidneys to relieve the manifestations of the UTI. However, another action is the priority.
   D. **CORRECT:** When prioritizing hypotheses, the nurse should identify that the greatest risk to the client is injury to the renal system and sepsis from the UTI. The priority intervention is to administer antibiotics.

   Ⓝ *NCLEX® Connection: Physiological Adaptation, Unexpected Response to Therapies*

3. A. **CORRECT:** When taking action, the nurse should identify that the client should avoid sitting in a wet bathing suit, which can increase the risk for a UTI by colonization of bacteria in a moist, warm environment.
   B. The client should wipe the perineal area from front to back after elimination to prevent contaminating the urethra with bacteria.
   C. **CORRECT:** The client should empty the bladder when there is an urge to void rather than retain urine for an extended period of time, which increases the risk for a UTI.
   D. The client should wear cotton underwear that absorbs moisture and keeps the perineal area drier, thus decreasing colonization of bacteria that can cause a UTI.
   E. **CORRECT:** The client should take a shower daily to promote good body hygiene and decrease colonization of bacteria in the perineal area that can cause a UTI.

   Ⓝ *NCLEX® Connection: Health Promotion and Maintenance, Health Promotion/Disease Prevention*

4. A. **CORRECT:** When analyzing cues, the nurse should identify that a client who is at 32 weeks of gestation is at risk for developing pyelonephritis because of increased pressure on the urinary system during pregnancy causing reflux or retention of urine.
   B. **CORRECT:** A client who has kidney calculi is at risk for pyelonephritis because stones harbor bacteria.
   C. The nurse should identify that the expected reference range for urine pH is 4.6 to 8.0. Alkaline urine promotes bacteria growth. The client who has a urine pH of 4.2 has acidic urine.
   D. **CORRECT:** The client who has a neurogenic bladder can retain urine, promoting bacterial growth and causing pyelonephritis.
   E. **CORRECT:** The client who has diabetes mellitus is at risk of pyelonephritis because glucose that can be in the urine promotes bacterial growth.

   Ⓝ *NCLEX® Connection: Physiological Adaptation, Alterations in Body Systems*

5. A. **CORRECT:** When generating solutions, the nurse should identify that the client requires adequate nutrition to promote healing.
   B. Encourage fluid intake of 2 L daily to maintain dilute urine.
   C. **CORRECT:** The nurse should plan to gently palpate the costovertebral angle for flank tenderness, which can indicate inflammation and infection.
   D. **CORRECT:** The nurse should monitor urinary output to determine that 1 to 3 L of urine is excreted daily, administer antibiotics to treat the bacteriuria and decrease progressive damage to the kidney, and encourage fluid intake of 2 L daily to maintain dilute urine.
   E. **CORRECT:** The nurse should monitor urinary output to determine that 1 to 3 L of urine is excreted daily, administer antibiotics to treat the bacteriuria and decrease progressive damage to the kidney, and encourage fluid intake of 2 L daily to maintain dilute urine.

   Ⓝ *NCLEX® Connection: Physiological Adaptation, Alterations in Body Systems*

6. **ACUTE PYELONEPHRITIS:** B, C, F;
   ACUTE GLOMERULONEPHRITIS: A, D, E, G

   When recognizing cues, the nurse should identify that clinical manifestations of acute pyelonephritis are costovertebral angle (CVA) tenderness, urinary frequency and urgency, and chills. Findings associated with acute glomerulonephritis include difficulty breathing, dark or cola-colored urine, weight gain, and edema of the face, hands, and other parts of the body.

   Ⓝ *NCLEX® Connection: Physiological Adaptation, Alterations in Body Systems*

Active Learning Scenario Key

Using the ATI Active Learning Template: System Disorder

ALTERATION IN HEALTH (DIAGNOSIS): Chronic pyelonephritis is a repetitive infection and inflammation of the kidney pelvis, calyces, and medulla, and generally begins from bacteria that ascends from a lower urinary tract infection.

COMPLICATIONS
- Septic shock caused by micro-organisms entering the bloodstream from the infected kidney
- Chronic kidney disease caused by inflammation, fibrosis, and scarring of the kidney filtration structure
- Hypertension (related to fluid and sodium retention) indicating chronic kidney disease caused by destruction of the filtration system of the kidney from infection

CLIENT EDUCATION
- Intake at least 2 L of fluids daily.
- Take all medications as prescribed.
- Notify the provider of acute, rapid onset of pain.
- Express any fears and anxiety.
- Balance between rest and activity.

Ⓝ *NCLEX® Connection: Physiological Adaptation, Alterations in Body Systems*

CHAPTER 56 *Renal Calculi*

Urolithiasis is the presence of calculi (stones) in the urinary tract. The majority of calculi are composed of calcium phosphate or calcium oxalate, but they can contain other substances (uric acid, struvite, cystine).

A diet high in calcium is not believed to increase the risk of calculi formation unless there is a preexisting metabolic disorder or renal tubular defect. Recurrence is increased in individuals who have a family history or whose first occurrence of renal calculi is prior to the age of 25.

Most clients can expel calculi without invasive procedures. Factors that influence whether a calculus will pass spontaneously or not include the composition, size, and location of the calculus.

DATA COLLECTION

RISK FACTORS

- Cause is unknown.
- Male assigned at birth
- Genetic predisposition
- Urinary tract lining that is damaged
- Urine flow that is decreased, concentrated, and contains particles (calcium)
- Metabolic defects
  - Increased intestinal absorption or decreased renal excretion of calcium
  - Increased oxalate production (genetic) or inability to metabolize oxalate from foods (black tea, spinach, beets, Swiss chard, chocolate, and peanuts)
  - Increased production or decreased clearance of purines (contributing to increased uric-acid levels)
- High alkalinity or acidity of urine
- Urinary stasis, urinary retention, immobilization, and dehydration
- Decreased fluid intake or increased incidence of dehydration among older adult clients Ⓒ

EXPECTED FINDINGS

- Severe pain (renal colic)
  - Pain intensifies as the calculus moves through the ureter.
  - Flank pain suggests calculi are located in the kidney or ureter.
  - Flank pain that radiates to the abdomen, scrotum, testes, or vulva suggests calculi in the ureter or bladder.
- Urinary frequency or dysuria (calculi in the bladder)
- Fever
- Diaphoresis
- Pallor
- Nausea/vomiting
- Tachycardia, tachypnea, increased blood pressure (pain), or decreased blood pressure (shock)
- Oliguria/anuria occurs with calculi that obstruct urinary flow. Urinary tract obstruction is a medical emergency and needs to be treated to preserve kidney function.
- Hematuria (rusty or smoky-looking urine) Ⓠ EBP

LABORATORY TESTS

Urinalysis

Urine is analyzed for pH (determines the type of calculi), specific gravity, and osmolarity (hydration status).
- Altered odor of the urine and increased urine turbidity if infection is present
- Increased RBCs, WBCs, and bacteria (presence of infection)
- Crystals noted on microscopic exam
- Abnormal blood calcium, phosphate, and uric-acid levels in the presence of metabolic disorders/defects
- Decreased pH: uric acid, cystine stones
- Increased pH: calcium or struvite stones

DIAGNOSTIC PROCEDURES

Radiology examination

X-ray of kidney, ureters, bladder (KUB), or intravenous pyelogram (IVP) is used to confirm the presence and location of calculi. IVP is contraindicated if there is a urinary obstruction.

CT or MRI of the abdomen and pelvis

A CT (noncontrast helical scan) or MRI is used to identify cystine or uric-acid calculi, which cannot be seen on standard x-rays.

Renal ultrasound or cystoscopy

These can confirm the diagnosis.

PATIENT-CENTERED CARE

NURSING CARE

- Report laboratory and diagnostic findings to the provider.
- Provide preoperative and postoperative care as indicated.
- Administer prescribed medications.
- Strain all urine to check for passage of the calculus, and save the calculus for laboratory analysis.
- Encourage increased oral intake to 3 L/day unless contraindicated.
- Encourage the use of hot baths and moist heat to promote comfort.
- Assist with the administration of IV fluids as prescribed.
- Encourage ambulation to promote passage of the calculus.
- Some clients can pass stones less than 5 mm without any interventions. Monitor the client closely during this period.

MONITOR:
- Pain status
- Intake and output
- Urinary pH

MEDICATIONS

Analgesics

Opioids
- Morphine sulfate can be used in the first 24 to 36 hr with the acute onset of calculi. It can be administered IV or IM.
- Opioid agents are used to treat moderate to severe pain. Activation of these receptors produces analgesia, respiratory depression, euphoria, sedation, and decreased GI motility.
- Use cautiously with clients who have asthma or emphysema due to the risk of respiratory depression.
- NURSING ACTIONS
  - Check the client frequently.
  - Watch for evidence of respiratory depression, especially in older adult clients. If respirations are 12/min or less, stop the medication and notify the provider immediately. Ⓖ
  - Monitor vital signs for hypotension and decreased respirations.
  - Monitor level of sedation (drowsiness, level of consciousness).
- CLIENT EDUCATION: Drink plenty of fluids to prevent constipation.

NSAIDs
- Ketorolac is used to treat mild to moderate pain, fever, and inflammation.
- There is a risk for decreased renal function and perfusion.
- NURSING ACTIONS: Observe for indications of bleeding.
- CLIENT EDUCATION
  - Watch for bleeding (dark stools, blood in stools).
  - Notify the provider if abdominal pain occurs, which can be due to gastric ulceration.

Spasmolytic medications

Oxybutynin alleviates pain by decreasing bladder spasms that can result due to renal calculi.

NURSING ACTIONS
- Check for history of glaucoma, as this medication increases intraocular pressure. Ⓠᴘᴄᴄ
- Monitor for dizziness and tachycardia.
- Monitor for urinary retention.

CLIENT EDUCATION
- Report palpitations and problems with voiding or constipation.
- Dizziness and dry mouth are common with the medication.
- Suck on hard candies to alleviate dry mouth.

Antibiotics

Gentamicin and cephalexin are used to treat UTIs.

NURSING ACTIONS
- Administer medication with food to decrease GI distress.
- Monitor for nephrotoxicity and ototoxicity for clients taking gentamicin.

CLIENT EDUCATION
- Urine can have foul odor related to the antibiotic.
- Report loose stools related to the medication.

Miscellaneous medications

Thiazide diuretics and allopurinol can be used to increase excretion of calculi and decrease the pH of the urine.

INTERPROFESSIONAL CARE

Urology services can be consulted for management of urolithiasis.

Nutritional services can be consulted for dietary modifications concerning foods related to calculi formation.

THERAPEUTIC PROCEDURES

Extracorporeal shock wave lithotripsy (ESWL)
- Uses sound, laser, or shock-wave energies to break calculi into fragments
- Requires moderate (conscious) sedation and ECG monitoring during the procedure

NURSING ACTIONS
- Preprocedure
  - Assist with obtaining informed consent for treatment.
  - Position the client in a flat position.
  - Assist with the application of a topical anesthetic over stone site 45 min prior to procedure.
  - Monitor for gross hematuria and strain urine following the procedure.
- Postprocedure
  - Strain all urine.
  - Monitor site.

CLIENT EDUCATION
- Bruising is normal at the site where waves are applied.
- There will be hematuria postprocedure.

Surgical interventions

Stenting is the placement of a small tube in the ureter during a ureteroscopy to dilate the ureter and allow passage of a calculus. An indwelling urinary catheter can be used to facilitate the passage of calculus.

Percutaneous ureterolithotomy/nephrolithotomy is the insertion of an ultrasonic or laser lithotripter into the ureter or kidney to grasp and extract the calculus using a basket and forceps.

Open surgery uses a surgical incision to remove the calculus. This surgery is used for large or impacted calculi (staghorn calculi) or for calculi not removed by other approaches.
- **Ureterolithotomy:** into the ureter
- **Pyelolithotomy:** into the kidney pelvis
- **Nephrolithotomy:** into the kidney

CARE AFTER DISCHARGE: Nutritional services can be consulted for dietary modifications concerning foods related to calculi formation.

CLIENT EDUCATION

Adhere to the diet and medications in the treatment for prevention of renal calculi.

Calcium phosphate

- Limit intake of food high in animal protein (reduction of protein intake decreases calcium precipitation).
- Limit sodium intake.
- Reduced calcium intake (dairy products) is individualized.

Medications
- Thiazide diuretics (hydrochlorothiazide) are used to increase calcium reabsorption.
- Orthophosphates are used to decrease urine saturation of calcium oxalate.
- Sodium cellulose phosphate is used to reduce the intestinal absorption of calcium.

Calcium oxalate

- Avoid oxalate sources: spinach, black tea, rhubarb, cocoa, beets, pecans, strawberries, peanuts, okra, chocolate, wheat germ, lime peel, and Swiss chard. ○PCC
- Limit sodium intake.

Struvite (magnesium ammonium phosphate)

Avoid high-phosphate foods: dairy products, red and organ meats, and whole grains.

Uric acid (urate)

- Decrease intake of purine sources: organ meats, poultry, fish, gravies, red wine, and sardines.
- Lemon or orange juice can be consumed to alkalinize the urine.

Medications
- Allopurinol is used to prevent the formation of uric acid.
- Potassium or sodium citrate or sodium bicarbonate is used to alkalinize the urine.

Cystine

Limit animal protein intake.

Medications
- Alpha mercaptopropionyl glycine (AMPG) is used to lower urine cystine.
- Captopril is used to lower urine cystine.

COMPLICATIONS

Obstruction

A calculus can block the passage of urine into the kidney, ureter, or bladder. Urinary output can be diminished or absent. This can predispose the client to hydroureter (enlargement of the ureter).

NURSING ACTIONS
- Notify the provider immediately.
- Prepare the client for removal of the calculus.

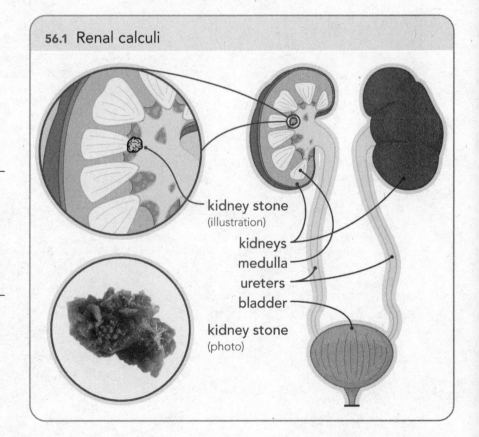

56.1 Renal calculi

kidney stone (illustration)

kidneys
medulla
ureters
bladder

kidney stone (photo)

Active Learning Scenario

A nurse is contributing to the plan of care for a client who has renal calculi and prescriptions for morphine and oxybutynin for pain control. What should the nurse take into consideration when administering these medications? Use the ATI Active Learning Template: Medication to complete this item.

THERAPEUTIC USES: Identify the rationale for administering morphine and oxybutynin.

COMPLICATIONS: Identify adverse effects the nurse should monitor for when administering each of these medications.

NURSING INTERVENTIONS: Identify nursing considerations and client education the nurse should plan to provide when administering each of these medications.

Application Exercises

1. A nurse is collecting data on a client who has renal calculi. Which of the following findings should the nurse expect?
   - A. Bradycardia
   - B. Nausea
   - C. Nocturia
   - D. Bradypnea

2. A nurse is reinforcing teaching with a client who is scheduled for extracorporeal shock wave lithotripsy (ESWL). Which of the following statements by the client indicates understanding of the instruction?
   - A. "I will be fully awake during the procedure."
   - B. "Lithotripsy will reduce my chances of having stones in the future."
   - C. "I will report any bruising that occurs to my doctor."
   - D. "Straining my urine following the procedure is important."

3. A nurse is reinforcing discharge instructions with a client who had spontaneous passage of a calcium phosphate renal calculus. Which of the following instructions should the nurse include? (Select all that apply.)
   - A. Limit intake of food high in protein.
   - B. Reduce sodium intake.
   - C. Strain urine for 48 hr.
   - D. Report burning with urination to the provider.
   - E. Increase fluid intake to 3 L/day.

4. A nurse is reinforcing discharge instructions with a client who has spontaneously passed a calcium oxalate calculus. To decrease the chance of recurrence, the nurse should instruct the client to avoid which of the following foods? (Select all that apply.)
   - A. Red meat
   - B. Peanuts
   - C. Cheese
   - D. Whole grains
   - E. Spinach

5. A nurse is caring for a client who has a left renal calculus and an indwelling urinary catheter. Which of the following data collection findings is the priority for the nurse to report to the provider?
   - A. Flank pain that radiates to the lower abdomen
   - B. Client report of nausea
   - C. Absent urine output for 1 hr
   - D. Blood WBC count 15,000/mm$_3$

Application Exercises Key

1. B. **CORRECT**: When recognizing cues, the nurse should identify that nausea (as well as vomiting) is a manifestation associated with a client who has renal calculi.

   Ⓝ *NCLEX® Connection: Physiological Adaptation, Basic Pathophysiology*

2. D. **CORRECT**: When taking actions, the nurse should instruct the client to strain their urine following lithotripsy to verify that the renal calculi has passed.

   Ⓝ *NCLEX® Connection: Reduction of Risk Potential, Therapeutic Procedures*

3. A, B, D, E. **CORRECT**: When taking actions, the nurse should reinforce teaching with the client who has passed a calcium phosphate renal calculus to limit intake of food high in protein, which contains calcium phosphate. When taking actions, the nurse should instruct the client to report burning with urination to the provider because this can indicate a urinary tract infection. When taking actions, the nurse should remind the client to increase their fluid intake to 2 to 3 L/day. A decrease in fluid intake can cause dehydration, which increases the risk for renal calculi.

   Ⓝ *NCLEX® Connection: Reduction of Risk Potential, Therapeutic Procedures*

4. B, E. **CORRECT**: When taking actions, the nurse should reinforce to the client who has passed a calcium oxalate renal calculus to avoid foods composed of calcium oxalate such as peanuts. Other foods composed of calcium oxalate include Swiss chard, parsley, strawberries and chocolate.

   Ⓝ *NCLEX® Connection: Physiological Adaptation, Alterations in Body Systems*

5. C. **CORRECT**: The nurse should analyze the findings and determine that the priority hypothesis is that the client is at greatest risk for damage to the kidney resulting in obstruction of urine flow as a result of the renal calculi. Therefore, the nurse should report absence of urinary output for 1 hr to the provider immediately.

   Ⓝ *NCLEX® Connection: Physiological Adaptation, Unexpected Response to Therapies*

Active Learning Scenario Key

Using the ATI Active Learning Template: Medication

THERAPEUTIC USES
- Morphine sulfate, an opioid, is administered during the first 24 hr to treat moderate to severe pain associated with acute renal calculi.
- Oxybutynin, a spasmolytic, is administered to provide pain relief by decreasing bladder spasms resulting from renal calculi.

COMPLICATIONS
- Morphine sulfate: respiratory depression, euphoria, sedation, decreased GI motility
- Oxybutynin: dizziness, tachycardia, urinary retention, dry mouth, constipation, nausea

NURSING INTERVENTIONS
- Morphine sulfate
  - Administer cautiously with clients who have asthma or emphysema due to the risk of respiratory depression.
  - Monitor frequently for respiratory depression, especially in older adults. If respirations are 12/min or less, stop the medication and notify the provider immediately.
  - Monitor vital signs frequently for hypotension.
  - Encourage the client to drink plenty of fluids to prevent constipation.
- Oxybutynin
  - Determine prior to administration if the client has a history of glaucoma, as this medication increases intraocular pressure.
  - Monitor for dizziness and tachycardia.
  - Monitor for urinary retention.
  - Instruct the client to report palpitations and problems with voiding or constipation.
  - Inform the client that dizziness and dry mouth are common with the medication.
  - Encourage the client to suck on hard candies to alleviate dry mouth and practice good oral hygiene measures.
  - Increase fiber or bulk in diet.

Ⓝ *NCLEX® Connection: Pharmacological Therapies, Expected Actions/Outcomes*

When reviewing the following chapters, keep in mind the relevant topics and tasks of the NCLEX outline.

Health Promotion and Maintenance

HEALTH PROMOTION/DISEASE PREVENTION: Participate in health screening or health promotion programs.

Reduction of Risk Potential

DIAGNOSTIC TESTS: Perform diagnostic testing.

LABORATORY VALUES: Compare client laboratory values to normal laboratory values.

THERAPEUTIC PROCEDURES: Reinforce client teaching on treatments and procedures.

POTENTIAL FOR ALTERATIONS IN BODY SYSTEMS: Monitor client output for changes from baseline.

POTENTIAL FOR COMPLICATIONS FROM SURGICAL PROCEDURES AND HEALTH ALTERATIONS: Monitor client responses to procedures and treatments.

CHAPTER 57 ## Diagnostic and Therapeutic Procedures for Reproductive Disorders

Screening tests can be used to aid in the early identification of certain cancers of the reproductive system. The American Cancer Society (ACS) recommends that clients who are considered average risk should make an informed decision with their provider about routine screening tests for the early detection of cancer (breast, testicular, prostate) after receiving information about the potential benefits, risks, and uncertainties of cancer screening tests. The client should only be screened after receiving this information. Clients at high risk should be highly encouraged to obtain routine screening examination/testing.

Laboratory testing can be used to identify unexpected findings and manage the client's condition. Diagnostic tests and therapeutic procedures are used to evaluate the structure, condition, and function of a client's reproductive tissues and organs. Biopsies can also serve as therapeutic purposes in identifying and removing suspected lesions or harmful tissue. Surgical removal of the affected organ may also be warranted.

SCREENING TESTS

BREAST EXAM

The ACS states clinical breast exams are not recommended for breast cancer screening among average-risk clients at any age. Clients who are considered average risk do not have a personal or have not family history of breast cancer, do not have genetic mutations (BRCA gene), or received chest radiation prior to 30 years of age. The ACS also suggests that these clinical and breast self-exams (BSE) be performed if the client is at high risk, stating there is little evidence to support that these tests assist with detecting breast cancer early when clients also get screening mammograms. Most unexpected findings (lumps, lesions) are detected when the client performs their routine ADLs. When a clinical breast exam is performed, the provider will inspect and palpate each breast. The client can be sitting and then asked to lie down and position their arms to their side or raise over their head. When performing a BSE, the client should inspect the size, shape, and coloration of each breast, and palpate in a systematic manner for any lesions or masses.

CLIENT EDUCATION
- Inform the client to become familiar with how their breasts look and feel.
- Notify the provider immediately of any unexpected findings.

PELVIC AND BIMANUAL EXAM

An examination performed by a provider to examine the external and internal reproductive organs. The client is placed in a lithotomy position while provided privacy (draping). Prior to examination, the environment should be comfortable, and adequate lighting should be provided. During an external pelvic examination, the provider can inspect and palpate the external genitalia for any unexpected findings (trauma, lesions, masses). During the internal pelvic examination, the provider inserts a warm, lubricated speculum into the client's vagina to examine the cervix. The provider can also perform cervical cancer screening test Papanicolaou test (Pap smear) and HPV testing, and cervical cultures for STIs during the internal examination. A bimanual exam is an internal exam in which the provider inserts two lubricated gloved fingers into the vagina and traps the reproductive structures between the fingers of the one hand and the fingers of the opposite hand that is on the abdomen and palpates the client's internal reproductive structures (cervix, uterus, ovaries, fallopian tubes) to identify any unexpected findings (masses, lesions).

CLIENT EDUCATION
- Inform client to schedule this examination 6-10 days after their last menstrual cycle (if present).
- Inform client to void prior to examination.
- During internal examination, inform client to take deep breaths and relax muscles and "bear down" while speculum is being inserted.

TESTICULAR EXAM

An exam by the provider in which each testicle is palpated separately for swelling, tenderness, and lumps (size and location). Most providers agree that a testicular exam should be part of the client's physical exam during their routine check-up. The ACS suggest that clients should make their own decision about performing self-testicular exams; however, if the client is at high risk, they should seriously consider monthly self-testicular exams.

CLIENT EDUCATION: Provide client with information about how to perform self-testicular exams.
- Perform the self-exam during or after bath or shower.
- Hold the penis out of the way and examine each testicle separately.
- Gently roll each testicle by holding it with your thumbs and fingers of both hands.
- Note any lumps or nodules (smooth round masses) or changes in the size, shape, or consistency of your testicles.

DIGITAL RECTAL EXAM (DRE)

DRE is done in an office or clinic in which a provider can examine the client's prostate, rectum, pelvis, and lower abdomen to identify any unexpected findings such as lesions or masses. The ACS recommends that a discussion for prostate cancer screening occur at the following intervals.
- Age 40 for clients who are at greatest risk (more than one first-degree relative (parent, sibling) who had prostate cancer at an early age).
- Age 45 for clients who are at high risk (clients who are African American, or clients who have a first-degree relative diagnosed with prostate cancer at an early age [less than 65 years of age])
- Age 50 for clients who are at average risk with a life expectancy of 10 or more years

After this discussion between the client and their provider occurs, the client should then decide and provide consent to screening and testing (DRE exam and prostate-specific antigen (PSA) blood test). The client is positioned by leaning over the examination table (or side-lying fetal position). The provider inserts their gloved and lubricated finger in the client's anus and can palpate the rectum, anus, or prostate. If the provider identifies any unexpected findings, the client may require further testing (ultrasounds, biopsies) to determine the exact finding.

CLIENT EDUCATION: May feel the urge to urinate during examination

LABORATORY TESTS

STI PANEL (BLOOD, CULTURE, URINE)

Syphilis

TYPE OF SCREENING TEST
- Darkfield exam and molecular testing directly from lesion drainage or tissue sample used for definitive diagnosis (CDC, 2021)
- Presumptive diagnosis: use of 2 laboratory blood test: nontreponemal tests: (Venereal Disease research Laboratory (VDRL) or Rapid Plasma Reagin (RPR), which is more sensitive)
- Treponemal tests: pallidum passive particle agglutination (TP-PA) assay, various EIAs, chemiluminescence immunoassays (CIAs) and immunoblots, or rapid treponemal assay
- Neurosyphilis: If clinical findings are present; may need to test CSF

INTERPRETATION OF FINDINGS
- Nonreactive (negative for syphilis) or reactive (positive for syphilis)
- Reactive (positive for syphilis) diagnosis should be confirmed using one of the following tests.
- Confirmation testing for reactive/positive results
- Fluorescent treponemal antibody absorption (FTA-ABS) or enzyme-linked immunosorbent assay (ELISA/EIA)
- If FTA-ABS or ELISA (non-reactive), provider may need to look for other conditions that cause positive (reactive) results.

SCREENING RECOMMENDATIONS ACCORDING TO CDC 2021
- Screen asymptomatic adults and females who have intercourse with females who have an increased risk for developing syphilis.
- Males who have sex with males (MSM): At least annually if sexually active or every 3-6 months if at increased risk
- LGBTQIA populations: Consider at least annual screening based upon the clients, report of sexual behaviors and exposure.
- Clients with HIV: For sexually active individuals, screen at first HIV evaluation, and at least annually thereafter; frequency will vary depending upon the client's individual risk behaviors and local epidemiology.

HIV

TYPE OF SCREENING TEST
- Blood sample: (new oral fluid, urine)
- Immunology: identifies antibodies developed as result of HIV1/HIV2 infection
- Virologic: identifies RNA (DNA) specific to HIV
- Nucleic acid amplification testing (NAAT): more expensive; detects HIV 11 days after infection

INTERPRETATION OF FINDINGS

- False positive results can occur, so further testing is needed.
- If results are positive, then confirmation testing should be performed.
- The Western blot assay and the immunofluorescence assay (IFA) are used to confirm the diagnosis of HIV. The IFA is more sensitive and can discriminate between HIV1/HIV2.

SCREENING RECOMMENDATIONS ACCORDING TO CDC 2021

- Encourage all male and female clients who are 13-64 years of age to receive screening, and clients who request evaluation for management for STIs should receive testing.
- CDC recommends annual screening if at high risk.
- Males who have sex with males (MSM): At least annually for sexually active if HIV status is unknown or negative and the client or their sex partner(s) have had more than one sex partner since most recent HIV test. Frequency can vary (every 3-6 months) for clients who are at increased risk for acquiring HIV infection.
- LGBTQIA populations: Discuss and offer screening to all clients; frequency of repeat screenings to be determined by the client's risk level.

Genital herpes (HSV)

TYPE OF SCREENING TEST: Diagnosis: Based on the client's history and physical examination

Confirmation

- Herpes viral culture: Fluid from a lesion is obtained using a swab and placed in a cup for culture. Low sensitivity especially for recurrent lesions that begin to heal; may need specific typing for HSV
- Polymerase chain reaction (PCR) test: Identifies genetic material of the virus. Cells from a lesion, blood, or other body fluids can be tested. Identifies type of virus (herpes simplex 1 [HSV 1] or herpes simplex 2 [HSV 2]).
- Antibody test: Blood is tested for antibodies to the virus. Some tests can identify the type of virus. An immunoblot and ELISA test can be used to differentiate between HSV 1 and HSV 2.

INTERPRETATION OF FINDINGS: Recurrences and subclinical shedding are much more frequent for HSV-2 genital herpes infection than for HSV-1 genital herpes (439,440). Therefore, prognosis and counseling depend on which HSV type is present.

SCREENING RECOMMENDATIONS ACCORDING TO CDC 2021

- Type-specific HSV serologic testing can be considered for male and female clients who present for an STI evaluation (especially for male and female clients who have multiple sex partners).
- Males who have sex with males (MSM): Type-specific serologic tests can be considered if infection status is unknown in MSM with previously undiagnosed genital tract infection.
- Clients with HIV: Type-specific HSV serologic testing can be considered for clients who present for an STI evaluation (especially for clients who have multiple sex partners).

Gonorrhea

TYPE OF SCREENING TEST

- Cultures/swabs: (endocervical/urethral, anal, oropharyngeal): NAAT, POC, NAAT
- Urine specimens

INTERPRETATION OF FINDINGS: Positive: Retest all clients 3 months after treatment if not feasible, then provider should provide retesting whenever the client seeks healthcare less than 12 months after initial treatment.

SCREENING RECOMMENDATIONS ACCORDING TO CDC 2021

- Females: Annually for sexually active females who are < 25 years of age; sexually active females who are > than 25 years of age if at increased risk (those who have a new sex partner, more than one sex partner, a sex partner with concurrent partners, or a sex partner who has an STI; pharyngeal and rectal screening can be considered in females based on reported sexual behaviors and exposure, through shared clinical decision between the client and their provider.
- Males who have sex with females: There is insufficient evidence for screening among heterosexual male clients who are at low risk for infection.
- Males who have sex with males (MSM): At least annually for sexually active MSM at sites of contact (urethra, rectum, pharynx (gonorrhea) regardless of condom use; frequency can vary (every 3-6 months) if at increased risk
- LGBTQIA populations: Screening recommendations should be adapted based on anatomy (i.e., annual, routine screening for gonorrhea in cisgender females < 25 years old should be extended to all transgender males and gender diverse people with a cervix. If over 25 years old, screen if at increased risk); pharyngeal/rectal screening can be considered based on the client's reported sexual behaviors and exposure.
- Clients with HIV: Screen at first HIV evaluation for clients who are sexually active, and at least annually thereafter; frequency will vary depending on individual risk behaviors and the local epidemiology.

Chlamydia

TYPE OF SCREENING TEST

- Cultures/swabs (DNA probes, NAAT): pharyngeal, endocervical/urethral
- Urine specimens: (NAAT) first voided urine
- Blood studies
- POC test for clients who are asymptomatic

INTERPRETATION OF FINDINGS: Positive: Retest all clients 3 months after treatment if not feasible, then provider should provide retesting whenever the client seeks healthcare less than 12 months after initial treatment

SCREENING RECOMMENDATIONS ACCORDING TO CDC 2021

- Females: Annually for sexually active females who are < 25 years of age; sexually active females who are > than 25 years of age if at increased risk (those who have a new sex partner, more than one sex partner, a sex partner with concurrent partners, or a sex partner who has an STI; rectal screening can be considered in females based on reported sexual behaviors and exposure, through shared clinical decision between the client and their provider
- Males who have sex with females: There is insufficient evidence for screening among heterosexual male clients who are at low risk for infection; chlamydia screening for young male clients can be considered in clinical setting with high prevalence (correctional facilities, STI/sex health clinics).
- Males who have sex with males (MSM): At least annually for sexually active MSM at sites of contact (urethra, rectum, pharynx (gonorrhea) regardless of condom use; frequency can vary (every 3-6 months) if at increased risk
- LGBTQIA populations: Screening recommendations should be adapted based on anatomy (i.e., annual, routine screening for gonorrhea in cisgender females < 25 years old should be extended to all transgender males and gender diverse people with a cervix. If over 25 years old, screen if at increased risk); pharyngeal/rectal screening can be considered based on the client's reported sexual behaviors and exposure
- Clients with HIV: Screen at first HIV evaluation for clients who are sexually active, and at least annually thereafter; frequency will vary depending on individual risk behaviors and the local epidemiology.

Trichomonas

TYPE OF SCREENING TEST

- Microscopic Wet-mount
- Females: NAAT (vaginal swabs, urine specimens) some liquid Pap smear cytology specimens can incidentally detect
- Males: Cultures: urethral swabs, urine sediment, semen

INTERPRETATION OF FINDINGS

- Positive: Testing for other STIs, including HIV, syphilis, gonorrhea, and chlamydia should be considered.
- Negative: Retesting for all females who are sexually active after 3 months of initial treatment; or retest whenever the client seeks healthcare in less than 12 months after initial treatment. Insufficient data to support retesting in clients who are male after treatment

SCREENING RECOMMENDATIONS ACCORDING TO CDC 2021

- Females: Consider annual screening for females receiving care in high-prevalence settings (e.g., STI clinics and correctional facilities) and for asymptomatic females at high risk for infection (e.g., female with multiple sex partners, transactional sex, drug misuse, or a history of STI or incarceration).
- Clients with HIV: For clients who are female and sexually active, recommend screening at first initial provider visit and at least annually thereafter.

Genital warts (HPV)

TYPE OF SCREENING TEST

- Visual inspection of lesions by a provider; cytology of cervical and anal lesions, HPV testing (DNA)
- In recent years, the HPV test has been approved as another screening test for cervical cancer. The HPV test looks for infection by high-risk types of HPV that are more likely to cause pre-cancers and cancers of the cervix. The HPV test can be used alone (primary HPV test) or at the same time as the Pap test (called a co-test).

INTERPRETATION OF FINDINGS: Clients who are 25-65 years of age should have primary HPV test every 5 years. If primary HPV testing is unavailable, screening can be done with a co-test that combines HPV test with Papanicolaou (Pap) test every 5 years or Pap test alone every 3 years.

SCREENING RECOMMENDATIONS ACCORDING TO CDC 2021

- Females: Females who are 21-29 years of age every 3 years with cytology; females who are 30-65 years every 3 years with cytology, or every 5 years with co-test (cytology and HPV) testing; American Cancer Society (ACS) (2021) recommends that clients who are 25-65 years of age (with a cervix): HPV co-test with Pap smear (cytology) every 5 years or with Pap test alone every 3 years
- Males who have sex with males (MSM): Digital anorectal rectal exam; routine anal cancer screening with anal cytology is not currently recommended due to insufficient data
- LGBTQIA populations: Screening for clients with a cervix should follow current screening guidelines for cervical cancer.
- Clients with HIV: Females who have HIV should be screened within 1 year of sexual activity using conventional or liquid-based cytology; testing should be repeated 6 months later. With 3 normal and consecutive Pap tests, screening should be every 3 years.

Hepatitis B

TYPE OF SCREENING TEST: Blood testing for hepatitis B surface antigen (HBsAg) or antibody (HBsAb) or core antibodies (HBcAb)

INTERPRETATION OF FINDINGS

- The presence of HBsAg and anti-HBc, with a negative test for IgM anti-HBc, indicates chronic HBV infection.
- The presence of total anti-HBc alone might indicate acute, resolved, or chronic infection or a false-positive result.

SCREENING RECOMMENDATIONS ACCORDING TO CDC 2021

- Females: Females at increased risk (having had more than one sex partner in the previous 6 months, evaluation, or treatment for an STI, past or current injection-drug use, and an HBsAg-positive sex partner)
- Males who have sex with females: Males at increased risk (i.e., by sexual or percutaneous exposure)
- Males who have sex with males (MSM): All MSM should be tested for HBsAg, HBV core antibody, and HBV surface antibody.
- Clients with HIV: Test for HBsAg and anti-HBc and/or anti-HBs.

Hepatitis C

TYPE OF SCREENING TEST

- Blood testing for HCV antibodies
- FDA-cleared test for antibody to HCV (i.e., immunoassay, EIA, or enhanced CIA and, if recommended, a supplemental antibody test) followed by NAAT to detect HCV RNA for those with a positive antibody.
- Clients who have HIV and low CD4+ T-cell count might require further testing by NAAT because of the potential for a false-negative antibody assay.

INTERPRETATION OF FINDINGS: Positive: (i.e., positive for HCV RNA) should be evaluated for treatment. Antibody to HCV remains positive after spontaneously resolving or successful treatment; therefore, subsequent testing for HCV reinfection among clients with ongoing risk factors should be limited to HCV RNA. Clients who have spontaneous resolution or who have undergone successful management are not immune to reinfection.

SCREENING RECOMMENDATIONS ACCORDING TO CDC 2021

- All clients who are greater than 18 years of age should be screened for hepatitis C except in settings where the hepatitis C infection (HCV) positivity is < 0.1%
- Clients with HIV: Serologic testing at initial evaluation; annual testing in MSM with HIV infection

Mammography

During a mammogram, the breasts are compressed vertically and horizontally by the mammography machine while radiologic pictures are taken of each breast. Traditional mammography images are stored on film while digital mammography takes an electronic image and can be more useful in clients who have dense breast tissue. Digital mammograms are more expensive.

Several organizations provide guidelines for screening mammograms, including the American Cancer Society and the U.S. Preventive Services Task Force. For current guidelines, see www.cancer.org and www.uspreventiveservicestaskforce.org. The ACS recommends the following guidelines for screening mammograms.

- Clients who are 40-44 years of age should have the have the option to start screening mammograms annually.
- Clients who are 45-54 years of age should obtain screening mammograms annually.
- Clients who are > 55 years of age can switch to a mammogram every other year, or they can choose to continue yearly mammograms. Routine screenings should continue for as long as the client is in good health and is expected to live at least 10 more years.
- All clients should be informed about the benefits, limitation, and potential harm of screening.

INDICATIONS

- Detect unexpected findings (cancers, lesions, tumors, cysts) prior to being palpable
- **Screening mammograms:** detect breast cancer lesions in clients who do not have manifestations. Screening mammograms decrease cancer death rates because the treatment options and outcomes are best when the cancer is detected early.
- **Diagnostic mammograms** are used when a screening mammogram reveals abnormal findings or when breast cancer manifestations are present. The diagnostic mammogram provides a more detailed picture and is more accurate than the screening mammogram.

CONSIDERATIONS

POTENTIAL CONTRAINDICATIONS

- Age less than 25
- Pregnancy (unless benefits are greater than risks)

	INDICATIONS	EXPECTED REFERENCE RANGES	INTERPRETATION OF FINDINGS	
			INCREASED VALUES	DECREASED VALUES
ESTROGEN (TOTAL)	Sexual maturity, menopause status, menstrual/fertility problems, fetal/placental well-being; evaluate gynecomastia and feminization syndrome.	N/A	Feminization syndrome, precocious puberty, ovarian/ testicular/adrenal tumors, normal pregnancy (E3), hyperthyroidism, liver necrosis	Turner syndrome, hyperpituitarism, menopause, anorexia nervosa, pregnancy complications (E3)
ESTRADIOL (E2)	Produced in ovaries primarily, commonly used to evaluate menstrual and fertility problems	Male: 10-50 pg/mL Female: 20-750* pg/mL Postmenopausal: < 20 pg/mL		
ESTRIOL (E3)	Major estrogen in pregnancy	N/A		
ESTRONE (E1)	Secreted by ovary, major circulating estrogen after menopause			
FOLLICLE-STIMULATING HORMONE (FSH)	Stimulates production of ovarian follicles; stimulates Sertoli cell development, maturation of the ovaries and testes, spermatogenesis. Aids in the identification of menopause, testicular dysfunction, evaluation of infertility	Male: 1.42-15.4 IU/L Female: 1.09-17.2* IU/L Postmenopausal: 19.3-100.6 U/L	Gonad failure, menopause, testicular dysgenesis, castration, hypogonadism, polycystic ovaries, precocious puberty, pituitary adenoma	Stress, pituitary/ hypothalamic failure, anorexia nervosa, nutritional deficiencies
LUTEINIZING HORMONE (LH)	LH produced in the anterior pituitary in response to stimulation by gonadotropin-releasing hormone (GnRH). LH stimulates testosterone production, spermatogenesis, stimulates follicular production estrogen, ovulation, and the formation of the corpus luteum. Aids in the identification of menopause, testicular dysfunction, evaluation of infertility	Male: 1.24-7.8 IU/L Female: 0.61-56.6* IU/L Postmenopausal: 14.2-52.3 IU/L		
PROGESTERONE	Used to evaluate clients who are having problems with becoming pregnant or maintain pregnancy. Progesterone initiates secretory phase of endometrium for the anticipation of implantation of fertilized ovum, evaluation ovulation.	Male: 10-50 ng/dL Female: < 50-2500* ng/dL Postmenopausal: < 40 ng/dL	Ovulation, pregnancy, luteal ovarian cysts, adrenocortical hyperplasia, ovarian choriocarcinoma, molar pregnancy	Preeclampsia, threatened miscarriage, placental failure, fetal demise, amenorrhea, ovarian neoplasm
PROLACTIN	Secreted by the anterior pituitary, promotes lactation, useful for monitoring pituitary adenomas	Male: 3-13 ng/mL Female: 3-27 ng/mL	Galactorrhea, amenorrhea, prolactin secreting pituitary tumor, hypothyroidism, stress, polycystic ovarian syndrome (PCO), kidney failure	Pituitary destruction by tumor
EARLY PROSTATE CANCER ANTIGEN (EPCA)	Determines the amount of protein in blood that is only produced by unexpected prostate cell to determine if biopsy is needed EPCA-2 is highly sensitive in detecting prostate cancer; some providers are using this test in place of a biopsy. Follow ACS recommendations for PSA.	< 30 ng/mL	Prostate cancer (values greater than 30 ng/mL)	

	INDICATIONS	EXPECTED REFERENCE RANGES	INTERPRETATION OF FINDINGS	
			INCREASED VALUES	DECREASED VALUES
TESTOSTERONE (TOTAL)	Evaluates for infertility, impotence, precocious puberty, ambiguous sex traits, virilizing syndrome	Male: 280 to 1080 ng/dL Female: Less than 70 ng/dL	Adrenocortical tumor, testicular or extragonadal tumor, hyperthyroidism, ovarian/adrenal tumor, polycystic ovaries, idiopathic hirsutism	Klinefelter syndrome, cryptorchidism, orchiectomy, Trisomy 21
PROSTATE SPECIFIC ANTIGEN (PSA)	Measures the amount of protein produced by prostate. Measured before DRE (palpation can cause elevated PSA levels). Test can detect prostate cancer and stage cancer of the prostate. The ACS recommends against having routine screening if the client is at average risk. Other recommendations by the ACS include: • If the client desires testing, and the initial PSA is less than 2.5 ng/mL, may only need to be retested every 2 years. • Screening should be done yearly for men whose PSA level is 2.5 ng/mL or higher. • Clients without symptoms of prostate cancer and a less than 10-year life expectancy should not be offered testing since they are not likely to benefit because prostate cancer grows slowly. • The client's overall health status, and not age alone, should be considered when making decisions about screening. • After a decision about testing has been made, the discussion about the risks and benefits of testing should be repeated as new information becomes available. Further discussions are also needed to consider changes in the client's health, values, and preferences.	Low: 0 to 2.5 ng/mL Slight-moderate elevated: 2.6 to 10 ng/mL Moderately elevated: 10.1 to 19.9 ng/mL Significantly elevated: Greater than 20 ng/mL	BPH, prostatitis, cancer of the prostate PSA levels increase with age. PSA greater than 4 ng/mL may require further evaluation depending upon the client's age/ The client can have an elevated PSA level for up to 6 weeks following a urinary tract infection.	

Other tests

COMPLETE BLOOD COUNT (CBC)	To evaluate any evidence of systemic infection or anemia from hematuria			

*Results can vary depending on client's phase of menstrual cycle when testing is performed.

CLIENT EDUCATION Q EBP

- Provide information about procedure (what to expect when getting a mammogram for breast cancer screening – what the test can and cannot do.
- Potential discomfort during procedure.
- Avoid the use of deodorant, lotion, or powders in the axillary region or on the breasts prior to the exam (could interfere with results of the examination).
- Examine and inspect the breasts regularly to detect changes.
- Follow the advice of the provider regarding when to return for a follow-up mammogram.

PREPROCEDURE

- Inform the client to disrobe from waist up.
- Instruct client to point to any areas of concern (these will be marked for further evaluation).

INTRAPROCEDURE

- Radiologic technicians are often the members of the health care team who perform mammograms.
- The client can feel slight, temporary discomfort when the breast is compressed.

POSTPROCEDURE

Allow client privacy while re-dressing.

Papanicolaou test (Pap test/smear)

During the pelvic examination, a provider obtains cervical fluid/cells by using a brush or spatula and sends the specimen off for cytology or pathology. The most common types of Pap smears include liquid-based, which uses a preservative, Thin Prep, and conventional, also known as CPT, with the use of slides). A co-test (Papanicolaou [Pap test/smear] and HPV testing can detect unexpected cervical findings (lesions, cancer, dysplasia, HPV). There are different recommended guidelines for cervical cancer screenings. The most common are from the American Cancer Society (ACS) and the U.S. Preventive Services Task Force (USPSTF). Refer to chart/table for Pap test screening recommendations from the ACS 62.2. Regardless, clients should be screened regularly for cervical cancer.

INDICATIONS

The Pap test is used to identify precancerous and cancerous cells of the cervix. The HPV test is used to identify HPV infections that can lead to cervical cancer. Screening tests offer the best chance to have cervical cancer found early when treatment can be most successful.

CONSIDERATIONS

POTENTIAL CONTRAINDICATIONS

- Client who is menstruating
- Client who has a vaginal infection
- Age greater than 65, with low risk
- Clients who have had a total hysterectomy (removal of the uterus and cervix) should stop screening (such as Pap tests and HPV tests) unless the hysterectomy was done as a treatment for cervical cancer or serious pre-cancer. Clients who have had a hysterectomy without removal of the cervix (called a supra-cervical hysterectomy) should continue cervical cancer screening according to the guidelines.

CLIENT EDUCATION Q EBP

- Schedule Pap smear testing at least 6 days after last menstrual cycle if indicated.
- Refrain from using vaginal medications, douching, or having sexual intercourse within 24 hours prior to examination which can alter test results.
- May experience mild cramping minimal during the examination and cervical bleeding after the examination,
- Follow up with the provider if there are any unexpected findings.

PREPROCEDURE

- Explain purpose of test.
- Ensure informed consent is obtained.
- Instruct client to empty bladder prior to testing (assists with provider when performing pelvic exam when palpating).
- Assist the client into a lithotomy position and drape appropriately.
- Gather supplies/equipment and ensure adequate lighting.
- Provide privacy.

57.2 PAP and HPV screening guidelines

25 YEARS OF AGE	Begin cervical cancer screening. If primary HPV testing is unavailable, screening can be done with a co-test that combines HPV test with Papanicolaou (Pap) test every 5 years or individual Pap test every 3 years. If the client has received HPV vaccine, the ACS recommends routine screening for HPV according to guidelines.
25-65 YEARS OF AGE (WITH CERVIX)	Primary HPV test every 5 years. If primary HPV testing is unavailable, screening can be done with a co-test that combines HPV test with Papanicolaou (Pap) test every 5 years or individual Pap test every 3 years. If the client has received HPV vaccine, the ACS recommends routine screening for HPV according to guidelines.
65 AND OLDER	If client has had regular screening in the past 10 years with normal results and no history of CIN2 or other serious diagnosis within the past 25 years, they should stop cervical cancer screening. Once stopped, it should not be started again.

Based on the recommendations by the American Cancer Society (ACS) 2020

INTRAPROCEDURE

- Remain with the client and provide support.
- Have ready the necessary equipment for the provider during procedure.
- Transfer specimens to appropriate containers (specimen containers or slides (apply fixative to slides).

POSTPROCEDURE

Provide the client with perineal pads and tissues (potential for bleeding after the procedure).

Abdominal/pelvic/ breast ultrasound

Noninvasive procedure that uses sound waves for evaluation of the scanned area. Can be performed in provider's office or radiology department. Used to evaluate tissue

INDICATIONS

- Identifying and monitoring of masses, cysts, and fibroids
- Guide needle directed biopsies of suspected tumor site
- Stage tumors
- Evaluate pregnancy and placenta, and fetal status and identify any unexpected findings (abdominal/pelvic)
- Detect abscesses and direct drainage
- Monitoring the effects of tumor-reducing treatment
- Evaluate trauma
- Identify causes of pain
- Follow-up of lesions noted during mammography (breast)

CONSIDERATIONS

POTENTIAL CONTRAINDICATIONS

Latex allergy: Ultrasound probe is covered by a latex sac. Therefore, it is important to check the client for a latex allergy prior to the procedure. (transvaginal). Qs

CLIENT EDUCATION QEBP

- A full/empty bladder will vary depending on type of ultrasound.
- For transvaginal ultrasound, a transducer probe will be inserted into the vagina.
- For breast ultrasound, the chest will be exposed.
- For internal (transvaginal or transrectal) ultrasound, mild discomfort can be experienced.
- For abdominal ultrasound, a full bladder can be required to promote better visualization of the internal organs.

PREPROCEDURE

- Explain procedure to client.
- Ensure informed consent is obtained (if a transducer is used or biopsy is planned).
- Fasting is dependent upon the organ being scanned (abdominal).
- Do not apply lotions or powders to the breast on day of exam (breast).

INTRAPROCEDURE

- Transducer gel lubricant is applied to the area overlying the organ to be evaluated.
- Place client in prone or supine position (dependent upon organ to be examined).

POSTPROCEDURE

Wipe transducer gel off area.

Transrectal ultrasound (TRUS) and prostate biopsy

TRUS is used to detect prostate cancer. A biopsy can be performed during TRUS if prostate cancer is suspected. This procedure can be performed in provider's office (urologist) or radiology department.

INDICATIONS

- If a client's PSA is elevated or has unexpected findings during a DRE, the provider may refer the client for a TRUS.
- Diagnosis of prostate cancer (staging/monitoring)
- Detection of perirectal abscesses
- Guide a prostate biopsy (biopsy needle is inserted into the transrectal area during TRUS and tissue specimens are obtained)

CONSIDERATIONS

POTENTIAL CONTRAINDICATIONS

- Clients who take anticoagulants (warfarin, aspirin) should discuss with provider if these medications should be withheld prior to procedure (biopsy).
- Latex allergy (a latex covering maybe used to cover the ultrasound probe) Qs

CLIENT EDUCATION Q_EBP

- Take enema 1 hour prior to the procedure (if prescribed).
- Instruct the client about breathing and relaxation techniques to be used during the procedure.
- Inform client if biopsy was performed, there could be mild discomfort, slight hematuria (urine pink-to light red), and scant rectal bleeding for a few days following procedure.
- Inform client to take mild analgesic for discomfort following biopsy.
- Notify provider of increased discomfort; fever; prolonged and heavy, bright red bleeding; dysuria; and swelling following biopsy.

PREPROCEDURE

- Explain procedure with client and allow the client to express concerns or potential fears.
- Ensure informed consent is obtained.
- Check for allergies to latex.
- Obtain urinalysis if indicated (check for UTI, may need to reschedule biopsy).

INTRAPROCEDURE

- DRE can be performed to check prostate or identify any tumors.
- Ultrasound probe (covered and lubricated) is inserted into the client's rectum.
- If biopsy is performed, assist the client into a side-lying knee-chest position.

POSTPROCEDURE

- Provide the client with items to cleanse perianal area (tissue, wipes).
- Refrain from strenuous activity (heavy lifting) for at least 24 hr following biopsy.

COMPLICATIONS

- Infection (biopsy)
- Hemorrhage (biopsy)

Hysterosalpingography

Visualization of the cervix, uterus, and fallopian tubes by fluoroscopic x-ray with injection of contrast dye. Performed 6-11 days following the client's last (decreases risk of pregnancy and avoids menstruation)

INDICATIONS

- Evaluation of fertility (fallopian tube patency/obstruction)
- Evaluation of anatomy following tubal ligation or reversal
- Evaluation of conditions (fibroids, fistulas, tumors)

CONSIDERATIONS

POTENTIAL CONTRAINDICATIONS

- Clients who have infections of reproductive system
- Clients who have uterine bleeding
- Clients who are pregnant

CLIENT EDUCATION Q_EBP

- Instruct client to take laxative the night prior to procedure (if prescribed).
- Vaginal discharge (bloody) can occur 1-2 days following procedure.
- Cramping and dizziness are expected findings following procedure.
- Notify the provider if signs of infection are present (fever, tachycardia, pain).

PREPROCEDURE

- Confirm date of client's last menstrual cycle.
- Check for allergy to iodine or shellfish.
- Ensure the client has provided informed consent.
- Administer enemas/suppositories the morning of the procedure (if prescribed).
- Administer sedatives/ antispasmodics (if prescribed).
- Ensure client voids prior to procedure.

INTRAPROCEDURE

- Remain with the client and provide support.
- Place the client in lithotomy position.
- Have ready the necessary equipment for the provider during the procedure.

POSTPROCEDURE

Provide client with items for perineal care (perineal pad and tissues).

COMPLICATIONS

- Infection: endometritis, salpingitis
- Perforation of uterus

Colposcopy and cervical biopsy

A colposcopy is the examination of cervix, vagina, vulva, and anus by using a colposcope (macroscope with light and magnifier lens). Allows for direct examination of unexpected lesions. During a colposcopy, the provider can perform an endocervical curettage (scraping of endometrial tissue) or cervical biopsy (sample of cervical tissue). The best time to perform the biopsy procedure is in the early phase of the menstrual cycle because the cervix is less vascular.

INDICATIONS

- Pap test results with atypical or unexpected findings (HPV, dysplasia)
- Determines need for cone biopsy (an extensive biopsy that removes cone-shaped sample of tissue from cervix to remove harmful cells). In some cases, anesthesia is used for the procedure. Margins of the excised tissue are examined to ensure removal of all harmful cells. The surgeon can destroy the cells using a scalpel, cryosurgery (extreme cold, which freezes the tissue), lasers, or loop electrosurgical excision (LEEP). LEEP uses an electric current, and the laser procedure uses a laser beam that vaporizes the abnormal tissue.

CONSIDERATIONS

POTENTIAL CONTRAINDICATIONS

Clients who have heavy menstrual flow

CLIENT EDUCATION QEBP

- Instruct client not to douche or use vaginal prep for at least 24-48 hours prior to the procedure.
- If a biopsy is performed, there could be minor discomfort and cramping that is temporary.
- Expect vaginal bleeding (if biopsy was performed).
- Rest for the first 24 hr after the procedure.
- Abstain from sexual intercourse and no insertion of items into vagina (douche, vaginal creams, or tampons) until confirmation of healing has occurred (approximately 2 weeks).
- Avoid lifting heavy objects for approximately 2 weeks to allow time for the cervix to heal.
- Use analgesics as directed by the provider, but avoid the use of aspirin because it can cause bleeding. Qs
- Report excessive bleeding, fever, or foul-smelling drainage to the provider.

PREPROCEDURE

- Ensure informed consent is obtained.
- Explain procedure.
- Provide psychological support.
- Preprocedural care is the same as that for a Pap test.

INTRAPROCEDURE

- Speculum is used to assist with locating the cervix.
- Acetic acid is applied to cervix for cleaning and identification of lesions (iodine or potassium iodine can be used).
- If unexpected findings (lesions) are present, biopsy can be performed.
- Assist with placing the client in a lithotomy position.

POSTPROCEDURE

Cervix is cleaned with normal saline solution and hemostasis is ensured. Provide client with items for perineal care (perineal pad and tissues).

COMPLICATIONS

- **Hemorrhage:** Monitor for heavy bleeding. Inform client to report this finding to provider.
- **Infection** (Monitor for fever, chills, severe pain, foul odor, or purulent vaginal discharge. Notify provider of unexpected findings.)
- **Vasovagal response** (cardiac conditions)

Endometrial biopsy

A thin, hollow tube is inserted through the cervix, and a curette or suction equipment is used to obtain a sample of endometrial tissue. Client can report unexpected or postmenopausal bleeding. Suction endometrial biopsy is commonly performed in the provider's office.

INDICATIONS

- Check for uterine cancer.
- Evaluate menstrual irregularities.
- Evaluate unexpected findings for uterine bleeding.
- Determine cause of infertility.

CONSIDERATIONS

POTENTIAL CONTRAINDICATIONS

- Clients who have infections
- Pregnancy

CLIENT EDUCATION QEBP

- Biopsy is performed while awake.
- There could be discomfort and cramping during procedure.
- Expect vaginal spotting or mild bleeding.
- Notify provider of heavy vaginal bleeding, fever, severe pain, or foul discharge.
- Abstain from sexual intercourse and no insertion of items into vagina (douche, vaginal creams, or tampons) until discharge has stopped (1–2 days).
- Follow up with provider for results of procedure (within 1–2 weeks).

PREPROCEDURE

- Ensure informed consent is obtained.
- Explain procedure.
- Obtain the client's menstrual history.
- Prepare client for pelvic examination.
- Administer any prescribed analgesics.
- Ensure client has empty bladder.

INTRAPROCEDURE

- Speculum is used to assist with locating the cervix.
- Assist with placing the client in a lithotomy position.

POSTPROCEDURE

- Provide client with items for perineal care (perineal pad and tissues).
- Ensure specimens are sent to lab.

COMPLICATIONS

- **Hemorrhage:** Monitor for heavy bleeding. Inform client to report this finding to provider.
- **Infection** (Monitor for fever, chills, severe pain, foul odor, or purulent vaginal discharge. Notify provider of unexpected findings)
- **Perforation of uterus**

Laparoscopy

Endoscopic procedure in which a laparoscope is inserted through the abdominal wall into the peritoneum. A camera is attached to scope, which allows direct visualization of the abdominal/pelvic organs on monitors. Procedure is performed in the OR.

INDICATIONS

- Evaluate acute/chronic pain abdominal/pelvic, unexplained infertility.
- Evaluate suspected abdominal mass or cancer.
- Diagnosis conditions: adhesions, tumors, cysts, tubal and uterine causes of infertility, endometriosis, ectopic pregnancy, ruptured cysts
- Used during other procedures such as oophorectomy, tubal ligation, myomectomy, endometriosis removal, GI surgery (appendectomy, cholecystectomy), liver biopsy, nephrectomy

CONSIDERATIONS

POTENTIAL CONTRAINDICATIONS

- Clients who have had multiple abdominal surgeries
- Clients who have suspected intra-abdominal hemorrhage

CLIENT EDUCATION Q EBP

- Notify provider of findings of fever and chills, severe abdominal pain.
- May experience discomfort in shoulder and ribs (gas) from carbon dioxide inserted during the procedure
- Avoid strenuous activity for at least 1 week following procedure.

PREPROCEDURE

- Inform client to be NPO after midnight the day prior to the procedure and how to perform bowel prep (enemas), if prescribed.
- Explain procedure with client.
- Ensure client has provided informed consent.
- Ensure client voids prior to procedure.
- Prepare client for anesthesia (general/regional).

INTRAPROCEDURE

- Client is initially placed in supine position; during procedure other positions can be used.
- Urinary catheter or nasogastric tube may be inserted after general anesthesia.
- Abdomen is cleansed with antiseptic solution.
- Trocar is used for the insertion of laparoscope.
- Carbon dioxide instilled into peritoneal area to separate abdominal wall from intra-abdominal structures (enhance visualization)
- Abdominal incision(s) closed (sutures) and covered with dressing (bandages)

POSTPROCEDURE

- Monitor client frequently for bleeding (tachycardia, hypotension) and perforation (abdominal tenderness and guarding hypoactive bowel sounds). Report unexpected findings to provider.
- Administer analgesic for discomfort.

COMPLICATIONS

- Infection
- Hemorrhage
- Perforation of intestines
- Hernias (umbilical/incisional

Hysteroscopy

Endoscopic procedure in which a fiberoptic telescope (hysteroscope) is inserted through cervix to visualize the internal contents of uterus. Procedure can be performed in outpatient center or provider office.

INDICATIONS

- Identify the cause of unexpected uterine bleeding.
- Infertility
- Repeated miscarriages
- Uterine adhesions, polyps, myomas (evaluation and removal)
- Misplaced intrauterine devices (IUD)
- Endometrial ablation (destruction of lining of uterus by use of laser)
- Confirm results of hysterosalpingography.

POTENTIAL CONTRAINDICATIONS

- Clients who have infection such as PID
- Clients who are pregnant
- Clients who have cervical or endometrial cancer

CLIENT EDUCATION Q_{EBP}

- Scant vaginal bleeding and cramping is expected for 1-2 days following procedure; can take mild analgesic for discomfort.
- Notify provider of findings of fever, moderate bleeding or vaginal discharge, and severe abdominal pain.
- May experience gas discomfort

PREPROCEDURE

- Explain procedure to client.
- Ensure client has given informed consent.
- Ensure client voids prior to procedure.
- Prepare client for anesthesia (general, spinal, or light sedation, paracervical block) if indicated.
- Client may need to be NPO for at least 8 hours prior to testing.

INTRAPROCEDURE

- Client is placed in a lithotomy position.
- Vaginal area is cleansed with antiseptic solution.
- Cervix may be dilated, and a liquid or gas can be released through hysteroscope to expand the uterus.
- Client may experience some cramping during procedure.

POSTPROCEDURE

Administer analgesic for mild pain or discomfort.

COMPLICATIONS

- Infection
- Perforation of uterus

Dilation and curettage (D&C)

A diagnostic or therapeutic procedure in which cervix is dilated by using a dilator and a curette is used to scrape the endometrium of the uterus. Can be performed in OR or outpatient surgical center. A hysteroscope can be used during this procedure.

INDICATIONS

- Obtain an endometrial tissue sample (cytologic examination).
- Identify cause of irregular bleeding.
- Temporarily cease irregular uterine bleeding.
- Therapeutic procedure to remove tissue of pregnancy (incomplete abortion, miscarriage, or retained products of conception following childbirth)

CLIENT EDUCATION Q_{EBP}

- Restrict activity (no heavy lifting, strenuous activity, driving, climbing stairs, sexual intercourse).
- Notify provider if experiencing heavy bleeding, fever, chills, incisional drainage, excessive pain, swelling in calf, burning upon urination).
- May experience menopausal symptoms if ovaries were removed
- If vaginal repair was also completed, the client can experience discomfort with intercourse; may use a water-based lubricants.
- May experience psychological reactions such as sadness, mood changes
- Refer client to support groups as needed.

PREPROCEDURE

- If experiencing discomfort, take mild analgesic.
- Notify provider of fever, abdominal pain, heavy bleeding, or foul-smelling vaginal discharge.
- Refrain from sexual intercourse or inserting items into vagina (tampons) for about 2 weeks.

INTRAPROCEDURE

Assist with placing the client in lithotomy position.

POSTPROCEDURE

- Provide the client with items for perineal care (wipes, perineal pad).
- Monitor and report excessive bleeding.

COMPLICATIONS

- Uterine perforation
- Hemorrhage
- Infection

Hysterectomy

A hysterectomy is the second most common gynecological procedure in which the uterus is removed. The uterus can be removed:

- Laparoscope: The surgeon can use a laparoscopic to remove the client's uterus.
- Robot: Newer method in which a surgeon can use a robot to assist with surgery
- Vaginally: surgeon removes the uterus through the client's vagina (Surgeon can use a laparoscope to assist, and this is called Laparoscopic Vaginal Hysterectomy).
- Abdomen: Surgeon removes the uterus through an incision on the client's abdomen.

There are several options available for a client who requires a hysterectomy and, in some cases, the decision regarding which procedure is based on the client's preference in conjunction with the surgeon's recommendation. There are also procedures in which the uterus is preserved in which the surgeon removes the unexpected finding (fibroids-myomectomy procedure). The types of procedures that correlate with the hysterectomy procedure include:

- Total hysterectomy: Uterus and cervix are removed.
- Supracervical, partial or subtotal hysterectomy: Uterus is removed; cervix is not.
- Radical hysterectomy: Uterus, cervix, upper part of the vagina, and adjacent tissue (including lymph nodes) are removed.
- Salpingo-oophorectomy: Removal of the ovary and fallopian tube (Bilateral salpingo-oophorectomy is the removal of both ovaries and fallopian tubes).

INDICATIONS

- Constant pain, uterine bleeding, emotional stress
- Uterine cancer
- Noncancerous conditions: infections, fibroids, endometriosis, pelvic organ prolapse,

CONSIDERATIONS

CLIENT EDUCATION Q EBP

- Inform client to withhold these medications as prescribed prior to surgery: anticoagulants, aspirin, nonsteroidal anti-inflammatory drugs (NSAIDs), or vitamin E.
- Scant vaginal bleeding and cramping is expected for 1-2 days following procedure; can take mild analgesic for discomfort.
- Reinforce post-op teaching with the client. (TCDB, leg exercises, breathing exercises [incentive spirometer], early ambulation).
- Restrict activity following surgery (no heavy lifting, strenuous activity, climbing stairs, sexual intercourse) for up to 6 weeks depending on type of surgery.
- Notify provider of findings of infection (temperature, purulent drainage, dysuria).
- If ovaries were removed, menopausal findings could develop. Be aware of issues related to hormonal therapy.

PREPROCEDURE

- Perform prescribed pre-op laboratory test (pregnancy test to rule out pregnancy, heme/platelet).
- Administer preoperative antibiotics.
- Apply antiembolism stockings or sequential compression sleeves.
- Check client's psychological condition.
- Ensure client has been NPO prior to surgery.
- Ensure that informed consent has been obtained.

INTRAPROCEDURE

- Client is initially placed in supine position; during procedure other positions can be used.
- Insert indwelling urinary catheter.

POSTPROCEDURE

- Check the client's pain frequently.
- Administer prescribed analgesics (PCA may be used).
- Administer antibiotics as prescribed.
- Administer IV fluids.
- Advance diet as tolerated (may need clear liquids until bowel sounds return).
- Monitor vital signs frequently (fever, hypotension).
- Check breath and bowel sounds (risk of atelectasis and paralytic ileus).
- Assist the client with dangling on side of bed or ambulation.
- Take thromboembolism precautions (sequential compression devices, administer anticoagulants, ambulation).
- Check incision site, dressing (bleeding, drainage, redness, warmth, dehiscence).
- Monitor vaginal bleeding: Excess bleeding is more than 1 saturated pad in 1 hr.
- Monitor heme/platelet and WBC count (determine client risk for anemia, bleeding, infection).
- Monitor intake and output (an indwelling urinary catheter may be present and removed within 24 hours following surgery).

COMPLICATIONS

Complications are similar to other general surgeries.
- Infection (fever, odorous drainage, drainage at incision site)
- Hemorrhage (blood loss can place client at risk for hypovolemic shock.)
  ○ Monitor vital signs and heme/plat count.
  ○ Check for excessive bleeding.
  ○ Provide fluid replacement (IVFs or blood products).
- Psychological reactions
  ○ Can occur months to years following surgery. Occasional sadness is expected; however, persistent sadness or depression requires intervention (counseling).
  ○ Encourage client to express feelings and focus on positive aspects of life.
  ○ Refer client to support groups as needed.

Active Learning Scenario

A nurse is contributing to the plan of care for a client who will have a total abdominal hysterectomy. Use the ATI Active Learning Template: Therapeutic Procedure to complete this item.

NURSING INTERVENTIONS (PRE, INTRA, POST): List at least four preprocedural and postprocedural nursing actions the nurse should recommend be included in the plan of care.

Application Exercises

1. A nurse is reinforcing information with a newly licensed nurse about laboratory and diagnostic tests for STIs. Match the STI to its corresponding type of laboratory/diagnostic test.

   A. Trichomonas   1. Pap smear

   B. Syphilis   2. Viral culture

   C. Chlamydia   3. Cervical culture

   D. HSV   4. VDRL

   E. HPV   5. Wet mount

2. A nurse is reinforcing information with a client about their prescribed laboratory test and the indications for each. Match the reproductive laboratory test to its corresponding indication.

   A. FSH

   B. Progesterone

   C. PSA

   D. Estradiol

   E. Testosterone

   1. Evaluates precocious puberty, ambiguous sex traits, infertility, impotence, virilizing syndrome

   2. Evaluates menstrual and fertility conditions

   3. Detects prostate cancer and used to stage cancer of the prostate

   4. Evaluate problems of pregnancy

   5. Aids in the identification of menopause, testicular dysfunction, and evaluation of infertility

3. A nurse is reinforcing instructions with a client prior to an initial mammogram. Which of the following information should the nurse provide prior to the procedure?

   A. "You should avoid taking aspirin products prior to the exam."

   B. "You should avoid applying deodorant the day of the exam."

   C. "You should avoid sexual intercourse the day before the exam."

   D. "You should avoid exercising prior to the exam."

4. A nurse is reinforcing teaching with a client prior to an initial Papanicolaou (Pap) test. Which of the following statements should the nurse make?

   A. "You should urinate immediately after the procedure is over."

   B. "You will not feel any discomfort."

   C. "You may experience some bleeding after the procedure."

   D. "You will be assisted to a prone position during the examination."

5. A nurse is reinforcing information with a client who is scheduled for a transrectal ultrasound (TRUS) with a potential biopsy. Which of the following information should the nurse include?

   A. "You may experience scant hematuria following biopsy."

   B. "The procedure is contraindicated if you have an allergy to eggs."

   C. "The procedure is performed under general anesthesia."

   D. "You should avoid having a bowel movement for 1 hr prior to the procedure."

6. A nurse is reinforcing teaching with a client who is scheduled for a colposcopy with a cervical biopsy. Which of the following statements should the nurse include? (Select all that apply.)

   A. "The procedure can cause mild discomfort."

   B. "Avoid heavy lifting for approximately 2 weeks after the procedure."

   C. "Heavy bleeding is common during the first 12 hours after the procedure."

   D. "Plan to rest for the first 72 hours after the procedure."

   E. "Avoid the use of tampons for 2 weeks after the procedure."

7. Match each procedure listed below to the appropriate position that the client will need to be placed in for the procedure (lithotomy, side lying knee to chest, supine, prone).

   A. Hysteroscopy

   B. TRUS

   C. Laparoscopy

   D. D&C

   E. Endometrial biopsy

   F. Pelvic sonogram

1. A, 5; B, 4; C, 3; D, 2; E, 1

   When recognizing cues, the nurse should identify that screening tests for HPV include the Pap smear, which can detect HPV lesions. HSV is viral culture of lesion. An endocervical culture is used to screen for chlamydia. A VDRL test is used to screen for syphilis. A wet mount is used to identify the presence of trichomonas.

   Ⓝ NCLEX® Connection: Health Promotion and Maintenance, Health Promotion/Disease Prevention

2. A, 5; B, 4; C, 3; D, 2; E, 1

   When taking action and providing the client with information about their laboratory testing, the nurse should provide the client the following information: Testosterone levels can evaluate precocious puberty, ambiguous sex traits, infertility, impotence, and virilizing syndrome; estradiol can evaluate menstrual and fertility conditions; PSA can detect prostate cancer; progesterone is used to evaluate problems of pregnancy; and FSH aids in the identification of menopause, and testicular dysfunction and the evaluation of infertility.

   Ⓝ NCLEX® Connection: Reduction of Risk Potential/ Laboratory Values

3. B. **CORRECT:** The client should be informed not to apply any deodorant prior to examination. This could interfere with the results of testing. Taking aspirin products, having sexual intercourse, or exercising does not alter the accuracy of a mammogram.

   Ⓝ NCLEX® Connection: Reduction of Risk Potential, Therapeutic Procedures

4. A. The nurse should inform the client to urinate prior to the procedure to ensure the bladder is empty.
   B. During the examination, the nurse will assist the client into a lithotomy position, and following the procedure, there could be mild cramping.
   C. **CORRECT:** When taking action and reinforcing teaching with the client about a PAP test, the nurse should inform the client that there could be potential bleeding after the procedure. Therefore, the nurse should provide the client with items for perineal care.
   D. During the examination, the nurse will assist the client into a lithotomy position, and following the procedure, there could be mild cramping.

   Ⓝ NCLEX® Connection: Reduction of Risk Potential, Therapeutic Procedures

5. A. **CORRECT:** When taking actions and reinforcing information with a client about a TRUS, the nurse should inform the client about the potential for bleeding following a prostate biopsy. The client can experience scant hematuria and rectal bleeding. If the bleeding is heavy after 2-3 days, the client should notify their provider.

   Ⓝ NCLEX® Connection: Reduction of Risk Potential, Potential for Complications From Surgical Procedures and Health Alterations

6. A, E. **CORRECT:** When taking action and reinforcing teaching with a client about a colposcopy, the nurse should inform the client that during a colposcopy with cervical biopsy, the client may experience temporary mild cramping and discomfort. The client should avoid inserting items into the vagina (except for a tampon) for about 2 weeks to promote healing and can decrease risk for infection. After the procedure, bleeding should be minimal, and the client should rest for at least 1 day following the procedure.

   Ⓝ NCLEX® Connection: Reduction of Risk Potential, Therapeutic Procedures

7. **LITHOTOMY:** A, D, E; **SIDE LYING KNEE TO CHEST:** B; **SUPINE:** C; **PRONE:** F

   Ⓝ NCLEX® Connection: Reduction of Risk Potential, Diagnostic Procedures

Active Learning Scenario Key

Using the ATI Active Learning Template: Therapeutic Procedure

NURSING ACTIONS (PRE, POST)

Preprocedure
- Perform prescribed pre-op laboratory test (pregnancy test to rule out pregnancy, heme/platelet).
- Administer preoperative antibiotics.
- Apply antiembolism stockings or sequential compression sleeves.
- Check client's psychological condition.
- Ensure client has been NPO prior to surgery.
- Ensure that informed consent has been obtained.

Postprocedure
- Check the client's pain frequently.
- Administer prescribed analgesics (PCA may be used).
- Administer antibiotics as prescribed.
- Administer IV fluids.
- Advance diet as tolerated (may need clear liquids until bowel sounds return).
- Monitor vital signs frequently (fever, hypotension).
- Check breath and bowel sounds (risk of atelectasis and paralytic ileus).
- Assist the client with dangling on side of bed or ambulation.
- Take thromboembolism precautions (sequential compression devices; administer anticoagulants; ambulation).
- Check incision site, dressing (bleeding, drainage, redness, warmth, dehiscence).
- Monitor vaginal bleeding: Excess bleeding is more than 1 saturated pad in 4 hr.
- Monitor heme/platelet and WBC count (determine client risk for anemia, bleeding, infection).
- Monitor intake and output (an indwelling urinary catheter may be present and removed within 24 hours following surgery).

Ⓝ NCLEX® Connection: Reduction of Risk Potential, Therapeutic Procedures

NCLEX® Connections

When reviewing the following chapters, keep in mind the relevant topics and tasks of the NCLEX outline.

Health Promotion and Maintenance

HEALTH PROMOTION/DISEASE PREVENTION: Assist client in disease prevention activities.

Reduction of Risk Potential

THERAPEUTIC PROCEDURES: Reinforce client teaching on treatments and procedures.

POTENTIAL FOR ALTERATIONS IN BODY SYSTEMS: Monitor client output for changes from baseline.

Physiological Adaptation

ALTERATIONS IN BODY SYSTEMS
Provide care to correct client alteration in body system.

Reinforce education to client regarding care and condition.

BASIC PATHOPHYSIOLOGY
Identify signs and symptoms related to an acute or chronic illness.

Apply knowledge of pathophysiology to monitoring client for alterations in body systems.

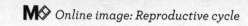
CHAPTER 58 **Reproductive Physiologic Processes**

There are various physiologic processes that occur in the reproductive system, such as the production and transportation of sperm, ovulation, menstruation, fertilization, and embryonic development. It is important to obtain a detailed history to determine how to assist the client. When collecting data on a client who has a menstrual disorder, the nurse should check the client's:

- Menstrual history (age of first menses, monthly cycle)
- Sexual history
- Nutritional history

Reproductive cycle

There are different components of a reproductive cycle, which are controlled by the pituitary gland and the hypothalamus. The ovarian cycle is responsible for development of follicular development of mature ovum. It has 2 phases (follicular and luteal). The follicular phase is the (first 14 days of a 28-day cycle. The luteal phase is the 15-28 days of a 28-day menstrual cycle. A complete menstrual cycle is approximately 28 days. This cycle affects the endometrium of the uterus and allows for implantation of fertilized ovum and menses. It has four phases: menstrual, proliferative, ovulation, and secretory.

Menstrual: the start of menstrual flow (sloughing of the endometrial lining of the uterus) and the process of maturation of the follicles begin

Proliferative: maturation of egg, thickening of the endometrium

Ovulation: occurs approximately 14 days prior to menses; pregnancy can occur; if no pregnancy, the corpus luteum resolves

Secretory: secretion of progesterone; endometrium thickens in response to estrogen and progesterone, or uterus prepares for fertilized ovum
The four criteria used to define bleeding are regularity, length, volume, and frequency and are based upon the client's bleeding pattern within the last 6 months.

Frequency: Expected is the onset of menstrual bleeding every 24–38 days.

Regularity: The number of days from the start (day 1) of one period until start (day 1) of the next period

Duration: The expected number of days in a single menstrual period is less than or equal to 8 days.

Volume: Varies, but an expected finding is less than or equal to 80 mL hr

The average age of menarche (first menses) is 12.4 years, but it can occur from 10 to 16 years. Data collection is indicated if an adolescent has not begun menstruation by 15 years of age. The first day of menstruation is day 1 of a menstrual cycle. Menstrual cycles continue until menopause or surgical removal of the uterus. Menopause is when ovulation ceases, and menstrual cycles become irregular and eventually stop. The median age of onset of menopause is 51 years.

Menstrual disorders

Dysmenorrhea

Painful menstruation, or dysmenorrhea, is common in adolescents and young clients. In many clients, this pain is significantly decreased after the birth of a child or as the client becomes older. Dysmenorrhea is classified as primary or secondary.
- **Primary:** occurs at least 6 months after menarche and is thought to be caused by the release of increased prostaglandins, which causes discomforting uterine contractions
- **Secondary:** caused by a pathological condition of the pelvic cavity (PID, endometriosis, tumors, fibroids)

DATA COLLECTION

EXPECTED FINDINGS

- **Primary**
  - Insomnia, backache, headache, cramping in pelvic area
- **Secondary**
  - Nausea, backache, dizziness, dull abdominal pain

DIAGNOSTIC PROCEDURES

- Pelvic examination by provider (identify unexpected pathological findings)
- Laparoscopy

PATIENT-CENTERED CARE

NURSING ACTIONS/CLIENT EDUCATION

- Provide information about the condition and provide reassurance as needed.
- Reinforce teaching and assist the client with using non–pharmacological pain relief measures (heating pad, massage, effleurage, pelvic rock).
- Low-fat diet with natural diuretics
- Provide information about the use of analgesics and heat therapy (combination therapy may provide more comfort).

THERAPEUTIC MANAGEMENT

Treat pathological cause (secondary)

MEDICATIONS

Prostaglandin inhibitors (NSAIDs)

- Inhibits production of prostaglandins
- Aids in treatment of pain and discomfort

Oral contraceptives

Assist with alleviating menstrual discomforts

Complementary and alternative therapy (CAM)

- Aromatherapy
- Meditation
- Herbal preparations

Premenstrual syndrome (PMS) and premenstrual dysphoric disorder (PMDD)

Premenstrual syndrome (PMS) is also known as ovarian syndrome. It is thought to be caused by an imbalance between estrogen and progesterone, which can cause psychological, physical, or behavioral manifestations. The manifestations can vary among clients and can vary for an individual from one cycle to the next.

Premenstrual dystrophic disorder (PMDD) is a severe form of PMS and is thought to be caused by unexpected serotonin response to estrogen levels during a menstrual cycle. It is seen in only a small number of clients, and it interferes with the ability to carry out daily activities.

DATA COLLECTION

EXPECTED FINDINGS

Manifestations begin a few days before the menstrual period and end a few days after the onset of the menstrual period for both conditions. PMDD will have more severe findings.

PMS and PMDD: Irritability, depression, poor concentration, mood swings, increased appetite, fluid retention (breast tenderness, bloating, weight gain), headache, and back pain

LABORATORY/DIAGNOSTIC TESTS

The provider will diagnose based upon the client's pattern of manifestations (for 3 months) (PMDD).

PATIENT-CENTERED CARE

NURSING ACTIONS/CLIENT EDUCATION

- Provide information about the condition and provide reassurance as needed.
- Check for suicidal ideations (PMDD).
- Assist with referring client for psychological counseling (PMDD).
- Decrease stress.
- Avoid caffeine, foods high in fat and sodium, and foods or beverages high in refined sugars.
- Consume diet that is well-balanced with whole grains and fruits and vegetables.
- Increase water intake if not contraindicated.
- Exercise regularly.

THERAPEUTIC MANAGEMENT

Medications

ORAL CONTRACEPTIVES: Can be used to decrease the severity of manifestations of PMS, PMDD

PROSTAGLANDIN INHIBITORS (NSAIDS: ibuprofen)
- Inhibits the production of prostaglandins
- Aids in treatment of pain and discomfort related to PMS and PMDD

SSRIS: (fluoxetine, sertraline): Used to manage the emotional and physical manifestations of PMS and PMDD

SPIRONOLACTONE: Aids in fluid retention related to PMS and PMDD

Conditions related to menses or bleeding

Amenorrhea

Amenorrhea: is the absence of menses. In a client who has had menstrual cycles, this can be an indication of pregnancy or a medical condition, such as thyroid disorder or structural disorders of the reproductive system. This condition is classified as primary or secondary.

- Primary amenorrhea (never started menstruation) is considered a delay in menarche (no secondary sex characteristics by 15 years of age or no menarche by 16 years of age).
- Secondary (started menstruation and then stopped) is the omission of menstruation for at least 3 cycles or 6 months after regular menarche.

Oligomenorrhea is infrequent or decreased menstrual periods.

DATA COLLECTION

RISK FACTORS

- **Primary**
  - Genetic and anatomical conditions
  - Turner syndrome
  - Anorexia
  - Polycystic ovarian syndrome
- **Secondary**
  - Pituitary conditions
  - Increased BMI
  - Decreased body fat
  - Breastfeeding
  - Menopause
  - Polycystic ovarian syndrome
  - Anorexia, bulimia
  - Participation in competitive sports

PATIENT-CENTERED CARE

NURSING ACTIONS/CLIENT EDUCATION

- Provide information about the condition and provide reassurance as needed.
- Inform client to document/record menstrual period.

THERAPEUTIC MANAGEMENT

Identify underlying cause and manage accordingly.

MEDICATIONS

Hormonal contraceptives

Can be used to induce menstruation or provide regularity

Menorrhagia/metrorrhagia

Menorrhagia is excessive menstrual bleeding (in amount and duration), possibly with clots that saturate more than one tampon or pad per hour. **Metrorrhagia, or "breakthrough bleeding,"** is bleeding between menstrual periods. It is more common in clients who are entering menopause and in adolescents. Menometrorrhagia is unexpected vaginal bleeding between menstrual periods and excessive vaginal bleeding during the menstrual period.

DATA COLLECTION

RISK FACTORS

Menorrhagia

- Malignancies
- Fibroids
- Hormone imbalances
- Von Willebrand disease
- Infections

Metrorrhagia

- Fibroids, polyps
- Trauma
- Malignancies

EXPECTED FINDINGS

- Epistaxis (menorrhagia)
- Report of breakthrough bleeding (while taking oral contraceptives)

LABORATORY TESTS

Hemoglobin and hematocrit can be below the expected reference range due to excessive blood loss.

PATIENT-CENTERED CARE

NURSING ACTIONS/CLIENT EDUCATION

- Encourage client to document findings about their menstrual cycle (amount of bleeding, findings, pad counts).
- Provide information about the condition and provide reassurance as needed.

THERAPEUTIC MANAGEMENT

Varies depending on underlying cause

MEDICATIONS

Tranexamic acid (menorrhagia)

- Reduces the breakdown of clots within the uterus
- Risk of thrombus formation

Hormonal contraceptives

Can be used to provide regularity of menstruation

Oral iron supplements

Used to manage anemia

Abnormal uterine bleeding (AUB)

Abnormal uterine bleeding, also known as dysfunctional uterine bleeding (DUB), can be caused by an anovulation or hormonal imbalance of decreased estrogen. It is the unexpected bleeding that is not related to regular menstrual period. It occurs at the beginning of menarche or during menopause. Vaginal bleeding in a client who is considered postmenopausal should be evaluated for cancer (cervical/uterine).

DATA COLLECTION

RISK FACTORS

- Thyroid conditions
- Polycystic ovarian syndrome
- Infection
- Trauma
- Neoplasm

LABORATORY TESTS

- **Hemoglobin and hematocrit** can be below the expected reference range due to excessive blood loss.
- Platelet count

DIAGNOSTIC PROCEDURES

- **Pelvic exam:** Provider will perform a pelvic exam to determine cause.
- **Endometrial biopsy** determines the relationship between menstrual flow and the hormone cycle, as well as possible pathologic reasons for bleeding, such as uterine cancer.

PATIENT-CENTERED CARE

NURSING ACTIONS/CLIENT EDUCATION

Provide information about the condition and provide reassurance as needed.

THERAPEUTIC MANAGEMENT

Medications

HORMONAL CONTRACEPTIVES: Three to six months of therapy (to decrease the severity of findings such as bleeding and provide regularity of menstruation)

CONJUGATED ESTROGENS: Manage or decrease bleeding

ORAL IRON SUPPLEMENTS: Used to manage anemia

THERAPEUTIC PROCEDURES

Dilatation and curettage: Used to diagnose and treat AUB. The cervix is dilated, and the wall of the uterus is scraped with a curette. Endometrium scraped from the uterine wall is sent to the laboratory for examination.

Perimenopause and menopause

Perimenopause is the transitional period (approximately 4 years) that precedes menopause. Hormonal imbalances occur as the ovarian function declines as ova slowly diminish. The menstrual cycle can be anovulatory, which can lead to irregular bleeding.

Menopause is also known as the "change of life" and is the cessation of menses for at least 12 months that occurs during 41–59 years of age. Menses will appear on an infrequent cycle, and the flow will decrease until there is complete cessation. Menopause is the result of hormonal changes such as decrease in production of estrogen. The client can have natural or surgically induced menopause.

Post-menopause is 1 year after the cessation of menses.

DATA COLLECTION

EXPECTED FINDINGS

- **Vasomotor manifestations:** Hot flashes (Feeling of warmth followed by diaphoresis causes sleep disturbances and fatigue.) (Both)
- **Genitourinary:** Atrophic vaginitis, shrinking of labia, dyspareunia, increased vaginal pH (decreased vaginal secretions and dryness), incontinence
- **Psychological:** Mood swings, changes in sleep patterns, decreased REM sleep
- **Skeletal:** Joint pain (perimenopause), decreased bone density
- **Dermatological:** Decreased skin elasticity, loss of genital hair
- **Neuro/cognitive:** Migraine headaches, forgetfulness (perimenopause)
- **Reproductive:** Breast tenderness (perimenopause), breast tissue changes and irregular menses

LABORATORY TESTS

- **Hormones:** Estrogen and progesterone decreased; FSH increased
- **Cholesterol:** LDL increased; HDL may decrease (menopause)

DIAGNOSTIC PROCEDURES

- **Pelvic examination with Papanicolaou (Pap) test** to rule out cancer in cases of abnormal bleeding
- **Endometrial biopsy** in cases of undiagnosed abnormal uterine bleeding in a client older than 40 years of age, or in a client whose menses has stopped for 1 year and bleeding has begun again
- **Bone mineral density measurement using dual-energy x-ray absorptiometry DXA)** to determine the client's risk for osteoporosis

PATIENT-CENTERED CARE

NURSING ACTIONS/CLIENT EDUCATION

- Provide education with the client about the condition and how to manage.
- Inform client to report vaginal bleeding
- **Management of clinical findings**
  - Atrophic vaginitis (vaginal burning and bleeding, pruritus, and painful intercourse) can improve with HT. Vaginal instillations of estrogen can be the best option because systemic absorption is reduced. Qpcc
  - Reinforce with client self-administration of HT.
  - Dyspareunia from vaginal dryness inform; client to use water-soluble lubricant, hormone cream (Refrain from inserting or using HT cream prior to intercourse, or the partner can absorb some of the product.)
- **Nutrition**
  - Encourage client to decrease calories and fat intake.
  - Increase fiber and whole grains.
  - Drink adequate water daily (6–8 glasses) if not contraindicated.
- **Encourage physical activity**
  - Encourage at least 30 minutes of physical activity at 3–4 times per week.
  - Weight-bearing exercises can prevent muscle and bone loss.
- **Health promotion**
  - Encourage routine health screenings (mammograms, colonoscopy, bone density fecal occult blood testing, gynecologic exam).
  - Encourage client to stop smoking immediately if applicable.

MEDICATIONS

Menopausal hormone therapy (HT)

Contains estrogen or estrogen and progesterone/progestin
- Used to manage findings of menopause (vasomotor) prevent atrophy of vaginal tissue, and decrease risk of fractures (osteoporosis)
- Based on their individual risk factors and health care needs, clients should discuss the risks and benefits of using HT with their providers.
- Start with low dose and consider short-term therapy.
- Available in vaginal creams, suppositories, transdermal patches, or PO
- For a client who has a uterus, HT includes estrogen and progestin. For a client who no longer has a uterus (following a hysterectomy), estrogen alone is prescribed.
- The risk associated with the use of HT depends on many factors (the age of the client, their personal/family history, the regimen prescribed). HT places clients at risk for several adverse conditions, including coronary heart disease, myocardial infarction, deep vein thrombosis, stroke, and breast cancer.

Contraindications: Clients with a history of breast cancer, liver impairment, thrombosis, uterine cancer, AUB

Oral contraceptives

Used for a client who is a nonsmoker and is perimenopausal to decrease severity of perimenopausal findings and pregnancy prevention

CAM therapies

Ask the client about their use of CAM: Research regarding their usefulness is inconsistent.
- Natural estrogens
- Black cohosh, ginseng, soy
- Aromatherapy, acupuncture, reflexology, yoga, breathing exercises
- Phytoestrogens interact with estrogen receptors in the body, which can result in a decrease in the manifestations of menopause. Vegetables such as dandelion greens, alfalfa sprouts, black beans, and soy beans contain phytoestrogens. QEBP
- Vitamins E and B6 are reported to decrease hot flashes in some clients.

COMPLICATIONS

OSTEOPOROSIS

Risk for decreased bone mass increases the risk for fractures.
- HT with estrogen to assist with enabling vitamin D to assist with calcium absorption
- Bisphosphonate, calcium therapy
- Weight-bearing exercises

EMBOLIC COMPLICATIONS

Risk increased by concurrent tobacco use
- Myocardial infarction, especially during the first year of therapy
- Stroke
- Venous thrombosis: Thrombophlebitis, especially during the first year of therapy

CANCER

- In some studies, long-term use of HT has been found to increase the risk for breast cancer.
- Some studies indicate that long-term use of estrogen-only HT increases the risk for ovarian and endometrial cancer.

Active Learning Scenario

A nurse is caring for a client who has a new diagnosis of premenstrual syndrome (PMS). Use the ATI Active Learning Template: Basic Concept to complete this item.

EXPECTED FINDINGS: Identify six manifestations and at least 4 nursing actions/client education the nurse should take for a client who has PMS.

Application Exercises

1. A nurse is reinforcing teaching about menstruation with an adolescent client. Which of the following statements should the nurse include? (Select all that apply.)
   A. "The average age of onset of menstruation is 10."
   B. "The typical menstrual cycle is approximately 28 days."
   C. "The first day of the menstrual cycle begins with the last day of the menstrual period."
   D. "Ovulation typically occurs around the 14th day of the menstrual cycle."
   E. "A menstrual period can last as long as 8 days."

2. A nurse is reviewing the medical record of a client who has premenstrual syndrome (PMS). The nurse should identify that which of the following medications are used in the therapeutic management of PMS? (Select all that apply.)
   A. Fluoxetine
   B. Spironolactone
   C. Ethinyl estradiol/drospirenone
   D. Ferrous sulfate
   E. Methylergonovine

3. A nurse in a provider's office is providing information to an older adult client who has abnormal uterine bleeding (AUB). Which of the following statements by the client indicates understanding of the information? (Select all that apply.)
   A. "My heavy bleeding can be related to a hormonal imbalance."
   B. "If I experience menstrual pain, I can take aspirin."
   C. "The use of oral contraceptives is contraindicated for this condition."
   D. "I may need a D&C to determine cause of this bleeding."
   E. "My condition is more common in clients who are in their 30s."

4. A nurse is reviewing the medical record of a client who is menopausal. Which of the following findings should the nurse expect? (Select all that apply.)
   A. Increased estrogen
   B. Decreased LDL level
   C. Report of increased vaginal secretions
   D. Report of dyspareunia
   E. Report of mood swings
   F. Report of hot flashes

Application Exercises Key

1. B, D, E. **CORRECT:** When taking actions and reinforcing teaching with an adolescent client about menstruation, the nurse should include that a complete menstrual cycle is about 28 days, menstruation can last up to 8 days, and ovulation occurs around day 14.

   Ⓝ *NCLEX® Connection: Physiological Adaptation, Alterations in Body Systems*

2. A. **CORRECT:** Medications used to treat PMS include SSRIs, NSAIDs, diuretics, and oral contraceptives. Fluoxetine is an SSRI that is used to manage the client's psychosocial findings.
   B. **CORRECT:** Spironolactone is a potassium-sparing diuretic that is used to manage fluid retention.
   C. **CORRECT:** Ethinyl estradiol/drospirenone is an oral contraceptive that is used to decrease severity of the manifestations of PMS.
   D. Ferrous sulfate is not indicated because there is no risk for anemia.
   E. Methylergonovine is used to prevent bleeding and manage conditions such as postpartum hemorrhage.

   Ⓝ *NCLEX® Connection: Pharmacological Therapies, Expected Actions/Outcomes*

3. A, D. **CORRECT:** To evaluate outcomes, the nurse should identify that the client understands the information provided when the client states heavy bleeding can be related to hormonal imbalance and the D&C is needed to determine the cause of the bleeding. AUB is caused by a potential hormonal imbalance. A D&C is a therapeutic procedure that can identify and manage the cause of AUB. The client should avoid aspirin because this can cause more bleeding.

   Ⓝ *NCLEX® Connection: Physiological Adaptation, Alterations in Body Systems*

4. D, E, F. **CORRECT:** Findings include vaginal dryness, and the laboratory results include decreased estrogen and increased LDL. Findings of menopause include client report of hot flashes, mood swings, and pain during sexual intercourse. These are caused by hormonal changes that occur during menopause, such as decreased estrogen.

   Ⓝ *NCLEX® Connection: Physiological Adaptation, Basic Pathophysiology*

Active Learning Scenario Key

Using the ATI Active Learning Template: Basic Concept

EXPECTED FINDINGS
- Irritability
- Depression
- Poor concentration
- Mood swings
- Increased appetite
- Breast tenderness
- Bloating
- Weight gain
- Headache
- Back pain

NURSING ACTIONS/CLIENT EDUCATION
- Provide information about the condition and provide reassurance as needed.
- Decrease stress.
- Avoid caffeine, foods high in fat and sodium, and foods or beverages high in refined sugars.
- Consume diet that is well-balanced with whole grains and fruits and vegetables.
- Increase water intake if not contraindicated.
- Exercise regularly.

Ⓝ *NCLEX® Connection: Physiological Adaptation, Basic Pathophysiology*

CHAPTER 59 # Disorders of Reproductive Tissue

Disorders of the reproductive tissue can encompass various conditions that can affect the breasts and genitourinary and reproductive system. Disorders can occur across the lifespan. It is important to reinforce education with the client about their condition and support with management.

Fibrocystic breast condition

Fibrocystic breast condition is a noncancerous breast condition. It is most common in young adult clients. It occurs less frequently in postmenopausal clients. The condition is thought to occur due to cyclic hormonal changes. Fibrosis (of connective tissue) and cysts (fluid-filled sacs) develop.

DATA COLLECTION

RISK FACTORS

Premenopausal status

EXPECTED FINDINGS

CLIENT MAY REPORT
- Breast pain, swelling
- Tender lumps Q EBP

PHYSICAL EXAMINATION FINDINGS: Palpable firm, hard, rubberlike lumps, usually in the upper, outer quadrant

DIAGNOSTIC PROCEDURES

Breast ultrasound is used to confirm the diagnosis.

Mammogram detects cancer.

Breast biopsy/fine-needle aspiration is used to confirm the diagnosis or to reduce pain due to fluid buildup.

PATIENT-CENTERED CARE

NURSING CARE/CLIENT EDUCATION

- Suggest that the client reduce the intake of salt before menses, wear a supportive bra, and apply either local heat or cold to temporarily reduce pain.
- Encourage client to become familiar with breast to identify changes. Notify provider promptly of identified changes.
- Inform the client that having fibrocystic breast condition does not increase the risk of breast cancer.

THERAPEUTIC MANAGEMENT

CONSERVATIVE
- Wear support bra.
- Apply local heat or cold therapy (compresses).
- Avoid caffeine.

MEDICATIONS

- **Over-the-counter analgesics** such as acetaminophen or ibuprofen (manage breast discomfort)
- **Oral contraceptives or hormonal medication therapy** if manifestations are severe to suppress estrogen/progesterone secretion
- **Selective estrogen modulators**: tamoxifen, danazol
- **Complementary/alternative therapies:** Vitamin E supplements, chamomile
- **Diuretics** to decrease breast engorgement

Gynecomastia

A benign condition that is characterized by an increase in the size of breast tissue by the proliferation of the glandular tissue. This condition is caused by increased hormonal ratios of estrogen to androgen. It can be physiologic or pathologic and occur bilateral or unilateral. The prevalence rate for gynecomastia is about 50% for adolescents and 25% for older adults. In adolescence, the condition may resolve spontaneously within 24 months.

DATA COLLECTION

RISK FACTORS

- **Assigned sex at birth:** male
- **Pathologic:** testicular tumors, CKD, hyperthyroidism
- **Medications:** Spironolactone

EXPECTED FINDINGS

CLIENT MAY REPORT: Tenderness upon touch to affected area

PHYSICAL EXAMINATION FINDINGS: Palpable mass (diameter < 0.5 cm) that could be tender

DIAGNOSTIC PROCEDURES

- Breast exam by provider (determine presence of condition and to distinguish with pseudogynecomastia)
- Breast ultrasound is used to confirm the diagnosis.
- Testicular exam to determine cause

PATIENT-CENTERED CARE

NURSING CARE/CLIENT EDUCATION

- Discuss condition with client.
- Encourage client to express their concerns or fears.
- Encourage client to become familiar with breast to identify changes. Notify provider promptly of identified changes.
- Monitor the client's psychosocial status.
- Interprofessional collaboration Qꜰᴄ
  - Mental health provider (Client may need a referral if having concerns with coping.)
  - Social worker

THERAPEUTIC MANAGEMENT

- Management depends on severity, cause, duration and presence or absence of tenderness.
- First-line of management
  - Identify potential cause and manage underlying cause.
    - If the cause is medication related, the provider will discontinue any medications that can cause the condition.
    - If the cause is related to other conditions (hyperthyroidism, hypogonadism), the provider will manage these.

MEDICATIONS

Medical therapy begins when breast is greater than 4 cm in diameter in younger clients and the client reports pain, tenderness, or embarrassment from condition. The provider can prescribe hormonal medications to assist with shrinking breast tissue.
- Selective estrogen receptor modulators (tamoxifen)
- Androgens (testosterone)

THERAPEUTIC PROCEDURES

- Surgical management (performed if client has symptoms greater than 12 months, fibrosis occurs, or if management of the condition was unsuccessful with medications)
  - Direct excision of glandular tissue, liposuction
  - Skin excision/cosmetic surgery
- Radiotherapy: improve discomfort and tenderness

Leiomyomas (fibroids)

Leiomyomas are also known as fibroids or myomas. These are benign tumors of the uterus in which their growth is affected by ovarian hormone stimulation. Each year, uterine fibroids cost the U.S. over $30 billion, and it affects 11 million clients. Fibroids can occur as a single or multiple tumors and in different origins (submucosal, subserosal, or intramural areas of the myometrium of the uterus). Morbidity from symptomatic fibroids can affect the client's employment. Some clients report absence from work, utilization of sick time, and lost wages because of the discomfort or bleeding.

DATA COLLECTION

RISK FACTORS

- Age 25-40
- Black ethnicity
- Early menarche
- Oral contraceptive use
- Genetic predisposition

EXPECTED FINDINGS

- Client can be asymptomatic.
- Abnormal uterine bleeding (AUB) (moderate with possible clots)
- Backache
- Dyspareunia
- Lower abdominal pressure
- Constipation
- Urinary frequency, retention, incontinence

PHYSICAL EXAMINATION FINDINGS: Palpable rubberlike lumps in the abdominal area, enlarged or distended abdomen

LABORATORY/DIAGNOSTIC PROCEDURES

- Hemoglobin, hematocrit (uterine bleeding)
- Pelvic exam by provider (identify unexpected findings)
- Ultrasound (identify presence and extent of condition)
- Hysteroscopy (identify presence and extent of condition)
- Endometrial biopsy (determine unexpected findings of the endometrial tissue)

PATIENT-CENTERED CARE

NURSING CARE/CLIENT EDUCATION

- Encourage client to express their fears or concerns. Qᴘᴄᴄ
- Provide support.
- Refer clients to a support group if needed.

THERAPEUTIC MANAGEMENT

- If asymptomatic, no treatment warranted. The provider will monitor the client's condition.
- If client is menopausal, the fibroids may shrink spontaneously (decreased estrogen and progesterone).
- Overall, management will vary and depend on the client's reproductive plans, size, and location of fibroid.

MEDICATIONS

- NSAIDs (discomfort)
- Oral contraceptives (control bleeding)
- Gonadotrophin releasing hormone analogues (GnRH): leuprolide (used to shrink the fibroid)
  - Client can receive monthly injections for about 6 months.
  - Can be prescribed prior to surgery management

THERAPEUTIC PROCEDURES

- **Uterine artery embolism (UAE):** An interventional radiologist will inject polyvinyl alcohol or gelatin-like pellets into the vascular of the uterus (uterine artery) via the femoral artery to restrict circulation to the fibroid and cause it to shrink.

CLIENT EDUCATION: No strenuous activities; expect scant vaginal discharge, cramping, and minor discomfort following

Hysterectomy: Refer to RN ADULT MEDICAL SURGICAL NURSING CHAPTER 64. Leiomyomas are the main reason a hysterectomy is performed.

Myolysis: Laser or electrosurgery to coagulate fibroid

Myomectomy: Excision of fibroid

Can be performed laparoscopic, hysteroscopic, with laser

Benign prostatic hyperplasia

As an adult male ages, the prostate gland enlarges. When the enlargement of the gland begins to cause urinary dysfunction, it is called benign prostatic hyperplasia (BPH). BPH is a very common condition of the older adult male. BPH can significantly impair the outflow of urine from the bladder, making a client susceptible to infection and retention. Excessive amounts of urine retained can cause reflux urine into the kidney, dilating the ureter and causing kidney infections that can lead to kidney damage. Client will require a referral to a urologist for management.

DATA COLLECTION

RISK FACTORS

- Genetic predisposition
- Black ethnicity
- Increased consumption of caffeine and coffee
- Increased age
- Smoking, chronic alcohol use
- Sedentary lifestyle, obesity
- Western diet (high-fat, -protein, -carbohydrate; low-fiber)
- Diabetes mellitus, heart disease

EXPECTED FINDINGS

- The International Prostate Symptom Score (I-PSS) is a data collection tool used to determine the severity of manifestations and their effect on the client's quality of life. The client rates the severity of lower urinary tract manifestations using a 0 to 5 scale and rates their quality of life as affected by urinary tract manifestations.
- The client may be asymptomatic with BPH; if symptoms are present, the client may report manifestations of lower urinary tract findings:
  - Urinary frequency, urgency, hesitancy, or incontinence, nocturia
  - Dribbling post-voiding, diminished force of urinary stream, incomplete emptying of bladder, straining with urination, and hematuria

LABORATORY TESTS

- Urinalysis and culture: WBCs elevated, hematuria, and bacteria present with urinary tract infection
- CBC: WBCs elevated if systemic infection present, RBCs possibly decreased due to hematuria
- BUN and creatinine: Elevated, indicating kidney damage
- Prostate-specific antigen: To rule out prostate cancer
- Culture and sensitivity of prostatic fluid: Can be performed if fluid is expressed during digital rectal examination

DIAGNOSTIC PROCEDURES

Digital rectal exam will reveal an enlarged, smooth prostate. Q EBP

Transrectal ultrasound with needle aspiration biopsy is performed to rule out prostate cancer in the presence of an enlarged prostate.

Early prostate cancer antigen blood test can be prescribed instead of a biopsy to rule out prostate cancer.

59.1 Therapeutic management: Medications

The goal of medication for BPH is to re-establish uninhibited urine flow out of the bladder.

MEDICATIONS	GENERAL CONSIDERATIONS	NURSING ACTIONS/CLIENT EDUCATION
5-alpha reductase inhibitor (5-ARI) (finasteride, dutasteride)	Lowers dihydrotestosterone (DHT) which decreases the production of testosterone in the prostate gland and causes a reduction in the size of the prostate.	Remind clients that it can take up to 6 months before effects of the medication are evident. Monitor for adverse effects of impotence, gynecomastia, and decrease in libido. Clients who are pregnant or who could become pregnant should avoid contact with finasteride tablets that are crushed or broken and with the semen of a client who is currently taking this medication because of teratogenicity. Qs
Alpha-adrenergic receptor antagonists (tamsulosin)	Cause relaxation of the smooth muscle of the bladder outlet and prostate gland. These agents decrease pressure on the urethra, thereby re-establishing a stronger urine flow.	Monitor for adverse effects of tachycardia, syncope, headache, and postural hypotension. Inform client to change positions slowly. Qs
Phosphodiesterase type 5 inhibitors (PDE5) (tadalafil)	Use for BHP or erectile dysfunction (causes vasodilation)	Do not take with grapefruit.
Complementary Therapies	Saw palmetto is commonly used; however, it is not recommended. Pygeum africanum (African plum) can provide an anti-inflammatory effect	Encourage client to discuss with their provider about the use of saw palmetto or any herbal medications.

59.2 Therapeutic management: Minimally invasive procedures

MINIMALLY INVASIVE THERAPEUTIC PROCEDURES	GENERAL CONSIDERATIONS	NURSING ACTIONS/CLIENT EDUCATION
Transurethral needle ablation (TUNA)	Radiofrequency needles are injected directly into the prostate, which cause coagulation of the prostate tissue	May experience mild hematuria for at least 1 week following the procedure. May need an indwelling urinary catheter for 1 week. Risk of developing complications (UTIs, bladder stones, urinary incontinence, and retention).
Transurethral microwave therapy (TUMT)	Heat is applied to the prostate, which causes coagulation of the tissue	May need an indwelling urinary catheter for 1 week. Take medications as prescribed (analgesics, antibiotics, anti-spasmodic agents).
Prostatic stent	Placed to keep the urethra patent, especially if the client is a poor candidate for surgery	Not frequently used.
Holmium laser enucleation of the prostate	Uses a laser to remove excess prostatic tissue that is obstructing the client's urethra. The tissue is then moved to the bladder, where the client eliminates it in the urine.	The client often has an indwelling urinary catheter that is left in place overnight. Bleeding is minimal.
Transurethral electro-vaporization of the prostate (TUVP)	High-frequency electrical current is used to vaporize and destroy prostate tissue	Risk of complications following procedure (hematuria, retrograde ejaculation).
Transurethral incision of the prostate (TUIP)	Involves incisions into the prostate to relieve constriction of the urethra. Tissue is not removed with this procedure. It is minimally invasive and typically performed in an outpatient setting.	

59.3 Therapeutic management: Invasive procedures

INVASIVE PROCEDURES	GENERAL CONSIDERATIONS	NURSING ACTIONS/ CLIENT EDUCATION
Prostatectomy (open, laparoscopic, robotic)	Removal of the entire prostate via (perineal, retropubic, or suprapubic). A robotic and laparoscopic approach is less invasive.	Risk of infection and erectile dysfunction. The client may have a long recovery time.

Transurethral resection of the prostate (TURP)	TURP is the most common surgical procedure for BPH. The provider uses a resectoscope (similar to a cystoscope) to trim excess prostatic tissue to enlarge the passageway of the urethra through the prostate gland. Since some of the prostate tissue is removed, the prostate can potentially continue to grow. Potential complications: Urethral trauma, urinary retention, bleeding, infection, and recurrence of the condition.	**PREOPERATIVE:** Ensure informed consent is obtained. **POSTOPERATIVE**
		• Monitor vital signs and urinary output.
		• Administer/provide increased fluids.
		• Monitor for bleeding (persistent bright-red bleeding unresponsive to increase in CBI and traction on the catheter or reduced Hgb levels) and report to the provider.
		• Assist the client to ambulate as soon as possible (decrease the risk of deep vein thrombosis (DVT) and other complications related to immobility).
		• Administer medications as prescribed:
		  ○ Analgesics (surgical manipulation or incisional discomfort)
		  ○ Antispasmodics (bladder spasms)
		  ○ Antibiotics (prophylaxis)
		  ○ Stool softeners (avoid straining)
		• **Continuous Bladder Irrigation (CBI)**
		  ○ Following TURP, the client could have placement of an indwelling three-way catheter which drains urine and allows for CBI with normal saline or another irrigating solution. This will keep the catheter patent.
		  ○ The catheter has a large balloon (30 to 45 mL). The catheter is taped tightly to the client's abdomen or thigh, creating traction so that the balloon will apply firm pressure to the prostatic fossa to prevent bleeding. This makes the client feel a continuous need to urinate. Instruct the client not to void around the catheter as this causes bladder spasms.
		  ○ The rate of the CBI is adjusted to keep the irrigation return pink or lighter. For example, if bright-red or ketchup-appearing (arterial) bleeding with clots is observed, notify the provider. May need to increase the CBI flow rate.
		• **Monitor urinary output:** Record the amount of irrigating solution instilled (generally very large volumes) and the amount of return. The difference equals urine output.
		• **Obstructed catheter (bladder spasms, reduced irrigation outflow):** Check for kinks in tubing, turn off the CBI, and irrigate (aseptic technique) with 50 mL irrigation solution using a large piston syringe or per facility or surgeon protocol. Contact the provider if unable to dislodge the clot. Avoid kinks in the tubing.
		• **Catheter removal**
		  ○ Monitor urinary output.
		  ○ The initial void can be uncomfortable, red in color, and contain clots. The color of the urine should progress toward amber in 2 to 3 days.
		  ○ Instruct the client that the expected output is 150 to 200 mL every 3 to 4 hours. The client should notify the provider if unable to void.

PATIENT-CENTERED CARE

NURSING ACTIONS/CLIENT EDUCATION

Remind clients that frequent ejaculation releases retained prostatic fluids, thereby decreasing the size of the prostate.

CLIENT EDUCATION FOLLOWING TURP PROCEDURE

- Avoid heavy lifting, strenuous exercise, straining, and sexual intercourse for the prescribed length of time (usually 2 to 6 weeks).
- Drink 12 or more 8-oz glasses of water each day unless contraindicated.
- Avoid nonsteroidal anti-inflammatory medications due to increased risk for bleeding.
- Avoid bladder stimulants (caffeine, alcohol). Qpcc
- If urine becomes bloody, then stop activity, rest, and increase fluid intake.
- Contact the surgeon for persistent bleeding or obstruction (less than expected output or distention).

THERAPEUTIC MANAGEMENT

CONSERVATIVE

For a client who has BPH the provider will prescribe or recommend behavioral management initially.

- Limit fluid intake prior to sleep.
- Avoid bladder stimulants (caffeine and alcohol).
- Avoid drinking large amounts of fluids at one time and urinate when the urge is initially felt.
- Avoid medications that cause decreased bladder tone (anticholinergics, decongestants, antihistamines).
- Avoid constipation.
- Increase physical activity (exercise regularly).
- Kegel exercises
- Scheduled voiding

COMPLICATIONS

- CKD
- Infection

Pelvic relaxation syndrome

Pelvic relaxation syndrome is also known as pelvic organ prolapse (POP) and can consist of various conditions (cystocele, rectocele, uterine prolapse). This is caused by the weakening of the pelvic structures (muscles, fascia, ligaments), which cause organs to displace towards the vaginal orifice. Decreased estrogen can cause the pelvic structures to weaken as well. Therapeutic management is based upon the client's severity of the condition. By 2030, the prevalence rate of uterine prolapse is expected to double because of an increase in the older adult population. The treatment of uterine prolapse costs about $1 billion yearly with about 200,000 surgical procedures performed. QEBP

HEALTH PROMOTION AND DISEASE PREVENTION

- Lose weight if obese and at risk.
- Eat high-fiber diets and drink adequate fluids to prevent constipation.

Polycystic ovarian syndrome (PCOS)

PCOS, also known as Stein-Leventhal syndrome, is a condition characterized by several ovarian cysts, caused by hormonal imbalance. The changes in the hypothalamus-pituitary and endocrine system can cause findings of chronic anovulation, hyperandrogenism, and multiple small cysts. According to the World Health Organization, PCOS affects over 116 million clients worldwide and is the leading cause of infertility in clients who are assigned the sex of female at birth. The prevalence rate is estimated at 10% -47% in the U.S.

DATA COLLECTION

RISK FACTORS QEBP

- Obesity
- Family history of PCOS
- Sedentary lifestyle (decreased exercise)
- Risk of developing the following
  - Infertility
  - Diabetes mellitus
  - Hyperlipidemia
  - Liver disease
  - Anxiety, depression
  - Endometrial cancer

EXPECTED FINDINGS

- Obesity
- Insulin resistance
- Glucose intolerance
- Irregular menses
- Hirsutism
- Infertility

LABORATORY TESTS/ DIAGNOSTIC PROCEDURES

Pelvic exam by provider identifies ovarian cysts.

LABORATORY FINDINGS: Increased testosterone and LH, decreased FSH

To determine a diagnosis of PCO, 2/3 of the following must be present. QEBP
- Hyperandrogenism
- Chronic anovulation
- Ultrasound identifies ovarian cysts.

NURSING CARE/CLIENT EDUCATION

Encourage the client to consider lifestyle modification (weight loss) if indicated. Weight loss can assist with improving hormonal imbalance and infertility.

THERAPEUTIC MANAGEMENT

MEDICATIONS

- Oral contraceptives or hormonal medication therapy to inhibit testosterone and LH production
- Ovulation stimulators if the client is desiring pregnancy

THERAPEUTIC PROCEDURES

Surgery: removal of cysts

Endometriosis

Chronic condition that affects about 7% of the clients who are of reproductive age. Implantation of benign lesions with endometrial tissue outside the uterine cavity. It is a major cause of infertility and chronic pelvic pain.

DATA COLLECTION

RISK FACTORS

- Nulliparity
- Family history
- Late childbearing
- Early menarche Q EBP
- Risk for infertility and ovarian cancer

EXPECTED FINDINGS

- Dysmenorrhea
- Dyspareunia
- Dyschezia (pain with defecation)
- Pelvic pain/discomfort
- Menorrhagia
- Depressed mood

DIAGNOSTIC PROCEDURES

- Bimanual pelvic examination by provider (uterus fixed, nodular, and tenderness noted)
- Laparoscopy is used to confirm the diagnosis.
- Ultrasound, MRI, and CT scans identify condition.

NURSING ACTIONS/CLIENT EDUCATION

- Provide client with information about condition. Q EBP
- Gather data (health history, medications, and future reproductive plans).
- Refer to support groups for endometriosis.
- Administer analgesics.

THERAPEUTIC MANAGEMENT

MEDICATIONS

- Analgesics (NSAIDs) provide comfort.
- GnRH agonists: suppress estrogen production and cause amenorrhea
  - Adverse effects: vaginal dryness, hot flashes
- Oral contraceptives provide pain relief and prevent the progression of condition.
- Androgens: (danazol) inhibit the release of gonadotrophin and cause endometrial atrophy and amenorrhea
  - Expensive
  - Adverse effects: fatigue, weight gain, hot flashes, vaginal atrophy
- Complementary and alternative therapy: aromatase inhibitors

THERAPEUTIC PROCEDURES

- Laparoscopy: (cut the implants of endometriosis)
- Laser ablation (coagulation and destruction of the implants of endometriosis)
- Laparotomy (surgical removal of individual implants of endometriosis)
- Hysterectomy (removal of entire uterus; abdominal method preferred)
- Oophorectomy (removal of ovary)

Prostatitis

Prostatitis is an inflammation of the prostate gland often associated with lower urinary tract findings. This condition is the most common diagnosis in clients who are less than 50 years, and the third most common diagnosis in clients who are greater than 50 years of age. Classified as:
- Type I (acute)
- Type II (chronic bacterial)
- Type III (chronic prostatitis and chronic pelvic pain syndrome); occurs most commonly
- Type IV (asymptomatic)

59.4 Data collection

	UTERINE PROLAPSE	CYSTOCELE	RECTOCELE
	Downward protrusion of the uterus through vaginal wall	Protrusion of bladder through vaginal wall	Protrusion of rectum through vaginal wall
RISK FACTORS	• Obesity • Aging • Hormone deficiency (loss of estrogen) • Genetic predisposition • Multiparity • Childbirth (trauma, strain) • Menopause • Previous pelvic surgery • Increased intrabdominal pressure • Physical exertion (heavy lifting) • Constipation		
EXPECTED FINDINGS	• Client may report "feeling of something falling out." • Dyspareunia • Backache • Pelvic pressure • Urinary incontinence or retention	• Urinary frequency and/or urgency • Stress incontinence • History of frequent urinary tract infections • Sense of vaginal fullness • Dyspareunia • Fatigue • Back and pelvic pain	• Constipation • Sensation of a mass in the vagina • Pelvic/rectal pressure or pain • Dyspareunia • Fecal incontinence • Uncontrollable flatus • Hemorrhoids
DIAGNOSTIC PROCEDURES	Bimanual and speculum examination by provider to identify presence of conditions • Bulging of the anterior wall when the client is instructed to bear down (cystocele) • Bulging of the posterior wall when the client is instructed to bear down (rectocele) Pelvic Organ Prolapse Quantification system: Provider can use this for staging the severity of condition.		
	• Perineal ultrasound • Postvoid residual urine volume	• Postvoid residual urine volume • Bladder ultrasound measures residual urine. • Urine culture and sensitivity is used to diagnose urinary tract infection associated with urinary stasis. • A cystography is performed to identify the degree of bladder protrusion. • An x-ray can help assess the degree of cystocele.	Rectal examination reveals the presence of a rectocele.

59.5 Pessary

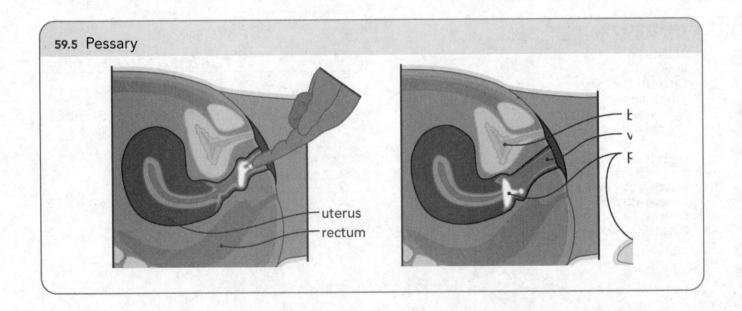

uterus
rectum

59.6 Therapeutic management: Non-surgical

PROCEDURE	GENERAL CONSIDERATIONS	NURSING ACTIONS/CLIENT EDUCATION
Pelvic floor muscle exercises (Kegels)	Exercises the client performs to strengthen the pelvic floor muscles, which results in reduction or prevention of pelvic organ prolapse and stress urinary incontinence.	• Perform the exercises. • Contract the circumvaginal and perirectal muscles. • Tighten pelvic muscles. • Gradually increase the contraction period to 10 seconds. • Follow each contraction period with a relaxation period of 10 seconds. • Perform exercise 30-80 times daily while lying down, sitting, and standing. • Keep abdominal muscles relaxed during contractions.
Pessary	An appliance device (hard rubber, silicone) that is fitted and inserted by a provider to raise the prolapse and provide pelvic structure support.	• Inform client how to insert, remove, and clean the device. • Ensure that the client does not have a latex allergy if a rubber pessary is prescribed. Qs • Routine checks by the provider are necessary to ensure proper fit, and to monitor for complications. • Notify the provider of pain, discomfort, or vaginal discharge.
Bladder training (emptying)		
• High fiber diet • Stool softeners • Laxatives • Increase fluids if not contraindicated	Actions to prevent constipation	
Estrogens	Intravaginal – prevents atrophy of pelvic muscles in clients who are postmenopausal	

59.7 Therapeutic management: Surgical

PROCEDURE	GENERAL CONSIDERATIONS	NURSING ACTIONS/CLIENT EDUCATION
Transabdominal repair with mesh	Abdominal mesh that forms a sling to support the pelvic floor.	• Adhere to postoperative restrictions, including avoidance of strenuous activity, lifting anything weighing greater than 5 pounds, and sexual intercourse, for 6 weeks. • Prevent recurrence by adhering to postoperative restrictions and avoiding smoking and straining with constipation
Anterior colporrhaphy	Using a vaginal or laparoscopic approach, the pelvic muscles are shortened and tightened, resulting in increased bladder support (cystocele).	• Provide routine postoperative care to prevent complications. • Indwelling urinary catheter for at least 24 hours following procedure • Teach how to turn, cough, and deep-breathe and splint abdomen • Notify provider of signs of infection (fever, consistent pain, purulent discharge • Keep all scheduled follow up appointments • Administer analgesics, antimicrobials, and stool softeners/laxatives as prescribed. • Avoid straining at defecation; sneezing; coughing; lifting; and sitting, walking, or standing for prolonged periods following surgery. • Adhere to postoperative restrictions, including avoidance of strenuous activity, lifting anything weighing greater than 5 pounds, and sexual intercourse, for 6 weeks. Qs
Posterior colporrhaphy	Using a vaginal/perineal approach, the pelvic muscles are shortened and tightened, resulting in a reduction of rectal protrusion into the vaginal canal (rectocele).	
Anterior-Posterior Repair	Surgical repair of both a cystocele and a rectocele.	
Hysterectomy	Can be performed at the same time as cystocele or rectocele repair.	

DATA COLLECTION

EXPECTED FINDINGS

Acute prostatitis

- Fever
- Urinary findings: dysuria, frequency, urgency, nocturia, hesitancy
- Pain and discomfort

Chronic prostatitis

Client can be asymptomatic.
- Pelvic pain
- Recurrent urinary infections
- Sexual dysfunction

PHYSICAL EXAMINATION FINDINGS

- Palpation of the prostate that can result in urethral discharge containing white blood cells
- Urethral discharge, boggy, tender prostate

DIAGNOSTIC PROCEDURES

Prostate specific antigen: Elevated

Prostate massage: allows for excretion of prostate fluid to obtain culture (risk of bacteremia)

Urinalysis

- If the condition is suspected, a midstream, clean-catch sample should be obtained.
- Urine for culture and sensitivity identifies the causative organism (bacteria) and determines the type of antibiotic to treat the infection.

White blood cell count increased due to infection and inflammation

PATIENT-CENTERED CARE

NURSING ACTIONS/CLIENT EDUCATION

- Use sitz baths, NSAIDS, and muscle relaxants if prescribed for promotion of comfort.
- Avoid alcohol, tea, coffee, and spicy foods that increase findings.
- Take medications as directed and complete the entire course of therapy.
- Sexual intercourse and masturbation can manage chronic prostatitis by reducing retention on the prostate.
- Prostatitis is not infectious or contagious.
- Keep follow-up appointments.
- Encourage fluid intake.
- Avoid sitting for extended periods.
- Report recurrence of symptoms to provider.

THERAPEUTIC MANAGEMENT

Overall management depends on the type of prostatitis.

CONSERVATIVE

- Biofeedback therapy
- Pelvic floor training
- Sitz baths Qpcc

MEDICATIONS

Antimicrobials: fluoroquinolones, trimethoprim-sulfamethoxazole

- Prescribed based on the results of the culture and sensitivity testing of urine
- Antimicrobial treatment can last weeks or months and can require hospitalization inpatient IV antibiotics.

Alpha-blocking agents: tamsulosin

- Alpha-adrenergic receptor antagonists cause relaxation of the bladder outlet and prostate gland.
- These agents decrease pressure on the urethra, thereby re-establishing a stronger urine flow.

Stool softeners

Used for prevention of straining and rectal irritation of the prostate during bowel movements

COMPLICATIONS

- Epididymitis: inflammation of the epididymis
- Cystitis: inflammation of the bladder
- Urinary tract infections
- Difficulty with sexual function

Epididymitis

Inflammation of the epididymis of the genitalia caused by infection or UTI. About 30 million clients experience ED with an incidence rate of 1:1,000 annually. It can also be related to STI (chlamydia) in younger clients.

DATA COLLECTION

RISK FACTORS

History of STI (chlamydia)
- Recent genitourinary surgery
- Enlarged prostrate
- Uncircumcised
- Chronic indwelling catheter

EXPECTED FINDINGS

CLIENT MAY REPORT:
- Pain and edema in the scrotum or groin
- Pyuria
- Urinary frequency, urgency, dysuria
- Fever, chills

PHYSICAL EXAMINATION FINDINGS: swollen epididymis, urethral discharge

DIAGNOSTIC PROCEDURES

Urinalysis detects presence of infection (culture to identify causative organism).

Urethral culture detects presence of infection (gonorrhea, chlamydia).

PATIENT-CENTERED CARE

NURSING ACTIONS/CLIENT EDUCATION

- Apply intermittent cold packs to affected area (decrease swelling and promote comfort).
- Apply local heat or encourage sitz bath (used later to decrease inflammation and promote comfort).
- Elevate scrotum with folded towel (promote drainage and provide comfort).
- Administer prescribed analgesics (relieve discomfort).
- Administer prescribed antibiotics.
- Encourage client to take all medications as prescribed.
- Educate client about condition and cause.
- Encourage testing for other STIs (HIV, syphilis).
- Avoid heavy lifting, straining, and sexual intercourse until infection has subsided up to 4 weeks.

THERAPEUTIC MANAGEMENT

Medications

- Over-the-counter analgesics such as acetaminophen or ibuprofen
- Antibiotics (depend on infectious agent); partner should receive treatment as well
- Local anesthetic injection (relieve pain/discomfort)

Erectile dysfunction (ED)

ED also known as impotence, is the inability to achieve or maintain an erection. ED affects 30 million older adult clients. The two major types of ED are organic and psychological.
- **Organic ED** involves a gradual reduction in function resulting from **other sources (diabetes, medications, vascular disease).**
- **Psychological ED** is a result of a psychological cause such as high stress, anxiety, fatigue, depression, decreased desire, and concerns with relationship.

DATA COLLECTION

RISK FACTORS

- Trauma (pelvic/genital)
- Surgery (prostatectomy)
- Vascular disease, such as hypertension
- Chronic neurologic conditions (multiple sclerosis, spinal cord injury, Parkinson's)
- Endocrine disorders (diabetes, thyroid disorders)
- Obesity
- Substance misuse disorder
- Smoking and alcohol consumption
- Medications such as antihypertensives, diuretics

EXPECTED FINDINGS

CLIENT MAY REPORT: Inability to achieve or maintain an erection for sexual intercourse

LABORATORY TEST/ DIAGNOSTIC PROCEDURES

- Glycosylated hemoglobin (DM), lipid panel, total testosterone, TSH (identify presence of contributing conditions)
- Penile Doppler ultrasonography (determines blood flow to the penis)
- Nocturnal penile tumescence test (sleep study that detects changes in the penis circumference)

PATIENT-CENTERED CARE

NURSING ACTIONS/CLIENT EDUCATION

- Provide education to the client about condition. Q EBP
- Encourage modifications to lifestyle (smoking cessation, weight loss).
- Suggest using a condom during sexual intercourse for a client who is receiving penile injections (prevent infection at injection site).
- This modality is used when other interventions fail.

Interprofessional collaboration

- Sex therapist (may need referral to discuss condition)
- Psychologist (manage psychologic causes)
- Support groups (may need referral)

THERAPEUTIC MANAGEMENT

Provider will determine the underlying cause of ED by conducting a thorough history and examination and prescribing and reviewing diagnostic testing and procedures. If an underlying cause is identified, the provider will manage this prior to initiating other measures for ED.

MEDICATIONS

Prior to medication therapy, a cardiovascular workup is recommended.

Phosphodiesterace-5 (PDE-5) inhibitors: (sildenafil, vardenafil, tadalafil); Relax the smooth muscles in the corpora cavernosa to increase penile blood flow while compressing the veins to prevent loss of blood.

- Take the medication 1 hour before sexual intercourse.
- Sildenafil and vardenafil, sexual stimulation is needed within 1/2 to 1 hour to promote the erection; tadalafil (sexual stimulation can occur for a longer period of time)
- Avoid nitrates (vasodilation that can cause hypotension and decrease blood flow), alcohol, or grapefruit (eating or drinking juice) when taking PDE-5 inhibitors.
- Potential adverse effects: heartburn, headaches, facial flushing, priapism

Vasodilators (penile injections): (alprostadil, papaverine, phentolamine, or a combination of these)

- Relaxes smooth muscle to increase blow flow to penis that results in an erection
- Injected into the penis about 20 minutes prior to intercourse and lasts for about 1 hour
- The client should alternate sides for injection.
- May cause penile discomfort and hypertension

THERAPEUTIC PROCEDURES

Vacuum constriction device (VCD)

- Creates erection by use of vacuum
- A cylinder is placed around the penis while a vacuum is created to draw blood into the penis.
- A rubber ring is then placed at the base of the penis to maintain an erection, and the cylinder is removed.

Penile implants

- This modality is used when other interventions fail.
- Implants can be flexible or rigid (rods, silicone, or an inflatable).
- The rigid implants will create semi-permanent to permanent erection. A three-piece inflatable device is implanted in the penis with the reservoir planted in the scrotum.

Penile suppository (alprostadil)

- Relaxes smooth muscle, increasing blood flow into the penis
- Inserted into the urethra 10 min before intercourse
- Erections can last up to 1 hr and can be used twice a day.
- Adverse effects include urethral and genital pain, risk of hypertension, and syncope.
- This medication is not recommended for use with pregnant partners.
- Oral contraceptives: Can be used

Application Exercises

1. A nurse is caring for a client who is at risk for developing leiomyomas. Which of the following information in the client's EMR should the nurse identify as a risk factor for leiomyomas? (Select all that apply.)

   A. 20 years of age
   B. Family history of fibroids
   C. Early menarche
   D. White ethnicity
   E. History of using oral contraceptives

2. A nurse is preparing to assist with providing care for a client following a TURP procedure. Which of the following actions should the nurse plan to take? (Select all that apply.)

   A. Encourage client to increase fluid intake.
   B. Provide intermittent urinary catheterization every 8 hours.
   C. Encourage the client to maintain bed rest for 72 hours.
   D. Administer antispasmodics as prescribed.
   E. Assist with continuous bladder irrigations.

3. A nurse is preparing to assist with the discharge of a client following an anterior and posterior colporrhaphy. Which of the following instructions should the nurse reinforce?

   A. "Do not bend over for at least 6 weeks."
   B. "You can lift objects as heavy as 10 pounds."
   C. "Do not engage in intercourse for at least 6 weeks."
   D. "You might have foul-smelling drainage for the first week after surgery."

4. A nurse is preparing to care for a client who has polycystic ovarian syndrome (PCOS). Which of the following findings should the nurse expect? (Select all that apply.)

   A. Report of irregular menses
   B. Hirsutism
   C. BMI less than 18
   D. Report of dysuria
   E. Hemoglobin A1C of 4%

5. A nurse is reinforcing teaching with a client who has ED about a new prescription for alprostadil penile injections. Which of the following statements by the client indicates an understanding?

   A. "The injection is painless."
   B. "This medication will last up to an hour."
   C. "I should self-inject on the same side."
   D. "This medication can cause low blood pressure."

Application Exercises Key

1. B, C, E. **CORRECT:** While recognizing cues when reviewing the client's EMR, the nurse should identify that genetic predisposition, early menarche, and the use of oral contraceptives are risk factors for leiomyomas.
   A. Other risk factors include 25-40 years of age and black ethnicity.
   D. Other risk factors include 25-40 years of age and black ethnicity.

   Ⓝ *NCLEX® Connection: Health Promotion and Maintenance, Health Promotion/Disease Prevention*

2. A. **CORRECT:** While generating solutions following a TURP procedure, the nurse should plan to encourage the client to increase their fluid intake, administer antispasmodics as prescribed, and assist with providing continuous bladder irrigations (CBI). Increasing fluids would provide hydration and assist with maintaining urinary output.
   B. Intermittent urinary catheterization is not recommended because of increased risk for infection, and the client will likely receive CBI.
   C. The nurse should encourage the client to ambulate following TURP to prevent DVT formation.
   D. **CORRECT:** While generating solutions following a TURP procedure, the nurse should plan to encourage the client to increase their fluid intake, administer antispasmodics as prescribed, and assist with providing continuous bladder irrigations (CBI). Administering antispasmodics would prevent bladder spasms, which could persist following a TURP procedure.
   E. **CORRECT:** While generating solutions following a TURP procedure, the nurse should plan to encourage the client to increase their fluid intake, administer antispasmodics as prescribed, and assist with providing continuous bladder irrigations (CBI). Assisting with providing continuous bladder irrigations would assist with preventing catheter obstruction.

   Ⓝ *NCLEX® Connection: Reduction of Risk Potential, Diagnostic Tests*

3. A. There are no restrictions about bending over.
   B. The client should avoid heavy lifting greater than 5 lb.
   C. **CORRECT:** While taking action, the nurse should reinforce instructions with the client about activity restrictions. The client should avoid heavy lifting greater than 5 lb and avoid sexual intercourse for 6 weeks following an anterior-posterior colporrhaphy. These actions would prevent injury, promote healing, and prevent complications.
   D. The nurse should also reinforce with the client to monitor for infection by reporting foul-smelling drainage or discharge following surgery.

   Ⓝ *NCLEX® Connection: Reduction of Risk Potential, Diagnostic Tests*

4. A, B. **CORRECT:** When recognizing cues, the nurse should expect a client who has PCOS to report irregular menses, and have hirsutism, BMI greater than 25, and Hemoglobin A1C of greater than 6%.
   D. Dysuria is not an expected finding of PCOS.

   Ⓝ *NCLEX® Connection: Reduction of Risk Potential, Diagnostic Tests*

5. A. When evaluating outcomes, it is important for the client to understand education provided about their medication, and its use, its adverse effects, and how to administer. The client may experience pain at injection site and hypertension following use.
   B. **CORRECT:** When evaluating outcomes, it is important for the client to understand education provided about their medication, and its use, its adverse effects, and how to administer. The client should understand that the medication will last up to 1 hour following administration.
   C. When evaluating outcomes, it is important for the client to understand education provided about their medication, and its use, its adverse effects, and how to administer. The client should alternate sides for injections to prevent injury.
   D. When evaluating outcomes, it is important for the client to understand education provided about their medication, and its use, its adverse effects, and how to administer. Alprostadil is a vasodilator that is used to manage erectile dysfunction.

   Ⓝ *NCLEX® Connection: Reduction of Risk Potential, Diagnostic Tests*

Active Learning Scenario

A nurse is preparing an educational session for a group of clients on medications used to treat fibrocystic breast condition and gynecomastia. Use the ATI Active Learning Template: Basic Concept to complete this item.

THERAPEUTIC USES: Identify 3 types of medications used to manage fibrocystic breast and 2 types of medications for gynecomastia. Include brief description of the purpose of the medications.

Active Learning Scenario Key

Using the ATI Active Learning Template: Basic Concept

FIBROCYSTIC BREAST
- Analgesics, such as acetaminophen or ibuprofen, are used to relieve pain.
- Oral contraceptives or hormonal medication therapy suppress estrogen/progesterone secretion.
- Diuretics decrease breast engorgement.

GYNECOMASTIA: The provider may prescribe hormonal medications to assist with shrinking breast tissue.
- Selective estrogen receptor modulators (tamoxifen)
- Androgens (testosterone)

Ⓝ *NCLEX® Connection: Physiological Adaptation, Basic Pathophysiology*

UNIT 9   REPRODUCTIVE DISORDERS
SECTION: REPRODUCTIVE DISORDERS

CHAPTER 60 # Infections of the Reproductive System

Infections of the reproductive system require prompt identification and treatment by a provider. These include general infections (candidiasis, bacterial vaginosis (BV), infections identified by type of lesion if present (human papillomavirus (HPV), herpes simplex virus (HSV), syphilis, infections identified by type of discharge if present (gonorrhea, chlamydia, trichomonas) and other infections (pelvic inflammatory disease, HIV and hepatitis B). Most STIs are preventable, and it's estimated that there are 20 million new cases of STIs in the U.S. each year. Healthy People 2030's overall goal for STIs is to "reduce STIs and their complications and improve access to quality STI care." Clients should be educated about STIs and their individual risks as well as the need to follow current recommendations for STI screenings. (Refer to PN AMS: CH 57: DIAGNOSTIC AND THERAPEUTIC PROCEDURES FOR REPRODUCTIVE DISORDERS.)

It is important that healthcare providers conduct a thorough client sexual history and suggest including primary prevention strategies into the plan of care. These measures will identify risks for STIs and allow for prompt intervention. According to the CDC (2021), some of the questions to ask while obtaining a client's sexual history are related to the 5 P's. Qᴘᴄᴄ

5 P'S

Practices

"What type of sexual contact do you have or have you had in the past?"

Protection from STIs

- "What protection methods do you use?"
- "Do you and your partner have conversations about prevention of STIs and getting tested?"

Past history of STIs

- "Have you been tested for STIs?"
- "Have you been diagnosed with any STIs?"

Pregnancy intention

- "What is your plan for having children?"
- "Are you using in contraceptives?"

Partners

- "Are you currently sexually active?" (Ask about the number of sex partners within recent months.)
- "What's the gender/sex of your partners?"

Primary prevention strategies
- Encourage vaccinations (HPV, HAV, HBV).
- Discuss the importance of use of external/internal condoms (decreased risk of STIs with persistent and proper usage).
- Discuss the importance of retesting after diagnosis (gonorrhea, chlamydia, trichomoniasis) and the importance of serologic testing for diagnosis (HIV, syphilis), and follow the recommended guidelines for follow-up testing.

General infections

Bacterial vaginosis (BV)

BV is prevalent, worldwide condition that is the common cause of vaginal discharge. It is caused by the replacement of the expected vaginal flora (hydrogen peroxide and lactobacilli) with anaerobic bacteria (*Gardnerella vaginalis, Mycoplasma hominis, Mobiluncus, Prevotella*).

COMPLICATIONS

If BV is left untreated, it can increase risk for the development of other STIs, including HIV and complications of pregnancy.

DATA COLLECTION

RISK FACTORS

- New or multiple sex partners
- Unprotected sexual practices
- Douching
- HSV2
- Increases during menses
- IUD use

EXPECTED FINDINGS

- Most clients are asymptomatic.
- Client may report thin or milky, white or gray discharge with a fish-like odor, especially after sex.

PHYSICAL EXAMINATION FINDINGS: Discharge in the vaginal vault, which can be sampled for microscopy

LABORATORY TESTS/ DIAGNOSTIC PROCEDURES

- **Wet prep:** microscopic examination of discharge that is placed on a slide with normal saline and 10% potassium hydroxide (KOH) (identifies the presence of clue cells, which could indicate presence of BV)
- Sample of the vaginal discharge applied to pH (nitrazine) paper (pH > 4.5 could indicate presence of BV.)
- Whiff test (The release of a fishy odor before or after the addition of KOH could indicate the presence of BV.)

PATIENT-CENTERED CARE

NURSING ACTIONS

CLIENT EDUCATION
- Encourage client to be tested for other STIs and HIV.
- Clindamycin intravaginal ovules can decrease the effectiveness of latex or rubber contraceptives (condoms, diaphragms). Clients should avoid using these products concurrently and within 72 hours following treatment.
- Sprinkle PO granules onto yogurt, pudding, or unsweetened applesauce prior to administration and ingestion followed by a glass of water to aid in swallowing.
- Avoid alcohol while taking metronidazole due to a disulfiram-like reaction (severe nausea and vomiting).
- Take all medications as prescribed.
- Understand the possibility of decreasing effectiveness of oral contraceptives.
- Treatment is not usually indicated for sex partners who are male.
- Adhere to safe sex practices.
- If findings reoccur, follow up with provider.

THERAPEUTIC MANAGEMENT

Medications

Recommended
- Metronidazole PO or intravaginal gel
- Clindamycin intravaginal cream

Alternatives
- Clindamycin PO
- Clindamycin intravaginal ovules
- Secnidazole (PO granules) or tinidazole PO

Other: Probiotic lactobacilli can be used for prevention of BV.

Candidiasis

Candidiasis, also known as vulvovaginal candidiasis (VVC) or yeast infection, is a fungal infection most often caused by *Candida albicans*, or other non-*Candida albicans* or yeast. According to the CDC (2021), 75% of clients who have a vagina will experience at least one incident of VVC. It is the second most common type of vaginal infection in the U.S. VVC is classified as uncomplicated (occasional episode of VVC) or complicated (3 or more episodes within 1 year).

COMPLICATIONS

May increase risk for developing other STIs in clients who are sexually active

DATA COLLECTION

RISK FACTORS

- **Medications:** oral contraceptive, corticosteroids, antibiotics
- **Personal hygiene:** frequent douching
- Pregnancy
- **Conditions:** systemic (diabetes mellitus) or immunocompromised (HIV)

EXPECTED FINDINGS

Client may report vulvar and vaginal pruritus; painful urination (due to the excoriation from itching); dyspareunia; and white, clumpy discharge.

PHYSICAL EXAMINATION FINDINGS
- **Speculum examination:** Thick, creamy, white, cottage cheese-like vaginal discharge, white patches on vaginal walls
- Vulvar and vaginal erythema and inflammation

LABORATORY/DIAGNOSTIC TESTS

- **Wet mount smear:** microscopic evaluation of vaginal discharge applied to slide and normal saline, and 10% potassium chloride (KOH) solution is applied to slide sample. If positive for candidiasis, yeast buds, hyphae, or pseudohyphae will be present.
- **pH testing:** Less than 5 may indicate candidiasis.
- Vaginal cultures
- PCR testing for clients who remain symptomatic after receiving treatment

PATIENT-CENTERED CARE

NURSING ACTIONS

CLIENT EDUCATION

- Medication therapy may weaken or decrease the effectiveness of rubber or latex contraceptives (condoms, diaphragms).
- All clients who have manifestations should be tested.
- Follow up with provider if experience recurrent findings.
- Avoid tight-fitting clothing, and wear cotton-lined underpants.
- Avoid douching.
- If infections are recurrent or frequent, diabetes should be ruled out.

THERAPEUTIC MANAGEMENT

Medications

Clients who have complicated findings of VVC or recurrent VVC may need longer duration of therapy or combination therapy.

Over-the-counter antifungals: used to manage uncomplicated findings of VVC; however, the provider should diagnose candidiasis initially. Available in topical preparations, intravaginal creams, suppositories, and ointments and can be taken up to 7 days
- Miconazole
- Clotrimazole

Prescribed antifungals: Available topically, intravaginally, and orally
- Terconazole
- Butoconazole
- Fluconazole (PO) as single dose

Infections identified by type of lesion if present

Herpes simplex virus (HSV)

HSV is a chronic, lifetime, double-strand DNA virus that has two types (HSV-1, HSV-2). HSV-1 affects the oral cavity and is associated with cold sores. However, according to CDC (2021), there is an increased proportion of anogenital HSV infections. HSV-2 affects the genital area and is associated with genital herpes. Genital herpes is spread by direct contact (mouth, oropharynx, or oral mucosa genitals, cervix, rectal) with lesions and can invade the nerve cells at the site of infection. HSV can remain dormant and flare up spontaneously. Reoccurrence will vary.

Healthy People 2030

Goal: Reduce proportion of adolescents with HSV2.

COMPLICATIONS

- May increase risk for developing other STIs in clients who are sexually active and vulnerable to HIV
- Aseptic meningitis
- Neonatal transmission
- Severe emotional stress

DATA COLLECTION

RISK FACTORS

Reoccurrences: stress, sun exposure, dental procedures, fatigue, decreased nutritional intake

EXPECTED FINDINGS

Client may initially report lesions and tender lymph nodes, pain and itching at infection site, dysuria. After lesions appear may report malaise, muscle aches, mild fever.

PHYSICAL EXAMINATION FINDINGS
Genital herpes (lesions) can be diagnosed by the provider based on appearance during physical examination.
- Lesions at the site of infection: initially macules or papules that progress to vesicles and ulcers. The vesicular lesions will rupture and ulcerate and eventually encrust within 2 weeks.
- Inguinal lymphadenopathy

LABORATORY/DIAGNOSTIC TESTS

- **Viral culture:** Obtained from sample of fluid from lesions
- **Virologic testing:** NAAT assays (highly sensitive)

PATIENT-CENTERED CARE

NURSING ACTIONS

CLIENT EDUCATION

- Reinforce with the client there is no cure and HSV is managed by reliving symptoms and decreasing reoccurrences.
- Encourage testing for other STIs such as HIV.
- Refrain from direct sexual activity while infection is active.
- Avoid sun exposure.
- Encourage the use of barrier contraceptives (condoms).
- Inform sex partners to receive evaluation.
- Refer for support services.
- Keep follow-up appointments.
- Take medications as prescribed (prevent reoccurrence).
- Take analgesics for pain or discomfort.
- Lesion care: Wash lesions with mild soap and water and dry gently.
- Wash hands after contact with lesions.
- Wear loose clothing if lesions are present.

THERAPEUTIC MANAGEMENT

Medications

There is no cure for HSV. Therefore, therapy involves managing symptoms and preventing reoccurrences and decreasing transmission to sex partners.

Antivirals: used to decrease the duration of lesions and prevent reoccurrence; recurrent infections may need suppressive therapy (take antiviral medications for longer duration)
- Acyclovir PO
- Valacyclovir PO
- Famciclovir PO

Other

Analgesics: manage discomfort

Human papilloma virus (HPV)

HPV is the most common STI in the U.S. There are over 14 million new cases annually and an estimated total of 79 million cases. There are several strains of the virus. HPV strain 6,11 can cause genital warts (condyloma acuminata). Other strains can affect the cervix and cause dysplasia, or cancer. HPV can spread through oral, vaginal, and anal sex (most commonly vaginal or anal routes). Prevention is key; therefore, encouraging routine recommended Pap test screening for females who are 21 to 65 years of age (and during pregnancy) can provide early detection. All clients who are eligible should be provided information about the HPV vaccine. The vaccine is indicated for all clients (male and female) who are 9-26 years of age and is routinely recommended for all clients 11 or 12 years of age to prevent the transmission of HPV (The Advisory Committee on Immunization Practices (ACIP) (2019).

Healthy People 2030 Goals

- Increase proportion of adolescents who get recommended doses of HPV vaccine.
- Reduce HPV infection types that are prevented by vaccine in young adults.

COMPLICATIONS

- May increase risk for developing other STIs in clients who are sexually active and increased vulnerability to HIV
- Increases risk for cervical, vulvar, vaginal, oropharyngeal, and penile cancer

DATA COLLECTION

RISK FACTORS

- Young age
- Multiple partners
- Unprotected sexual practices

EXPECTED FINDINGS

Client reports lesions/bumps in the genital area that might not itch or hurt, vaginal discharge, dyspareunia, and bleeding after intercourse.

Physical examination findings

Genital warts (lesions) can be diagnosed by the provider based on appearance during physical examination.

Small papules (that are white or color of the client's skin tone) that can appear as growths on the genital area. They can appear in a cluster and grow into a cauliflower mass-like appearance.

LABORATORY/DIAGNOSTIC TESTS

- Pap test with or without HPV co-testing (can follow screening recommendations per American Cancer Society and American College of Obstetricians and Gynecologists guidelines) detects unexpected findings on the cervix (dysplasia, lesions, HPV).
- 3-5% acetic acid application to affected area (causes lesion to turn white)
- Colposcopy (with possible cervical biopsy) can further examine unexpected finding from Pap test.

PATIENT-CENTERED CARE

NURSING ACTIONS

CLIENT EDUCATION

- Consider abstinence or safe sex practices (mutual monogamy; correct, consistent condom use).
- Inform clients about condition and the potential for reoccurrences after receiving treatment.
- Provide information about any prescribed topical medications and how to administer.

- Encourage client to receive routine recommended Pap smear screenings.
- HPV can remain present and still be transmitted to partners after warts are gone.
- Inform partner(s) of diagnosis of genital warts.
- Encourage testing for other STIs such as HIV.

THERAPEUTIC MANAGEMENT

There is no cure for HPV, and the management focuses on the client's lesions and decreasing their severity of symptoms.

Medications

Topical agents: applied by provider directly to lesions
- Trichloroacetic acid (TCA) application or bichloroacetic acid (BCA) application
- Podophyllin resin with benzoin

Topical agents: applied by the client directly to lesions
- Podofilox
- Imiquimod
- Sinecatechins (green-tea extract)

PROCEDURES

- Cryotherapy
- Surgical removal (scissor or shave excision)
- Laser therapy

Syphilis

Syphilis is an acute or chronic STI that is caused by the spirochete *Treponema pallidum*. Syphilis has three stages (primary, secondary, tertiary). It can be transmitted through oral, vaginal, or anal sex, as well as transmitted by birth parent to fetus during pregnancy (congenital).

Healthy People 2030 Goal/objective

Reduce the rate of syphilis in clients who are female and men who have sex with men.

COMPLICATIONS

- If untreated, can cause brain and eye problems and increase the likelihood of developing and transmitting HIV. Condom use, screening, and early treatment of clients and their sexual partner(s) can decrease rate.
- Infection of the eyes (leading to blindness) or nervous system (headache, numbness, paralysis, dementia)

DATA COLLECTION

RISK FACTORS

- Individuals of Black and Pacific Islander cultures are at increased risk.
- Multiple partners
- Unprotected sexual practices

EXPECTED FINDINGS (RELATED TO STAGE)

Primary stage

Within at least 2 weeks after inoculation, a client may notice a chancre lesion appears at the site of infection (genitals, oral cavity). A chancre is a small, painless papule with raised margins. After 3-7 days, the chancre lesion can ulcerate to weeping lesion. The chancre can spontaneously resolve within 3-12 weeks, with or without treatment.

Secondary stage

After the appearance of the chancre lesion, within 1 week-6 months, the client may develop generalized findings. The client may notice a reddish-brown maculopapular skin rash on the palmar surface of the hands and the soles of the feet. Other findings include lymphadenopathy, malaise, weight loss, meningitis, and arthritis.

Latent (phase)

The client does not have any expected findings of syphilis present.

Tertiary stage

This is the final stage of syphilis that is noted 1-20 years after infection. The client can experience damage to multiple organs. Findings can include neurosyphilis, psychosis, dementia, stroke, and meningitis. A soft tumor known as "gumma" can appear on internal organs and cause multiple unexpected findings.

PHYSICAL EXAMINATION FINDINGS
Chancre lesion on genital area, reddish-brown maculopapular skin rash on palms of hands and soles of the feet and lymphadenopathy

LABORATORY/DIAGNOSTIC TESTS

Serology tests

Nontreponemal: used often for initial screening. Venereal Disease Research Laboratory (VDRL) or rapid plasma regain (RPR)

Treponemal: If client has a positive or reactive nontreponemal test, then a treponemal test is performed to determine definite diagnosis of syphilis. This test can detect specific antibodies for syphilis.
- Fluorescent treponemal antibody absorption (FTA-ABS)
- Enzyme immunoassay, immunoassays

Microscopic: Darkfield examination of sample of primary lesion (diagnostic of syphilis as well)

PATIENT-CENTERED CARE

NURSING ACTIONS

CLIENT EDUCATION

- Abstain from sexual contact until lesions are completely healed.
- Inform client that their sex partner(s) should be tested and treated.
- Adhere to safe sex practices.
- All states have a reportable diseases list. Syphilis is a commonly reported condition. It is the responsibility of the provider to report cases of these diseases to the local health department.
- After treatment, report headache, fever, tachycardia, and myalgia. This could be indicative of Jarisch-Herxheimer reaction and should be reported to the provider.

THERAPEUTIC MANAGEMENT

Medications

Antibiotics: used to decrease the duration of lesions and prevent reoccurrence

- Benzathine penicillin G (IM) single dose if duration of condition known; if duration is unknown, the client may require 3 injections at 1-week intervals
- Doxycycline or tetracycline PO (if client has penicillin allergy)

Infections identified by type of discharge if present

Chlamydia

Chlamydia is a bacterial infection caused by *Chlamydia trachomatis* and is the most frequent and commonly reported STI in America. The infection can be difficult to diagnose because the client rarely has manifestations. Chlamydia is transmitted by direct sexual contact or during birth to newborn. The Centers for Disease Control and Prevention (CDC) recommends yearly screening of all sexually active females younger than 25 years, as well as older females who have risk factors.

Healthy People 2030

Goal: Increase the proportion of clients who are female and are sexually active to be screened for chlamydia.

Complications: If chlamydia is untreated, can cause:
- Pelvic inflammatory disease (PID)
- Increased risk of ectopic pregnancy
- Increased risk for infertility
- Conjunctivitis

DATA COLLECTION

RISK FACTORS

- Multiple or new sexual partners
- Unprotected sex
- Female

EXPECTED FINDINGS

Male

Often asymptomatic
- Penile discharge (watery or mucus)
- Dysuria, urinary frequency
- Testicular edema or pain

Female

Can be asymptomatic
- Vulvar itching
- Gray-white or yellowish discharge
- Dysuria, urinary frequency
- Spotting, bleeding between menstrual periods, or postcoital bleeding

PHYSICAL EXAMINATION FINDINGS
- Mucopurulent (yellowish green) endocervical discharge
- Easily induced endocervical bleeding

LABORATORY/DIAGNOSTIC TESTS

- Swab culture of discharge
- Urine culture specimen

PATIENT-CENTERED CARE

NURSING ACTIONS

CLIENT EDUCATION

- Instruct client to take all medication as prescribed.
- Inform client that their sex partners should be tested and treated.
- Retest within 3 months after treatment is complete.
- Encourage safe sex practices (mutual monogamy; correct, consistent condom use).
- Abstain from sexual intercourse until sex partners are treated.
- Encourage annual recommended screening according to guidelines.
- Encourage testing for other STIs (gonorrhea, syphilis, HIV).
- Doxycycline may decrease the effectiveness of oral contraceptives.
- If continued sexual activity is desired, be aware of the sexually transmitted infection status of any sexual partner(s) and use a barrier contraceptive each time you have sex.
- All states have a reportable diseases list. Chlamydia is a commonly reported condition. It is the responsibility of the provider to report cases of these diseases to the local health department.

THERAPEUTIC MANAGEMENT

Medications

Antibiotics
- Doxycycline PO up to 7 days (recommended)
- Azithromycin PO single dose
- Levofloxacin PO

Gonorrhea

Gonorrhea is the 2nd most reported STI with over 1 million new cases annually. *Neisseria gonorrhoeae* is the causative agent of gonorrhea. Gonorrhea is a bacterial infection that is primarily spread by genital-to-genital contact. However, it also can be spread by anal-to-genital or oral-to-genital contact. It can also be transmitted to a newborn during birth. Females frequently have no manifestations. The CDC recommends yearly screening for all sexually active females younger than 25 years as well as older females who have risk factors (new or multiple sex partners).

Healthy People 2030

Goal: Reduce gonorrhea in clients who are male.

Complications: If gonorrhea is untreated, can cause:
- Scarring of fallopian tubes and lead to pelvic inflammatory disease (PID)
- Increased risk of ectopic pregnancy
- Increased risk for infertility
- Chronic pelvic pain
- Epididymitis

DATA COLLECTION

RISK FACTORS

- Multiple sexual partners
- Unprotected sexual practices
- Age less than 25, if sexually active

EXPECTED FINDINGS

Rectal: Client may report purulent discharge, rectal pain or bleeding, and diarrhea.

Male

- Dysuria
- Testicular edema or pain
- Penile discharge (purulent or white), sometimes profuse

Female

Often no manifestations, but can experience:
- Dysuria
- Vaginal bleeding between periods
- Dysmenorrhea

PHYSICAL EXAMINATION FINDINGS
- Yellowish-green vaginal discharge
- Easily induced endocervical bleeding

LABORATORY/DIAGNOSTIC TESTS

- Swab specimen of discharge for cultures: (endocervical, anal, oral)
- Urine cultures

PATIENT-CENTERED CARE

NURSING ACTIONS

CLIENT EDUCATION
- Instruct client to take all medication as prescribed.
- Inform client that their sex partners (within last 60 days) should be tested and treated.
- Retest within 3 months after treatment is complete.
- Provide client with information regarding infection transmission.
- Encourage safe sex practices (mutual monogamy; correct, consistent condom use).
- Abstain from sexual intercourse until sex partners are treated.
- Encourage annual screening.
- Medications used to manage gonorrhea may decrease the effectiveness of oral contraceptives.
- If continued sexual activity is desired, be aware of the sexually transmitted infection status of any sexual partner(s) and use a barrier contraceptive each time you have sex.
- All states have a reportable diseases list. Gonorrhea is a commonly reported condition. It is the responsibility of the provider to report cases of these diseases to the local health department.

THERAPEUTIC MANAGEMENT

Medications

CDC recommends treatment for chlamydia as well for those who test positive for gonorrhea.

Antibiotics
- Dual therapy is the recommended first-line treatment: Azithromycin PO single dose and ceftriaxone IM administered concurrently on the same day
- Alternatives: Gentamicin IM and azithromycin PO or cefixime PO
- Single IM dose of ceftriaxone (infection of oropharynx)

Trichomoniasis

Trichomoniasis is a STI caused by the protozoan parasite *Trichomonas vaginalis.* There are about 3.7 million cases annually in the U.S. It can be spread penis-to-vagina or vagina-to-vagina.

Complications: If trichomoniasis is untreated, can cause:
- Complications of pregnancy
- Increased risk for development of PID
- Infertility
- Increased risk of contracting HIV from a partner who is infected

DATA COLLECTION

RISK FACTORS

- Black older adult clients who are female
- Multiple sex partners
- History of chlamydia within the past 12 months
- Incarceration

EXPECTED FINDINGS

Male

- Urethral draining, itching, or irritation
- Dysuria or pain with ejaculation

Female

- Yellow-green, frothy vaginal discharge with foul odor
- Dyspareunia and vaginal itching
- Dysuria

PHYSICAL EXAMINATION FINDINGS
- Speculum examination: discharge in the vaginal vault (which can be sampled for microscopy); strawberry spots on the cervix (tiny petechiae)
- A cervix that bleeds easily

LABORATORY/DIAGNOSTIC TESTS

- Wet mount saline prep microscopically detects the presence of trichomonad(s).
- Cultures, urine specimens (POC, molecular testing, NAAT, rapid tests)
- Pap smear can incidentally detect the presence of trichomonads.

PATIENT-CENTERED CARE

NURSING ACTIONS

CLIENT EDUCATION
- Instruct client to take all medication as prescribed.
- Inform client that their sex partners should be tested and treated.
- Retest clients who are female within 3 months after treatment is complete (no data to support retesting of clients who are male).

- Provide client with information regarding infection transmission.
- Encourage client to receive testing for presence of other STIs (HIV, syphilis, gonorrhea, chlamydia).
- Encourage safe sex practices (mutual monogamy; correct, consistent condom use).
- Abstain from sexual intercourse until treatment is complete and sex partner(s) are treated.
- Avoid alcohol consumption while taking metronidazole (can cause disulfiram-like reaction of severe nausea and vomiting).

THERAPEUTIC MANAGEMENT

Medications

CDC recommends treatment for chlamydia as well for those who test positive for gonorrhea.

Antibiotics
- Metronidazole: PO single dose or BID for 7 days (recommended)
- Tinidazole: PO single dose (more expensive)

Other Infections

Pelvic inflammatory disease (PID)

PID is an inflammatory condition that affects the reproductive tract. It can begin as cervicitis and can spread to uterus, fallopian tubes, ovaries, pelvic vascular or peritoneum. Infections can be acute, subacute, recurrent, or chronic. It can be localized or widespread. It can be caused by bacteria, parasite, virus, or fungus; however, gonorrhea and chlamydia most common factor. Routine screenings for clients who are sexually active for gonorrhea and chlamydia can reduce risk.

Healthy People 2030

Goal: Reduce PID in adolescent clients who are female.

COMPLICATIONS

- Scarring or obstruction of fallopian tubes
- Increased risk of infertility, ectopic pregnancy
- Recurrent infections, pelvic pain
- Tubo-ovarian abscess, peritonitis, strictures,
- Recurrent infections
- Pelvic adhesions

DATA COLLECTION

RISK FACTORS

- Multiple sexual partners
- Early age of first sex
- Unprotected sexual practices
- Frequent sexual intercourse
- History of other STIs or pelvic infections
- Invasive procedures (endometrial biopsies, hysteroscopy)
- Intrauterine device (IUD)

EXPECTED FINDINGS

Could be asymptomatic or have findings that are non-specific

- Vaginal discharge (odorous, purulent), dysuria, dyspareunia, pelvic pain or tenderness, bleeding after intercourse
- Fever, malaise, anorexia, nausea, vomiting, headache

PHYSICAL EXAMINATION FINDINGS
Pelvic exam: tenderness (cervical, adnexal, uterine)

LABORATORY/DIAGNOSTIC PROCEDURES

- Increased ESR, C-reactive protein
- Gonorrhea/chlamydia positive
- Swab specimen of discharge for cultures: (endocervical, anal, oral)
- Urine cultures
- Laparoscopy (salpingitis)
- Endometrial biopsy (endometritis)
- Transvaginal sonogram

PATIENT-CENTERED CARE

NURSING ACTIONS

CLIENT EDUCATION
- Instruct client to take all medication as prescribed.
- Inform client that their sex partner(s) (within last 60 days) may need testing and treatment (depending on causative findings).
- Retest within 3 months after treatment is complete (if positive for gonorrhea or chlamydia).
- Provide client with information regarding infection transmission.
- Encourage safe sex practices (mutual monogamy; correct, consistent condom use).
- Encourage client to receive testing for presence of other STIs (HIV, syphilis, gonorrhea, chlamydia).
- If IUD is present, may need removal.
- Abstain from sexual intercourse until both client and sex partners are treated (completed treatment).
- Encourage recommended annual screening for gonorrhea and chlamydia.

THERAPEUTIC MANAGEMENT

Clients are managed outpatient, but inpatient management may be indicated depending on severity of symptoms. Treatment may be initiated as soon as presumptive diagnosis of PID is known.

Medications

Antibiotics: Broad spectrum/combination therapy to provide treatment for various causative organisms

IV therapy
- Ceftriaxone IV, doxycycline IV/PO, and metronidazole PO/IV
- Cefotetan IV and doxycycline IV
- Cefoxitin IV and doxycycline PO/IV
- Alternate parenteral therapy: Ampicillin-sulbactam IV and doxycycline PO/IV; clindamycin IV and gentamicin IV

IM/PO therapy
- Ceftriaxone IM, doxycycline PO, and metronidazole PO
- Cefoxitin and probenecid PO and doxycycline PO, metronidazole PO
- Other third generation cephalosporin IM, plus doxycycline PO and metronidazole PO

Analgesics: Manage discomfort

HIV/AIDS

HIV is a retrovirus that attacks and causes destruction of T lymphocytes. It causes immunosuppression in a client. Clients who are severely immunosuppressed develop acquired immunodeficiency syndrome (AIDS). HIV screening should be voluntary and free from coercion and clients should provide informed consent. Clients should not be tested without their knowledge. (Refer to **PN AMS: CHAPTER 86: PREOPERATIVE NURSING CARE** for Comprehensive Information regarding HIV/AIDS.)

Healthy People 2030

- Reduce the number of new HIV infections for adolescent clients.
- LBGTQIA populations: increase knowledge of HIV status, reduce number of new HIV cases, increase linkage to HIV medical care, and increase viral suppression.

GENERAL CONSIDERATIONS

- ART should be initiated ASAP regardless of the client's CD4 count.
- All states have a reportable diseases list, and HIV is condition that requires mandatory reporting. It is the responsibility of the provider to report cases of these diseases to the local health department.
- Determine need for additional support (psychosocial, medical) and help with obtaining.
- Screen clients for other STIs (gonorrhea, chlamydia, syphilis, hepatitis B).
- Encourage safe sex practices (mutual monogamy; correct, consistent condom use).
- Encourage client to receive testing for presence of other STIs (HIV, syphilis, gonorrhea, chlamydia).

Hepatitis B

Hepatitis B is a virus that is transmitted by contact via blood or sexual intercourse. It can also be transmitted to fetus during pregnancy. (Refer to **PN AMS: CHAPTER 55** for comprehensive information regarding Hepatitis infection.)

Healthy People 2030

- Reduce rate of deaths with hepatitis B and C as the cause.
- Reduce the rate of hepatitis A, B, C.
- Increase the proportion of clients who know they have chronic hep B.
- Increase the proportion of clients who no longer have hepatitis C.

GENERAL CONSIDERATIONS

- Encourage clients to receive HBV and HBA vaccine according to current recommended schedule guidelines if not previously vaccinated.
- Encourage household members, sexual partners, and injectable-substance-use partners to be tested for susceptibility for HBV. All susceptible clients may require vaccination.
- Encourage clients to limit or avoid alcohol consumption to prevent additional harm to liver.
- To prevent the risk of transmitting to others.
  - Encourage safe sex practices (correct, consistent condom use).
  - Keep open cuts and lesions covered.
  - Avoid donating blood, semen.
  - Avoid sharing of household items (razor, toothbrush).
- All states have a reportable diseases list, and if a client tests positive for HBsAg, the provider is responsible for reporting this to the state or local health department.
- Encourage client to be retested to determine the presence of chronic infection with HBV.
- If positive for chronic HBV, client will require referral to specialist provider.
- Provide supportive care; no specific therapy for HBV infection.
- Determine need for additional support (psychosocial, medical) and help with obtaining.

1. A nurse is caring for a client who has vulvovaginal candidiasis infection. Which of the following findings in the client's EMR should the nurse identify as a risk factor for candidiasis infection?
   - A. Multiparity
   - B. Recent antibiotic use
   - C. History of UTI
   - D. Unprotected sex with monogamous partner

2. A nurse is reinforcing teaching with client who has a new diagnosis of genital herpes (HSV2). Which of the following client statements indicates teaching was effective? (Select all that apply.)
   - A. "I will take acyclovir to prevent reoccurrence."
   - B. "I can apply imiquimod cream to my genitals."
   - C. "I will not have herpes once I finish taking all of my medication."
   - D. "I should take 3 doses of the herpes vaccine."
   - E. "I should keep the lesions clean and dry."

3. A nurse has collected data from two clients who are reporting a genital lesion. Which of the following client findings should the nurse identify as findings for genital wart (HPV) or syphilis? Sort the findings to indicate either HPV or syphilis.
   - A. Ulceration
   - B. Papule
   - C. Chancre-like lesion
   - D. Condyloma

4. A nurse is caring for a client who has a positive test result for chlamydia. Which of the following medications should the nurse anticipate a prescription for by the provider?
   - A. Metronidazole
   - B. Doxycycline
   - C. Fluconazole
   - D. Podophyllin

5. A nurse is assisting with the admission of a client who has PID. Which of the following findings should nurse expect the client to report? (Select all that apply.)
   - A. Purulent discharge
   - B. Nausea
   - C. Dizziness
   - D. Fever
   - E. Pain during intercourse

Active Learning Scenario

A nurse is planning care for a client who has syphilis. Use the ATI Active Learning Template: System Disorder to complete this item.

RISK FACTORS: List 3 risk factors.

LABORATORY/DIAGNOSTIC TESTS: Explain the different diagnostic tests.

THERAPEUTIC MANAGEMENT: Discuss the medications used to manage the condition.

CLIENT EDUCATION: Provide 5 educational points to discuss with client.

Active Learning Scenario Key

Using the ATI Active Learning Template: System Disorder

RISK FACTORS:
- Individuals from Black and Pacific Islander cultures are at increased risk.
- Multiple partners
- Unprotected sexual practices

LABORATORY/DIAGNOSTIC TESTS: Serology tests
- Nontreponemal: used often for initial screening
  - Venereal Disease Research Laboratory (VDRL) or rapid plasma regain (RPR)
- Treponemal: If client has a positive or reactive nontreponemal test, then a treponemal test is performed to determine definite diagnosis of syphilis. This test can detect specific antibodies for syphilis.
  - Fluorescent treponemal antibody absorption (FTA-ABS)
  - Enzyme immunoassay, immunoassays
- Microscopic: Darkfield examination of sample of primary lesion (diagnostic of syphilis as well)

MEDICATIONS:
- There is no cure for HSV. Therefore, therapy involves managing symptoms and preventing reoccurrences.
- Antibiotics: used to decrease the duration of lesions and prevent reoccurrence
- *Benzathine penicillin G (IM) single dose if duration of condition known; if duration is unknown, the client may require 3 injections at 1-week intervals
- *Doxycycline or tetracycline PO (if client has penicillin allergy)

CLIENT EDUCATION:
- Abstain from sexual contact until lesions are completely healed.
- Inform client that their sex partners should be tested and treated.
- Adhere to safe sex practices.
- All states have a reportable diseases list. Syphilis is a commonly reported condition. It is the responsibility of the provider to report cases of these diseases to the local health department.
- After treatment, report headache, fever, tachycardia, and myalgia. This could be indicative of Jarisch-Herxheimer reaction and should be reported to the provider.

Ⓝ *NCLEX® Connection: Physiological Adaptation, Alterations in Body Systems*

Application Exercises Key

1. B. **CORRECT:** When analyzing cues from the client's manifestations, the nurse should identify that risk factors for vulvovaginal candidiasis include recent antibiotic use, which could affect the expected flora of the vagina. Other risk factors include conditions such as diabetes and immunosuppression, pregnancy, and use of contraceptives or corticosteroids.

Ⓝ *NCLEX® Connection: Health Promotion and Maintenance, Health Promotion/Disease Prevention*

2. A, E. **CORRECT:** The reinforcing of teaching is effective when the client states, "I will take acyclovir to prevent reoccurrence," and "I should keep my lesions clean and dry." Acyclovir is an antiviral medication that decreases the severity of symptoms with HSV2 and prevents reoccurrence. The client should keep the lesions clean and dry to promote healing. Applying imiquimod cream is used for a client who has genital warts. Herpes is a virus, which means that the client will still have the condition, but it can remain dormant in the body or flare up at any time. There is no vaccine for herpes.

Ⓝ *NCLEX® Connection: Physiological Adaptation, Alterations in Body Systems*

3. **HPV2:** B, D; **SYPHILIS:** A, C

By recognizing cues, the nurse should identify that a lesion with the appearance of an ulceration and chancre could indicate syphilis. A lesion that looks like a papule or condyloma could indicate HPV or genital wart.

Ⓝ *NCLEX® Connection: Physiological Adaptation, Basic Pathophysiology*

4. B. **CORRECT:** The nurse should anticipate a prescription for doxycycline, which is the recommended antibiotic that is used to treat chlamydia. The nurse should recognize metronidazole, fluconazole, and podophyllin are medications that can be prescribed to manage other infections. Metronidazole can be prescribed to treat infections such as bacterial vaginosis and trichomoniasis. Fluconazole may be prescribed to treat candida infections. Podophyllin can be prescribed and applied by the provider to treat genital warts (HPV2).

Ⓝ *NCLEX® Connection: Pharmacological Therapies, Expected Actions/Outcomes*

5. A, B, D, E. **CORRECT:** When recognizing cues from a client who has PID, the nurse can expect the client to report a purulent vaginal discharge, nausea, fever, and pain during intercourse.

Ⓝ *NCLEX® Connection: Physiological Adaptation, Alterations in Body Systems*

ⓝ NCLEX® Connections

When reviewing the following chapters, keep in mind the relevant topics and tasks of the NCLEX outline.

Basic Care and Comfort

ASSISTIVE DEVICES: Contribute to the care of the client using assistive device.

MOBILITY/IMMOBILITY: Identify signs and symptoms of venous insufficiency and intervene to promote venous return.

NONPHARMACOLOGICAL COMFORT INTERVENTIONS
Provide nonpharmacological measures for pain relief.

Apply therapies for comfort and treatment of inflammation/swelling.

Reduction of Risk Potential

POTENTIAL FOR ALTERATIONS IN BODY SYSTEMS
Identify the client with an increased risk for insufficient blood circulation.

Apply and check proper use of compression stockings and/or sequential compression devices.

POTENTIAL FOR COMPLICATIONS OF DIAGNOSTIC TESTS/ TREATMENTS/PROCEDURES: Use precautions to prevent injury and/or complications associated with a procedure or diagnosis.

POTENTIAL FOR COMPLICATIONS FROM SURGICAL PROCEDURES AND HEALTH ALTERATIONS: Monitor client responses to procedures and treatments.

Physiological Adaptation

ALTERATIONS IN BODY SYSTEMS
Perform wound care and/or dressing change.

Remove wound sutures or staples.

Reinforce education to client regarding care and condition.

MEDICAL EMERGENCIES: Notify primary health care provider about client unexpected response/emergency situation.

CHAPTER 61 *Musculoskeletal Diagnostic Procedures*

Imaging studies are the primary diagnostic procedures for musculoskeletal disorders. Muscle weakness is an indication for evaluating the conduction of electrical impulses. Arthroscopy monitors the condition of a joint and allows the repair of tears and other joint defects.

Musculoskeletal diagnostic procedures that nurses should be knowledgeable about include arthroscopy, nuclear scans (bone scan, gallium scan, thallium scan), dual-energy x-ray absorptiometry scans (DXA), electromyography (EMG), and nerve conduction studies. Other diagnostic procedures that help detect joint problems and identify musculoskeletal structures are x-ray studies, ultrasounds (US), computed tomography (CT) scans, and magnetic resonance imaging (MRI). Informed consent should be obtained prior to certain procedures and tests.

Arthroscopy

- Arthroscopy allows visualization of the internal structures of a joint through the use of an endoscope. It is most commonly used to evaluate the knee and shoulder joints and is performed in the operating room under sterile conditions using local or general anesthesia.
- Number and placement of incisions depend on the area of the joint undergoing visualization and the extent of the repair.
- Infection in the joint and a lack of joint mobility are contraindications for arthroscopy.

INDICATIONS

POTENTIAL DIAGNOSES: A client who has a joint injury can undergo arthroscopy to ascertain the extent of damage, during which the provider can use the arthroscope to repair a torn ligament or meniscus or perform a synovial biopsy.

CLIENT PRESENTATION
- Joint swelling, pain, and crepitus
- Joint instability

CONSIDERATIONS

PREPROCEDURE

NURSING ACTIONS: Ensure the client signed the informed consent form.

CLIENT EDUCATION: The provider might require performing postoperative joint exercises (straight-leg raises, quadriceps setting isometrics).

POSTPROCEDURE

NURSING ACTIONS
- Provide postoperative care; specific actions and recovery time depend on type of sedation used. The procedure is usually done in an outpatient setting.
- Monitor neurovascular status and dressings on the client's limb every hour or per the facility's protocol. Qs
- Administer mild analgesia for mild pain; opioids can be required if the operation was corrective.

CLIENT EDUCATION
- Apply ice for the first 24 hours to control edema.
- Elevate the extremity for 12 to 24 hours.
- Maintain activity restrictions.
- Monitor the color and temperature of the extremity, as well as pain and sensation.
- Notify the provider of any changes, such as swelling, increased joint pain, thrombophlebitis, or infection (redness, swelling, purulent drainage, fever).

COMPLICATIONS

Infection

Complications are uncommon after this procedure, but infection can occur as with any procedure that disrupts the integrity of the skin.

CLIENT EDUCATION: Notify the provider immediately of swelling, redness, or fever.

Nuclear scans

Bone scans

Bone scans evaluate the entire skeletal system.
- A radionuclide test involves a radioactive isotope via IV injection 2 to 3 hours before scanning. Areas of abnormal bone formation will appear brighter when later scanned.
- Bone scans can detect hairline bone fractures, tumors, fractures, and diseases of the bone (osteomyelitis, osteoporosis, vertebral compression fractures).

Gallium and thallium scans

- The radioisotope migrates to tissues of the brain, liver, and breast and helps detect disease in these organs.
- The client receives the radionuclide injection.
- The scan takes 30 to 60 minutes and can require sedation to help the client lie still during that time. Repeat scanning occurs at 24, 48, and 72 hours as needed.

INDICATIONS

POTENTIAL DIAGNOSES
- Degenerative bone diseases and their progression
- Osteomyelitis
- Stress or vertebral compression fractures, or nonhealing fractures
- Osteoporosis
- Primary or metastatic bone cancer
- Bone pain of unknown origin
- Aseptic necrosis

CLIENT PRESENTATION: Bone pain

CONSIDERATIONS

PREPROCEDURE

NURSING ACTIONS
- Inform the client about the procedure.
- Monitor for allergy to radioisotope or conditions that would prevent performing the procedure (pregnancy, lactation, kidney disease).

CLIENT EDUCATION
- Remain still during the entire procedure.
- Empty the bladder before the procedure to promote visualization of pelvic bones. ◯EBP

POSTPROCEDURE

CLIENT EDUCATION
- Following the procedure, radioactive precautions no longer need to be taken.
- Drink fluids to increase excretion of radioisotope in the urine and feces.

Dual-energy x-ray absorptiometry

- DEXA scans estimate the density of bone mass—usually in the hip or spine—and the presence/extent of osteoporosis.
- A DEXA scan uses two beams of radiation. A computer analyzes the findings, and a radiologist interprets them. Clients do not receive contrast material. Clients receive a score that relates their amount of bone density to that of other people with demographic similarities.
- Clients lie on an x-ray table during scanning of the hip or spine.

Note: These scores are not sex-specific.

INDICATIONS

POTENTIAL DIAGNOSES
- Osteoporosis
- Postmenopausal state
- Baseline testing: females ages 40–49 years

CLIENT PRESENTATION
- Loss of height
- Bone pain
- Fractures

CONSIDERATIONS

PREPROCEDURE CLIENT EDUCATION: Stay dressed but remove metallic objects.

POSTPROCEDURE CLIENT EDUCATION: Follow up with the provider to discuss possible supplements and medications if bone loss is present.

Electromyography and nerve conduction studies

EMG and nerve conduction studies determine the presence and cause of muscle weakness.

EMG

- Clients undergo EMG at the bedside or in an EMG laboratory.
- The technician places thin needles in the muscle under study. Electrodes attach the needles to an oscilloscope, which records activity during a muscle contraction.

Nerve conduction study

- The technician attaches surface or needle electrodes to the skin.
- Low electrical currents go through the electrodes, producing a recording of the muscle response to the stimulus.

INDICATIONS

POTENTIAL DIAGNOSES
- Neuromuscular disorders
- Motor neuron disease
- Peripheral nerve disorders (carpal tunnel)

CONSIDERATIONS

PREPROCEDURE

NURSING ACTIONS
- Inform the client about what to expect.
- Determine whether the client takes an anticoagulant, because anticoagulation is a contraindication for this procedure due to the risk of bleeding within the muscle with needle insertion.
- Check for any skin infections in the area of data collection. Infection is a contraindication for this procedure due to the risk for transmission of the infection to the muscle. Qs
- Ask whether the client takes any muscle relaxants. The provider might discontinue these prior to the procedure to ensure accurate test results.
- Ensure the client signed the consent form.
- Inform the client that fasting is not usually required for an EMG; however, they should avoid smoking and consuming stimulants at least 3 hours prior to the test.
- Inform the client that premedication and sedation is generally avoided for an EMG because the client needs to follow commands during the test.

CLIENT EDUCATION
- Discomfort is possible during needle insertion and when the electrical current goes through the electrodes.
- You might be asked to flex certain muscles during needle insertion.

POSTPROCEDURE

CLIENT EDUCATION
- Bruising can occur at needle insertion sites.
- Report swelling or tenderness at any of the sites to the provider.
- Apply ice to prevent hematoma formation at the needle insertion sites and to reduce swelling. Apply warm compresses to relieve residual discomfort.

CT scan, resonance imaging, radiography, ultrasonography

- Provide detailed images of the body structures, bone density, and texture as well as surgical hardware
- Magnetic resonance imaging (MRI), ultrasound (US) and computed tomography (CT) provide visualization of soft tissues.

INDICATIONS

POTENTIAL DIAGNOSES
- Injuries to tendons and ligaments
- Fractures of bony structures of the chest and pelvis
- Skull and vertebral fracture or herniated disc

CLIENT PRESENTATION
- Bone pain
- Joint instability

NURSING ACTIONS
- **CT scan:** If contrast media is prescribed, monitor for allergy, and ensure client has adequate fluid intake following testing. Qs
- **MRI:** Determine whether the client has metal in the body (pacemakers) and be sure to remove exterior metal (jewelry, hair clips). Qs

DIAGNOSTIC PROCEDURES

EMG

Evaluates muscle weakness and differentiates muscle diseases from neurologic conditions. Ensure the client has not ingested stimulants or muscle relaxants prior to the procedure.

DEXA

Determines bone mineral content and bone density. Ensure the client removes all metallic objects prior to the test.

Gallium scan

Used to detect metastatic tumors, locate infection or inflammation, and monitor response to treatments. Precautions against radioactive exposure are not necessary.

Bone scan

Used to identify pathologic bone conditions and metastatic bone cancer. Encourage the client to drink several glasses of water between the isotope injection and scan.

Arthroscopy

Endoscopic procedure used to examine a joint. Ensure the client has been NPO after midnight the day of the procedure.

CT scan

Used to evaluate pain, trauma, mass, or possible bone fracture. If contrast is injected, the client may feel warmth or flushing.

Application Exercises

1. A nurse is reinforcing preoperative teaching for a client who is to undergo an arthroscopy to repair a shoulder injury. Which of the following statements should the nurse include? (Select all that apply.)

   A. "Avoid damage or moisture to the cast on your arm."

   B. "Inspect your incision daily for indications of infection."

   C. "Apply ice packs to the area for the first 24 hours."

   D. "Keep your arm in a dependent position."

   E. "Perform isometric exercises."

2. A nurse is contributing to the plan of care for a client who is postoperative following an arthroscopy of the knee. Which of the following nursing actions are appropriate? (Select all that apply.)

   A. Monitor color and temperature of the extremity.

   B. Apply warm compresses to incision sites.

   C. Place pillows under the extremity.

   D. Administer analgesic medication.

   E. Monitor pulse and sensation in the foot.

3. A nurse is reinforcing teaching with a client who is going to have a bone scan. Which of the following statements should the nurse include?

   A. "You will receive an injection of a radioactive isotope when the scanning procedure begins."

   B. "You will be inside a tube-like structure during the procedure."

   C. "You will need to take radioactive precautions with your urine for 24 hours after the procedure."

   D. "You will have to urinate just before the procedure."

4. A nurse is reinforcing teaching with clients at a health fair about dual-energy x-ray absorptiometry (DXA) scans. Which of the following information should the nurse include? (Select all that apply.)

   A. The test requires the use of contrast material.

   B. The hip and spine are the usual areas the device scans.

   C. The scan detects osteoarthritis.

   D. Bone pain can indicate a need for a scan.

   E. Females should have a baseline scan during ages 40-49 years.

5. A nurse is contributing to the plan of care for a client who will undergo an electromyography (EMG). Which of the following actions should the nurse include? (Select all that apply.)

   A. Assess for bruising.

   B. Administer aspirin prior to the procedure.

   C. Determine whether the client takes a muscle relaxant.

   D. Instruct the client to flex muscles during needle insertion.

   E. Expect swelling, redness, and tenderness at the insertion sites.

Application Exercises Key

1. **B, C, E. CORRECT:** When taking action, the nurse should tell the client to inspect the incision for evidence of infection (redness, swelling, purulent drainage). The client should apply ice packs to the affected area for the first 24 hours to reduce swelling and discomfort. The client should perform isometric exercises as prescribed by the provider. The nurse should identify that a cast is not typically required following arthroscopy. The client should elevate the affected extremity for 12 to 24 hours to reduce swelling.

   Ⓝ *NCLEX® Connection: Reduction of Risk Potential, Therapeutic Procedures*

2. **A, C, D, E. CORRECT:** When generating solutions, the nurse should plan to monitor color and temperature of the affected extremity to help identify alterations in circulation. When planning care, the nurse should identify that elevating the leg will help decrease swelling and pain in the affected extremity. Administering analgesic medication helps relieve joint pain in the affected extremity. Monitoring the pulse and sensations of the affected extremity helps identify alterations in circulation. The nurse should plan to apply cold compresses on the incisional site for the first 24 hours help decrease swelling and pain.

   Ⓝ *NCLEX® Connection: Physiological Adaptation, Alterations in Body Systems*

3. **D. CORRECT:** The nurse should inform the client that they will need to urinate prior to the procedure. An empty bladder promotes visualization of the pelvic bones. The client should be informed that the radioactive isotope is either injected intravenously (IV) or administered orally 2 to 3 hours before the scanning. Inform the client that the procedure does not use a tube-like structure as for an MRI. The client should be told that radioactive precautions for their urine are not necessary following the procedure.

   Ⓝ *NCLEX® Connection: Reduction of Risk Potential, Therapeutic Procedures*

4. **B, D, E. CORRECT:** When taking action, the nurse should inform the client that the most common areas for a DEXA scan are the hip and spine for more clear visualization of a large area of bone. The nurse should tell the client that bone pain, loss of height, and fractures are findings that can indicate the need for a DEXA scan. Inform the client that a baseline scan for females ages 40-49 years is helpful for comparison with a scan during the postmenopausal period. When reinforcing teaching with the client, tell them that a DEXA scan detects osteoporosis, not osteoarthritis, and that a DEXA scan does not require contrast material.

   Ⓝ *NCLEX® Connection: Reduction of Risk Potential, Therapeutic Procedures*

5. **A, C, D. CORRECT:** When generating solutions, the nurse should identify that some bruising can occur at the needle insertion sites. The nurse should check the client's medications to determine if they take a muscle relaxant, which can decrease the accuracy of the test results. The nurse should ask the client to flex their muscles for an easier insertion of the needle into the muscle. The client should withhold any anticoagulant medication prior to the procedure to reduce the risk of bleeding. The nurse should instruct the client to report swelling, redness, and tenderness at the insertion sites to the provider because this can indicate an infection.

   Ⓝ *NCLEX® Connection: Reduction of Risk Potential, Diagnostic Tests*

Active Learning Scenario

A nurse is reinforcing teaching with a client who is having a gallium scan. What information should the nurse include? Use the ATI Active Learning Template: Diagnostic Procedure to complete this item.

DESCRIPTION OF PROCEDURE

INDICATIONS: List three.

NURSING INTERVENTIONS (PRE, INTRA, POST): List two preprocedure and one postprocedure.

Active Learning Scenario Key

Using the ATI Active Learning Template: Diagnostic Procedure

DESCRIPTION OF PROCEDURE: A gallium scan involves a radioisotope called radioactive gallium that is injected into the client before the scan to view the client's bones. The radionuclide also migrates to the tissues of the brain, liver, and breast and is used to detect disease of these organs.

INDICATIONS: Detect fractures, osteoporosis, bone lesions, osteomyelitis, and arthritis

NURSING INTERVENTIONS (PRE, INTRA, POST)

Preprocedure
- Monitor for allergy to radioisotopes.
- Monitor for existing conditions (pregnancy, kidney disease) that are contraindications for the procedure.
- Have the client empty their bladder before the procedure.

Postprocedure: Inform the client to increase fluid intake to promote the excretion of the radioisotope in the urine and feces.

Ⓝ *NCLEX® Connection: Reduction of Risk Potential, Diagnostic Tests*

UNIT 10   MUSCULOSKELETAL DISORDERS
SECTION: DIAGNOSTIC AND THERAPEUTIC PROCEDURES

CHAPTER 62 *Arthroplasty*

Most musculoskeletal surgical procedures are performed to repair damaged joints, particularly the knees and the hips.

Arthroplasty refers to the surgical removal of a diseased joint due to osteoarthritis, osteonecrosis, rheumatoid arthritis, trauma, or congenital anomalies, and replacement with prosthetics or artificial components made of metal (stainless steel, titanium) and/or plastic.

Total joint arthroplasty, also called total joint replacement, involves replacement of all components of an articulating joint.

Total knee arthroplasty involves the replacement of the distal femoral component, the tibia plate, and the patellar button. Total knee arthroplasty is a surgical option when conservative measures fail. (62.1)

Unicondylar knee replacement is done when a client's joint is diseased in one compartment of the joint.

Total hip arthroplasty involves the replacement of the acetabular cup, femoral head, and femoral stem. (62.2)

Hemiarthroplasty refers to half of a joint replacement. Fractures of the femoral neck can be treated only with the replacement of the femoral component.

INDICATIONS

The goal of both hip and knee arthroplasty is to eliminate pain, restore joint motions, and improve a client's functional status and quality of life.

POTENTIAL DIAGNOSES: Knee and hip arthroplasty treats degenerative disease (osteoarthritis, rheumatoid arthritis). Q EBP

CLIENT PRESENTATION
- Pain when bearing weight on the joint (walking, running)
- Joint crepitus and stiffness
- Joint swelling (primarily occurs in the knees)

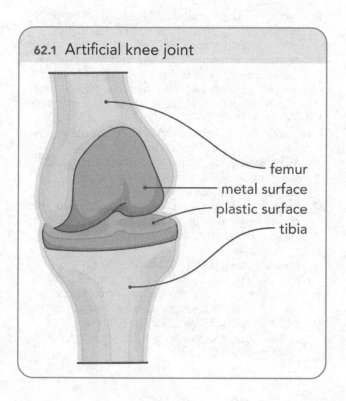

62.1 Artificial knee joint

- femur
- metal surface
- plastic surface
- tibia

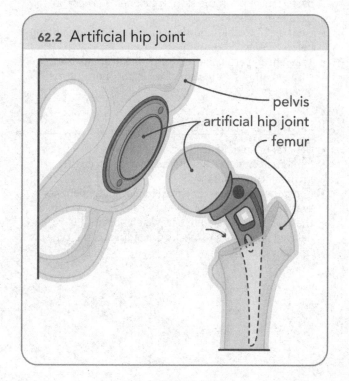

62.2 Artificial hip joint

- pelvis
- artificial hip joint
- femur

CONSIDERATIONS

CONTRAINDICATIONS

- Recent or active infection (urinary tract infection), which can cause micro-organisms to migrate to the surgical area and cause the prosthesis to fail
- Arterial impairment to the affected extremity
- Client inability to follow the postsurgical regimen
- A comorbid condition (uncontrolled diabetes mellitus or hypertension, advanced osteoporosis, progressive inflammatory condition, unstable cardiac or respiratory conditions)

PREPROCEDURE

NURSING ACTIONS: Review diagnostic test results.
- Complete blood count (CBC), urinalysis, electrolytes, blood urea nitrogen (BUN), and creatinine: Check surgical readiness, and rule out anemia, infection, or organ failure.
- Chest x-ray: Rule out pulmonary surgical contraindications (infection, tumor).
- Electrocardiogram (ECG): Gather baseline rhythm to identify cardiovascular surgical contraindications (dysrhythmia).

CLIENT EDUCATION

- Expectations for postoperative care: incentive spirometry, transfusion, surgical drains, dressing, pain control, transfer, exercises, and activity limitations
- Consider autologous blood donation. The client donates blood prior to the procedure to be used during or after the procedure.
- Scrub the surgical site with a prescribed antiseptic soap the night before and the morning of surgery to decrease bacterial count on the skin, which helps lower the chance of infection. Qᴘᴄᴄ
- Wear clean clothes and sleep on clean linens the night before surgery.
- Take antihypertensive and other medications the surgeon allows with a sip of water the morning of surgery.

INTRAPROCEDURE

- General or spinal anesthesia can be used.
- Joint components are removed and replaced with artificial components.
- Components can be cemented in place. Components that do not use cement allow the bone to grow into the prosthesis to stabilize it. Weight-bearing is delayed a few days to weeks depending on the type of implant used.

POSTPROCEDURE

CLIENT EDUCATION

- Extensive physical therapy is required to regain mobility. The client is discharged to home or to an acute rehabilitation facility. If discharged home, outpatient or in-home therapy is provided.
- Monitor for evidence of incisional infection (fever, increased redness, swelling, purulent drainage).
- Care for the incision (clean daily with soap and water).
- Monitor for deep vein thrombosis (swelling, redness, pain in calf), pulmonary embolism (shortness of breath, chest pain), and bleeding (if taking an anticoagulant).

KNEE ARTHROPLASTY

NURSING ACTIONS

- Provide postoperative care, and prevent postoperative complications (anemia, infection, neurovascular compromise, or venous thromboembolism that manifests as a deep vein thrombosis [DVT] or pulmonary embolism).
- Older adult clients are at a higher risk for medical complications related to chronic conditions, including hypertension, diabetes mellitus, coronary artery disease, and obstructive pulmonary disease.
- A continuous passive motion (CPM) machine can be prescribed to promote motion in the knee, promote circulation, and prevent scar tissue formation. CPM is usually placed and initiated immediately after surgery. CPM provides a passive range of motion from full extension to the prescribed amount of flexion. Follow the prescribed duration of use, but turn it off during meals.
- Positions of flexion of the knee are limited to avoid flexion contractures.
  - Avoid placing pillows behind the knee or positioning the mattress to create a knee gatch. Place one pillow under the lower calf and foot to cause a slight extension of the knee joint and to prevent flexion contractures. The knee can also rest flat on the bed.
- To prevent pressure injury on the heels, place a small blanket or pillow slightly above the ankle area to keep heels off the bed.
- Provide medications as prescribed. This promotes client participation in early ambulation.
  - **Analgesics:** Opioids (epidural, patient-controlled analgesic [PCA], IV, oral), non-steroidal anti-inflammatory drugs (NSAIDs)
  - **Antibiotics:** Prophylaxis is generally administered 30 min before the surgical incision is made and continued for 24 hr postoperatively to prevent infection.
  - **Anticoagulant:** Warfarin, fondaparinux, rivaroxaban, or low-molecular-weight heparin (enoxaparin). The client can have a prescription for sequential compression devices, foot pumps, and/or anti-embolism stockings to prevent venous thromboembolism formation that can develop into DVT.

- Apply ice or cold therapy to the incisional area to reduce postoperative swelling.
- Monitor the neurovascular status of the surgical extremity (movement, sensation, color, pulse, capillary refill) every 2 to 4 hours, and compare it with the other extremity.
- Check frequently for overt bleeding and manifestations of hypovolemia (hypotension, tachycardia).
- Monitor the compression bandage and wound suction device for excessive drainage.

INTERPROFESSIONAL CARE: Physical therapy, to assist with mobility on the first postoperative day with a knee immobilizer in place. Degree of weight-bearing is determined by the provider.

CLIENT EDUCATION: Dislocation is not common following total knee arthroplasty. However, kneeling and deep-knee bends are limited indefinitely.

HIP ARTHROPLASTY

NURSING ACTIONS
- Provide postoperative care and prevent complications.
- Check the dressing site frequently, noting any evidence of bleeding. Monitor and record drainage from surgical drains.
- Monitor daily laboratory values, including hemoglobin (Hgb) and hematocrit (Hct) levels. Hgb and Hct can continue to drop for 48 hours after surgery. Autologous blood from pre-surgery donation can be used for postoperative blood replacement.
- Monitor the neurovascular status of the surgical extremity (movement, sensation, color, pulse, and capillary refill, and compare with contralateral extremity) every 2 to 4 hours.
- Assist with the provision of medications as prescribed.
  - **Analgesics:** Opioids (epidural, PCA, IV, oral), NSAIDs. Monitor for respiratory depression with opioid use
  - **Antibiotics:** Generally administered 30 min before the surgical incision is made as a prophylaxis, and continued for 24 hr postoperatively to prevent infection
  - **Anticoagulant:** Warfarin, dalteparin, fondaparinux, rivaroxaban, or low-molecular-weight heparin (enoxaparin)

- Provide early ambulation.
  - Transfer the client out of bed from their unaffected side into a chair or wheelchair.
  - Weight-bearing status is determined by the orthopedic surgeon and by choice of cemented (usually partial/full weight-bearing as tolerated) vs. non-cemented prostheses (usually only partial or minimal weight-bearing [toe touch] until after a few weeks of bone growth).
  - Use assistive (walker) and adaptive (raised toilet seat, grab bars, and shower chairs) devices when caring for the client. Qs
  - Apply ice to the surgical site following ambulation as a nonpharmacological measure to decrease pain and discomfort.
- Place the client supine with the head slightly elevated and the affected leg in a neutral position. Place a pillow or abduction device between the legs when turning to the unaffected side. The client should not be turned to the operative side, which could cause hip dislocation.
- Use total hip precautions (maintain abduction, neutral rotation, limited flexion) to prevent dislocation of the new joint.
- Monitor for new joint dislocation: acute onset of pain, reports of hearing "a pop," internal or external rotation of the affected extremity, and shortened affected extremity.

CLIENT EDUCATION
- Use raised toilet seats and assistive items (long-handled shoehorn, dressing sticks) to prevent strain on the prosthesis/flexion > 90 degrees.
- Follow position restrictions to avoid dislocation.
  - Use straight chairs with arms.
  - Use an abduction pillow or regular pillow, if prescribed, between the legs while in bed (and with turning, if restless, or in an altered mental state).
  - Externally rotate the toes.
  - Avoid hip flexion greater than 90°.
  - Avoid low chairs.
  - Do not cross the legs.
  - Do not internally rotate the toes.
  - Avoid turning to the operative side, unless prescribed.
  - Anticoagulant medications (warfarin, aspirin) can be required for several weeks after surgery.

COMPLICATIONS

Venous thromboembolism

Can manifest as a deep vein thrombosis (DVT) or pulmonary embolism, a life-threatening complication after total hip arthroplasty

- Older adult clients are at the greatest risk for a potentially life-threatening complication (venous thromboembolism that manifests as a DVT and/or pulmonary emboli) due to age and compromised circulation before surgery.
- Clients who are obese or who have a history of venous thromboembolism formation are also at increased risk for developing DVT or pulmonary emboli.

NURSING ACTIONS

- Monitor for manifestations of pulmonary embolism, including acute dyspnea, tachycardia, and pleuritic chest pain.
- Follow venous thromboembolism prophylaxis to include pharmacological management, anti-embolic stockings, and sequential compression devices or foot pumps while in bed.
- Encourage plantar flexion, dorsiflexion, and circumduction exercises to prevent clot formation.
- Encourage early ambulation with physical and occupational therapy.

Joint dislocation, infection, anemia, neurovascular compromise

Older adult clients are at an increased risk for medical complications related to chronic conditions (hypertension, diabetes mellitus, coronary artery disease, obstructive pulmonary disease). Ⓖ

NURSING ACTIONS

- Monitor for bleeding.
- Maintain aseptic technique during dressing changes.
- Monitor incision site for manifestations of infection.
- Follow prescriptions regarding mobility and positioning to protect the joint and prosthesis.
- Monitor neurovascular status of operative extremity (color, temperature, capillary refill, presence of edema, quality of pulses, sensation).

Active Learning Scenario

A nurse is assisting with planning an in-service to a group of newly licensed nurses about arthroplasty. Identify the following information that should be included in the teaching. Use the ATI Active Learning Template: Therapeutic Procedure to complete this item.

INDICATIONS: List two.

POTENTIAL COMPLICATIONS: List four.

CLIENT EDUCATION: List four.

Application Exercises

1. A nurse is collecting data from a client who is scheduled to undergo a right knee arthroplasty. The nurse should expect which of the following findings? (Select all that apply.)
   - A. Skin reddened over the joint
   - B. Pain when bearing weight
   - C. Joint crepitus
   - D. Swelling of the affected joint
   - E. Limited joint motion

2. A nurse is reviewing the health record of a client who is to undergo total joint arthroplasty. The nurse should recognize which of the following findings as a contraindication to this procedure?
   - A. Age 55 years
   - B. History of cancer
   - C. Previous joint replacement
   - D. Bronchitis 2 weeks ago

3. A nurse working on an orthopedic unit is caring for a client following a total knee replacement. Which of the following actions should the nurse take? (Select all that apply.)
   - A. Check continuous passive motion device settings.
   - B. Palpate dorsal pedal pulses.
   - C. Place a pillow behind the knee.
   - D. Request a referral for outpatient physical therapy.
   - E. Apply heat therapy to the incision.

4. A nurse is providing postoperative care for a client who has a total hip arthroplasty. Which of the following actions should the nurse take? (Select all that apply.)
   - A. Provide a raised toilet seat for the client.
   - B. Place client in a low reclining chair.
   - C. Instruct the client to roll onto the operative hip.
   - D. Use an abductor pillow when turning the client.
   - E. Instruct the client on the use of an incentive spirometer.

5. A nurse is reinforcing teaching with a client who had a total hip arthroplasty. Which of the following information should the nurse include? (Select all that apply.)
   - A. Perform calf and leg exercises every 2 hr.
   - B. Turn toes inward when sitting or lying.
   - C. Remain at a 90 degree angle when sitting.
   - D. Bend at the waist when putting on socks.
   - E. Use a raised toilet seat.

1. B, D, E. **CORRECT:** The nurse should recognize the cues from the client's data collection and determine pain when bearing weight, swelling of the affected joint, and limited joint motion are expected findings for a client who requires arthroplasty of the affected joint.

Ⓝ NCLEX® Connection: *Physiological Adaptation, Basic Pathophysiology*

2. D. **CORRECT:** The nurse should analyze the cues from the client's health record and determine that a recent infection such as bronchitis can cause failure of the prosthesis if the micro-organisms are still present in the body and migrate to the surgical site.

Ⓝ NCLEX® Connection: *Reduction of Risk Potential, Potential for Complications of Diagnostic Tests/Treatments/Procedures*

3. A, B, D. **CORRECT:** When taking actions, the nurse should check the continuous passive motion settings to ensure the settings are as prescribed. The nurse should monitor the strength of the pedal pulses of both lower extremities to determine adequate circulation. The nurse should also request a referral for outpatient physical therapy to continue exercises of range of motion of the operated joint.

Ⓝ NCLEX® Connection: *Reduction of Risk Potential, Potential for Complications From Surgical Procedures and Health Alterations*

4. A, D, E. **CORRECT:** When taking actions, the nurse should provide a raised toilet seat for the client to avoid hip flexion of 90 degrees, which can cause dislocation of the operated hip. The nurse should place an abductor pillow in between the client's legs when turning to prevent dislocation of the operated hip. The nurse should also instruct the client to perform incentive spirometry exercises to promote alveolar expansion and avoid postoperative respiratory complications.

Ⓝ NCLEX® Connection: *Reduction of Risk Potential, Therapeutic Procedures*

5. A, C, E. **CORRECT:** When taking actions, the nurse should reinforce teaching the client to perform calf and leg exercises every 2 hr to promote circulation and prevent clot formation. The client should remain at no more than a 90 degree angle flexion when sitting and externally rotate the toes to avoid dislocation of the hip. The client should use a raised toilet seat to prevent extreme flexion of the hip, which can cause dislocation.

Ⓝ NCLEX® Connection: *Reduction of Risk Potential, Potential for Complications of Diagnostic Tests/Treatments/Procedures*

Active Learning Scenario Key

Using the ATI Active Learning Template: Therapeutic Procedure

INDICATIONS
- Degenerative disease (osteoarthritis, rheumatoid arthritis)
- Relief of pain
- Restore joint motions and improve functional status and quality of life.

POTENTIAL COMPLICATIONS
- Venous thromboembolism
- Joint dislocation
- Infection
- Anemia
- Neurovascular compromise

CLIENT EDUCATION
- Extensive physical therapy is required to regain mobility.
- Monitor the incision for evidence of infection (fever, increased redness, swelling, purulent drainage).
- Cleanse the incision daily with soap and water.
- Monitor for evidence of deep vein thrombosis (swelling, redness, pain in the calf) or pulmonary embolism (shortness of breath, chest pain).
- Monitor for bleeding if taking an anticoagulant medication (aspirin, warfarin, fondaparinux, rivaroxaban, enoxaparin).
- Specifically for hip arthroplasty
  ○ Use raised toilet seats and assistive items (long-handled shoehorn, dressing sticks) to prevent strain on the prosthesis.
  ○ Follow position restrictions to avoid dislocation.

Ⓝ NCLEX® Connection: *Reduction of Risk Potential, Therapeutic Procedures*

CHAPTER 63 *Amputations*

Amputation is the removal of a body part, most commonly an extremity. Amputations can be elective due to complications of peripheral vascular disease and arteriosclerosis, congenital deformities, chronic osteomyelitis, or malignant tumor; or traumatic due to an accident.

In the United States:

- 2.1 million individuals currently have had loss of a limb.

- 185,000 individuals each year undergo amputations.

- 507 individuals each day have amputations.

- 35% of amputees have upper limb losses.

- 65% of amputees have lower limb losses.

- Greater than 50% of lower limb losses are related to complications of peripheral artery disease and diabetes mellitus.

Amputations are described in regard to the extremity and whether they are located above or below the designated joint. The term disarticulation describes an amputation performed through a joint.

The higher the level of amputation, the greater the amount of effort that will be required to use a prosthesis. The level of the amputation is determined by the presence of adequate blood flow needed for healing.

Significant changes to body image occur after an amputation and should be addressed during the perioperative and rehabilitative phases.

UPPER EXTREMITY AMPUTATIONS

Upper extremity amputations include above- and below-the-elbow amputations, wrist and shoulder disarticulations, and finger amputations.

LOWER EXTREMITY AMPUTATIONS

- Lower extremity amputations include above- and below-the-knee amputations, hip and knee disarticulations, Syme's amputation (removal of foot with ankle saved), and mid-foot and toe amputations.
- Peripheral vascular disease is the cause of most lower extremity amputations.
- Every effort is made to save as much of the extremity as possible. Even loss of the big toe can significantly affect balance, gait, and push-off ability during ambulation. Salvage of the knee with a below-the-knee amputation also improves function vs. an above-the-knee amputation.

HEALTH PROMOTION AND DISEASE PREVENTION

- Clients who have diabetes mellitus should monitor blood glucose and maintain it within the expected reference range.
- Use safety measures when working with heavy machinery or in areas where there is a risk of electrocution or burns.
- Encourage clients to quit or not start smoking, maintain a healthy weight, and exercise regularly.
- Tell clients to maintain good foot care and to seek early medical attention for non-healing wounds.

DATA COLLECTION

RISK FACTORS

- Traumatic injury: motor vehicle crashes, industrial equipment, war-related injuries
- Thermal injury: frostbite, electrocution, burns
- Malignancy

CHRONIC DISEASE PROCESSES
- Older adult clients have a higher risk of peripheral vascular disease and diabetes mellitus resulting in decreased tissue perfusion and peripheral neuropathy. Both conditions place older adult clients at risk for lower extremity amputation. Ⓖ
- Peripheral vascular disease resulting in ischemia/gangrene
- Diabetes mellitus resulting in peripheral neuropathy and peripheral vascular disease
- Infection (osteomyelitis)

EXPECTED FINDINGS

Decreased tissue perfusion
- Clients might report pain.
- History of injury or disease process precipitating amputation
- Altered peripheral pulses compared with the client's expected skin tone (can use a Doppler if needed)
- Differences in temperature of extremities (Note the level of the leg at which temperature becomes cool.)
- Altered color of extremities (pallor, cyanosis, or gangrenous skin)
- Presence of infection and open wounds
- Lack of sensation in the affected extremity

NURSING ACTIONS

- Monitor capillary refill by comparing the extremities. In older adult clients, capillary refill can be difficult to monitor due to thickened and opaque nails. ⓖ
- Observe for edema, necrosis, and lack of hair distribution of the extremity due to inadequate peripheral circulation.
- Monitor peripheral pulses bilaterally.

DIAGNOSTIC PROCEDURES

To determine blood flow at various levels of an extremity

Angiography: Allows visualization of peripheral vasculature and areas of impaired circulation

Doppler laser and ultrasonography studies: Measures speed of blood flow in an extremity

Transcutaneous oxygen pressure (TcPO₂): Measures oxygen pressures in an extremity to indicate blood flow in the extremity, which is a reliable indicator for healing

Ankle–brachial index: Measures difference between ankle and brachial systolic pressures

PATIENT-CENTERED CARE

MANAGEMENT OF TRAUMATIC AMPUTATION

- Activate the medical emergency system (EMS).
- Apply direct pressure using gauze, if available, or clean cloth to prevent life-threatening hemorrhage.
- Elevate the extremity above the heart to decrease blood loss.
- Wrap the severed extremity in dry, sterile gauze (if available) or in a clean cloth, and place in a sealed plastic bag or watertight container. Submerge the bag/container in ice water (one part ice and three parts water), and send with the client.

NURSING CARE

- Prevent postoperative complications (hypovolemia, pain, edema, infection).
- Monitor dressings and surgical site for bleeding. Monitor vital signs frequently.
- Monitor tissue perfusion of end of residual limb.
  - Palpate residual limb for warmth. Heat can indicate infection.
  - Compare pulse most proximal to incision with pulse in other extremity. ꞯPCC
- Monitor for manifestations of infection and non-healing of incision. Infection can lead to osteomyelitis.
  - Elevate the stump, if ordered, to increase circulation and decrease pain and swelling.
  - Administer antibiotics and change dressings as prescribed if open amputation was performed.
  - Record characteristics of drainage (amount, color, and odor).
  - Keep a surgical tourniquet at the beside.
  - Change positions frequently.

63.1 Case study

Part 1

A nurse is driving home from work and witnesses a motor vehicle collision between two cars. The nurse parks their car on the side of the road, ensures the scene is safe, then begins to approach the cars. The driver and passengers of one car are out of the vehicle and report no injuries.

Scene 1

The nurse then sees a person who has been ejected from the other car bleeding profusely from a traumatic amputation above the left ankle.

Part 2

The client was transported to the emergency department and prepared for surgery. The surgeon was unable to reattach the severed ankle and foot and performed a closed below-the-knee amputation of the left lower extremity in the operating room.

Scene 2

A nurse on the medical-surgical unit is contributing to the plan of care for the client following the surgical below-the-knee amputation. The client has a rigid dressing to the left lower extremity, which is elevated on a pillow, and reports pain in the left foot.

Part 3

The client and family have received teaching from the interprofessional team in preparation for the client's discharge to their home.

Scene 3

The client states they are still concerned about developing complications. The nurse reinforces discharge teaching with the client.

Case study exercises

1. The nurse returns to their own car to retrieve clean gloves and towels and asks a few witnesses for help. Place in order the steps the nurse should take in the management of the traumatic amputation.

   A. Ask a witness to don gloves and hold the victim's leg above their heart.

   B. Use clean towels to apply pressure to the site of the amputation.

   C. Call 911.

   D. Wrap the amputated foot in a clean cloth and place in a zippered bag a witness retrieved from a nearby store.

2. Which suggestions for the plan of care should the nurse make for this client? (Select all that apply.)

   A. Administer analgesics for phantom limb pain.

   B. Delay range-of-motion exercises for 48 hours following surgery.

   C. Record amount, color, and odor of wound drainage.

   D. Reinforce education with the client to avoid the prone position.

   E. Compare pulses in the affected extremity with pulses in the other extremity.

   F. Discontinue elevation of the extremity after 24 hours.

3. Discuss three measures the nurse should reinforce with the client about preventing contractures of the affected extremity.

PAIN

- Monitor and treat pain.
- Differentiate between phantom limb and incisional pain.

Incisional pain is treated with analgesics or PCA pump.

Phantom limb pain

- The sensation of pain in the location of the extremity following the amputation
- Related to severed nerve pathways and is a frequent complication in clients who experienced chronic limb pain before the amputation
- Often described as deep and burning, tingling, cramping, shooting, or aching
- Treated much differently from incisional pain
  - Administering antiepileptics (gabapentin or pregabalin) can relieve sharp, stabbing, and burning phantom limb pain.
  - Recognize the pain is real and manage it accordingly.
  - Might need referral to pain clinic for management
  - Alternative treatment for phantom limb pain can include nonpharmacological methods (massage, heat, transcutaneous electrical nerve stimulation [TENS], ultrasound therapy, biofeedback, acupuncture, relaxation therapy).
  - Reinforce with the client how to push the residual limb down toward the bed while supported on a soft pillow. This helps reduce phantom limb pain and prepare the limb for a prosthesis.

CLIENT PERCEPTION AND FEELINGS REGARDING AMPUTATION

- Allow for the client and family to grieve for the loss of the body part and change in body image.
- Feelings can include depression, anger, withdrawal, and grief.
- Monitor the psychosocial well-being of the client. Check for feelings of altered self-concept and self-esteem and willingness and motivation for rehabilitation.
- Facilitate a supportive environment for the client and family so grief can be processed. Refer the client to religious/spiritual adviser, social worker, or counselor.
- Rehabilitation should include adaptation to a new body image and integration of prosthetic and adaptive devices into self-image.
- Offer visitation by another amputee.

RESIDUAL LIMB PREPARATION AND PROSTHESIS FITTING

Residual limb must be shaped and shrunk in preparation for prosthetic training.

SHRINKAGE INTERVENTIONS

- Wrap the residual limb up to three times daily, using elastic bandages (figure-eight wrap) to prevent restriction of blood flow and decrease edema.
- After bandages are removed, check the skin for breakdown.
- Use a residual limb shrinker sock (easier for the client to apply).
- Use an air splint (plastic inflatable device) inflated to protect and shape the residual limb and for easy access to inspect the wound.

CLIENT EDUCATION

- Care for and wrap the residual limb, and perform limb-strengthening exercises.
- Properly apply and care for the prosthesis.
- Safely transfer and use mobility devices and adaptive aids. Qs
- Manage phantom limb pain.

THERAPEUTIC PROCEDURES

Closed amputation: This is the most common technique used. A skin flap is sutured over the end of the residual limb, closing the site. A compression dressing is applied after surgery to decrease swelling and prevent infection.

Open amputation: This technique is used when an active infection is present. A skin flap is not sutured over the end of the residual limb, allowing for drainage of infection. The skin flap is closed at a later date.

CLIENT EDUCATION

Stump care

- Inspect all areas of the stump daily. Can use a mirror if needed
- Perform stump care as directed.
- Do not alter or adjust prosthesis.
- Yearly appointments for prosthesis evaluation

INTERPROFESSIONAL CARE

Intensive efforts by the interprofessional team are necessary to facilitate successful rehabilitation.

- A certified prosthetic orthotist will fit client with prosthesis after the wound is healed and the residual limb has shrunk.
- A physical therapist will train the client in the application and care of the prosthesis and mobility aids.
- An occupational therapist can assist the client with performing ADLs.
- A psychologist can be needed to help with adjustment to loss of the extremity.
- A social worker will assist the client who has financial issues and can refer the client to resources and a support group or organization for people who have had amputations.

COMPLICATIONS

FLEXION CONTRACTURES

Flexion contractures are more likely with the hip or knee joint following amputation due to improper positioning.

- Prevention includes range-of-motion (ROM) exercises and proper positioning immediately after surgery.
- To prevent hip or knee flexion contracture, some providers do not advocate elevating the residual limb on a pillow. However, other providers allow elevation for the first 24 hr to reduce swelling and discomfort. **Qpcc**

NURSING ACTIONS

- Have the client lie prone for 20 to 30 min several times a day to help prevent hip flexion contractures.
- Discourage prolonged sitting.
- Perform active and passive ROM exercises.
- Turn and reposition frequently.
- Encourage participation with physical therapy.

CLIENT EDUCATION

- Practice exercises that will prevent contractures.
- Stand using good posture with residual limb in extension. This also will aid in balance.

INFECTION

Increased risk for infection or delayed wound healing (diabetics, older adult, and PVD)

NURSING ACTIONS

- Monitor for manifestations of infection (such as redness, edema, heat, purulent drainage, increased pain, fever, and chills) and report to provider.
- Provide good skin hygiene.
- Maintain aseptic technique during dressing changes.
- Assist with administration of postoperative antibiotics as ordered.

DELAYED WOUND HEALING

Increased risk for delayed wound healing (diabetes mellitus, older adult, and PVD)

NURSING ACTIONS

- Notify provider of manifestations of delayed wound healing (such as if residual limb is cool to touch).
- Monitor dressing and output from wound drain.

Active Learning Scenario

A nurse is assisting with discharge planning for a client who had an amputation. What members of an interprofessional team should the nurse include in the discharge planning process? Use the ATI Active Learning Template: Basic Concept to complete this item.

RELATED CONTENT: List three members of the interprofessional team and describe the principal purpose of each member.

Active Learning Scenario Key

Using the ATI Active Learning Template: Basic Concept
RELATED CONTENT

- Certified prosthetic orthotist fits the client with the prosthesis following healing and shrinking of the stump.
- Physical therapist provides training for applying the prosthesis, assists in mobility training, and reviews mobility aids.
- Occupational therapist assists with teaching clients how to perform ADLs.
- Psychologist assists the client and family in adjusting to the loss of an extremity.
- Social worker provides referral information for financial assistance, resources and support groups, or organizations to help adjust to life-changing physical conditions.

Ⓝ *NCLEX® Connection: Coordinated Care, Collaboration with Multidisciplinary Team*

When reviewing the following chapters, keep in mind the relevant topics and tasks of the NCLEX outline.

Basic Care and Comfort

ASSISTIVE DEVICES: Contribute to the care of the client using assistive device.

NONPHARMACOLOGICAL COMFORT INTERVENTIONS
Provide nonpharmacological measures for pain relief.

Apply therapies for comfort and treatment of inflammation/swelling.

NUTRITION AND ORAL HYDRATION: Reinforce client teaching on special diets based on client diagnosis/nutritional needs and cultural considerations.

Health Promotion and Maintenance

HEALTH PROMOTION/DISEASE PREVENTION
Assist client in disease prevention activities.

Identify risk factors for disease/illness.

Reduction of Risk Potential

POTENTIAL FOR ALTERATIONS IN BODY SYSTEMS: Apply and check proper use of compression stockings and/or sequential compression devices.

POTENTIAL FOR COMPLICATIONS OF DIAGNOSTIC TESTS/ TREATMENTS/PROCEDURES: Use precautions to prevent injury and/or complications associated with a procedure or diagnosis.

Physiological Adaptation

ALTERATIONS IN BODY SYSTEMS
Provide care to correct client alteration in body system.

Perform wound care and/or dressing change.

Reinforce education to client regarding care and condition.

MEDICAL EMERGENCIES: Notify primary health care provider about client unexpected response/emergency situation.

BASIC PATHOPHYSIOLOGY: Identify signs and symptoms related to an acute or chronic illness.

CHAPTER 64 *Osteoporosis*

Osteoporosis is a common chronic metabolic bone disorder resulting in low bone density. It's estimated that more than 10 million people in the United States have osteoporosis. Osteoporosis occurs when the rate of bone resorption (osteoclast cells) exceeds the rate of bone formation (osteoblast cells), resulting in fragile bone tissue, and can lead to fractures. More than 1.5 million fractures from osteoporosis occur yearly. Common sites of osteoporotic fractures include the wrists, hips, and the spine, although any bone can sustain a fracture. Osteoporosis is classified as primary (genetic or environmental factors) or secondary (medical conditions or chronic medication use).

Osteopenia, the precursor to osteoporosis, refers to low bone mineral density relative to the client's age and sex. Bone mineral density peaks between the ages of 18 to 30. After peak years, bone density decreases, with a significant increase in the rate of loss in postmenopausal clients due to estrogen loss.

HEALTH PROMOTION AND DISEASE PREVENTION

- Consume adequate amounts of calcium and vitamin D from food or supplements, especially during young adulthood. Ensure to read food labels for sources of calcium.
  - Foods rich in vitamin D are most fish, egg yolks, fortified milk, and cereal.
  - Foods rich in calcium are milk products; green, leafy vegetables; fortified orange juice and cereals; red and white beans; and figs. Some soy and rice products are fortified with vitamin D and calcium.
- Spend time outdoors to increase the body's production of vitamin D. Exposure to the sun for any length of time should include wearing sunscreen to avoid getting a sunburn.
- Tobacco cessation
- Limit consumption of alcohol.
- Consider engaging in weight-bearing exercises (walking, lifting weights, climbing stairs). These activities promote bone rebuilding and maintenance. Qpcc

DATA COLLECTION

RISK FACTORS

- Ethnicity: Asian American and White American
- Age greater than 50
- Family history and thin, lean body build are precursors to low bone density.
- Females (sex assigned at birth) have a higher risk for primary osteoporosis. The decline in estrogen levels following menopause or ovary removal increases the rate of bone resorption.
- Males (sex assigned at birth) have a higher risk for secondary osteoporosis; a decrease in testosterone can lead to decreased bone mass.
- History of low calcium intake with suboptimal levels of vitamin D decreases bone formation (causes calcium to be removed from bones).
- Clients who limit protein have a reduced ability to use calcium because up to 50% of calcium is bound to protein. Clients who follow a high-protein, low-carbohydrate diet can eliminate important nutrients (calcium-rich foods).
- Tobacco smoke exposure (active or passive) and high alcohol intake (three or more drinks per day) causes decreased bone formation and increased bone absorption.
- Excess caffeine consumption causes excretion of calcium in the urine.
- History of malabsorption disorders (anorexia nervosa, celiac disease, bariatric surgery) limits the amount of calcium available.
- Lack of physical activity or prolonged immobility increases risk because bones need the stress of weight-bearing activity for bone rebuilding and maintenance.
- Secondary osteoporosis results from medical conditions.
  - Co-morbidities (hyperparathyroidism, hyperthyroidism, diabetes mellitus, Cushing's syndrome, rheumatoid arthritis, bone cancer, female hypogonadism, growth hormone deficiency, chronic airway disorders that affect calcium absorption and bone development [COPD, asthma])
  - Medication use over a prolonged period (loop diuretics, corticosteroids, thyroid medications, anticonvulsants) affects calcium absorption and bone metabolism.
  - Long-term lack of weight-bearing (spinal cord injury, sedentary lifestyle)
- Older adult clients have an increased risk of falls related to impaired balance, generalized weakness, gait changes, and impaired vision and hearing. Adverse medication effects can cause orthostatic hypotension, urinary frequency, or confusion, which can also raise the risk for falls. The body also does not absorb and use calcium as efficiently, but it does excrete calcium more readily than it occurs in the younger adult. Ⓖ
- High phosphorus intake increases the rate of calcium loss. Drinking more than 40 oz/day of carbonated beverages increases osteoporosis risk due to the amount of phosphorus consumed.

EXPECTED FINDINGS

- Reduced height of 5 to 7.5 cm (2 to 3 in)
- Acute back pain after lifting or bending (worse with activity, relieved by rest)
- Restriction in movement and spinal deformity
- History of fractures (wrist, femur, thoracic spine)
- Thoracic (kyphosis) of the dorsal spine
- Pain upon palpation over affected area

LABORATORY TESTS

- Blood calcium, vitamin D, phosphorus, hematocrit, ESR, and alkaline phosphatase levels are drawn to rule out other metabolic bone diseases (Paget's disease or osteomalacia). Blood calcium and vitamin D should be checked yearly for females (sex assigned at birth) at high risk and yearly after age 50 for males (sex assigned at birth) at high risk.
- 24-hr urine can evaluate the rate of calcium excretion.
- Bone turnover markers measure bone formation and resorption activity.

DIAGNOSTIC PROCEDURES

Radiography

Radiographs of the spine and long bones reveal low bone density and fractures.

Dual-energy x-ray absorptiometry (DEXA)

- A DEXA scan is used to screen for early changes in bone density and is usually done on the hip or spine.
- A peripheral DEXA scan is used to check the bone density of the heel, forearm, or finger.
- DEXA uses two beams of radiation. Findings are analyzed by a computer and interpreted by a radiologist. Clients receive a score that relates their amount of bone density to that of young, healthy adults (T score). Another reading, a Z score, compares the client's readings with those of a group of age-matched clients who serve as a control.
- The client will lie on an x-ray table while a scan of a selected area is done. Although clothing is not removed for the test, metallic objects that might interfere with the scanning procedure should be removed.

Peripheral quantitative ultrasound (pQUS)

- An ultrasound, usually of the heel, tibia, and patella, is performed.
- pQUS is an inexpensive, portable, and low-risk method to determine osteoporosis and monitor for risk of fracture, especially in males (sex assigned at birth) over the age of 70 years.

Quantitative computed tomography

Quantitative computer tomography, as well as CT-based absorptiometry, is used to measure bone density, especially in the vertebral column.

- Used to predict spinal or hip fractures
- Requires more radiation than DEXA scanning

Magnetic resonance imaging (MRI) and magnetic resonance spectroscopy (MRS)

- These provide information about bone density without exposing the client to radiation.
- Areas of osteoporosis show decreased perfusion.
- Fat marrow content is higher if the client has reduced bone mineral density.
- MRS provides a graph to quantify bone marrow adipose tissue.

PATIENT-CENTERED CARE

NURSING CARE

- Instruct the client and family regarding dietary calcium food sources.
- Provide information regarding calcium and vitamin D supplementation. (Take with food.)
- Reinforce the need for exposure to vitamin D (moderate sun exposure using sunscreen, fortified milk).
- Encourage weight-bearing exercises (at least 30 min, three to five times a week) to improve strength and reduce bone loss.
- Check the home environment for safety (remove throw rugs, provide adequate lighting, clear walkways) to prevent falls, which can result in fractures. **Qs**
  - Reinforce the use of safety equipment and assistive devices.
  - Clearly mark thresholds, doorways, and steps.

CLIENT EDUCATION

- Limit excess caffeine, alcohol, and carbonated beverages, which increase bone loss.
- Consume adequate amounts of protein, magnesium, vitamin K, and other trace minerals needed for bone formation.
- Avoid slippery surfaces and wear rubber-bottomed shoes. **Qs**
- Exercise, under guidance from the provider, to reduce the risk for vertebral fractures.
  - Isometric exercises can help with strengthening the core.
  - Avoid activities that would increase body stress (jarring activities, strenuous lifting).

MEDICATIONS

Medications (calcium and vitamin D) can slow or prevent osteoporosis. A combination of several of these medications can be used.

Thyroid hormone

Calcitonin (salmon)

- THERAPEUTIC USES: Decreases bone resorption by inhibiting osteoclast activity for treatment of osteoporosis, hypercalcemia, and Paget's disease of the bone
- NURSING ACTIONS
  - Calcitonin human can only be administered subcutaneously.
  - Calcitonin salmon can be administered subcutaneously, intramuscularly, and intranasally.

Teriparatide

- Medication is contraindicated for hypercalcemia, history of bone cancer, radiation, or Paget's disease.
- Adverse effects include nausea, back pain and arthralgia, and leg cramps.
- Orthostatic hypotension can occur up to 4 hr after receiving the medication.

THERAPEUTIC USES

- A parathyroid hormone that stimulates osteoblasts to increase new bone formation to increase bone mass
- Stimulates calcium absorption
- Limited use in clients who are at high risk for fractures and those who have prolonged corticosteroid use

NURSING ACTIONS: Administer only subcutaneously.

CLIENT EDUCATION: Teriparatide can only be used for 2 years, and then bisphosphonates are started.

Estrogen hormone supplements

Estrogen, medroxyprogesterone: Estrogen should be given along with progesterone in clients who still have their uterus.

- THERAPEUTIC USES: Replaces estrogen lost due to menopause or surgical removal of ovaries
- CLIENT EDUCATION
  - Potential complications include breast and endometrial cancers and deep vein thrombosis (DVT).
  - Perform monthly breast self-examinations.

Selective estrogen receptor modulators (estrogen agonist/antagonist)

Raloxifene

- THERAPEUTIC USES
  - Decreases osteoclast activity, subsequently decreasing bone resorption and increasing bone mineral density
  - Prevents and treats postmenopausal osteoporosis and breast cancer
- NURSING ACTIONS
  - Avoid for clients who have a history of DVT.
  - Monitor liver function tests.
  - Discontinue use 72 hr before prolonged bed rest.
- CLIENT EDUCATION
  - Report unusual calf pain or tenderness, acute migraine, insomnia, urinary tract infection, or vaginal burning/itching to the provider. Qs
  - Take calcium and vitamin D supplements.

Calcium supplement

Calcium carbonate, calcium citrate

- THERAPEUTIC USES: Supplements calcium consumed in food products to promote healthy bones (not to slow osteoporosis)
- NURSING ACTIONS
  - Give with food in divided doses with 6 to 8 oz of water.
  - Calcium supplements can cause GI upset.
  - Monitor for constipation and of hypercalcemia.

Vitamin D supplement

Vitamin D is a fat-soluble vitamin, so toxicity can occur. Findings of toxicity include weakness, fatigue, nausea, constipation, and kidney stones.

THERAPEUTIC USES

- Increases absorption of calcium from the intestinal tract and availability of calcium in the blood needed for remineralization of bone
- Needed by individuals who are not exposed to adequate amounts of sunlight or who do not meet its daily requirements

Bisphosphonates

Alendronate, ibandronate, risedronate, zoledronic acid, pamidronate

- THERAPEUTIC USES: Decreases number and actions of osteoclasts, subsequently inhibiting bone resorption for prevention and treatment of osteoporosis, hypercalcemia, and Paget's disease of the bone
- NURSING ACTIONS
  - Monitor calcium levels in clients receiving IV preparations.
  - There is a risk for esophagitis and esophageal ulcers with oral preparations. Report early manifestations of indigestion, chest pain, difficulty swallowing, or bloody emesis to the provider immediately.
  - Take with 8 oz water in the early morning before eating.
  - Remain upright for 30 min after taking oral medication.
  - Clients using IV preparations should have dental examinations and preventative treatment prior to starting therapy to minimize the risk of osteonecrosis of the jaw.

Receptor activator of nuclear factor Kappa-B Ligand (RANKL inhibitors)

Denosumab

- Contraindicated for clients who have hypocalcemia
- Clients should have dental examinations and preventative treatment prior to starting therapy to minimize the risk of osteonecrosis of the jaw.
- THERAPEUTIC USES
  - Reduces bone resorption and increases bone density
  - Limited use in clients who are at high risk for fractures

- **NURSING ACTIONS**
  - Monitor calcium levels.
  - Administer subcutaneously into the upper arm, upper thigh, or abdomen.
- **CLIENT EDUCATION:** Notify the provider if manifestations of infection develop.

THERAPEUTIC PROCEDURES

Orthotic devices

Orthotic devices are available for immobilization of the spine immediately after a compression fracture of the spine (a trunk orthosis or lumbosacral corset).
- The device provides support and decreases pain.
- A physical therapist fits the device for the client and teaches them how to apply it.

CLIENT EDUCATION
- Check for skin breakdown under the orthotic device.
- Use good posture and body mechanics.
- Log roll when getting out of bed.
- Use heat and back rubs to promote muscle relaxation. Qpcc

Joint repair or joint arthroplasty

Can be necessary to repair or replace a joint weakened by osteoporosis. This is most often the hip joint.

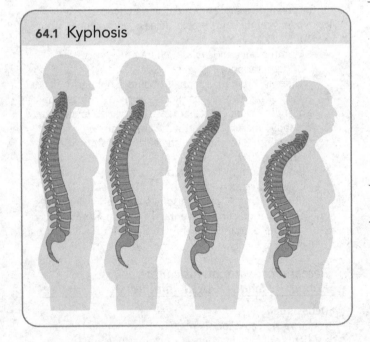

64.1 Kyphosis

Vertebroplasty or kyphoplasty

Minimally invasive procedures performed by a surgeon or radiologist. Used after other conservative measures to treat the fractures have proven ineffective
- Bone cement is injected into the fractured space of the vertebral column with or without balloon inflation.
- Balloon inflation of the fracture is to contain the cement and add height to the fractured vertebra.
- Mild sedation is used.
- Client lies in a supine position for 1 to 2 hr following procedure. The client might be discharged within 4 hr.

NURSING ACTIONS
- Monitor vital findings for shortness of breath and the puncture site for bleeding.
- Complete a neurologic data collection.
- Apply cold therapy to the injection site.

CLIENT EDUCATION
- Avoid driving for 24 hr following the procedure.
- Keep the dressing dry. Remove it the day following the procedure.
- Monitor the site for findings of infection.
- Resume activities (walking) the day following the procedure and gradually increase activity level as tolerated.
- Encourage the client to increase fluid intake and consume foods high in fiber to prevent constipation.

INTERPROFESSIONAL CARE

- Physical therapy can be used to establish an exercise regimen: 20 to 30 min of aerobic exercise (such as walking) at least three times per week in addition to weight lifting.
- Clients can need rehabilitation if fractures cause immobilization or disability.
- Most hip fractures are due to osteoporosis. Joint repair or joint arthroplasty requires physical therapy for a full recovery.

COMPLICATIONS

FRACTURES

Fractures are the leading complication of osteoporosis. Early recognition and treatment is essential.

NURSING ACTIONS: Support the client's knees in a flexed position to relieve back pain.

CLIENT EDUCATION: Move the trunk as a unit and avoid twisting to relieve pain from vertebral fractures.

Application Exercises

1. A nurse is reinforcing dietary teaching about calcium-rich foods with a client who has osteoporosis. Which of the following foods should the nurse include in the instructions?

   A. White bread

   B. Broccoli

   C. Apples

   D. Brown rice

2. A nurse is assisting with performing health screenings at a health fair. Which of the following clients have a risk factor for osteoporosis? (Select all that apply.)

   A. A 40-year-old client who has been taking prednisone for 1 month

   B. A 30-year-old client who jogs ½ of a mile daily

   C. A 45-year-old client who has been taking phenytoin for 20 years

   D. A 65-year-old client who has been taking furosemide for 15 years

   E. A 50-year-old client who has smoked tobacco for 5 years

3. A nurse is reviewing the electronic health record (EHR) of a client who has suspected osteoporosis. Which of the following findings should the nurse identify as a risk factor for osteoporosis? (Select all that apply.)

   A. History of consuming 3 alcoholic beverages daily

   B. Loss in height of 2 in (5.1 cm)

   C. Body mass index (BMI) of 28

   D. History of hyperthyroidism

   E. Age less than 45

4. A nurse is planning discharge teaching on home safety for a client who has osteoporosis. Which of the following information should the nurse include in the teaching? (Select all that apply.)

   A. Remove throw rugs in walkways.

   B. Use prescribed assistive devices.

   C. Remove clutter from the environment.

   D. Wear soft-bottomed shoes.

   E. Maintain lighting of doorway areas.

5. A nurse is assisting with the care of a client following a vertebroplasty of the thoracic spine. Which of the following actions should the nurse take?

   A. Apply heat to the puncture site.

   B. Ensure client maintains a supine position.

   C. Turn the client every 1 hr.

   D. Assist the client with ambulation within the first hour postprocedure.

Active Learning Scenario

A nurse is administering raloxifene to a client who has osteoporosis. What should the nurse consider before administering the medication? Use the ATI Active Learning Template: Medication to complete this item.

THERAPEUTIC USES: List two.

NURSING INTERVENTIONS: Describe two.

EVALUATION OF MEDICATION EFFECTIVENESS: Describe one.

Active Learning Scenario Key

Using the ATI Active Learning Template: Medication

THERAPEUTIC USES: Selective estrogen receptor modulator (estrogen agonist/antagonist)
- Decreases bone resorption and increases bone density
- Treatment of postmenopausal osteoporosis
- Treatment of breast cancer

NURSING INTERVENTIONS
- Avoid administering to a client who has a history of deep vein thrombosis (DVT).
- Instruct the client to report unusual calf pain or tenderness and manifestations of DVT.
- Check liver function tests periodically.
- Review need for calcium and vitamin D supplements when taking the medication.

EVALUATION OF MEDICATION EFFECTIVENESS
- Improved bone mineral density
- No further loss in height

Ⓝ *NCLEX® Connection: Pharmacological Therapies, Medication Administration*

Application Exercises Key

1. B. **CORRECT:** When taking action to reinforce dietary teaching for a client who has osteoporosis, the nurse should include food choices that are high in calcium such as dairy products and green leafy vegetables (broccoli, kale, mustard greens). Food choices such as white bread, apples, and brown rice may have some calcium; however, the content of calcium is not very high.

Ⓝ *NCLEX® Connection: Basic Care and Comfort, Nutrition and Oral Hydration*

2. C, D, E. **CORRECT:** While assisting with performing health screenings, the nurse recognizes risks for osteoporosis include chronic use of certain medications such as anticonvulsants or loop diuretics, age greater than 50, and tobacco smoke. Therefore, the clients who are at risk for developing osteoporosis include the 45-year-old client who has been taking phenytoin for 20 years, the 65-year-old client who has been taking furosemide for 15 years, and the 50-year-old client who has smoked tobacco for 5 years.

Ⓝ *NCLEX® Connection: Health Promotion and Maintenance, Health Promotion/Disease Prevention*

3. A, B, D. **CORRECT:** When recognizing cues, the nurse should identify after reviewing the client's EHR that a history of consuming 3 or more alcoholic beverages daily, loss in height of 2 in (5.1 cm), and a history of hyperthyroidism are risk factors for osteoporosis. Other risk factors include age greater than 50.

Ⓝ *NCLEX® Connection: Health Promotion and Maintenance, Health Promotion/Disease Prevention*

4. A, B, C, E. **CORRECT:** The nurse should plan to include information to promote a safe environment and prevent falls, such as removing throw rugs in walkways, using prescribed assistive devices, removing clutter, wearing rubber-bottomed shoes, and maintaining good lighting in doorway areas.

Ⓝ *NCLEX® Connection: Safety and Infection Control, Home Safety*

5. B. **CORRECT:** When taking action while assisting with the care of a client following vertebroplasty, the nurse should ensure the client maintains a supine position for at least 1 hour to prevent injury. Applying heat, turning every 1 hour, and ambulating within the first hour are contraindicated because the client should remain in a supine position for at least an hour.

Ⓝ *NCLEX® Connection: Reduction of Risk Potential, Therapeutic Procedures*

CHAPTER 65 *Musculoskeletal Trauma*

A fracture is a break in a bone secondary to trauma or a pathological condition. Fractures caused by trauma are the most common type of bone fracture. Pathological fractures can be caused by metastatic cancer, osteoporosis, or Paget's disease.

Bone is continually going through a process of remodeling as osteoclasts (cells that resorb or dissolve bone) release calcium from the bone and osteoblasts (cells that form new bone) build up the bone. Remodeling of bone occurs at equal rates until an individual reaches their thirties. From this age on, the activity of the osteoclasts outpace the osteoblasts, increasing an individual's risk of osteoporosis. This process significantly increases following menopause. Subsequently, these clients experience fractures secondary to osteoporosis about a decade earlier than clients who do not enter menopause.

Fractures

- A **closed (simple) fracture** does not break through the skin surface.
- An **open (compound) fracture** disrupts the skin integrity, causing an open wound and tissue injury with a risk of infection.
- Open fractures are graded based upon the extent of tissue injury.
- A **complete fracture** goes through the entire bone, dividing it into two distinct parts. An **incomplete fracture** goes through part of the bone.
- A **simple fracture** has one fracture line, while a **comminuted fracture** has multiple fracture lines splitting the bone into multiple pieces.
- A **displaced fracture** has bone fragments that are not in alignment, and a **non-displaced fracture** has bone fragments that remain in alignment.

- A **fatigue (stress) fracture** results when excess strain occurs from recreational and athletic activities.
- A **pathological (spontaneous) fracture** occurs to bone that is weak from a disease process (bone cancer or osteoporosis).
- **Compression fracture** occurs from a loading force pressing on cancellous bone. This condition is common among older adult clients who have osteoporosis.

COMMON TYPES OF FRACTURES

Comminuted: Bone is fragmented.

Oblique: Fracture occurs at oblique angle and across bone.

Spiral: Fracture occurs from twisting motion (common with physical abuse).

Impacted: Fractured bone is wedged inside opposite fractured fragment.

Greenstick: Fracture occurs on one side (cortex) but does not extend completely through the bone (most often in children).

Hip fractures are the most common injury in older adults and are usually associated with falls.

HEALTH PROMOTION AND DISEASE PREVENTION

- Ensure recommended intake of calcium for developmental stage in life.
- Ensure adequate intake of vitamin D and/or exposure to sunlight.
- Monitor for development of osteoporosis, especially in postmenopausal clients and clients who have a thyroid disorder.
- Engage in weight-bearing exercise on a regular basis.
- Take a bisphosphonate if prescribed to slow bone resorption and treat osteoporosis.
- Use caution to prevent falls or accidents.
- Prevent injury with the use of seat belts and helmets.

65.1 X-ray of leg fracture

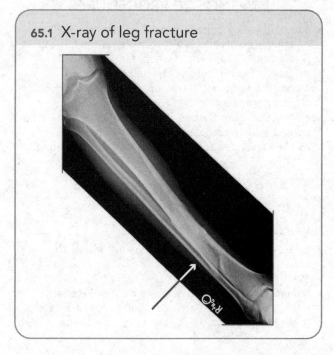

DATA COLLECTION

RISK FACTORS

- Osteoporosis
- Falls
- Motor vehicle crashes
- Substance use disorder
- Diseases (bone cancer, Paget's disease)
- Contact sports and hazardous recreational activities (football, skiing)
- Physical abuse
- Lactose intolerance
- Age, as bone becomes less dense with advancing age Ⓖ

EXPECTED FINDINGS

- History of trauma, metabolic bone disorders, chronic conditions, and possible use of corticosteroid therapy
- Pain and reduced movement manifest at the area of fracture or the area distal to the fracture.
- Crepitus (a grating sound created by the rubbing of bone fragments)
- Deformity: Internal or external rotation of extremity, shortened extremity, visible bone with open fracture, asymmetrical appearance of the affected limb (compared with the other side of the body)
- Muscle spasms due to the pulling forces of the bone when not aligned
- Edema (swelling) from trauma
- Ecchymosis (bleeding into underlying soft tissues) from trauma

LABORATORY TESTS

- CBC can help detect bleeding (decreased hemoglobin, hematocrit) or infection (increased WBC).
- ESR can be increased if inflammation is present.

DIAGNOSTIC PROCEDURES

- Standard radiographs, computed tomography (CT) imaging scan used to detect fractures of the hip and pelvis, and/or magnetic resonance imagery (MRI)
  - Identify the type of fracture and location.
  - Indicate pathological fracture resulting from tumor or mass.
  - Determine soft tissue damage around fracture (MRI).
- Bone scan using radioactive material determines hairline fractures and complications/delayed healing.

PATIENT-CENTERED CARE

INITIAL NURSING CARE

- Assist with the provision of emergency care at time of injury.
- Maintain ABCs.
- Monitor vital signs and neurologic status because injury to vital organs can occur due to bone fragments (fractures of pelvis, ribs).

- Stabilize the injured area, including the joints above and below the fracture, by using a splint and avoiding unnecessary movement. Ⓠᴇʙᴘ
- Ask the client about the cause of the injury, to determine if other internal injuries are possible.
- Maintain proper alignment of the affected extremity.
- Elevate the limb above the heart and apply ice.
- Check for bleeding and apply pressure, if needed.
- Cover open wounds with a sterile dressing.
- Remove clothing and jewelry near the injury or on the affected extremity.
- Keep the client warm.
- Collect data regarding pain frequently and follow pain management protocols, both pharmacological and nonpharmacological.
- Continue neurovascular checks at least every hour. Immediately report any change in status to the provider.
- Prepare the client for any immobilization procedure appropriate for the fracture.
- Provide nonpharmacological pain control (ice or heat packs, electrical stimulation, iontophoresis [delivery of dexamethasone through electrodes on the skin]).

PATIENT-CENTERED CARE

NURSING CARE

Neurovascular check

Neurovascular checks are essential throughout immobilization. Data collection is performed every hour for the first 24 hr and every 1 to 4 hr thereafter following initial trauma to monitor neurovascular compromise related to edema and/or the immobilization device. Neurovascular checks include the following.

Pain: Collect data regarding pain level, location, and frequency. Determine pain using a 0 to 10 pain rating scale, and have the client describe the pain. Immobilization, ice, and elevation of the extremity with the use of analgesics should relieve most of the pain.

Sensation: Check for numbness or tingling of the extremity. Loss of sensation can indicate nerve damage.

Skin temperature: Check the temperature of the affected extremity. The extremity should be warm (not cool) to touch. Cool skin can indicate decreased arterial perfusion.

Capillary refill: Press nail beds of affected extremity until blanching occurs. Blood return should be within 3 seconds. Prolonged refill indicates decreased arterial perfusion. Nail beds that are cyanotic can indicate venous congestion.

Pulses: Pulses should be palpable and strong. Pulses should be equal to the unaffected extremity. Edema can make it difficult to palpate pulses, so Doppler ultrasonography might be required.

Movement: Client should be able to move affected extremity in active motion.

Nutrition

- Provide diet high in protein and calcium to facilitate bone healing.
- If the client experienced blood loss, encourage foods high in iron.

CLIENT EDUCATION: Vitamin and mineral supplements promote healing.

MEDICATIONS

Analgesics
- Opioid and non-opioid analgesics as needed to control pain
- NSAIDs decrease associated tissue inflammation.
- Long-term intake of NSAIDS can delay bone healing.

Muscle relaxants: Relieve muscle spasms

Stool softener: To prevent constipation

Antibiotic: Prophylactic antibiotics to decrease the risk of infection for open fractures

THERAPEUTIC PROCEDURES

Immobilizing interventions

Immobilization secures the injured extremity in order to:
- Prevent further injury
- Promote healing/circulation
- Reduce pain
- Correct a deformity

TYPES OF IMMOBILIZATION DEVICES
- Braces
- Casts
- Splints/immobilizers
- Traction
- External fixation
- Internal fixation
- Orthopedic shoes and boots

Closed reduction

A pulling force (traction) is applied manually to realign the displaced fractured bone fragments. Once the fracture is reduced, immobilization is used to allow the bone to heal.

Splint and immobilizer use

Splints and immobilizers provide support, control movement, reduce pain, correct a deformity, and prevent additional injury.
- Splints are removable and allow for monitoring of skin swelling or integrity.
- Splints can support fractured/injured areas until casting occurs and swelling is decreased. Casting is then used for post-paralysis injuries to avoid joint contracture.
- Immobilizers are prefabricated and typically fasten with hook-and-loop fastener straps.

CLIENT EDUCATION
- Adhere to application protocol regarding full-time or part-time use.
- Observe for skin breakdown at pressure points.

Cast application

Casts are more effective than splints or immobilizers because the client is unable to remove.
- Casts, as circumferential immobilizers, are applied once the swelling has subsided (to avoid compartment syndrome). If the swelling continues after cast application and causes unrelieved pain, the cast can be split on one side (univalve) or on both sides (bivalved).
- A window can be placed in an area of the cast to allow for skin inspection (such as a client who has a wound under the cast), wound drainage, or checking the pulse.
- Moleskin is used over any rough area of the cast that can rub against the client's skin.
- A fitted stockinette is placed under the plaster cast.

TYPES OF CASTS
- Short and long arm and leg casts
- Walking cast (A rubber walking pad on the sole of the cast assists the client in ambulating when weight-bearing is allowed.)
- Spica casts (a portion of the trunk and one or two extremities; typically used on children who have congenital hip dysplasia)
- Body casts (encircle the trunk of the body)

CASTING MATERIALS
- Plaster of Paris casts are heavy, not water-resistant, and can take 24 to 72 hr to dry.
- Synthetic fiberglass casts are light, stronger, water-resistant, dry very quickly (in 30 min), and are most commonly used.

NURSING ACTIONS
- Monitor neurovascular status every hour for first 24 hr and collect data regarding pain. Qs
- Apply ice for 24 to 48 hr.
- Handle a plaster cast with the palms, not fingertips, until the cast is dry to prevent denting the cast.
- Avoid setting the cast on hard surfaces or sharp edges.
- Prior to casting, the area is cleaned and dried. Tubular cotton web roll is placed over the affected area to maintain skin integrity. The casting material is then applied.
- After cast application, position the client so that warm, dry air circulates around and under the cast (support the casted area without pressure under or directly on the cast) for faster drying and to prevent pressure from changing the shape of the cast. Use gloves to touch the cast until it is completely dry.
- Elevate the cast during the first 24 to 48 hr to prevent edema of the affected extremity. Use a cloth-covered pillow instead of plastic while cast is drying. Elevate arm casts above heart level; elevate leg cast on several pillows when resting.
- Ensure that cast is not too tight; there should be room for one finger between the skin and cast.
- Document presence of drainage and report sudden increase in drainage. Circling drainage on cast is an unreliable indicator of drainage amount and can increase client anxiety.

- Older adult clients have an increased risk for impaired skin integrity due to the loss of elasticity of the skin and decreased sensation (comorbidities). Ⓖ
- Provide assistive devices (sling to support the weight of an arm cast, cast shoes/boots to facilitate walking).
- Inspect the cast every 8 to 12 hr.
- Monitor for drainage, and report increased drainage to the provider.

CLIENT EDUCATION

- To avoid trauma to the skin, do not to place any foreign objects inside the cast. Relieve itching under the cast by blowing cool air from a hair dryer into the cast.
- Cover the cast with plastic if needed to avoid soiling from urine or feces.
- Cover the cast with a plastic bag before baths and showers to keep the cast dry.
- Report any areas under the cast that are painful, have a "hot spot," have increased drainage, are warm to the touch, or have an odor, which can indicate infection.
- Report change in mobility and complications (shortness of breath, skin breakdown, constipation).
- Casts often become too loose after swelling subsides and need to be replaced.

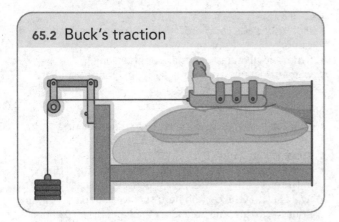

65.2 Buck's traction

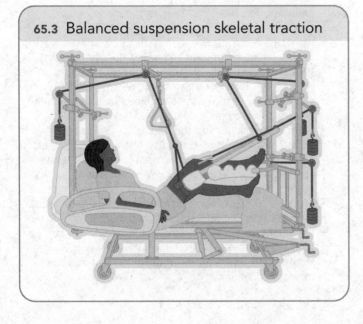

65.3 Balanced suspension skeletal traction

Traction

- Traction uses a pulling force to promote and maintain alignment of the injured area.
- Traction prescriptions should include the type of traction, amount of weight, and whether traction can be removed for nursing care. Qᴇʙᴘ

GOALS OF TRACTION

- Prevent soft tissue injury.
- Realign of bone fragments.
- Decrease muscle spasms and pain.
- Correct or prevent further deformities.

TYPES OF TRACTION

- **Manual:** A pulling force is applied by the hands of the provider for temporary immobilization, usually with sedation or anesthesia, in conjunction with the application of an immobilizing device.
- **Straight or running:** The counter traction is provided by the client's body by applying a pulling force in a straight line. Movement of the client's body can alter the traction provided.
  - **Skin:** Primary purpose is to decrease muscle spasms and immobilize the extremity prior to surgery. The pulling force is applied by weights that are attached by rope to the client's skin with tape, straps, boots, or cuffs. Examples include Bryant's traction (used for congenital hip dislocation in children) and Buck's traction (used preoperatively for hip fractures for immobilization in adult clients). (63.2) Uses light (7 to 10 lb) weights
- **Balanced suspension:** The counter traction is produced by devices (slings or splints) to support the fractured extremity off the bed while pulling with ropes and weights. The client's body can move without altering the traction.
  - **Skeletal:** Screws are inserted into the bone (such as halo traction). Can use heavier weights (15 to 30 lb) and longer traction time to realign the bone. Provide frequent pin site care to prevent infection. Qₛ

NURSING ACTIONS

- Perform a neurovascular check of the affected body part every hour for 24 hr and every 4 hr after that.
- Maintain body alignment and realign if the client seems uncomfortable or reports pain.
- Avoid lifting or removing weights.
- Ensure that weights hang freely and are not resting on the floor.
- If the weights are accidentally displaced, replace the weights. If the problem is not corrected, notify the provider.
- Ensure that pulley ropes are free of knots, fraying, loosening, and improper positioning at least every 8 to 12 hr.
- Notify the provider if the client experiences severe pain from muscle spasms unrelieved with medications or repositioning.
- Move the client in halo traction as a unit, without applying pressure to the rods. This will prevent loosening of the pins and pain.

- Routinely monitor skin integrity and document.
- Use heat/massage as prescribed to treat muscle spasms.
- Use therapeutic touch and relaxation techniques.

PIN SITE CARE
- Pin care is done frequently throughout immobilization (skeletal traction and external fixation methods) to prevent and to monitor for manifestations of infection.
  - Drainage and redness (color, amount, odor)
  - Loosening of pins
  - Tenting of skin at pin site (skin rising up pin)
- Pin care protocols (chlorhexidine) are based on provider preference and facility policy. A primary concept of pin care is that one cotton swab is designated for each pin to avoid cross-contamination.
- Pin care is provided usually once a shift, one to two times per day, or per facility protocol. Increase the frequency of care if an increased amount of drainage is noted or infection is suspected.

External fixation

External fixation involves fracture immobilization using percutaneous pins and wires that are attached to a rigid external frame.

USED TO TREAT
- Comminuted fracture or nonunion fractures with extensive soft tissue damage
- Leg length discrepancies from congenital defects
- Bone loss related to tumors or osteomyelitis

ADVANTAGES
- Immediate fracture stabilization
- Minimal blood loss occurring in comparison with internal fixation
- Allowing for early mobilization and ambulation
- Maintaining alignment of closed fractures that could not be maintained in cast or splint
- Permitting wound care with open fractures

DISADVANTAGES
- Risk of pin site infection leading to osteomyelitis
- Potential overwhelming appearance to client
- Noncompliance issues

NURSING ACTIONS
- Elevate extremity.
- Monitor neurovascular status and skin integrity.
- Collect data regarding body image.
- Perform pin care frequently. Monitor site for drainage, color, odor, and redness. Expect weeping or drainage of clear fluid for the first 48 to 72 hr.
- Observe for manifestations of fat and pulmonary embolism.
- Provide anti-embolism stockings and sequential compression device to prevent deep vein thrombosis (DVT).

CLIENT EDUCATION
- Perform pin care as prescribed.
- Clothing might need to be altered to cover the device.
- If activity is restricted, perform deep breathing and leg exercises and other techniques to prevent complications to immobilization (pneumonia or thrombus formation).

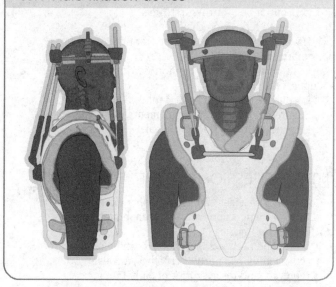

65.4 Halo fixation device

Open reduction and internal fixation

- Open reduction refers to visualization of a fracture through an incision in the skin and internal fixation with plates, screws, pins, rods, and prosthetics as needed.
- After the bone heals, the hardware might be removed, depending on the location and type of hardware.
- Circular external fixation: Technique to promote new bone growth for malunion and nonunion fracture. Device is turned four times per day to pull apart the cortex of the bone and stimulate growth.

NURSING ACTIONS
- Prevent dislocation, especially of hip. Qᴘᴄᴄ
- Monitor skin integrity.
- Ensure heels are off bed at all times and inspect bony prominence every shift.
- Perform a neurovascular check.
- Observe the cast or dressing for postoperative drainage. The cast can have a window cut in it through which the incision can be viewed. An elastic wrap is used to keep the window block cover in place to decrease localized edema.
- Monitor for manifestations of fat and pulmonary embolism.
- Provide anti-embolism stockings and a sequential compression device to prevent DVT and administer prescribed anticoagulants.
- Monitor the client's pain level.
  - Administer analgesics, antispasmodics, and/or anti-inflammatory medication (NSAIDs) and determine relief.
  - Position for comfort and with ice on the surgical site.
- Monitor for manifestations of infection.
  - Monitor vital signs, observing for fever, tachycardia, incisional drainage, redness, and odor.
  - Monitor laboratory values (WBC, ESR).
  - Provide surgical aseptic wound care.

- Increase physical mobility as appropriate.
  - Monitor orthostatic blood pressure when the client gets out of bed for the first time.
  - Turn and reposition the client every 2 hr.
  - Have the client get out of bed from the unaffected side.
  - Position the client for comfort (within restrictions).
- Support nutrition.
  - Encourage increased calorie intake.
  - Ensure use of calcium supplements.
  - Encourage small, frequent meals with snacks.
  - Monitor for constipation.

INTERPROFESSIONAL CARE

- Counseling services can assist clients experiencing anxiety or depression from long rehabilitation or life-altering injuries. Q PCC
- Physical and occupational therapy can be required for ambulation, particularly if crutches, a walker, or a cane is required, and for activities of daily living.
- Physical therapy can help restore range of motion, review strengthening exercises, and assist the client with accepting the injury.
- Case management can coordinate discharge planning, especially if inpatient rehabilitative care will be required (more common for older adults and clients who have multiple injuries). Q TC
- Social workers assist with financial concerns, especially if a long recovery period is expected.
- Home health care can provide follow-up care and assist with ADLs.
- A vocational counselor if the injury affects the client's ability to return to prior employment

COMPLICATIONS

Compartment syndrome

- Compartment syndrome usually affects extremities and occurs when pressure within one or more of the muscle compartments (covered with fascia) compromises circulation, resulting in an ischemia-edema cycle.
- Increased edema causes pressure on the nerve endings, resulting in pain. Blood flow is further reduced and ischemia persists, resulting in compromised neurovascular status.
- Pressure can result from external sources (a tight cast or a constrictive bulky dressing).
- Internal sources (an accumulation of blood or fluid within the muscle compartment) can cause pressure as well.

MANIFESTATIONS

- Compartment syndrome is identified by using the five P's (pain, paralysis, paresthesia, pallor, and pulselessness).
  - Increased pain unrelieved with elevation or by pain medication. Intense pain when passively moved.
  - Paresthesia or numbness, burning, and tingling are early manifestations.
  - Paralysis, motor weakness, or inability to move the extremity indicate major nerve damage and are late manifestations.
  - Pallor of the affected tissue, and nail beds are cyanotic
  - Pulselessness is a late manifestation of compartment syndrome.
  - Palpated muscles are hard and swollen from edema.
- If untreated, tissue necrosis can result. Neuromuscular damage occurs within 4 to 6 hr.
- Surgical treatment is a fasciotomy, which is a surgical incision.
- A surgical incision is made through the subcutaneous tissue and fascia of the affected compartment to relieve the pressure and restore circulation.
- After the fasciotomy, the open wounds require sterile packings and dressings until secondary closure occurs. Skin grafts might be necessary. Negative pressure wound therapy can be used to reduce edema.

NURSING ACTIONS
Prevention includes the following.
- Perform a neurovascular check frequently.
- Notify the provider when compartment syndrome is suspected.
- The provider will cut the cast on one side (univalve) or both sides (bivalve).
- Loosen the constrictive dressing or cut the bandage or tape.

CLIENT EDUCATION
- Report pain not relieved by analgesics or pain that continues to increase in intensity.
- Report numbness, tingling, or a change in color of the extremity.

Fat embolism

- Adults aged 70 to 80 and those assigned male at birth between 20 and 40 years are at increased risk.
- Most common following hip fracture; other cases are within 72 hr following pelvic fracture or surgery.
- Fat embolism can occur after the injury, usually within 12 to 48 hr following long bone fractures or with total joint arthroplasty.
- Fat globules from the bone marrow are released into the vasculature and travel to the small blood vessels, including those in the lungs, resulting in acute respiratory insufficiency and impaired organ perfusion. Careful diagnosis should differentiate between fat embolism and pulmonary embolism.

65.5 Case study

Part 1

Day 1: James is a nurse on a medical-surgical floor assisting with the care of Joe Smith. The client fractured their left tibia and fibula in a motor vehicle accident. They are post-operative following an open reduction, external fixation of a fracture of the left tibia and fibula.

Part 2

Day 3: James is assisting with the discharge of Joe Smith, who is post-operative following an open reduction, external fixation of a fracture of the left tibia and fibula.

Part 3

Day 14: Amy is assisting with the care of Joe Smith. The client developed osteomyelitis 2 weeks following an open reduction, external fixation of a left tibia and fibula fracture. The client is postoperative following a wound debridement for osteomyelitis.

Case study exercises

1. The nurse is collecting data on the client who had an external fixation device applied 2 hr ago for a fracture of the left tibia and fibula. Which of the following findings is a manifestation of compartment syndrome? (Select all that apply.)

   A. Report of pain of a 10 on a scale of 0 to 10 when the client's affected foot is passively moved

   B. Capillary refill of 2 sec on the toes of the client's affected foot

   C. Hard, swollen muscle palpated on the client's affected leg

   D. Report of tingling on the client's affected foot

   E. 2+ pedal pulses on the client's affected foot

2. The nurse is reinforcing teaching with the client how to manage an external fixation device upon discharge. Which of the following statements by the client indicates an understanding?

   A. "I will expect to have white-colored drainage around the pin sites."

   B. "I will clean each pin with sterile water."

   C. "I will tighten the pins if they become loose."

   D. "I will remove crusts if they form around the pin site."

3. The nurse is reinforcing discharge teaching with the client who had a wound debridement for osteomyelitis. Which of the following information should the nurse include?

   A. Antibiotic therapy should continue for one month.

   B. Relief of pain indicates the infection is eradicated.

   C. Airborne precautions are used during wound care.

   D. Expect paresthesia distal to the wound.

Manifestations

EARLY MANIFESTATIONS
- Dyspnea, increased respiratory rate, decreased oxygen saturation
- Headache
- Decreased mental acuity related to low arterial oxygen level
- Respiratory distress
- Tachycardia
- Confusion
- Chest pain

LATE MANIFESTATION: Cutaneous petechiae: pinpoint-sized subdermal hemorrhages that occur on the neck, chest, upper arms, and abdomen (from the blockage of the capillaries by the fat globules). This is a discriminating finding from pulmonary embolism.

NURSING ACTIONS
- Maintain the client on bed rest.
- Prevention includes immobilization of fractures of the long bones and minimal manipulation during turning if immobilization procedure has not yet been performed.
- Treatment includes oxygen for respiratory compromise, corticosteroids for cerebral edema, vasopressors, and fluid replacement for shock, as well as pain and antianxiety medications as needed.

Venous thromboembolism

Deep vein thrombosis and pulmonary embolism: Deep vein thrombosis is a common complication following trauma, surgery, or disability related to immobility.

NURSING ACTIONS
- Encourage early ambulation.
- Apply anti-embolism stockings, sequential compression device.
- Administer anticoagulants as prescribed.
- Encourage intake of fluids to prevent hemoconcentration.
- Monitor for manifestations (swollen, reddened calf).

CLIENT EDUCATION: Rotate feet at the ankles and perform other lower extremity exercises as permitted by the particular immobilization device. Q EBP

Osteomyelitis

Osteomyelitis is an infection of the bone that begins as an inflammation within the bone secondary to penetration by infectious organisms (virus, bacteria, or fungi) following trauma or surgical repair of a fracture.

MANIFESTATIONS
- Bone pain that is constant, pulsating, localized, and worse with movement
- Erythema and edema at the site of the infection
- Fever: Older adults might not have an elevated temperature. Ⓖ
- Leukocytosis and possible elevated sedimentation rate
- Many of these manifestations will disappear if the infection becomes chronic.

DIAGNOSTIC PROCEDURES

- Bone scan using radioactive material to diagnose osteomyelitis, and MRI can also facilitate a diagnosis
- Cultures are performed for detection of possible aerobic and anaerobic organisms.
- If septicemia develops, blood cultures will be positive for offending microbes.

TREATMENT

- Long course (at least 4 to 6 weeks) of IV and oral antibiotic therapy
- Surgical debridement can be indicated. If a significant amount of the bone requires removal, a bone graft can be necessary.
- Hyperbaric oxygen treatments can promote healing in chronic cases of osteomyelitis.
- Surgically implanted antibiotic beads in bone cement are packed into the wound as a form of antibiotic therapy.
- Unsuccessful treatment can result in amputation.

NURSING ACTIONS

- Administer antibiotics as prescribed to maintain a constant blood level.
- Administer analgesics as needed.
- Conduct neurovascular checks if debridement is done.
- If the wound is left open to heal, standard precautions are adequate, and clean technique can be used during dressing changes.

Avascular necrosis

- Avascular necrosis results from the circulatory compromise that occurs after a fracture. Blood flow is disrupted to the fracture site, and the resulting ischemia leads to tissue (bone) necrosis.
- Commonly found in hip fractures or in fractures with displacement of a bone.
- Risk factors for developing avascular necrosis include long-term corticosteroid use, radiation therapy, rheumatoid arthritis, and sickle cell disease.
- Replacement of damaged bone with a bone graft or prosthetic replacement can be necessary.

Failure of fracture to heal

A fracture that has not healed within 6 months of injury is considered to be experiencing delayed union.
- **Malunion:** Fracture heals incorrectly.
- **Nonunion:** Fracture that never heals
  - Electrical bone stimulation and bone grafting can treat nonunion.
  - Low intensity pulse ultrasound can promote healing to treat nonunion.
  - Can occur more frequently in older adult clients due to impaired healing process ⑥
- Malunion or nonunion can cause immobilizing deformity of the bone involved.

Hemorrhage

Because bones are highly vascular, bleeding is always a risk following fracture. Hemorrhage can progress to hypovolemic shock.

NURSING ACTIONS

- Monitor for bruising and swelling at the injury site with increased pain.
- Monitor for indications of blood loss (hypotension and tachycardia).

Complex regional pain syndrome (CRPS)

- Severe chronic pain, usually following musculoskeletal trauma
- More common in the feet and hands
- Can develop if acute pain is not well managed
- Triad of manifestations includes motor changes (muscle spasms, paresis), autonomic nervous system changes (temperature, sensitivity, diaphoresis), and sensory changes (intractable burning sensation).
- Can progress to osteoporosis

Carpal tunnel syndrome

Compression of the median nerve in the wrist from swollen or thickened synovium, causing pain and numbness

DATA COLLECTION

RISK FACTORS

- Some metabolic and connective tissue diseases (rheumatoid arthritis [synovitis] and diabetes mellitus [reduced circulation])
- Occupational injury from repetitive stress of hand activities (pinching or grasping during wrist flexion [computer users])
- Repetitive sports injury (tennis)
- Children and adolescents due to use of computers and handheld devices
- Growth of a space occupying lesion (a ganglia or lipoma)

EXPECTED FINDINGS

- Diagnosis is made based on history and report of pain and numbness in affected hand.
- Pain is often worse at night and can radiate to the arm, shoulder, and neck or chest.
- Paresthesia (painful tingling): Sensory changes occur weeks or months before motor.
- Phalen's maneuver (positive in most clients who have carpal tunnel syndrome)
  - Ask the client to place the back of their hands together and flex both wrists at the same time.
  - Tinel's sign: Tap lightly over the median nerve area of the wrist.
  - A positive result is paresthesia in the median nerve distribution (palmer side of thumb, index, middle and half of ring finger).

PATIENT-CENTERED CARE

NURSING CARE

- Medication therapy
  - NSAIDs for relief of pain and inflammation
  - Corticosteroid injections directly into the carpal tunnel
- Splint or hand brace to immobilize the wrist: can use during the day, during the night, or both
- Laser or ultrasound therapy
- Yoga and exercise
- Surgery can relieve the pressure by decompressing the pressure on the nerve, if nonsurgical methods are ineffective
  - Endoscopic carpal tunnel release: less invasive but a longer recovery period of postoperative pain and numbness
  - Open carpal tunnel release

POSTOPERATIVE CARE

- Monitor vital signs and check dressing for drainage and tightness.
- Elevate hand above the heart to reduce swelling.
- Check neurovascular status of fingers every hour and encourage the client to move them frequently.
- Offer pain medications.
- The client might need assistance with personal care.

CLIENT EDUCATION

- Hand movements and heavy lifting might be restricted 4 to 6 weeks.
- Expect weakness and discomfort for weeks or months.
- Report any changes in neurovascular status, including increase in pain to surgeon immediately.

Sprains and strains

Strain

- Excessive stretching or pulling of a muscle or tendon that is weak or unstable
- Often caused by falls, lifting a heavy item, and exercise

CLASSIFICATIONS OF STRAINS

- **First-degree (mild) strain** causes mild inflammation and little bleeding. There can be swelling, ecchymosis, and tenderness.
- **Second-degree (moderate) strain** involves partial tearing of the muscle or tendon fibers. Involves impaired muscle function
- **Third-degree (severe) strain** involves a ruptured muscle or tendon with separation of muscle from muscle, tendon from muscle, or tendon from bone. Causes severe pain and immobility.

Sprain

- Excessive stretching of a ligament. Twisting motions from a fall or sports activity can be the cause of the injury.
- Classification of sprains are according to severity.

PATIENT-CENTERED CARE

Management of strain

- Cold and heat application, exercise, and activity limitations
- Anti-inflammatory medications and muscle relaxants to decrease inflammation and pain
- Surgical repair if needed for third-degree strains to repair ruptured muscle or tendon

Management of sprain

- RICE (rest, ice, compression, elevation) for mild sprains.
- Second-degree sprains require immobilization and partial weight bearing while the tear heals.
- Immobilization for 4 to 6 weeks is necessary for third-degree sprains. Arthroscopic surgery if needed.
- Apply ice for the first 24 to 72 hr after injury.

Application Exercises

1. A nurse is assisting with teaching a class about types of fractures. Match the type of fracture with the associated characteristics.

   A. Greenstick
   B. Impacted
   C. Spiral
   D. Oblique
   E. Comminuted

   1. Bone is fragmented.
   2. Fracture occurs at an angle and across bone
   3. Fracture that winds around the bone.
   4. Fractured bone is wedged inside another bone fragment.
   5. Fracture occurs on one side of the bone but does not extend completely through the bone.

2. A nurse is assisting with teaching a class about types of tractions. Sort the following characteristics into those associated with skin traction and those associated with skeletal traction.

   A. Screws are inserted into bone.
   B. Weights are attached to a boot.
   C. Uses 5 to 10 lb weights
   D. Uses 15 to 30 lb weights

3. A nurse is collecting data on a client who has a casted compound fracture of the femur. What findings are manifestations of a fat embolus?

Active Learning Scenario

A nurse is performing a neurovascular check on a client who has a cast applied following a right arm fracture. What interventions should the nurse take? Use the ATI Active Learning Template: Basic Concept to complete this item.

RELATED CONTENT: Identify the purpose of neurovascular check.

UNDERLYING PRINCIPLES: Identify the components of a neurovascular check.

NURSING INTERVENTIONS: Describe a nursing intervention related to each of the components.

Active Learning Scenario Key

Using the ATI Active Learning Template: Basic Concept

RELATED CONTENT: A neurovascular check is performed to monitor for any compromise in the affected extremity caused by edema and or immobilization device.

UNDERLYING PRINCIPLES

- Pain: Monitor pain level, location, and frequency. Monitor pain using a 0 to 10 pain rating scale, and have the client describe the pain.
- Sensation: Monitor for numbness or tingling of the extremity. Loss of sensation can indicate nerve damage.
- Skin temperature: Check the temperature of the affected extremity. The extremity should be warm (not cool) to the touch.
- Skin color: Pale (restricted blood), blue (impaired oxygenation), bruised (bleeding into tissues), or red (infection)
- Capillary refill: Press nail beds of affected extremity until blanching occurs. Blood return should be within 3 seconds.
- Pulses: Should be palpable and strong. Pulses should be equal to the unaffected extremity.
- Movement: Client should have movement of affected extremity and the area distal to the injury in active motion.

NURSING INTERVENTIONS: Immobilize, apply ice, and elevate the extremity to reduce swelling, relieve pain, increase sensation, improve circulation, and increase movement.

Ⓝ *NCLEX® Connection: Reduction of Risk Potential, Potential for Alterations in Body Systems*

Application Exercises Key

1. A, 5; B, 4; C, 3; D, 3; E, 1

   When taking actions, the nurse should instruct that a comminuted fracture is a fracture in which bone is broken into many fragments. An oblique fracture is a fracture that occurs at an angle across the bone. A spiral fracture is a fracture that winds around the bone. This type of fracture is seen in physical abuse. An impacted fracture is a fracture in which a bone is wedged or impacted inside another bone fragment. A greenstick fracture is a fracture that occurs on one side of the bone but does not extend completely through the bone. This type of fracture is seen in children.

   Ⓝ *NCLEX® Connection: Basic Care and Comfort, Mobility/ Immobility*

2. **SKIN TRACTION:** B, C; **SKELETAL TRACTION:** A, D

   When taking actions, the nurse should instruct that light weights are attached to a boot with skin traction to reduce muscle spasms in hip and proximal femur fractures. Screws are inserted into the bone, and heavy weights are used with skeletal traction to provide longer traction time.

   Ⓝ *NCLEX® Connection: Basic Care and Comfort, Mobility/ Immobility*

3. When recognizing cues, the nurse should identify early manifestations of a fat emboli include dyspnea, increased respiratory rate, decreased oxygen saturation, headache, confusion and decreased mental acuity related to low arterial oxygen level, respiratory distress, tachycardia, and chest pain. Late manifestations of fat emboli include cutaneous petechiae (pinpoint-sized subdermal hemorrhages that occur on the neck, chest, upper arms, and abdomen). Petechiae is caused by the blockage of the capillaries by fat globules. This is a discriminating finding from pulmonary embolism.

   Ⓝ *NCLEX® Connection: Basic Care and Comfort, Mobility/ Immobility*

Case Study Exercises Key

1. A, C, D. **CORRECT:** When analyzing cues, the nurse should identify that manifestations of compartment syndrome include intense pain of the affected foot when passively moved; hard, swollen muscle on the affected extremity; and burning and tingling of the affected foot. These manifestations are due to edema and nerve ischemia near the injury.

   Ⓝ *NCLEX® Connection: Reduction of Risk Potential, Potential for Complications From Surgical Procedures and Health Alterations*

2. B. **CORRECT:** When evaluating outcomes, the nurse should identify that the client understands to clean each pin with sterile water to decrease the risk of pin site infection.

   Ⓝ *NCLEX® Connection: Basic Care and Comfort, Mobility/ Immobility*

3. A. **CORRECT:** When taking actions, the nurse should instruct the client that oral and/or IV antibiotic therapy will need to continue for at least 4 to 6 weeks to eradicate the infection.

   Ⓝ *NCLEX® Connection: Reduction of Risk Potential, Potential for Complications from Surgical Procedures and Health Alterations*

CHAPTER 66 *Osteoarthritis and Low-Back Pain*

Osteoarthritis (OA), or degenerative joint disease (DJD), is a disorder characterized by progressive deterioration of the articular cartilage. It is a noninflammatory (unless localized), nonsystemic disease. It is no longer thought to be only a wear-and-tear disease associated with aging, but rather a process in which new tissue is produced as a result of cartilage destruction within the joint. The destruction outweighs the production. The cartilage and bone beneath the cartilage erode, and osteophytes (bone spurs) form, resulting in narrowed joint spaces. The changes within the joint lead to pain, immobility, muscle spasms, and potential inflammation. Early in the disease process of OA, it can be difficult to distinguish from rheumatoid arthritis (RA).

Low-back pain (LBP) occurs along the lumbosacral area of the vertebral column. LBP can be acute (less than 4 weeks) or chronic (longer than 3 months or repeated episodes of pain). LBP can be related to an injury, fall, or heavy lifting. LBP is a common cause of absence from work. Acute pain results from muscle spasm or strain, ligament sprains, or disk herniation or degeneration. Spinal stenosis (narrowing of spinal canal or other spaces) can cause back pain.

Osteoarthritis

HEALTH PROMOTION AND DISEASE PREVENTION

- Encourage the client to use joint-saving measures (good body mechanics, labor-saving devices).
- Encourage the client to maintain a healthy weight to decrease joint degeneration of the hips and knees.
- Encourage the client to avoid or limit repetitive strain on joints (jogging, contact sports, risk-taking activities).
- Recommend wearing well-fitted shoes with supports to prevent falls.

DATA COLLECTION

RISK FACTORS

- Aging
- Genetic factors
- Joint injury due to acute or repetitive stress on joints
- Obesity

66.1 Characteristics of osteoarthritis and rheumatoid arthritis

	Osteoarthritis	*Rheumatoid arthritis*
Disease process	Cartilage destruction with bone spur growth at joint ends; degenerative	Synovial membrane inflammation resulting in cartilage destruction and bone erosion; inflammatory
Findings	Pain with activity that improves at rest	Swelling, redness, warmth, pain at rest or after immobility (morning stiffness)
Effusions	Localized inflammatory response	All joints
Body size	Usually overweight	Usually underweight
Nodes	Heberden's and Bouchard's nodes	Swan neck and boutonnière deformities of hands
Systemic involvement	No: articular	Yes: lungs, heart, skin, and extra-articular
Symmetrical	No	Yes
Diagnostic tests	X-rays	X-rays and positive rheumatoid factor

EXPECTED FINDINGS

- Joint pain and stiffness
- Pain with joint palpation or range of motion (Observe for muscle atrophy, loss of function, limp when walking, and restricted activity due to pain.)
- Crepitus in one or more of the affected joints
- Enlarged joint related to bone hypertrophy
- Heberden's nodes enlarged at the distal interphalangeal joints
- Bouchard's nodes located at the proximal interphalangeal joints (OA is not a symmetrical disease, but these nodes can occur bilaterally.) Nodes can be inflamed and painful
- Limping gait due to hip or knee pain.
- Back pain due to OA of the spine

LABORATORY TESTS

Laboratory tests are usually normal with OA. Erythrocyte sedimentation rate and high-sensitivity C-reactive protein can be increased slightly related to secondary synovitis.

DIAGNOSTIC PROCEDURES

Radiographs (x-ray): to determine changes to joints

PATIENT-CENTERED CARE

NURSING CARE

- Inspect gait, joints, and ROM.
- Assist the client with pharmacological and nonpharmacological pain relief.
- Have the client determine an acceptable level of pain as a goal to measure progress (a rating of 3 or less on a 0 to 10 scale).
- Determine the psychosocial impact of OA for the client (body image changes or altered ability to perform self-care or maintain employment).

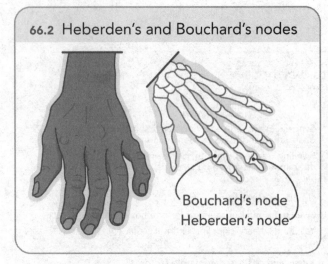

66.2 Heberden's and Bouchard's nodes

Bouchard's node
Heberden's node

- Reinforce with the client about joint protection: using large joints rather than small ones, using two hands to hold objects, bending the knees when reaching down rather than bending the waist.
- Determine the need for assistive or adaptive devices (mobility aids, splints, clothing with Velcro closures).
- Warn the client about using so-called cures for osteoarthritis and to talk with the provider before trying any new therapies to reduce the risk of harm.

CLIENT EDUCATION

- Balance activity with rest.
- Heat can help with joint tenderness and muscle stiffness. Use hot baths and showers or hot packs and moist heating pads to promote comfort, but avoid high temperatures to prevent burns.
- Achieve and maintain a healthy weight to reduce stress on the joints.
- Follow the prescribed exercise regime consistently. Active exercises are more beneficial than passive.
- On days when pain is increased, attempt exercise, but reduce the number of repetitions and avoid resistance exercises.
- Use nonpharmacological measures for pain relief such as relaxation, meditation, and distraction, which can promote comfort and reduce muscle tension.

MEDICATIONS

Acetaminophen

The medication of choice for managing OA

NURSING ACTIONS

- Limit administration of acetaminophen to a maximum of 4,000 mg/24 hr. Some experts recommend a maximum daily dose of 3,000 mg/day when used long-term to prevent liver toxicity.
- Monitor liver function tests. ⓆEBP

Topical medications

- Topical salicylates (gels, patches, or creams) and topical buspirone cream can be used.
- Limit use to 3 to 4 times a day. Stop use if irritation occurs.

Nonsteroidal anti-inflammatory drugs (NSAIDs)

- Analgesics and anti-inflammatories (celecoxib, naproxen, ibuprofen) are used to relieve pain unrelieved by acetaminophen and topical agents and synovitis if present.
- Baseline liver and kidney function tests and CBC are needed if NSAIDs are to be given.
- Topical NSAID (diclofenac epolamine patch) can be used and is non-systemic.

NURSING ACTIONS: Monitor kidney function
(BUN, creatinine).

CLIENT EDUCATION

- NSAIDs are nephrotoxic and should be taken as prescribed.
- Report evidence of black, tarry stool; indigestion; and shortness of breath.

COMPLEMENTARY AND ALTERNATIVE THERAPIES

Massage, aromatherapy, acupuncture

- Used to relieve discomfort and maintain mobility associated with OA
- Assist with referring client as needed.

Topical capsaicin

Provides temporary pain relief by blocking some pain impulses
- Cream is applied topically 3 to 4 times daily.
- Causes brief burning sensation after applications; avoid touching face and eyes

CLIENT EDUCATION

- Wear gloves during application and wash the hands immediately afterwards. If application site is the hands, leave on for 30 min without touching anything else, then wash the hands.
- A burning sensation of the skin after application is normal and should subside. Burning sensation becomes less frequent the more the cream is used.

Glucosamine and chondroitin supplements

- Glucosamine and chondroitin are natural substances that aid in repair and maintenance of cartilage.
- Glucosamine assists in reducing inflammation, and chondroitin helps strengthen the cartilage.
- Adverse effects of glucosamine include GI upset, rash, headache, and drowsiness.
- There is an increased risk for bleeding if the client takes anticoagulants and chondroitin.

CLIENT EDUCATION

- Consult the provider regarding use and dosage, which should be based on weight.
- Do not take glucosamine if you have hypertension, are pregnant, or are lactating.
- Monitor for bleeding if taking chondroitin, especially if also taking an anticoagulant.
- Inform the provider regarding concurrent use of chondroitin, NSAIDs, heparin, and warfarin.

INTERPROFESSIONAL CARE

- Physical therapy to assist with comfort therapies (diathermy, ultrasonography, paraffin dips)
- Case manager or home health nurse to determine home modifications (handrails, raised or lowered counters)

THERAPEUTIC PROCEDURES

Intra-articular injections

- Glucocorticoids are used to treat localized inflammation. One joint can be injected no more than 4 times a year.
- Hyaluronic acid is sometimes used to replace the body's natural hyaluronic acid, which is destroyed by joint inflammation. Evidence supporting the benefits is unclear.

Total joint arthroplasty or replacement

When other measures fail, the client can choose to undergo total joint arthroplasty of synovial joints to relieve the pain and improve mobility and quality of life.
- Joint replacement is contraindicated with any type of infection, advanced osteoporosis, or rapidly progressive inflammation.
- Complications include infection, nerve damage, and thromboembolism.

Low-back pain

HEALTH PROMOTION AND DISEASE PREVENTION

- Exercise to keep back healthy and strong (swimming, walking).
- Use body mechanics and proper lifting techniques (ergonomics).
- Maintain correct posture.
- Wear low-heeled shoes.
- Maintain a healthy weight.
- Smoking cessation, as smoking is linked to disk degeneration Ⓠ EBP
- Avoid prolonged sitting/standing.
- Healthy diet including adequate calcium and vitamin D

DATA COLLECTION

RISK FACTORS

- Family history of back pain or history of a back injury
- History of spine problems, back surgery, or compression fracture
- Job or occupation that requires heavy lifting, twisting, or repetitive motion
- Smoking (linked to disk degeneration)
- Overweight
- Having poor posture
- Osteoarthritis

EXPECTED FINDINGS

- Muscle spasms, cramping, and stiffness, often in a location closest to the affected disk
- Pain that radiates to the buttock
- Sciatic nerve compression causes severe pain when leg is straightened and held up and limping when walking.
- Numbness/tingling of the leg (paresthesia); burning or stabbing pain in the leg or foot

DIAGNOSTIC PROCEDURES

Radiographs (x-ray): to determine changes to joints

CT scan and magnetic resonance imaging: to visualize bones, nerves, disks, ligaments, spinal cord and nerves, muscles and disks

Bone scan: provides visualization of increased vascularity indicating tumor or infection

Myelogram and post-myelogram CT scan: show nerve root lesions or other lesions, masses, or infection

Electromyography (EMG) with nerve conduction studies: to determine whether motor neuron issues or peripheral neuropathies are the cause

PATIENT-CENTERED CARE

Evidence-based practice recommendations include nonpharmacological interventions with an interprofessional approach as initial management strategies.

NURSING CARE

- Assist with management of acute back pain. Inform the client that unmanaged acute pain can lead to chronic pain.
- Assist the client to change positions frequently to minimize pain.
- Discourage prolonged time in bed and assist the client to perform stretching exercises as soon as possible.
- Encourage stress relief.

CLIENT EDUCATION
- Heat therapy can help reduce pain.
- Acetaminophen is usually not helpful for lower back pain.
- Semi-Fowler's position with a pillow under flexed knees can alleviate pain associated with LBP from a herniated disk. Q EBP
- When sitting in a recliner, elevate the legs, or when in bed, use pillows to elevate the head and legs.
- Avoid twisting or turning the vertebral column while changing position.
- Sleep on a firm mattress.
- No heavy lifting.
- Ice packs after the first 48 hr to decrease spasms.
- If prolonged standing is required, shoe insoles or floor pads can provide relief.
- Avoid wearing shoes with high heels.
- Achieve and maintain a healthy weight.

MEDICATIONS

Nonsteroidal anti-inflammatory drugs

Over-the-counter or prescription NSAIDs can be helpful.

Mild opioids

Tramadol can be used if NSAIDs are ineffective.

Oral corticosteroids

Decrease inflammation

Muscle relaxants

Decrease muscle spasms

COMPLEMENTARY AND ALTERNATIVE THERAPIES

Massage, spinal manipulation, mindfulness, progressive muscle relaxation, yoga, and acupuncture can be helpful.

INTERPROFESSIONAL CARE

- Pain management specialists can assist with long-term management.
- Physical therapy can assist the client in creating an individualized exercise plan; can include water therapy.

THERAPEUTIC PROCEDURES

Transcutaneous electrical nerve stimulator (TENS) unit

Can help minimize pain

Minimally invasive surgery

Microscopic endoscopic diskectomy or percutaneous endoscopy diskectomy: Fluoroscopy is used to guide a tubular device through which the herniated disk is removed by cutting it out or suctioning out the center of the disk.

Laser-assisted laparoscopic lumbar diskectomy: Laparoscope and laser are used to treat the herniated disks.

Open surgical procedures

Open diskectomy: removal of the herniated disk

Laminectomy: removal of part of the laminae and facet joints

Surgery for tumors or infection

Arthrodesis/spinal fusion: surgery to join or fuse two or more vertebrae. Often required if the spine is unstable or multiple laminectomies are required
- A bone graft from the pelvic bone or bone bank is used to make a bridge between vertebrae that are next to each other.
- Metal implants can also be used.

Interbody cage fusion: implantation of a cagelike device following disk removal

PREPROCEDURE NURSING ACTIONS
- Assist with collecting baseline neurological data.
- Reinforce with the client and family on methods to change position following surgery.
- Ensure informed consent is signed. Special consent might be needed if donor bone is used for grafting.

POSTPROCEDURE NURSING ACTIONS
- Provide standard postoperative care.
- Perform neurologic checks with vital sign measurement.
- Check for numbness, tingling, and muscle strength.
- Ensure the client is able to void. Inability can indicate damage to the bladder muscles.
- Check incisions for bleeding and drainage.

- Check for pain. Administer analgesia as needed. Patient-controlled analgesia (PCA) can be used following open procedures.
- If a surgical drain is present, empty every shift. The surgeon removes the drain after about 24 to 36 hr.
- Do not place an overhead trapeze on the client's bed; use can damage the surgical area.
- Provide a straight-back chair for the client and ensure feet rest on the floor when sitting.
- Expect the client to be discharged within 24 to 48 hr.
- Turn the body as a unit (log roll).

CLIENT EDUCATION
- Initiate prescribed exercise plan following discharge.
- Report new sensory changes (increased numbness, decreased movement) for any extremity to the provider immediately.
- A back orthotic can be required for 4 to 6 weeks following surgery. Follow provider instructions for wearing and when removal is allowed.
- Activity limitations following minimally invasive surgery can range from 2 days to 3 weeks. Following open surgery, restrictions are in place for 4 to 6 weeks.

COMPLICATIONS

Include nerve injury, disk inflammation, and tears to the dura covering the spinal cord

Cerebrospinal fluid leakage

Examine wound dressing drainage for a halo–like appearance. Other manifestations include sudden headache and bulging of the incision.

Active Learning Scenario

A nurse is providing information on collaborative and nonpharmacological therapies for a client who is having continual joint pain from osteoarthritis. What information should the nurse include? Use the ATI Active Learning Template: Basic Concept to complete this item.

RELATED CONTENT: Describe two activities each for collaborative care involving physical therapy and nutrition therapy.

NURSING INTERVENTIONS: Describe three actions the nurse could add to reinforce teaching for this client.

Application Exercises

1. A nurse is collecting data from a client who has osteoarthritis of the knees and fingers. Which of the following manifestations should the nurse expect to find? (Select all that apply.)
   A. Heberden's nodes
   B. Swelling of all joints
   C. Small body frame
   D. Enlarged joint size
   E. Limp when walking

2. A nurse is reinforcing teaching with a client who has osteoarthritis of the hip and knee. Which of the following information should the nurse include? (Select all that apply.)
   A. Apply heat to joints to alleviate pain.
   B. Ice inflamed joints for 30 min following activity.
   C. Reduce the amount of exercise done on days with increased pain.
   D. Elevate the knees with a pillow while in bed.
   E. Massage can alleviate pain of joints.

3. A nurse is reinforcing teaching about capsaicin cream with a client who reports continuous knee pain from osteoarthritis. Which of the following information should the nurse include?
   A. Continuous pain relief is provided.
   B. Put on gloves before applying the cream to other parts of the body.
   C. Remove cream if burning sensation occurs.
   D. Apply the medication every 2 hr during the day.

4. A nurse is caring for a client who injured their lower back due to a fall and reports sharp pain in their back and down their left leg. In which of the following positions should the nurse place the client to attempt to decrease their pain?
   A. Prone without use of pillows
   B. Semi-Fowler's with a pillow under the knees
   C. High-Fowler's with the knees flat on the bed
   D. Supine with the head flat

5. A nurse is reinforcing teaching with a client who has a history of low-back injury. Which of the following instructions should the nurse provide the client to prevent future problems with low-back pain? (Select all that apply.)
   A. Engage in regular exercise, including walking.
   B. Sit for up to 10 hr each day to rest the back.
   C. Maintain weight within 25% of ideal body weight.
   D. Create a smoking cessation plan.
   E. Wear low-heeled shoes.

Active Learning Scenario Key

Using the ATI Active Learning Template: Basic Concept

RELATED CONTENT: Physical therapy
- Apply heat, diathermy, and ultrasound.
- Perform stretching and strengthening exercises.
- Use transcutaneous electrical nerve stimulation (TENS).

NURSING INTERVENTIONS
- Balance rest with activity.
- Identify need for assistive devices and mobility aids.
- Apply thermal therapies (heat or cold).
- Reinforce with the client to use the large joints rather than the small ones.
- Help the client set a pain goal.

Ⓝ *NCLEX® Connection: Basic Care and Comfort, Nonpharmacological Comfort Interventions*

Application Exercises Key

1. A, D, E. **CORRECT:** The nurse should recognize the cues from the client's data collection and expect Heberden's nodes, which are enlarged nodules on the distal interphalangeal joints of the hand and feet of a client who has osteoarthritis. The nurse should expect the client's joints to be enlarged due to bone hypertrophy. The nurse should also expect the client who has osteoarthritis to limp when walking due to pain from inflammation of the localized joint.

   Ⓝ *NCLEX® Connection: Physiological Adaptation, Basic Pathophysiology*

2. A, C, E. **CORRECT:** When taking actions, the nurse should instruct the client to apply heat to their joints, which can provide temporary relief of pain. The nurse should instruct the client to reduce the amount of exercise done on days of increased pain to prevent harm to their joints. The nurse should also instruct the client that massage can alleviate pain of their joints.

   Ⓝ *NCLEX® Connection: Physiological Adaptation, Alterations in Body Systems*

3. B. **CORRECT:** When taking action, the nurse should instruct the client to put on gloves before applying cream to parts of the body other than the hands. Capsaicin can cause a burning sensation.

   Ⓝ *NCLEX® Connection: Pharmacological Therapies, Medication Administration*

4. B. **CORRECT:** When taking actions, the nurse should place the client in semi-Fowler's position with their knees flexed by pillows. This position has been shown to relieve low-back pain caused by a bulging disk and nerve root involvement.

   Ⓝ *NCLEX® Connection: Basic Care and Comfort, Nonpharmacological Comfort Interventions*

5. A, D, E. **CORRECT:** When taking actions, the nurse should instruct the client to engage in regular exercise, including walking or swimming, which can prevent low-back pain. The nurse should instruct the client in stopping or limiting the amount of smoking, which can decrease problems with low-back pain, as smoking can cause disk degeneration as a result of poor oxygenation. The nurse should also instruct the client to wear low-heeled shoes. Wearing low-heeled, well-fitting shoes can prevent low-back pain. The client should avoid high-heeled shoes, which cause stress on the back.

   Ⓝ *NCLEX® Connection: Reduction of Risk Potential, Potential for Alterations in Body Systems*

When reviewing the following chapters, keep in mind the relevant topics and tasks of the NCLEX outline.

Reduction of Risk Potential

DIAGNOSTIC TESTS: Perform diagnostic testing.

POTENTIAL FOR ALTERATIONS IN BODY SYSTEMS: Reinforce client teaching on methods to prevent complications associated with activity level/diagnosed illness/disease.

POTENTIAL FOR COMPLICATIONS FROM SURGICAL PROCEDURES AND HEALTH ALTERATIONS: Monitor client responses to procedures and treatments.

THERAPEUTIC PROCEDURES: Reinforce client teaching on treatments and procedures.

CHAPTER 67 *Integumentary Diagnostic Procedures*

Integumentary diagnostic procedures involve identification of pathogenic micro-organisms. The most accurate and definitive way to identify micro-organisms and cell characteristics is by examining blood, body fluids, and tissue samples under a microscope.

Skin lesions or changes in the skin can need confirmation by microscope to determine if the cause is viral, fungal, or bacterial.

Always use standard precautions when handling skin that is not intact.

Skin diagnostic studies

Wood's light examination

- For clients who have dark skin tones, changes in skin color (changes in underlying red tones or presence of bluish-gray undertones) are best detected using bright lighting. For clients who have light skin tones, or who have areas of hypopigmentation, color changes are best detected using the Wood's light examination.
- The room is darkened, and ultraviolet light is used to produce specific colors to reveal a skin infection and discern between dermal and epidermal lesions and to differentiate normal skin from hypopigmented and hyperpigmented areas.

Diascopy

A glass slide or lens is pressed down over the skin area to be examined to test for blanchability. It is painless and used to determine whether the lesion is vascular (inflammatory) or nonvascular (nevus) or hemorrhagic (petechiae or purpura). Hemorrhagic and nonvascular lesions do not blanch, but inflammatory lesions do.

Skin culture and sensitivity

- **Culture** refers to isolation of the pathogen on culture media. Q̄EBP
- **Sensitivity** refers to the effect that antimicrobial agents have on the micro-organism.
  ○ If the micro-organism is killed by the antimicrobial, the microbe is considered to be sensitive to that medication.
  ○ If tolerable levels of the medication are unable to kill the microbe, the microbe is considered to be resistant to that medication.
- A culture and sensitivity can be done on a sample of purulent drainage from a skin lesion.
- Cultures should be done prior to initiating antimicrobial therapy.
- Results of a culture and sensitivity test usually are available preliminarily within 24 to 48 hr and final results in 72 hr.

INDICATIONS

CLIENT PRESENTATION

- Skin lesions, which can be infectious, can appear raised, reddened, edematous, and/or warm.
- There can be purulent drainage and/or fever.

CONSIDERATIONS

PREPROCEDURE

NURSING ACTIONS
- Use standard precautions when collecting and handling specimens. Q̄s
- Most specimens will be collected by the nurse or provider.

INTRAPROCEDURE

Bacterial or viral specimens

Bacterial

NURSING ACTIONS
- Culturette tubes are specific for specimen collection and contain a sterile cotton-tipped applicator and a fixative that is released after the infectious exudate is applied to the applicator and inserted in the tube.
- A specimen obtained for a viral culture is immediately placed on ice and sent to the laboratory. If laboratory is not readily available, the collected specimen tube should be refrigerated.

Viral
- A cotton-tipped applicator is used to obtain vesicle fluid from intact lesions for culture.
- A specimen obtained for a viral culture is immediately placed on ice and sent to laboratory. If laboratory is not readily available, the collected specimen tube should be refrigerated.

Fungal specimen

NURSING ACTIONS

- Requires a sufficient quantity of scales collected using a wooden tongue depressor to scrape the skin and place the specimen in a clean container
- If a fungal culture is needed because of inconclusive results due to a deeper fungal infection, a punch biopsy is performed.
- Specimens must be properly labeled and delivered to the laboratory promptly for appropriate storage and analysis.

INTERPRETATION OF FINDINGS

The microbe responsible for the infection is identified in the culture, and the antimicrobials that are sensitive to that microbe are listed.

POTASSIUM HYDROXIDE (KOH) TEST

- The test confirms a fungal skin lesion.
- A microscopic examination of the scales scraped off a lesion is mixed with KOH. Specimen is positive for fungus if there is the presence of fungal hyphae (threadlike filaments).

Biopsy

Biopsy is the removal of a sample of tissue by excision or needle aspiration for cytological (histological) examination.

- Biopsy confirms or rules out malignancy.
- Skin biopsies are performed under local anesthesia and can be a punch, shave, or excisional biopsy. Punch biopsy is the most common technique.

Punch biopsy: A small plug of tissue approximately 2 to 6 mm is removed with a specific cutting instrument, with or without sutures to close the site. Most skin biopsies are obtained using the punch.

Shave biopsy: Removal of only the part of the lesion that is raised above the surrounding tissue using a scalpel or razor blade with no suturing

Excisional biopsy: A larger and deeper specimen is obtained, and suturing is required.

INDICATIONS

POTENTIAL DIAGNOSES: A biopsy is commonly performed to establish an exact diagnosis or to rule out diseases (cancer).

CLIENT PRESENTATION: Evidence of skin lesion can include an area of discoloration that is thickened, thinned, raised, flat, rough, painful, open, dry, and/or itchy.

CONSIDERATIONS

PREPROCEDURE

NURSING ACTIONS

- Ensure that the client has signed the informed consent form.
- Inform the client that a scar can form after the biopsy.

INTRAPROCEDURE

NURSING ACTIONS

- Establish a sterile field. Qs
- Place the tissue sample in a container containing appropriate solution, label, and send to the laboratory.
- Apply pressure to the biopsy site to control bleeding as appropriate.
- Place a sterile dressing over the biopsy site.

POSTPROCEDURE

Post-biopsy discomfort usually is relieved by mild analgesics.

NURSING ACTIONS: Monitor the biopsy site for bleeding.

CLIENT EDUCATION

- Check the biopsy site daily. Report excessive bleeding or evidence of infection (redness, warmth, drainage, fever) to the provider. Qs
- Dressings can be removed after 8 hr. Use tap water and 0.9% sterile sodium chloride to clean the biopsy site of dried blood or crusts.
- If prescribed, apply an antibacterial topical medication to prevent infection.
- If sutures are used, return to the provider for removal in 3 to 10 days depending on the biopsy site.
- It could take several days for the results of the biopsy.

INTERPRETATION OF FINDINGS

After a biopsy is completed, the tissue sample is sent to pathology for interpretation.

Application Exercises

1. A nurse in a clinic is preparing to assist with obtaining a skin specimen from a client who has a suspected herpes infection. Which of the following actions should the nurse take?

   A. Scrape the site with a wooden tongue depressor.

   B. Use a razor to cut the scabbed area to obtain the specimen.

   C. Use a cotton-tipped applicator to obtain fluid from the lesion.

   D. Place specimen in a potassium hydroxide (KOH) solution tube.

   E. Place collected specimen tube immediately on ice.

2. A nurse is caring for a client who has a suspected fungal skin lesion. Which of the following diagnostic procedures should the nurse prepare the client for to confirm diagnosis?

   A. Potassium hydroxide (KOH) test

   B. Diascopy

   C. Tzanck smear

   D. Shave biopsy

3. A nurse is reinforcing discharge instructions with a client who had a skin biopsy with sutures. Which of the following statements by the client indicates an understanding of the instructions?

   A. "I can expect redness around the site for 5 to 7 days."

   B. "I will most likely have a fever for the first few days."

   C. "I should clean the site with a sterile saline solution."

   D. "I will make a return appointment in 2 days for removal of my sutures."

Active Learning Scenario

A nurse is caring for a client who will have a biopsy of a skin lesion. What should the nurse consider in planning for the procedure? Use the ATI Active Learning Template: Basic Concept to complete this item.

UNDERLYING PRINCIPLES: List and describe the three types of integumentary biopsies.

NURSING INTERVENTIONS: Describe two intraprocedure nursing actions.

Active Learning Scenario Key

Using the ATI Active Learning Template: Basic Concept

UNDERLYING PRINCIPLES
- Punch biopsy: A 2 to 6 mm plug of tissue is removed from the skin lesion, followed with or without suturing.
- Shave biopsy: A scalpel or razor blade removes only the raised area of the lesion, with no suturing.
- Excisional biopsy: A large, deep specimen of tissue is obtained, followed with suturing.

NURSING INTERVENTIONS
- Assist with setting up materials for placement of a local anesthetic.
- Apply pressure to the biopsy site to control bleeding.
- Prep biopsy skin area accordingly.
- Label all specimens.
- Place a sterile dressing over the biopsy site if needed.

Ⓝ *NCLEX® Connection: Reduction of Risk Potential, Potential for Complications of Diagnostic Tests/Treatments/Procedures*

Application Exercises Key

1. C, E. **CORRECT:** When generating solutions, the nurse should assist with planning to collect a sample from a viral lesion by using a sterile cotton-tipped applicator to obtain fluid from the lesion. The nurse should refrigerate the specimen if not able to transport to lab immediately. The specimen should be placed on ice soon after specimen has been collected and sent to laboratory immediately.

Ⓝ *NCLEX® Connection: Reduction of Risk Potential, Diagnostic Tests*

2. A. **CORRECT:** When analyzing cues for a client who has a suspected fungal skin lesion, the nurse should assist with preparing the client for potassium hydroxide testing. This test is used to confirm the diagnosis of fungal skin lesions.

Ⓝ *NCLEX® Connection: Reduction of Risk Potential, Diagnostic Tests*

3. C. **CORRECT:** After a biopsy procedure, the client is at risk for infection. Therefore, it is important for the nurse to reinforce signs of infection and how to prevent infection. The client should clean the site with a 0.9% sterile sodium chloride solution as needed to remove dried blood and crustations.

Ⓝ *NCLEX® Connection: Reduction of Risk Potential, Potential for Complications of Diagnostic Tests/Treatments/Procedures*

When reviewing the following chapters, keep in mind the relevant topics and tasks of the NCLEX outline.

Reduction of Risk Potential

POTENTIAL FOR ALTERATIONS IN BODY SYSTEMS: Reinforce client teaching on methods to prevent complications associated with activity level/diagnosed illness/disease.

POTENTIAL FOR COMPLICATIONS FROM SURGICAL PROCEDURES AND HEALTH ALTERATIONS: Monitor client responses to procedures and treatments.

THERAPEUTIC PROCEDURES: Reinforce client teaching on treatments and procedures.

Physiological Adaptation

ALTERATIONS IN BODY SYSTEMS
Identify signs and symptoms of an infection.

Perform wound care and/or dressing change.

BASIC PHYSIOLOGY: Identify signs and symptoms related to an acute or chronic illness.

CHAPTER 68 *Skin Disorders*

Psoriasis is a skin disorder characterized by scaly dermal patches and caused by overproduction of keratin. This overproduction can occur at a rate up to seven times the rate of normal cells. It is thought to be an autoimmune disorder and has periods of exacerbations and remissions. Although lesions can appear anywhere, they are commonly present on the elbows, knees, trunk, scalp, sacrum, and the lateral aspects of extremities. Psoriasis can be classified as psoriasis vulgaris, exfoliative, or palmoplantar pustulosis. In some clients, psoriasis affects the joints, causing arthritis-type changes and pain.

Dermatitis is an inflammation of the skin resulting from exposure to allergens (internal or external) that causes changes in the skin structure or tissue destruction. Manifestations of dermatitis can be nonspecific and include itching, lesions without distinct borders, and different distribution patterns. Rashes can evolve from acute to chronic and place the client at increased risk for bacterial infection resulting from breaks in the skin caused by scratching. Dermatitis can be classified as nonspecific eczematous, contact, or atopic.

Infections of the skin can be of bacterial, viral, or fungal origin. Prevention is the key; therefore, it's important for the nurse to educate clients about the importance of appropriate personal hygiene (daily bathing/showering and handwashing).

Psoriasis

DATA COLLECTION

RISK FACTORS

- Infections (severe streptococcal throat infection, Candida infection, upper respiratory infection)
- Skin trauma (recent surgery, sunburn)
- Genetics
- Stress (related to overstimulation of the immune system)
- Seasons (warm weather improves manifestations)
- Hormones (puberty or menopause)
- Medications (lithium, beta blocker, indomethacin)
- Obesity

EXPECTED FINDINGS

- **Psoriasis vulgaris** presents as reddened, thickened skin with silvery white scales with bilateral distribution.
- **Exfoliative psoriasis** displays as erythema and scaling from a severe inflammatory reaction with no obvious lesions. The reaction can cause dehydration and hypothermia or hyperthermia.
- **Palmoplantar pustulosis** manifests as reddened hyperkeratotic areas (accelerated maturation of epidermal cells) due to an inflammatory disorder. Plaques form, and pustules turn brown, peel, and form a crust on the palms of the hands and soles of the feet. The course of the disease is cyclic.
- Exacerbation and remission of pruritic lesions

CLASSIFICATION OF LESIONS
- Mild: less than 5% of body surface area (BSA)
- Moderate: 5% to 10% of BSA
- Severe: greater than 10% of BSA

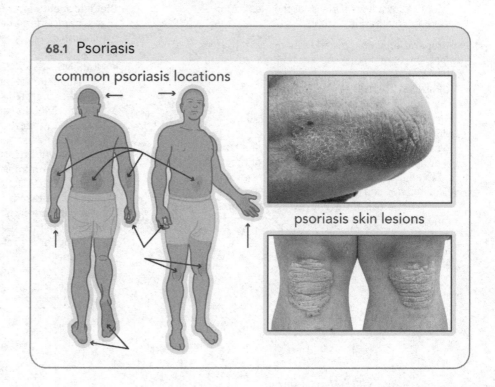

68.1 Psoriasis

common psoriasis locations

psoriasis skin lesions

PHYSICAL FINDINGS
- Scaly patches
- Bleeding stimulated by removal of scales
- Pruritic skin lesions primarily on the scalp, elbows and knees, sacrum, and lateral areas of the extremities (psoriasis vulgaris)
- Pitting, crumbling nails

PATIENT-CENTERED CARE

MEDICATIONS

There is no cure for psoriasis. Treatment is aimed at decreasing the severity of the manifestations and decreasing the turnover rate of the epidermal cells.

Topical therapies

Corticosteroids (triamcinolone, betamethasone) reduce secondary inflammatory response of lesions and suppress cellular division/proliferation.
- NURSING ACTIONS
  - Observe skin for thinning, striae, or hypopigmentation with high-potency corticosteroids.
  - Instruct client on proper application.
- CLIENT EDUCATION
  - Apply high-potency corticosteroids as prescribed to prevent adverse effects and take periodic medication vacations.
  - The provider might recommend warm, moist, occlusive dressings of plastic wrap (gloves, plastic garments, booties) after applying the topical medication. These can be left in place up to 8 hr each day.
  - Avoid application of high-potency medication on face or into skin folds. Medication can be applied to the scalp.
  - Monitor for adverse effects of the medication (hypopigmentation, atrophy).

Tar preparations: Coal tar and tars made from trees (juniper, birch, and pine) suppress cellular division/proliferation and reduce inflammation.
- NURSING ACTIONS
  - Monitor skin for irritation.
  - Instruct the client on proper application.
- CLIENT EDUCATION
  - Tar applications can cause stinging and burning.
  - Tar applications can cause staining of the skin and hair.
  - Due to odor and staining, apply this product at night and cover areas of the body with old pajamas, gloves, and socks.

Vitamin D analogs (calcipotriene, calcitriol) prevent cellular proliferation and regulate skin cell division.
- NURSING ACTIONS
  - Monitor for itching, irritation, and erythema.
  - Monitor for hypercalcemia (elevated blood calcium, muscle weakness, fatigue, anorexia).
- CLIENT EDUCATION
  - Limit sun exposure due to increased risk of developing skin cancer.
  - Adhere to proper application. Do not put on face.
  - Monitor for cancerous lesions.

Vitamin A (tazarotene) slows cellular division and reduces inflammation and causes sloughing of skin cells.
- NURSING ACTIONS
  - Medication is contraindicated during pregnancy. Qpcc
  - Monitor for localized reactions, burning sensation, inflammation, and desquamation of the skin.
  - Instruct clients on proper application.
- CLIENT EDUCATION: Avoid exposure to sun or artificial UV light.

Systemic medications

Cytotoxic medications (methotrexate, acitretin) reduce turnover of epidermal cells; used for severe, intractable cases.
- NURSING ACTIONS
  - Monitor liver and renal function tests for toxicity if methotrexate or acitretin therapy is being used.
  - Methotrexate can cause bone marrow suppression (leukopenia, thrombocytopenia, anemia).
  - Medication is contraindicated during pregnancy and can cause fetal death or congenital anomalies.
- CLIENT EDUCATION
  - Avoid alcohol while taking these medications.
  - These medications can decrease the effectiveness of contraceptives.

Biologic agents for moderate to severe plaque psoriasis that suppress immune function (adalimumab, etanercept, ustekinumab, alefacept, and infliximab) and suppress the stimulation of the keratinocytes
- NURSING ACTIONS
  - Evaluate for latent tuberculosis and hepatitis B virus.
  - Inspect prefilled syringe for particles or discoloration.
  - Rotate injection sites, and do not rub after administration.
  - Protect medication from light.
  - Implement infection control measures. Client is at risk for immunosuppression.
- CLIENT EDUCATION
  - Do not to take if pregnant or breastfeeding.
  - Properly administer subcutaneous medication.
  - Report manifestations of infection.
  - Treatment is lifelong, and there is an increased risk of cancer.
  - Do not receive any live vaccines while taking the medication.

Cyclosporine and azathioprine: Immunosuppressant medications are administered when lesions do not respond to other therapies.

- Nephrotoxicity occurs and increases the risk of infections.
- These are used for short-term therapy (less than 6 months).
- CLIENT EDUCATION: Monitor blood pressure throughout therapy. Medication can cause hypertension.

THERAPEUTIC PROCEDURES

Photochemotherapy and ultraviolet light (PUVA therapy)

- A psoralen photosensitizing medication (methoxsalen) is administered, followed by long-wave ultraviolet A (UVA) to decrease proliferation of epidermal cells.
- Methoxsalen is given orally 2 hr before UV treatments.
- Treatments are given two to three times per week, avoiding consecutive days.

- NURSING ACTIONS
  - Monitor the client's response.
  - Ensure that the client wears eye protection during treatment and for 24 hr following a treatment (indoors and outside). Qs
- CLIENT EDUCATION
  - Notify the provider of extreme redness, swelling, or discomfort.
  - Long-term effects include premature skin aging, cataracts, and skin cancer.
  - Obtain regular eye examinations.
  - Avoid direct sunlight for 8 to 12 hr following treatment.
  - Protect the skin with the use of sunscreen.

Narrow-band ultraviolet B light therapy can be implemented without medication application and requires fewer treatments.

Laser light therapy is used for mild to moderate psoriasis to target lesions directly and decrease exposure to surrounding skin.

68.2 Assessment/patient-centered care

	EXPECTED FINDINGS	MEDICATION MANAGEMENT	NURSING ACTIONS/ CLIENT EDUCATION
BACTERIAL (FURUNCLES, CARBUNCLES, CELLULITIS, MRSA)	• May report fever, malaise, chills, pain depending on causative organism • Multiple or single lesions (pustules, papules, nodular) • Lesions can be erythematous, edematous, painful, and warm to touch.	• Superficial skin infections are treated with topical antibacterial cream or ointment. • Extensive bacterial skin infections involving the lymphatic system, or if cellulitis is present, are treated with systemic antibiotic therapy (cephalosporin or penicillin). • If client is allergic to cephalosporin and penicillin, the provider can prescribe tetracycline, erythromycin, azithromycin, or tobramycin. • If the skin lesion is cultured as having methicillin-resistant *Staphylococcus aureus*, IV vancomycin or oral linezolid or clindamycin is prescribed.	• Bathe daily using an antibacterial soap. • Do not squeeze bacterial lesions but remove the crusted exudate so the antibacterial topical medication can penetrate the lesion. • Apply warm compresses to the affected area to promote comfort (furuncles/cellulitis). QEBP • Always use good hand hygiene. • Do not share personal items. • Position clients on bed rest for optimal air circulation to the area and to avoid occlusive dressings or garments.
VIRAL (HERPES: SIMPLEX/ ZOSTER)	• May report itching, pain, or stinging • Vesicular-like lesions that can progress to pustules that ulcerate and crust • Location: face, oral mucosa, genitalia, trunk of body (anterior/posterior)	• Antivirals: acyclovir, valacyclovir, or famciclovir can be prescribed to decrease the number of active viruses on the surface of the skin and reduces the discomfort associated with a herpetic infection or lesion. • Apply compress of Burow's solution (aluminum acetate in water) for 20 min three times a day to promote the formation of a crust and healing.	• Avoid triggers (UV light, stress). • Use soothing measures such as applying warm compresses or anti-itching creams/ lotions (calamine lotion). • Avoid tight, restrictive clothing that can irritate a lesion. • Allow a lesion to dry between treatments and avoid lying on the lesion to promote circulation and comfort. • Use good hand hygiene to prevent cross-contamination of the infection. • Avoid sharing personal items (combs, brushes, clothing, footwear).
FUNGAL (TINES/MYCOSIS) (CANDIDIASIS)	• Reports itching or burning • Single or multiple lesions • Oral: white plaques on oral mucosa • Body cavity: erythematous and moistened lesions	Antifungals (ointments/ creams/powders): nystatin, clotrimazole, miconazole	• Skin must be clean and dry before applying topical antifungals. • Avoid sharing personal footwear and clothing (tinea). • Turn and reposition frequently to increase airflow to skin.

NURSING INTERVENTIONS

- Instruct lifestyle modifications and coping strategies.
- Discuss treatment plan with the client.

CLIENT EDUCATION

- Use comfort measures (baths with emollients, oatmeal baths, emollient creams) to soften scales.
- Do not scratch or pick lesions.

Dermatitis

HEALTH PROMOTION AND DISEASE PREVENTION

Avoid exposure to harsh chemicals.

DATA COLLECTION

RISK FACTORS

- External skin exposure to allergens
- Internal exposure to allergens and irritants
- Stress (eczematous dermatitis)
- Genetic predisposition (eczematous dermatitis)
- Specific cause not always known

EXPECTED FINDINGS

Nonspecific eczematous dermatitis

- Development of thickened areas of skin
- Can appear dry or moist and crusted
- Pruritus
- Symmetrical involvement anywhere on the body

Contact dermatitis

- Contact dermatitis is caused by direct exposure to allergen, chemical, or mechanical irritation.
- Rash is well-demarcated and localized.
- Distribution varies depending upon the cause and the exposure to the allergen.

Atopic dermatitis

- Chronic rash
- Can be caused by allergens or chronic skin disease
- Development of thickened areas of skin along with scaling and desquamation
- Pruritus, which can be intense
- Distribution including face, neck, and upper torso along with skin folds (antecubital, popliteal)

PATIENT-CENTERED CARE

Avoidance therapy if cause identified

MEDICATIONS

Steroid therapy: topical, intralesional, systemic (hydrocortisone, betamethasone, triamcinolone, prednisone)

- Reduce secondary inflammatory response of lesions
- NURSING ACTIONS
  - Monitor for adrenal suppression.
  - Instruct client about proper application.
- CLIENT EDUCATION Qpcc
  - If using steroids for long periods, taper doses when discontinuing medication.
  - Avoid using topical steroids on lesions that are infected.
  - Warm, moist dressings can be used over topical application to increase absorption of medication.
  - Avoid the use of occlusive dressings over rash after applying topical steroid medications.

Antihistamines: topical, systemic (diphenhydramine, cetirizine, fexofenadine)

- Relief of redness, pruritus, and edema
- NURSING ACTIONS: Monitor for urinary retention with the use of systemic medications.
- CLIENT EDUCATION
  - Product can cause photosensitivity.
  - Avoid operating machinery and driving while taking systemic antihistamine.
  - Take systemic form at bedtime, as product can cause drowsiness.

Topical immunosuppressants: tacrolimus, pimecrolimus

- For use in treatment of eczematous dermatitis that has been resistant to glucocorticoid treatment
- Relieves inflammation
- NURSING ACTIONS
  - Instruct client on application of medication.
  - Monitor for erythema, burning sensation.
  - Avoid the use of occlusive dressings.
- CLIENT EDUCATION
  - Avoid use if infection is present.
  - Discontinue use when rash clears.
  - Avoid direct sunlight and the use of tanning beds.

Infections

HEALTH PROMOTION AND DISEASE PREVENTION

- Avoid organisms that can cause infection.
- Use appropriate skin hygiene (showers/bathing).
- Perform appropriate handwashing techniques.

Application Exercises

1. A nurse is reviewing information about a new prescription for corticosteroid cream with a client who has mild psoriasis. Which of the following instructions should the nurse include? (Select all that apply.)

   A. Apply an occlusive dressing after application.

   B. Apply three to four times per day.

   C. Wear gloves after application to lesions on the hands.

   D. Avoid applying in skin folds.

   E. Use medication continuously over a period of several months.

2. A nurse is reinforcing teaching with a client about photochemotherapy and ultraviolet light (PUVA) treatments who has a history of psoriasis. Which of the following instructions should the nurse include?

   A. Apply vitamin A cream before each treatment.

   B. Administer a psoralen medication before the treatment.

   C. Use this treatment every evening.

   D. Remove the scales gently following each treatment.

3. A nurse is reinforcing teaching with the guardian of a child who has contact dermatitis. Which of the following information should the nurse include?

   A. Use fabric softener dryer sheets when drying the child's clothing.

   B. Apply a warm, dry compress to the rash area.

   C. Place the child in a bath with colloidal oatmeal.

   D. Leave the child's hands uncovered during the night.

4. A nurse is reinforcing teaching with a client who has a new prescription for clotrimazole topical cream. Which of the following statements should the nurse include?

   A. "This cream reduces the discomfort for viral lesions."

   B. "This cream is for treating bacterial infections."

   C. "Apply the topical medication for up to 2 weeks after the lesions are gone."

   D. "Apply the cream to lesions while they are moist."

5. A nurse is reinforcing discharge instructions with a client who has a bacterial infection of the skin. Which of the following instructions should the nurse include?

   A. Bathe daily with moisturizing soap.

   B. Apply antibacterial topical medication to the crusted exudate.

   C. Apply warm compresses to the affected area.

   D. Cover affected area with snug-fitting clothing.

Active Learning Scenario

A nurse is reviewing information with a client who has a prescription for pimecrolimus to treat severe eczematous dermatitis. What information should the nurse include? Use the ATI Active Learning Template: Medication to complete this item.

THERAPEUTIC USES

NURSING INTERVENTIONS: Describe two.

CLIENT EDUCATION: Describe two instruction points.

Active Learning Scenario Key

Using the ATI Active Learning Template: Medication

THERAPEUTIC USES: Relieves itching associated with atopic dermatitis

NURSING INTERVENTIONS
- Instruct client on application of medication.
- Monitor for erythema, burning sensation.
- Avoid the use of occlusive dressings.

CLIENT EDUCATION
- Discontinue use when rash clears.
- Avoid direct sunlight and the use of tanning beds.

Ⓝ *NCLEX® Connection: Pharmacological Therapies, Medication Administration*

Application Exercises Key

1. A, C, D. **CORRECT:** The nurse should discuss with the client who has a prescription for a topical corticosteroid cream that an application of an occlusive dressing or gloves to hand lesions after application of the medication can enhance efficacy of medication on lesion. The client should avoid applying to skin folds because this increases the risk for fungal infections.

   Ⓝ *NCLEX® Connection: Pharmacological Therapies, Medication Administration*

2. B. **CORRECT:** When taking action, the nurse should reinforce with the client that PUVA treatments involve the administration of psoralen because this would enhance photosensitivity. PUVA treatment does not involve the use of vitamin A cream and is two to three times per week on non-consecutive days.

   Ⓝ *NCLEX® Connection: Reduction of Risk Potential, Therapeutic Procedures*

3. C. **CORRECT:** When taking action, the nurse should reinforce teaching with the guardian of a child who has contact dermatitis to place child in a bath with colloidal oatmeal. This would relieve itching.

   Ⓝ *NCLEX® Connection: Pharmacological Therapies, Expected Actions/Outcomes*

4. C. **CORRECT:** When taking action, the nurse should reinforce with the client that clotrimazole is a medication used to treat a fungal infection and is applied to the affected area for 1 to 2 weeks after the infection is resolved.

   Ⓝ *NCLEX® Connection: Pharmacological Therapies, Medication Administration*

5. C. **CORRECT:** When taking action for a client who has a suspected bacterial infection of the skin, the nurse should reinforce with the client to apply warm compresses to the affected area to promote comfort.

   Ⓝ *NCLEX® Connection: Reduction of Risk Potential, Therapeutic Procedures*

CHAPTER 69 *Burns*

Dry heat, moist heat, direct contact with hot surfaces, chemicals, electricity, and ionizing radiation can cause burns, which result in cellular destruction of the skin layers and underlying tissue. The type and severity of the burn affect the treatment plan.

In addition to destruction of body tissue, a burn injury results in the loss of temperature regulation, sweat and sebaceous gland function, and sensory function. When the dermis is destroyed, skin can no longer regrow over the affected area. Metabolism increases to maintain body heat as a result of burn injury and tissue damage. Every body system can be affected following major burns.

TYPES OF BURNS

Dry heat injuries result from open flames and explosions.

Moist heat injuries result from contact with hot liquid or steam. Scald injuries are more common in older adults and younger children.

Contact burns occur when hot metal, tar, or grease contacts the skin.

Chemical burns result from exposure to a caustic agent. Cleaning agents in the home (drain cleaner, oven cleaner, bleach) and agents in the industrial setting (caustic soda, sulfuric acid) can cause chemical burns.

Electrical burns result when an electrical current passes through the body and can cause severe damage, including loss of organ function, tissue destruction with subsequent need for amputation of a limb, and cardiac or respiratory arrest.

Thermal burns result when clothes ignite from heat or flames that electrical sparks produce.

Flash (arc) burns result from contact with an electrical current that travels through the air from one conductor to another.

Conductive electrical injury results when a person touches electrical wiring or equipment.

Radiation burns most often result from therapeutic treatment for cancer or from sunburn.

SEVERITY OF THE BURNS

Percentage of total body surface area (TBSA): Use standardized charts for age groups to identify the extent of the injury and calculate medication doses, fluid replacement volumes, and caloric needs. ⓠEBP

Depth of the burn: Classify burns according to the layers of skin and tissue involved: superficial, partial, full, and deep full thickness.

Body location of the burn: In areas where the skin is thinner, there is more damage to underlying tissue (any part of the face, hand, perineum, feet).

Age: Young clients and older adult clients have less reserve capacity to deal with a burn injury. Skin thins with aging, so more damage to underlying tissue can occur. Ⓖ

Causative agent: Thermal, chemical, electrical, or radioactive

Presence of other injuries: Fractures or other injuries increase the risk of complications.

Involvement of the respiratory system: Inhalation of deadly fumes, smoke, steam, and heated air can cause respiratory failure or airway edema. Carbon monoxide poisoning also can occur, especially if the injury took place in an enclosed area.

Overall health of the client: A client who has a chronic illness has a greater risk of complications and a worse prognosis.

HEALTH PROMOTION AND DISEASE PREVENTION

- Ensure that the number and placement of fire extinguishers, smoke alarms, and carbon monoxide detectors in the home are adequate and operable. Family members should know how to use the extinguishers.
- Keep emergency numbers near the phone. ⓠs
- Have a family exit and meeting plan for fires. Reinforce that no one should ever re-enter a burning building.
- Follow the principles of "stop, drop, and roll" to extinguish fire on clothing or skin.
- Store matches and lighters out of reach and out of sight of children and adults who lack the ability to protect themselves.
- Reduce the setting on water heaters to 48.9° C (120° F).
- Have an annual professional inspection and cleaning of the chimney and fireplace.
- Turn handles of pots and pans to the side, or use back burners.
- Don't leave hot cups on the edge of the counter.
- Cover electrical outlets.
- Keep flammable objects away from heat sources (candles, space heaters).
- Wear gloves when handling chemicals and keep chemicals out of reach of children.
- Wear protective clothing during sun exposure and use sunscreen.

- Avoid using tanning beds.
- Avoid smoking in bed and when under the influence of alcohol or sedating medications.
- Do not smoke or have open flames in a room where oxygen is in use.
- Never add flammable substances (gasoline, lighter fluid, kerosene) to an open flame.

DATA COLLECTION

RISK FACTORS

Exposure to sources of heat, flame, explosion, hot liquids, chemicals, or radiation

OLDER ADULTS ©
- Higher risk for damage to subcutaneous tissue, muscle, connective tissue, and bone because of thinner skin
- Higher risk for complications from burns because of chronic illnesses (diabetes mellitus, cardiovascular disease)

EXPECTED FINDINGS

Report of burn agent (dry heat, moist heat, chemical, electrical, ionizing radiation)
- Inhalation damage findings include singed nasal hair, eyebrows, and eyelashes; sooty sputum; hoarseness; wheezing; edema of the nasal septum; and smoky-smelling breath. Indications of the impending loss of the airway include hoarseness, brassy cough, drooling or difficulty swallowing, and audible wheezing, crowing, and stridor. Qs
- Carbon monoxide inhalation (from burns in an enclosed area) findings include headache, weakness, dizziness, confusion, erythema (pink or cherry red skin), and upper airway edema, followed by sloughing of the respiratory tract mucosa.
- Hypovolemia and shock can result from fluid shifts from the intercellular and intravascular space to the interstitial space. Additional findings include hypotension, tachycardia, and decreased cardiac output.

METHODS OF BURN DATA COLLECTION

Rule of nines: Quick method to approximate the extent of burns by dividing the body into multiples of nine. The sum equals the TBSA.

Lund and Browder method: A more exact method estimating the extent of burn by the percentage of surface area of specific anatomic parts, particularly the head and legs.

Palmar method: Quick method to approximate scattered burns using the palm of the client's hand. The palm of the hand (including the fingers) is equal to 1% TBSA.

LABORATORY TESTS

Resuscitation phase: Initial fluid shift (occurs in the first 12 hr and continues for 24 to 36 hr) after the burn injury with peak approximately 6 to 8 hours after the burn injury
- **Hct and Hgb:** elevated (hemoconcentration) due to the loss of fluid volume and the fluid shift into the interstitial space (third spacing)
- **Glucose:** elevated due to stress
- **BUN:** elevated due to fluid loss
- Electrolytes
  - **Sodium:** decreased due to third spacing (hyponatremia)
  - **Potassium:** increased due to cell destruction (hyperkalemia)
  - **Chloride:** increased due to fluid volume loss and chlorine reabsorption in urine
- **Carboxyhemoglobin:** more than 10% strongly indicates smoke inhalation
- **Plasma lactate:** elevated if the client has cyanide toxicity
  - **Other:** total protein and blood albumin (decreased), ABGs (possible metabolic acidosis), liver enzymes (alterations due to hepatic edema, apoptosis, and insulin resistance), urinalysis, and clotting studies (rare decrease in platelets and prolonged clotting times in severe burns)

Fluid remobilization (starts at about 24 hr; diuretic stage begins at 48 to 72 hr after injury)
- **Hgb and Hct:** decreased (hemodilution) due to the fluid shift from the interstitial space back into vascular fluid
- **Sodium:** remains decreased due to renal and wound loss
- **Potassium:** decreased due to renal loss and movement back into cells (hypokalemia)
- **WBC count:** initial increase then decrease with left shift
- **Blood glucose:** elevated due to the stress response
- **ABGs:** slight hypoxemia and metabolic acidosis
- **Total protein and albumin:** low due to fluid loss

DIAGNOSTIC PROCEDURES

Diagnostic studies can include renal scans, computed tomography, ultrasonography, bronchoscopy, and magnetic resonance imaging to determine the extent of the burn injury.
- Indirect calorimetry can help determine calorie needs (on admission to a burn center and weekly).
- Evaluation of burn depth using indocyanine green video angiography and laser Doppler imaging. Thermography is not as reliable.

69.1 Depth of injury

	Superficial thickness	Superficial partial thickness	Deep partial thickness	Full thickness	Deep full thickness
Area involved	Damage to epidermis	Damage to the entire epidermis and some parts of the dermis	Damage to entire epidermis and deep into the dermis	Damage to the entire epidermis and dermis Can extend into the subcutaneous tissue Nerve damage	Damage to all layers of skin Extends to muscle, tendons, and bones
Appearance	Pink to red No blisters Mild edema No eschar	Pink to red Blisters Mild to moderate edema No eschar	Red to white Blisters rare Moderate edema Eschar soft and dry	Red, black, brown, yellow, or white No blisters Severe edema Eschar hard and inelastic	Black No blisters No edema Eschar hard and inelastic
Sensation/ Healing	Painful/tender Sensitive to heat Heals within 3 to 6 days No scarring	Painful Heals within 2 to 3 weeks No scarring but minor pigment changes	Painful and sensitive to touch Heals in 2 to 6 weeks Scarring likely Possible grafting	Sensation minimal or absent Heals within weeks to months Scarring Grafting	No pain Heals within weeks to months Scarring Grafting
Example	Sunburn Flash burn (sudden intense heat)	Flash flame and scalds Brief contact with hot object	Flame and scalds Grease, tar, or chemical burns Prolonged exposure to hot objects	Scalds Grease, tar, chemical, or electrical burns Prolonged exposure to hot objects	High-voltage or prolonged electrical burns Flames

69.2 Burn staging

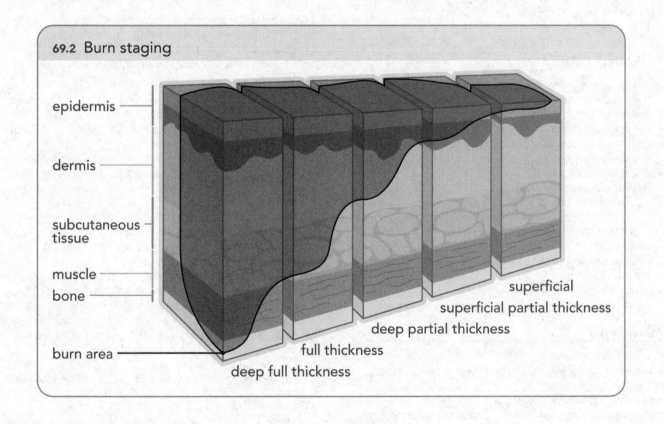

epidermis
dermis
subcutaneous tissue
muscle
bone
burn area

superficial
superficial partial thickness
deep partial thickness
full thickness
deep full thickness

PATIENT-CENTERED CARE

PHASES OF BURN CARE

Emergent (resuscitative phase)

- This phase begins with the injury and continues for 24 to 48 hr.
- Phase ends with completion of fluid resuscitation.
- Priorities include securing the airway, supporting circulation and organ perfusion by fluid replacement, managing pain, preventing infection through wound care, maintaining body temperature, and providing emotional support.

Acute

- This phase begins 48 to 72 hr after injury when the fluid shift resolves.
- Phase ends with closure of the wound.
- Priorities include data collection and maintenance of the cardiovascular, respiratory, and gastrointestinal systems (including nutrition); wound care; pain control; and psychosocial interventions.

Rehabilitative

- This phase begins when most of the burn area has healed.
- Phase ends when the client achieves the highest level of functioning possible.
- Priorities include psychosocial support; prevention of scars and contractures; and resumption of activities, including work, family, and social roles.
- This phase can last for years.

NURSING CARE

Stop the burning process. Q_{EBP}

- If providing care at the burn scene, extinguish flames or remove the source of fire.
- Remove clothing or jewelry that might conduct heat.
- Apply cool water soaks or run cool water over injury; do not use ice.
- Chemical burns
  - Wear gloves if available
  - Liquid chemicals: Flush with a large volume of water.
  - Dry chemicals: Brush dry chemicals from skin before flushing with large amounts of water.
- Cover the burn with a clean cloth to prevent contamination and hypothermia.
- Provide warmth.
- Perform an ABCDE primary survey and provide treatment.

Minor burns

- Provide analgesics.
- Cleanse with mild soap and tepid water. (Avoid excess friction.)
- Use antimicrobial ointment.
- Apply a dressing (nonadherent, hydrocolloid) if clothing is irritating the burn.

- Encourage the family to avoid using greasy lotions or butter on the burn.
- Reinforce teaching with the family to observe for evidence of infection.
- Determine the need for a tetanus immunization.

Moderate and major burns

During the initial (resuscitation) phase (from the time of injury to up to 48 hr later) following a major burn, sympathetic nervous system manifestations (tachycardia, increased respiratory rate, decreased gastrointestinal motility, increased blood glucose) are expected findings.

Respiratory system

- Monitor respiratory rate and depth. Monitor chest expansion during respiration to ensure that eschar or chest dressings on chest, neck, and back do not restrict movement.
- Upper airway edema becomes pronounced 8 to 12 hr after the beginning of fluid resuscitation. Crowing, stridor, or dyspnea requires nasal or oral intubation.
- Provide humidified supplemental oxygen.
- Support the airway and ventilation. Mechanical ventilation and paralytic medications (atracurium or vecuronium) can become necessary if the PaO_2 is less than 60 mm Hg. A tracheotomy can be required when long-term intubation is expected.
- Monitor and maintain chest tubes.
- Perform chest physiotherapy and have the client cough, breathe deeply, and use incentive spirometry.
- Suction (endotracheal or nasotracheal) every hour or as needed. Consider the need for additional analgesics.

Cardiovascular system: Monitor central and peripheral pulses, capillary refill, pulse oximetry, invasive or noninvasive blood pressure and for electrocardiographic changes or the presence of edema.

Fluid replacement

- Third spacing (capillary leak syndrome) is a continuous leak of plasma from the vascular space into the interstitial space, which results in electrolyte imbalance and hypotension.
- Ensure the initiation of IV access using a large-bore needle. If burns cover a large area of the body, the client requires insertion of a central venous catheter or intraosseous catheter.
- Fluid resuscitation meets individual clients' needs (TBSA of burn, burn depth, inhalation injury, associated injuries, age, urine output, cardiac output, blood pressure, status of electrolytes).
- Ensure the administration of half of the total 24-hr IV fluid volume within the first 8 hr from the time the burn occurred and the remaining volume over the next 16 hr. Q_{EBP}
- Assist with the infusion of isotonic crystalloid solutions (0.9% sodium chloride or lactated Ringer's).
- Ensure colloid solutions (albumin or synthetic plasma expanders) are infused by an RN after the first 24 hr of burn recovery.
- Monitor vital signs.
- Monitor for fluid overload: edema, engorged neck veins, rapid and thready pulse, lung crackles, and wheezes.

- Weigh the client daily.
- Monitor urine hourly for color, specific gravity, protein, and maintain urine output of 0.5 mL/kg/hr, which is around 30 mL/hr for the average client.
- Administration of blood products can be needed.
- Monitor for manifestations of shock.
  - Alterations in sensorium (confusion)
  - Increased capillary refill time
  - Urine output less than 30 mL/hr
  - Rapid elevations of temperature
  - Decreased bowel sounds
  - Blood pressure average or low
- If urine output is below the expected reference range, request the RN to inquire about a prescription to increase fluid replacement, and do not administer diuretics.

Comfort management

- Monitor pain and the effectiveness of pain treatment.
- Avoid routes other than IV during the resuscitation phase due to decreased absorption from other routes.
- IV opioid analgesics can be administered for pain as needed (morphine, hydromorphone, and fentanyl or anesthetics [ketamine, nitrous oxide]). Q EBP
- Monitor for respiratory depression when opioids have been administered. Qs
- The use of patient-controlled analgesia (PCA) is appropriate for some clients. PCA helps manage pain, and the client benefits from having a sense of control.
- Administer pain medication prior to dressing changes and procedures.
- Use nonpharmacologic methods for pain control (guided imagery, music therapy, and therapeutic touch) to enhance the effects of analgesic medications and manage pain more effectively.
- Provide a restful environment and nonpainful touch to help increase comfort (massage of non-burned areas) and promote rest.
- Involve the client in decision-making (mutually agreeing on how long painful procedure will take), which can reduce pain-related anxiety.
- Provide relief for pruritus, which can be highly stressful for the client. Administer oral antipruritics, keep skin lubricated, and provide diversions.
- Instruct the client to pat rather than scratching to relieve itching.

Thermoregulation

- The skin helps control the body's temperature. With skin injury, the body loses heat. Decreased temperatures can occur in the first few hours following burn injury.
- For decreased temperature, use warm, inspired air, a warm room, warming blankets, and warmers for infusing fluids. Keep wounds covered or work quickly when wounds must be exposed.
- Low-grade fever can occur later after the first few hours following injury due to increased metabolism, and the temperature can remain increased for several weeks.

Gastrointestinal system

- Clients might need NG tube insertion to reduce the risk of aspiration or for bowel decompression. Some clients experience gastroparesis and vomiting.
- Monitor stool, vomitus, and gastric secretions for blood.
- Monitor for hypomotility and for tolerance of feedings.

Urinary system

- Insert an indwelling urinary catheter.
- Monitor I&O.
- Monitor for red-tinged urine as an indication of damage to red blood cells or muscles.
- Glycosuria is expected due to breakdown of glycogen as part of the stress response.

Infection prevention

- Maintain a protective environment.
- Restrict plants and flowers due to the risk of contact with *Pseudomonas aeruginosa*.
- Check facility policy regarding consumption of fresh fruits and vegetables, which can be restricted.
- Limit visitors; do not allow sick individuals, small children, or other clients to visit.
- Monitor for manifestations of infection and report them to the provider.
- Use client-dedicated equipment (blood pressure cuffs, thermometers).
- Administer tetanus toxoid.
- Administer antibiotics to treat infection. Monitor peak and trough levels.
- Use strict asepsis with wound care.

Nutritional support

- A loss of 10% or more body weight indicates a need for additional calorie intake.
- Large burn areas create a hypermetabolic and hypercatabolic state, requiring 5,000 calories/day. Caloric needs double or triple 4 to 12 days after the burn.
- Increase caloric intake to meet increased metabolic demands and prevent hypoglycemia.
- Increase protein intake to prevent tissue breakdown and promote healing, and provide high carbohydrates (55% to 60% of intake) to decrease protein catabolism.
- Decreased gastrointestinal motility and increased caloric needs require enteral therapy or total parenteral nutrition.
- Perform a calorie count daily.

Restoration of mobility

- Maintain correct body alignment, splint extremities, and facilitate position changes to prevent contractures.
- Maintain active and passive range of motion.
- Assist with ambulation as soon as the client is stable.
- Apply pressure dressings to prevent contractures and scarring.
- Monitor areas at high risk for pressure sores (heels, sacrum, back of the head).

Psychological support of client and family

- Provide emotional support. Q PCC
- Assist with coping.
- The client might require antianxiety medications.
- Address body image with the client and discuss any concerns about altered appearance.
- Assist client through the stages of grieving.
- Provide peer support, with the client's approval.

MEDICATIONS

Silver nitrate 0.5%

Apply with a gauze dressing.

ADVANTAGES
- Reduces fluid evaporation
- Bacteriostatic
- Inexpensive

DISADVANTAGES
- Does not penetrate eschar
- Stains clothing and linen
- Depletes sodium and potassium

Silver sulfadiazine 1%

Apply a thin layer with a clean glove.

ADVANTAGES
- Usually pain-free
- Effective against gram-negative bacteria, gram-positive bacteria, and yeast

DISADVANTAGES
- Can cause transient neutropenia
- Sulfa allergy, which is a contraindication
- Penetrates eschar minimally
- Can cause a gray or blue-green discoloration
- Decreases granulocyte formation

Mafenide acetate

Apply twice daily.

ADVANTAGES
- Penetrates eschar and goes into underlying tissues
- Bacteriostatic against gram-negative and gram-positive bacteria

DISADVANTAGES
- Painful to apply and remove
- Can cause metabolic acidosis

Polymyxin B-bacitracin

Apply every 2 to 8 hr to keep the burn moist.

ADVANTAGES
- Bacteriostatic against gram-positive organisms
- Painless and easy to apply

DISADVANTAGES: Hypersensitivity can develop.

Mannitol

Used following some electrical burns when obstruction of the renal tubules with protein myoglobin hinders urine output

Other medications

- Antianxiety and antipruritic medications
- Antimicrobial ointment
- Electrolyte replacement

THERAPEUTIC PROCEDURES

Wound care

NURSING ACTIONS Q PCC
- Premedicate the client with an analgesic.
- Remove all previous dressings.
- Note any odors, drainage, and discharge. Monitor for sloughing, eschar, bleeding, and new skin-cell regeneration.
- Cleanse the wound thoroughly, removing all previous ointments.
- Assist with debridement.
  - **Mechanical:** Scissors and forceps are used to cut away the dead tissue during the hydrotherapy treatment.
  - **Hydrotherapy:** Assist the client into a warm tub of water or use warm running water, as if to shower, to cleanse the wound.
    - Use mild soap or detergent to wash burns gently, and then rinse with room-temperature water.
    - Encourage the client to exercise the joints during hydrotherapy treatment.
  - **Chemical:** Apply a topical enzyme to break down and remove dead tissue.
    - Apply topical enzyme agents (collagenase) to the wound during a daily dressing change.
- Use surgical asepsis while applying a thin layer of topical antibiotic ointment and cover it with a dressing.

Escharotomy

Incision through the eschar relieves pressure from the constricting force of fluid buildup under circumferential burns on the extremity or chest and improves circulation.

Fasciotomy

Incision through eschar and fascia relieves tissue pressure when escharotomy alone does not.

Skin coverings

Biologic skin coverings temporarily promote healing of large burns. Additionally, biologic skin coverings promote the retention of water and protein and provide coverage of nerve endings, thus reducing pain. The provider stipulates whether to leave skin coverings open or protect them with a dressing.

- Allograft (homograft): Skin donations from human cadavers for partial- and full-thickness burn wounds
- Xenograft (heterograft): Skin from animals (pigs) for partial-thickness burn wounds
- Amnion: From human placenta; requires frequent changes
- Artificial skin: Two layers of skin made from beef collagen and shark cartilage

Synthetic skin coverings are made from plastic or silicone and are usually clear. They allow for wound visualization and reduce pain.

Biosynthetic dressings contain both synthetic and biological materials.

- Used for superficial partial-thickness burns or donor site dressing
- Allows exudate to drain through the wound

Wound grafting can be the treatment of choice for burns covering large areas of the body.

- Autografts: Skin from another area of the client's body
  - Sheet graft: Sheet of skin for covering the wound
  - Mesh graft: Sheet of skin in which a mesher has created small slits, so the graft can stretch over large areas of the burn
- Artificial skin: Synthetic product for faster healing of partial- and full-thickness burns
- Cultured epithelium: Epithelial cells to use for clients who have few grafting sites; biopsies are taken from client's unburned skin and small sheets of skin are grown

NURSING ACTIONS

- Maintain immobilization of graft sites.
- Elevate extremities.
- Provide wound care to the donor site.
- Administer analgesics.
- Monitor for infection before and after applying skin coverings or grafts. Q EBP
  - Discoloration of unburned skin surrounding burn wound
  - Green subcutaneous fat
  - Degeneration of granulation tissue
  - Development of subeschar hemorrhage
  - Hyperventilation indicating systemic involvement of infection
  - Unstable body temperature
- Determine the client's level of pain, and provide additional measures to control donor site pain.

CLIENT EDUCATION

- Keep the extremity elevated.
- Report manifestations of infection.
- Continue to perform range-of-motion exercises and work with a physical therapist to prevent contractures.
- Observe the wound for infection and perform wound care.

Excision of wound tissue or surgical debridement

Removal of thin layers of necrotic tissue until bleeding occurs, which indicates viable tissue. Can be replaced throughout the restoration process

Cosmetic or reconstructive surgeries

The client might elect to have these procedures following recovery, which might be years after the injury.

INTERPROFESSIONAL CARE

- Recommend referrals to a dietitian, social worker (for community support services), psychological counselor, and physical therapist.
- Respiratory therapy can help improve pulmonary function.
- Recommend consultation with a case manager to coordinate the client's postdischarge care, and assist the client with reintegration into the community, work, or school.
- Recommend a referral for home health nursing care. Q TC
- Recommend a referral to occupational therapy for evaluation of the home environment and assistance to relearn how to perform ADLs.
- Specialists can evaluate vision and hearing if eyes and ears are affected.
- Speech therapy can be indicated.
- Prosthetics might be required.

CLIENT EDUCATION

- Infection control precautions are extremely important to prevent harm.
- In the acute phase, it is common to experience many feelings (confusion, anxiety, fear). Talk about these feelings with the provider and people you care about.
- Peer or support groups can be helpful in coping.
- Anticipate changes in appearance from wounds or surgical procedures, and understand that scarring and discoloration will occur.
- Wear compression dressings and garments as prescribed (usually 23 hr daily) to minimize scarring and prevent difficulty with mobility.
- Massage scars with moisturizers daily.
- Avoid tight clothing over burned areas. Loose-fitting clothing from dye-free fabric is best.
- Participate in sexual activity as desired.
- Use splints and assistive devices as instructed.
- Follow-up appointments are often required for 2 years following burn injury.

COMPLICATIONS

Airway injury

- Thermal injuries to the airway can result from steam or chemical inhalation, aspiration of scalding liquid, and external explosion while breathing. If the injury took place in an enclosed space, suspect carbon monoxide poisoning.
- Effects might not manifest for 24 to 48 hr. They include progressive hoarseness, brassy cough, difficulty swallowing, drooling, copious secretions, adventitious breath sounds, and expiratory sounds that include audible wheezes, crowing, and stridor.

NURSING ACTIONS: Support the airway and ventilation, and administer supplemental oxygen.

CLIENT EDUCATION: Perform airway management (deep breathing, coughing, and elevating the head of the bed).

Fluid imbalances

Hypovolemic shock is possible with inadequate fluid replacement. Excessive or rapid replacement can lead to heart failure.

NURSING ACTIONS
- Monitor for indications of inadequate perfusion, confusion, hypotension, or decreased urine output.
- Monitor for indications of excessive hydration (bounding pulse, lung crackles, persistent edema, venous distention).

Sepsis

Most common cause of death following burn injury

NURSING ACTIONS
- Monitor for discoloration, edema, odor, and drainage.
- Monitor for fluctuations in temperature and heart rate.
- Obtain specimens for wound culture.
- Administer antibiotics.
- Monitor laboratory results, observing for anemia and infection.
- Use surgical aseptic technique with dressing changes.
- Reinforce education with the client and family about the importance of infection control.

Impaired muscle and joint mobility

Scarring and contractures: Deep burns can limit movement of bones and joints. Scar tissue can form and cause shortening and tightening of skin, muscles, and tendons (contractures).

NURSING ACTIONS
- Assist with active or passive range-of-motion exercises at least three times daily.
- Encourage neutral positions with limited flexion. Encourage the use of splints.
- Encourage ambulation as soon as possible.
- Use compression dressings for up to 24 months to increase mobility and reduce scarring.

Compartment syndrome

Can develop as edema increases and the skin has lost elasticity due to damage

NURSING ACTIONS: Monitor peripheral circulation on affected extremities, and report adverse findings to the provider.

Paralytic ileus

NURSING ACTIONS
- Monitor bowel sounds and for abdominal distention.
- Provide NG decompression until motility returns.
- Report paralytic ileus to the provider because it can be an indicator of systemic infection.

Posttraumatic stress disorder

NURSING ACTION: Encourage the client to discuss feelings regarding the event. Recommend referral to a mental health professional.

Active Learning Scenario

A nurse is reviewing the care of a client who has an autograft skin covering over a burn injury with a nurse who will assume care of the client at the end of the day. What should the nurse include in the review? Use the ATI Active Learning Template: Therapeutic Procedure to complete this item.

DESCRIPTION OF PROCEDURE

NURSING INTERVENTIONS: Describe at least four.

Application Exercises

1. A nurse in a provider's office is collecting data from a client who has a severe sunburn. Which of the following classifications should the nurse use to document this burn?

   A. Superficial thickness

   B. Superficial partial thickness

   C. Deep partial thickness

   D. Full thickness

2. A nurse is caring for a client who has sustained burns over 35% of total body surface area. The client's voice has become hoarse, a brassy cough has developed, and the client is drooling. The nurse should identify these findings as indications that the client has which of the following?

   A. Pulmonary edema

   B. Bacterial pneumonia

   C. Inhalation injury

   D. Carbon monoxide poisoning

3. A nurse is collecting data from a client who sustained deep partial-thickness and full-thickness burns over 40% of the body 24 hr ago. Which of the following findings are common during this phase? (Select all that apply.)

   A. Hypoglycemia

   B. Decreased blood urea nitrogen

   C. Hyperkalemia

   D. Hyponatremia

   E. Decreased hematocrit

4. A nurse is caring for a burn client whose calculated 24-hour intravenous fluid requirements are determined to be 5,000 mL. What is the total volume (mL) that the nurse should infuse after the first 8 hours of fluid resuscitation has infused?

5. A nurse is assisting with the care of a client who sustained deep partial-thickness and full-thickness burns over 60% of their body 24 hr ago and is requesting pain medication. The nurse should ensure the medication is administered using which of the following routes to administer the medication?

   A. Subcutaneous

   B. Oral

   C. Intravenous

   D. Transdermal

6. A nurse is contributing to the plan of care for an adult client who sustained severe burn injuries. Which of the following interventions should the nurse recommend for inclusion in the plan of care? (Select all that apply.)

   A. Assign the client to a private room.

   B. Perform a 24-hour calorie count once a week.

   C. Increase dietary protein intake.

   D. Instruct the client to consume 2,000 calories/day.

   E. Restrict fresh flowers in the client's room.

7. Identify whether the following skin coverings are used as temporary or permanent grafts.

   A. Allograft

   B. Autograft

   C. Cultured epithelium

   D. Xenograft

Active Learning Scenario Key

Using the ATI Active Learning Template: Therapeutic Procedure

DESCRIPTION OF PROCEDURE: An autograft is donor skin from another area of the client's body. This is a permanent skin covering and used for burns on larger areas of the body.

NURSING INTERVENTIONS

- Maintain immobilization of the graft site.
- Elevate the extremity.
- Provide wound care to the donor site.
- Administer analgesics.
- Monitor for evidence of infection before and after skin coverings or grafts are applied.
  - Discoloration of unburned skin surrounding burn wound
  - Green color to subcutaneous fat
  - Degeneration of granulation tissue
  - Development of subeschar hemorrhage
  - Hyperventilation indicating systemic involvement of infection
  - Unstable body temperature

Ⓝ *NCLEX® Connection: Physiological Adaptation, Alterations in Body Systems*

Application Exercises Key

1. A. **CORRECT:** The nurse should recognize the cues from the client's data collection and document a sunburn as a superficial thickness burn. Superficial burns damage the epidermis.

   Ⓝ *NCLEX® Connection: Physiological Adaptation, Basic Pathophysiology*

2. C. **CORRECT:** When recognizing cues, the nurse should identify wheezing and hoarseness indicate inhalation injury with impending loss of the airway.

   Ⓝ *NCLEX® Connection: Physiological Adaptation, Basic Pathophysiology*

3. A. The nurse should expect glucose to be elevated due to the stress response, and the client would demonstrate hyperglycemia.
   B. The client's blood urea nitrogen (BUN) is elevated due to fluid loss from shift of fluid from the intravascular to interstitial spaces.
   C. **CORRECT:** The nurse should recognize the cues from the client's data collection and expect hyperkalemia, which occurs during the initial phase following a burn as a result of leakage of fluid from the intracellular space.
   D. **CORRECT:** Hyponatremia occurs during the initial phase of a burn as a result in sodium retention in the interstitial space.
   E. **CORRECT:** The hematocrit (Hct) increases during the initial phase of a burn due to hemoconcentration.

   Ⓝ *NCLEX® Connection: Physiological Adaptation, Fluid and Electrolyte Imbalances*

4. The nurse should prepare to administer half of the total 24-hr IV fluid volume within the first 8 hr from the time the burn occurred (2,500 mL) and the remaining volume over the next 16 hr (2,500 mL).

   Ⓝ *NCLEX® Connection: Pharmacological Therapies, Medication Administration*

5. C. **CORRECT:** When taking actions, the nurse should identify the intravenous route should be used to administer pain medication for rapid absorption and fast pain relief during the resuscitation phase.

   Ⓝ *NCLEX® Connection: Pharmacological Therapies, Pharmacological Pain Management*

6. A, C, E. **CORRECT:** The nurse should contribute to the plan of care to decrease the risk of infection by assigning the client to a private room. The nurse should increase the client's protein intake, which promotes wound healing and prevents tissue breakdown. Flowers should not be in the client's room due to the bacteria they carry, which increases the risk for infection.

   Ⓝ *NCLEX® Connection: Physiological Adaptation, Basic Pathophysiology*

7. **TEMPORARY:** A, D; **PERMANENT:** B, C

   Allografts and xenografts are temporary grafts that are used to promote healing. Allografts are from cadavers, and xenografts come from animals (pigs). Autografts and cultured epithelium are used for permanent grafts as the skin or cells come from the burned client.

   Ⓝ *NCLEX® Connection: Physiological Adaptation, Basic Pathophysiology*

When reviewing the following chapters, keep in mind the relevant topics and tasks of the NCLEX outline.

Reduction of Risk Potential

LABORATORY VALUES

Notify primary health care provider about client laboratory test results.

Monitor diagnostic or laboratory test results.

THERAPEUTIC PROCEDURES: Reinforce client teaching on treatments and procedures.

CHAPTER 70 # *Endocrine Diagnostic Procedures*

Disorders of the endocrine system relate to either the excess or deficiency of a hormone or to a defect in a receptor site for a hormone. Laboratory tests for evaluating endocrine function vary according to the organ or system under analysis.

Many of these tests are blood, urine, or saliva tests that determine an excess or lack of a particular hormone in the body. Some of these tests stimulate a reaction in the body that will facilitate diagnosis of a particular disorder.

Stimulation testing involves giving hormones to stimulate the target gland to determine if the gland is capable of normal hormone production. Suppression testing involves giving medications or substances to evaluate the body's ability to suppress excessive hormone production.

Posterior pituitary gland

The posterior pituitary gland secretes the hormone vasopressin (antidiuretic hormone [ADH]). ADH increases permeability of the renal distal tubules, causing the kidneys to reabsorb water.
- A deficiency of ADH causes diabetes insipidus, which is the excretion of a large quantity of dilute urine.
- Excessive secretion of ADH causes the syndrome of inappropriate antidiuretic hormone (SIADH). With SIADH, the kidneys retain water, urine becomes concentrated, urinary output decreases, and extracellular fluid volume increases.
- Diagnostic tests for the posterior pituitary gland include the water deprivation test, ADH, blood and urine electrolytes and osmolality, and urine specific gravity.

INDICATIONS

Water deprivation test

The water deprivation test deprives the client of fluids and measures the kidneys' ability to concentrate urine in light of an increased plasma osmolality and a low blood ADH level. It requires a controlled setting with careful observation of the client for complications of dehydration.

This test helps identify causes of polyuria, including diabetes insipidus (DI).
- Nephrogenic DI
- Central (neurogenic) DI
- Psychogenic polydipsia: compulsive fluid intake, associated with conditions (schizophrenia)

Tests that diagnose SIADH

ADH, blood and urine electrolytes and osmolality, and urine-specific gravity tests identify SIADH.

CONSIDERATIONS

Water deprivation test

PREPROCEDURE
- The client is either asked to withhold fluids the night before the test or when the test begins. No intake is allowed during the test. Total fluid deprivation time can be 8 to 12 hr.
- Monitor closely to identify and intervene for severe dehydration.

INTRAPROCEDURE
- The client's weight is measured hourly.
- Measure the client's urine osmolality every hour, until three separate checks show an increase of less than 30 mOsm/kg (ensures the client is adequately dehydrated).
- At that point, measure the blood osmolality.
- If blood osmolality is greater than 288 mOsm/kg, a dose of ADH (vasopressin) is administered subcutaneously.
- Measure the urine osmolality 30 to 60 min later after the administration of vasopressin.

POSTPROCEDURE: Assist with rehydration, and monitor for orthostatic hypotension.

ADH

- The client should fast and avoid stress for 12 hr prior to the test.
- Some medications (including acetaminophen, antidepressants, diuretics, opioids, phenytoin) can interfere with the test. Review medications with the provider.
- Collect a blood sample and transport it to the laboratory within 10 min.

Blood electrolyte levels

- No preprocedure or postprocedure care is necessary.
- The laboratory analyzes samples of blood for electrolyte components.

Urine osmolality

Determines the amount of dissolved particles for the concentration of urine

- No preprocedure or postprocedure care is necessary for random urine sampling.
- Clients can be required to fast from fluids for 12 to 14 hr prior to testing and to consume a high-protein diet for 3 days prior to testing.
- Urine osmolality is a better indicator of urine concentration than specific gravity.

Urine specific gravity

- Measures the concentration of particles in urine
- Performed by laboratory

Urine sodium

- No preprocedure or postprocedure care is necessary.
- Can be random urine sample or 24-hr test

INTERPRETATION OF FINDINGS

Water deprivation test

- Clients who have nephrogenic DI have little to no increase in urine osmolality during the test or following ADH administration, due to the kidneys' inability to concentrate urine.
- Clients who have neurogenic DI have a rise in osmolality of more than 9% following administration of vasopressin.
- Clients who have psychogenic polydipsia have minimal increase or no increase in urine osmolality during the test or following DH administration and take longer to become dehydrated during the test than clients who have neurogenic DI.

ADH

- Increased ADH indicates SIADH, nephrogenic DI.
- Decreased ADH can indicate neurogenic DI.

EXPECTED REFERENCE RANGE: 1 to 5 pg/mL (1 to 5 ng/L)

Electrolytes

Low sodium and chloride are expected with SIADH.

EXPECTED REFERENCE RANGE
- **Sodium:** 136 to 145 mEq/L
- **Potassium:** 3.5 to 5.0 mEq/L
- **Chloride:** 98 to 106 mEq/L
- **Magnesium:** 1.3 to 2.1 mEq/L

Urine

- Increased urine osmolality indicates SIADH.
- Decreased urine osmolality is an expected finding of diabetes insipidus.

EXPECTED REFERENCE RANGE
- **Urine osmolality:** 50 to 1,200 mOsm/kg H_2O for a random sample, depending on fluid intake; greater than 850 mOsm/kg H_2O if fluid restriction prior to testing

Urine specific gravity

- An increase in urine specific gravity is an expected finding of SIADH.
- Decreased urine specific gravity is an expected finding of diabetes insipidus.

EXPECTED REFERENCE RANGE: 1.010 to 1.025

Urine sodium

Increase in SIADH

EXPECTED REFERENCE RANGE: **Urine sodium:** 40 to 220 mEq/24 hr in a 24-hr collection; greater than 20 mEq/L in random sampling

COMPLICATIONS

Water deprivation test

Dehydration can occur due to a decrease in vascular volume.

NURSING ACTIONS: Monitor closely for early indications of dehydration, including postural hypotension, tachycardia, and dizziness. Discontinue the test if the client's weight decreases by 2 kg (4.4 lb) or a specific amount of body weight.

Adrenal cortex

- A hyperfunctioning adrenal cortex and an excess production of cortisol characterize Cushing's disease and Cushing's syndrome (hypercortisolism).
- Hypofunctioning of the adrenal cortex and a consequent lack of adequate amounts of blood cortisol characterize Addison's disease.
- Diagnostic tests for the adrenal cortex include the dexamethasone suppression test, plasma and salivary cortisol, 24-hr urine for cortisol, adrenocorticotropic hormone (ACTH), and ACTH stimulation tests.
- A CT scan and an MRI identify atrophy of the adrenal glands, causing hypofunction.
- Certain medications, stress, exercise, and pregnancy can affect testing related to the adrenal cortex. Check individual testing requirements and notify the provider of any concerns.

INDICATIONS

Dexamethasone suppression test

This test determines whether dexamethasone, a synthetic steroid similar to cortisol, has an effect on cortisol levels.

ACTH

Determines how well the adrenal glands respond to the presence of ACTH. Used in determination of both Cushing's and Addison's diseases

CONSIDERATIONS

Dexamethasone suppression test

- Obtain baseline weight prior to testing.
- For rapid testing, the client takes a dose of dexamethasone before sleeping, and a blood sample for cortisol is obtained after waking and before getting out of bed. For clients who sleep during the night, dexamethasone is administered at 11 p.m. and the blood cortisol drawn at 8 a.m.
  - If there is no decrease in blood cortisol level, the test is repeated again with a higher dose.
- Prolonged testing involves baseline 24-hr urine cortisol and blood cortisol prior to 2 continuous days of urine collection while dexamethasone is administered every 6 hr.
- Following testing, monitor the client's blood glucose and potassium levels for adverse effects.

Blood cortisol

Cortisol varies according to the time (higher levels are present in the early morning, and the lowest levels occur around midnight, or 3 to 5 hr after the onset of sleep). The provider determines the best time for testing, usually with blood sampling at 8 a.m. and again at 4 p.m.

Salivary cortisol

- Salivary cortisol testing is preferred over blood or urine for mild Cushing's syndrome.
- Midnight is the usual time for salivary collection; they should be lowest at this time for the client who sleeps at night.
- The client should not brush teeth before providing the specimen and should not eat or drink for 15 min prior.
- The test pad is dropped from the container directly into the client's mouth for the prescribed time to collect the saliva.

Urinary cortisol

- The laboratory measures cortisol in a 24-hr urine collection.
- Report signs of physical stress prior to testing.

ACTH

- ACTH is most accurate if drawn toward the end of the sleep cycle when the level is at its peak (between 4 to 8 a.m. with the typical sleep pattern).
- The client should be fasting prior to testing and screened for stress factors, which could affect the results.

ACTH stimulation test

Rapid testing: Obtain baseline blood cortisol level, then wait 30 min. Assist with administering cosyntropin IV or IM, and obtain specimens for blood cortisol levels drawn at 30 min and 1 hr.

Extended testing can be required for clients who do not pass the rapid screening test and can last 1 to 3 days.

INTERPRETATION OF FINDINGS

Dexamethasone suppression test

EXPECTED FINDINGS: In clients who have functioning adrenals, pituitary, and hypothalamus, the administration of dexamethasone should suppress ACTH, evidenced by decreased blood cortisol level on the latter blood sample.

- Cushing's disease: Blood cortisol levels will decrease only after the higher dose of dexamethasone is administered (at least a 50% decrease, along with increased ACTH).
- Adrenal adenoma/carcinoma: No change with low or high dosing; ACTH is below the expected range or undetectable
- ACTH-producing tumor: No change with low or high dosing; ACTH is within or above the expected range

Blood cortisol

- Cushing's disease: increased
- Addison's disease: decreased

EXPECTED REFERENCE RANGE: The 4 p.m. value should be 1/3 to 2/3 of the 8 a.m. value. For the client who works days and sleeps at night, the values might be opposite.
- 8 a.m.: 5 to 23 mcg/dL
- 4 p.m.: 3 to 13 mcg/dL

Salivary cortisol

- Cushing's disease: increased
- Addison's disease: decreased; diagnosis cannot be confirmed by salivary testing

EXPECTED REFERENCE RANGE
- 11 p.m. to midnight: < 100 ng/dL (< 2 ng/mL)
- If results are elevated, confirmatory testing is required.

Urinary cortisol

- Cushing's disease: increased
- Addison's disease: decreased

EXPECTED REFERENCE RANGE: Less than 100 mcg/day in a 24-hr urine collection

ACTH

- Cushing's disease: increased or decreased
- Addison's disease: increased

EXPECTED REFERENCE RANGE:
- Female: 6 to 58 pg/mL
- Male: 7 to 69 pg/mL

ACTH stimulation test

An increase in cortisol after administration of ACTH is expected.

EXPECTED REFERENCE RANGE: Rapid testing: an increase of > 7 mg/dL; 24-hr or 3-day testing: an increase of > 40 mcg/dL
- If the response is at or below the expected level, it indicates Cushing's disease due to a tumor or chronic steroids, or it indicates primary adrenal insufficiency.
- If the response is exaggerated, it indicates Cushing's due to adrenal hyperplasia or secondary adrenal insufficiency.

Adrenal medulla

Disorders of the adrenal medulla (tumor) can cause hypersecretion of catecholamines (epinephrine and norepinephrine), resulting in stimulation of a sympathetic response (tachycardia, hypertension, diaphoresis). These tests determine whether the cause of a client's unrelieved hypertension is a pheochromocytoma.

- Diagnostic tests for the adrenal medulla include plasma-free metanephrine testing and the clonidine suppression test (Pheochromocytoma suppression test).
- Pheochromocytoma provocative testing is done less often due to the risk of dangerously high blood pressure and involves administration of a substance that will trigger catecholamine release (glucagon, metoclopramide, naloxone).
- Some medications, stress, and exercise can affect test results.

INDICATIONS

Plasma-free metanephrine test

- Identification of a pheochromocytoma often indicated as follow-up testing if catecholamine level test results are unclear
- The laboratory tests blood samples for both metanephrine and normetanephrine.

Clonidine suppression test

- This test is an identification of a pheochromocytoma.
- The laboratory measures plasma catecholamines levels prior to and 3 hr after administration of clonidine.
- Hypovolemia is a contraindication due to the risk for severe hypotension.

CONSIDERATIONS

Plasma-free metanephrine test

- The client can be required to lie down for 15 to 30 min prior to testing.
- Caffeine and alcohol can affect results and might be restricted prior to testing.

Clonidine suppression test

- The client must rest for 30 min prior to specimen collection.
- Continue monitoring blood pressure for at least 1 hr following the procedure.

INTERPRETATION OF FINDINGS

Plasma-free metanephrine test

- Elevation of both metanephrine and normetanephrine above the expected reference range indicates a pheochromocytoma.
- If only one of these catecholamines is elevated, a pheochromocytoma is probable.
- If results are unclear, urine catecholamine testing can facilitate diagnosis, although different catecholamines are measured.

Clonidine suppression test

- If a client does not have a pheochromocytoma, clonidine suppresses catecholamine release and decreases the level of catecholamines (decreases blood pressure).
- If the client has a pheochromocytoma, the clonidine has no effect on blood pressure.

Carbohydrate metabolism

Insulin deficiency and insulin resistance can alter carbohydrate metabolism, resulting in hyperglycemia.

- Diagnostic tests to evaluate carbohydrate metabolism include blood glucose testing (fasting or casual), glucose tolerance testing, and glycosylated hemoglobin (HbA1c).
- Many medications, stress, and caffeine can affect glucose levels and alter test results.
- Elevated glucose results on a single test should be confirmed by a second test on a different day.

CONSIDERATIONS

Fasting blood glucose

- Ensure that the client has fasted (no food or beverages other than water) for the 8 hr prior to blood sampling.
- The client should postpone taking antidiabetes medications until after the blood sampling.

Casual (random) blood glucose

- Refers to any time of day without regard to mealtime
- No preprocedure or postprocedure care necessary; requires obtaining a random blood sample

Glucose tolerance test

- This test determines the ability to metabolize a standard amount of glucose.
- Instruct the client to consume a balanced diet for 3 days prior to the test and fast for 10 to 12 hr prior to the test.
- The technician will obtain a specimen for a fasting blood glucose level and urine specimen at start of the test.

- The client then consumes a prescribed amount of glucose (weight-based). Glucose can be administered IV rather than orally, if needed.
- The technician obtains blood samples at 30 min, 1 hr, 2 hr, 3 hr, and sometimes 4 hr after the client consumes glucose. Urinalysis can be performed every hour.
- Observe for dizziness, weakness, sweating, or giddiness, and obtain a blood glucose level if seen.

Glycosylated hemoglobin (HbA1c)

No preprocedure or postprocedure care is necessary. The test requires obtaining a random blood sample.
- HbA1c is the best indicator of an average blood glucose level for the past 120 days.
- Assists in evaluating treatment effectiveness and adherence to the diet plan, medication regimen, and exercise schedule

INTERPRETATION OF FINDINGS

Fasting blood glucose

- Fasting blood glucose greater than 126 mg/dL on two different occasions can indicate diabetes mellitus.
- Fasting blood glucose levels 100 to 125 mg/dL can indicate prediabetes.

EXPECTED REFERENCE RANGE
- 70 to 110 mg/dL for adults and children older than 2 years
- 82 to 115 mg/dL for adults 60 to 90 years
- 75 to 121 mg/dL for adults over 90 years

Casual (random) blood glucose

EXPECTED REFERENCE RANGE: Less than 200 mg/dL

Glucose tolerance test

Elevated blood glucose at 2 hr following glucose ingestion can indicate diabetes. The test can be repeated on another day to check results.

EXPECTED REFERENCE RANGE
- Less than 180 mg/dL 1 hr following glucose ingestion
- Less than 140 mg/dL 2 hr following glucose ingestion
- 70 to 115 mg/dL 3 or 4 hr following glucose ingestion

Glycosylated hemoglobin (HbA1c)

- Increased levels support new diagnosis of diabetes mellitus when paired with other increased glucose testing results or poor glucose control for clients who have existing diabetes mellitus.
- Decreased levels can be present if the client has anemia or blood loss or chronic kidney disease.

EXPECTED REFERENCE RANGE
- HbA1c 5.9% or less indicates no diabetes mellitus.
- HbA1c less than 7% indicates good diabetes control.
- HbA1c 8% to 9% indicates fair diabetes control.
- HbA1c 9% or greater indicates poor diabetes control.

Thyroid and anterior pituitary gland

Hyperthyroidism and hypothyroidism are disorders in which there are inappropriate amounts of the thyroid hormones triiodothyronine (T_3) and thyroxine (T_4) circulating. These inappropriate amounts of T_3 and T_4 cause an increase or decrease in metabolic rate that affects all body systems.
- Diagnostic tests to evaluate the function of the thyroid and anterior pituitary glands include T_3 (triiodothyronine), T_4 (thyroxine), TSH, thyrotropin-releasing hormone (TRH) stimulation test, and radioactive iodine uptake. In many facilities, immunoassay testing for the presence of antithyroid antibodies has replaced the need for TRH stimulation testing.
- The anterior pituitary gland secretes thyroid stimulating hormone (TSH), which prompts the thyroid to release T_3 and T_4. Hyposecretion of TSH can lead to secondary hypothyroidism, and hypersecretion of TSH can cause secondary hyperthyroidism.
- Ultrasounds and CT scans determine the size, shape, and presence of nodules and masses on these glands.

INDICATIONS

TSH, T_3, and T_4

Results help monitor thyroid replacement therapy and differentiate types of thyroid disorders.

Thyroid scan

- This test evaluates size, shape, position and ability of the thyroid gland to function following an oral dose of 123I.
- Whole body scanning using the same method can detect metastasis of thyroid cancer.

CONSIDERATIONS

TSH, T_3, and T_4

- Obtain an accurate medication list, because numerous medications can affect the accuracy of the test.
- No preprocedure or postprocedure care is necessary for these tests.
- The laboratory requires a random blood sample.

Thyroid scan

- The client receives an oral dose of radioactive isotope, and an external probe or counter measures the amount the thyroid absorbed. Areas where the isotope was absorbed are noted as hot or warm and areas of decreased absorption as cold.
- Pregnancy and recent exposure to iodine-containing dye are contraindications. Thyroid or iodine-containing medications must be withheld for 6 weeks prior to testing.
- Explain to the client that the radioactive substance has a very short half-life; thus, radiation precautions are not necessary for this test unless high doses are required.

INTERPRETATION OF FINDINGS

T_3 and T_4

- Low and high levels of each indicate hypothyroidism and hyperthyroidism, respectively.
- A high level of T_3 is a better indicator of hyperthyroidism than T_4.

EXPECTED REFERENCE RANGE

- **T_3:** 70 to 205 ng/dL in adults ages 20 to 50
  - 40 to 180 ng/dL in clients older than 50
- **T_4 (total):** 4 to 12 mcg/dL up to 60 years old
  - 5 to 11 mcg/dL over 60 years old

TSH

- An increased value indicates primary hypothyroidism due to thyroid dysfunction or thyroiditis.
- A decreased value indicates hyperthyroidism (Graves' disease) or secondary hypothyroidism (due to pituitary or hypothalamus dysfunction).

EXPECTED REFERENCE RANGE: 0.3 to 5 microunits/mL

Thyroid scan

- Non-functioning areas of the thyroid can indicate the presence of lymphoma, thyroiditis, a cyst, or other carcinoma.
- Functioning thyroid nodules can also represent toxic goiter or a benign adenoma.

Active Learning Scenario

A nurse is contributing to the plan of care for a client who will undergo a clonidine suppression test. What should the nurse include in the plan of care? Use the ATI Active Learning Template: Diagnostic Procedure to complete this item to include the following.

INDICATIONS

INTERPRETATION OF FINDINGS

NURSING INTERVENTIONS: Describe one intraprocedure.

Application Exercises

1. A nurse is comparing the pathophysiology of diabetes insipidus (DI) with the pathophysiology of syndrome of inappropriate antidiuretic hormone (SIADH). Sort the manifestations below into manifestations of DI and manifestations of SIADH.

   A. Excessive urinary output

   B. Fluid retention

   C. Hypernatremia

   D. Hyponatremia

   E. Weight gain

   F. Tachycardia

2. A nurse is reviewing the laboratory findings for a client who has SIADH. Which of the following findings should the nurse anticipate? (Select all that apply.)

   A. Low sodium

   B. High potassium

   C. Increased urine osmolality

   D. High urine sodium

   E. Increased urine specific gravity

3. A nurse is collecting data on a client during a water deprivation test. For which of the following complications should the nurse monitor the client?

   A. Orthostatic hypotension

   B. Bradycardia

   C. Neck vein distention

   D. Crackles in the lungs

4. A nurse is caring for a client who has primary adrenal insufficiency and is preparing to undergo an ACTH stimulation test. Which of the following findings should the nurse expect after an IV injection of cosyntropin?

   A. No change in plasma cortisol

   B. Elevated fasting blood glucose

   C. Decreased sodium

   D. Increased potassium

5. A nurse is caring for a client who asks why the provider bases the medication regime on HbA1c results instead of the log of morning fasting blood glucose levels. Which of the following responses should the nurse make?

   A. "HbA1c measures how well insulin is regulating your blood glucose between meals."

   B. "HbA1c indicates how well you have regulated your blood glucose over the past 120 days."

   C. "HbA1c is the first test your provider prescribed to determine if you have diabetes."

   D. "HbA1c determines how well your insulin regulates your blood glucose."

Application Exercises Key

1. **DIABETES INSIPIDUS (DI):** A, C, F;
   SYNDROME OF INAPPROPRIATE ANTIDIURETIC HORMONE (SIADH): B, D, E

   In the presence of DI, there is a decreased amount of antidiuretic hormone, which results in excessive amounts of urine. Most of the manifestations of DI are related to dehydration; therefore, hypernatremia and tachycardia occur. In the presence of SIADH, which is the opposite of DI, there is fluid retention, which leads to hyponatremia and weight gain.

   (N) *NCLEX® Connection: Reduction of Risk Potential, Laboratory Values*

2. A, C, D, E. **CORRECT:** The nurse should anticipate the client's sodium to be low (dilutional hyponatremia), the urine osmolality to be increased due to a decrease in urine volume, and the urine sodium and urine specific gravity to be elevated due to increased urine concentration. Potassium is unaffected by SIADH.

   (N) *NCLEX® Connection: Physiological Adaptation, Basic Pathophysiology*

3. A. **CORRECT:** The water dehydration test can lead to severe dehydration (fluid volume deficit). Manifestations for clients who experience fluid volume deficit include orthostatic hypotension and tachycardia.
   B. The water dehydration test can lead to severe dehydration (fluid volume deficit). Manifestations for clients who experience fluid volume deficit include orthostatic hypotension and tachycardia.
   C. Manifestations for clients who have fluid volume excess include neck vein distension and crackles in the lungs.
   D. Manifestations for clients who have fluid volume excess include neck vein distension and crackles in the lungs.

   (N) *NCLEX® Connection: Physiological Adaptation, Basic Pathophysiology*

4. A. **CORRECT:** The ACTH stimulation test evaluates the adrenal gland's response to ACTH administration. Cosyntropin is a synthetic analog of ACTH. If the cortisol level does not increase, primary adrenal insufficiency is confirmed. Although low fasting blood glucose and decreased sodium levels can occur in clients with adrenal insufficiency, this finding is not related to ACTH stimulation testing. Although an increase in potassium can occur in clients who have adrenal insufficiency, this finding is not related to ACTH stimulation testing.

   (N) *NCLEX® Connection: Reduction of Risk Potential, Potential for Complications of Diagnostic Tests/Treatments/Procedures*

5. B. **CORRECT:** HbA1c measures blood glucose control of blood glucose over the last 120 days; thus, its findings are the best way to make adjustments to the medication regime. Two tests are used to diagnose diabetes mellitus; a fasting glucose test and a glucose tolerance tests Capillary glucose monitoring evaluates how well insulin regulates blood glucose between meals and makes an overall determination of how well insulin regulates blood glucose.

   (N) *NCLEX® Connection: Reduction of Risk Potential, Laboratory Values*

Active Learning Scenario Key

Using the ATI Active Learning Template: Diagnostic Procedure

INDICATIONS: Confirms a pheochromocytoma

INTERPRETATION OF FINDINGS
- If client does not have a pheochromocytoma, clonidine suppresses catecholamine release and decreases the blood level of catecholamines (decreases blood pressure).
- If client has a pheochromocytoma, clonidine has no effect on blood pressure.

NURSING ACTIONS: Monitor the client for hypotension.

(N) *NCLEX® Connection: Reduction of Risk Potential, Potential for Complications of Diagnostic Tests/Treatments/Procedures*

When reviewing the following chapters, keep in mind the relevant topics and tasks of the NCLEX outline.

Reduction of Risk Potential

THERAPEUTIC PROCEDURES: Reinforce client teaching on treatments and procedures.

Physiological Adaptation

FLUID AND ELECTROLYTE IMBALANCES

Provide care for a client with a fluid and electrolyte imbalance.

Identify signs and symptoms of client fluid and/or electrolyte imbalances.

BASIC PATHOPHYSIOLOGY

Identify signs and symptoms related to an acute or chronic illness.

Apply knowledge of pathophysiology to monitoring client for alterations in body systems.

MEDICAL EMERGENCIES

Respond and intervene to a client life-threatening situation.

Notify primary health care provider about client unexpected response/ emergency situation.

CHAPTER 71 *Pituitary Disorders*

The pituitary gland (hypophysis) is known as the "master gland" due to its regulation of many bodily functions. Located underneath the hypothalamus, at the base of the skull, the pituitary gland is regulated by the hypothalamus. It is divided into two lobes: anterior (adenohypophysis) and posterior (neurohypophysis), which secrete regulatory hormones. The anterior pituitary gland secretes six hormones while the posterior pituitary secretes two hormones.

The hormones associated with the posterior pituitary are produced in the hypothalamus and stored in the posterior pituitary, where they are released into the circulation as needed.

HORMONES

Anterior pituitary

Thyroid-stimulating hormone: Stimulation of the thyroid gland

Adrenocorticotropic hormone (ACTH): Stimulation of the adrenal glands to secrete glucocorticoids

Luteinizing hormone: Stimulates maturation of ova/ovulation and the production of testosterone

Follicle-stimulating hormone: Stimulates growth of ovarian follicles and estrogen secretion and sperm production

Prolactin: Stimulates breast milk production during lactation

Growth hormone (GH): Stimulates protein synthesis and growth of muscle and bone

Posterior pituitary

Antidiuretic hormone (ADH) (vasopressin): Increases resorption of water in the kidneys

Oxytocin (OT)
- Stimulates contraction of uterus following delivery
- Stimulates ejection of breast milk during lactation

DISORDERS

Altered function of the pituitary gland can be caused by disease of the pituitary gland or the hypothalamus, trauma, tumor, or vascular lesion. Hyperfunction or hypofunction of the anterior and posterior pituitary gland can occur independently of one another.
- Oversecretion of ACTH from the anterior pituitary gland results in Cushing's disease.
- Oversecretion of GH results in gigantism in children and acromegaly in the adult client. In the adult client, acromegaly manifests as enlargement of body parts without affecting the client's height.
- Undersecretion of GH in children results in dwarfism.
- Insufficient secretion of hormones in the anterior pituitary typically affects all the hormones, termed panhypopituitarism. It affects the target organs of the hormones produced in the anterior pituitary, including the thyroid, adrenal cortex, and gonads.
- A deficiency of ADH causes diabetes insipidus (DI). DI is characterized by the excretion of a large quantity of diluted urine.
- Excessive secretion of ADH causes the syndrome of inappropriate antidiuretic hormone (SIADH). In SIADH, the kidneys retain water, urine output decreases, and extracellular fluid volume is increased.
- Posterior pituitary disorders result in fluid and electrolyte imbalances.

Acromegaly

Acromegaly is characterized by excess growth hormone in adults, which causes an increase in size of body parts but not height. Manifestations are widespread, including overgrowth of the skin; bones of the forehead, jaw, feet and hands; and enlargement of organs, including the liver and the heart. If left untreated, acromegaly can cause hypertension, diabetes mellitus, and heart problems. Onset is gradual and can progress for years before becoming noticeable.

DATA COLLECTION

RISK FACTORS

- Age (adulthood)
- Benign tumors (pituitary adenoma)

EXPECTED FINDINGS

- Severe headaches
- Thick lips with coarse facial structures
- Joint pain, muscle weakness
- Enlarged hands and feet
- Hyperglycemia
- Lower jaw protrusion
- Bulging of forehead
- Sweating
- Hypertension

LABORATORY TESTS

Growth hormone suppression test

Growth hormone level is measured as a baseline following administration of glucose. Elevated glucose levels are expected to suppress GH; however, clients who have acromegaly will show only a slight decrease or no decrease at all in GH levels.

NURSING ACTIONS

- Obtain baseline GH and glucose levels.
- Administer prescribed glucose.
- Obtain GH and blood glucose levels at 10, 60, and 120 min after glucose administration.

CLIENT EDUCATION: Consume nothing but water for 6 to 8 hr preceding the test.

DIAGNOSTIC PROCEDURES

X-rays of the skull: Identify abnormalities of the sella turcica, the location of the pituitary gland within the skull.

CT or MRI of the head: Identify soft tissue lesions.

Cerebral angiography: Evaluate for the presence of vascular malformation or aneurysms.

PATIENT-CENTERED CARE

NURSING CARE

- Check the client's self-concept related to physical manifestations of disorder.
- Reinforce instructions with the client regarding medications or other treatment options.

MEDICATIONS

Dopamine agonists (bromocriptine mesylate, cabergoline) inhibit the release of GH.

CLIENT EDUCATION: Notify the provider immediately if chest pain, dizziness, or watery nasal discharge occurs while taking bromocriptine. This can indicate cardiac dysrhythmia, coronary artery spasms, or leakage of CSF. Qs

Somatostatin analogs (octreotide, lanreotide) inhibit GH release.

Growth hormone receptor blocker (pegvisomant) prevents GH receptor activity and blocks production of insulin-like growth factor.

THERAPEUTIC PROCEDURES

Hypophysectomy

Removal of the pituitary gland through an endoscopic transnasal or oronasal (transsphenoidal) approach. If these approaches do not provide access to the tumor, a craniotomy is indicated.

PREOPERATIVE CLIENT EDUCATION: Do not brush teeth, blow the nose, or bend at the waist postoperatively. These actions can increase intracranial pressure. Qs

POSTOPERATIVE NURSING ACTIONS

- Monitor neurologic status.
- Monitor vital signs frequently.
- Monitor drainage to mustache dressing (nasal drip pad).
- Notify provider of the presence of a clear watery drainage that could be indication of glucose in the drainage (indication of leakage of cerebrospinal fluid).
- Maintain the client in a semi- to high-Fowler's position.
- Monitor fluid balance, especially greater output than intake (DI).
- Encourage deep breathing exercises, but limit coughing as this increases intracranial pressure and can cause a leak of cerebrospinal fluid (CSF).
- Monitor for manifestations of meningitis.
- Reinforce with the client that nasal packing will remain for 2 to 3 days following procedure.
- Encourage the client to breathe through their mouth.
- Note and report any change in vision or mental status.
- Monitor client after receiving replacement hormones.

CLIENT EDUCATION

- Hormone replacement therapy will be lifelong.
- Avoid activities that increase intracranial pressure.
- Report postnasal drip or increased swallowing.
- Rinse mouth frequently to minimize effects of mouth breathing.
- Use oral rinses and flossing to clean teeth. Avoid brushing teeth due to risk of trauma to the operative site.
- Consume a diet high in fiber to minimize straining to defecate.

Radiation therapy

Shrinks pituitary tumor over a period of time

Diabetes insipidus (DI)

Diabetes insipidus results from a deficiency of ADH. Decreased ADH reduces the ability of the distal renal tubules in the kidneys to collect and concentrate urine, resulting in excessive diluted urination, excessive thirst, electrolyte imbalance, and excessive fluid intake.

TYPES OF DIABETES INSIPIDUS

Neurogenic: A lack of ADH production or release, caused by defects in the hypothalamus or pituitary gland, brain surgery, or head trauma

Nephrogenic: Renal tubules that do not react to ADH, can be inherited, the result of kidney damage, or an adverse medication effect (lithium carbonate)

DATA COLLECTION

RISK FACTORS

- Head injury, tumor or lesion, surgery or irradiation near or around the pituitary gland, or cancer
- Taking lithium carbonate or demeclocycline

EXPECTED FINDINGS

- Polyuria (abrupt onset of excessive urination, urinary output of 3 to 20 L/day of dilute urine): failure of the renal tubules to collect and reabsorb water
- Polydipsia (excessive thirst, consumption of 2 to 20 L/day)
- Older adult clients are at higher risk for dehydration due to lower water content of the body, decreased thirst response, decreased ability of the kidneys to concentrate urine, increased use of diuretics, swallowing difficulties, or inadequate food intake. ⓒ

PHYSICAL FINDINGS
- Tachycardia
- Hypotension
- Loss or absence of skin turgor
- Dry mucous membranes
- Weak, poor peripheral pulses
- Decreased cognition
- Constipation
- Nocturia
- Weight loss
- Fatigue
- Muscle weakness
- Dilute urine

LABORATORY TESTS

Urine testing: Think DILUTE. As urine volume increases, urine osmolality decreases.
- Decreased urine specific gravity (less than 1.005)
- Decreased urine osmolality (less than 200 mOsm/L)
- Decreased urine pH, sodium, potassium
- As urine volume increases, urine osmolality decreases.

Blood testing: Think CONCENTRATED. As blood volume decreases, the blood osmolality increases.
- Increased blood osmolality (greater than 300 mOsm/L)
- Increased blood sodium and potassium

DIAGNOSTIC PROCEDURES

Water deprivation test (ADH stimulation test)

- This is an easy and reliable diagnostic test. Dehydration is induced by withholding fluids.
- A subcutaneous injection of vasopressin produces urine output with an increased specific gravity and osmolality.
- If there is an increase in urine osmolality of more than 9%, this is indicative of neurogenic DI; if there is little or no increase in urine osmolality, this is indicative of nephrogenic DI.

PATIENT-CENTERED CARE

Treatment for neurogenic DI is different than nephrogenic DI.

NURSING CARE

- Monitor vital signs, urinary output, central venous pressure, strict I&O, specific gravity, and laboratory studies (potassium, sodium, BUN, creatinine, specific gravity, osmolarity).
- Weigh the client daily.
- Promote the prescribed diet (regular diet with restriction of foods that exert a diuretic effect [caffeine]).
- IV therapy: Hydration (I&O must be matched to prevent dehydration) and electrolyte replacement
- Implement fall precautions. Qs
- Add bulk foods and fruit juices to the diet if constipation develops. A laxative might be needed.
- Check skin turgor and mucous membranes.
- Provide skin and mouth care using a soft toothbrush and mild mouthwash to avoid trauma to the oral mucosa. Use alcohol-free skin care products and apply emollient lotion after baths.
- Encourage the client to drink fluids in response to thirst and to match the volume of urine output.

CLIENT EDUCATION

- Weigh daily, eat a high-fiber diet, wear a medical alert wristband, and monitor fluid I&O.
- Monitor for indications of dehydration (weight loss; dry, cracked lips; confusion; weakness).
- Restrict fluids as prescribed to prevent water intoxication and avoid consumption of alcohol.

MEDICATIONS

ADH replacement agents (or neurogenic DI)

- Desmopressin (DDAVP), which is a synthetic ADH or aqueous vasopressin that is administered intranasally, orally, or parenterally. Vasopressin can be administered intranasally or by injection.
- This results in increased water absorption from kidneys and decreased urine output.
- Chlorpropamide and thiazide diuretics facilitate vasopressin action (for clients who have neurogenic DI).
- Clients who have nephrogenic DI are prescribed prostaglandin inhibitors and thiazide diuretics and mild salt depletion.

NURSING ACTIONS
- Dose can be adjusted depending on urine output.
- Give vasopressin cautiously to clients who have coronary artery disease because the medication can cause vasoconstriction.
- Monitor for a severe headache, confusion, drowsiness, abdominal cramps, or other indications of water intoxication.

CLIENT EDUCATION

- For neurogenic DI, lifelong self-administration of vasopressin therapy is required. Qpcc
- To administer intranasal vasopressin, clear nasal passage and sit upright prior to inhalation.
- Monitor weight daily and notify the provider of a gain greater than 0.9 kg (2 lb) in 24 hr.
- Restrict fluids if directed and notify the provider of headache or confusion.

INTERPROFESSIONAL CARE

Home assistance for fluid, medication, and dietary management might be required.

COMPLICATIONS

Dehydration, hyperosmolarity, hypernatremia, circulatory collapse, unconsciousness, central nervous system damage, and seizures because of excessive urine output from untreated DI

NURSING ACTIONS: Monitor fluid balance and prevent dehydration by providing proper fluid intake.

CLIENT EDUCATION: Seek early medical attention for any indications of DI, and follow care instructions.

Syndrome of inappropriate antidiuretic hormone (SIADH)

SIADH, or Schwartz-Bartter syndrome, is an excessive release of ADH, also known as vasopressin, secreted by the posterior lobe of the pituitary gland (neurohypophysis). Excess ADH leads to renal reabsorption of water and fluid retention, which can lead to hyponatremia. Fluid shifts within compartments cause decreased blood osmolarity.

DATA COLLECTION

RISK FACTORS

Conditions that stimulate the hypothalamus to hypersecrete ADH include malignant tumors, increased intrathoracic pressure (positive pressure ventilation), head injury, meningitis, and medications (barbiturates, anesthetics, or diuretics, chemotherapy agents, TCAs, SSRIs, opioids, fluoroquinolone antibiotics).

EXPECTED FINDINGS

- Early manifestations include headache, weakness, anorexia, and weight gain (without edema because water, not sodium, is retained).
- As the blood sodium level decreases, the client experiences personality changes, hostility, sluggish deep tendon reflexes, nausea, vomiting, diarrhea, and oliguria with dark-yellow concentrated appearance and an increase in urine osmolarity.

PHYSICAL FINDINGS

- Confusion, lethargy, and Cheyne-Stokes respirations herald impending crisis. When the blood sodium level drops further, seizures, coma, and death can occur.
- Manifestations of fluid volume excess include tachycardia, bounding pulses, possible hypertension, crackles in lungs, distended neck veins, taut skin, and weight gain without edema. Intake is greater than output.
- Older adults are at increased risk for hyponatremia because certain medications can decrease kidney function. ©

LABORATORY TESTS

Urine testing: Think CONCENTRATED. As urine volume decreases, urine osmolarity increases.
- Increased urine specific gravity
- Increased urine osmolarity
- Increased urine sodium

Blood testing: Think DILUTE. As blood volume increases, blood osmolarity decreases.
- Decreased blood sodium (dilutional hyponatremia)
- Decreased blood osmolarity (less than 270 mEq/L)
- Decrease in BUN, Hgb, Hct, creatinine clearance

PATIENT-CENTERED CARE

Management includes addressing the underlying cause and implementing fluid restriction.

NURSING CARE

- Restrict oral fluids to 500 to 1,000 mL/day to prevent further hemodilution (first priority). During fluid restriction, provide comfort measures for thirst (mouth care, ice chips, lozenges, staggered water intake).
- Use 0.9% sodium chloride, instead of water, to flush enteral tubes and to mix medications or dilute feedings administered enterally. Qebp
- Monitor and maintain strict I&O. Report decreased urine output.
- Monitor vital signs for increased blood pressure, tachycardia, and hypothermia.
- Auscultate lung sounds to monitor for pulmonary edema (can develop rapidly and is a medical emergency).
- Monitor for decreased blood sodium/osmolarity and elevated urine sodium/osmolarity.
- Weigh the client daily. A weight gain of 1 kg (2.2 lb) indicates a gain of 1 L of fluid. Report this to the provider.
- Report altered mental status (headache, confusion, lethargy, seizures, coma).
- Reduce environmental stimuli and position the client as needed.
- Provide a safe environment for clients who have altered levels of consciousness. Maintain seizure precautions. Qs
- Monitor for indications of heart failure, which can occur from fluid overload. Use of a loop diuretic can be indicated.

MEDICATIONS

Tetracycline derivative (demeclocycline)

- Unlabeled use to correct fluid and electrolyte imbalances in mild SIADH by stimulating urine flow
- Contraindicated in clients who have impaired kidney function

NURSING ACTIONS: Monitor for effective treatment (increased blood sodium/osmolarity and decreased urine sodium osmolarity).

CLIENT EDUCATION

- Avoid taking demeclocycline at the same time as calcium, iron, magnesium supplements, antacids containing aluminum, or milk products.
- Monitor for indications of a yeast infection (a white, cheese-like film inside the mouth).
- Avoid prolonged exposure to sunlight. Protective clothing and sunscreen should be used.
- Notify the provider if diarrhea develops.

Vasopressin antagonists (tolvaptan, conivaptan)

Promote water excretion without causing sodium losses; used in an acute (inpatient) setting because they rapidly increase sodium levels

NURSING ACTIONS Qpcc

- Monitor blood glucose levels.
- Monitor blood sodium levels.
- Monitor intake and output.
- Monitor bowel patterns.

CLIENT EDUCATION: Perform frequent oral care.

Loop diuretic (furosemide)

Used to increase water excretion from the kidneys

NURSING ACTIONS: Use with caution because loop diuretics cause sodium excretion and can worsen hyponatremia.

CLIENT EDUCATION

- Change positions slowly in case of postural hypotension.
- Notify the provider of findings of hyponatremia (nausea, decreased appetite, vomiting).

THERAPEUTIC PROCEDURES

Hypertonic sodium chloride IV fluid

The goal is to elevate the sodium level enough to alleviate neurologic compromise.

NURSING ACTIONS

- In severe hyponatremia/water intoxication, administer 200 to 300 mL hypertonic IV fluid (3% sodium chloride).
- Monitor for fluid overload and heart failure (distended neck veins, crackles in lungs).

CLIENT EDUCATION

- Report difficulty breathing or shortness of breath, which can indicate heart failure.
- Obtain daily weights, wear a medical alert wristband, and restrict fluid intake.
- Monitor for indications of hypervolemia (weight gain, difficulty breathing) or any neurologic changes (tremors, disorientation), which can lead to seizures. Qs
- Notify the provider of indications of hyponatremia (nausea, decreased appetite, vomiting).
- Avoid consumption of alcohol.

INTERPROFESSIONAL CARE

Home care can be required for fluid, medication, and dietary management.

COMPLICATIONS

Water intoxication, cerebral/pulmonary edema, and severe hyponatremia

Without prompt treatment, SIADH can lead to these complications, which can result in coma and death.

NURSING ACTIONS

- Monitor for early manifestations of water intoxication (lung crackles, distended neck veins, changes in neurologic state [confusion, headaches, twitching, disorientation], edema, and decreased urinary output).
- Maintain seizure precautions.
- Monitor blood sodium level.

CLIENT EDUCATION: Follow fluid restrictions to prevent worsening of the condition.

Active Learning Scenario

A nurse is planning care for a client who has SIADH and a new prescription for demeclocycline. What should the nurse include in the plan of care? Use the ATI Active Learning Template: Medication to complete this item.

THERAPEUTIC USES

NURSING INTERVENTIONS: Describe one.

CLIENT EDUCATION: Describe two.

Application Exercises

1. A nurse is collecting data from a client who has acromegaly. Which of the following findings should the nurse expect? (Select all that apply.)

   A. Thick lips

   B. Lower jaw protrusion

   C. Report of joint pain

   D. Moon face

   E. Enlarged hands

2. A nurse is assisting with the plan of care for a client who has acromegaly and is postoperative following a hypophysectomy. Which of the following actions should the nurse recommend including in the client's plan of care?

   A. Keep the head of the client's bed flat.

   B. Encourage the client to cough frequently.

   C. Assist the client to brush their teeth when awake and alert.

   D. Monitor nasal dressing for watery drainage.

3. A nurse is reviewing the laboratory findings for a client who has diabetes insipidus. Which of the following urinalysis findings should the nurse expect?

   A. Presence of glucose

   B. Decreased specific gravity

   C. Presence of ketones

   D. Presence of red blood cells

4. A nurse is collecting data from a client who has syndrome of inappropriate antidiuretic hormone. Which of the following findings should the nurse expect? (Select all that apply.)

   A. Increased urine osmolarity

   B. Bradycardia

   C. Polyuria

   D. Weight gain

   E. Distended neck veins

5. A nurse is reinforcing teaching with a client who has a new prescription for demeclocycline to treat syndrome of inappropriate antidiuretic hormone (SIADH). Which of the following statements should the nurse make?

   A. "You should notify the provider if you experience diarrhea."

   B. "You should take this medication with an antacid if you develop GI distress."

   C. "You should avoid using sunscreen while taking this medication."

   D. "You should change positions carefully while taking this medication."

Application Exercises Key

1. A, B, C, E. **CORRECT:** Acromegaly is the excessive secretion of growth hormone. The nurse should expect findings of coarse facial feature, thickening of the lips, lower jaw protrusion, enlarged hands and feet, and client report of joint pain. Moon face is a finding that occurs with Cushing's, a condition that is caused by excessive secretion of cortisol.

    Ⓝ *NCLEX® Connection: Physiological Adaptation, Basic Pathophysiology*

2. A. The nurse should keep the head of the bed elevated to reduce the risk of increased intracranial pressure.
    B. The nurse should encourage the client to avoid coughing because this increases the pressure in the incisional area and can lead to cerebral spinal fluid (CSF) leakage.
    C. The client should avoid brushing their teeth because this interferes with the healing process; however, the client can use dental floss and mouthwash.
    D. **CORRECT:** The nurse should recommend monitoring the nasal dressing for watery drainage, which could indicate cerebrospinal leakage.

    Ⓝ *NCLEX® Connection: Reduction of Risk Potential, Potential for Complications from Surgical Procedures and Health Alterations*

3. B. **CORRECT:** When analyzing cues for a client who has diabetes insipidus, secretion of ADH is insufficient, which causes water to be excreted and therefore, the nurse should expect dilute urine with a low specific gravity.

    Ⓝ *NCLEX® Connection: Reduction of Risk Potential, Laboratory Values*

4. A, D, E. **CORRECT:** In the presence of SIADH, too much ADH is produced, resulting in fluid retention. Therefore, hyponatremia is an expected finding (dilutional hyponatremia). Increased fluid volume leads to tachycardia, weight gain, and distended neck veins, as well as crackles in the lungs. Water retention causes a decrease in urine output and urine osmolarity to increase.

    Ⓝ *NCLEX® Connection: Physiological Adaptation, Fluid and Electrolyte Imbalances*

5. A. **CORRECT:** The tetracyclines, including demeclocycline, can cause bacterial superinfection of the bowel, which can result in severe diarrhea; therefore, the client should inform the provider if diarrhea is experienced.
    B. Because antacids reduce the absorption of tetracyclines, the client should avoid taking an antacid for GI distress. If GI distress occurs, the client can take the medication with food. However, taking the medication with food also decreases absorption.
    C. This medication increases the sensitivity of the skin to ultraviolet light; therefore, the client should avoid prolonged exposure to sunlight, wear protective clothing, and apply sunscreen.
    D. Furosemide, a loop diuretic that can be used to treat SIADH, causes dizziness due to orthostatic hypotension. However, dizziness is not an adverse effect of this demeclocycline.

    Ⓝ *NCLEX® Connection: Pharmacological Therapies, Adverse Effects/Contraindications/Side Effects/Interactions*

Active Learning Scenario Key

Using the ATI Active Learning Template: Medication

THERAPEUTIC USES: Demeclocycline is a derivative of tetracycline and is used to treat SIADH.

NURSING INTERVENTIONS: Monitor effectiveness of treatment (increased blood sodium/osmolarity and decreased urine sodium osmolarity).

CLIENT EDUCATION
- Avoid taking demeclocycline at the same time as calcium, iron, magnesium supplements, antacids containing aluminum, or milk products.
- Monitor for indications of a yeast infection (a white, cheese-like film inside the mouth).
- Avoid prolonged exposure to sunlight. Protective clothing and sunscreen should be used.
- Notify the provider if diarrhea develops.

Ⓝ *NCLEX® Connection: Pharmacological Therapies, Expected Actions/Outcomes*

When reviewing the following chapters, keep in mind the relevant topics and tasks of the NCLEX outline.

Reduction of Risk Potential

THERAPEUTIC PROCEDURES: Reinforce client teaching on treatments and procedures.

Physiological Adaptation

FLUID AND ELECTROLYTE IMBALANCES
Provide care for a client with a fluid and electrolyte imbalance.

Identify signs and symptoms of client fluid and/or electrolyte imbalances.

BASIC PATHOPHYSIOLOGY
Identify signs and symptoms related to an acute or chronic illness.

Apply knowledge of pathophysiology to monitoring client for alterations in body systems.

MEDICAL EMERGENCIES
Respond and intervene to a client life-threatening situation.

Notify primary health care provider about client unexpected response/ emergency situation.

CHAPTER 72 *Hyperthyroidism*

The thyroid gland produces three hormones: thyroxine (T_4), triiodothyronine (T_3), and thyrocalcitonin (calcitonin). Secretion of T_3 and T_4 is regulated by the anterior pituitary gland through a negative feedback mechanism.

When blood T_3 and T_4 levels decrease, thyroid-stimulating hormone (TSH) is released by the anterior pituitary. This stimulates the thyroid gland to secrete more hormones until normal levels are reached. T_3 and T_4 affect all body systems by regulating overall body metabolism and energy production and controlling tissue use of fats, proteins, and carbohydrates. When the thyroid is functioning appropriately, the term euthyroid is used.

Calcitonin inhibits mobilization of calcium from bone and reduces blood calcium levels. Dietary intake of protein and iodine is necessary for the production of thyroid hormones.

Hyperthyroidism is a clinical syndrome caused by excessive circulating thyroid hormones. Because thyroid activity affects all body systems, excessive thyroid hormone exaggerates normal body functions and produces a hypermetabolic state.

DATA COLLECTION

RISK FACTORS

- Sex assigned at birth: female
- Age: 30-50

Causes of hyperthyroidism

- Graves' disease (toxic diffuse goiter) is the most common cause. Autoimmune antibodies result in hypersecretion of thyroid hormones.
- Thyroiditis
- Toxic adenoma
- Toxic nodular goiter, a less common form of hyperthyroidism, is caused by overproduction of thyroid hormone due to the presence of thyroid nodules.

- Exogenous hyperthyroidism is caused by excessive dosages of thyroid hormone.
- Drug-induced: Iodine-induced – can occur after administration of supplemental iodine to those with prior iodine deficiency or after pharmacologic doses of iodine (contrast media, medications) in those with underlying nodular goiter; amiodarone – has a high iodine content, which is primarily responsible for producing a hyperthyroid state, although the medication itself may induce autoimmune thyroid disease; antineoplastic agents – may cause thyroid dysfunction in 20-50% of clients

EXPECTED FINDINGS

- Nervousness, irritability, hyperactivity, emotional lability, decreased attention span, change in mental or emotional status
- Weakness, easy fatigability, exercise intolerance
- Muscle weakness
- Heat intolerance
- Weight change (usually loss) and increased appetite
- Insomnia and interrupted sleep
- Frequent stools and diarrhea
- Menstrual irregularities (amenorrhea or decreased menstrual flow) and decreased fertility
- Libido decreases as the condition progresses.
- Warm, sweaty, flushed skin with velvety-smooth texture
- Hair thins and develops a fine, soft, silky texture
- Tremor, hyperkinesia, hyperreflexia
- Exophthalmos (Graves' disease only) due to edema in the extraocular muscles and increased fatty tissue behind the eye. Often causes blurred or double vision and tiring of eyes due to pressure on the optic nerve
- Excessive tearing and bloodshot appearance of eyes
- Vision changes
  - Eyelid retraction (lag), which can cause an unblinking staring appearance
- Goiter (common in Graves' disease)
- Tachycardia, palpitations, and dysrhythmias
- Elevated systolic blood pressure and widened pulse pressure
- Dyspnea
- Pretibial myxedema: dry, waxy swelling of the front surfaces of the lower legs that resembles benign tumors (Graves' disease only)
- Findings in older adult clients can be vague or assumed to be caused by age-related changes (weight loss, fatigue, change in bowel habit) or can be a single manifestation (atrial fibrillation, angina or heart failure). ©

LABORATORY TESTS

Blood TSH level: Decreased in the presence of Graves' disease (can be elevated in secondary or tertiary hyperthyroidism)

Free T_4 index, T_4 (total), T_3: Elevated in the presence of disease

Thyroid-stimulating immunoglobulins: Elevated in Graves' disease, normal in other types of hyperthyroidism

Thyrotropin receptor antibodies: Elevation most indicative of Graves' disease

DIAGNOSTIC PROCEDURES

Ultrasound: Used to produce images of the thyroid gland and surrounding tissue

Electrocardiogram: Used to evaluate the effects of excessive thyroid hormone on the heart (tachycardia, dysrhythmias). ECG changes include atrial fibrillation and changes in the P and T waveforms.

Thyroid scan: Nuclear medicine test
- This test clarifies size and function of the gland.
- The uptake of a radioactive isotope, administered orally 6 to 24 hr prior to the test, is measured.
- An elevated uptake is indicative of hyperthyroidism.

NURSING ACTIONS
- Confirm that the client is not pregnant prior to the scan.
- Take a medication history to determine the use of iodides or medications that could affect results (oral contraceptives, vitamins).
- Inform the provider if the client received any iodine contrast recently or had other radiography testing.

CLIENT EDUCATION: Some foods and medications need to be avoided before testing, sometimes up to 6 weeks. Follow directions from the provider.

PATIENT-CENTERED CARE

NURSING CARE
- Minimize the client's energy expenditure by assisting with activities as necessary and by encouraging the client to alternate periods of activity with rest.
- Promote a calm environment.
- Monitor mental status and decision-making ability. Intervene as needed to ensure safety.
- Monitor nutritional status. Provide increased calories, protein, and other nutritional support as necessary.
- Monitor I&O and the client's weight.
- Provide eye protection (patches, eye lubricant, tape to close eyelids) for a client who has exophthalmos.
- Monitor vital signs and hemodynamic parameters.
- Reduce room temperature.
- Provide cool shower/sponge bath to promote comfort.
- Provide linen changes as necessary.
- Report a temperature increase of 1° F or more to the provider immediately, because this may indicate an impending thyroid crisis.
- Monitor ECG for dysrhythmias.
- Reinforce with the client and their significant others that any abrupt changes in their behavior are likely disease-related and should subside with antithyroid therapy.
- Avoid excessive palpation of the thyroid gland.
- Administer antithyroid medications as prescribed.

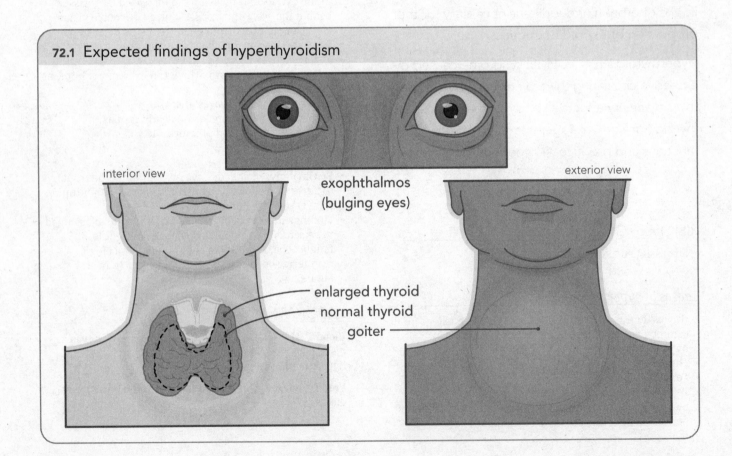

72.1 Expected findings of hyperthyroidism

interior view

exterior view

exophthalmos (bulging eyes)

enlarged thyroid
normal thyroid
goiter

MEDICATIONS

Thionamides

- Methimazole and propylthiouracil inhibit the production of thyroid hormone.
- Thionamides are used to treat Graves' disease, as an adjunct to radioactive iodine therapy, to decrease hormone levels in preparation for surgery and to treat thyrotoxicosis.

NURSING ACTIONS

- Monitor for manifestations of hypothyroidism (intolerance to cold, edema, bradycardia, increase in weight, depression).
- Monitor CBC for leukopenia or thrombocytopenia.
- Monitor for indications of hepatotoxicity.
- Monitor T_3 and T_4 levels prior to and during therapy.

CLIENT EDUCATION

- Take the medication with meals in divided doses at regular intervals to maintain an even therapeutic medication level. Do not stop taking abruptly.
- Report fever, sore throat, jaundice, or bruising to the provider.
- Follow the provider's instructions about dietary intake of iodine.
- Methimazole should be stopped (under guidance from the provider) if pregnancy occurs.

Beta-adrenergic blockers

Propranolol, atenolol, and metoprolol treat sympathetic nervous system effects (tachycardia, palpitations). These medications counteract the effects of increased thyroid hormones but do not alter the levels of the hormones.

NURSING ACTIONS

- Monitor blood pressure, heart rate, and ECG.
- Monitor for hypoglycemia in clients who have diabetes mellitus.

CLIENT EDUCATION

- Change positions slowly, because the medication can cause dizziness.
- Check pulse prior to taking each dose. Notify the provider if heart rate falls below 60/min.
- Discontinue the medication only on the advice of the provider.

Iodine/potassium solutions

Lugol's solution is a nonradioactive 5% elemental iodine in 10% potassium iodine, and saturated solution of potassium iodine (SSKI) inhibits the release of thyroid hormone. These medications are for short-term use only and can be prescribed for at least 10 days prior to therapeutic procedures for the thyroid.

CLIENT EDUCATION

- Take iodine solution 1 hr after an antithyroid medication.
- These medications should not be used during pregnancy.
- Mix the medication solution with juice or other liquid to mask the taste. Use a straw to avoid staining teeth. Take with food. ○EBP
- Caution with breastfeeding because these medications can pass into breast milk and can have undesirable effects on the infant.
- Notify the provider of fever, sore throat, metallic taste, and mouth ulcers.

THERAPEUTIC PROCEDURES

Radioactive iodine (ablation) therapy

Radioactive iodine is administered orally and taken up by the thyroid gland to destroy some of the hormone-producing cells (^{131}I).
- One dose can be sufficient, but a second or third dose might be needed.
- The degree of thyroid destruction varies and can require lifelong thyroid replacement.

NURSING ACTIONS

- Radioactive iodine therapy is contraindicated in clients who are pregnant or lactating.
- Monitor for manifestations of hypothyroidism (edema, intolerance to cold, bradycardia, increase in weight, depression).

CLIENT EDUCATION ○s

- The effects of therapy might not be evident for 6 to 8 weeks.
- Continue taking antithyroid medication as directed.
- Stay at least 1 m away from pregnant individuals, infants, or small children for the first week following treatment. Limit contact to no more than 1 hr daily.
- Depending on the dosage received during therapy, the client may need to take precautions to prevent radiation exposure to others, which can include the following.
  - Do not use the same toilet as others for 2 weeks.
  - Sit down to urinate to prevent splashing of urine.
  - Flush the toilet three times after urinating or defecating.
  - Take a laxative 2 to 3 days after treatment to help rid the body of stool contaminated with radiation.
  - Wear clothing that is washable, wash clothing separate from clothing of others, and run the washing machine for a full cycle after washing contaminated clothing.
  - Avoid contamination from saliva, do not share a toothbrush, and use disposable food service items (paper plates).

Thyroidectomy

The surgical removal of part or all of the thyroid gland

- **Subtotal thyroidectomy** can be performed for the treatment of hyperthyroidism when medication therapy fails or radiation therapy is contraindicated. It can also be used to correct diffuse goiter and thyroid cancer. After a subtotal thyroidectomy, the remaining thyroid tissue usually supplies enough thyroid hormone for normal function.
- If a **total thyroidectomy** is performed, the client will need lifelong thyroid hormone replacement therapy.
- The client might need to follow a high-protein, high-carbohydrate diet prior to surgery.

PREPROCEDURE NURSING ACTIONS

- Reinforce the purpose of the thyroidectomy to the client.
- The client usually receives propylthiouracil or methimazole 4 to 6 weeks before surgery.
- The client should receive iodine for 10 to 14 days before surgery. This reduces the gland's size and prevents excess bleeding.
- Notify the provider immediately if the client does not follow the medication regimen.

CLIENT EDUCATION

- Support the neck when performing deep breathing and coughing exercises postoperatively.
- Some medications help prepare the body for surgery.
- Expect to have a neck incision covered with a dressing and a possible drain.
- Hoarseness and sore throat can occur following intubation.
- Notify the nurse if tingling of the mouth, extremities, or muscle twitching occurs.

POSTPROCEDURE NURSING ACTIONS

- Keep the client in a semi-Fowler's position. Support head and neck with pillows. Avoid neck extension. **Qs**
- Following protocols, monitor vital signs typically every 15 min until stable, then every 30 min.
- Assist with deep breathing exercises every 30 to 60 min.
- Ensure oral and tracheal suction is provided as needed.
- Check the surgical dressing and back of the neck for excessive bleeding.
- Respiratory distress can occur from compression of trachea due to hemorrhage, which is most likely to occur in the first 24 hr. Respiratory distress also can occur due to edema. Ensure that tracheostomy supplies are immediately available. Humidify air, assist to cough and deep breathe, and ensure oral and tracheal suction is provided if needed.
- Check for laryngeal nerve damage by asking the client to speak as soon as awake from anesthesia and every 2 hr thereafter.
- Administer medication to manage pain. Reassure the client that discomfort will resolve within a few days.
- Check for indications of hypocalcemia or tetany, which can result from parathyroid damage intraoperatively (perioral or extremity tingling, muscle twitching for positive Chvostek's and Trousseau's signs).
  - Ensure that IV calcium gluconate or calcium chloride are immediately available.
  - Keep emergency equipment near the bedside. **Qs**

CLIENT EDUCATION

- Support the neck while performing coughing exercises or changing positions.
- Do not manipulate the surgical drain, and prevent pulling.
- Report incisional drainage, swelling, or redness which can indicate infection.
- Monitor for manifestations of hypothyroidism (hypothermia, lethargy, weight gain).
- Take all medications as directed. Following a total thyroidectomy, lifelong thyroid replacement medications will be required.
- Check with the provider prior to taking over-the-counter medications.
- Report fever, increased restlessness, palpitations, or chest pain.

INTERPROFESSIONAL CARE

An endocrinologist, radiologist, pharmacist, and dietitian can collaborate in providing care for the client.

COMPLICATIONS

Hemorrhage

Due to a loosened surgical tie, excessive coughing, or movement, this can occur at the incision or in the tissues, leading to respiratory distress.

NURSING ACTIONS

- Inspect the surgical incision and dressing for drainage and bleeding, especially at the back of the neck, and change the dressing as directed.
- Monitor blood pressure and pulse.
- Monitor surgical drain if present. A moderate amount of drainage is expected.
- Monitor for voice hoarseness or vocal changes which could indicate bleeding or compression of the trachea.
- Report suspected bleeding to the provider.

Thyroid storm/crisis (thyrotoxicosis)

Thyroid storm/crisis results from a sudden surge of large amounts of thyroid hormones into the bloodstream, causing an even greater increase in body metabolism. This is a medical emergency with a high mortality rate.

- Precipitating factors include uncontrolled hyperthyroidism occurring most often with Graves' disease, infection, trauma, emotional stress, diabetic ketoacidosis, and digitalis toxicity, all of which increase demands on body metabolism. It also can occur following a surgical procedure or a thyroidectomy as a result of manipulation of the gland during surgery.
- Findings are hyperthermia, hypertension, delirium, vomiting, abdominal pain, tachydysrhythmias, chest pain, dyspnea, and palpitations.

NURSING ACTIONS

- Assist with transferring client to ICU.
- Ensure a patent airway is maintained.
- Assist with monitoring vital signs frequently.
- Ensure continuous cardiac monitoring for dysrhythmias is provided.
- Administer acetaminophen to decrease temperature.

> **!** Salicylate antipyretics (aspirin) are contraindicated because they release thyroxine from protein-binding sites and increase free thyroxine levels.

- Provide cool sponge baths, or apply ice packs to decrease fever. If fever continues, obtain a prescription for a cooling blanket for hyperthermia.
- Client may receive thionamides (methimazole, propylthiouracil), sodium iodine, and beta-adrenergic blockers. Monitor the effects of these medications.
- Assist with administering IV fluids to provide adequate hydration and prevent vascular collapse. Fluid volume deficit can occur due to increased fluid excretion by the kidneys or excessive diaphoresis. Monitor intake and output hourly to prevent fluid overload or inadequate replacement.
- Administer supplemental O_2 to meet increased oxygen demands.

CLIENT EDUCATION: Notify the provider of fever, increased restlessness, palpitations, and chest pain.

Airway obstruction

Hemorrhage, tracheal collapse, tracheal mucus accumulation, laryngeal edema, and vocal cord paralysis can cause respiratory obstruction, with sudden stridor and restlessness.

NURSING ACTIONS

- Keep a tracheostomy tray and suction equipment available at all times during the immediate recovery period. Qs
- Maintain the bed in a high-Fowler's position to decrease edema and swelling of the neck.
- Alert the Rapid Response team and provider immediately if respiratory manifestations occur. Qtc
- Provide humidified air.
- Medicate as prescribed to reduce swelling.

Hypocalcemia and tetany

Damage to parathyroid gland causes hypocalcemia and tetany.

NURSING ACTIONS

- Monitor for indications of hypocalcemia (tingling of the fingers and toes, carpopedal spasms, convulsions).
- Have IV calcium gluconate available for emergency administration. Qs
- Maintain seizure precautions.

Nerve damage

- Nerve damage can lead to vocal cord paralysis and vocal disturbances.
- Incisional damage or swelling can cause nerve damage.

NURSING ACTIONS

- Monitor the client's ability to speak every 2 hr.
- Monitor the client's voice tone and quality, and compare it with the preoperative voice.
- Document findings, and report adverse findings to the provider.

CLIENT EDUCATION: Notify the nurse of any tingling sensation of the mouth, tingling of distal extremities, or muscle twitching.

1. A nurse is reviewing the manifestations of hyperthyroidism with a client. Which of the following findings should the nurse include? (Select all that apply.)

   A. Anorexia

   B. Heat intolerance

   C. Constipation

   D. Palpitations

   E. Weight loss

   F. Bradycardia

2. A nurse is reviewing the electronic health record (EHR) of a client who has Graves' disease and findings of exophthalmos. Which of the following locations should the nurse expect to find exophthalmos?

   A. Top of head

   B. Over right or left eye

   C. Over the heart

3. A nurse is reviewing the electronic health record of a client who has Graves' disease. Which of the following laboratory findings should the nurse expect?

   A. Decreased thyrotropin receptor antibodies

   B. Decreased thyroid-stimulating hormone (TSH)

   C. Decreased free thyroxine index

   D. Decreased triiodothyronine

4. A nurse is reinforcing instructions with a client who has Graves' disease and has a new prescription for propranolol. Which of the following information should the nurse include?

   A. "An adverse effect of this medication is jaundice."

   B. "Take your pulse before each dose."

   C. "The purpose of this medication is to decrease production of thyroid hormone."

   D. "You should stop taking this medication if you have a sore throat."

5. A nurse is contributing to the plan of care for a client who has a new diagnosis of Graves' disease and a new prescription for methimazole. Which of the following interventions should the nurse include in the plan of care? (Select all that apply.)

   A. Monitor CBC.

   B. Monitor triiodothyronine (T_3).

   C. Instruct the client to increase consumption of shellfish.

   D. Advise the client to take the medication at the same time every day.

   E. Inform the client that an adverse effect of this medication is iodine toxicity.

6. A nurse is preparing to assist with the care of a client who is postoperative following a thyroidectomy. Which of the following items should the nurse ensure is available? (Select all that apply.)

   A. Suction equipment

   B. Humidified oxygen

   C. Flashlight

   D. Tracheostomy tray

   E. Chest tube tray

Application Exercises Key

1. B, D, E. **CORRECT:** Hyperthyroidism increases the client's metabolism, leading to heat intolerance, palpitations, and weight loss. Diarrhea, not constipation, is an expected finding for the client who has hyperthyroidism. Hyperthyroidism increases the client's metabolism, causing tachycardia, not bradycardia.

Ⓝ *NCLEX® Connection: Physiological Adaptation, Basic Pathophysiology*

2. B. **CORRECT:** Exophthalmos is abnormal protrusion of the eyeball, which is due to edema in the extraocular muscles and increased fatty tissue behind the eye.

Ⓝ *NCLEX® Connection: Physiological Adaptation, Basic Pathophysiology*

3. B. **CORRECT:** In the presence of Graves' disease, low TSH is an expected finding. The pituitary gland decreases the production of TSH when thyroid hormone levels are elevated. In the presence of Graves' disease, elevated thyrotropin receptor antibodies, elevated free thyroxine index, and elevated triiodothyronine are expected findings.

Ⓝ *NCLEX® Connection: Reduction of Risk Potential, Laboratory Values*

4. A. Yellowing of the skin is an adverse effect of methimazole.
   B. **CORRECT:** Propranolol can cause bradycardia. The client should take their pulse before each dose. If there is a significant change, they should withhold the dose and consult the provider.
   C. The purpose of propranolol is to suppress tachycardia, diaphoresis, and other effects of Graves' disease.
   D. Sore throat is not an adverse effect of this medication. The client should not discontinue taking this medication because this action can result in tachycardia and dysrhythmias.

Ⓝ *NCLEX® Connection: Pharmacological Therapies, Expected Actions/Outcomes*

5. A. **CORRECT:** Methimazole can cause several hematologic effects, including leukopenia and thrombocytopenia, so it is important to monitor the CBC.
   B. **CORRECT:** Because methimazole reduces thyroid hormone production, the nurse should also monitor the T₃.
   C. Because methimazole reduces thyroid hormone production by blocking iodine, the nurse should instruct the client to limit iodine-containing foods (shellfish).
   D. **CORRECT:** To maintain blood levels, instruct the client to take the methimazole at the same time every day.
   E. Iodine toxicity is an adverse effect of potassium iodide solution.

Ⓝ *NCLEX® Connection: Pharmacological Therapies, Expected Actions/Outcomes*

6. A. **CORRECT:** The client can require oral or tracheal suctioning. The nurse should ensure that suctioning equipment, supplemental oxygen, and a tracheostomy tray are available at the bedside.
   B. **CORRECT:** The client can also require supplemental oxygen due to respiratory complications. Humidified oxygen thins secretions and promotes respiratory exchange. The nurse should ensure that suctioning equipment, supplemental oxygen, and a tracheostomy tray are available at the bedside.
   C. A flashlight is used to measure the reaction of the pupils to light for a client who has an intracranial disorder. Checking pupil reaction with a flashlight is not indicated for this client.
   D. **CORRECT:** The client can experience respiratory obstruction due to laryngeal edema. The nurse should ensure that suctioning equipment, supplemental oxygen, and a tracheostomy tray are available at the bedside.
   E. A chest tube tray would be used for a client who develops a hemothorax or pneumothorax. This is not an expected complication of a thyroidectomy. This equipment is not indicated for this client.

Ⓝ *NCLEX® Connection: Reduction of Risk Potential, Potential for Complications from Surgical Procedures and Health Alterations*

Active Learning Scenario

A nurse is reinforcing teaching with a client who will have radioactive iodine therapy. What should the nurse review? Use the ATI Active Learning Template: Therapeutic Procedure to complete this item.

DESCRIPTION OF PROCEDURE: Provide a brief description of the procedure.

CLIENT EDUCATION: Identify three client instructions the nurse should include.

Active Learning Scenario Key

Using the ATI Active Learning Template: Therapeutic Procedure

DESCRIPTION OF PROCEDURE: Radioactive iodine is administered orally. While it is used for thyroid scan, it is a small amount for testing. For therapy, larger amounts are given for cell destruction. The thyroid absorbs the radiation, which results in destruction of cells that produce thyroid hormone.

CLIENT EDUCATION
- The effects of the therapy might not be evident for 6 to 8 weeks.
- Take medication as directed.
- Follow precautions to prevent radiation exposure to others.
- Follow directions from the provider, which can include the following.
  ○ Do not use same toilet as others for 2 weeks.
  ○ Sit down to urinate.
  ○ Flush the toilet three times after use.
  ○ Take a laxative 2 to 3 days after treatment to rid the body of stool contaminated with radiation.
  ○ Wear clothing that is washable, wash clothing separate from clothing of others, and run the washing machine for a full cycle after washing contaminated clothing.
  ○ Avoid close contact with infants, young children, and pregnant individuals for the first week following treatment.
  ○ Do not share a toothbrush, and use disposable food service items (paper plates).

Ⓝ *NCLEX® Connection: Reduction of Risk Potential, Therapeutic Procedures*

UNIT 12 ENDOCRINE DISORDERS
SECTION: THYROID DISORDERS

CHAPTER 73 *Hypothyroidism*

Hypothyroidism is a condition in which there is an inadequate amount of circulating thyroid hormones triiodothyronine (T3) and thyroxine (T4), causing a decrease in metabolic rate that affects all body systems. Thyroid function can decline slowly or rapidly (myxedema).

Because hypothyroidism can have manifestations that mimic the aging process, hypothyroidism is often undiagnosed in older adult clients. This can lead to potentially serious adverse effects from medications (sedatives, opiates, anesthetics). ©

CLASSIFICATIONS BY ETIOLOGY

Primary hypothyroidism stems from dysfunction of the thyroid gland. This is the most common type of hypothyroidism and is caused by the following.
- Disease: autoimmune thyroiditis
- Use of medications that decrease the synthesis of thyroid hormone
- Loss of the thyroid gland: iodine deficiency, radioactive iodine or radiation treatment, surgical removal of the gland

Secondary hypothyroidism is caused by failure of the anterior pituitary gland to stimulate the thyroid gland or failure of the target tissues to respond to the thyroid hormones (pituitary tumors).

Tertiary hypothyroidism is caused by failure of the hypothalamus to produce thyroid-releasing hormone.

Secondary and tertiary hypothyroidism is sometimes called central hypothyroidism.

Congenital hypothyroidism is a severe lack of TH in utero, leading to growth failure (cretinism).

DATA COLLECTION

RISK FACTORS

- Females 30 to 60 years old are affected 7 to 10 times more often than males
- Use of certain medications (examples: lithium, amiodarone, thalidomide, rifampin, phenobarbital, phenytoin, carbamazepine)
- Inadequate intake of iodine
- Radiation therapy to the head and neck

EXPECTED FINDINGS

Hypothyroidism is often characterized by vague and varied findings that develop slowly over time. Manifestations can vary and are related to the severity of the condition.
- Fatigue, lethargy (sleeping up to 16 hr/day)
- Irritability
- Intolerance to cold
- Constipation
- Weight gain without an increase in caloric intake
- Pallor
- Thick, brittle fingernails
- Depression and apathy
- Joint or muscle pain
- Bradycardia, hypotension, dysrhythmias
- Slow thought processes and speech
- Hypoventilation, pleural effusion
- Thickening of the skin
- Hair loss
- Thinning of hair on the eyebrows
- Dry, flaky skin, brittle nails
- Swelling in face and tongue, hands, and feet (myxedema [non-pitting, mucinous edema])
- Decreased acuity of taste and smell
- Hoarse, raspy speech due to myxedema affecting the larynx
- GI symptoms resulting from decreased peristalsis, possibly leading to paralytic ileus
- Abnormal menstrual periods (menorrhagia/amenorrhea)
- Decreased libido, impotence
- Many individuals who have mild hypothyroidism are frequently undiagnosed, but the hormone disturbance can contribute to an acceleration of atherosclerosis or complications of medical treatment (intraoperative hypotension, cardiac complications following surgery)
- Delayed physical and mental growth in children

LABORATORY TESTS

EXPECTED RESULTS WITH HYPOTHYROIDISM
- **T_3, T_4:** Decreased
- **Blood thyroid–stimulating hormone (TSH)**
  - Increased with primary hypothyroidism
  - Decreased or within the expected reference range in secondary hypothyroidism
- **Blood cholesterol:** Increased
- **Antithyroid antibodies:** Present in some cases

DIAGNOSTIC PROCEDURES

Thyroid scan: Clients who have hypothyroidism have a low uptake of the radioactive preparation.

ECG: Sinus bradycardia, dysrhythmias

PATIENT-CENTERED CARE

Clients older than 80 years of age are not prescribed treatment for low thyroid hormone levels unless experiencing manifestations. ©

NURSING CARE

- Monitor for cardiovascular changes (low blood pressure, bradycardia, dysrhythmias). Monitor for chest pain for clients who have chronic hypothyroidism because it can lead to cardiovascular disease. Check for peripheral edema.
- Monitor the client's weight.
- If mental status is compromised, orient the client periodically, and provide safety measures. Qs
- Increase the client's activity level gradually, and provide frequent rest periods to avoid fatigue and decrease myocardial oxygen demands.
- Apply anti-embolism stockings, and elevate the client's legs to assist venous return.
- Monitor respiratory status including rate, depth, pattern, oximetry, and arterial blood gases. Encourage the client to cough and breathe deeply to prevent pulmonary complications.
- Consult with a dietitian. Provide a low-calorie, high-bulk diet, and encourage fluids and activity to prevent constipation and promote weight loss.
- Administer cathartics and stool softeners as needed. Avoid fiber laxatives, which interfere with absorption of levothyroxine. Qтc
- Provide meticulous skin care. Turn and reposition the client every 2 hr as prescribed bed rest. Use alcohol-free skin care products and an emollient lotion after bathing.
- Provide extra clothing and blankets for clients who have decreased cold tolerance. Dress the client in layers, adjust room temperature, and encourage intake of warm liquids if possible.
- Caution the client against using electric blankets or other heating devices because the combination of vasodilation, decreased sensation, and decreased alertness can result in unrecognized burns. Qs
- Encourage the client to verbalize feelings and fears about changes in body image. Return to the euthyroid (normal thyroid gland function) state takes time. Reassure the client that most physical manifestations are reversible.
- Use caution with medications due to alteration in metabolism. Qs
  - CNS depressants (barbiturates or sedatives) are used with caution due to the risk of respiratory depression. If prescribed, the dose should be significantly decreased.
  - Hypothyroidism alters metabolism and excretion of medications. The provider uses caution in prescribing medications to clients who have this condition.

CLIENT EDUCATION

- Report chest pain or discomfort immediately.
- Take thyroid replacement as prescribed without changing timing, dose, or brand, unless the provider is consulted.

MEDICATIONS

Thyroid hormone replacement therapy

Levothyroxine
- A synthetic thyroid hormone replacement, the most common medication prescribed.
- Levothyroxine increases the effects of warfarin and can increase the need for insulin and digoxin.
- Many other medications can affect the therapeutic effectiveness of levothyroxine.
- Use caution when starting thyroid hormone replacement with older adult clients and those who have coronary artery disease to avoid coronary ischemia because of increased oxygen demands of the heart. It is preferable to start with much lower doses and increase gradually. Ⓒ

NURSING ACTIONS
- Monitor for cardiovascular compromise (chest pain, palpitations, rapid heart rate, shortness of breath).
- Inform the client that fiber supplements, calcium, iron, and antacids interfere with absorption. Before taking any over-the-counter medications, the client must consult with the provider.

CLIENT EDUCATION
- Treatment begins slowly and the dosage will be increased every 2 to 3 weeks until the desired response is obtained. Blood TSH is monitored at scheduled times to ensure correct dosage.
- Take the dose prescribed. Do not stop taking the medication or change the dose or brand name.
- Take the medication on an empty stomach, typically 30 to 60 min before breakfast.
- Monitor for and report manifestations of hyperthyroidism (irritability, tremors, tachycardia, palpitations, heat intolerance, rapid weight loss).
- Treatment is considered to be lifelong, requiring ongoing medical assessment of thyroid function.

INTERPROFESSIONAL CARE

A home health nurse might need to visit the client and monitor for adverse effects during the first few weeks of therapy.

COMPLICATIONS

Myxedema coma

Myxedema coma is a life-threatening condition that occurs when hypothyroidism is untreated, poorly managed, or when a stressor (acute illness, surgery, chemotherapy, discontinuing thyroid replacement therapy, use of sedatives/opioids) affects a client who has hypothyroidism.

MANIFESTATIONS

- Respiratory failure
- Hypotension
- Hypothermia
- Bradycardia, dysrhythmia
- Hyponatremia
- Hypoglycemia
- Coma

NURSING ACTIONS

- Monitor mental status.
- Cover the client with warm blankets.
- Monitor body temperature and blood pressure hourly until stable.
- Assist with fluid replacement with 0.9% sodium chloride IV.
- Monitor I&O and daily weights. With treatment, urine output should increase, and body weight should decrease. Failure to do so should be reported to the provider.
- Treat hypoglycemia with glucose.
- Assist with the administration of corticosteroids.
- Adhere to aspiration precautions.
- Check for possible sources of infection (blood, sputum, urine) that might have precipitated the coma. Treat any underlying illness.

Active Learning Scenario

A nurse is reinforcing teaching about hypothyroidism with a client. What information should the nurse reinforce? Use the ATI Active Learning Template: System Disorder to complete this item.

ALTERATION IN HEALTH (DIAGNOSIS): Provide a brief description of the disorder.

RISK FACTORS: Identify two risk factors.

DIAGNOSTIC PROCEDURES: Identify two laboratory tests that are used to diagnose hypothyroidism.

Application Exercises

1. A nurse is collecting data from a client who has hypothyroidism. Which of the following findings should the nurse expect? (Select all that apply.)

    A. Diarrhea

    B. Slurred speech

    C. Dry skin

    D. Increased libido

    E. Hoarseness

2. A nurse is reviewing laboratory results of a client who is being evaluated for secondary hypothyroidism. Which of the following laboratory findings should the nurse expect?

    A. Elevated T_4

    B. Decreased T_3

    C. Elevated thyroid stimulating hormone

    D. Decreased cholesterol

3. A nurse is reinforcing teaching with a client who has a new prescription for levothyroxine who has hypothyroidism. Which of the following information should the nurse include in the teaching? (Select all that apply.)

    A. Weight gain is expected while taking this medication.

    B. Medication should not be discontinued without the advice of the provider.

    C. Follow-up blood TSH levels should be obtained.

    D. Take the medication on an empty stomach.

    E. Use fiber laxatives for constipation.

4. A nurse is collecting data from a client who recently began taking levothyroxine who has hypothyroidism. Which of the following findings should indicate to the nurse that the client may require a decrease in the dosage of the medication?

    A. Hand tremors

    B. Bradycardia

    C. Pallor

    D. Slow speech

5. A nurse is contributing to the plan of care for a client who has myxedema coma. Which of the following actions should the nurse include? (Select all that apply.)

    A. Provide warming measures.

    B. Administer IV fluid replacement therapy.

    C. Monitor blood pressure.

    D. Initiate aspiration precautions.

    E. Anticipate IV glucose to be administered.

Active Learning Scenario Key

Using the ATI Active Learning Template: System Disorder

ALTERATION IN HEALTH (DIAGNOSIS): Hypothyroidism is a condition in which there is an inadequate amount of circulating thyroid hormones triiodothyronine (T_3) and thyroxine (T_4), causing a decrease in metabolic rate that affects all body systems.

RISK FACTORS
- Female clients age 30 to 60 years
- Use of lithium or amiodarone

LABORATORY TESTS
- Blood T_3
- Blood T_4
- Free T_4 index
- Thyroid antibodies
- TSH
- Blood cholesterol

Ⓝ *NCLEX® Connection: Physiological Adaptation, Alterations in Body Systems*

Application Exercises Key

1. B, C, E. **CORRECT:** When recognizing cues, the nurse should identify slurred speech, slow thought processes, dry skin and hoarseness are manifestations of hypothyroidism.

   Ⓝ *NCLEX® Connection: Physiological Adaptation, Basic Pathophysiology*

2. B. **CORRECT:** When recognizing cues, the nurse should identify decreased levels of T3 in the blood is an expected finding for a client who has secondary hypothyroidism due to an impairment of the function of the parathyroid or hypothalamus gland.

   Ⓝ *NCLEX® Connection: Reduction of Risk Potential, Laboratory Values*

3. B, C, D. **CORRECT:** When taking actions, the nurse should instruct the client that levothyroxine should not be discontinued without the notification of the provider. Changes in level of hormone can be dangerous. The client should schedule follow-up blood TSH levels to be checked to monitor the efficacy of the medication. Levothyroxine should be taken on an empty stomach to promote absorption.

   Ⓝ *NCLEX® Connection: Pharmacological Therapies, Medication Administration*

4. A. **CORRECT:** When recognizing cues, the nurse should expect hand tremors are a manifestation of hyperthyroidism that can result from thyroid hormone replacement therapy. The nurse should notify the client's provider adjust the dose of levothyroxine.

   Ⓝ *NCLEX® Connection: Pharmacological Therapies, Expected Actions/Outcomes*

5. A. **CORRECT:** When generating solutions, the nurse should provide warming measures such as a warming blanket because hypothermia can be a manifestation myxedema coma condition.
   B. **CORRECT:** The nurse should anticipate administering IV fluid replacement therapy because hyponatremia can be a manifestation of myxedema coma.
   C. **CORRECT:** The nurse should monitor the client's blood pressure because hypotension is a manifestation of myxedema coma.
   D. **CORRECT:** The nurse should initiate aspiration precautions because myxedema coma is a severe complication of hypothyroidism that can lead to compromised airway.
   E. The nurse should anticipate IV glucose to be administered because hypoglycemia is a manifestation of myxedema coma.

   Ⓝ *NCLEX® Connection: Physiological Adaptation, Medical Emergencies*

When reviewing the following chapters, keep in mind the relevant topics and tasks of the NCLEX outline.

Reduction of Risk Potential

THERAPEUTIC PROCEDURES: Reinforce client teaching on treatments and procedures.

Physiological Adaptation

FLUID AND ELECTROLYTE IMBALANCES
Provide care for a client with a fluid and electrolyte imbalance.

Identify signs and symptoms of client fluid and/or electrolyte imbalances.

BASIC PATHOPHYSIOLOGY
Identify signs and symptoms related to an acute or chronic illness.

Apply knowledge of pathophysiology to monitoring client for alterations in body systems.

MEDICAL EMERGENCIES
Respond and intervene to a client life-threatening situation.

Notify primary health care provider about client unexpected response/emergency situation.

CHAPTER 74 # *Adrenal Disorders*

Cushing's disease (hypercortisolism) and Cushing's syndrome are caused by an oversecretion of the hormones the adrenal cortex produces. Cushing's disease can be the result of a tumor in the pituitary gland, resulting in release of the hormone ACTH. The ACTH then stimulates the adrenal cortex to increase the secretion of the glucocorticoid hormone cortisol. It can also be the result of hyperplasia of the adrenal cortex. Cushing's syndrome results from long-term use of glucocorticoids to treat other conditions (asthma or rheumatoid arthritis).

Addison's disease is an adrenocortical insufficiency. It is caused by damage or dysfunction of the adrenal cortex. With Addison's disease, the production of mineralocorticoids and glucocorticoids is diminished, resulting in decreased aldosterone and cortisol. Acute adrenal insufficiency, also known as Addisonian crisis, has a rapid onset. It is a medical emergency. If it is not quickly diagnosed and properly treated, the prognosis is poor. Older adult clients are less able to tolerate the complications of Addison's disease and acute adrenal insufficiency and need more frequent monitoring. ©

Cushing's disease/syndrome

ADRENAL CORTEX HORMONES

Mineralocorticoids: Aldosterone increases sodium absorption and causes potassium excretion in the kidney.

Glucocorticoids: Cortisol affects glucose, protein, and fat metabolism; the body's response to stress; and the body's immune function.

Sex hormones: Androgens and estrogens

HEALTH PROMOTION AND DISEASE PREVENTION

- Following an adrenalectomy, hormone therapy replacement is lifelong.
- Follow health promotion recommendations and obtain an annual influenza immunization.
- Wear a medical alert bracelet that lists Cushing's as a condition and the medications you are taking.
- Monitor blood glucose and blood pressure and report unexpected findings.

DATA COLLECTION

RISK FACTORS

Females between the ages of 30 and 50 years

Cushing's disease

ENDOGENOUS CAUSES OF INCREASED CORTISOL
- Adrenal hyperplasia
- Adrenocortical carcinoma
- Pituitary carcinoma that secretes adrenocorticotropic hormone (ACTH)
- Carcinomas of the lung, gastrointestinal (GI) tract, or pancreas (these tumors can secrete ACTH)

Cushing's syndrome

EXOGENOUS CAUSES OF INCREASED CORTISOL:
Therapeutic use of glucocorticoids for the following.
- Organ transplant
- Chemotherapy
- Autoimmune diseases
- Asthma
- Allergies
- Chronic fibrosis

EXPECTED FINDINGS

- Weakness, fatigue, sleep disturbances
- Back and joint pain
- Altered emotional state (irritability, depression)
- Decreased libido

PHYSICAL FINDINGS
- Evidence of decreased immune function and decreased inflammatory response (infections without fever, swelling, drainage, erythema)
- Thin, fragile skin
- Bruising and petechiae (fragile blood vessels)
- Hypertension (sodium and water retention)
- Tachycardia
- Gastric ulcers due to oversecretion of hydrochloric acid
- Weight gain and increased appetite
- Irregular, scant menses
- Dependent edema
- Changes in fat distribution (characteristic fat distribution of moon face, truncal obesity, fat collection on the back of the neck [buffalo hump])
- Fractures (osteoporosis)

- Bone pain and fractures with an increased risk for falls Qs
- Muscle wasting (particularly in the extremities)
- Impaired glucose tolerance
- Frequent infections, poor wound healing
- Hirsutism
- Acne
- Red cheeks
- Striae (reddish purple lines on the abdomen, upper arms, thighs)
- Clitoral hypertrophy
- Thinning, balding hair
- Hyperglycemia
- Emotional lability

LABORATORY TESTS

Elevated blood cortisol levels in the absence of acute illness or stress indicate Cushing's disease/syndrome.

Urine (24-hr urine collection) contains elevated levels of free cortisol.

Plasma adrenocorticotropic hormone (ACTH) levels
- Hypersecretion of ACTH by the anterior pituitary results in elevated ACTH levels.
- Disorders of the adrenal cortex or medication therapy results in decreased ACTH levels.

Salivary cortisol elevations confirm the diagnosis of Cushing's disease.

Blood potassium and calcium levels: Decreased

Blood glucose level: Increased

Blood sodium level: Increased

Lymphocytes: Decreased

Dexamethasone suppression tests: Tests vary in length and amount of dexamethasone to administer. Clients might have to stay overnight and the medication is administered orally in the evening or at bedtime. 24-hr urine collections show suppression of cortisol excretion in clients who do not have Cushing's disease. Nonsuppression of cortisol excretion indicates Cushing's disease. Clients should stop taking medications and try to reduce stress prior to and during testing. False positive results can occur for clients who have acute illnesses and alcohol use disorder.

DIAGNOSTIC PROCEDURES

- X-ray, magnetic resonance imaging, arteriography, and CT scans identify lesions of the pituitary gland, adrenal gland, lung, GI tract, and pancreas.
- Radiological imaging determines the source of adrenal insufficiency (tumor, adrenal atrophy).

74.1 Case study

Part 1

Matt is a nurse caring for Annie, a client who has hypercortisolism and has been admitted to determine the cause of this anomaly.

Part 2

Testing reveals that Annie has Cushing's disease.

Part 3

Matt reviews the laboratory results from Annie.

Part 4

Matt is collecting data from Annie to obtain and prioritize information regarding her new diagnosis.

Case study exercises

1. Matt is caring for Annie who has hypercortisolism. Sort the conditions that cause increased cortisol. (Endogenous conditions (Cushing's disease), Exogenous (Cushing's syndrome))

   A. Asthma

   B. Adrenal carcinoma

   C. Chemotherapy

   D. Adrenal hyperplasia

2. Matt is contributing to the plan of care for Annie who has Cushing's disease. Matt should identify that clients who have Cushing's disease are at increased risk for which of the following? (Select all that apply.)

   A. Infection

   B. Peptic ulcer

   C. Renal calculi

   D. Bone fractures

   E. Dysphagia

3. Matt is reviewing the laboratory findings for Annie who has Cushing's disease. Which of the following findings should Matt expect to find? (Select all that apply.)

   A. Increased sodium

   B. Increased potassium

   C. Increased calcium

   D. Increased blood glucose

   E. Decreased lymphocytes

4. Matt is collecting data from Annie who has Cushing's disease. Which of the following findings is the priority?

   A. Weight gain

   B. Fatigue

   C. Fragile skin

   D. Joint pain

PATIENT-CENTERED CARE

NURSING CARE

- Monitor I&O and daily weight.
- Monitor for indications of hypervolemia (edema, distended neck veins, shortness of breath, adventitious breath sounds, hypertension, tachycardia).
- Maintain a safe environment to minimize the risk of pathological fractures and skin trauma. Qs
- Prevent infection by performing frequent hand hygiene.
- Encourage physical activity within the client's limitations.
- Provide meticulous skin care.
- Change the client's position at least every 2 hr.
- Monitor for and protect against skin breakdown and infection.
- Use surgical asepsis when performing dressing changes and any invasive procedures.
- Monitor WBC count with differential daily.

CLIENT EDUCATION

- Take medications and watch for adverse reactions. The need for medication therapy can be lifelong.
- Eat foods high in calcium and vitamin D.
- Assistance might be needed at home due to residual muscle weakness.
- Monitor weight every day and report weight gain of more than 2 lb over a 24 hr period or 3 lb over a week.

MEDICATIONS

Treatment depends on the cause. For Cushing's syndrome, taper glucocorticoids and manage manifestations as needed.

Ketoconazole

- An adrenal corticosteroid inhibitor, ketoconazole is an antifungal agent that inhibits adrenal corticosteroid synthesis in high dosages.
- Ketoconazole supplements radiation or surgery.

NURSING ACTIONS

- Monitor liver enzymes and for indications of liver toxicity (yellow sclera, dark-colored urine).
- Monitor fluids and electrolytes for clients who have gastric effects.

CLIENT EDUCATION

- The medication can cause nausea, vomiting, fatigue, skin changes, and dizziness.
- Relief is temporary. Findings will return after stopping taking the medication.
- Take the medication with food to relieve gastric effects. Qs

Mitotane

Produces selective destruction of adrenocortical cells

NURSING ACTIONS

- Mitotane treats inoperable adrenal carcinoma.
- Monitor for indications of shock, renal damage, and hepatotoxicity.
- Monitor for orthostatic hypotension.

CLIENT EDUCATION

- The purpose of the medication is to reduce the size of the tumor.
- Notify the provider for adverse effects (visual disturbances, hematuria).
- Use caution when driving or operating heavy machinery.
- Lifelong replacement with glucocorticoids is likely.

Hydrocortisone

For replacement therapy for clients who have adrenocortical insufficiency as a result of the treatment of Cushing's disease

NURSING ACTIONS

- This medication can be used in conjunction with ketoconazole to avoid adrenal insufficiency.
- Monitor potassium and glucose levels.
- Measure daily weight. Notify the provider of weight gain greater than 2.3 kg (5 lb)/week.
- Monitor blood pressure and pulse.
- Monitor for manifestations of infection (increased temperature, increased WBC).

CLIENT EDUCATION

- Carry emergency identification about corticosteroid use.
- Report abdominal pain or black, tarry stools.
- Notify the provider for any manifestations of infection.
- Take the medication without skipping any doses.
- Consult the provider before taking any OTC medications or supplements.
- Avoid infection by using good hygiene and avoiding crowds or individuals who have an infection.

THERAPEUTIC PROCEDURES

Chemotherapy

With cytotoxic agents for Cushing's disease resulting from a tumor

Hypophysectomy

Surgical removal of the pituitary gland (depending on the cause of Cushing's disease)

NURSING ACTIONS

- Monitor and correct electrolytes, especially sodium, potassium, and chloride. Monitor and adjust glucose levels. Monitor ECG.
- Protect the client from developing an infection by using good hand hygiene and making sure the client avoids contact with individuals who have infections. Use caution to prevent a fracture by providing assistance getting out of bed and raising side rails.

- Monitor for bleeding. Monitor nasal drainage for a possible cerebrospinal fluid (CSF) leak. Observe drainage for the presence of glucose or a halo sign (yellow on the edge and clear in the middle), which can indicate CSF.
- Ensure neurologic status is assessed every hour for the first 24 hr and then every 4 hr.
- Administer glucocorticoids before, during, and after surgery to prevent an abrupt drop in cortisol level.
- Administer stool softeners to prevent straining.
- Maintain a high caloric and protein diet.

CLIENT EDUCATION
- Use caution preoperatively to prevent infection or fractures.
- The surgeon will perform a transsphenoidal hypophysectomy through the sphenoid sinus via the nasal cavity or under the upper lip, and expect nasal packing postoperatively. There will be a drip pad under the nose for bloody drainage, so breathing must be through the mouth. Avoid coughing, blowing the nose, and sneezing.
- Numbness at the surgical site and a diminished sense of smell can occur for 3 to 4 months after surgery.
- Avoid bending over at the waist and straining to prevent increased intracranial pressure. If picking up an object or to tying shoes, bend at the knees.
- Avoid brushing teeth for 2 weeks, and floss and rinse the mouth with warm water. Qᴱᴮᴾ
- Notify the provider of increased swallowing, drainage that makes a halo (yellow on the edge and clear in the middle), or clear drainage from the nose, which can indicate a CSF leak. Another indication is a headache.
- Notify the provider of excessive bleeding, confusion, or headache.
- To avoid constipation, which contributes to increased intracranial pressure, eat high-fiber food and take docusate.

Adrenalectomy

Surgical removal of the adrenal gland can be unilateral (one gland) or bilateral (both glands).

NURSING ACTIONS
- Inform the client that they will be monitored closely in the ICU.
- Provide glucocorticoid and hormone replacement.
- Monitor for adrenal crisis due to an abrupt drop in cortisol level. Findings include hypotension, tachycardia, tachypnea, nausea, and headache.
- Monitor vital signs and hemodynamic levels initially every 15 min.
- Monitor fluids and electrolytes.
- Monitor the incision site for bleeding.
- Monitor bowel sounds.
- Provide pain medication. Administer stool softeners.
- Slowly reintroduce foods.
- Observe the abdomen for distention and tenderness. Monitor the incision site for redness, discharge, and swelling.

CLIENT EDUCATION
- Perform postoperative pain management, deep breathing, and anti-embolism care.
- Take glucocorticoids, mineralocorticoids, and hormone replacements.

COMPLICATIONS

Infection due to immunosuppression

Immunosuppression and reduced inflammatory response occur due to elevated glucocorticoid levels.

NURSING ACTIONS
- Monitor for subtle indications of infection (fatigue, fever, localized swelling or redness).
- Monitor WBC counts and sources for infection (urine, skin).

CLIENT EDUCATION
- Minimize exposure to infectious organisms. (Avoid people who are ill. Avoid crowds. Use hand hygiene.) Qs
- Report indications of infection to the provider.

Adrenal crisis (acute adrenal insufficiency)

Sudden drop in corticosteroids is due to the following.
- Sudden tumor removal
- Stress of illness, trauma, surgery, or dehydration
- Abrupt withdrawal of steroid medication

PHYSICAL FINDINGS
- Hypotension
- Hypoglycemia
- Hyperkalemia
- Abdominal pain
- Weakness
- Weight loss

NURSING ACTIONS
- Administer glucocorticoids for treatment of acute adrenal insufficiency.
- Administer insulin with dextrose, a potassium-binding and -excreting resin (sodium polystyrene sulfonate), or loop or thiazide diuretics to treat hyperkalemia.
- Ensure glucagon or glucose are administered via IV bolus to treat hypoglycemia.
- Monitor vital signs and glucose levels.
- Monitor ECG.

CLIENT EDUCATION
- Taper the medication.
- During times of stress, additional glucocorticoids might be needed to prevent adrenal crisis.

Addison's disease

PRODUCED BY THE ADRENAL CORTEX

Mineralocorticoids: Aldosterone increases sodium absorption and causes potassium excretion in the kidney.

Glucocorticoids: Cortisol affects glucose, protein, and fat metabolism; the body's response to stress; and the body's immune function.

Sex hormones: Androgens and estrogens

DATA COLLECTION

RISK FACTORS

CAUSES OF PRIMARY ADDISON'S DISEASE
- Idiopathic autoimmune dysfunction (majority of cases)
- Tuberculosis
- Histoplasmosis
- Adrenalectomy
- Cancer with metastasis
- Radiation therapy of the abdomen

CAUSES OF SECONDARY ADDISON'S DISEASE
- Steroid withdrawal
- Hypophysectomy
- Pituitary neoplasm
- High dose radiation of pituitary gland or entire brain

ACUTE ADRENAL INSUFFICIENCY is a life-threatening event in which the need for cortisol is greater than the body's supply and if left untreated can lead to death. Factors that precipitate acute adrenal insufficiency are the following.
- Sepsis
- Trauma
- Stress (myocardial infarction, surgery, anesthesia, hypothermia, volume loss, hypoglycemia)
- Adrenal hemorrhage
- Steroid withdrawal

EXPECTED FINDINGS

Manifestations of chronic Addison's disease develop slowly, and manifestations of acute adrenal insufficiency develop rapidly.
- Weight loss
- Craving for salt
- Hyperpigmentation of the skin and mucous membranes
- Weakness and fatigue
- Nausea, anorexia, and vomiting
- Abdominal pain
- Constipation or diarrhea
- Dizziness with orthostatic hypotension
- Severe hypotension (acute adrenal insufficiency)
- Dehydration
- Hyponatremia
- Hyperkalemia
- Hypoglycemia
- Hypercalcemia

LABORATORY TESTS

Blood electrolytes: increased K⁺, increased WBC, decreased Na⁺, and increased calcium

BUN and creatinine: increased

Blood glucose: normal to decreased

Blood/salivary cortisol: decreased

Adrenocorticotropic hormone (ACTH) stimulation test (provocation test): ACTH is infused, and the cortisol response is measured 30 min and 1 hr after the injection. With primary adrenal insufficiency, plasma cortisol levels do not rise. With secondary adrenal insufficiency, plasma cortisol levels are increased. ACTH test cannot be performed if the client is experiencing an acute crisis.

DIAGNOSTIC PROCEDURES

Electrocardiogram (ECG)

Used to determine ECG changes or dysrhythmias associated with electrolyte imbalance.

X-ray, CT scan, and MRI scan

Radiological imaging to determine source of adrenal insufficiency (a tumor or adrenal atrophy)

PATIENT-CENTERED CARE

NURSING CARE

- The primary goal of care is preventing circulatory shock.
- Monitor for fluid and electrolyte imbalances.
- Assist with the administration of saline infusions to restore fluid volume. Observe for dehydration. Measure orthostatic vital signs. Monitor daily weights.
- The RN will administer hydrocortisone IV bolus and a continuous infusion or intermittent IV bolus.
- Monitor for and treat hyperkalemia.
  - Measure blood potassium and obtain an ECG.
  - Administer sodium polystyrene sulfonate, insulin, calcium, glucose, and sodium bicarbonate.
  - Obtain vital signs frequently, and monitor for dysrhythmias.
- Monitor for and treat hypoglycemia.
- Maintain a safe environment. Qs

MEDICATIONS

Hydrocortisone, prednisone, and cortisone

Glucocorticoids are used as adrenocorticoid replacement for adrenal insufficiency and as an anti-inflammatory.

NURSING ACTIONS
- Monitor weight, blood pressure, and electrolytes.
- Increase dosage during periods of stress or illness if necessary.
- Taper dose if discontinuing to avoid acute adrenal insufficiency.
- Administer with food to reduce gastric effects.

CLIENT EDUCATION

- Avoid discontinuing the medication abruptly. Qᴘᴄᴄ
- Report manifestations of Cushing's syndrome (round face, edema, weight gain).
- Take the medication with food.
- Report manifestations of adrenal insufficiency (fever, fatigue, muscle weakness, anorexia).
- Report acute illness to the provider.

OTHER MEDICATIONS

Vasopressors: Used for clients who have persistent hypotension

Antibiotics: Used to treat infections

INTERPROFESSIONAL CARE

Home assistance for fluid, medication, and dietary management can be required.

CLIENT EDUCATION

- Monitor for adverse reactions.
- Avoid using alcohol and caffeine. Qᴘᴄᴄ
- Monitor for indications of gastric bleeding (coffee-ground emesis; tarry, black stool).
- Monitor for hypoglycemia (diaphoresis, shaking, tachycardia, headache).
- Report manifestations of adrenal insufficiency (fever, fatigue, muscle weakness, dizziness, anorexia).
- To prevent acute adrenal insufficiency, increase corticosteroid doses as prescribed during times of stress.
- Medication therapy can be lifelong.
- Keep an emergency kit with hydrocortisone in case Addisonian crisis occurs; administer injection and seek immediate medical care.
- Avoid stress and strenuous activity in hot weather.
- Replace sodium lost during episodes of nausea and vomiting.

COMPLICATIONS

Acute adrenal insufficiency (Addisonian crisis)

Acute adrenal insufficiency (Addisonian crisis) occurs when there is an acute drop in adrenocorticoids due to sudden discontinuation of glucocorticoid medications or when induced by severe trauma, infection, or stress. Qᴇʙᴘ

NURSING ACTIONS
- Monitor electrolytes.
- Position the client in a recumbent position with legs elevated.

CLIENT EDUCATION
- Notify the provider of any infection, trauma, or stress that can increase the need for adrenocorticoids.
- Do not discontinue the medication abruptly. Qs

Hypoglycemia

Insufficient glucocorticoid causes increased insulin sensitivity and decreased glycogen, which leads to hypoglycemia.

NURSING ACTIONS
- Monitor glucose levels.
- Administer glucagon as needed.

CLIENT EDUCATION
- Monitor for hypoglycemia. Manifestations can include diaphoresis, shaking, tachycardia, and headache.
- Have a 15 g carbohydrate snack readily available. Qᴇʙᴘ

Hyperkalemia/Hyponatremia

Decrease in aldosterone levels can cause an increased excretion of sodium and a decreased excretion of potassium.

NURSING ACTIONS
- Monitor electrolytes and ECG.
- Administer kayexalate, or loop diuretics.
- Assist the RN with insulin (IV) administration.

CLIENT EDUCATION: Report indications of hyperkalemia (muscle weakness, tingling sensation, irregular heartbeat). Qs

---

Application Exercises

1. A nurse is reinforcing teaching with a client who has a prescription for prednisone. Which of the following instructions should the nurse include?

   A. Do not abruptly stop taking the medication.

   B. You will need to have the dosage decreased during times of stress.

   C. Take the medication on an empty stomach.

   D. An adverse effect of this medication is weight loss.

Active Learning Scenario

A nurse is reinforcing teaching with a client who has a new prescription for hydrocortisone following an adrenalectomy. Use the ATI Active Learning Template: Medication to complete this item.

THERAPEUTIC USES: Explain why the client needs to take this medication.

CLIENT EDUCATION: Identify three instructional points to include about this medication.

Case Study Exercises Key

1. **ENDOGENOUS CONDITIONS (CUSHING'S DISEASE):** B, D; **EXOGENOUS (CUSHING'S SYNDROME):** A, C

   When recognizing cues, Matt should identify that both Cushing's disease and Cushing's syndrome are caused by hypercortisolism. Cushing's disease is caused by excess secretion of cortisol due to an adrenal, pituitary, lung, or pancreatic tumor (Endogenous), while the most common cause of Cushing's syndrome is long term use of glucocorticoids to treat conditions such as asthma, allergies, or the use of chemotherapy.

   Ⓝ *NCLEX® Connection: Physiological Adaptation, Basic Pathophysiology*

2. **A, B, D. CORRECT:** When generating solutions and contributing to the plan of care for Annie, Matt should identify that clients who have Cushing's disease are at risk for gastrointestinal problems, including anorexia, nausea, vomiting, and abdominal pain. Matt should also identify that excessive cortisol causes suppression of immunity which places the client at risk for infection. The overproduction of cortisol inhibits the production of a protective mucus lining in the stomach and causes an increase in the amount of gastric acids which can lead to peptic ulcers. Clients who have Cushing's disease are also at risk for bone fracture because decreased calcium absorption leads to osteoporosis.

   Ⓝ *NCLEX® Connection: Physiological Adaptation, Alterations in Body Systems*

3. **A, D, E. CORRECT:** When evaluating the laboratory values of Annie who has hypercortisolism, Matt should expect to fine an increase in sodium and glucose, and decreased calcium, potassium, and lymphocytes.

   Ⓝ *NCLEX® Connection: Physiological Adaptation, Alterations in Body Systems*

4. **A. CORRECT:** The nurse should analyze the findings and determine that the priority hypothesis is that the client is at greatest risk for fluid retention, which can lead to pulmonary edema, hypertension, and heart failure; therefore, weight gain is the priority finding.

   Ⓝ *NCLEX® Connection: Physiological Adaptation, Alterations in Body Systems*

Application Exercises Key

1. **A. CORRECT:** When taking action and reinforcing teaching with a client about prednisone, the nurse should instruct the client not to stop taking the medication suddenly because this action could cause adrenal insufficiently, which has the potential to be life threatening.

   Ⓝ *NCLEX® Connection: Pharmacological Therapies, Expected Actions/Outcomes*

Active Learning Scenario Key

Using the ATI Active Learning Template: Medication

THERAPEUTIC USES: Hydrocortisone is a glucocorticoid that treats adrenal insufficiency resulting from adrenalectomy surgery.

CLIENT EDUCATION
- Carry emergency identification about corticosteroid use.
- Report abdominal pain or black, tarry stools.
- Notify the provider for any manifestations of infection.
- Take the medication without skipping any doses.
- Consume a diet high in calcium and vitamin D.
- Consult the provider before taking any OTC medications or supplements.

Ⓝ *NCLEX® Connection: Pharmacological Therapies, Medication Administration*

When reviewing the following chapters, keep in mind the relevant topics and tasks of the NCLEX outline.

Reduction of Risk Potential

THERAPEUTIC PROCEDURES: Reinforce client teaching on treatments and procedures.

Physiological Adaptation

FLUID AND ELECTROLYTE IMBALANCES
Provide care for a client with a fluid and electrolyte imbalance.

Identify signs and symptoms of client fluid and/or electrolyte imbalances.

BASIC PATHOPHYSIOLOGY
Identify signs and symptoms related to an acute or chronic illness.

Apply knowledge of pathophysiology to monitoring client for alterations in body systems.

MEDICAL EMERGENCIES
Respond and intervene to a client life-threatening situation.

Notify primary health care provider about client unexpected response/ emergency situation.

CHAPTER 75 *Diabetes Mellitus Management and Complications*

Diabetes mellitus is a metabolic disorder resulting from either an inadequate production of insulin (type 1) or an inability of the body's cells to respond to insulin that is present (type 2).

Type 1 diabetes mellitus is an autoimmune dysfunction involving the destruction of beta cells, which produce insulin in the islets of Langerhans of the pancreas. Immune system cells and antibodies are present in circulation and can also be triggered by certain genetic tissue types or viral infections.

Type 2 diabetes mellitus is a progressive condition due to increasing inability of cells to respond to insulin (insulin resistance) and decreased production of insulin by the beta cells. It is linked to obesity, sedentary lifestyle, and heredity. Metabolic syndrome, a combination of conditions, that include abdominal obesity, hyperglycemia, hyperlipidemia, and hypertension, often precedes type 2 diabetes mellitus.

Diabetes mellitus has wide ranging systemic effects and is a contributing factor to development of cardiovascular disease, hypertension, kidney disease, neuropathy, retinopathy, peripheral vascular disease, and stroke.

Diabetes mellitus is significantly more prevalent in African American, Indigenous Peoples, and Hispanic populations.

Diabetic ketoacidosis (DKA) is an acute, life-threatening condition characterized by uncontrolled hyperglycemia (greater than 250 mg/dL), metabolic acidosis, and an accumulation of ketones in the blood and urine. The onset is rapid, and the mortality rate is up to 10%.

Hyperglycemic hyperosmolar state (HHS) is an acute, life-threatening condition characterized by profound hyperglycemia (greater than 600 mg/dL), hyperosmolarity that leads to dehydration, and an absence of ketosis. Onset generally occurs gradually over several days, and if left untreated can lead to coma and death.

HEALTH PROMOTION AND DISEASE PREVENTION

- Diabetes mellitus type 1 cannot be prevented. Lifestyle modifications can reduce the risk of diabetes mellitus type 2 and minimize the risk of complications for clients who develop diabetes mellitus.
- Try to maintain weight appropriate for body build and height.

Diabetic screening

- Screen clients who have a BMI of 25 or above and one or more of these factors.
  - A first-degree relative who has diabetes mellitus
  - Age 45 years or older
  - Report of sedentary lifestyle
  - History of vascular disease, polycystic ovary syndrome, gestational diabetes, or giving birth to an infant weighing more than 9 lb
  - Reports African, Hispanic, Asian, American Indian, or Pacific Islander heritage
  - Has a blood pressure consistently greater than 140/90 mm Hg
  - HgA1C greater than 5.7%, impaired fasting glucose, or impaired glucose tolerance
  - HDL level less than 35 mg/dL or triglyceride level greater than 250 mg/dL
- Screening is done with fasting blood glucose levels, oral glucose tolerance test, or glycosylated hemoglobin (A1C).

CLIENT EDUCATION

- Exercise and good nutrition are necessary for preventing or controlling diabetes.
  - Carbohydrates: 45% of total daily intake
  - Protein: 15% to 20% of total daily intake, depending upon kidney function
  - Total fats: 20% to 35% of total daily intake
- Consistency in the amount of food consumed and regularity in meal times promotes blood glucose control.

- Consume a diet low in saturated fats to decrease low-density lipoprotein (LDL), assist with weight loss for secondary prevention of diabetes, and reduce risk of heart disease.
- Modify the diet to include sources of omega-3 fatty acids and fiber to lower cholesterol, improve blood glucose for clients who have diabetes, for secondary prevention of diabetes, and to reduce the risk of heart disease.
- Perform physical activity at least three times per week (150 min/week).

DATA COLLECTION

Clients are considered to have prediabetes when the glucose level is above the expected range and below levels that indicate diabetes mellitus (impaired fasting glucose or impaired glucose tolerance).

RISK FACTORS

Metabolic syndrome
The presence of at least three factors that increase the client's risk for cardiovascular events and developing diabetes mellitus type 2
- Central obesity: waist circumference greater than 100 cm (40 in) for males (sex assigned at birth); greater than 88 cm (35 in) for females (sex assigned at birth)
- Hyperlipidemia: triglyceride level greater than 150 mg/dL or taking medication for triglycerides; decreased HDL level (less than 50 mg/dL for females (sex assigned at birth); less than 40 mg/dL for males (sex assigned at birth))
- Blood pressure consistently greater than 130 mm Hg systolic, or 85 mm Hg diastolic; taking medication for hypertension
- Hyperglycemia (fasting blood glucose at or greater than 100 mg/dL, or taking medication for hyperglycemia)

Insulin resistance: Impaired fasting glucose levels 100 to 125 mg/dL, impaired glucose tolerance 140 mg/dL, or A1C level 5.7% to 6.4%

Age
- Older adult clients might not be able to drive to the provider's office, grocery store, or pharmacy. Determine support systems available for older adult clients. Ⓒ
- Older adults are at risk for altered metabolism of medication due to decreased kidney and liver function because of the aging process.
- Older adults can have vision alterations (yellowing of lens, decreased depth perception, cataracts), which can affect ability to read information and administer mediation.
- Vision and hearing deficits can interfere with the understanding of instruction, reading of materials, and preparation of medications.
- Tissue deterioration secondary to aging can affect the client's ability to prepare food, care for self, perform ADLs, perform foot/wound care, and perform glucose monitoring.
- A fixed income can mean that there are limited funds for buying diabetic supplies, wound care supplies, insulin, and medications. This can result in complications.

EXPECTED FINDINGS

Polyuria: Excess urine production and frequency from osmotic diuresis

Polydipsia: Excessive thirst due to dehydration
- Loss of skin turgor, skin warm and dry
- Dry mucous membranes
- Weakness and malaise
- Rapid weak pulse and hypotension

Polyphagia: Excessive hunger and eating caused from inability of cells to receive glucose (because of a lack of insulin or cellular resistance to available insulin) and the body's use of protein and fat for energy (which causes ketosis)

The client can display weight loss.

Kussmaul respirations: Increased respiratory rate and depth in attempt to excrete carbon dioxide and acid due to metabolic acidosis

Recurrent infections: Ask clients about the occurrence of vaginal yeast infections.

OTHER MANIFESTATIONS: Acetone/fruity breath odor (due to accumulation of ketones), headache, nausea, vomiting, abdominal pain, inability to concentrate, fatigue, weakness, vision changes, slow healing of wounds, decreased level of consciousness, seizures leading to coma

LABORATORY TESTS

Diagnostic criteria for diabetes include two findings (on separate days) of at least one of the following.
- Manifestations of diabetes plus casual blood glucose concentration greater than 200 mg/dL (without regard to time since last meal)
- Fasting blood glucose greater than 126 mg/dL (no caloric intake within 8 hr of testing)
- 2-hr glucose greater than 200 mg/dL with oral glucose tolerance test
- Glycosylated hemoglobin (A1C) greater than 6.5%

Fasting blood glucose

NURSING ACTIONS: Postpone administration of antidiabetic medication until after the level is drawn.

CLIENT EDUCATION: Fast (no food or drink other than water) for the 8 hr prior to the blood test.

Oral glucose tolerance test

- This is not generally used for routine diagnosis.
- A fasting blood glucose level is drawn at the start of the test. The client is then instructed to consume a specified amount of glucose. Blood glucose levels are obtained at 1 and 2 hr after the ingestion of glucose. The clients must be monitored for hypoglycemia throughout the procedure.
- The fasting glucose should be less than 110 mg/d; less than 180 mg/dL at 1 hr; and less than 140 mg/dL at 2 hr.

CLIENT EDUCATION

- Consume a balanced diet for 3 days prior to the test. Then, fast for 10 to 12 hr prior to the test.
- Only water can be taken during the testing period. Food or other liquids will affect the test results.

Glycosylated hemoglobin (HbA1c)

- The expected reference range is 5.5% to 7% but an acceptable reference range for clients who have diabetes can be 6.5% to 8%, with a target goal of 7% or less.
- HbA1c is the best indicator of the average blood glucose level for the past 120 days. It assists in evaluating treatment effectiveness and compliance.

CLIENT EDUCATION

- The test evaluates treatment effectiveness and compliance.
- The test is recommended quarterly or twice yearly depending on the glycemic levels.

Urine ketones

- Ketones accumulate in the blood due to breakdown of fatty acids when insulin is not available.
- High ketones in the urine associated with hyperglycemia (exceed 300 mg/dL) is a medical emergency.

Lipid profile

Obtain a baseline measurement at diagnosis, then every 1 to 2 years.

Other laboratory testing

C-peptide levels, autoantibodies for insulin, islet cells, and glutamic acid decarboxylase

DIAGNOSTIC PROCEDURES

Self-monitored blood glucose (SMBG)

NURSING ACTION: Ensure that the client follows the proper procedure for blood sample collection and use of a glucose meter. Supplemental short-acting insulin can be prescribed for elevated premeal glucose levels.

CLIENT EDUCATION

- Check the accuracy of the strips with the control solution provided.
- Use the correct code number in the meter to match the strip bottle number.
- Store strips in the closed container in a dry location.
- Obtain an adequate amount of blood sample when preforming the test.
- Perform appropriate hand hygiene.
- Use fresh lancets, and avoid sharing glucose monitoring equipment to prevent infection.
- Keep a record of the SMBG that includes time, date, blood glucose level, insulin dose, food intake, and other events that can alter glucose metabolism (activity level, illness).

MEDICATIONS

Antidiabetic medications are started at a low dose and increased every few weeks until effective control or maximum dosage is reached. Additional medications are added as needed.

- Insulin regimens are established for clients who have type 1 diabetes mellitus.
  - More than 1 type of insulin: rapid-, short-, intermediate-, and long-acting
  - Given two or more times a day based on blood glucose results
- Insulin can be required by some clients who have type 2 diabetes or gestational diabetes if glycemic control is not obtained with diet, exercise, and oral hypoglycemic agents.
  - Continuous infusion of insulin can be accomplished using a small pump that is worn externally. The pump is programmed to deliver insulin through a needle in subcutaneous tissue. The needle should be changed at least every 2 to 3 days to prevent infection.
  - Complications of the insulin pump are accidental cessation of insulin administration, obstruction of the tubing/needle, pump failure, and infection.
- Insulin pens are prefilled cartridges of 150 to 300 units of insulin in a programmable device with disposable needles.
  - Convenient for travel
  - Used for clients who have vision impairment or problems with dexterity
- Oral antidiabetic medications are used, along with diet and exercise, by clients who have type 2 diabetes to regulate blood glucose.

Insulin

Also see the **PN PHARMACOLOGY REVIEW MODULE: CHAPTER 34: DIABETES MELLITUS**.

A normally functioning pancreas releases insulin continuously (basal) and as needed following carbohydrate intake (prandial). Insulin therapy is prescribed to mimic the pancreas.

Therapy can range from a single daily injection containing an intermediate- to long-acting insulin, to two injections daily with combination insulins, to an intense regime of a basal insulin dose and subsequent injections for meal intake and glucose levels.

Rapid-acting insulin: Insulin lispro, insulin aspart, insulin glulisine, inhaled human insulin

- Administer before meals to control postprandial rise in blood glucose.
- Onset is rapid (< 15 min), depending on which insulin is administered.
- Administer in conjunction with intermediate- or long-acting insulin to provide glycemic control between meals and at night.

75.1 Case study

Part 1

John is a nurse on a medical-surgical floor assisting with the care of Sue. Sue is admitted to the health care facility with a new diagnosis of diabetes mellitus. Sue has a prescription for insulin aspart.

Part 2

John, a nurse on a medical-surgical floor, is assisting with the care of Sue who has diabetes mellitus. On morning rounds, John finds Sue lethargic, but arousable. John obtains a fingerstick glucose which is 52 mg/dL (<200 mg/dL).

Part 3

John, a nurse on a medical-surgical floor, is assisting with the care of Sue who has a new diagnosis of diabetes mellitus. John is reinforcing teaching Sue about foot care and nutrition.

Case study exercises

1. The nurse is preparing to administer insulin aspart to the client who has type 1 diabetes mellitus. Which of the following actions should the nurse plan to take?

   A. Administer the insulin in a muscle.

   B. Give the insulin 10 min before a meal.

   C. Shake the insulin vial before loading the syringe.

   D. Expect the insulin to peak in 6 hrs.

2. The nurse is assisting with the care of the client who has a blood glucose of 52 mg/dL. The client is lethargic but arousable. Which of the following actions should the nurse perform first?

   A. Recheck the client's blood glucose in 15 min.

   B. Give the client a protein snack.

   C. Provide the client with 177 mL (6 oz) of juice.

   D. Report the client findings to the RN.

3. The nurse is reinforcing teaching foot care to the client who has diabetes mellitus. Which of the following information should the nurse include in the teaching? (Select all that apply.)

   A. Remove calluses using over-the-counter remedies.

   B. Apply lotion between toes.

   C. Test water temperature with the wrist before bathing.

   D. Trim toenails straight across.

   E. Wear closed-toe shoes.

Short-acting insulin: Regular insulin
- Administer 15 to 60 min before meals to control postprandial hyperglycemia.
- Regular insulin is available in two concentrations.
  - U-500 is reserved for the client who has insulin resistance. It is administered subcutaneous and never administered IV.
  - U-100 is prescribed for most clients and can be administered subcutaneous or IV.

Intermediate-acting insulin: NPH insulin
- Administered for glycemic control 30 to 60 min before between meals and at night
- Not administered before meals to control postprandial rise in blood glucose
- Contains protamine (a protein), which causes a delay in the insulin absorption or onset and extends the duration of action of the insulin
- Administer NPH insulin subcutaneous only and as the only insulin to mix with short-acting insulin

Long-acting insulin: Insulin glargine, insulin detemir
- Administer once or twice daily, anytime during the day but always at the same time each day.
- Glargine insulin forms microprecipitates that dissolves slowly over 24 hr and maintains a steady blood sugar level with no peaks or troughs.
- Insulin detemir has an added fatty-acid chain that delays absorption. Although it does not have a peak, duration is dose-dependent (12 to 24 hr).
- Administer glargine insulin and insulin detemir subcutaneous only. Never administer IV.

Ultra long-acting insulin: U-300 insulin glargine, insulin degludec
- Duration is longer than 24 hr.
- Both medications are available only as a prefilled pen.
- U-300 insulin glargine is three times more concentrated than standard insulin glargine. It is useful for clients who do not receive 24 hr effective glucose with the standard concentration.
- Insulin degludec comes in U-100 and U-200 concentrations.

NURSING ACTIONS
- Observe the client perform self-administration of insulin, and offer additional instruction as indicated.
- Monitor for hypoglycemic reactions (sweating, weakness, dizziness, confusion, headache, tachycardia, slurred speech) at insulin peak times.
- Dosage can be adjusted when the client is scheduled for procedures that require fasting.

75.2 Hypoglycemia and hyperglycemia manifestations and management

Hypoglycemia

- Reinforce teaching with the client about measures to take in response to manifestations of hypoglycemia (mild shakiness, mental confusion, sweating, palpitations, headache, lack of coordination, blurred vision, seizures, and coma). When glucose declines slowly, manifestations relate to the central nervous system (headache, confusion, fatigue, drowsiness). With rapid glucose decline, the sympathetic nervous system is affected (tachycardia, diaphoresis, nervousness).
- If the client is unconscious, place the client in a lateral position to prevent aspiration and administer glucagon subcataneous or IM, and notify the provider. Repeat in 10 min if the client is still unconscious.
- Glucagon or IV 50% dextrose is appropriate for clients who cannot swallow.
- To avoid hypoglycemia, avoid excess insulin, exercise, and alcohol consumption on an empty stomach, and eat about the same amounts and at the same time periods daily.
- Measure blood glucose level if manifestations occur; if it confirms hypoglycemia (below 70 mg/dL), follow the steps below, or other protocol outlined by the provider.
  - Provide 15 to 20 g of a readily absorbable carbohydrate (4 to 6 oz of fruit juice or regular soft drink, glucose tablets or glucose gel per package instructions, 6 to 10 hard candies, or 1 tbsp of honey). 10 g of glucose will increase the blood glucose by 40 mg/dL over 30 min.
  - Recheck the blood glucose 15 min following intervention, and retreat the client if manifestations continue or the glucose is not above 70 mg/dL.
  - If blood glucose is within the expected reference range, have a snack containing a carbohydrate and protein (if the next meal is more than 1 hr away).
  - Once consciousness occurs and the client is able to swallow, have the client ingest oral carbohydrates.

Hyperglycemia

- Reinforce teaching with the client about manifestations of hyperglycemia (hot, dry skin, and fruity breath) and measures to take in response to hyperglycemia.
- Encourage oral fluid intake of sugar-free fluids to prevent dehydration.
- Administer insulin as prescribed.
- Test urine for ketones and report if outside of the expected reference range.
- Consult the provider if manifestations progress.

CLIENT EDUCATION

- Perform self-administration of subcutaneous insulin injections.
  - Rotate injection sites (to prevent lipohypertrophy) within one anatomic site (to prevent day-to-day changes in absorption rates).
  - Inject at a 90° angle (45° angle if the client is thin). Aspiration for blood is not necessary.
  - When mixing a rapid- or short-acting insulin with a longer-acting insulin, draw up the shorter-acting insulin into the syringe first and then the longer-acting insulin. This reduces the risk of introducing the longer-acting insulin into the shorter-acting insulin vial.

75.3 Insulin pen

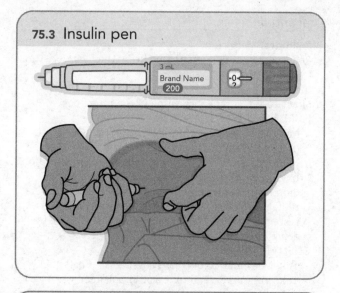

75.4 Insulin subcutaneous injection sites

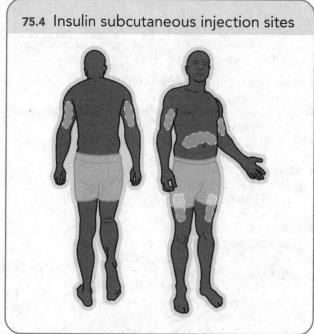

- Perform self-administration of inhaled human insulin.
  - Inhaled insulin is contraindicated in clients who have chronic lung diseases, such as COPD or asthma, because it can cause bronchospasms.
  - Cartridges containing the powdered insulin are available in 4, 8, or 12 units.
  - Use multiple cartridges if needed to administer the prescribed dose.
- Eat at regular intervals, avoid alcohol intake, and adjust insulin to exercise and diet to avoid hypoglycemia.
- Wear a medical identification wristband.

Oral antidiabetics

Biguanides: Metformin
- Reduces the production of glucose by the liver (gluconeogenesis)
- Increases tissue sensitivity to insulin
- Slows carbohydrate absorption in the intestines
- NURSING ACTIONS
  - Monitor significance of gastrointestinal (GI) effects (flatulence, anorexia, nausea, vomiting).
  - Monitor for lactic acidosis, especially in clients who have kidney disorders or liver dysfunction.
  - Stop medication for 48 hr before any type of elective radiographic test with iodinated contrast dye and restart 48 hr after (can cause lactic acidosis due to acute kidney injury).
- CLIENT EDUCATION
  - Take with food to decrease adverse GI effects.
  - Take vitamin B_{12} and folic acid supplements.
    - Avoid alcohol consumption while taking metformin to reduce the risk for lactic acidosis.
  - Contact the provider if manifestations of lactic acidosis develop (myalgia, sluggishness, somnolence, and hyperventilation).

Second-generation sulfonylureas: Glipizide, glimepiride, glyburide
- Stimulates insulin release from the pancreas causing a decrease in blood sugar levels
- Increases tissue sensitivity to insulin following long-term use
- NURSING ACTIONS
  - Monitor for hypoglycemia.
  - Beta blockers can mask tachycardia typically seen during hypoglycemia.
- CLIENT EDUCATION
  - Administer 30 min before meals.
  - Monitor for hypoglycemia and report frequent episodes to the provider.
  - Avoid alcohol due to disulfiram effect.
  - Avoid alcohol consumption while taking metformin to reduce the risk for lactic acidosis.

Meglitinides: Repaglinide, nateglinide
- Stimulates insulin release from pancreas
- Administered for post-meal hyperglycemia
- NURSING ACTIONS: Monitor for hypoglycemia.
- CLIENT EDUCATION
  - Take within 30 min before meals.
  - Omit the dose if skipped a meal to prevent hypoglycemic crisis.

Thiazolidinediones: Pioglitazone
- Reduces the production of glucose by the liver (gluconeogenesis)
- Increases tissue sensitivity to insulin
- NURSING ACTIONS
  - Monitor for fluid retention, especially in clients who have a history of heart failure.
  - Monitor for elevation of ALT, LDH, and triglycerides levels.
  - Monitor for hepatotoxicity.

- CLIENT EDUCATION
  - Report rapid weight gain, shortness of breath, decreased exercise tolerance, jaundice, or dark urine.
  - Use additional contraception methods because the medication reduces the blood levels of oral contraceptives and stimulate ovulation.
  - Have liver function tests at baseline and every 3 to 6 months thereafter.

Alpha-glucosidase inhibitors: Acarbose, miglitol
- Slow carbohydrate absorption from the intestinal tract
- Reduces post-meal hyperglycemia
- NURSING ACTIONS
  - Monitor liver function every 3 months.
  - Treat hypoglycemia with glucose, not table sugar (prevents table sugar from breaking down).
- CLIENT EDUCATION
  - Have liver function tests performed every 3 months or as prescribed.
  - Take the medication with the first bite of each meal in order for the medication to be effective.
  - GI discomfort (abdominal distention, cramps, excessive gas, diarrhea) is common with these medications.

Dipeptidyl peptidase-4 (DPP-4) inhibitors: Sitagliptin, saxagliptin, linagliptin, alogliptin
- Augments naturally occurring intestinal incretin hormones, which promote release of insulin and decrease secretion of glucagon
- Lowers fasting and postprandial glucose levels
- Few adverse effects, but upper respiratory manifestations (nasal and throat inflammation) and pancreatitis can occur.
- CLIENT EDUCATION
  - Report persistent upper respiratory manifestations.
  - Report severe abdominal pain, with or without emesis.
  - Medication only works when blood sugar is rising.

Sodium-glucose cotransporter 2 inhibitors: Canagliflozin, dapagliflozin
- Blocks reabsorption of glucose by kidneys, thus increasing urinary glucose excretion so that glucose is excreted in the urine
- NURSING ACTIONS
  - Monitor for development of urinary tract infections and genital yeast infection.
  - Monitor for postural hypotension in older adult clients, especially if taking diuretics concurrently.
- CLIENT EDUCATION
  - Take the medication before the first meal of the day.
  - Change positions slowly.
  - Monitor and report genital burning, itching, or increased drainage.

Non-insulin injectable medications

Incretin mimetic: Exenatide, liraglutide
- Mimics the function of intestinal incretin hormone by decreasing glucagon secretion, promoting insulin release, and gastric emptying
- Decreases insulin demand by reducing fasting and postprandial hyperglycemia

- NURSING ACTIONS
  - Administer exenatide subcutaneously 60 min before morning and evening meal.
  - Monitor for gastrointestinal distress.
- CLIENT EDUCATION
  - Do not administer after a meal.
  - Oral medications should never be taken within 1 hr of oral exenatide or 2 hr after an injection of exenatide because it will decrease effectiveness. Use caution, particularly with oral contraceptives and antibiotics.
  - Decreased appetite and weight loss can occur.
  - Report severe abdominal pain, with or without emesis, as a possible indication of pancreatitis.

Amylin mimetic: Pramlintide
- A synthetic amylin hormone found in the beta cells of the pancreas, suppresses glucagon secretion and controls postprandial blood glucose levels.
- Used for clients who are taking insulin, to provide more effective glucose control.
- The provider should reduce the premeal doses of rapid- or short-acting insulins by 50% when pramlintide therapy begins to reduce risk of hypoglycemia.
- NURSING ACTIONS
  - Administer subcutaneously immediately before each major meal.
  - Do not administer if client has hypoglycemia unawareness, or noncompliance/poor adherence to treatment regimens and self-monitoring blood glucose.
- CLIENT EDUCATION
  - Monitor and report frequent periods of hypoglycemia.
  - Administer the injection at least 5 cm (2 in) from any insulin injection given at the same time. Monitor for injection site reactions.

PATIENT-CENTERED CARE

NURSING CARE

- Monitor the following.
  - Blood glucose levels and factors affecting levels (other medications)
  - I&O and weight
  - Skin integrity and healing status of any wounds for presence of recurrent infections (feet and folds of the skin should be monitored)
  - Sensory alterations (tingling, numbness)
  - Visual alterations
  - Dietary practices
  - Exercise patterns
  - SMBG skill proficiency
  - Self-medication administration proficiency
- Instruct the client about the management of hyperglycemia and hypoglycemia.

- Vision and hearing deficits can impair communication between the nurse and client regarding diabetes mellitus and treatment. Use additional communication methods as needed to facilitate client understanding (written materials, interpreter).
- Provide information regarding self-administration of insulin. **(75.2)**
- Instruct the client to follow facility policies or recommendations of a podiatrist for nail care. Some protocols allow for trimming toenails straight across with clippers and filing edges with an emery board or nail file to prevent soft tissue injury. If clippers or scissors are contraindicated, the client should file the nails straight across.

CLIENT EDUCATION
- Practice appropriate techniques for SMBG, including obtaining blood samples, recording and responding to results, and correctly handling supplies and equipment.
- Perform self-administration of insulin.
- Rotate injection sites to prevent lipohypertrophy (increased swelling of fat) or lipoatrophy (loss of fat tissue) within one anatomic site (prevents day-to-day changes in absorption rates).

Foot care

CLIENT EDUCATION
- Inspect feet daily. Wash feet daily with mild soap and warm water. Test water temperature with the arms or a thermometer before washing feet. Do not soak the feet.
- Pat feet dry gently, especially between the toes, and avoid lotions between toes to decrease excess moisture and prevent infection.
- Use mild foot powder (powder with cornstarch) on sweaty feet.
- Do not use commercial remedies for the removal of calluses or corns, which can increase the risk for tissue injury and infection.
- Consult a podiatrist.
- Avoid open-toe, open-heel shoes. Leather shoes are preferred to plastic. Wear shoes that fit correctly. Wear slippers with soles. Do not go barefoot.
- Wear clean, absorbent socks or stockings that are made of cotton or wool and have not been mended. Wear socks at night if the feet get cold.
- Do not use hot water bottles or heating pads to warm feet. Wear socks for warmth.
- Avoid prolonged sitting, standing, and crossing of legs.
- Cleanse cuts with warm water and mild soap, gently dry, and apply a dry dressing. Monitor healing and seek intervention promptly.

Nutritional guidelines

CLIENT EDUCATION
- Participate in referring clients and their family to a dietitian for collaborative education on meal planning to include food intake, weight management, and lipid and glucose management. Q℡
- Assist with planning meals to achieve accurate timing of food intake, activity, onset, and peak of insulin. Calories and food composition should be similar each day. Eat at regular intervals, and do not skip meals.

- Count grams of carbohydrates consumed for glycemic control.
- 15 g carbohydrates is equal to 1 carbohydrate exchange.
- Restrict calories and increase physical activity if needed to facilitate weight loss (for clients who are overweight or obese) or to prevent obesity.
- Include fiber in the diet to increase carbohydrate metabolism and to help control cholesterol levels.
- Use artificial sweeteners. If caloric sweeteners are used, add this to daily carbohydrate intake.
- Read and interpret fat content information on food labels. Reduce intake of saturated and trans fats.

Exercise

CLIENT EDUCATION

- Only exercise when glucose levels are between 80 to 250 mg/dL; do not exercise if ketones are present in the urine.
- If more than 1 hr has passed since eating and high-intensity exercise is planned, consume a carbohydrate snack first.
- Wear comfortable shoes, and always carry identification information regarding diabetic status.
- Check blood glucose more often 24 hr after intensive exercise; a reduced medication dose might be required.

Illness

CLIENT EDUCATION

- Notify the provider when ill.
- Monitor blood glucose every 2 to 4 hr.
- Continue to take insulin or oral hypoglycemic agents.
- Meet carbohydrate needs through soft food (custard, cream soup, gelatin, graham crackers) six to eight times per day, if possible. If not, consume liquids equal to usual carbohydrate content.
- Test urine for ketones if blood sugar level is 300 mg/dL or higher. Report to the provider if they are outside the expected reference range.
- Rest.
- Call the provider for the following.
  ○ Presence of urine ketones
  ○ Blood glucose greater than 200 mg/dL that does not resolve with treatment
  ○ Fever greater than 38.6° C (101.5° F), does not respond to acetaminophen, or lasts more than 24 hr
  ○ Feeling disoriented or confused
  ○ Experiencing rapid breathing
  ○ Persistent nausea, vomiting, or diarrhea
  ○ Inability to tolerate liquids
  ○ Illness that lasts longer than 2 days

INTERPROFESSIONAL CARE

Recommend a referral for the client to a diabetes educator for comprehensive education in diabetes management.

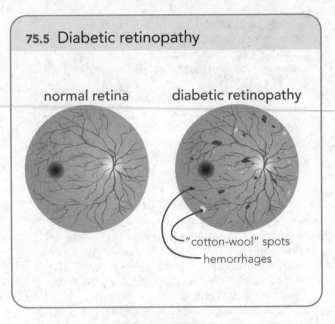

75.5 Diabetic retinopathy

normal retina   diabetic retinopathy

"cotton-wool" spots
hemorrhages

COMPLICATIONS

Consistent maintenance of blood glucose within the expected reference range is the best protection against the complications of diabetes mellitus. Expected reference ranges can vary.

Cardiovascular and cerebrovascular disease

Hypertension, myocardial infarction, and stroke

NURSING ACTIONS

- Ensure the client's blood pressure is measured at each visit; the target blood pressure is less than 140/90 mm Hg, or less than 130/80 mm Hg for young adult clients.
- Facilitate tobacco cessation.
- Promote adherence to prescriptions for lipid-lowering medications and aspirin.

CLIENT EDUCATION

- Perform checks of cholesterol (HDL, LDL, and triglycerides) yearly and HbA1c every 3 months.
- Participate in regular activity for weight loss and control.
- Consume a diet of low-fat meals that are high in fruits, vegetables, and whole grains.
- Report shortness of breath, headaches (persistent and transient), swelling of feet, and infrequent urination.

Diabetic retinopathy

Impaired vision and blindness

CLIENT EDUCATION

- Perform eye exams every 1 to 2 years to ensure the health of the eyes and to protect vision.
- Conduct management of blood glucose levels.
- Hypoglycemia causes temporary blurred vision; report other vision changes that do not fluctuate with glucose levels.

Diabetic neuropathy

Caused from damage to sensory nerve fibers resulting in numbness and pain

- Peripheral neuropathy includes focal neuropathies, caused by acute ischemic damage or diffuse neuropathies, which are more widespread and involve slow, progressive loss. This can lead to complications (foot deformities, ulcers).
- Autonomic neuropathy can affect nerve conduction of the heart (exercise intolerance, painless myocardial infarction, altered left ventricular function, syncope), gastrointestinal system (gastroparesis, reflux, early satiety), and urinary tract (decreased bladder sensation, urinary retention). It affects the autonomic nervous system, which minimizes manifestations of hypoglycemia (diaphoresis, tremors, palpitations), which can be dangerous for the client.

NURSING ACTIONS

- Monitor for tolerance to activity and other indicators of cardiac insufficiency.
- Administer medications to promote gastric motility as prescribed (metoclopramide).
- Check for urinary retention.
- Provide foot care.

CLIENT EDUCATION

- Obtain annual exams by a podiatrist.
- Practice regular follow-up with provider to monitor and treat neuropathy.
- Report numbness and tingling, joint problems, or difficulties with digestion or urinary elimination.
- Traditional indication of a heart attack might not be present (chest, back, or jaw pain). Monitor for and report other manifestations.
- If there is reduced awareness of hypoglycemia, monitor blood glucose more carefully.

Diabetic nephropathy

Damage to the kidneys from prolonged elevated blood glucose levels and dehydration. The blood vessels near the kidneys become more permeable, allowing fluids to escape and can become scarred over time.

NURSING ACTIONS

- Monitor hydration and kidney function (I&O, blood creatinine level).
- Report an hourly output less than 30 mL/hr.
- Monitor blood pressure.

CLIENT EDUCATION

- Conduct yearly urine analysis, BUN, microalbumin, and blood creatinine level.
- Avoid soda, alcohol, and toxic levels of acetaminophen or NSAIDs.
- Consume 2 to 3 L/day of fluid from food and beverages with artificial sweetener, and drink an adequate amount of water.
- Report decrease in output to the provider.

Sexual dysfunction

Damage to nerve and vascular tissue of the sexual organs

Males can experience retrograde ejaculation or erectile dysfunction.

NURSING ACTIONS: Discuss sexual concerns and recommend options or referral, if the client desires.

CLIENT EDUCATION: Report concerns or difficulties with the provider.

Other complications

Periodontal disease, integumentary disorders (infections, patchy color changes, sclerosing)

DATA COLLECTION

RISK FACTORS

Diabetic ketoacidosis

- Lack of sufficient insulin related to undiagnosed or untreated type 1 diabetes mellitus or nonadherence to a diabetic regimen
- Reduced or missed dose of insulin (insufficient dosing of insulin or error in dosage)
- Any condition that increases carbohydrate metabolism (physical or emotional stress, illness)
- Infection is the most common cause
- Increased hormone production (cortisol, glucagon, epinephrine) that stimulates the liver to produce glucose and decreases the effect of insulin

Hyperglycemic hyperosmolar state

Common in clients who have type 2 diabetes mellitus.

- Sustained osmotic diuresis results in dehydration and a hyperglycemic hyperosmolar state, resulting from one of the following.
  - Lack of sufficient insulin related to undiagnosed or poorly managed diabetes mellitus. There is sufficient endogenous insulin present to prevent the development of ketosis, but not enough to prevent hyperglycemia.
  - Inadequate fluid intake or poor kidney function.
- Most common in older adult clients due to greater risk for dehydration. Older adult clients often seek medical attention later when much sicker and have age-related changes that affect the body's ability to recover (decreased ability for urine concentration, decreased thirst perception).
- Other factors that contribute to the development of HHS include infection, stress, medical conditions (myocardial infarction, cerebral vascular injury, sepsis), and some medications (glucocorticoids, thiazide diuretics, phenytoin, beta blockers, calcium channel blockers).

EXPECTED FINDINGS

	DKA	HHS
Polyuria: Osmotic diuresis resulting in excess urine production	✓	✓
Polydipsia (excess thirst): Osmotic diuresis causing excess loss of fluids resulting in dehydration and increased thirst	✓	✓
Polyphagia: Cell starvation due to inability to receive glucose resulting in increased appetite	✓	✓
Weight loss: Cells are unable to use glucose because of insulin deficiency. The body is placed in a catabolic state.	✓	✓
GI effects (nausea, vomiting, abdominal pain): Increased ketones and acidosis lead to nausea, vomiting, and abdominal pain	✓	
Blurred vision, headache, weakness: Fluid volume depletion caused from osmotic diuresis resulting in dehydration	✓	✓
Orthostatic hypotension: Fluid volume depletion caused by osmotic diuresis resulting in dehydration	✓	✓
Fruity odor of breath: Elevated ketone bodies (small fatty acids) used for energy that collect in the blood, which leads to metabolic acidosis	✓	
Kussmaul respirations: Deep rapid respirations occur in an attempt to excrete carbon dioxide and acid when in metabolic acidosis	✓	
Metabolic acidosis: Breakdown of stored glucose, protein, and fat to produce ketone bodies	✓	
Mental status changes: Lack of glucose circulating to the brain can cause neuron dysfunction and even cell death of the brain. The brain cannot produce or store glucose.	✓	✓
Seizures, myoclonic jerking: Related to blood osmolarity greater than 350 mOsm/L		✓
Reversible paralysis: Related to how elevated the blood osmolarity becomes (coma occurs once blood osmolarity is greater than 350 mOsm/L)		✓

LABORATORY TESTS

Therapeutic management is guided by serial laboratory analysis.

Blood glucose

DKA: Greater than 250 mg/dL (up to 800 mg/dL is typical)

HHS: Greater than 600 mg/dL

Blood electrolytes: Sodium (Na⁺) and potassium (K⁺)

DKA
- **Na⁺:** below, within, or above the expected reference range
- **K⁺:** elevated initially due to potassium leaving the cells. Following treatment with fluids and insulin, potassium re-enters cells causing hypokalemia.

HHS
- **Na+:** normal or low
- **K+:** normal to high as a result of dehydration; must monitor for decrease when treatment started

Ketones: Blood and urine

DKA: Present in blood and urine

HHS: Absent in blood and urine

Blood osmolarity

DKA: High

HHS: Greater than 320 mOsm/L

Arterial blood gases

DKA
- Metabolic acidosis with respiratory compensation (Kussmaul respirations)
- pH less than 7.35

HHS
- Absence of acidosis
- pH greater than 7.30

PATIENT-CENTERED CARE

NURSING CARE

- Check vital signs every 15 min until stable, then every 4 hr.
- Check for indications of dehydration (weight loss, decreased skin turgor, oliguria, rapid, weak pulse).
- Always treat the underlying cause (infectious process).
- Physiological changes in cardiac and pulmonary function can place older adult clients at greater risk for fluid overload (precipitate heart failure exacerbation) from fluid replacement therapy. Ⓒ
- The RN will initiate a rapid infusion of 0.9% sodium chloride for the first 2 to 3 hr, followed with a hypotonic fluid (0.45% sodium chloride) to continue to correct sodium and fluid losses.
- When blood glucose levels decrease to 250 mg/dL, the IV solution should be changed to one containing 5% dextrose to prevent hypoglycemia.
- Regular insulin is administered to treat hyperglycemia.
- Monitor blood potassium levels. Potassium levels might initially be increased because potassium has been pulled out of the cells, but with insulin therapy potassium will shift into cells, and the client will need to be monitored for hypokalemia.
  - Provide potassium replacement therapy.
  - Ensure cardiac rhythm is monitored constantly. Monitor for weak pulse, shallow respirations, malaise, muscle weakness, and confusion.
  - Make sure urinary output is adequate before administering potassium.
- Monitor for and report changes in neurologic status in clients who have HHS. Ⓠs
- Reinforce education to prevent recurrence.

OLDER ADULT CLIENTS ⓖ

- Instruct older adult clients to monitor blood glucose every 1 to 4 hr when ill.
- Emphasize the importance of not skipping an insulin dose when ill.
- Maintain hydration because older adult clients can have a diminished thirst sensation.
- Changes in mental status can prevent older adult clients from seeking treatment.

CLIENT EDUCATION

- Wear a medical alert bracelet.
- Take measures to decrease the risk of dehydration.
  - Unless contraindicated by other health problems, consume 2 to 3 L/day of fluid from food and beverages with artificial sweetener, and drink an adequate amount of water.
  - If blood glucose levels are low, consume liquids with sugar.
- Monitor glucose every 2 to 4 hr when ill and continue to take insulin.
- Check urine for ketones if blood glucose is greater than 300 mg/dL
- Consume liquids with carbohydrates and electrolytes (sports drinks) when unable to eat solid food.
- Notify the provider for the following.
  - Illness that lasts longer than 24 hr
  - Blood glucose greater than 200 mg/dL
  - Inability to tolerate food or fluids
  - Ketones in urine for more than 24 hr
  - Temperature of 38.6° C (101.5° F) for 24 hr

Application Exercises

1. A nurse is assisting with teaching a client about manifestations of Hypoglycemia and hyperglycemia. Sort the following findings into those associated with Hypoglycemia and those associated with Hyperglycemia.

   A. Blurred vision

   B. Clammy skin

   C. Fruity breath

   D. Dry skin

   E. Cool skin

   F. Warm skin

2. The nurse is reinforcing teaching the client who has diabetes mellitus about nutrition. What information should the nurse include?

3. A nurse is reviewing characteristics of diabetic ketoacidosis (DKA) and hyperglycemic hyperosmolar state (HHS) with a group of newly licensed nurses. Sort the following characteristics into those that occur in either DKA or HHS.

   A. Fruity odor of breath

   B. Seizure activity

   C. Nausea

   D. Occurs primarily in client's who have type 2 diabetes mellitus

Active Learning Scenario

A nurse is reviewing guidelines with a client who has type 1 diabetes mellitus about self-care during illness. What information should the nurse review with the client? Use the ATI Active Learning Template: System Disorder to complete this item.

LABORATORY TESTS: Discuss parameters for testing urine and notifying the provider.

CLIENT EDUCATION: Describe six review points.

Application Exercises Key

1. **HYPOGLYCEMIA**: A, B, E; **HYPERGLYCEMIA**: C, D, F

   When taking actions, the nurse should instruct manifestations of hypoglycemia include cool, clammy skin, and blurred vision. Manifestations of hyperglycemia include warm, dry skin, and fruity breath.

   Ⓝ *NCLEX® Connection: Physiological Adaptation, Unexpected Response to Therapies*

2. When taking actions, the nurse should instruct the client to consult a dietitian for collaborative education with the client and family on meal planning to include food intake, weight management, and lipid and glucose management. Plan meals to achieve optimal timing of food intake, activity, onset, and peak of insulin. Calories and food composition should be similar each day. Eat at regular intervals, and do not skip meals. Count grams of carbohydrates consumed for glycemic control. (15 g carbohydrates is equal to 1 carbohydrate exchange.) Restrict calories and increase physical activity if required to facilitate weight loss (for clients who are overweight or obese) or to prevent obesity. Include fiber in the diet to increase carbohydrate metabolism and to control cholesterol levels. Use artificial sweeteners. If caloric sweeteners are used, add this to daily carbohydrate intake. Read and interpret fat content information on food labels. Reduce intake of saturated and trans fats.

   Ⓝ *NCLEX® Connection: Health Promotion and Maintenance, Health Promotion/Disease Prevention*

3. **DKA**: A, C; **HHS**: B, D

   When taking actions, the nurse should reinforce that a fruity odor of the breath and nausea are characteristics of DKA due to ketosis and acidosis. Characteristics of HHS include seizure activity and it occurs primarily in client's who have type 2 diabetes mellitus.

   Ⓝ *NCLEX® Connection: Physiological Adaptation, Unexpected Response to Therapies*

Active Learning Scenario Key

Using the ATI Active Learning Template: System Disorder

LABORATORY TESTS: Test urine for ketones if blood sugar level is 300 mg/dL or higher and report if outside of the expected reference range.

CLIENT EDUCATION
- Monitor blood glucose every 2 to 4 hr.
- Continue to take insulin as prescribed.
- Call the provider if unable to tolerate liquids.
- If unable to eat soft foods, consume liquids equal to usual carbohydrate content.
- Call the provider for illness longer than 2 days, if unable to take fluids, and the blood glucose remains greater than 200 mg/dL despite treatment.
- Call the provider for fever that is greater than 38.8° C (101.2° F) or increasing.

Ⓝ *NCLEX® Connection: Physiological Adaptation, Alterations in Body Systems*

Case Study Exercises Key

1. B. **CORRECT:** When generating solutions, the nurse should plan to administer insulin aspart 10 min before a meal. Insulin aspart is a rapid acting insulin that peaks in 1 to 3 hrs.

   Ⓝ *NCLEX® Connection: Pharmacological Therapies, Medication Administration*

2. C. **CORRECT:** When prioritizing hypothesis, the greatest risk to the client is injury from hypoglycemia. Therefore, the first action the nurse should take is to administer 15 to 20 g of a rapidly absorbed carbohydrate, such as fruit juice, to the client.

   Ⓝ *NCLEX® Connection: Physiological Adaptation, Unexpected Response to Therapies*

3. C, D, E. **CORRECT:** When taking actions, the nurse should instruct the client to test water temperature with a wrist before bathing, to reduce the risk of burning feet in hot water. The client should trim toenails straight across to reduce the risk of a cut that can lead to an infection. The client should wear closed-toe shoes to reduce the risk of injury.

   Ⓝ *NCLEX® Connection: Health Promotion and Maintenance, Health Promotion/Disease Prevention*

When reviewing the following chapters, keep in mind the relevant topics and tasks of the NCLEX outline.

Basic Care and Comfort

NUTRITION AND ORAL HYDRATION: Reinforce client teaching on special diets based on client diagnosis/nutritional needs and cultural considerations.

Health Promotion and Maintenance

HEALTH PROMOTION/DISEASE PREVENTION: Check results of client health screening tests.

Physiological Adaptation

ALTERATIONS IN BODY SYSTEMS: Notify primary health care provider of a change in client status.

Reduction of Risk Potential

LABORATORY TESTS: Compare client laboratory values to normal laboratory values.

POTENTIAL FOR COMPLICATIONS OF DIAGNOSTIC TESTS/ TREATMENTS/PROCEDURES: Use precautions to prevent injury and/or complications associated with a procedure or diagnosis.

CHAPTER 76 *Immune and Infectious Disorders Diagnostic Procedures*

Diagnostic procedures for immune and infectious disorders involve identification of pathogenic micro-organisms. The most accurate and definitive way to identify micro-organisms and cell characteristics is by examining blood, body fluids, and tissue samples under a microscope. Effective treatment of infectious disease begins with identification of the pathogenic micro-organism.

White blood cells

- WBCs, or leukocytes, stimulate the inflammatory response and offer protection against various types of infection and foreign antigens.
- There are five types of WBCs—neutrophils, lymphocytes, monocytes, eosinophils, and basophils—used in laboratory analysis. Circulating WBCs is the differential, which lists the percentages of the types of WBCs for a total of 100%. The percentages represent the proportion of each type of cell in a sample of WBCs. If the percentage of one type of cell increases, the percentages of other types decrease accordingly.

INTERPRETATION OF FINDINGS

The expected reference range for WBCs is 5,000 to 10,000/mm^3.

Leukopenia is a total WBC count less than 4,000/mm^3. It can indicate drug toxicity, autoimmune disease, bone marrow failure, and some overwhelming infections.

Leukocytosis is a total WBC count greater than 10,000/mm^3. It can indicate inflammation, infection, some malignancies, trauma, dehydration, stress, steroid use, and thyroid storm. The WBCs involved in inflammation are neutrophils, macrophages, eosinophils, monocytes, and basophils.
- A client who has had a splenectomy can have a persistently increased WBC count.
- Older adult clients can have a severe bacterial infection without leukocytosis. Manifestations of infection, such as fever, can be absent in an older adult who has an infection. The nurse should monitor older adult clients carefully for infection risks. ©

Neutropenia is a neutrophil count less than 2,000/mm^3. Neutropenia occurs in clients who have viral infections, overwhelming bacterial infections, or are undergoing radiation or chemotherapy. A client who has neutropenia is at an increased risk for infection.
- The absolute neutrophil count (ANC) of a client who has neutropenia can help determine severity of the client's risk for infection. Multiplying the total WBC count by the percentage of neutrophils plus the percentage of bands determines the ANC.
- An ANC less than 1,000 means that neutropenic precautions are essential.
- Neutropenic precautions (a protective environment) include the following.
  ○ Restricting visitors
  ○ Prohibiting visits by people who have an infection
  ○ Restricting exposure to live (cut or potted) plants
  ○ Ensuring that all fruits and vegetables are well washed prior to eating
  ○ Avoiding contamination from the client's own bacterial flora by avoiding the measurement of rectal temperature and administering IM injections Qᴘᴄᴄ

Left shift is an increase in immature neutrophils (bands or stabs) that occurs with an acute infection. Neutrophil production increases, allowing the release of immature neutrophils that are not capable of phagocytosis (ingesting and destroying bacteria).

TYPES OF WBCS

Neutrophils

The majority of neutrophils are segmented (mature) with others being banded (not fully mature). Percentage and number of circulating neutrophils is used to measure a client's risk for infection.

PERCENTAGE OF CIRCULATING NEUTROPHILS: 55% to 70%

INCREASED WITH
- Acute bacterial infection
- Myelocytic leukemia
- Trauma
- Rheumatoid arthritis

DECREASED WITH
- Sepsis
- Radiation therapy, aplastic anemia, chemotherapy
- Influenza

Lymphocytes (T cells and B cells)

- T-lymphocytes initiate cell–mediated immunity.
- B-lymphocytes initiate humoral immunity.

PERCENT OF CIRCULATING LYMPHOCYTES: 20% to 40%

INCREASED WITH
- Chronic bacterial or viral infection
- Viruses (mononucleosis, mumps, measles)
- Bacteria such as hepatitis
- Lymphocytic leukemia, multiple myeloma

DECREASED WITH
- Leukemia
- Sepsis

Monocytes

PERCENT OF CIRCULATING MONOCYTES: 2% to 8%

INCREASED WITH
- Chronic inflammation
- Protozoal infections
- Tuberculosis
- Viral infections such as mononucleosis

DECREASED WITH
- Corticosteroid therapy
- Aplastic anemia
- Hairy cell leukemia

Eosinophils

Eosinophils are active against infection and limit inflammatory response.

PERCENT OF CIRCULATING EOSINOPHILS: 1% to 4%

INCREASED WITH
- Allergic reactions
- Parasitic infection
- Eczema
- Leukemia
- Autoimmune diseases

DECREASED WITH
- Stress
- Corticosteroids

Basophils

Basophils stimulate general inflammation and the response of allergy and hypersensitivity reactions.

PERCENT OF CIRCULATING BASOPHILS: 0.5% to 1%

INCREASED WITH: Leukemia

DECREASED WITH
- Acute allergic/hypersensitivity reactions
- Hyperthyroidism
- Stress reactions

Blood allergy test (IgE antibody test)

Blood allergy testing can determine sensitivity to various allergens. The technician mixes specific allergens with the blood and incubates it with radiolabeled anti-IgE antibodies. Blood allergy testing can complement skin testing or be an alternative when the risk of a hypersensitivity reaction to an allergen exists. The radioallergosorbent test (RAST) is one form of blood allergy testing. **Q**EBP

ADVANTAGES
- Will not precipitate a dangerous allergic reaction
- Quicker than skin testing

DISADVANTAGES
- Usually only tests for a small amount of allergens at a time, such as a panel for meat allergens, or panel for fruit allergens
- Can be less sensitive than skin testing

INDICATIONS

POTENTIAL DIAGNOSES: Environmental and food allergies

EXPECTED FINDINGS
- Report of hypersensitivity reactions
- Hives, asthma, gastrointestinal (GI) dysfunction, rhinitis, dermatitis, angioedema

CONSIDERATIONS

- Clients who have a condition that raises IgG levels can have falsely negative test results.
- Taking corticosteroids prior to testing can elevate IgE levels.

INTRAPROCEDURE: Obtain a blood sample.

INTERPRETATION OF FINDINGS

Results reflect allergen-specific IgE levels and thus the degree of sensitivity on a 0 to 6 scale.

Skin testing for allergens

- Skin testing for allergens involves the use of intradermal injections or scratching the superficial layer (scratch or prick test) of the skin with small amounts of potential allergens.
- Intradermal testing runs a higher risk of hypersensitivity reactions and follows inconclusive scratch-test results.

INDICATIONS

POTENTIAL DIAGNOSES: Environmental and food allergies

EXPECTED FINDINGS: Hives, asthma, GI dysfunction, rhinitis, dermatitis, angioedema

INTERPRETATION OF FINDINGS

- A localized reaction (wheal and flare) to an allergen is a positive reaction to that allergen.
- The larger the reaction, the more severe the allergy.

CONSIDERATIONS

PREPROCEDURE

NURSING ACTIONS
- Prepare the skin on the client's back or forearm for application of various allergens using soap and water.
- Use alcohol to remove any oil.
- Have equipment available to treat anaphylaxis. **Q**s

CLIENT EDUCATION: Prior to testing, withhold corticosteroids and antihistamines for 48 hr to 2 weeks, as instructed by the provider.

INTRAPROCEDURE

NURSING ACTIONS
- Scratch or prick the skin with a needle after applying a drop of an allergen.
- Use a standard pattern of application to help identify the allergen. Q EBP
- Apply control drops (substances that should not produce a reaction, such as 0.9% sodium chloride irrigation, and substances that should produce a reaction, such as histamine).
- Monitor for reactions after 15 to 20 min.

POSTPROCEDURE

NURSING ACTIONS
- Observe skin for areas of reaction, and document the allergen that is responsible.
- Remove all solutions from the skin.
- Recommend an antihistamine or topical corticosteroid if skin itches after testing.

CLIENT EDUCATION Q PCC
- Follow instructions for desensitizing and avoidance therapies for allergens.
- Follow a diet that eliminates some allergens (gluten-free).

Application Exercises

1. A nurse is caring for a client who has a WBC count of 20,000/mm³. The nurse should conclude that the client has which of the following?
   - A. Neutropenia
   - B. Leukocytosis
   - C. Left shift
   - D. Leukopenia

2. A nurse is reviewing the laboratory findings of a client who has measles. The nurse should expect to find an increase in which of the following types of WBCs?
   - A. Neutrophils
   - B. Basophils
   - C. Lymphocytes
   - D. Eosinophils

3. A nurse is preparing to administer a scratch test to a client who has possible food and environmental allergies. Which of the following actions should the nurse perform prior to the procedure? (Select all that apply.)
   - A. Cleanse the client's skin with povidone-iodine.
   - B. Ask the client about previous reactions to allergens.
   - C. Ask the client about medications taken over the past several days.
   - D. Inform the client to expect itching at one site.
   - E. Obtain emergency resuscitation equipment.

Active Learning Scenario

A nurse is caring for a client who will have a radioallergosorbent test (RAST). Use the ATI Active Learning Template: Diagnostic Procedure to complete this item.

INDICATIONS: List two.

INTERPRETATION OF FINDINGS: Describe one.

NURSING INTERVENTIONS (PRE, INTRA, POST): Describe one intraprocedure nursing action.

Active Learning Scenario Key

Using the ATI Active Learning Template: Diagnostic Procedure

INDICATIONS
- Possible environmental and food allergies
- Report of hypersensitivity reactions
- Hives, asthma, gastrointestinal dysfunction, rhinitis, dermatitis, angioedema

INTERPRETATION OF FINDINGS: The technician mixes specific allergens with the blood and incubates it with anti-IgE antibodies. Results reflect allergen-specific IgE levels and thus the degree of sensitivity on a 0 to 6 scale.

NURSING INTERVENTIONS (PRE, INTRA, POST): Obtain a blood sample.

Ⓝ *NCLEX® Connection: Reduction of Risk Potential, Diagnostic Tests*

Application Exercises Key

1. A. Neutropenia is a neutrophil count less than 2,000/mm³.
   B. **CORRECT:** During data collection, it is important for the nurse to recognize cues and identify that a WBC count greater than 10,000/mm³ indicates inflammation or infection (leukocytosis).
   C. A left shifts means that there is an increase in immature neutrophils.
   D. Leukopenia is a total WBC count of less than 4,000/mm³.

   Ⓝ *NCLEX® Connection: Reduction of Risk Potential, Laboratory Values*

2. A. Neutrophils increase with an acute bacterial infection.
   B. Basophils increase with leukemia.
   C. **CORRECT:** During data collection, it is important for the nurse to compare client findings to expected findings. Lymphocytes increase with viral infections (measles, mumps, mononucleosis).
   D. Eosinophils increase with allergic reactions, leukemia, eczema, and parasitic infections.

   Ⓝ *NCLEX® Connection: Reduction of Risk Potential, Laboratory Values*

3. B, C, D, E. **CORRECT:** When the nurse is planning or generating solutions, it is important to identify evidence-based nursing actions for all procedures. The nurse should wash the skin with soap and water prior to the procedure; povidone-iodine is not used as it could elicit an allergic response. The nurse should ask about any previous reactions to allergens and if any medications such as antihistamines or corticosteroids have been taken as these can suppress allergic reactions. Emergency equipment should be readily available even if the client denies any previous anaphylactic reactions.

   Ⓝ *NCLEX® Connection: Reduction of Risk Potential, Diagnostic Tests*

CHAPTER 77 *Immunizations*

Administration of a vaccine causes production of antibodies that prevent illness from a specific microbe. Vaccines can be made from killed viruses or live, attenuated (weakened) viruses.

For additional information, refer to **PHARMACOLOGY REVIEW MODULE, CHAPTER 36: IMMUNIZATIONS.**

IMMUNITY

ACTIVE IMMUNITY is an adaptive process that allows the body to make antibodies in response to the entry of antigens into the body. Active immunity develops over several weeks to months and is long-lasting.

- **Active-natural immunity** develops when the body produces antibodies in response to exposure to a live pathogen that enters the body naturally. ⃝**EBP**
- **Active-artificial immunity** develops after a vaccine is given and the body produces antibodies in response to exposure to a killed or attenuated virus.

PASSIVE IMMUNITY develops when antibodies that are created by another human or animal are transferred to the client. Because the client does not independently develop antibodies, passive immunity is temporary.

- **Passive-natural immunity** occurs when antibodies are passed from the mother to the fetus/newborn through the placenta and breast milk.
- **Passive-artificial immunity** occurs after administration of antibodies in the form of immune globulins to an individual who requires immediate protection against a disease when re exposure has already occurred, such as following a bite from a poisonous snake or an animal who has rabies. The individual's protection from the disease will only extend for several weeks or months.

ADMINISTRATION

The Centers for Disease Control and Prevention (CDC) immunization recommendations for adults (19 years and older) follows. Go to the CDC's website for updates.

Tetanus, diphtheria (Td) booster: Give booster every 10 years. For adults 19 and older who did not receive a dose of tetanus, diphtheria, pertussis (Tdap) previously, substitute one dose with Tdap.

Measles, mumps, and rubella (MMR) vaccine: Follow recommendations for administering one or two doses to clients between the ages of 19 and 49 who lack documentation of immunization or prior infection, or laboratory proof of immunity. People born before 1957 are considered immune to measles and mumps.

- Anaphylactic-like reaction to gelatin or neomycin is also a contraindication for not administering the MMR vaccine.
- Use caution when administering to a client who has history of thrombocytopenia or thrombocytopenic purpura.

Varicella vaccine: Give two doses to adults who do not have evidence of a previous infection (or one dose, depending on the type of zoster vaccine). Give a second dose to adults who have had only one previous dose.

- Varicella vaccine is contraindicated for clients who have some cancers or have hypersensitivity to neomycin and gelatin.
- The vaccine is not recommended for clients who have HIV, congenital immune deficiencies, or those taking immunosuppressive medications.

Pneumococcal vaccine

Pneumococcal polysaccharide vaccine (PPSV23) and pneumococcal conjugate vaccine (PCV-15 and PVC-20). Follow recommendations for administration to adults who are immunocompromised, have specific chronic diseases, smoke cigarettes, live in long-term care facilities, or received previous doses of PCV13 and or PPSV23.

- PPSV23 is not effective in children younger than 2 years old.
- For adults who have not been immunized with a pneumococcal conjugate vaccine, either administer one dose PCV15 , then give PPSV23 in12 months, or administer one dose PCV20. ⃝**G**
- 13-valent pneumococcal conjugate vaccine (PCV-13) is recommended for infants and children.

Hepatitis A

2 to 3 doses depending on vaccine type.
One month after the first dose of hepatitis A vaccine, 94% to 100% of adults and children develop a protective level of antibodies. Adults who receive the second dose have 100% protective levels of antibodies after 1 month.

Hepatitis B: 2, 3, or 4 doses depending on vaccine type or medical condition. There must be at least 1 month between doses one and two, and at least 2 months between doses two and three. A minimum of 4 months are required between doses one and three.

- Clients have greater than 85% protection after the second dose of hepatitis B vaccine and more than 90% after the third dose.
- The antibody duration of protection is 5 to 7 years.

Influenza vaccine

- Recommended for all adults annually.
- Inactivated influenza vaccine (IIV) is approved for clients who are pregnant.
- Recombinant influenza vaccine (RIV) is approved for adults 18 years and older.

- The live attenuated vaccine (LAIV), given as a nasal spray, is indicated only for clients ages 2 to 49, who are not immunocompromised.
- Clients who have a severe allergy to chicken eggs, such as respiratory distress, should receive the influenza vaccine under medical supervision. Clients who had a previous severe reaction to the influenza vaccine should not receive the influenza vaccine.
- Precautions: Occurrence of Guillain-Barré syndrome within 6 weeks of prior influenza vaccine.
- Administration recommendations can change yearly, because the vaccine is created with different influenza strains each year. The vaccine is typically available beginning in early fall.

Meningococcal (MenACWY, MenB)
- **MenACWY:** 2 doses are recommended for children (1 dose at 11-12 years of age, 2 dose (booster) at 16 years of age.
- **MenACWY:** Administer to clients greater than 16 years of age who are at high risk (history sickle cell disease, history of HIV, travel outside the US frequently to hyperendemic areas or live in high-risk areas, military, college student living in dorms. Two doses recommended if not vaccinated previously. Adults who are at high risk should receive reimmunization every 5 years.
- MenB is recommended for those who are at increased risk for meningococcal disease (history sickle cell disease, military, college student), 2 doses between 16-23 years of age at least 1 to 6 months apart . Can reimmunize every 2-3 years for clients who remain at high risk.

Human papilloma virus vaccine
- There are three types of vaccines; only the 9-valent vaccine is available for use in the U.S.
- 9-valent human papillomavirus (9vHPV) prevents HPV 6, 11, 16, 18, plus HPV 31, 33, 45, 52, and 58 noninfectious virus-like particles (VLP). Administered to adolescents as young as age 9 years but usually at ages 11 to 12 years.
- If initial dose is administered before age 15, only 2 doses are required, and the second should be given 6 to 12 months after the first.
- If the initial dose is administered after the 15th birthday, 3 doses are required. The second dose is recommended 1 to 2 months after the first, and the third dose 6 months from the first.
- Recommend a 2-3 dose series depending on age of initial dose. Do not restart if vaccine schedule was interrupted.
  - 9-14 years of age for initial dose: 2 dose series at (0, 6-12 months)
  - Greater than 15 years of age for initial dose: 3 dose series (0, 1-2 months, 6 months)
- Vaccine is not recommended for clients who are older than 26 years of age. Can be administered to clients 27-45 years of age after shared decision making with provider.

Zoster vaccine: Recommended as a one-time dose for all adults older than 60 years. ⓒ
- Clients who are immunocompromised should receive the vaccine at age 19.

COVID-19
- Refer to CDC guidelines for various age groups
- Not recommended for children less than 6 months of age.
- Administer IM
- **Current Recommendations are as follows:**
- **mRNA vaccine and protein subunit vaccine:**
  - 2-Primary doses: given 3-8 weeks apart.
  - 1-dose of bivalent mRNA booster recommended to clients ages 12 to 18 years and older at least 2 months following other monovalent boosters and to replace other booster recommendations.
  - Clients who are immunocompromised: 3 primary doses: 1 and 2 given 3-8 weeks apart, dose 3, at least 4 weeks later. Followed by 1-dose of bivalent mRNA booster at least 2 months later.
- **Adenovirus vector vaccine** (Use of adenovirus vector vaccine is restricted):
  - For clients who have previously received a primary dose, administer 1-dose of bivalent mRNA booster at least 2 months later.

PURPOSE

EXPECTED PHARMACOLOGICAL ACTION

Immunizations produce antibodies that provide active immunity. Immunizations can take months to have an effect, but they provide long-lasting protection against infectious diseases.

THERAPEUTIC USES

- Eradication of infectious diseases
- Prevention of childhood and adult infectious diseases and their complications (tetanus, pneumococcal pneumonia, hepatitis)

CONTRAINDICATIONS/PRECAUTIONS

- An anaphylactic reaction to a vaccine is a contraindication to further doses of that vaccine. Qs
- An anaphylactic reaction to a vaccine is a contraindication to use of other vaccines containing the same substance.
- Moderate or severe illnesses with or without fever are precautions to receiving immunizations. The common cold and other minor illnesses are not contraindications.
- Do not administer live virus vaccines, such as varicella or MMR, to a client who is severely immunocompromised.
- Precautions to immunizations require the provider to analyze data and weigh the risks that come with and without immunizations.

Td, DTaP, Tdap

ADVERSE EFFECTS
- Mild: Redness, swelling, and tenderness at the injection site; low fever; behavioral changes (drowsiness, irritability, anorexia)
- Moderate: Fever 40.6° C (105° F) or greater; seizures (with or without fever); shock-like state
- Severe: Acute encephalopathy (rare)

CONTRAINDICATIONS: Occurrence of encephalopathy within 7 days following prior dose of the vaccine

PRECAUTIONS
- Occurrence of Guillain-Barré syndrome within 6 weeks of prior dose of tetanus toxoid
- Progressive neurologic disorders; uncontrolled seizures
- Fever within 48 hr of prior dose
- Shock-like state within 48 hr of prior dose
- Seizures within 3 days of prior dose

MMR

ADVERSE EFFECTS
- Mild: Local reactions (rash; fever; swollen glands in cheeks or neck)
- Moderate: Joint pain and stiffness lasting for days to weeks, febrile seizure, low platelet count
- Severe: Transient thrombocytopenia

PRECAUTIONS
- Transfusion with blood product containing antibodies within the prior 11 months
- Simultaneous tuberculin skin testing

Varicella

ADVERSE EFFECTS
- Mild: Tenderness and swelling at injection site, fever, rash (mild) for up to 1 month after immunization
- Moderate: Seizures
- Severe: Pneumonia, low blood count (extremely rare), severe brain reactions (extremely rare)

CONTRAINDICATIONS: Pregnancy, severe immunodeficiency

PRECAUTIONS
- Transfusion with blood product containing antibodies within the prior 11 months
- Treatment with antiviral medication within 24 hr prior to immunization (avoid taking antivirals for 14 days following immunization)
- Extended use (2 weeks or longer) of corticosteroids or other medications that affect the immune system
- Cancer

Pneumococcal conjugate

ADVERSE EFFECTS
- Swelling, redness and tenderness at site of injection
- Fever
- Irritability
- Drowsiness
- Anorexia

CONTRAINDICATIONS: Anaphylactic reaction to any vaccine containing diphtheria toxoid

Pneumococcal polysaccharide

ADVERSE EFFECTS
- Redness and tenderness at site of injection
- Fever
- Myalgia

Hepatitis A

ADVERSE EFFECTS
- Local reaction at injection site
- Headache
- Loss of appetite
- Mild fatigue

CONTRAINDICATIONS: Hypersensitivity after previous dose or components of vaccine (neomycin)

Hepatitis B

ADVERSE EFFECTS
- Local reaction at injection site
- Temperature of 37.7° C (99.9° F) or greater

CONTRAINDICATIONS: Severe allergy (anaphylaxis) to yeast

Inactivated influenza

ADVERSE EFFECTS
- Swelling, redness, and tenderness at the injection site
- Hoarseness
- Fever
- Malaise
- Headache
- Cough
- Aches
- Increased risk for Guillain-Barré syndrome

PRECAUTIONS: Occurrence of Guillain-Barré syndrome within 6 weeks of prior influenza vaccine

Live, attenuated influenza

ADVERSE EFFECTS
- Vomiting, diarrhea
- Cough
- Fever
- Headache
- Myalgia
- Nasal congestion/runny nose

CONTRAINDICATIONS: Age 50 years or older

PRECAUTIONS
- Occurrence of Guillain-Barré syndrome within 6 weeks of prior influenza vaccine
- Treatment with antiviral medication within 48 hr prior to immunization (avoid taking antivirals for 14 days following immunization)
- Some chronic conditions

  Clients who have a history of a severe egg allergy, having any manifestation of allergy other than hives, should receive the immunization where a provider is present and emergency equipment is available.

Meningococcal MenACWY

CONTRAINDICATIONS: Reaction to tetanus toxoid vaccine

ADVERSE EFFECTS
- Mild local reaction and rare risk of allergic response
- Possible mild fever

Zoster

ADVERSE EFFECTS
- Local reaction at injection site
- Headache

CONTRAINDICATIONS: Existing herpes zoster infection

COVID-19

ADVERSE EFFECTS
- Pain, redness and swelling at the injection site
- Fatigue, headache, muscle pain, chills, fever, nausea
- Severe allergic reaction (rare)

CONTRAINDICATIONS
- Severe allergic reaction (anaphylaxis) following a previous dose to a component of the COVID-19 vaccine
- Known diagnosed allergy to a component of the COVID-19 vaccine

PRECAUTIONS
- Moderate or severe acute illness
- History of an immediate allergic reaction to any non-COVID-19 vaccine or injectable therapy

Human papilloma virus (9vHPV)

ADVERSE EFFECTS
- Mild local reaction and fever
- Mild to moderate fever
- Headache
- Fainting shortly after receiving vaccine

CONTRAINDICATIONS: Severe allergy (anaphylaxis) to yeast

INTERACTIONS

None significant

NURSING ADMINISTRATION

- Have emergency medications and equipment on standby in case the client experiences an allergic response such as anaphylaxis (rare) or serious reaction at injection site. Qs
- Follow storage and reconstitution directions.
- Provide written vaccine information sheets (VIS), and review the content with clients. Document the publication date of each VIS given to the client.
- Administer antipyretic for fever, apply cool compress for localized tenderness, and mobilize the affected extremity.
- Instruct clients to observe for complications and to notify the provider if adverse effects occur.
- Document administration of vaccines including date, route, site, type, manufacturer, lot number, and expiration date. Include the name, address, and title of the person administering the vaccine, and the address of the facility where the permanent record is located. Qι

ADULTS

- Give subcutaneous immunizations in outer aspect of the upper arm or anterolateral thigh.
- Give IM immunizations into the deltoid muscle.
- Report any unusual or serious adverse effects to the Vaccine Adverse Event Reporting System (VAERS) by calling 800-822-7967, using the reporting form which can be printed from the FDA website (www.fda.gov), or the CDC website (www.cdc.gov).

NURSING EVALUATION OF MEDICATION EFFECTIVENESS

Depending on therapeutic intent, effectiveness can be evidenced by development of immunity.

1. A nurse is assisting with teaching a class on immunity. Sort the following into either an example of Active or Passive immunity.

   A. Antibodies are passed from the mother to the fetus.

   B. Antibodies are produced after exposure to a killed virus.

   C. Antibodies are produced after an infection.

   D. Antibodies are administered in the form of immune globulins.

2. A nurse is reinforcing teaching with a client who is receiving an injection of hepatitis B immune globulin. Which of the following statements should the nurse make?

   A. "This vaccine is contraindicated in clients who are allergic to eggs."

   B. "This vaccine requires one single injection."

   C. "This vaccine provides you with passive immunity."

   D. "This vaccine contains a live attenuated virus."

3. A nurse is assisting with teaching a class about vaccines. Match the following clients with the recommended vaccines.

A. Clients, age 50 or older	1. Meningococcal vaccine
B. Pregnant women	2. Tetanus, diphtheria, and pertussis vaccine
C. Students living in dormitories	3. Zoster vaccine

4. A nurse is assisting with teaching a class about vaccines. Sort the following vaccines into those that are contraindicated in clients who are Pregnant and those that are contraindicated in clients who are Severely allergic to neomycin.

   A. Varicella

   B. Live attenuated influenza

   C. Hepatitis A

   D. MMR

5. A nurse is preparing to document administration of a meningococcal vaccine to a client. What information should the nurse plan to include in the documentation?

A nurse at a community health clinic is assisting with administering influenza vaccines for a group of clients. What information should the nurse take into consideration when selecting the type of vaccine to administer? Use the ATI Active Learning Template: Medication to complete this item.

NURSING INTERVENTIONS: Identify the three types of influenza vaccine and the available routes of administrations for each of the three types.

Active Learning Scenario Key

Using the ATI Active Learning Template: Medication

NURSING INTERVENTIONS

- Inactivated influenza vaccine (IIV) given IM with the exception of Fluzone, which is administered intradermal.
- Recombinant influenza vaccine (RIV) given IM.
- The live attenuated vaccine (LAIV) given as a nasal spray.

Ⓝ *NCLEX® Connection: Pharmacological Therapies, Medication Administration*

Application Exercises Key

1. **ACTIVE:** B, C; **PASSIVE:** A, D

   When taking actions, the nurse should instruct examples of active immunity include when antibodies are produced after exposure to a killed virus, and when antibodies are produced following an infection. Antibodies that are passed from a mother to a fetus and antibodies that are administered in the form of immune globulins are examples of passive immunity.

   Ⓝ *NCLEX® Connection: Physiological Adaptation, Basic Pathophysiology*

2. C. **CORRECT:** When taking actions, the nurse should instruct the client that this vaccine provides passive-artificial immunity to protect against the hepatitis B virus.

   Ⓝ *NCLEX® Connection: Pharmacological Therapies, Expected Actions/Outcomes*

3. A, 3; B, 2; C, 1

   When taking actions, the nurse should instruct that students who live in dormitories should receive the meningococcal vaccine to protect them from meningococcal disease. Pregnant women should receive the tetanus, diphtheria, and pertussis vaccine to protect the newborn infant from pertussis. Clients, age 50 or older, should receive the zoster vaccine to protect them from herpes zoster.

   Ⓝ *NCLEX® Connection: Pharmacological Therapies, Adverse Effects/Contraindications/Side Effects/Interactions*

4. **PREGNANT:** A, B, D; **SEVERE NEOMYCIN ALLERGY:** C

   When taking actions, the nurse should instruct that pregnancy is a contraindication for the varicella, live attenuated influenza, and the MMR vaccines. Hepatitis A vaccine is contraindicated in clients who are severely allergic to neomycin.

   Ⓝ *NCLEX® Connection: Pharmacological Therapies, Adverse Effects/Contraindications/Side Effects/Interactions*

5. When taking actions, the nurse should instruct that pregnancy is a contraindication for the varicella, live attenuated influenza, and the MMR vaccines. Hepatitis A vaccine is contraindicated in clients who are severely allergic to neomycin.

   Ⓝ *NCLEX® Connection: Pharmacological Therapies, Adverse Effects/Contraindications/Side Effects/Interactions*

When reviewing the following chapters, keep in mind the relevant topics and tasks of the NCLEX outline.

Basic Care and Comfort

NONPHARMACOLOGICAL COMFORT INTERVENTIONS: Assist in planning comfort interventions for client with impaired comfort.

NUTRITION AND ORAL HYDRATION: Reinforce client teaching on special diets based on client diagnosis/nutritional needs and cultural considerations.

Health Promotion and Maintenance

HEALTH PROMOTION/DISEASE PREVENTION
Assist client in disease prevention activities.

Gather data on client health history and risk for disease.

Identify risk factors for disease/illness.

Pharmacological Therapies

ADVERSE EFFECTS/CONTRAINDICATIONS/SIDE EFFECTS/ INTERACTIONS: Identify potential and actual incompatibilities of client medications.

EXPECTED ACTIONS/OUTCOMES: Use resources to check on purposes and actions of pharmacological agents.

PHARMACOLOGICAL PAIN MANAGEMENT: Monitor and document client response to pharmacological interventions.

Physiological Adaptation

ALTERATIONS IN BODY SYSTEMS
Provide care to correct client alteration in body system.

Reinforce education to client regarding care and condition.

Identify signs and symptoms of an infection.

Notify primary health care provider of a change in client status.

BASIC PATHOPHYSIOLOGY: Identify signs and symptoms related to an acute or chronic illness.

Safety and Infection Control

STANDARD PRECAUTIONS/TRANSMISSION-BASED PRECAUTIONS/SURGICAL ASEPSIS: Protect immunocompromised client from exposure to infectious diseases/organisms.

CHAPTER 78 *HIV/AIDS*

Human immunodeficiency virus (HIV) is a retrovirus that is transmitted through blood and body fluids (semen, vaginal secretions).

HIV targets CD4+ lymphocytes, also known as T-cells or T-lymphocytes. T-cells work in concert with B-lymphocytes. Both are part of specific acquired (adaptive) immunity. HIV integrates its RNA into host cell DNA through reverse transcriptase, reshaping the host's immune system.

HIV is found in feces, urine, tears, saliva, cerebrospinal fluid, cervical cells, lymph nodes, corneal tissue, and brain tissue, but epidemiologic studies indicate that these are unlikely sources of infection.

All clients who are pregnant should be screened for HIV. Q EBP

DISEASE PROCESS STAGES

HIV infection is one continuous disease process with three stages.

Progression of HIV infection

- Manifestations occur within 2 to 4 weeks of infection.
- Manifestations are similar to those of influenza and can include a rash and a sore throat.
- Manifestations of acute HIV infection can include the following: fever, night sweats, chills, headaches, muscle aches, sore throat, and rash. The findings are temporary and resolve with the client returning to previous level of health.
- This stage is marked by a rapid rise in the HIV viral load, decreased CD4+ cells, and increased CD8 cells.
- The resolution of manifestations coincides with the decline in viral HIV copies.
- Lymphadenopathy persists throughout the disease process.

Chronic asymptomatic infection

- This stage can be prolonged and clinically silent (asymptomatic).
- The client can remain asymptomatic for 10 years or more.
- Anti–HIV antibodies are produced (HIV positive).
- Over time, the virus begins active replication using the host's genetic machinery.
  - CD4+ cells are destroyed.
  - The viral load increases.
  - Dramatic loss of immunity begins.

AIDS

- This stage is characterized by life-threatening opportunistic infections.
- This is the end stage of HIV infection. Without treatment, death occurs within 5 years.
- All people with AIDS have HIV, but not all people who have HIV have AIDS.

78.1 HIV infection stages

A confirmed case classification meets the laboratory criteria for a diagnosis of HIV infection and one of the four HIV infection stages.

To read more about HIV, go to the CDC's website.

Stage 1

DEFINING CONDITIONS: None

CD4+ T-LYMPHOCYTE COUNT: 500 cells/mm³ or more

CD4+ T-LYMPHOCYTE PERCENTAGE OF TOTAL LYMPHOCYTES: 29% or more

Stage 2

DEFINING CONDITIONS: None

CD4+ T-LYMPHOCYTE COUNT: 200 to 499 cells/mm³

CD4+ T-LYMPHOCYTE PERCENTAGE OF TOTAL LYMPHOCYTES: 14% to 28%

Stage 3 (AIDS)

Documentation of an AIDS-defining condition supersedes a CD4+ T-lymphocyte count of 200 cells/mm³ or more and a CD4+ T-lymphocyte percentage of total lymphocytes of more than 14%.

DEFINING CONDITIONS: One or more of the following.

- Candidiasis of the esophagus, bronchi, trachea, or lungs
- Herpes simplex: Chronic ulcers (more than 1 month duration)
- HIV-related encephalopathy
- Disseminated or extrapulmonary histoplasmosis
- Kaposi's sarcoma
- Burkitt's lymphoma
- Mycobacterium tuberculosis of any site
- *Pneumocystis jirovecii* pneumonia
- Recurrent pneumonia
- Progressive multifocal leukoencephalopathy
- Recurrent salmonella septicemia
- Wasting syndrome attributed to HIV

CD4+ T-LYMPHOCYTE COUNT: Less than 200 cells/mm³

CD4+ T-LYMPHOCYTE PERCENTAGE OF TOTAL LYMPHOCYTES: Less than 14%

Stage 4

No information available

HEALTH PROMOTION AND DISEASE PREVENTION

- Reinforce teaching with the client regarding virus transmission and ways to prevent infection, such as the use of condoms, abstinence, and avoiding sharing needles. (Refer to **FUNDAMENTALS FOR NURSING REVIEW MODULE: CHAPTER 34: SELF CONCEPT AND SEXUALITY.**)
- Encourage the client to maintain up-to-date immunizations, including yearly seasonal influenza and pneumococcal polysaccharide vaccine.
- Providers should use standard precautions when caring for the client.

DATA COLLECTION

RISK FACTORS

- Unprotected sex (vaginal, anal, oral)
- Multiple sex partners
- Occupational exposure (health care workers)
- Perinatal exposure
- Blood transfusions (not a significant source of infection in the U.S.)
- IV drug use with a contaminated needle
- Older adult clients
  - HIV infection can go undiagnosed in older adult clients due to the similarity of its manifestations to other illnesses that are common in this age group.
  - Older adults are more susceptible to fluid and electrolyte imbalances, malnutrition, skin alterations, and wasting syndrome than younger adults.
  - Older adult females experience vaginal dryness and thinning of the vaginal wall, increasing their susceptibility to HIV infection.

EXPECTED FINDINGS

- Chills
- Rash
- Anorexia, nausea, weight loss
- Weakness and fatigue
- Headache and sore throat
- Night sweats

LABORATORY TESTS

CBC and differential: Abnormal (anemia, thrombocytopenia, leukopenia)

Platelet count: Decreased less than 150,000/mm3

DIAGNOSTIC PROCEDURES

- CDC Recommends that everyone between the ages of 13 and 64 get tested for HIV at least once as part of routine health care; for people with certain risk factors, CDC recommends getting tested at least once a year.
- A positive result from an HIV antibody screening test (enzyme-linked immunosorbent assay [ELISA]) confirmed by a positive result from a supplemental HIV antibody test (Western blot or indirect immunofluorescence assay [IFA]).

- Home test kits are also available using a drop of blood. These provide anonymous registration and counseling before the test via a telephone call. (Refer to **FUNDAMENTALS FOR NURSING REVIEW MODULE: CHAPTER 34: SELF CONCEPT AND SEXUALITY.**)
- Two noninvasive tests are available using either mucosal fluid or urine.
- Clients who have a positive result from a confirmatory test (such as Western blot) should then be tested for viral load.

HIV RNA quantification (HIV viral load test)

- Determines viral load before beginning treatment
- Can be repeated at intervals to monitor disease progression, identify compliance with treatment and determine HIV medication resistance

HIV drug resistance testing (HIV genotype or HIV tropism)

- Guides changes in medication therapy when resistance occurs
- Useful with CD4 counts fall despite therapy

Liver profile, biopsies, and testing of stool for parasites

NURSING ACTIONS: Prepare the client for the test.

CLIENT EDUCATION Qpcc
- Understand the details of the test, such as length and what to expect.
- A positive Western blot or IFA test means the client has been exposed to and has the AIDS virus in their body, but this does not mean the client has clinical AIDS.
- Ask questions or express emotions.
- Understand and adhere to safe sexual practices.

Brain or lung MRI or CT scan

Detailed image of the brain or lung to detect abnormalities

NURSING ACTIONS: Prepare the client for the procedure.

CLIENT EDUCATION: Be aware of the length of time the test takes (up to 1 hr).

PATIENT-CENTERED CARE

NURSING CARE

- Collect data on risk factors (sexual practices, IV drug use).
- Monitor fluid intake/urinary output.
- Obtain daily weights to monitor weight loss.
- Monitor nutritional intake.
- Monitor electrolytes.
- Monitor skin integrity (rashes, open areas, bruising).
- Monitor pain status.
- Monitor vital signs (especially temperature).
- Check lung sounds/respiratory status (diminished lung sounds).
- Check neurologic status (confusion, dementia, visual changes).
- Encourage activity alternated with rest periods.

- Administer supplemental oxygen as needed.
- Provide analgesia as needed.
- Provide skin care as needed.

MEDICATIONS

Highly active antiretroviral therapy involves using three to four HIV medications in combination with other antiretroviral medications to reduce medication resistance, adverse effects, and dosages.

Fusion inhibitors: Enfuvirtide blocks the fusion of HIV with the host cell.

Entry inhibitors: Maraviroc blocks the CCR5 receptor on the CD4 T cell to prevent further progression of the infection.

Nucleoside reverse transcriptase inhibitors: Zidovudine interferes with the virus's ability to convert RNA into DNA.

Non-nucleoside reverse transcriptase inhibitors: Delavirdine and efavirenz inhibit viral replication in cells.

Protease inhibitors: Atazanavir, nelfinavir, saquinavir, and indinavir inhibit an enzyme needed for the virus to replicate.

Integrase inhibitors: Raltegravir and dolutegravir inhibit viral replication by stopping the HIV enzyme integrase from inserting into the host cell DNA.

Antineoplastic medication: Interleukin is an immunostimulant that enhances the immune response and reduces the production of cancer cells (used commonly with Kaposi's sarcoma).

NURSING ACTIONS

- Monitor laboratory results (CBC, WBC, liver function tests). Antiretroviral medications can increase alanine aminotransferase, aspartate aminotransferase, bilirubin, mean corpuscular volume, high-density lipoproteins, total cholesterol, and triglycerides. Qᴇʙᴾ
- Monitor total CD4+ T lymphocyte count as well as CD4 percentage and ratio of CD4 to CD8 cells.
  - Normal CD4-to-CD8 ratio is 2:1. A ratio of less than 1 indicates more severe disease manifestations.
  - Low CD4 T lymphocyte counts and steadily decreasing counts indicate poor prognosis or medication resistance.

CLIENT EDUCATION Qᴾᶜᶜ

- Be aware of the adverse effects of the medications and ways to decrease the severity of adverse effects.
- Take medications on a regular schedule and do not miss doses. Missed medication doses can cause drug resistance.

INTERPROFESSIONAL CARE

- Infectious disease services can be consulted to manage HIV.
- Respiratory services can be consulted to improve respiratory status and provide portable oxygen.
- Nutritional services can be consulted for dietary supplementation. Food services can be indicated for clients who are homebound and need meals prepared.

- Rehabilitation services can be consulted for strengthening and improving the client's level of energy.
- Recommend a referral the client to local AIDS support groups as appropriate. Qᴛᶜ
- Home health services can be indicated for clients who need help with strengthening and assistance regarding ADLs. Home health services can also provide assistance with IVs, dressing changes, and total parenteral nutrition (TPN).
- Long-term care facilities can be indicated for clients who have chronic HIV.
- Hospice services can be indicated for clients who have a late stage of HIV.

Alternative therapy

Vitamins, herbal products, and shark cartilage can help alleviate manifestations of HIV. Ask the client if they are taking herbal products. These can alter the effects of prescribed medications.

CLIENT EDUCATION

- Practice good hygiene and frequent hand hygiene to reduce the risk of infection.
- Avoid crowded areas or traveling to countries with poor sanitation.
- Avoid raw foods (fruits, vegetables) and undercooked foods (meat, fish, eggs).
- Avoid cleaning pet litter boxes to reduce the risk of toxoplasmosis.
- Keep the home environment clean and avoid being exposed to family and friends who have colds or flu viruses.
- Wash dishes in hot water using a dishwasher if available.
- Bathe daily using antimicrobial soap.
- Express understanding of the following instructions. Qᴾᶜᶜ
  - Transmission, infection control measures, and safe sex practices
  - Importance of maintaining a well-balanced diet
  - Self-administration of prescribed medications and potential adverse effects
  - Findings that need to be reported immediately (infection)
- Adhere to the antiretroviral dosing schedules.
- Conduct frequent follow-up monitoring of CD4+ and viral load counts.
- Perform constructive coping mechanisms.
- Identify primary support systems.
- Report manifestations of infection immediately to the provider.

COMPLICATIONS

Opportunistic infections

- **Bacterial diseases,** such as tuberculosis, bacterial pneumonia, and septicemia (blood poisoning, nocardiosis)
- **HIV-associated malignancies,** such as Kaposi's sarcoma, lymphoma, Hodgkin's lymphoma, non–Hodgkin's lymphoma, invasive cell carcinoma, and squamous cell carcinoma
- **Viral diseases,** such as those caused by cytomegalovirus, herpes simplex, and herpes zoster virus
- **Fungal diseases**, such as pneumocystis jiroveci pneumonia (PCP), candidiasis, cryptococcosis, coccidioidomycosis, and penicilliosis
- **Protozoal diseases**, such as PCP, toxoplasmosis, microsporidiosis, cryptosporidiosis, isosporiasis, giardiasis, and leishmaniasis

NURSING ACTIONS
- Implement and maintain antiretroviral medication therapy as prescribed.
- Assist with the administration of antineoplastics, antibiotics, analgesics, antifungals, and antidiarrheals.
- Administer appetite stimulants (to enhance nutrition).
- Monitor for skin breakdown.
- Maintain fluid intake.
- Maintain nutrition.

CLIENT EDUCATION: Report indications of infection immediately to the provider. Qᴘᴄᴄ

Wasting syndrome

NURSING ACTIONS
- Maintain nutrition orally or by TPN if indicated.
- Monitor weight, calorie counts, and I&O.
- Provide between–meal supplements/snacks.
- Decrease fat content of foods to prevent complications of fat intolerance.
- Rinse the client's mouth several times daily with saline or sodium bicarbonate and sterile water to reduce mouth pain and increase appetite.
- Serve at least six small feedings with high protein value. Qᴇʙᴘ

Fluid/electrolyte imbalance

NURSING ACTIONS
- Monitor fluid/electrolyte status.
- Report abnormal laboratory data promptly.
- Encourage the client to drink 2,000 to 3,000 mL of fluid daily.
- Make dietary adjustments to reduce diarrhea.

Seizures (HIV encephalopathy)

NURSING ACTIONS
- Maintain client safety.
- Implement seizure precautions. Qs

Application Exercises

1. A nurse is collecting data from a client suspected of having HIV. The nurse should identify that which of the following are risk factors associated with this virus? (Select all that apply.)
   - A. Perinatal exposure
   - B. Pregnancy
   - C. Monogamous partner
   - D. Older adult female
   - E. Occupational exposure

2. A nurse in the outpatient clinic is collecting data from a client who reports night sweats, fatigue, cough, nausea, diarrhea and has a temperature of 38.1° C (100.6° F). The client is concerned about the possibility of having HIV. Which actions should the nurse take? (Select all that apply.)
   - A. Perform physical data collection.
   - B. Ask the client when the symptoms began.
   - C. Provide the client with a pamphlet about HIV transmission.
   - D. Collaborate with the RN to determine if blood should be drawn for HIV testing.
   - E. Obtain a sexual history.

3. A nurse is caring for a client who is suspected of having HIV. The nurse should identify that which of the following diagnostic and laboratory values are used to confirm HIV infection? (Select all that apply.)
   - A. HIV antibody test
   - B. Immunofluorescence assay
   - C. CD4+ T-lymphocyte count
   - D. HIV RNA quantification test
   - E. Cerebrospinal fluid (CSF) analysis

4. A nurse is reinforcing teaching for a client who has stage 3 HIV disease. Which of the following client statements indicate an understanding of the teaching?
   - A. "I will wear gloves while changing the pet litter box."
   - B. "I should avoid using antibacterial soap as it will dry my skin."
   - C. "I will wear a cloth mask when I am around family members who are ill."
   - D. "I need to wash all fruits and vegetables well before eating."

5. A nurse is reinforcing teaching to a client with stage 2 HIV disease and is having difficulty maintaining a normal weight. Which of the following statements made by the client indicates an understanding of the teaching?
   - A. "I should eat a diet high in fats to promote weight gain."
   - B. "It is a good idea to eat three large meals each day."
   - C. "I only need about one liter of fluids each day."
   - D. "I should increase my intake of protein at every meal."

Application Exercises Key

1. A, D, E. **CORRECT:** When recognizing cues, the nurse should identify perinatal exposure of the HIV virus can occur across the placenta due to the infant's exposure to blood and vaginal secretions. Older adult women experience vaginal dryness and thinning of the vaginal wall, increasing their susceptibility to HIV infection. Needlesticks are the primary means of occupational exposure for healthcare workers.

   Ⓝ *NCLEX® Connection: Health Promotion and Maintenance, Health Promotion/Disease Prevention*

2. A, B, D, E. **CORRECT:** When generation solutions, the nurse should recognize the client's manifestations that can occur with multiple infections, including HIV, therefore, physical data collection is required at this time. The nurse should also gather more data about the timing of the start of symptoms as HIV manifestations can occur at two to four weeks post exposure. The nurse should obtain a sexual history as HIV is transmitted by genital, anal, or oral sexual contact. The nurse should collaborate with the RN to determine if a blood specimen is needed at this time. The CDC recommends that individuals between the ages of 13 and 64 get tested for HIV at least once as part of routine health care and those with risk factors get tested more frequently.

   Ⓝ *NCLEX® Connection: Physiological Adaptation, Alterations in Body Systems*

3. A, B. **CORRECT:** When analyzing cues the nurse should recognize a HIV antibody test along with an indirect immunofluorescence assay are standard tests to confirm the presence of the HIV antibody.

   Ⓝ *NCLEX® Connection: Reduction of Risk Potential, Laboratory Values*

4. D. **CORRECT:** When generating solutions, the nurses should instruct the client who has stage 3 HIV to wash all fruits and vegetable prior to eating to remove bacteria to avoid the risk of infection.

   Ⓝ *NCLEX® Connection: Reduction of Risk Potential, Potential for Alterations in Body Systems*

5. D. **CORRECT:** When recognizing cues, the nurse should identify the client understands the teaching by responding to increase their intake of protein at every meal. Protein is needed to make antibodies.

   Ⓝ *NCLEX® Connection: Reduction of Risk Potential, Potential for Alterations in Body Systems*

Active Learning Scenario

A nurse is contributing to the plan of care for a client who has AIDS. Use the ATI Active Learning Template: System Disorder to complete this item.

NURSING CARE: Describe at least three nursing actions.

Active Learning Scenario Key

Using the ATI Active Learning Template: System Disorder
NURSING CARE
- Collect data on risk factors (sexual practices, IV drug use).
- Monitor fluid intake/urinary output.
- Obtain daily weights to monitor weight loss.
- Monitor nutritional intake.
- Monitor electrolytes.
- Monitor skin integrity (rashes, open areas, bruising).
- Monitor pain status.
- Monitor vital signs (especially temperature).
- Check lung sounds/respiratory status (diminished lung sounds).
- Check neurologic status (confusion, dementia, visual changes).

Ⓝ *NCLEX® Connection: Physiological Adaptation, Alterations in Body Systems*

When reviewing the following chapters, keep in mind the relevant topics and tasks of the NCLEX outline.

Basic Care and Comfort

NONPHARMACOLOGICAL COMFORT INTERVENTIONS: Assist in planning comfort interventions for client with impaired comfort.

NUTRITION AND ORAL HYDRATION: Reinforce client teaching on special diets based on client diagnosis/nutritional needs and cultural considerations.

Health Promotion and Maintenance

HEALTH PROMOTION/DISEASE PREVENTION
Assist client in disease prevention activities.

Gather data on client health history and risk for disease.

Identify risk factors for disease/illness.

Pharmacological Therapies

ADVERSE EFFECTS/CONTRAINDICATIONS/SIDE EFFECTS/ INTERACTIONS: Identify potential and actual incompatibilities of client medications.

EXPECTED ACTIONS/OUTCOMES: Use resources to check on purposes and actions of pharmacological agents.

PHARMACOLOGICAL PAIN MANAGEMENT: Monitor and document client response to pharmacological interventions.

Physiological Adaptation

ALTERATIONS IN BODY SYSTEMS
Provide care to correct client alteration in body system.

Reinforce education to client regarding care and condition.

Identify signs and symptoms of an infection.

Notify primary health care provider of a change in client status.

BASIC PATHOPHYSIOLOGY: Identify signs and symptoms related to an acute or chronic illness.

Safety and Infection Control

STANDARD PRECAUTIONS/TRANSMISSION-BASED PRECAUTIONS/SURGICAL ASEPSIS: Protect immunocompromised client from exposure to infectious diseases/organisms.

CHAPTER 79 *Lupus Erythematosus, Gout, and Fibromyalgia*

Lupus erythematosus (lupus) is an autoimmune disorder in which an atypical immune response results in chronic inflammation and destruction of healthy tissue. Other autoimmune disorders include rheumatoid arthritis, vasculitis, multiple sclerosis, scleroderma (including Raynaud's phenomenon), and psoriasis.

In autoimmune disorders, small antigens can bond with healthy tissue. The body then produces antibodies that attack the healthy tissue. This can be triggered by toxins, medications, bacteria, and viruses. Control of manifestations and a decrease in the number and frequency of exacerbations is the goal of treatment, because there is no cure for autoimmune disorders. Occurrence of autoimmune disorders increases with age. ©

Gout, also known as gouty arthritis, is a systemic disorder caused by hyperuricemia (increase in serum uric acid). Urate levels can be affected by medications, diet, and overproduction in the body. This can cause uric crystal deposits to form in the joints, and a gout attack can occur.

Fibromyalgia is a chronic pain syndrome that involves stiffness, sleep disturbance, generalized muscle weakness, and chronic fatigue. People who have fibromyalgia have another form of a rheumatologic disorder, such as RA or SLE.

Lupus erythematosus

- Lupus varies in severity and progression. It is generally characterized by periods of exacerbations (flares) and remissions. Lupus can be difficult to diagnose because of the vague nature of early manifestations. The incidence of lupus is 1.8–7.6 per 100,000 individuals.
- Lupus is classified as discoid or systemic. A temporary form of lupus can be medication-induced.
  - **Systemic lupus erythematosus (SLE)** affects the connective tissues of multiple organ systems and can lead to major organ failure.
  - **Discoid lupus erythematosus (DLE)/cutaneous lupus erythematosus** only affects the skin.
  - **Medication-induced lupus erythematosus** can be caused by medications (procainamide, hydralazine, minocycline). Findings resolve when the medication is discontinued.

DATA COLLECTION

RISK FACTORS

- Genetic predisposition
- Females (sex assigned at birth) who are 20–40 years of age
- Ethnicity: African American, Asian, Hispanic, or Indigenous Peoples
- Triggers for exacerbations of lupus include trauma, infection, certain medications, UV light exposure, stress
- Diagnosis of lupus can be delayed in older adult clients because many of the manifestations mimic other disorders or can be associated with reports common to the normal aging process. Joint pain and swelling can significantly limit ADLs in older adult clients who have comorbidities. ©

EXPECTED FINDINGS

- Fatigue/malaise
- Alopecia
- Blurred vision
- Pleuritic pain
- Anorexia/weight loss
- Depression
- Joint pain, swelling, tenderness
- Weakness

PHYSICAL ASSESSMENT FINDINGS Q_{EBP}

- Fever (also a major indication of exacerbation)
- Anemia
- Lymphadenopathy
- Pericarditis (presence of a cardiac friction rub or pleural friction rub)
- Raynaud's phenomenon (arteriolar vasospasm in response to cold/stress)
- Erythematous "butterfly" rash on the nose and cheeks (raised, dry, scaly)
- Discoid: coin shaped lesions on body areas exposed to sun (face, scalp)
- Oral lesions
- Few to no manifestations if lupus is in remission
- With exacerbation of lupus, multiple body systems are often affected (kidney, heart, lungs, gastrointestinal tract, vasculature)

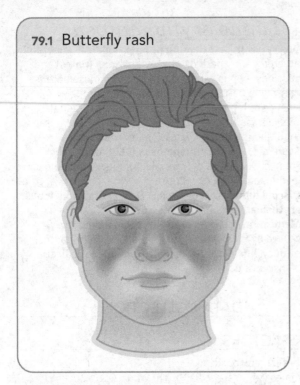

79.1 Butterfly rash

LABORATORY TESTS

Skin biopsy: Used to diagnose DLE by confirming the presence of lupus cells and cellular inflammation

Immunologic tests: Used to diagnose SLE
- Antinuclear antibodies (ANAs): antibodies produced against one's own DNA; positive titers in 95% of clients who have lupus
  - SLE prep
  - dsDNA (very specific for SLE; assists with differentiation between SLE and medication-induced lupus)
  - ssDNA
  - Anti-DNP
- Serum complement (C4): decreased
  - The complement system is made of proteins (there are nine major complement proteins). These proteins affect the immune system's development of inflammation. C4 are diagnostic for SLE because the exaggerated immune response in SLE depletes C4, leading to a decrease from the expected amount.
- Erythrocyte sedimentation rate (ESR): elevated due to systemic inflammation
- Anti-SS-a
- Anti-SS-b
- Anti-Smith
- Antiextractable nuclear antigens (Anti-ENAs)

BUN and blood creatinine: Increased (with kidney involvement)

Urinalysis: Positive for protein and RBCs (kidney involvement)

CBC: Pancytopenia

PATIENT-CENTERED CARE

NURSING CARE

- Monitor the following.
  - Pain, mobility, and fatigue
  - Vital signs (especially blood pressure)
  - Systemic manifestations
    - Hypertension and edema (renal compromise)
    - Urine output (renal compromise)
    - Diminished breath sounds (pleural effusion)
    - Tachycardia and sharp inspiratory chest pain (pericarditis)
    - Rubor, pallor, and cyanosis of hands/feet (vasculitis/vasospasm, Raynaud's phenomenon)
    - Arthralgias, myalgias, and polyarthritis (joint and connective tissue involvement)
    - Changes in mental status that indicate neurologic involvement (psychoses, paresis, seizures)
    - BUN, blood creatinine level, and urinary output for renal involvement
    - Nutritional status
- Provide small, frequent meals if anorexia is a concern. Offer between-meal supplements. Ⓠ EBP
- Encourage the client to limit salt intake for fluid retention secondary to steroid therapy.
- Provide emotional support to the client and family.

MEDICATIONS

NSAIDs

- Used to reduce inflammation and arthritic pain
- Contraindicated for clients who have impaired kidney function

NURSING ACTIONS: Monitor for NSAID-induced hepatitis.

Corticosteroids

Prednisone is used for immunosuppression and to reduce inflammation.

NURSING ACTIONS: Monitor for fluid retention, hypertension, and impaired kidney function.

CLIENT EDUCATION
- Do not stop taking steroids abruptly. Gradually taper the dosage as prescribed.
- Older adult clients are at an increased risk for fractures if corticosteroid therapy is used.

Immunosuppressant agents

- Methotrexate and azathioprine are used to suppress the immune response. Ⓠ PCC
- Belimumab is a human monoclonal antibody administered with other medications for SLE that inhibits the stimulation of B-cells, reducing the autoimmune response.

NURSING ACTIONS: Monitor for toxic effects and infection (bone marrow suppression, increased liver enzymes).

CLIENT EDUCATION: Avoid live vaccine administration for 30 days before beginning immunosuppressant therapies.

Antimalarial

Hydroxychloroquine is used for its anti-inflammatory properties and the suppression of synovitis, fever, and fatigue, and decreases the risk of developing skin lesions from the absorption of ultraviolet light from sun exposure.

NURSING ACTIONS: Encourage frequent eye examinations.

INTERPROFESSIONAL CARE

- Physical and occupational therapy services can be used for strengthening exercises and adaptive devices as needed.
- Ophthalmologists monitor client for visual deficits if taking hydroxychloroquine
- Recommend a referral for clients to support groups as appropriate.

CLIENT EDUCATION

- Wear a wide-brimmed hat, long-sleeve shirt, and long pants when outdoors.
- Avoid UV and prolonged sun exposure. Use sunscreen when outside and exposed to sunlight.
- Use mild protein shampoo and avoid harsh hair treatments.
- Use steroid creams for skin rash.
- Report peripheral and periorbital edema promptly.
- Report evidence of infection related to immunosuppression.
- Avoid crowds and individuals who are sick, because illness can precipitate an exacerbation.
- Understand the risks of pregnancy with lupus and treatment medications. Qs
- Cleanse skin with mild soap and inspect for open areas and rashes daily.
- Apply lotion to dry skin.
- Avoid applying drying agents to skin, such as powder or rubbing alcohol.
- Pat skin dry rather than rubbing.
- Understand the effect of the disease on lifestyle.

COMPLICATIONS

Lupus nephritis

Clients whose SLE cannot be managed with immunosuppressants, and corticosteroids can experience chronic kidney disease, resulting in the possible need for a kidney transplant. Lupus nephritis is the leading cause of death related to SLE.

NURSING ACTIONS: Monitor for periorbital and lower extremity swelling and hypertension. Monitor renal status (creatinine, BUN).

CLIENT EDUCATION
- Take immunosuppressants and corticosteroids as prescribed.
- Avoid stress and illness.

Pericarditis and myocarditis

Inflammation of the heart, its vessels, and the surrounding sac can occur secondary to SLE.

NURSING ACTIONS: Monitor for chest pain, fatigue, arrhythmias, and fever.

CLIENT EDUCATION
- Report chest pain.
- Take immunosuppressants and corticosteroids as prescribed.
- Avoid stress and illness.
- Report chest pain to the provider.

Gout

Gout or gouty arthritis is the most common inflammatory arthritis and has a prevalence rate of greater than 3%. Gout is a systemic disease caused by a disruption in purine metabolism in which uric acid crystals are deposited in joints and body tissues. Gout is classified as either primary or secondary.

Primary gout

- Most common.
- Primary gout has three stages: asymptomatic hyperuricemia, acute gouty arthritis, and chronic gout.
- Uric acid production is greater than excretion of it by the kidneys.
- Can have genetic component.
- Middle and older adult males (sex assigned at birth) and postmenopausal clients

Secondary gout

- Caused by another disease or condition (chronic kidney failure, some carcinomas, excessive diuretic use) that causes excessive uric acid in the blood.
- Treatment is based on treating the underlying condition.
- Can affect people of any age.

DATA COLLECTION

RISK FACTORS

- BMI greater than 30
- Heredity
- Trauma
- Alcohol ingestion
- Starvation dieting
- Diuretic use
- Some chemotherapy agents
- Chronic kidney failure

EXPECTED FINDINGS

- Severe joint pain, especially in the metatarsophalangeal joint of the great toe that could be very painful when touched or moved
- Redness, swelling, and warmth of affected joint
- Appearance of tophi (deposits of sodium urate crystals under the skin) with chronic gout

LABORATORY TESTS

Erythrocyte sedimentation rate (ESR): Elevated

Blood uric acid: Repeated measurements obtained because of dietary intake on results. Consistent elevation above 6.8 mg/dL is associated with gout.

Urinary uric acid: Elevated

Blood urea nitrogen (BUN), blood creatinine: Elevated

DIAGNOSTIC PROCEDURE

Aspiration of synovial fluid for analysis or uric acid crystals in affected joints

PATIENT-CENTERED CARE

NURSING CARE

Monitor the following.
- Pain
- Redness/swelling of affected joint
- Blood uric acid levels

MEDICATIONS

Acute gout

Antigout agent
- Colchicine (PO or parenteral) is used to decrease pain and inflammation.
- Use cautiously in clients who have impaired kidney function.

NSAIDs
- Indomethacin or ibuprofen is used to decrease pain and inflammation.
- Contraindicated for clients who have impaired kidney function.

CLIENT EDUCATION: Do not take on an empty stomach.

Corticosteroids: Prednisone used to treat inflammation.

NURSING ACTIONS: Monitor for fluid retention, hypertension, and impaired kidney dysfunction.

CLIENT EDUCATION: Do not stop taking the medication abruptly. Gradually taper dosage as prescribed.

Chronic gout

Xanthine oxidase inhibitor: Allopurinol or febuxostat is used as a maintenance medication to promote uric acid excretion and decrease its production.

CLIENT EDUCATION: Take after meals and with a full glass of water. Increase fluid intake.

Uricosuric: Probenecid is used as a maintenance medication to promote uric acid excretion.

NURSING ACTIONS: Monitor uric acid levels.

CLIENT EDUCATION: Do not use aspirin because it will decrease the effectiveness of the medication.

Enzymes
- Enzyme treatment is used with refractory gout, when acute or chronic gout does not respond to other medication treatment.
- Pegloticase is administered as an IV dose every other week. It converts uric acid to allantoin, so it can be excreted by the kidneys.

NURSING ACTIONS: Monitor closely for allergic reaction or anaphylaxis. The risk is increased because of the protein component in the medication.

CLIENT EDUCATION: Report allergic reaction to health care provider immediately.

Combination medications: Probenecid and colchicine are available as a combination medication.

CLIENT EDUCATION

- Stay on a low-purine diet, which includes no organ meats or shellfish. ⓠEBP
- Limit alcohol intake.
- Avoid starvation diets, aspirin, and diuretics.
- Limit physical or emotional stress.
- Increase fluid intake.
- Practice medication adherence.
- Use stress-management techniques.

Fibromyalgia

Fibromyalgia, also known as fibromyalgia syndrome, is a chronic pain syndrome which manifests as pain, stiffness, and tenderness at trigger points in the body. The pain is typically described as a burning, gnawing pain that can be elicited by palpating trigger points. Fibromyalgia affects about 5 million individuals in the United States.
- The client can also experience chronic fatigue, sleep disturbances, and functional impairment.
- Pain and tenderness vary depending on stress, activity, and weather conditions.

DATA COLLECTION

RISK FACTORS

- Females (sex assigned at birth) who are between the ages of 30 and 60 years of age
- History of stressors: trauma, infection, autoimmune disease, and genetic history
- Deep sleep deprivation

EXPECTED FINDINGS

- Moderate to severe fatigue
- Sleep disturbances
- Numbness/tingling of extremities
- Sensitivity to noxious smells, loud noises, and bright lights
- Headaches
- Jaw pain
- Depression
- Concentration and memory difficulties
- GI manifestations: abdominal pain, heartburn, constipation, diarrhea
- Genitourinary manifestations: frequency, urgency, dysuria, pelvic pain
- Visual changes

PATIENT-CENTERED CARE

NURSING CARE

- Monitor pain, mobility, and fatigue.
- Provide emotional support to the client and family.

MEDICATIONS

Serotonin-norepinephrine reuptake inhibitors (SNRIs) and anticonvulsants

Pregabalin (anticonvulsant) and duloxetine (SNRI) are used to increase the release of serotonin and norepinephrine, resulting in decreased nerve pain.

CLIENT EDUCATION
- Do not drink alcohol while taking this medication.
- SNRIs can cause drowsiness/sleepiness.

NSAIDs

- Used to decrease pain and inflammation
- Contraindicated for clients who have impaired kidney function

CLIENT EDUCATION: Do not take on an empty stomach.

Tricyclic antidepressants

Amitriptyline, nortriptyline, and trazodone are used to help induce sleep and decrease pain.
- Amitriptyline and nortriptyline can cause confusion and orthostatic hypotension in older adult clients.
- Trazodone is often the medication of choice for the older adult clients due to decreased adverse effects. Ⓖ

Combination medications

Tramadol has tricyclic and opioid components to reduce pain. Opioid component can lead to physical or psychological dependence or tolerance over time.

Other therapies

- Cognitive/behavior therapy
- CAM therapies: acupuncture

INTERPROFESSIONAL CARE

- Physical therapy can be helpful to decrease pain.
- Recommend a referral for the client to national foundations and local support groups.

CLIENT EDUCATION

- Limit intake of caffeine, alcohol, and other substances that interfere with sleep.
- Develop a routine for sleep.
- Engage in regular, low-impact exercise.
- Complementary and alternative therapies can be helpful (acupuncture, stress management, tai chi, hypnosis).

Active Learning Scenario

A nurse is reinforcing teaching with a client who has a new diagnosis of fibromyalgia. What should the nurse include in the discussion? Use the ATI Active Learning Template: System Disorder to complete this item.

ALTERATION IN HEALTH (DIAGNOSIS)

RISK FACTORS: Describe two.

EXPECTED FINDINGS: Include three findings.

MEDICATIONS: Identify two types of medications used to treat fibromyalgia along with their purpose and specific nursing considerations.

Application Exercises

1. A nurse is collecting data from a client who has a new diagnosis of SLE. Which of the following findings should the nurse expect?
   A. Client report of weight gain
   B. Petechiae on thighs
   C. Systolic murmur
   D. Client report of fatigue

2. A nurse assisting with the admission of a client who has systemic lupus erythematous (SLE). The client reports fatigue, joint tenderness, swelling, and difficulty urinating. Which of the following laboratory findings should the nurse anticipate? (Select all that apply.)
   A. Positive ANA titer
   B. Increased hemoglobin
   C. 2+ urine protein
   D. Increased blood C3 and C4
   E. Elevated BUN

3. A nurse is reinforcing self-care instructions with a client who has SLE. Which of the following statements by the client indicates an understanding of the instruction?
   A. "I should limit my time to 10 minutes in the tanning bed."
   B. "I should apply a powder to any skin rash."
   C. "I should use a mild soap for my personal hygiene."
   D. "I will inspect my skin monthly for rashes."

4. A nurse is reinforcing education with a client who is concerned about developing gout. Which of the following findings should the nurse identify as risk factors for gout? (Select all that apply.)
   A. Diuretic use
   B. BMI greater than 30
   C. Deep sleep deprivation
   D. Depression
   E. Excessive alcohol consumption

5. A nurse is assisting with providing care for a client who has new diagnosis of fibromyalgia. Which of the following classification of medications should nurse anticipate a prescription by the provider?
   A. Tricyclic antidepressants
   B. Calcium channel blockers
   C. Loop diuretics
   D. Beta blocker

Application Exercises Key

1. D. **CORRECT:** When recognizing cues while collecting data for a client who has new diagnosis of SLE, the nurse should expect the client to report/exhibit the following findings of fever, joint pain, malaise, weight loss, alopecia, facial rash with a butterfly appearance, and reports of fatigue.

Ⓝ *NCLEX Connection: Physiological Adaptation, Alterations in Body Systems*

2. A. **CORRECT:** When recognizing cues, the nurse anticipates that a client who has SLE could have a positive ANA titer, proteinuria, and elevated BUN. Since SLE is an autoimmune disorder, the ANA would be elevated because this indicates the presence of antibodies produced against the client's own DNA.
   B. A client who has SLE is expected to have pancytopenia, and decreased levels of C3 and C4.
   C. **CORRECT:** When recognizing cues, the nurse anticipates that a client who has SLE could have a positive ANA titer, proteinuria, and elevated BUN. Proteinuria and elevated BUN is an expected finding in SLE due to kidney damage.
   D. A client who has SLE is expected to have pancytopenia, and decreased levels of C3 and C4.
   E. **CORRECT:** When recognizing cues, the nurse anticipates that a client who has SLE could have a positive ANA titer, proteinuria, and elevated BUN. Proteinuria and elevated BUN is an expected finding in SLE due to kidney damage.

Ⓝ *NCLEX® Connection: Reduction of Risk Potential, Laboratory Values*

3. A. Clients with SLE should avoid prolonged sun exposure and the use of tanning beds and avoid applying topical powders or creams; steroid creams are typically suggested
   B. Clients with SLE should avoid prolonged sun exposure and the use of tanning beds and avoid applying topical powders or creams; steroid creams are typically suggested
   C. **CORRECT:** When evaluating outcomes for a client who has SLE and has received self-care instructions, the nurse should inform the client to avoid skin and scalp irritants and use mild soaps and shampoo for their personal hygiene.
   D. A client with SLE needs to inspect their skin daily for rashes or open areas.

Ⓝ *NCLEX® Connection: Physiological Adaptation, Alterations in Body Systems*

4. A, B, E. **CORRECT:** The risk factors for gout include diuretic use, BMI greater than 30, and the excessive consumption of alcohol. Alcoholic beverages can contain purines can cause exacerbations of gout and decrease kidney function.

Ⓝ *NCLEX Connection: Health Promotion and Maintenance, Health Promotion/Disease Prevention*

5. A. **CORRECT:** A client who has fibromyalgia may experience pain, stiffness, and sleep deprivation. Therefore, medications such as amitriptyline and trazodone, which are tricyclic antidepressants, can be prescribed to manage the client manifestations.

Ⓝ *NCLEX Connection: Pharmacological Therapies, Expected Actions/Outcomes*

Active Learning Scenario Key

Using the ATI Active Learning Template: System Disorder

ALTERATION IN HEALTH (DIAGNOSIS)
- Fibromyalgia, also known as fibromyalgia syndrome, is a chronic pain syndrome which manifests as pain, stiffness, and tenderness at certain "trigger points" in the body.
- The pain is typically described as a gnawing pain that can be elicited by palpating "trigger points".
- The client can also experience chronic fatigue, sleep disturbances, and functional impairment.
- Pain and tenderness vary depending on stress, activity, and weather conditions.

RISK FACTORS
- Females between ages of 26 and 60 years
- History of stressors: trauma, infection, autoimmune disease, family history
- Deep sleep deprivation

EXPECTED FINDINGS
- Moderate to severe fatigue
- Sleep disturbances
- Numbness/tingling of extremities
- Sensitivity to noxious smells, loud noises, and bright lights
- Headaches
- Jaw pain
- Depression
- Concentration and memory difficulties
- GI manifestations: abdominal pain, heartburn, constipation, diarrhea
- Genitourinary manifestations: frequency, urgency, dysuria, pelvic pain
- Visual changes

MEDICATIONS

Serotonin-norepinephrine reuptake inhibitors (SNRIs) and anticonvulsants
- Pregabalin (anticonvulsant) and duloxetine (SNRI) are used to increase the release of serotonin and norepinephrine, resulting in decreased nerve pain.
- Nursing Actions: Can cause drowsiness/sleepiness.
- Client Education: Do not drink alcohol while on this medication.

NSAIDs
- Used to decrease pain and inflammation.
- Nursing Actions: Contraindicated for clients who have impaired kidney function.
- Client Education: Do not take on an empty stomach.

Tricyclic antidepressants
- Amitriptyline, nortriptyline, and trazodone are used to help induce sleep and decrease pain.
- Nursing Actions: Amitriptyline and nortriptyline can cause confusion and orthostatic hypotension in older adult clients. Trazodone is often the medication of choice for the older adult client due to decreased adverse effects.

Ⓝ *NCLEX® Connection: Physiological Adaptation, Alterations in Body Systems*

UNIT 13   **IMMUNE SYSTEM AND CONNECTIVE TISSUE DISORDERS**
SECTION: CONNECTIVE TISSUE DISORDERS

CHAPTER 80 *Rheumatoid Arthritis*

Rheumatoid arthritis (RA) is a chronic, progressive inflammatory disease that can affect tissues and organs but principally attacks the joints, producing an inflammatory synovitis. It involves joints bilaterally and symmetrically, and typically affects several joints at one time.

RA is an autoimmune disease that is precipitated by WBCs attacking synovial tissue. The WBCs cause the synovial tissue to become inflamed and thickened. The inflammation can extend to the cartilage, bone, tendons, and ligaments that surround the joint. Joint deformity and bone erosion can result from these changes, decreasing the joint's range of motion and function.

RA is also a systemic disease that can affect any connective tissue in the body. Common structures affected are the blood vessels, pleura surrounding the lungs, and pericardium. Iritis and scleritis can also develop in the eyes.

The natural course of the disease is one of exacerbations and remissions. If RA is diagnosed and treated early, it is possible to avoid permanent joint damage.

HEALTH PROMOTION AND DISEASE PREVENTION

- Use adaptive devices that prevent development of deformity of inflamed joints during ADLs.
- Continue using affected joints and ambulating to maintain function and range of motion.

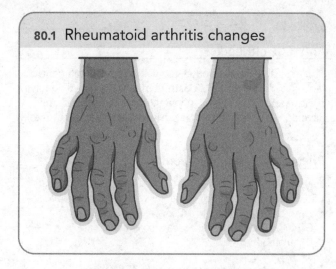

80.1 Rheumatoid arthritis changes

DATA COLLECTION

RISK FACTORS

- Female sex
- Age 30 to 50 years
- Genetic predisposition
- Bacterial or viral infection
- Environmental factors
- Older age

EXPECTED FINDINGS

Findings depend on the area affected by the disease process.
- Pain with movement
- Morning stiffness ⓠEBP
- Pleuritic pain (pain upon inspiration)
- Xerostomia (dry mouth)
- Anorexia/weight loss
- Fatigue
- Paresthesias
- Recent illness/stressor
- Joint pain
- Lack of function
- Joint swelling and deformity
  - Joint deformities are late manifestations of RA.
  - Joint swelling, warmth, and erythema are common.
  - Finger, hands, wrists, knees, and foot joints are generally affected.
  - Finger joints affected are the proximal interphalangeal and metacarpophalangeal joints.
  - Joints can become deformed merely by completing ADLs.
  - Ulnar deviation, swan neck, and boutonnière deformities are common in the fingers.
- Subcutaneous nodules
- Fever (generally low-grade)
- Early manifestations of RA (fatigue, joint discomfort) are vague and can be attributed to other disorders in older adult clients. ⓒ

LABORATORY TESTS

Anti-CCP antibodies

This test detects antibodies to cyclic citrullinated peptide (anti-CCP). The result is positive in most people who have rheumatoid arthritis, even years before manifestations develop. The test is more sensitive for RA than rheumatoid factor (RF) antibodies.

Rheumatoid factor antibody

Diagnostic level for rheumatoid arthritis is greater than 1:80 (expected reference range less than 60 units/mL).
- High titers correlate with severe disease.
- Other autoimmune diseases also can increase RF antibody.

Erythrocyte sedimentation rate (ESR)

Elevated ESR is associated with the inflammation or infection in the body.

Other autoimmune diseases also can increase ESR antibody.

C-reactive protein (CRP)

- This test can be done in place of ESR.
- This test is useful for diagnosing disease or monitoring disease activity, and for monitoring the response to anti-inflammatory therapy.
- Elevated levels indicate inflammation in the body (expected reference range is less than 1.0 mg/dL).

Antinuclear antibody (ANA) titer

Antibody produced against one's own DNA
- A positive ANA titer is associated with RA.
- Other autoimmune diseases also can increase ANA.

Elevated WBCs

- WBC count can be elevated during an exacerbation secondary to the inflammatory response.
- Decreased RBCs due to anemia.

DIAGNOSTIC PROCEDURES

Arthrocentesis

Arthrocentesis is synovial fluid aspiration by needle. With RA, increased WBCs and RF are present in fluid.

NURSING ACTIONS: Monitor for bleeding or a synovial fluid leak from the needle biopsy site.

CLIENT EDUCATION
- Take acetaminophen for pain.
- Apply ice.
- Avoid strenuous use of the joint over several days.

X-ray

X-rays are used to determine the degree of joint destruction and monitor its progression. They can provide adequate visualization and reveal bony erosions and narrowed joint spaces.

NURSING ACTIONS: Assist the client into position.

CLIENT EDUCATION: Minimize movement during the procedure.

PATIENT-CENTERED CARE

NURSING CARE

- Assist with and encourage physical activity to maintain joint mobility (within the capabilities of the client).
- Monitor for indications of fatigue.
- Reinforce with the client measures to do the following.
  ○ Maximize functional activity.
  ○ Minimize pain.
  ○ Monitor skin closely.
- Provide a safe environment. Qs
  ○ Provide referrals for physical therapy and occupational therapy.
  ○ Provide information for support organizations.
  ○ Facilitate the use of assistive devices.
  ○ Remove unnecessary equipment and supplies.
- Monitor for medication effectiveness (reduced pain, increased mobility)

Nutritional education

Eat small, frequent meals. Q EBP

MEDICATIONS

Acetaminophen

NSAIDs

- NSAIDs provide analgesic, antipyretic, and anti-inflammatory effects.
- NSAIDs can cause considerable gastrointestinal (GI) distress.
- Decreased dosages are recommended for older adult clients.

NURSING ACTIONS
- Request a concurrent prescription for a GI-acid lowering agent (histamine2-receptor antagonist, proton pump inhibitor) if GI distress is reported.
- Monitor for fluid retention, hypertension, and renal dysfunction.

CLIENT EDUCATION
- Take the medication with food or with a full glass of water or milk. If taking routinely, an H_2-receptor antagonist can also be prescribed.
- Observe for GI bleeding (coffee-ground emesis; dark, tarry stools).
- Avoid alcohol, which can increase the risk of GI complications.

COX-2 enzyme blockers, 770

- Cause less GI distress but carry a risk of cardiac disease.
- COX-2 inhibiting medications, such as celecoxib, are not recommended if the client has a history of myocardial infarction.

Corticosteroids

Corticosteroids (prednisone) are strong anti-inflammatory medications that can be given for acute exacerbations or advanced forms of the disease. They are not given for long-term therapy due to significant adverse effects (osteoporosis, hyperglycemia, immunosuppression, cataracts).

NURSING ACTIONS
- Observe for Cushingoid changes.
- Monitor weight and blood pressure.

CLIENT EDUCATION
- Observe for changes in vision; blood glucose; impaired healing; black, tarry stools; or weight gain.
- Avoid crowds.
- Follow the prescription (alternate-day dosing, tapering, discontinuing medication).

Disease modifying anti-rheumatic drugs (DMARDs)

DMARDs work in a variety of ways to slow the progression of RA and suppress the immune system's reaction to RA that causes pain and inflammation. Relief of manifestations might not occur for several weeks.
- **Antimalarial agent**: Hydroxychloroquine
- **Antibiotic**: Minocycline
- **Sulfonamide:** Sulfasalazine
- **Biologic response modifiers**: Etanercept, infliximab, adalimumab, and chelator penicillamine
- **Cytotoxic medications:** Methotrexate, leflunomide, cyclophosphamide, and azathioprine can cause severe adverse effects.

NURSING ACTIONS
- Monitor for allergic reactions and low WBC counts.
- Monitor lab results for decreased WBCs and platelets, and increased liver enzymes for clients taking leflunomide.

CLIENT EDUCATION
- Avoid crowds, which increase the risk of infection.
- Monitor for an allergic reaction.
- If taking leflunomide, report hair loss or diarrhea to the provider.
- Leflunomide is contraindicated during pregnancy, because it increases the risk of fetal birth defects .
- Many DMARDs can affect the liver; avoid alcohol consumption to prevent additional harm to the liver.

THERAPEUTIC PROCEDURES

Total joint arthroplasty

Surgical repair and replacement of a joint can be done for a severely deformed joint that has not responded to medication therapy.

Synovectomy

Surgical removal of the synovial membrane surrounding the affected joints

INTERPROFESSIONAL CARE

- Refer the client to support groups as appropriate.
- Refer the client to occupational therapy for adaptive devices that can facilitate carrying out ADLs and prevent deformities.
- A home health aide can be necessary for assistance with ADLs.

CLIENT EDUCATION

- Apply heat or cold to the affected areas as indicated based on client response.
  - Morning stiffness (hot shower)
  - Pain in hands/fingers (heated paraffin)
  - Edema (cold therapy)
- Conserve energy (space out activities, take rest periods, ask for additional assistance when needed).
- Follow routine health screenings.
- Use progressive muscle relaxation.
- Report manifestations that can indicate early or late exacerbation of the RA that need to be reported immediately (fever, infection, pain upon inspiration, pain in the substernal area of the chest). Q EBP
- Express feelings regarding effects of the disease on body image and self-esteem.
- Use nonpharmacologic pain relief through therapies (hypnosis, acupuncture, imagery, music therapy, spiritual practices).

Active Learning Scenario

A nurse is providing information about rheumatoid arthritis (RA) to a client who has a new diagnosis of RA. Use the ATI Active Learning Template: System Disorder and the ATI Pharmacology Review Module to complete this item.

CLIENT EDUCATION: List five instructions for the client regarding self-management of RA.

Application Exercises

1. A nurse is caring for a client who has rheumatoid arthritis. Which of the following tests are used to diagnose this disease? (Select all that apply.)

   A. Erythrocyte Sedimentation Rate

   B. Red Blood Cell count

   C. White blood Cell count

   D. Antinuclear antibody titer

   E. Potassium level

2. A nurse is collecting data about pain in a client who has rheumatoid arthritis. Which question should the nurse ask first?

   A. Where is your pain?

   B. What does it feel like?

   C. How does it change with time?

   D. How severe is your pain?

3. A nurse is reinforcing education with a client who has an acute exacerbation of rheumatoid arthritis about a new prescription of prednisone. Which of the following should the nurse include in the education? (Select all that apply.)

   A. You may have confusion while taking the medication

   B. This medication will be prescribed for long-term treatment

   C. Avoid crowds while taking this medication

   D. Your blood glucose may increase while taking this medication

   E. Drink plenty of fluids while taking this medication

   F. Visual changes should be reported if they occur

Active Learning Scenario Key

Using the ATI Active Learning Template: System Disorder

CLIENT EDUCATION

- Use heat therapy (hot shower, paraffin treatments) or cold to relieve discomfort.
- Remain physically active to promote joint mobility.
- Report indications of an acute exacerbation of RA (fever, infection, pain with breathing or in the center of the chest).
- Consider other nonpharmacological pain strategies (hypnosis, acupuncture, imagery, music therapy, progressive relaxation) with the provider's approval.
- Conserve energy (space out activities, take rest periods, ask for additional assistance when needed).
- Follow routine health screenings.
- Use progressive muscle relaxation.

Ⓝ *NCLEX® Connection: Physiological Adaptation, Alterations in Body Systems*

Application Exercises Key

1. A, C, D. **CORRECT:** When analyzing cues, the nurse should identify that a client who is suspected of having rheumatoid arthritis would have the erythrocyte sedimentation rate, white blood cell count, and antinuclear antibody titer evaluated to diagnose rheumatoid arthritis. Red blood cell count and potassium levels do not assist with diagnosing rheumatoid arthritis.

   Ⓝ *NCLEX® Connection: Reduction of Risk Potential, Diagnostic Tests*

2. A. **CORRECT:** When recognizing cues, it is important to identify where the pain is located to address the pain. The first question to ask the client is where their pain is located. The nurse should then ask the client to describe how their pain feels, followed by how their pain changes with time and the severity of their pain.

   Ⓝ *NCLEX® Connection: Pharmacological Therapies, Pharmacological Pain Management*

3. C, D, F. **CORRECT:** When taking actions, the nurse should identify that a client receiving prednisone should be advised to avoid crowds as prednisone suppresses inflammation and the normal immune response; blood glucose and intraocular pressure may increase while taking prednisone. Prednisone does not generally cause confusion in adults; it should not be taken for long-term treatment. Fluids should not be increased while taking prednisone.

   Ⓝ *NCLEX® Connection: Pharmacological Therapies, Adverse Effects/Contraindications/Side Effects/Interactions*

When reviewing the following chapters, keep in mind the relevant topics and tasks of the NCLEX outline.

Basic Care and Comfort

NONPHARMACOLOGICAL COMFORT INTERVENTIONS: Assist in planning comfort interventions for client with impaired comfort.

NUTRITION AND ORAL HYDRATION: Reinforce client teaching on special diets based on client diagnosis/nutritional needs and cultural considerations.

Health Promotion and Maintenance

HEALTH PROMOTION/DISEASE PREVENTION
Assist client in disease prevention activities.

Gather data on client health history and risk for disease.

Identify risk factors for disease/illness.

Pharmacological Therapies

ADVERSE EFFECTS/CONTRAINDICATIONS/SIDE EFFECTS/ INTERACTIONS: Identify potential and actual incompatibilities of client medications.

EXPECTED ACTIONS/OUTCOMES: Use resources to check on purposes and actions of pharmacological agents.

PHARMACOLOGICAL PAIN MANAGEMENT: Monitor and document client response to pharmacological interventions.

Physiological Adaptation

ALTERATIONS IN BODY SYSTEMS
Provide care to correct client alteration in body system.

Reinforce education to client regarding care and condition.

Identify signs and symptoms of an infection.

Notify primary health care provider of a change in client status.

BASIC PATHOPHYSIOLOGY: Identify signs and symptoms related to an acute or chronic illness.

Safety and Infection Control

STANDARD PRECAUTIONS/TRANSMISSION-BASED PRECAUTIONS/SURGICAL ASEPSIS: Protect immunocompromised client from exposure to infectious diseases/organisms.

CHAPTER 81 *General Principles
of Cancer*

Cancer is a neoplastic disease process that involves abnormal cell growth and differentiation. Normal body cells grow, divide, and die in an orderly fashion. In cancer, dying cells grow and form new abnormal cells and can form new blood vessels to provide nourishment for continued growth. Genetic mutations are responsible for abnormal cancerous growth. These mutations are either inherited or caused by something external. Viruses, physical and chemical agents, hormones, familial history, and lifestyle are thought to be factors that trigger abnormal cell growth.

Cancer cells can invade surrounding tissues and spread to other areas of the body through lymph and blood vessels (metastasis). No matter where cancer spreads, it is named based on the origin in which it started. For example, colon cancer that spreads to the liver is called metastatic colon cancer. Metastasis is usually diagnosed when there is onset of new findings (bone pain indicative of bone metastasis; change in bowel or bladder tone indicative of nervous system involvement).

Cancer impacts more than 1.8 million individuals in the United States. Cancer has an incidence rate of 442.4/100,000 and a mortality rate of 158.2/100,000. The most common types of cancer in the U.S. include breast, bladder, kidney, liver, lung, melanoma, lymphoma, leukemia, colorectal, prostate, pancreas, and thyroid. Screening and early diagnosis are important aspects of health education and care. The nurse should prevent, recognize, and treat complications associated with carcinoma. The incidence and risk of death differs among certain races and ethnicities. Qpcc

A tumor is an abnormal collection of cells, but not all tumors are cancers. Noncancerous tumors are benign. They do have the potential of pressing on healthy organs and tissues as they grow, but they do not invade other tissues and they do not metastasize.

BODY TISSUES

Cancers can arise from almost any tissue in the body. Cancerous cells decrease the functional ability of the tissue in which they are located.
- Epithelial tissue: carcinomas
- Glandular organs: adenocarcinomas
- Mesenchymal tissue: sarcomas
- Blood-forming cells: leukemias
- Lymph tissue: lymphomas
- Plasma cells: myelomas

HEALTH PROMOTION AND DISEASE PREVENTION

- Consume a healthy diet (low-fat with increased consumption of fruits, vegetables, and lean protein).
- Limit intake of sugar, salt, nitrates, nitrites, and processed and red meats.
- Maintain a healthy body weight/body mass index.
- Avoid use of tobacco products.
- Limit alcohol consumption to one drink per day for females (assigned female at birth) and two drinks per day for males (assigned male at birth).
- Avoid risky lifestyle choices (recreational drug use, needle sharing, unprotected sexual intercourse).
- Avoid exposure to environmental hazards (radiation, chemicals). Use personal protective equipment when available.
- Engage in physical activity or exercise routinely.
- Protect skin and eyes from UVA and UVB rays.
- Remove at-risk tissue such as moles to prevent conversion to skin cancer.
- Chemoprevention is the use of medications or other substances to disrupt cancer development.
- Aspirin and celecoxib to reduce the risk of colon cancer
- Vitamin D and tamoxifen to reduce the risk of breast cancer
- Immunization to prevent human papilloma virus (HPV), which is associated with cervical, vulvar, and vaginal cancers in females and anal cancer and genital warts in females.
- Immunization for Hepatitis B to prevent liver disease, which can progress to liver cancer.

DATA COLLECTION

RISK FACTORS

Age: Highest incidence of cancer occurs in older adults. ⓖ
- Females (sex assigned at birth) most commonly develop colorectal, breast, lung, pancreatic, and ovarian cancers.
- Males (sex assigned at birth) most commonly develop lung, colorectal, prostate, pancreatic, and gastric cancers.

Immune function: Cancer incidence increases among clients who are immunosuppressed.

Chronic irritation and tissue trauma: Incidence of skin cancer is higher in people who have burn scars or other types of severe skin injury.

Race Ⓠᴘᴄᴄ
- Non-Hispanic white American clients are at an increased risk for testicular cancer than any other group.
- African American clients are at increased risk for prostate, colorectal and pancreatic cancer than any other group.
- Mexican American clients have a high occurrence rate of liver cancer.

Genetic predisposition

Exposure to chemicals, tobacco, and alcohol

Exposure to some viruses and bacteria
- Liver cancer can develop after many years of infection with hepatitis B or hepatitis C.
- Infection with human T-cell leukemia virus increases the risk of lymphoma and leukemia.
- Infection with Epstein-Barr virus has been linked to an increased risk of lymphoma.
- HPV infection is the main cause of cervical cancer.
- HIV increases the risk of lymphoma and Kaposi's sarcoma.
- Helicobacter pylori can increase the risk of stomach cancer and lymphoma of the stomach lining.

Diet: A diet high in fat, red meat, processed meat, preservatives, and additives, and low in fiber

Sun, ultraviolet light, or radiation exposure: Ionizing (radon, x-ray) and UV (sun, tanning beds)

Sexual lifestyles: Multiple sexual partners or STIs

Poverty, obesity, and chronic GERD

Chronic disease

Air pollution

EXPECTED FINDINGS

- Benign tumors are often slower growing, have cells that closely resemble the surrounding area, and primarily have localized effects unless they compress blood vessels or nerves.
- Malignant tumors have cells that are different from the cells around them and can grow very rapidly if they are more abnormal. These cells continually proliferate toward the outer edges of the tumor, so that they can take over other tissue and access vasculature and lymphatics.
- The findings associated with the presence of a tumor are dependent on the tissue in which they are located; clients will report pain and possible physiological changes if organ or tissue function has been disrupted.

Laboratory tests

Laboratory testing can help identify cancerous tumors. Tests include tumor markers and tests used for screening, such as CA-125.

Diagnostic procedures

Diagnostic procedures can determine the size and location of tumors and can include imaging tests used for screening in addition to biopsy and other types of imaging (MRI, CT scan, fluoroscopy, PET scan, nuclear imaging).

Staging of cancer

The tumor-node-metastasis (TNM) system is used to stage cancer.

TUMOR (T)
- **TX**: Unable to evaluate the primary tumor
- **TØ**: No evidence of primary tumor
- **Tis**: Tumor in situ
- **T1, T2, T3, and T4**: Size and extent of tumor

NODE (N)
- **NX**: Unable to evaluate regional lymph nodes
- **NØ**: No evidence of regional node involvement
- **N1, N2, and N3**: Number of nodes that are involved and/or extent of spread

METASTASIS (M)
- **MX**: Unable to evaluate distant metastasis
- **MØ**: No evidence of distant metastasis
- **M1**: Presence of distant metastasis

Grading Ⓠᴇʙᴘ

Grading is needed because some cancer cells are more malignant than others. Well-differentiated means the cells look much like normal cells and tend to grow slowly. Undifferentiated, or poorly differentiated, means the cells do not look like normal cells and tend to grow quickly and spread.
- **GX**: Grade cannot be determined.
- **G1**: Tumor cells are well differentiated.
- **G2**: Tumor cells are moderately differentiated.
- **G3**: Tumor cells are poorly differentiated, but the tissue of origin can be established.
- Tumor cells are poorly differentiated, and determination of the tissue of origin is difficult.

Prognosis

- Early diagnosis of cancer usually results in a better prognosis. Many cancers spread or metastasize before any manifestations are noted.
- For the client who has successful cancer treatment, the nurse should help create a survivorship plan. The client will need to continue prevention and screening for new cancer or recurrence of the original cancer, as well as watch for manifestations of metastasis. The client might require ongoing therapy for the effects of cancer and cancer treatment, such as pain management or fertility treatments. The nurse should assist with management and help the client coordinate care among various providers.

COMPLICATIONS

Malnutrition

Clients who have cancer are at increased risk for weight loss and anorexia.

- The presence of carcinoma in the body increases the amount of energy required for metabolic function.
- Cancer can impair the body's ability to ingest, digest, and absorb nutrients.
- Adverse effects of cancer treatment can affect the desire for food or the ability to eat. Findings include nausea, vomiting, changes in taste, anorexia, pain, diarrhea, early satiety, dry mouth, thickened saliva, and irritation to the gastrointestinal tract.

NURSING ACTIONS

- Administer antiemetics and antacids as prescribed.
- Monitor relevant laboratory data (albumin, ferritin, and transferrin).
- Encourage frequent oral hygiene.
- Incorporate client preferences into meal planning when possible.
- Avoid early satiety by limiting liquids during meals.
- Instruct the client to collaborate with dietary services. Qtc

CLIENT EDUCATION

- Understand how to manage the expected effects of treatment.
- Consume adequate protein, carbohydrates, and calories.

Constipation/gastric stasis/intestinal obstruction

NURSING ACTIONS

- Can be related to cancer or cancer treatment.
- Opioids can cause delayed emptying, slowed bowel motility.
- Administer stool softener or laxative as needed.
- Encourage fluids, fiber, and activity as tolerated.

ONCOLOGIC EMERGENCIES Qs

Hypercalcemia

A common complication of breast, lung, head, and neck cancers; leukemias and lymphomas; multiple myelomas; and bony metastases of any cancer

MANIFESTATIONS: Anorexia, nausea, vomiting, shortened QT interval, kidney stones, bone pain, and changes in mental status

NURSING ACTIONS: Monitor the client while receiving 0.9% sodium chloride IV, furosemide, pamidronate, and phosphates as prescribed.

Superior vena cava syndrome

Results from obstruction (metastases from breast or lung cancers) of venous return and engorgement of the vessels from the head and upper body

MANIFESTATIONS: Periorbital and facial edema, erythema of the upper body, dyspnea, cough, wheezing, hypotension

NURSING ACTIONS

- Position the client in a semi-Fowler's position initially to facilitate lung expansion.
- Use high-dose radiation therapy for emergency temporary relief.

Hematologic disorders

Hematologic problems can be caused by the cancer itself or chemotherapy.

Anemia: When cancer invades the bone marrow, it decreases the number of red blood cells, platelets (thrombocytopenia) and white blood cells (neutropenia).

Disseminated intravascular coagulation: Secondary to leukemia or adenocarcinomas

NURSING ACTIONS

- Observe for bleeding, and apply pressure as needed.
- Monitor the client while receiving blood clotting factors that have been lost through bleeding and need to be replaced with plasma transfusions. Heparin also can be used to slow the cascade of events that makes the body overuse its blood clotting factors.

Sepsis

- Pathogens in the body can lead to septicemia and septic shock, which are life-threatening.
- Clients who are neutropenic are at an increased risk.

NURSING ACTIONS: Assist and monitor resuscitation measures, including obtaining blood cultures, measuring blood lactate, and administering antibiotics and crystalloid fluids. Vasopressors can be required if fluid administration is insufficient.

Spinal cord compression

Occurs when vertebrae degrade secondary to cancer, or tumors invade the spinal column. Without immediate intervention, permanent neurologic damage can occur.

MANIFESTATIONS: Changes in sensation, muscle strength, reduced deep tendon reflexes, worsening back pain, and bowel or bladder retention

NURSING ACTIONS
- Plan to administer high-dose IV corticosteroids to reduce inflammation around the spinal cord.
- Prepare the client for possible radiation therapy or surgery to relieve cord compression.

CLIENT EDUCATION: An MRI usually confirms diagnosis.

Tumor lysis syndrome (TLS)

TLS occurs when tumors are rapidly destroyed, releasing intracellular content into the bloodstream faster than the body can process them. This rapid release causes hyperkalemia, hyperphosphatemia, and hyperuricemia. Without correction, TLS leads to kidney injury and changes in cardiac function that can lead to death. Older age increases risk, as well as certain chemotherapy agents and types of cancer.

MANIFESTATIONS: Gastrointestinal distress, flank pain muscle cramps and weakness, seizures, and mental status changes

NURSING ACTIONS
- Monitor the administration of IV fluids and encourage fluid intake of 3 L daily, including consumption of alkaline fluids to lower uric acid levels.
- Assist with administering medications (diuretics, allopurinol, sodium polystyrene) to reduce potassium, uric acid, and phosphorus levels.

CLIENT EDUCATION: Hemodialysis and intensive care might be required.

Application Exercises

1. A nurse is reviewing the pathology report on a client who had a biopsy to stage and grade ovarian cancer. The report states the tumor is graded G1 and staged T2-N3-MX. The nurse should interpret which of the following information based on the pathology report?
   - A. The tumor is moderate in size.
   - B. The cancer has not spread to the lymph nodes.
   - C. The tumor cells are poorly differentiated.
   - D. The cancer has metastasized to other areas in the body.

2. A nurse is assisting with the plan of care for a client who has malnutrition due to cancer. What interventions should the nurse recommend including in the plan?

3. A nurse is assisting with collecting data on a client who has cancer and is experiencing superior vena cava syndrome. Which of the following findings should the nurse expect? (Select all that apply.)
   - A. Facial edema
   - B. Wheezing
   - C. Cough
   - D. Client report of nausea
   - E. Increased urine specific gravity

4. A nurse is assisting with teaching a class about nursing interventions for oncologic emergencies. Match the nursing intervention with the oncologic emergency.

A. Spinal cord compression	1. Encourage fluid intake of 3 L (12.7 c) daily
B. Hypercalcemia	2. Obtain blood cultures
C. Sepsis	3. Administer a bisphosphonate
D. Tumor lysis syndrome	4. Administer high-dose IV corticosteroids

Active Learning Scenario

A nurse is assisting with preparing an in-service about identifying risk factors for cancer to a group of adults at a community health fair. What information should the nurse include in the in-service? Use the ATI Active Learning Template: System Disorder to complete this item.

RISK FACTORS
- Identify two types of cancer with increased incidence in female older adults.
- Identify two types of cancer with increased incidence in male older adults.
- Identify one type of cancer with a risk factor related to racial background.
- Describe three diet-related risk factors.
- Describe at least three lifestyle-related risk factors.

PATHOPHYSIOLOGY RELATED TO CLIENT PROBLEM: Describe at least three viruses/bacteria and the type of cancer they can cause.

Application Exercises Key

1. A. **CORRECT**: When analyzing cues, the nurse should identify that T2 indicates the tumor is moderate in size, N3 indicates high lymph node involvement, MX indicates no metastasis is detected, and G1 indicates well differentiated tumor cells.

   Ⓝ *NCLEX® Connection: Reduction of Risk Potential, Laboratory Values*

2. When generating solutions, the nurse should plan to administer antiemetics and antacids as prescribed. Monitor the client's laboratory data, such as albumin, ferritin, and transferrin, to monitor the client's nutritional status. Encourage the client perform frequent oral hygiene before and after meals to promote salivation and improve taste perception. Incorporate client preferences into meal planning when possible. Encourage the client to limit drinking fluids with meals because fluids can cause early satiety and decrease adequate intake of food. Instruct the client to collaborate with dietary services and to eat nutrient-dense foods first to increase adequate nutritional intake to treat malnutrition.

   Ⓝ *NCLEX® Connection: Basic Care and Comfort, Nutrition and Oral Hydration*

3. A, B, C. **CORRECT**: When recognizing cues, the nurse should identify manifestations of superior vena cava syndrome includes facial edema, wheezing, and cough. The client report of nausea and an increase in urine specific gravity could be related to excessive fluid.

   Ⓝ *NCLEX® Connection: Physiological Adaptation, Basic Pathophysiology*

4. A, 4; B, 3; C, 2; D, 1

   When taking actions, the nurse should instruct to encourage clients who have tumor lysis syndrome to drink at least 3 L (12.7 c) of fluid daily. This intervention can reduce the risk of uric acid build up in the kidneys that can result in acute kidney injury. The nurse should instruct to obtain blood cultures on clients who have sepsis to identify the pathogen causing the infection and to determine the required treatment. The nurse should instruct to administer a bisphosphonate to clients who have hypercalcemia to block resorption of calcium in the bone and decrease serum calcium level. The nurse should instruct to administer high-dose corticosteroids to clients who have spinal cord compression to reduce inflammation in the spinal cord.

   Ⓝ *NCLEX® Connection: Physiological Adaptation, Basic Pathophysiology*

Active Learning Scenario Key

Using the ATI Active Learning Template: System Disorder

RISK FACTORS
- Older adult females: Colorectal, breast, lung, pancreatic, and ovarian cancers
- Older adult males: Lung, colorectal, prostate, pancreatic and gastric cancers
- Risk related to racial background:
  - Non-Hispanic white American clients are at an increased risk for testicular cancer than any other group.
  - African American clients are at increased risk for prostate, colorectal and pancreatic cancer than any other group.
  - Mexican American clients have a high occurrence rate of liver cancer.
- Diet-related: Diet high in fat and red meat, low in fiber
- Lifestyle-related
  - Multiple sexual partners or STIs
  - Sun, ultraviolet light, and radiation exposure
  - Use of tobacco and alcohol

PATHOPHYSIOLOGY RELATED TO CLIENT PROBLEM
- Hepatitis B or C: Liver cancer
- Human T-cell leukemia virus: Lymphoma and leukemia
- Epstein-Barr virus: Lymphoma
- Human papillomavirus: Cervical cancer
- HIV: Lymphoma and Kaposi's sarcoma
- Helicobacter pylori: Stomach cancer and lymphoma of the stomach lining

Ⓝ *NCLEX® Connection: Health Promotion and Maintenance, Health Promotion/Disease Prevention*

CHAPTER 82

Cancer Screening and Diagnostic Procedures

Screening and diagnostic procedures provide objective and subjective client data. The nurse should ensure that the client understands all tests and procedures and ensure that the client gives informed consent. Screening and diagnosis for cancer can involve the use of hands-on data collection techniques, invasive procedures, radiography and imaging studies, and laboratory testing. The type and location of the suspected cancer dictate which methods are used. Identification of tumor cells is required for definitive diagnosis and the development of a targeted treatment plan.

SCREENING RECOMMENDATIONS

Instruct clients to discuss benefits and risks for each screening exam with their provider to determine when screening should take place. Clients who are at increased risk for specific cancer types may need to start screenings earlier or have them performed more frequently. For clients who have a strong family history of breast or colon cancer, a screening for gene mutations can be performed. Clients, who are at average risk, starting at 50 years of age, every 2 years (varies)

DATA COLLECTION

CLIENT PRESENTATION

Cancer

- Altered body function (fatigue, weakness, anorexia)
- Change in body structure (weight loss, masses)
- Change in body symmetry or onset of recent findings (pain, nausea, vomiting)
- Unexpected bleeding or discharge
- Non-healing lesion
- Unexpected change in bowel or urinary habits
- Unexpected lump
- Persistent cough
- Difficulty swallowing

82.1 American Cancer Society cancer screening recommendations, 2020

Breast

- 40-44 years of age: Start screening mammograms yearly if desired
- 45-54 years of age should receive annual mammograms
- > 55 years of age: mammograms every other year or yearly if desired. Continue screenings for a long as client's condition is good and has life expectancy of 10 or more years
- Average risk: Clinical breast exams are no longer recommended

Colorectal

- Average risk
  - 45 years of age (initiation) up to 75 years of age should receive stool screening/visual examination (based upon if the client has 10 or more years of life expectancy)
  - 76-85 years of age: decision for screening is dependent upon the client's personal preference, life expectancy, general condition, and previous screening history
  - > 85 years of age: screening no longer required
- Stool
  - Fecal immunochemical test (FIT) or guaiac based fecal occult blood test (gFOBT) annually
  - Stool DNA (every 3 years)
- Visual
  - Colonoscopy every 10 years
  - CT colonoscopy (virtual) every 5 years
  - Flexible sigmoidoscopy every 5 years

Prostate

- Clients should be given the opportunity to make an informed decision with their provider after receiving information about the benefits, risks, and uncertainty related to prostate screening. The discussion with their provider about screening should occur at the following recommended age intervals:
  - 40 years of age for those who are at highest risk
  - 45 years of age for those who are at higher risk
  - 50 years of age for those who are at average risk
- Prostate specific antigen (PSA) digital rectal examination (DRE) (if desired)
- Retesting every 2 years if PSA less than 2.5 ng/mL,
- PSA > than 2.5 ng/mL (provider should discuss the pros and cons of testing and consider the client's health, preference and beliefs).

Cervical

- 25 years of age (initiation) up to 65 years of age
- Papanicolaou (Pap) test with co-test for HPV every 5 years
- Papanicolaou (Pap) test without co-test for HPV every 3 years

Lung

- Client who are a current smoker, fair condition of health, 20 pack per year smoking history or quit within past 15 years:
- 50-80 years of age yearly low-dose helical CT (LCDT)
- Receive counseling to quit if currently smoke and talked about benefits, limits, and harms of screening, can go to center that has experience in lung cancer screening and treatment.
- Client should also receive counseling, if desired, to quit smoking and provider should discuss benefits, limitations, and potential harms of screening test.

For more information https://www.cancer.org/

Metastasis

- Secondary sites of discomfort
- Swelling and/or tenderness of lymph nodes or areas of the body
- Presence of masses
- Altered function of another body system
- Bone pain

PATIENT CENTERED CARE

NURSING ACTIONS

- Assist with obtaining a health history and physical examination including client report of findings and family history of cancer or genetic disorder.
- Inspect for changes in color, symmetry, movement, or body function.
- Auscultate for adventitious sounds that indicate altered body system function.
  - Heart, lung, and bowel sounds
  - Masses or areas of discomfort
- Palpate to detect masses or tissue abnormalities.
- Report unexpected findings.
- Reinforce explanations when there is need for further testing or evaluation of unexpected findings.

CLIENT EDUCATION

- Perform self-examination (breast and testicular) practices at home, if desired.
- Understand the general findings that could indicate cancer. If found, notify the provider for further screening.
  - Change in bowel or bladder habits, change in shape or texture of a body or skin region
  - Difficulty eating, chewing, swallowing, or decreased appetite
  - Non-healing sores or wounds, or a cough or hoarseness that does not go away
  - Unexplained pain, night sweats, fatigue, weight loss, or weight gain
  - Unusual bleeding

THERAPEUTIC MANAGEMENT

Biopsy

Provides definitive diagnosis indicating the site of origin (specific cell type) and cell characteristics (specific receptors on cell surface). **QEBP**

Can be obtained during other procedures (endoscopy, laparoscopy, thoracotomy).

Shave biopsy (basal or squamous cell skin cancer): Sampling of outer skin layers (raised lesions) using a scalpel or razor blade.

Needle biopsy (fine or core): Aspiration of tumor close to the skin surface for fluid and tissue sampling. Bone marrow aspiration is a form of needle biopsy used to diagnose leukemia and lymphoma.

Incisional or excisional (open) biopsy: Cutting through skin to remove part (incisional) or all (excisional) of a tumor. Punch biopsy is a form of excisional biopsy used to diagnose skin cancer. A circular instrument punches a 2 to 6 mm sample of subcutaneous fat.

Sentinel lymph node biopsy: Biopsy of lymph node closest to the cancer. A dye or colloid is used to create a map of affected nodes.

- If the lymph node is negative, the lymph nodes in the surrounding area are assumed to be cancer-free.
- If the lymph node is positive, surgical excision of lymph nodes in the area is performed (lymph node dissection).

NURSING ACTIONS

- Verify a signed informed consent form from the client.
- Assemble supplies and facilitate aseptic technique.
- Prevent bleeding. Withhold anticoagulants as prescribed. Monitor findings of coagulation studies.
- Monitor for bleeding (visible staining of dressing, hypotension, tachycardia).
- Provide a safe environment until effects of sedation are minimal. (Maintain bed rest. Withhold oral intake.)
- Ensure adequate oxygenation during the recovery period.
- Position the client in a recovery position appropriate to the procedure (lay on right side following liver biopsy).

LABORATORY TESTS

Performed to check for possible cancer or effects on the body (electrolyte imbalance, altered function)

CBC: elevated WBCs and blast cells could indicate leukemia

Liver function tests: Elevation can indicate primary liver cancer or metastasis of another cancer (colorectal cancer).

Tumor marker assays: Detect the presence of expected body proteins at higher than expected levels (carcinoembryonic antigen (CEA), prostate-specific antigen [PSA], alpha fetoprotein).

- Samples of urine, stool, tissue, blood, or other body fluids are tested for an excess of specific proteins or DNA patterns.
- Used to detect cancer, measure the severity of cancer, or monitor for a positive response to the cancer treatment regimen (expected finding is a decrease in the tumor marker or return to expected reference range).

Other testing: Can be done in addition to biopsy to identify tumor cell type (sputum analysis, cytology of fluid sampling).

NURSING ACTIONS: Reinforce explanations of the purpose of testing, as appropriate.

CLIENT EDUCATION: Laboratory testing can continue throughout treatment (to monitor progress) and following treatment (to screen for return of cancer).

DIAGNOSTIC TESTS

Common imaging techniques (CT scan, MRI, PET scan, ultrasound, x-ray) are used as secondary tools to assist in the treatment of cancer. Imaging is completed around the time of diagnosis to measure the severity of cancer.

- Provide visualization of tumors and their borders.
- Detect metastasis to organs and other body structures.
- Clients can be given dye (IV pyelogram) or contrast (barium enema) to enhance visualization.
- Monitor the client during remission.

DIGITAL IMAGING

- Usually more accurate.
- Digital storage of images and results allows for information to be easily shared among members of the interprofessional treatment team. Qℓ

X-rays

- Provide visualization of body structures (chest x-ray, mammogram).
- With angiography, the client is injected with dye and then x-rays are taken to map vascular structures, such as arterial, venous, or lymphatic mapping.

NURSING ACTIONS
Monitor for allergic reaction to contrast dye (dyspnea, tachycardia, restlessness).

Computerized axial tomography (CT) scanning

- Combines x-ray images taken from different angles and uses computer processing to create cross-sectional images.
- Can be performed with or without contrast. Contrast can be administered orally or intravenously.

MRI

- Uses magnetic field and radio waves rather than radiation to generate pictures of tissue and organs.
- Contrast can be added to enhance the images. Clients who have any type of metal inside the body (clips, pacemaker, metal implants) should not have an MRI.

Ultrasound

- High-energy sound waves bounce off internal tissues and organs to produce an echo pattern that can be seen as an ultrasound image.
- A biopsy can be performed during the ultrasound.

Nuclear imaging

- Evaluates the function of organs and structures by detecting the presence of radiation in the body after the client is given a radioactive tracer (IV or oral).
- Used for detection and staging of cancer. Cancerous tissues can absorb more or less tracer than expected. These tissues are distinguishable by nuclear imaging.

82.2 Case study

Scenario introduction

0700: Amy is a nurse in a preoperative holding area and is assisting with the care of Ms. Anne Smith. Ms. Smith is scheduled for a biopsy of a right breast mass. Nurse Amy has completed the introduction and has collected data from Ms. Smith, including her personal preferences.

Part 1

- Nurse Amy: "Ms. Smith, can you tell me what type of procedure you will be having today?"
- Ms. Smith: "Yes. I am having a biopsy of a mass in my right breast."
- Nurse Amy: "How are you feeling about having this procedure?"
- Ms. Smith: "I am very nervous. My mother died from breast cancer."

Part 2

Nurse Amy: "This must be very scary for you."

Ms. Smith: "Yes, I am afraid of what the biopsy will show."

Part 3

Nurse Amy: "Ms. Smith, it's understandable to have these feelings. I will stay with you during the procedure if you like."

Ms. Smith: "That is fine, thank you."

Nurse Amy: "Your surgeon will be in soon to talk to you about the procedure."

Ms. Smith: "Okay."

Scenario conclusion

Nurse Amy documents the following information:

0715:
- Temperature 36° C (96.8° F)
- Heart rate 62/min
- Respiratory rate 20/min
- Blood pressure 104/56 mm Hg (right arm supine)
- Oxygen saturation 98% (room air)
- Client is awake, alert, and oriented, bilateral breath sounds clear and present throughout. Client reports anxiety about the possible diagnosis. The surgeon discussed genetic testing with the client.

Positron emission tomography (PET)

Measures positrons released with tissue uptake of radioactive sugar (more rapid in cancer). Mammography (PEM) can be performed this way. CT can be used with PET scans.

Electrocardiogram, echocardiogram, or multi gated acquisition scan

Used to evaluate heart function prior to cancer treatment or to identify damage following chemotherapy or radiation to the upper body.

Other types of imaging

Bone scan, gallium scan, and thyroid scan

Endoscopy

Permits visualization inside the body using flexible scopes and cameras. Tumors can be visualized in the joints (arthroscopy), respiratory system (laryngoscopy, bronchoscopy), body cavity (mediastinoscopy, thoracoscopy), or gastrointestinal system (enteroscopy, sigmoidoscopy). Organs can be visualized as well (hysteroscopy, cystoscopy).

NURSING ACTIONS

- Verify signed informed consent form.
- Prepare the client as indicated for the type of procedure to be performed.
- Provide a safe environment until effects of sedation are minimal (maintain bed rest, withhold oral intake).
- Ensure adequate oxygenation during the recovery period.

INTERPRETATION OF FINDINGS

- Findings that indicate or increase suspicion of cancer must be further evaluated.
- A variety of imaging and laboratory tests can be used to detect the following.
  - Degree of tumor involvement
  - Type of tumor
  - Areas of metastasis
  - Complications of cancer

NURSING ACTIONS

- Instruct the client about routine cancer screenings as part of health promotion and disease prevention.
- Provide care before, during, and after the procedure as indicated by procedure type.
- Reinforce teaching and provide resources for client about self-care in the home environment.

Active Learning Scenario

A nurse is discussing data collection as part of screening for cancer with a newly licensed nurse. What information should the nurse include in the discussion? Use the ATI Active Learning Template: Diagnostic Procedure to complete this item.

INTERPRETATION OF FINDINGS

- Describe at least three findings indicating the presence of metastasis.

- Describe three data collection techniques and possible findings.

CLIENT EDUCATION: Identify two self-assessment techniques that can identify data.

Active Learning Scenario Key

Using the ATI Active Learning Template: Diagnostic Procedure
INTERPRETATION OF FINDINGS

Metastasis
- Discomfort at secondary sites
- Swelling and/or tenderness of lymph nodes or areas of the body
- Presence of masses
- Altered function of another body system
- Bone pain

Data collection techniques
- Inspection for changes in color, symmetry, movement, or body function
- Auscultation for adventitious sounds, which can indicate altered body system function
- Palpation to detect masses or tissue abnormalities

CLIENT EDUCATION: Testicular and breast self-examinations if desired

Ⓝ *NCLEX® Connection: Coordinated Care, Referral Process*

Application Exercises

1. A nurse is assisting with teaching a class about screening prevention for cancer. Match the following tests with the recommended screening guideline.

   A. PSA
   B. Pap test
   C. Colonoscopy
   D. Mammogram

   1. Clients who are 45 to 54 years of age, every year
   2. Clients who are at average risk, every 10 years, beginning at age 45
   3. Client who are 25-65 years of age, every 3 years
   4. Clients, who are at average risk, starting at 50 years of age, every 2 years (varies)

2. A nurse is collecting data to screen for cancer on several clients. Which of the following findings is a possible manifestation of cancer? (Select all that apply.)

   A. Temperature 36° C (96.8° F)
   B. Sore that does not heal
   C. Difficulty swallowing
   D. Blood in the urine
   E. Rhinitis

3. A nurse is assisting with teaching a class about diagnostic procedures for cancer. Match the following types of biopsies with the associated procedure.

   A. Sentinel lymph node biopsy
   B. Incisional biopsy
   C. Needle biopsy
   D. Shave biopsy

   1. Samples of outer skin layers are obtained
   2. Aspiration of tumor for fluid or tissue sampling
   3. Skin is cut to remove part of a tumor
   4. Uses a dye to locate affected areas

4. The nurse is assisting with the care of the client who is having an incisional biopsy for a breast mass. What actions should the nurse take?

5. A nurse is assisting with teaching a newly licensed nurse about imaging studies. Match the study with the associated procedure.

   A. Echocardiogram
   B. Nuclear imaging
   C. Ultrasound
   D. MRI

   1. Uses a magnetic field to produce an image
   2. High-energy sound waves are used to produce an image
   3. A radioactive substance is used to locate cancer tissue
   4. Used to evaluate heart function

Application Exercises Key

1. A, 4; B, 3; C, 2; D, 1

   When taking actions, the nurse should include the following recommendations for screening: mammogram every year for clients who are 45-54 years of age, colonoscopy every 10 years starting at 45 years of age for client who are at average risk. Pap test every 3 years for clients who are 25- 65 years of age, PSA for clients who 50 years of age and considered to be at average risk every 2 years depending upon the results of the PSA.

   Ⓝ *NCLEX® Connection: Health Promotion and Maintenance, Health Promotion/Disease Prevention*

2. B, C, D. **CORRECT**: When recognizing cues, the nurse should identify that a sore that does not heal, difficulty swallowing, and blood in the urine are possible manifestations of cancer and require further actions to determine the cause.

   Ⓝ *NCLEX® Connection: Health Promotion and Maintenance, Health Promotion/Disease Prevention*

3. A, 4; B, 3; C, 2; D, 1

   When taking actions, the nurse should instruct that samples of outer skin layers are obtained during a shave biopsy. A tumor is aspirated for fluid or tissue sampling during a needle biopsy. Skin is cut to remove part of a tumor during an incisional biopsy. Dye is used to locate affected nodes during a sentinel lymph node biopsy.

   Ⓝ *NCLEX® Connection: Health Promotion and Maintenance, Health Promotion/Disease Prevention*

4. When taking actions, the nurse should ensure that an informed consent has been obtained, assemble supplies and maintain aseptic technique. The nurse should withhold anticoagulants as prescribed and monitor findings of coagulation studies to reduce the risk of bleeding. Following the biopsy, the nurse should monitor the client for manifestations of bleeding, such as sanguineous drainage on the dressing, hypotension, and tachycardia. The nurse should provide a safe environment for the client, such as maintaining bed rest, and withholding oral fluids, until effects of sedation are minimal. The nurse should monitor the client's airway, breath sounds, and oxygen saturation, to ensure adequate oxygenation during the recovery period.

   Ⓝ *NCLEX® Connection: Physiological Adaptation, Basic Pathophysiology*

5. A, 4; B, 3; C, 2; D, 1

   When taking actions, the nurse should instruct that an MRI uses a magnetic field to produce an image. An ultrasound uses high-energy sound waves to produce an image. Nuclear imaging uses a radioactive substance to locate cancer tissue. An echocardiogram is used to evaluate heart function.

   Ⓝ *NCLEX® Connection: Health Promotion and Maintenance, Health Promotion/Disease Prevention*

CHAPTER 83

Cancer Treatment Options

Cancer treatment is based on the cell of origin of the cancer. When metastasis occurs, treatment is still based on the primary tumor origin even though the malignancy is located elsewhere in the body. Many cancers are curable when diagnosed early.

Cancer treatment options focus on removing or destroying cancer cells and preventing the continued abnormal cell growth and differentiation. Treatment can be curative or palliative. The treatment plan is guided by client factors (age, childbearing desire, pregnancy, current state of health, expected lifespan) and can involve several treatment methods.

Adjuvant treatment is what is given in addition to the primary treatment standard and can include hormone, radiation, and targeted therapies; immunotherapy; and chemotherapy.

Nursing care for clients who have cancer should include collaboration with supportive therapies and services, counseling, and transfer of care to another provider at discharge. Qᴛᴄ

PROCEDURES

Cancer treatment includes manipulation or removal of the tumor.

Tumor reduction can be done through topical procedures (cryosurgery, laser therapy, ablation) or by destruction of the main arteries that provide blood flow to the tumor (artery embolization).

Tumor excision can be open or endoscopic (curettage and electro dissection for skin cancer).

- The tumor and tissue immediately surrounding it (tumor margin) are removed. The goal is that all of the surrounding outermost tissue that was removed does not contain cancer cells (a negative margin).
- Surgery can be done for biopsy (diagnosis and staging), or relief (palliation) based on findings.

Lymph node dissection or sentinel lymph node biopsy is done to determine if the cancer has spread or there is added risk of spread.

Prophylactic surgery involves removing precancerous tissue, or noncancerous tissue, for a client at high risk for developing cancer.

Rehabilitative or reconstructive surgeries improve appearance or functional ability for clients following cancer treatment.

More extensive surgeries (tumors involving multiple organs or structures, lymph node involvement, deep lesions) increase the risk of complications and typically require longer recovery periods. Intensive care can be required.

NURSING ACTIONS
- Provide perioperative care as indicated by tumor location and procedure type.
- Prevent general postoperative complications (infection, fluid or electrolyte imbalance, hemorrhage, thromboembolism, inadequate oxygenation, shock).
- Prevent and treat pain as prescribed using pharmacological and nonpharmacological measures.
- Reinforce teaching with the client on care for drains, wounds, and implanted devices.
- Provide psychological support to the client to facilitate coping with diagnosis and body image changes following surgery.
- Assist the client to develop strategies to compensate for loss of function of organs, tissue, or limbs.

CLIENT EDUCATION: Monitor for complications after discharge.

INTERPROFESSIONAL COLLABORATION

- Support groups for clients who have cancer, as well as their family and friends.
- Therapy services as indicated for the client's condition, such as physical, speech, respiratory, and occupational therapies.

Chemotherapy

Chemotherapy involves administration of systemic or local cytotoxic medications that damage a cell's DNA or destroy rapidly dividing cells.

- Chemotherapeutic agents are often selected in relation to their effect on various stages of cell division. Subsequently, combinations of anticancer medications are used to enhance destruction of cancer cells.
- Most chemotherapy agents are cytotoxic. The adverse effects of these agents are related to the unintentional harm done to normal rapidly proliferating cells, such as those found in the mucous membranes of the gastrointestinal (GI) tract, hair follicles, and bone marrow.
- For some cancer medications, agents that protect healthy cells (cytoprotectants or chemoprotectants) are given before or with chemotherapy to decrease the effect on noncancerous tissues. Examples include amifostine and mesna.

- Chemotherapy can be administered in a health care setting, provider's office, clinic, or home.
- Most chemotherapy medications, including oral, are absorbed through the skin and mucous membranes. Anyone preparing, giving, or disposing of these medications must wear proper personal protective equipment.
- Return unused chemotherapeutic agents to the dispensary or dispose of them per agency policy. Do not dispose of medications in the regular trash or sewage system.

ROUTE

- Depending on the agent, it can be given by the topical (for skin lesions); oral; parenteral; IV; intra-arterial; intraventricular (into the ventricles of the brain); intracavitary, which includes intraperitoneal (into the abdominal cavity); intravesicular (into the bladder); intrapleural (into the pleural space); or intrathecal (into the spinal cavity) route. Specialized training/certification is necessary for the administration of some agents.
- Oral anticancer medications are just as toxic to the client taking the medication and the nurse handling the medication as are standard chemotherapy medications.
- Oral medications should not be crushed, split, broken, or chewed.

CATHETERS

- A central catheter is usually placed for IV chemotherapy administration or blood testing.
- Some medications can cause serious damage to the skin and muscle tissue if they leak outside a vein (vesicants). Getting these through a central venous catheter rather than a short-term peripheral IV reduces the risk that the medication will leak and damage tissues. Many different types of central venous catheters can be used. Two of the more commonly used included the peripherally inserted central catheter and implanted port. (Refer to **PN ADULT MEDICAL SURGICAL NURSING CHAPTER 25: CARDIOVASCULAR DIAGNOSTIC AND THERAPEUTIC PROCEDURES.**)
- A port is implanted when therapy is intended to be given on a long-term basis. The port is comprised of a small reservoir that is covered by a thick septum.

CATEGORIES OF MEDICATIONS

- There are several categories of chemotherapy medications based on how they work and the chemical structure. Medications are selected based on the sensitivity of cancer cells to the medications and the stage of the cancer. Understanding the mechanism of the medication's action can help with predicting possible adverse effects.
- Categories include alkylating agents, antimetabolites, antimitotic agents, antitumor antibiotics, topoisomerase inhibitors, and other miscellaneous medications.

NURSING ACTIONS

- Instruct the client/family in the proper use of vascular access devices.
- Instruct family to dispense oral medications directly into a cup and not to touch pills or liquids with the hands.
- Closely monitor IV infusions and notify the charge nurse to provide immediate treatment for extravasation. Care includes identifying the antidote (neutralizing solution) for the specific medication the client is receiving.

INTRACAVITARY CHEMOTHERAPY

Involves the administration of chemotherapy directly into a body cavity (abdomen, pleural space, or bladder)
- A small catheter can be used.
- Local irritation might be increased, but systemic adverse effects are usually prevented.
- In some cases, the medication can be removed following a dwell time.

CLIENT EDUCATION

- Some discomfort can be present during infusion.
- Monitor for evidence of infection at the site of administration.

INDICATIONS

- Chemotherapy can be used to cure a disease, help control its progression, or as palliative treatment for individuals who have a terminal disease.
- Chemotherapy is often used for treatment of cancer. It can also be used for other disorders (autoimmune diseases).

CONSIDERATIONS

PREPROCEDURE

- Administration of chemotherapeutic medications is limited to certified individuals. Management of adverse effects is the primary focus of health care personnel.
- Instruct the client to immediately report findings that indicate potential complications. The client should report findings immediately.

COMPLICATIONS

Immunosuppression/neutropenia

- Due to bone marrow suppression by cytotoxic medications.
- A significant adverse effect of chemotherapy.
- Clients who have neutropenia might not develop a high fever or have purulent drainage, even when an infection is present.
- The risk of serious infection increases as the absolute neutrophil count (ANC) falls. An ANC less than 1,000/mm³ indicates a weak immune system and the need to initiate neutropenic/protective precautions.

NURSING ACTIONS

- Monitor temperature, white blood cell (WBC) count, and ANC.
- Report a fever greater than 37.8° C (100° F) to the provider immediately. Qs
- Monitor skin and mucous membranes for infection (breakdown, fissures, and abscess).
- Obtain prescribed cultures prior to initiating antimicrobial therapy.

NEUTROPENIC PRECAUTIONS

- Ensure the client is assigned to a private room. Have the client remain in the room unless they need to leave for a diagnostic procedure or therapy. In this case, place a mask on the client during transport.
- Protect the client from possible sources of infection (live plants, stagnant water, contaminated equipment).
- Have client, staff, and visitors perform frequent hand hygiene. Restrict visitors who are ill.
- Avoid invasive procedures that could cause a break in tissue (rectal temperatures, injections, indwelling urinary catheters) unless necessary.
- Keep dedicated equipment (blood pressure machine, thermometer, stethoscope) in the client's room.
- Administer colony-stimulating factors (filgrastim, safgramostim) as prescribed to stimulate WBC production.
- Follow agency policy regarding prohibitions of fresh flowers and plants in the client's room.

CLIENT EDUCATION

- Avoid crowds while undergoing chemotherapy.
- Take temperature daily. Report elevated temperature to the provider.
- Avoid people who are ill.
- Avoid food sources that could contain bacteria (fresh fruits and vegetables; undercooked meat, fish, and eggs; pepper and paprika).
- Avoid yard work, gardening, or changing a pet's litter box. Wear disposable gloves when working with house plants or doing outdoor gardening.
- Discard liquid beverages that have been sitting at room temperature for longer than 1 hr.
- Wash all dishes in hot, soapy water or a dishwasher. Wash glasses and cups after each use.
- Wash toothbrush daily in the dishwasher or rinse in a bleach solution.
- Do not share toiletry or personal hygiene items with others.
- Report manifestations of bacterial or viral infections immediately to the provider.
- Wash hands with antimicrobial soap before eating, after coming home from leaving the house, after using the toilet, after touching a pet, or shaking hands.
- Encourage client to bathe/shower with antimicrobial soap.
- Examine mouth for lesions or other unexpected findings daily and perform frequent oral care.

Nausea, vomiting, anorexia

- Many medications used for chemotherapy are emetogenic (induce vomiting) or cause anorexia and an altered taste in the mouth.
- A combination of medications can reduce chemotherapy-induced nausea and vomiting (CINV). These include:
  - Serotonin blockers (ondansetron, palonosetron) QEBP
  - Neurokinin receptor antagonists (aprepitant)
  - Corticosteroids (dexamethasone, methylprednisolone)
  - Dopamine antagonists (promethazine, prochlorperazine)
  - Proton pump inhibitors (omeprazole)
  - Histamine2 antagonists (cimetidine)
  - Prokinetic agents (metoclopramide)
  - Benzodiazepines (lorazepam)
  - Cannabinoids (dronabinol, nabilone)
  - Neurokinin-1 receptor antagonists (netupitant)

NURSING ACTIONS

- Ensure antiemetics are given before chemotherapy and repeated based on the response and duration of CINV.
- Administer antiemetic medications for several days after each treatment, even when CINV appears to be controlled.
- Remove vomiting cues, such as odor and emesis basins.
- Implement nonpharmacological methods to reduce nausea (visual imagery, relaxation, acupuncture, distraction).
- Perform calorie counts to determine intake. Provide liquid nutritional supplements as needed. Add protein powders to food or tube feedings.
- Administer megestrol to increase appetite if prescribed.
- Monitor for findings of dehydration or fluid and electrolyte imbalance.
- Perform mouth care prior to serving meals to enhance appetite.

CLIENT EDUCATION

- Some antiemetics can provide prophylactic treatment if given before meals.
- Eat several small meals a day if better tolerated. Low-fat dry foods (crackers, toast) and avoiding drinking liquids during meals can prevent nausea.
- Select foods that are served cold and do not require cooking. Cooking food can emit odors that stimulate nausea.
- Encourage consumption of high-protein, high-calorie, nutrient-dense foods and avoidance of low- or empty-calorie foods. Use meal supplements as needed.
- Use plastic eating utensils, suck on hard candy, and avoid consuming red meats to prevent or reduce the sensation of metallic taste.
- Create a food diary to identify items that can trigger nausea.

Alopecia

An adverse effect of certain chemotherapeutic medications that is usually temporary. The amount of hair lost can vary and can occur anywhere on the body.

NURSING ACTIONS
- Discuss the effect of alopecia on self-image.
- Discuss options (hats, turbans, wigs) to deal with hair loss. The American Cancer society has information on a variety of products. Recommend clients select a head covering prior to treatment. Qpcc
- Reinforce that hair should return about 1 month after chemotherapy is discontinued. The new hair can differ from the original hair in color, texture, and thickness.

CLIENT EDUCATION
- Hair loss occurs 7 to 10 days after treatment begins (for some agents).
- Avoid the use of damaging hair care measures (electric rollers, curling irons, hair dye, permanent waves). A soft hairbrush or wide-tooth comb for grooming is preferred.
- Consider cutting the hair short before treatment to decrease weight on the hair follicle.
- Consider collaborating with a hairdresser to assist with wig selection. Wearing a wig before therapy begins can reduce appearance changes.
- After hair loss, protect the scalp from sun exposure and use a diaper rash ointment/cream for itching. Qs
- Use head coverings to reduce body heat loss and protect skin while wearing helmets, headphones, headsets, or wigs.
- The oncologist might prescribe a cold cap during treatment to decrease hair loss. The cold caps cause vasoconstriction and decrease circulation to hair follicles.

Hypersensitivity

A client taking chemotherapy medication has an increased risk for hypersensitivity reactions. Reactions can occur as early as 1 hr following infusion but are also possible after several doses.

NURSING ACTIONS
- Stop the medication immediately if manifestations of a hypersensitivity reaction occur.
- Assist with the administration of emergency treatment, following facility protocol for hypersensitivity reactions.

CLIENT EDUCATION
- Watch for and report indications of a hypersensitivity reaction immediately.
- If hypersensitivity occurs, desensitization to the medication might be required so that the client can continue to receive the treatment most effective to combat the cancer.

Oral effects

Mucositis refers to inflammation in the mucous lining of the upper GI tract from the mouth to the stomach.

Stomatitis refers to inflammation of tissues in the oral cavity (gums, tongue, roof and floor of mouth, inside lips and cheeks).

NURSING ACTIONS
- Examine the client's mouth several times a day, and inquire about the presence of oral lesions.
- Document the location and size of lesions. For new lesions, obtain a specimen for culture and report them to the provider.
- Avoid using glycerin-based mouthwashes or mouth swabs for client care. Nonalcoholic, anesthetic mouthwashes are recommended. Qebp
- Administer a topical anesthetic prior to meals.
- Discourage consumption of salty, acidic, or spicy foods.
- Offer oral hygiene before and after each meal. Use lubricating or moisturizing agents to counteract dry mouth.

CLIENT EDUCATION
- Rinse the mouth with a solution of 0.9% sodium chloride, room-temperature tap water, or salt and soda water. Frequency is guided by the intensity of the mucositis.
- Perform gentle flossing and brushing using a soft-bristled toothbrush or foam swabs to avoid traumatizing the oral mucosa.
- Rinse the mouth before and after meals. Avoid mouthwash that contains alcohol or other irritants.
- Take medications to control infection as prescribed (nystatin suspension, acyclovir).
- Follow recommendations regarding the use of coating agents, topical analgesics, topical anesthetics, or oral or parenteral analgesics that can be prescribed.
- Choose soft, bland foods and supplements that are high in calories (mashed potatoes, scrambled eggs, cooked cereal, milk shakes, ice cream, frozen yogurt, bananas, and breakfast mixes). Avoid spicy, salty, acidic, rough, or hard food.
- Avoid drinking alcohol and the use of tobacco.
- Drink at least 2 L of water per day, if there is no fluid restriction prescribed by the provider.

Anemia and thrombocytopenia

Secondary to bone marrow suppression (myelosuppression)

Anemia
- **NURSING ACTIONS**
  - Monitor for fatigue, pallor, dizziness, and shortness of breath.
  - Help the client manage anemia-related fatigue by scheduling activities with rest periods in between and using energy saving measures (sitting during showers and ADLs).
  - Administer erythropoietic medications (darbepoetin alfa, epoetin alfa) and antianemic medications (such as ferrous sulfate) as prescribed.
  - Monitor Hgb values to determine response to medications. Be prepared to assist with the administration of blood if prescribed.

Thrombocytopenia

- NURSING ACTIONS
  - Monitor for petechiae, ecchymosis, bleeding of the gums, nosebleeds, and occult or frank blood in stools, urine, or vomitus.
  - Institute bleeding precautions.
    - Avoid IVs and injections. When needlesticks are necessary, use the smallest gauge needle possible.
    - Apply pressure for approximately 10 min after blood is obtained.
    - Handle client gently and avoid trauma.
    - To avoid bruising, do not over inflate the blood pressure cuff.
  - Administer thrombopoietic medications such as oprelvekin to stimulate platelet production. Monitor platelet count and be prepared to assist with the administration of platelets if the count falls below 20,000/mm³.
- CLIENT EDUCATION
  - Understand how to manage active bleeding.
  - Understand measures to prevent bleeding (use electric razor and soft-bristled toothbrush, avoid blowing nose vigorously, ensure that dentures fit appropriately). Avoid participation in contact sports or any activity in which injury is likely.
  - Avoid the use of NSAIDs.
  - Understand how to prevent injury when ambulating (wear closed-toes shoes, remove tripping hazards in the home) and apply cold if injury occurs. Qs

Chemotherapy-induced peripheral neuropathy

Loss of sensory or motor function of peripheral nerves is caused by exposure to certain anticancer medications. Higher doses of medication lead to greater neuropathy.

NURSING ACTIONS

- Monitor for loss of sensation in hands and feet, orthostatic hypotension, loss of taste, and constipation.
- Monitor for orthostatic hypotension.
- Monitor for early manifestations including numbness, tingling, and redness.
- Reinforce teaching how to prevent injury, including falls.
- Inform the client about the risk of erectile dysfunction and treatment options.

CLIENT EDUCATION

- Protect the skin because loss of sensation makes the client unaware of heat, cold, or pressure.
- Inspect the feet daily for any open areas.

Cognitive impairment

Cognitive changes occurring during and after chemotherapy treatment, including difficulty learning, decreased concentration, and memory loss.

NURSING ACTIONS: Support the client who reports cognitive changes by providing cognitive training resources.

CLIENT EDUCATION

- Avoid behaviors that could contribute to cognitive dysfunction, including excessive intake of alcohol, recreational drug use, and activities that are high-risk for head injury.
- Engage in strategies to improve memory and concentration (repeating challenging tasks).

Radiation therapy

Radiation therapy involves high-energy radiation to target tissues and destroy cells. Some cells are not destroyed but might become weakened and unable to divide, while others might be able to recover from the radiation damage.

- Radiation therapy is usually given as a series of divided small doses on a daily basis for a set period of time. The dose of radiation the client receives is determined by considering the duration of exposure, the intensity of the radiation, and the distance the radiation source is from the target cells.
- Radiation therapy might be given preoperatively to decrease the size of a tumor.
- Adverse effects on tissues within the radiation path include skin changes, hair loss, and stomatitis. Systemic effects can include debilitating fatigue, anorexia, and bone marrow suppression. Radiation effects can also cause long-term changes for the client.
- Radiation therapy can be administered internally (brachytherapy) with an implant or externally (teletherapy) with a radiation beam. The type used depends on the health of the client and shape, size, and location of the tumor.
- External beam radiation therapy.
- Delivers radiation from an external source to the client. The client does not retain the radiation and, therefore; is not at risk to spread the radiation to others.
- Internal radiation causes body fluids to be contaminated with radiation. Body wastes are radioactive and should be disposed of properly, as directed by the facility.
- Cytoprotectants (amifostine) are sometimes used to protect against harmful effects of radiation therapy, such as dryness of the mouth caused by radiation treatment for head and neck cancer.
- Radiation exposure to health care personnel and visitors is reduced by limiting indirect contact time, maintaining indicated distances from sources of radiation, and preventing direct contact with the source.

Internal radiation therapy

Brachytherapy describes internal radiation that is placed close to the target tissue. This is done via placement in a body orifice (vagina) or body cavity (abdomen) or delivered via IV such as with radionuclide iodine, which is absorbed by the thyroid.

- Brachytherapy provides radiation to the tumor and a limited amount to surrounding noncancerous tissues.
- Most clients remain in a medical facility until brachytherapy is complete. Clients who receive seed implants might go home with the implants.
- The client's excretions are radioactive until the isotope are eliminated from the body. Ensure no on touches the client's excretions.

NURSING ACTIONS

- Place the client in a private room. Keep the door closed as much as possible.
- Place a sign on the door warning of the radiation source. Qs
- Wear a dosimeter film badge that records personal amount of radiation exposure.
- Limit visitors to 30-min visits, and have visitors maintain a distance of 6 feet from the source.
- Individuals who are pregnant, trying to conceive, or under the age of 16 years should not enter the client's room.
- Wear a lead apron while providing care, keeping the front of the apron facing the source of radiation.
- Keep a lead container in the client's room if the delivery method could allow spontaneous loss of radioactive material. Tongs are available for placing radioactive material into this container.
- Follow protocol for proper removal of dressings and bed linens from the room. In most cases, all linens and dressings are kept in the client's room until the radiation source is removed, to ensure it is not lost in the trash or laundry.

CLIENT EDUCATION

- Remain in the position prescribed by the provider to prevent dislodgement of the radiation implant.
- Call the nurse for assistance with elimination.
- Follow radiation precautions in health care and home environments.

External beam radiation therapy

External beam radiation (EBRT) or teletherapy is delivered in relatively small doses over the course of several weeks and aimed at the body from an external source. Unlike internal radiation, the client is not radioactive and is not hazardous to others. Three-dimensional imaging facilitates visualization of the tumor for more effective treatment delivery.

- Intensity-modulated radiation therapy involves delivering radiation from several angles so that it is intense at the tumor but has minimal damage to the surrounding tissue.
- Stereotactic body radiotherapy (SBRT) is effective for deep tumors and involves high radiation doses gingiva in a short time span. A treatment that normally occurs 5 days a week for 6 to 8 weeks can be given in 1 to 5 days using SBRT.
- Proton therapy involves the use of charged protons to transfer energy to deep tumors with minimal effects on the tissue above the tumor, and minimal transfer of energy beyond the tumor.

NURSING ACTIONS

- The skin over the targeted area is marked with "tattoos" that guide the positioning of the external radiation source.
- Provide a well-balanced diet that does not contain red meat. Radiation can cause dysgeusia (altered taste), making foods such as red meat unpalatable.
- Help the client manage fatigue by scheduling activities with rest periods in between and using energy-saving measures (sitting during showers and ADLs).
- Monitor for radiation injury to skin and mucous membranes and implement a skin care regimen.
  - Skin: blanching, erythema, desquamation, sloughing, hemorrhage
  - Mouth: mucositis, xerostomia (dry mouth)
  - Neck: difficulty swallowing
  - Abdomen: gastroenteritis
- Monitor CBC (possible decreased platelets and WBCs).

CLIENT EDUCATION

- Adverse effects depend on which part of the body is being exposed to the radiation and how much radiation is being administered.
- If mucositis occurs:
  - Avoid spicy, salty, acidic foods.
  - Try eating foods that are cold rather than hot.
- Gently wash the skin over the irradiated area with mild soap and water. Dry the area thoroughly using patting motions. Use the hand to clean the skin rather than a washcloth. QEBP
- Do not remove or wash off radiation tattoos (markings) used to guide therapy. Do not apply powders, ointments, lotions, deodorants, or perfumes to the irradiated skin.
- Wear soft clothing. Avoid tight or constricting clothes.
- Do not expose the irradiated skin to sun or a heat source.
- Inspect skin for evidence of damage and report to the provider.

Hormone therapy

Hormone therapy is effective against tumors that are supported or suppressed by hormones, such as in breast or prostate cancer.

- By giving a similar hormone, uptake of the support hormone is blocked, or production reduced. Luteinizing hormone-releasing hormone (LH–RH) agonists like leuprolide and goserelin are effective against tumors that require a particular hormone for support.
  - The use of androgenic hormones in a client who has estrogen-dependent cancer can suppress growth of this type of cancer.
  - The use of estrogenic hormones for a testosterone-dependent cancer can suppress growth of this type of cancer.
- Hormone antagonists compete with the support hormone for binding sites on or in the tumor cell and are effective against tumors that require a particular hormone for support.
  - The use of an anti-estrogen hormone in a client who has estrogen-dependent cancer can suppress growth of this type of cancer. The same is true for anti-testosterone hormones.

LH–RH agonists

NURSING ACTIONS: Monitor cardiac status and blood pressure and for pulmonary edema.

CLIENT EDUCATION
- If assigned male at birth, understand the effect on sexual functions (decreased libido, erectile dysfunction) and feminizing effects of hormone therapy (gynecomastia, hot flashes, bone loss). Qpcc
- Increase intake of calcium and vitamin D.
- If assigned female at birth, understand the masculinizing effects (chest and facial hair growth, amenorrhea, decreased breast tissue).

Androgen antagonists (bicalutamide)

NURSING ACTIONS: Monitor laboratory findings (CBC [anemia], calcium, increased liver enzymes).

CLIENT EDUCATION
- If assigned male at birth, understand the feminizing effects of hormone therapy (gynecomastia, erectile dysfunction).
- Notify the provider of sore throat or bruising.

Estrogen receptor down-regulators

Estrogen receptor down-regulators (such as fulvestrant) induce degradation of estrogen receptors.

Estrogen antagonists

Tamoxifen, anastrozole, trastuzumab

NURSING ACTIONS
- Monitor CBC, clotting times, lipid profiles, calcium and cholesterol blood levels, and liver function for medication-related changes.
- Monitor neurologic and cardiovascular functioning for changes.

CLIENT EDUCATION
- Understand the adverse effects, which include nausea, vomiting, hot flashes, weight gain, vaginal bleeding, and increased risk of thrombosis.
- Understand the need for yearly gynecologic exams and the need to take calcium and vitamin D supplements.

Immunotherapy

Immunotherapy (biotherapy) alters a client's biological response to cancerous tumor cells. Antibodies, cytokines, and other immune substances normally produced by the immune system are administered to increase the body's defense against cancer. Immunotherapy includes biological response modifiers (BRM), monoclonal antibody targeted therapy, and cancer vaccines.

- The most common types of BRM are interleukins and interferons.
- **Interleukins** help coordinate the inflammatory and immune responses of the body, particularly the lymphocytes.
- **Interferons**, when stimulated, can exert an antitumor effect by activating a variety of responses.
- Monoclonal antibodies are a type of targeted therapy that binds to cancer cell proteins to inhibit cell division, make the cells more sensitive to treatment, and improve the body's ability to attack the cancer cells.
- Cancer vaccines can prevent infections that predispose a client to cancer (HPV), stop cancer from developing further, or kill cancer cells. Sipuleucel-T is the only FDA-approved therapeutic cancer vaccine and is appropriate for males who have metastatic prostate cancer that does not respond to other treatments.

NURSING ACTIONS
- **Interleukins:** Monitor for generalized edema, which can impair organ function. The client might require intensive care monitoring.
- **Interferons:** Monitor for peripheral neuropathy that can affect vision, hearing, balance, and gait.
- Take precautions for orthostatic hypotension.
- Monitor the client receiving BRM therapy for manifestations of inflammation (rigors, chills, malaise, fever, nausea, diarrhea, and anorexia).
- Observe for indication of neurologic effects of BRM therapy (agitation, hallucinations, sleep disorders, nightmares, mood swings, somnolence).
- Check the client's skin while taking BRM therapy for peeling, pruritus, or dryness. Protect the skin from sunlight and use mild cleansers and moisturizers.

CLIENT EDUCATION
- Report influenza-like manifestations or changes consistent with peripheral neuropathy immediately.
- Use a perfume-free moisturizer can be helpful in managing skin discomfort.
- Avoid sun exposure and swimming if skin manifestations develop.

Targeted therapy

- Target therapy acts on components produced by cancer cells and includes small molecule medications and monoclonal antibodies (discussed in the prior section). A targeted therapy that is effective for one client might not be effective for another client.
- Small molecule inhibitor targeted therapies are effective in affecting mainly cancer cells while not affecting healthy cells. These agents affect the replication process of cancer cells.
- Targeted therapy agents are classified based upon their mechanism of action (tyrosine kinase inhibitors, epidermal growth factor/receptor inhibitors, vascular endothelial growth factor/receptor inhibitors, multikinase inhibitors, protease inhibitors, and angiogenesis inhibitors).

NURSING ACTIONS: Monitor for adverse effects specific to type of agent administered.

CLIENT EDUCATION: Reinforce the importance of taking oral antineoplastic agents as prescribed.

Photodynamic therapy

Photodynamic therapy involves injection of a photosensitizing agent that is absorbed by all cells in the body. 1 to 3 days later when the agent remains in only the cancer cells, the tumor is exposed to a specific wavelength of light via an endoscope. Cells are subsequently destroyed, and tumors are eliminated or reduced in size.

- Used to treat esophageal cancer, ocular tumors, upper airway tumors, and nonmelanoma skin cancer.
- Adverse effects are related to the area of the body being treated.

NURSING ACTIONS

- Photodynamic therapy is contraindicated for clients who have a tumor with known major blood vessel involvement. When the tumor rapidly dies, the client might begin bleeding.
- Use caution for clients who have a history of radiation therapy or coagulation disorders.

CLIENT EDUCATION: Avoid sun exposure for 6 weeks. (Limit time outdoors, and wear sunglasses.)

Supportive treatment

In addition to cancer treatment, the client can require assistance for altered body function or to meet emotional and spiritual needs.

- Facilitate safe activity, providing assistive devices when necessary for clients who have altered mobility or require assistance with self-care activities. Qs
- Assist with the transfer of client care to home health, hospice, or a tertiary care setting (rehabilitation center) as appropriate.
- Provide alternate means of communication for clients who have cancer affecting the mouth, throat, larynx, or vocal cords.
- Use assistive aids and devices for clients who have visual or hearing impairments.
- Recommend a consultation with physical therapy and genetic or other counseling services as indicated.
- Recommend a consultation with pain management for persistent or uncontrolled pain. (See **CHAPTER 83: PAIN MANAGEMENT FOR CLIENTS WHO HAVE CANCER.**)
- Monitor client's nutritional intake and weight. Consult a dietitian or nutritionist if indicated and provide meal supplements.
- Determine whether the client has body image concerns and assist the client in promoting a positive body image (touching affected body areas, use of prosthetics, choosing clothing, head coverings, or makeup).
- Discuss common effects of treatment on sexual function. Assist the client with discussing any concerns, and arrange for counseling, if desired.
- Instruct the client about medications to promote erection or manage pain sensation.
- Check the client's coping ability, and help the client use prior positive coping mechanisms or to identify new ones.
- Inquire about whether the client uses complementary or alternative therapies to prevent or treat cancer, or the associated manifestations. Ensure the client is aware of any safety issues and recommend inclusion of the client's preferred strategies into the plan of care when possible. Qpcc

Application Exercises

1. A nurse is assisting with the plan of care for a client who is receiving chemotherapy and is at risk for nausea and mucositis. Sort the following nursing interventions into those implemented for Nausea and those implemented for Mucositis.

   A. Provide the client with several small meals during the day

   B. Have the client rinse their mouth with a solution of sodium chloride

   C. Instruct the client to avoid strong odors

   D. Advise the client to use a soft-bristle toothbrush

   E. Advise the client to avoid drinking fluids during meals

   F. Advise the client to use oral topical anesthetic prior to meals

2. A nurse is assisting with the plan of care for a client who is receiving chemotherapy. Match the adverse effect of chemotherapy with the possible pharmacological treatment.

   A. Anorexia   1. Filgrastim

   B. Nausea   2. Epoetin alfa

   C. Anemia   3. Ondansetron

   D. Neutropenia   4. Megestrol

3. A nurse is assisting with the plan of care for a client who is receiving chemotherapy and is at risk for myelosuppression. Sort the following nursing interventions into those implemented for Neutropenia and those implemented for Thrombocytopenia.

   A. Place the client in a private room

   B. Apply prolonged pressure to puncture site after blood sampling

   C. Have client-specific equipment remain in the room

   D. Advise the client to use an electric razor to shave

   E. Have the client wear a mask when leaving the room

   F. Administer a stool softener

4. A nurse is assisting with the plan of care for a client who has cervical cancer and is scheduled for brachytherapy. What actions should the nurse plan to take?

5. A nurse is reinforcing teaching about skin care to a client who is receiving external beam radiation therapy. Which of the following instructions should the nurse include?

   A. "Use your hand, rather than a washcloth, to clean your skin."

   B. "Remove ink markings when cleaning your skin."

   C. "Scrub skin with a towel, when drying."

   D. "Expose irradiated skin to the sun each day."

Active Learning Scenario

A nurse is reinforcing teaching with a client who is receiving chemotherapy and has alopecia. What should the nurse include when reinforcing the teaching? Use the Active Learning Template: System Disorder to complete this item.

PATHOPHYSIOLOGY RELATED TO CLIENT PROBLEM

CLIENT EDUCATION: Identify at least four instructional points.

NURSING CARE: Identify at least two nursing actions.

Active Learning Scenario Key

Using the Active Learning Template: System Disorder

PATHOPHYSIOLOGY RELATED TO CLIENT PROBLEM: Alopecia occurs as an adverse effect of chemotherapy medications. The medications interfere with the life cycle of rapidly proliferating cells, such as those found in hair follicles, resulting in hair loss.

CLIENT EDUCATION

- Wear head coverings to protect the skin when using headphones, or wearing helmets or wigs.
- Avoid the use of damaging hair-care measures (electric rollers, curling irons, hair dye, permanent waves).
- Use a soft hair brush or wide-tooth comb for grooming.
- Avoid sun exposure. Use a diaper rash ointment or cream for itching.
- Alopecia is usually temporary, and hair will return when chemotherapy is discontinued.

NURSING CARE

- Discuss the effect of alopecia on self-image. Encourage the client to express feelings.
- Recommend use of information from the American Cancer Society on managing alopecia.
- Provide referral to a cancer support group.

Ⓝ *NCLEX® Connection: Physiological Adaptation, Alterations in Body Systems*

Application Exercises Key

1. **NAUSEA:** A, C, E; **MUCOSITIS:** B, D, F

   When generating solutions, the nurse should plan to provide the client who has nausea with several small meals during the day to reduce nausea. The nurse should instruct the client to avoid strong odors and drinking fluids during meals to increase appetite and reduce nausea. The nurse should plan to have the client who has mucositis to rinse their mouth with a solution of 0.9% sodium chloride, use a soft-bristle toothbrush, and use an oral topical anesthetic prior to meals to reduce the discomfort.

   Ⓝ *NCLEX® Connection: Physiological Adaptation, Alterations in Body Systems*

2. A, 4; B, 3; C, 2; D, 1

   When generating solutions, the nurse should identify that filgrastim is administered to treat neutropenia. Epoetin alfa is administered to treat anemia. Ondansetron is administered to treat nausea. Megestrol is administered to treat anorexia.

   Ⓝ *NCLEX® Connection: Pharmacological Therapies, Expected Actions/Outcomes*

3. **NEUTROPENIA:** A, C, E; **THROMBOCYTOPENIA:** B, D, F

   When generating solutions, the nurse should plan to place the client who has neutropenia in a private room, have client-specific equipment remain in the client's room, and have the client wear a mask when leaving the room, to protect the client from acquiring an infection. The nurse should plan to apply prolonged pressure to puncture sites after blood sampling, advise the client to use an electric razor to shave, and administer a stool softener to the client who has thrombocytopenia to reduce the risk of bleeding.

   Ⓝ *NCLEX® Connection: Reduction of Risk Potential, Therapeutic Procedures*

4. When generating solutions, the nurse should plan to place the client in a private room, place a sign on the door to the client's room warning of the radiation source, and keep the door closed as much as possible to reduce the risk of exposure to others to radiation. The nurse should wear a dosimeter film badge that records personal amount of radiation exposure and wear a lead apron while providing care, keeping the front of the apron facing the source of radiation. Visitors should be limited to 30-min visits and stay at least 6 feet away from the source. Individuals who are pregnant, trying to conceive, or under the age of 16 years should not enter the client's room. The nurse should keep a lead container in the client's room in case of spontaneous loss of radioactive material. Tongs should be available for placing radioactive material into this container. The nurse should follow protocol for proper removal of dressings and bed linens from the client's room. In most cases, all linens and dressings are kept in the client's room until the radiation source is removed, to ensure it is not lost in the trash or laundry. The nurse should instruct the client to remain in the position prescribed by the provider to prevent dislodgement of the radiation implant and call the nurse for assistance with elimination.

   Ⓝ *NCLEX® Connection: Physiological Adaptation, Alterations in Body Systems*

5. A. **CORRECT:** When taking actions, the nurse should instruct the client to use their hand, rather than a washcloth, with mild soap and water, to clean the irradiated skin to reduce the risk of skin irritation.

   Ⓝ *NCLEX® Connection: Physiological Adaptation, Alterations in Body Systems*

CHAPTER 84 *Cancer Disorders*

The various types of cancer share general cancer principles: abnormal cell growth, tumor formation, and potential for invasion to other locations. Each type of cancer has distinguishing characteristics related to risk, manifestations, screening, and diagnosis. The prognosis and treatment can vary by type. The most common cancers in the US include bladder, breast, colorectal, endometrial, kidney, leukemia, liver, lung, melanoma, pancreas, prostate, and thyroid.

Skin cancer

Sunlight exposure is the leading cause of skin cancer. The most effective strategy for prevention of skin cancer is avoidance or reduction of skin exposure to ultraviolet light from sunlight and synthetic sources. Precancerous skin lesions, called actinic keratoses, can appear as scaly pink or reddish brown macules or papules and are common in clients who have chronically sun-damaged skin, such as older adults. Ⓖ These lesions should be removed promptly because of risk of developing squamous cell carcinoma.

TYPES OF SKIN CANCER

Squamous cell (epidermis)

CHARACTERISTICS
- Initially appears as a rough, scaly lesion with central ulceration and crusting
- Bleeding (possible)
- Usually present on sun-exposed areas

COURSE: Localized; can metastasize

Basal cell (basal epidermis or nearby dermal cells)

CHARACTERISTICS
- Open lesion that does not heal within 4 weeks
- Small waxy nodule with superficial blood vessels, well-defined borders
- Erythema and ulcerations
- Usually present on sun-exposed areas

COURSE: Invades local structures (nerves, bone, cartilage, lymphatic and vascular tissue); rarely metastatic but high rate of recurrence

Malignant melanoma (cancer of melanocytes)

CHARACTERISTICS
- Irregular shape and borders with multiple colors; can have elevated nodules and ulcerations
- New moles or change in an existing mole (can occur in intestines or any other body structure that contains pigment cells)
- Itching, cracks, ulcerations, or bleeding (possible)
- Common on upper back and lower legs and on palms and soles for clients who have dark skin

COURSE: Rapid invasion and metastasis with high morbidity and mortality

HEALTH PROMOTION AND DISEASE PREVENTION

- Limit exposure to sunlight, especially between 1000 and 1600.
- Apply sunscreen when near reflective surfaces (sand, snow, water, concrete).
- Use sunblock that has an SPF of at least 15, with both UVA and UVB protection. Apply 30 min before exposure to sun. Sunblock should be reapplied at least every 2 hr.
- Wear protective clothing, hats, sunglasses, and lip balm that has an SPF of at least 15.
- Avoid indoor tanning (tanning beds, booths, sunlamps).
- Reinforce with clients the "ABCDE" system to evaluate moles.
  ○ **A: Asymmetry:** One side does not match the other
  ○ **B: Borders:** Ragged, notched, irregular, or blurred edges
  ○ **C: Color:** Lack of uniformity in pigmentation (shades of tan, brown, or black)
  ○ **D: Diameter:** Width greater than 5 mm, or about the size of a pencil eraser or a pea
  ○ **E: Evolving:** Change in appearance (shape, size, color, height, texture) or condition (bleeding, itching)
- Because of the cumulative effects of sun damage over the lifespan, screening for suspicious lesions is an essential part of the routine physical data collection of older adult clients. Ⓖ

DATA COLLECTION

RISK FACTORS

- Occupational history of chemical carcinogens
- Exposure to ultraviolet light (natural light or indoor tanning) over long periods of time
- Ethnicity: non-Hispanic white
- Presence of several large or many small moles
- Genetic predisposition
- Older adult clients

EXPECTED FINDINGS

See types of skin cancers for expected findings. Client should report of change in appearance of mole or lesion

DIAGNOSTIC PROCEDURES

Examination (self or clinician)

EXPECTED FINDINGS
- New or suspicious lesions
- Recent changes in size, color, or sensation of any mole, birthmark, wart or scar

CLIENT EDUCATION: Develop a body map (diagram of scars or lesions) and monitor monthly for changes. Inspect skin between fingers and toes and on scalp.

Biopsy (punch, shave, or excisional)

EXPECTED FINDINGS: Cancerous cells

CLIENT EDUCATION
- Monitor for infection.
- Conduct wound care, including care of sutures (punch, excisional biopsy).

Lymph node biopsy/dissection

EXPECTED FINDINGS: Tissue examined microscopically for the spread of cancer

NURSING ACTIONS
- Monitor site of lymph node biopsy or removal for bleeding or infection.
- If melanoma is diagnosed, blood tests are prescribed (CBC, CMP, liver) to check for organ involvement.

PATIENT-CENTERED CARE

THERAPEUTIC PROCEDURES

Chemotherapy

Interferon therapy
For postoperative treatment of melanomas.

NURSING ACTIONS: Report and provide relief for adverse or toxic effects of chemotherapy.

CLIENT EDUCATION
- Perform adequate nutrition and fluid intake.
- Understand the self-injection procedure.

Targeted therapy

- Blocks or slows the spread of cancer by interfering with specific molecules (targets) that are involved in growth, progression, and spread of cancer. ⓠEBP
- Vemurafenib is an oral medication used for targeted therapy to treat melanoma.

Biotherapy

Monoclonal antibody therapy: Stimulates T-cell lymphocyte activity, which can produce antitumor immune response

Radiation

- Limited to older clients who have large, deeply invasive tumors and those who are poor surgical candidates.
- Melanoma is relatively resistant to radiation therapy.

Cryosurgery

- Freezes and destroys isolated lesions by applying liquid nitrogen (–200° C).
- Skin becomes edematous and tender.

CLIENT EDUCATION: Cleanse and apply a topical antimicrobial until healed.

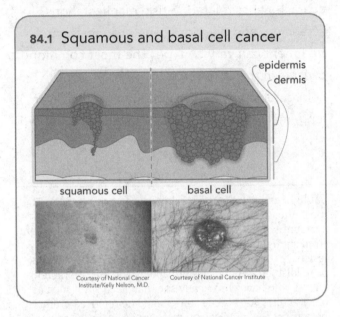

84.1 Squamous and basal cell cancer

epidermis
dermis

squamous cell   basal cell

Courtesy of National Cancer Institute/Kelly Nelson, M.D.   Courtesy of National Cancer Institute

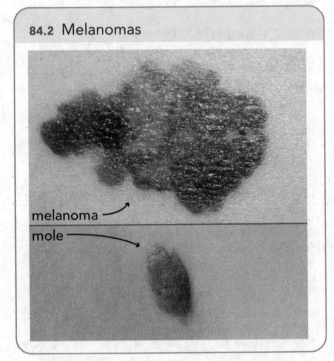

84.2 Melanomas

melanoma
mole

Curettage and electrodessication

Removes cancerous cells with the use of a curette to scrape away cancerous tissue, followed by the application of an electric probe to destroy remaining tumor tissue

Excision

The incision will be closed with sutures if possible. A skin graft can be necessary for large areas.

CLIENT EDUCATION: Perform postoperative wound care and care of the skin graft if used.

Mohs surgery

- Used with basal and squamous cell carcinoma
- Conserves more normal tissue and is used to determine the extent of nonmelanoma skin cancer
- Tissue is sectioned horizontally in layers and each layer is examined for presence of residual cancer; the process is continued until the samples are free of cancer

COMPLICATIONS: Skin abscess and cellulitis

84.3 Cancer therapies at a glance

Chemotherapy

Chemotherapy uses anti-cancer drugs administered orally or intravenously to destroy cancer cells.

Photodynamic therapy

Photodynamic therapy involves the injection of a photosensitizing agent that is absorbed by all the cells in the body. One to three days later when the agent remains in only the cancer cells, the tumor is exposed to a laser light via an endoscope. Cells are subsequently destroyed and tumors are eliminated or reduced in size. Used with small, noninvasive lesions.

Radiation

With extensive disease, radiation is combined with chemotherapy.

Brachytherapy is radiation delivered inside the body.

External beam radiation therapy (EBRT) uses radiation from a source outside of the body to destroy cancer cells.

Targeted therapy

Targeted therapy is a newer molecular-based medication therapy that targets specific receptors or other processes that produce cancer cells. Because this therapy has specific targets, it often causes less adverse effects than regular cancer chemotherapy, which typically kills large numbers of normal cells along with cancer cells.

Examples of targeted therapy includes biologic response modifiers, monoclonal antibodies, cytokines, growth factors, and gene therapy.

Immunotherapy (biotherapy) uses biologic response modifiers (BRMs), which alter a client's biological response to cancerous tumor cells. Cytokines work to enhance the immune system. They help the client's immune system recognize cancer cells and use the body's natural defenses to destroy them. Interleukins and interferons are the two primary cytokines (immune response modulators) used in immunotherapy.

- Interleukins help coordinate the inflammatory and immune responses of the body, in particular, the lymphocytes.
- Interferons, when stimulated, can exert an antitumor effect by activating a variety of responses.
- Tumor necrosis factor

Leukemias and lymphomas

Leukemias are cancers within the bone marrow that causes an increase production of immature WBCs. In leukemia, the white blood cells are not functional. They invade and destroy bone marrow, and they can metastasize to the liver, spleen, lymph nodes, testes, and brain. The goal of treatment is to eliminate all leukemic cells. The exact cause of leukemia is not known. The overgrowth of leukemic cells prevents growth of other blood components (platelets, erythrocytes, mature leukocytes). Qs

- Lack of mature leukocytes leads to immunosuppression. Infection is the leading cause of death among clients who have leukemia.
- Lack of platelets increases the client's risk of bleeding.

Leukemias are divided into acute (acute lymphocytic leukemia (ALL) and acute myelogenous leukemia (AML) and chronic (chronic lymphocytic leukemia (CLL) and chronic myelogenous leukemia (CML) and are further classified by the type of white blood cells primarily affected.

- ALL: Occurs most frequently in children. Various factors influence the prognosis for children, but the 5-year survival rate is approximately 91% (age at diagnosis, gender, cell type involved); 68% survival rate of children and adults combined.
- AML: Most common leukemia among adults; prognosis is poor. The 5-year survival rate is 26%.
- CLL: Most cases involve people older than 50 years of age. This is the most common adult leukemia.
- CML: Most prevalent after age 50 years. The disease is uncommon in children. Three phases: chronic (slow growing with mild manifestations); accelerated (more rapid growing with severe manifestations and failure to respond to therapy); and blast (very aggressive with metastasis to organs).

Lymphomas are cancers of lymphocyte cells. The lymphocyte cells overgrow and multiply and causes tumors within the lymph nodes (which produce antibodies and fight infection). Lymphomas can metastasize to almost any organ. The types of lymphoma include Hodgkin's lymphoma (HL) and non-Hodgkin's lymphoma (NHL).

Hodgkin's lymphoma

Also known as Hodgkin's disease

- Peaks in two age groups: teens and young adults; adults in their 50s and 60s.
- Possible causes include viral infections and exposure to chemical agents.
- Typically starts in a single node or chain of nodes that contain the Reed–Sternberg cell. HL spreads predictably from one group of lymph nodes to the next.
- One of the most treatable types of cancer with a survival rate of 86% at 5 years.

Non-Hodgkin's lymphoma

- More common in males (sex assigned at birth) and older adults.
- Possible causes include viral infections and autoimmune disease.
- There is an increased incidence in clients exposed to pesticides, insecticides, and dust.

HEALTH PROMOTION AND DISEASE PREVENTION

- Use protective equipment, such as a mask, and ensure proper ventilation while working in environments that contain carcinogens or particles in the air.
- Influenza and pneumonia vaccinations are important for all clients who are immunosuppressed.

DATA COLLECTION

RISK FACTORS

- Immunosuppression
- Exposure to chemotherapy agents or medications that suppress bone marrow
- Genetic factors (hereditary)
- Ionizing radiation (radiation therapy, environmental)
- Viral infections (Epstein-Barr virus, human T-cell leukemia/lymphoma virus, human immune deficiency virus)

OLDER ADULT CLIENTS Ⓖ

- Often have diminished immune function and decreased bone marrow function, which increase the risk of complications of leukemia and lymphoma.
- Have decreased energy reserves and can tire easily during treatment. Safety is a concern with ambulation.

EXPECTED FINDINGS

Acute leukemia

- Bone pain
- Joint swelling
- Enlarged liver and spleen
- Weight loss
- Fever
- Poor wound healing (infected lesions)
- Manifestations of anemia (fatigue, pallor, tachycardia, dyspnea on exertion)
- Evidence of bleeding (ecchymoses, hematuria, bleeding gums)
- Headaches, behavior changes, decreased attention

Hodgkin's and non-Hodgkin's lymphoma

- Lymphadenopathy: painless, enlarged lymph node (usually in the neck with HL), which is a typical finding.
- Other possible manifestations include fever, night sweats, unplanned weight loss, fatigue, and infections.
- Client may report abdominal fullness and prolonged swelling of lymph nodes.

DIAGNOSTIC PROCEDURES

Staging of lymphoma involves extensive testing to ensure proper treatment is prescribed.

CBC with differential

EXPECTED FINDINGS
- WBC can be high, low, or normal (leukemia)
- Blast cells increased (leukemia)
- Hemoglobin, hematocrit, and platelets decreased

Biopsy of bone marrow (core or fine-needle aspiration)

EXPECTED FINDINGS
- Large quantities of immature leukemic blast cells (confirms diagnosis)
- Typing of protein markers (to differentiate myeloid or lymphoid leukemia)

NURSING ACTIONS
- Administer pain medication as prescribed.
- Apply pressure for 5 to 10 min, then a pressure dressing.
- Monitor for bleeding and infection for 24 hr.

CT scan (used for HL staging)

EXPECTED FINDINGS: Guide for lymphoma staging procedures: identify presence, size, and shape of nodes, tumors.

Biopsy of lymph nodes

EXPECTED FINDINGS
- **Hodgkin's lymphoma**: presence of Reed–Sternberg cells (cancerous B-lymphocytes) (definite)
- **Non-Hodgkin's lymphoma**: any other lymph node malignancy

Chest x-ray, CT scan, PET scan, bone scan

EXPECTED FINDINGS: Confirms diagnosis or metastatic disease

PATIENT-CENTERED CARE

NURSING CARE

- Monitor for evidence of infection. Monitor for other physiological indicators of infection (lung crackles, cough, urinary frequency or urgency, oliguria, lesions of skin or mucous membrane).
- Prevent infection. (Implement neutropenic precautions.) These interventions are especially important during chemotherapy induction and for clients who have received a bone marrow transplant. Qs
  - Frequent, thorough hand hygiene is a priority intervention.
  - Place the client in a private room.
  - Allow only healthy visitors; when unavoidable, visitors who are ill must wear a mask.
  - Screen visitors carefully.
  - Restrict foods that can be contaminated with bacteria (no fresh or raw fruits, vegetables).
  - Monitor WBC.
  - Prevent transmission of bacteria and viruses (high-efficiency particulate air [HEPA] filtration). Eliminate standing water (humidifiers, denture cups, vases) to prevent bacteria breeding. Live plants and flowers might not be allowed in the client's room, depending on facility policy.
  - Encourage good personal hygiene.
  - Avoid crowds.
- Prevent injury.
  - Monitor platelets.
  - Monitor frequently for obvious and occult bleeding.
  - Protect the client from trauma (avoid injections and venipunctures, apply firm pressure, increase vitamin K intake).
  - Reinforce with the client how to avoid trauma (use electric shaver, soft bristled toothbrush, avoid contact sports).
- Conserve the client's energy.
  - Encourage rest, adequate nutrition, and fluid intake.
  - Ensure the client gets adequate sleep.
  - Monitor the client's energy resources/capability.
  - Plan activities to conserve energy.

THERAPEUTIC PROCEDURES

Chemotherapy

- Chemotherapy can be used to treat lymphoma in combination with other therapies.
- There are three phases of chemotherapy used to treat leukemia.

CLIENT EDUCATION: Report manifestations of infection or illness immediately to the provider.

Colony-stimulating medications

Medications such as filgrastim stimulate the production of leukocytes.

NURSING ACTIONS: Monitor for report of bone pain. Monitor CBC twice weekly to check leukocytes. Use cautiously with clients who have bone marrow cancer.

CLIENT EDUCATION: Report bone discomfort.

Immunotherapy

Monoclonal antibodies are man-made proteins that attack a specific target to treat lymphoma.

Targeted therapy

Radiation

- External lymph node radiation is the primary form of treatment for early stage HL. Radiation therapy or radiolabeled antibodies can be used as part of treatment for NHL.
- With extensive disease, radiation is combined with chemotherapy.
- Radiation is not typically a treatment used for clients who have leukemia.

84.4 Phases of chemotherapy to treat leukemia

	GOAL	PROCEDURE	LENGTH OF TIME
Induction therapy: intensive combination therapy	Induce remission: absence of all findings of leukemia, including less than 5% blasts in bone marrow.	Aggressive treatment (possible continuous infusion); IV infusion; CNS and CSF infusion prophylaxis (ALL).	4 to 6 weeks (hospitalization required due to increased risk for infection and hemorrhage)
Consolidation or intensification therapy	Cure by eradicating any residual leukemic cells.	Same medications as induction phase at lower dosage or different combination of medications	About 6 months
Maintenance therapy	Prevent relapse.	Lower doses of oral or IV chemotherapy	Months to years
Reinduction therapy: for a client who relapses	Place the client back in remission.	Combinations of chemotherapy used to achieve remission.	Probability of relapse occurring decreases over time

Hematopoietic stem cell (bone marrow) transplantation (HSCT)

Bone marrow is destroyed or ablated using radiation or chemotherapy and later replaced with healthy stem cells. The body will resume normal production of blood cells.

- Autologous cells are the client's own cells that are collected before chemotherapy.
- Matching of donor to recipient stem cells compares certain human leukocyte antigens (HLA) to reduce risk of rejection.
  - Syngeneic cells are donated from the client's identical twin (HLA identical).
  - Allogeneic cells are obtained from an HLA-matched donor, such as a relative or from umbilical cord blood (closely matched HLA).
- Following transplantation, the client is at high risk for infection and bleeding until the transfused stem cells begin producing white blood cells again.

COMPLICATIONS

Pancytopenia

Decrease in white and red blood cells and platelets
- Neutropenia secondary to disease or treatment greatly increases the client's risk for infection.
- The nurse should implement neutropenic precautions, including placing the client in a private room.

NURSING ACTIONS
- Maintain a hygienic environment.
- Practice frequent hand hygiene.
- Monitor vital signs every 4 hr.
- Monitor for infection (WBC, cough, alterations in breath sounds, urine, or feces). Report temperature greater than 37.8° C (100° F).
- Administer antimicrobial, antiviral, and antifungal medications as prescribed.
- Assist with the administration of blood products (granulocytes) as needed.

Thrombocytopenia

- Secondary to disease and/or treatment; greatly increases the client's risk for bleeding.
- The greatest risk is at platelet counts less than 50,000/mm³, and spontaneous bleeding can occur at less than 20,000/mm³. Qs

NURSING ACTIONS
- Monitor for petechiae, ecchymosis, bleeding of the gums, nosebleeds, and occult or frank blood in stool, urine, or vomitus.
- Institute bleeding precautions. (Avoid IVs and injections; apply pressure for approximately 10 min after blood is obtained; and handle client gently and avoid trauma.)
- Minimize the risk of trauma (safe environment).
- Assist with the administration of blood products (platelets) if platelet count is less than 20,000/mm³.

Hypoxemia

Anemia secondary to disease or treatment significantly increases the client's risk for hypoxemia.

NURSING ACTIONS
- Instruct client to cough and deep breath every hr to promote gas exchange.
- Monitor oxygen saturation.
- Plan client care to balance rest and activity and use assistive devices, as indicated.
- Monitor RBC.
- Provide a diet high in protein and carbohydrates.
- Administer colony-stimulating factors, such as epoetin alfa, as prescribed.
- Assist with the administration of blood products (packed red blood cells) as needed.

HSCT complications

Graft-versus-host disease (graft rejection)

NURSING ACTIONS: Administer immunosuppressants as prescribed.

Thyroid cancer

As thyroid tumors increase in size or spread, they impact the function of surrounding structures (larynx, pharynx, esophagus). The types of cancer include follicular, papillary, medullary, and anaplastic. Papillary is the most common type that of thyroid cancer. Only 5-10% of nodules are cancerous.

HEALTH PROMOTION AND DISEASE PREVENTION

- Avoid or stop smoking.
- Wear a thyroid guard to protect the neck during upper body x-rays.

DATA COLLECTION

RISK FACTORS

- Female sex (assigned at birth)
- Radiation exposure
- Family history

EXPECTED FINDINGS

- Dyspnea
- Dysphagia and vocal changes
- Change in size, shape of thyroid
- Palpable nodule(s) in neck area (painless)
- Other findings include weight changes, tiredness, depressed mood

DIAGNOSTIC PROCEDURE

Blood thyroglobulin

EXPECTED FINDINGS: Elevated

CLIENT EDUCATION: The result can indicate remaining cancer cells after treatment or return of cancer.

TSH, T₃, T₄

Indicates function of the thyroid

EXPECTED FINDINGS: T_3, T_4 levels, and TSH are usually normal in thyroid cancer.

CLIENT EDUCATION: Results indicate the function of the thyroid. Consider additional testing needed.

Biopsy (fine-needle plus open or core, if indicated)

EXPECTED FINDINGS: To identify presence of cancer cells in thyroid nodules or lymph nodes

NURSING ACTIONS
- Instruct client that lesions greater than 1 cm and suspicious lymph nodes are tested.
- Administer pain medication as prescribed.
- Apply pressure for 5 to 10 min, then a pressure dressing.
- Monitor for bleeding and infection for 24 hr.

Ultrasound

EXPECTED FINDINGS
- Used to guide biopsy
- Reveals whether nodules are fluid-filled (typically benign) or solid (typically cancerous)

Radioiodine scan

EXPECTED FINDINGS
- Presence of radioactive cells (cells that retained radioiodine)
- Not useful with medullary carcinoma

CLIENT EDUCATION: Dye will be administered (injection or oral) then the thyroid and other suspicious areas are scanned.

PATIENT-CENTERED CARE

NURSING CARE

- Monitor airway patency in client who has a tumor affecting or compressing the trachea.
- Monitor swallowing in client who has a tumor affecting or compressing the esophagus.

MEDICATIONS

Thyroid suppression therapy

- Involves administration of synthetic thyroxine (T_4, levothyroxine sodium).
- Suppression therapy replaces T_4 needed for body function. It also prevents or slows growth of cancerous thyroid cells.
- Therapy is typically prescribed for several months following thyroid surgery.

CLIENT EDUCATION
- Never stop taking levothyroxine sodium, unless instructed by the provider. Qs
- Take levothyroxine sodium on an empty stomach.

THERAPEUTIC PROCEDURES

Radiation

Used to treat anaplastic carcinoma

Radioactive iodine (RAI) therapy (ablation)

Used to destroy papillary or follicular carcinoma and can be used to treat hyperthyroidism
- RAI therapy works similarly to radioactive scanning (used to diagnose thyroid cancer).
- The client ingests RAI in liquid or tablet form, which is absorbed by thyroid cells which are then destroyed.
- Client can benefit from RAI therapy following thyroid suppression therapy.

NURSING ACTIONS
- Reinforce with the client about radioactive precautions to reduce risk of radiation exposure.
- Provide information on nutrition supplements for client experiencing altered taste. Consult nutrition services.
- Instruct client to expect nausea, dry mouth, neck tenderness, and altered taste.

CLIENT EDUCATION: Chew gum or suck on hard candy to relieve dry mouth or reduced salivation.

Surgical interventions

Papillary, follicular, and medullary carcinoma are treated surgically.
- **Thyroidectomy** (total or partial) or thyroid lobectomy is the treatment of choice for papillary carcinoma that is limited to the thyroid gland.
- Involved lymph nodes in the neck are removed during surgery.
- During surgery, the parathyroid glands or laryngeal nerve can be damaged.
- A wound drain can be placed intraoperatively.
- Refer to **CHAPTER 72: HYPERTHYROIDISM** for information on thyroidectomy surgery.

CLIENT EDUCATION

Take thyroid replacement therapy as prescribed. It is lifelong therapy for those who have had thyroidectomy surgery.

Lung cancer

Lung cancer is one of the leading causes of cancer-related deaths for all genders. In the U.S., there are about 228,000 new diagnosis of lung cancer and more than 135,000 deaths from lung cancer annually. Prognosis of lung cancer is poor because it is often diagnosed in an advanced stage after metastasis has occurred. Palliative care is often the focus at the advanced stage (III, IV).

- Most lung cancers arise from bronchogenic carcinomas (arising from the bronchial epithelium).
- Most lung cancers are non-small cell lung cancer (NSCLC), which includes squamous, adeno, and large cell carcinomas.
- Small cell lung cancer (SCLC) is fast-growing and is consistently linked to a history of cigarette smoking.

HEALTH PROMOTION AND DISEASE PREVENTION

- Promote smoking cessation, avoid beginning smoking, and avoid exposure to second/third-hand smoke Instruct the client that the safety of electronic nicotine devices is unknown, and there could be risk from inhaling the vapor of these devices. Over the counter and prescription nicotine replacement therapies are available to assist clients in smoking cessation.
- Use protective equipment (mask) and ensure proper ventilation while working in environments that can contain carcinogens or particles in the air.
- Screening (annual CT) for early detection for those at high risk for lung cancer development.

DATA COLLECTION

- Determine the pack-year history (number of packs of cigarettes smoked per day times the number of years smoked) for clients who smoke. ⃝EBP
- Evaluate use of other tobacco products (cigars, pipes, and chewing tobacco).
- Ask about exposure to secondhand smoke.
- Monitor for a cough that changes in pattern.

RISK FACTORS

- Age older than 40
- Smoking tobacco
- Exposure to second/third hand tobacco smoke
- Radiation exposure
- Chronic exposure to inhaled environmental irritants (air pollution, asbestos, coal, other talc dusts)
- History of lung conditions (COPD, tuberculosis)

EXPECTED FINDINGS

Clients can experience few manifestations early in the disease. Monitor for manifestations that often appear late in the disease.

- Fatigue, weight loss, or anorexia
- Persistent cough, with or without hemoptysis (rust-colored or blood-tinged sputum)
- Hoarseness
- Altered breathing pattern: dyspnea, prolonged exhalation alternated with shallow breaths (obstruction), rapid, shallow breaths (pleuritic chest pain, elevated diaphragm)
- Altered breath sounds (wheezing)
- Diminished or absent breath sounds (obstruction)
- Chest pain or tightness
- Chest wall masses
- Increased work of breathing (retractions, use of accessory muscle, stridor, nasal flaring)

DIAGNOSTIC PROCEDURES

Cytologic testing

EXPECTED FINDINGS: Sputum specimen contains cancer cells.

CLIENT EDUCATION
- Conduct sputum specimen collection.
- Cancer cells might not always be found in sputum specimens when cancer is present.

Thoracoscopy, bronchoscopy, mediastinoscopy

EXPECTED FINDINGS
- Presence of cancer cells
- Can include biopsy of tumor or lymph nodes

NURSING ACTIONS
- Keep client NPO after midnight and 4 to 8 hr prior to test.
- Provide throat lozenges or sprays for report of a sore throat once the gag reflex returns following procedure.
- Monitor for bleeding and check breath sounds. Chest x-ray following procedure might be required if a pneumothorax is suspected.

X-ray, CT scan

Most lung lesions are first found on chest x-ray.

EXPECTED FINDINGS: Presence of tumor

Thoracentesis with pleural biopsy; MRI, PET scan

EXPECTED FINDINGS: Presence of cancer and metastatic disease

Pulmonary function tests and arterial blood gases

EXPECTED FINDINGS: Compromised respiratory status'

PATIENT-CENTERED CARE

NURSING CARE

- Monitor nutritional status, weight loss, and anorexia.
  - Promote adequate nutrition to provide needed calories for increased work of breathing and prevention of infection.
  - Encourage fluids to promote adequate hydration.
- Maintain a patent airway and suction as needed.
- Position the client in Fowler's position to maximize ventilation.

MEDICATIONS

Bronchodilators and corticosteroids can be given to help decrease inflammation and to dry secretions.

THERAPEUTIC PROCEDURES

Chemotherapy

Chemotherapy is frequently used to treat lung cancers. It is often used in combination with radiation and/or surgery. Platinum compounds, such as cisplatin, are commonly used.

Photodynamic therapy

Photodynamic therapy is performed through bronchoscopy to treat small, accessible tumors.

Radiation therapy

Radiation therapy is effective for lung cancer that has not spread beyond the chest wall and is used as an adjuvant therapy.

Radiofrequency ablation

Most commonly used with NSCLC

Targeted therapy

Commonly used to treat non-small cell lung cancer

Surgical interventions

- The goal of surgery is to remove all tumor cells, including involved lymph nodes.
- Often involves removal of a lung (pneumonectomy), lobe (lobectomy), segment (segmentectomy), or peripheral lung tissue (wedge resection).
- Surgery is reserved for early-stage lung cancer (I or II) with no metastasis.

NURSING ACTIONS

- Monitor vital signs, oxygenation (SaO_2, ABG values), and for evidence of hemorrhage.
- Manage the client's chest tube. Clients who have a pneumonectomy might have a clamped chest tube on the operative side without a drainage system. For other lung surgeries, the chest tube should have a drainage system attached. (Refer to **CHAPTER 16: RESPIRATORY AND DIAGNOSTIC THERAPEUTIC PROCEDURES**.)
- Administer oxygen and manage the ventilator if appropriate.
- Manage pain. Reinforce teaching with the client regarding PCA use if prescribed.

CLIENT EDUCATION: Understand the surgical procedure and chest tube placement.

Palliative procedures

Oxygen therapy to correct hypoxemia

INTERPROFESSIONAL CARE

- Respiratory services should be consulted for inhalers, breathing treatments, and suctioning for airway management.
- Rehabilitation care can be consulted if the client has prolonged weakness and needs assistance with increasing the level of activity.
- Reinforce provided information for psychosocial support, particularly for clients who have a poor prognosis. Qpcc

CLIENT EDUCATION
- Take rest periods as needed.
- Eat high-calorie foods to promote energy.
- Consider cessation if smoking tobacco or using tobacco products.

COMPLICATIONS

Empyema

Presence of purulent fluid collecting in the pleural space

Oral cavity and oropharyngeal cancer

In the U.S., approximately 53,000 people will develop oral cancer and 11,000 will die from oral cancer annually. Treatment is effective for oral and pharyngeal carcinoma if detected early.

Main types of oropharyngeal cancer

Squamous cell carcinoma is the most common oral cancer and can be present on the lips, tongue, buccal mucosa, and oropharynx.

Basal cell carcinoma affects the lips and skin around the mouth.

Kaposi's sarcoma is a form of cancer that affects the endothelial cells of small blood vessels. Oropharyngeal lesions can be found on the hard palate, gums, tongue, or tonsils. Lesions can also occur on the skin, and in the gastrointestinal tract and lungs. Lesions appear as raised, purple nodules or plaques.

HEALTH PROMOTION AND DISEASE PREVENTION

- Schedule dental visits twice yearly for cleaning and inspection of mouth tissues.
- Limit exposure to ultraviolet rays (mid-day sun exposure, indoor tanning).
- Eliminate tobacco use, including smokeless tobacco and vaping.
- Limit alcohol consumption.
- Human papilloma virus vaccine is encouraged for children and adults who are of recommended age.
- Mouth lesions that do not heal within 2 weeks might be cancerous and should be reported to a provider.

DATA COLLECTION

RISK FACTORS

- Male sex (assigned at birth)
- Tobacco use (smokeless, pipe) QEBP
- Alcohol consumption (alcohol use combined with tobacco use significantly increases risk)
- Radiation exposure, including x-rays of head and neck
- Inadequate oral hygiene
- Lack of fruits and vegetables in the diet
- Occupation in textile, coal, metal, and plumbing industries
- Age greater than 40
- Genetic predisposition
- Human papilloma virus (HPV16) infection
- Periodontal disease with mandibular bone loss
- Weakened immune system

EXPECTED FINDINGS

- Mucosal erythroplasia (red or darkened, raised, eroded patches): earliest finding
- Color changes in the mouth
- Oral bleeding
- Difficulty chewing or swallowing
- Speech changes
- Palpable masses or thickening lump in the cheek
- Lesions that do not heal within 2 weeks
- Lesions in the buccal mucosa and gingiva for clients who smoke pipes or cigars, or use smokeless tobacco
- Lesions in the floor of the mouth, soft palate complex, or ventrolateral tongue in clients who smoke cigarettes and drink alcohol

DIAGNOSTIC PROCEDURES

Biopsy: fine-needle, incisional, excisional

EXPECTED FINDINGS: Presence of cancer

MRI, CT scan

EXPECTED FINDINGS

- Presence of cancer
- Thickness of lesion
- Presence of nerve involvement
- Possible metastasis

PATIENT-CENTERED CARE

Protecting the airway and providing adequate nutrition are priority interventions in managing oropharyngeal cancer. Qs

NURSING CARE

- Monitor for adequate clearance of secretions (have the client turn, cough, deep breathe; suction as needed).
- Auscultate for adventitious lung sounds: wheezes (due to aspiration) or stridor (due to obstruction).
- Consult respiratory therapy to provide chest physiotherapy, as indicated.
- Position the client in semi- or high-Fowler's position to promote chest expansion.
- Use a cool mist face tent to promote clearance of secretions and reduce inflammation.
- Monitor for difficulty swallowing.

MEDICATIONS

- Medications that block growth factor receptors prevent tumor growth (cetuximab, erlotinib).
- Antibiotics for infection as indicated.

INTERPROFESSIONAL CARE

- Provide alternate means of communication for clients who have impaired communication (pen and paper, picture boards). Consult speech therapy, as indicated.
- Consult nutrition services to determine swallowing and provide nutrition recommendations, as needed.

THERAPEUTIC PROCEDURES

Radiation and/or chemotherapy is used to treat oral lesions.

Chemotherapy

Used in conjunction with other treatments

Targeted therapy

Radiation (external, implanted, or both)

Commonly used prior to surgery to reduce tumor size.
- **External radiation** is used cautiously to minimize radiation dose to the brain and spinal cord.
- **Implanted radiation** is used to cure early lesions on the floor of the mouth or anterior tongue.
- Hospitalization is typically required until radiation dosing is complete.
- Place client on radiation transmission precautions. See **CHAPTER 83: CANCER TREATMENT OPTIONS**.
- Provide tracheostomy care if needed. Tracheostomy can be required due to edema and increased oral secretions.

Tumor excision

Used to remove lesions through the inside of the mouth or through external entry into the head and neck
- The larger the tumor, the greater the risk to the client for disfigurement and loss of function.
- Composite resections are the most extensive form of oral carcinoma surgery. They can include partial or total glossectomy and partial mandibulectomy.
- Combined neck dissection, mandibulectomy, and oropharyngeal resection can be used.
- Radical neck dissection can include removal of the sternocleidomastoid muscle, internal jugular vein, cranial nerve XI (accessory nerve), and all cervical lymph nodes on the affected side.
- Surgery to remove large lesions can also include placement of a tracheostomy or wound drain.

NURSING ACTIONS
- Maintain NPO status until intraoral suture lines heal (clients who have large tumors).
- Provide routine tracheostomy care and suctioning, as appropriate.
- Monitor wounds, incision sites, and donor grafting sites for evidence of infection.
- Consult a speech language pathologist for clients who have slurred speech or difficulty speaking.
- Provide comfort to clients who have permanent loss of voice or disfigurement. Make a referral to counseling services, as indicated.
- Monitor for effective swallowing and adequate nutrition once oral intake begins.

CLIENT EDUCATION
- Alternate means of communication, such as message boards, might be required following surgery.
- Keep the head of the bed elevated to reduce edema.
- Follow up regularly with the provider to screen for other disorders, due to an increased risk of cancer of the lung, mouth, or throat.

Gastric cancer

Most gastric cancers are adenocarcinomas that stem from the mucosal cells of the inner lining of the stomach. Gastric cancer account for 6% of all cancers worldwide and accounts for 1.5% of new cancers in the U.S. There are approximately 27,000 new diagnoses for stomach cancer and 11,000 people will die from this condition annually, in the U.S. Gastric cancer is often asymptomatic in early stages. Metastasis frequently occurs due to extensive vascular and lymph access to the stomach, often to liver, peritoneum, bones, lungs, and brain. Gastric cancer might spread to nearby organs, such as liver, pancreas, and transverse colon. *Helicobacter pylori* (*H. pylori*) infection is a primary risk factor for developing gastric cancer. Total gastrectomy might be indicated for clients who have hereditary diffuse gastric cancer.

HEALTH PROMOTION/ DISEASE PREVENTION

- Consume a diet rich in fresh fruits and vegetables, and avoid excessive intake of processed, pickled, and smoked foods.
- Screening (upper endoscopy) might be indicated for clients who have inherited cancer syndromes, such as Lynch syndrome or familial adenomatous polyposis.
- Maintain a healthy weight and participate in regular exercise.
- Avoid or reduce alcohol intake.
- Avoid use of tobacco.

DATA COLLECTION

RISK FACTORS

- Excessive intake of salty, pickled foods, and foods that contain nitrates (processed foods)
- Minimal intake of fruits and vegetables
- Infection with *H. pylori*
- History of gastritis
- Pernicious anemia
- Gastric polyps
- Achlorhydria (inability to produce hydrochloric acid)
- Tobacco use
- Obesity
- Previous gastric surgery
- First-degree relative who had gastric cancer
- Race: Black, non-Hispanic white, indigenous

EXPECTED FINDINGS

Early-stage gastric cancer
- Dyspepsia
- Abdominal discomfort
- Epigastric or back pain
- Abdominal fullness, indigestion

Advanced-stage gastric cancer
- Unexplained weight loss
- Decreased appetite
- Nausea and vomiting
- Iron deficiency anemia
- Palpable epigastric mass
- Enlarged lymph nodes
- Blood in stool
- Fatigue

DIAGNOSTIC PROCEDURES

Esophagogastroduodenoscopy (EGD) with biopsy

EXPECTED FINDINGS: Visualization and location of tumor and/or metastasis

NURSING ACTIONS
- Procedure is performed under moderate sedation. Informed consent is required.
- Monitor client's respirations and oxygen saturation.
- Keep client NPO until gag reflex returns.
- Monitor for perforation (bleeding, pain, dyspnea)

CLIENT EDUCATION
- Instruct clients to avoid NSAIDs or anticoagulants for a few days prior to test.
- Client should be NPO for 6 to 8 hr prior to exam.
- A local anesthetic spray will be used to suppress the client's gag reflex.
- After the procedure, swallowing might be difficult until anesthetic wears off. Client might have a sore throat, a hoarse voice, and might experience bloating and belching postprocedure.

Endoscopic ultrasound

Performed during endoscopy to determine depth of tumor and lymph node involvement

Barium swallow

NURSING ACTIONS: Check swallowing reflex prior to procedure.

CLIENT EDUCATION: Client should be NPO for 6 to 8 hr prior to exam.

CT, MRI

EXPECTED FINDINGS: Visualization and location of tumor and/or metastasis

Carcinoembryonic antigen (CEA)

EXPECTED FINDINGS: Positive (denotes malignancy; not specific to gastric cancer)

PATIENT-CENTERED CARE

THERAPEUTIC PROCEDURES

Chemotherapy

Combination chemotherapy can include fluorouracil, carboplatin, cisplatin, and/or oxaliplatin. It is used alone or along with surgery.

Targeted medication therapy

Given to treat advance gastric cancer. Can include trastuzumab, fluorouracil, cisplatin.

Radiation therapy

Radiation therapy is used to treat advanced gastric cancer to slow tumor growth. It is used alone or along with chemotherapy and surgery. Radiation can be used as a palliative measure to control pain, hemorrhage, or obstruction.

Surgical interventions

Billroth I (Gastroduodenostomy): Removal of lower portion of the stomach (antrum).

Billroth II (Gastrojejunostomy): Removal of 75% of stomach.

Subtotal gastrectomy: Used to treat tumors in the middle or distal area of the stomach.

Total gastrectomy: Removal of the stomach, lymph nodes, and omentum. Esophagus is reattached to the duodenum or jejunum.

PREOPERATIVE CLIENT EDUCATION
- Instruct about preoperative diet (clear liquids several days prior to surgery).
- Complete bowel prep with cathartics as prescribed.
- Nasogastric tube (NGT) might be inserted preoperatively for clients who are scheduled for open abdominal surgery, NGT should remain in place for a few days postoperative to decompress the stomach.
- Nutritional supplements might be required preoperative and postoperative via enteral nutrition or total parenteral nutrition.

POSTOPERATIVE NURSING ACTIONS
- Elevate the client's head of bed.
- Monitor breath sounds, encourage pulmonary exercises.
- Monitor bowel sounds.
- Monitor for bleeding (sanguineous drainage on operative site, tachycardia, hypotension).
- Monitor for infection (swelling, redness, fever).
- Manage pain and instruct the client regarding PCA.
- Maintain nasogastric suction (decompression).

POSTOPERATIVE CLIENT EDUCATION
- Understand the care of the incision, activity limits.
- Monitor for pernicious anemia (Beefy, glossy tongue, fatigue, weight loss).
- Avoid heavy lifting. Plan to resume normal activity in 1 to 2 weeks following laparoscopy, or 4 to 6 weeks following open surgery.

INTERPROFESSIONAL CARE

- Dietitian referral to promote nutritional intake and prevent dumping syndrome.
- Case manager or social worker for ongoing client and family support

COMPLICATIONS

Dumping syndrome

- Occurs due to a rapid bolus of food into the small intestines.
- Manifestations include abdominal pain, nausea, tachycardia, syncope, diaphoresis, and palpitations.

NURSING ACTIONS: Provide frequent small meals, drink fluids between meals instead of during meals, provide high protein, high fat, low carbohydrate diet.

Pernicious anemia

Due to lack of intrinsic factor following a total gastrectomy.

NURSING ACTIONS: Injection of vitamin B_{12}

Colorectal cancer

Colorectal cancer (CRC) is cancer of the rectum or colon. Healthy People 2030 goal is to decrease reduction of CRC and incidence of invasion. Most CRCs are adenocarcinoma, a tumor that occurs in the epithelial layer of the colon. Adenocarcinoma begins as a polyp and is benign in the early stages. If left untreated, the polyp will grow and the risk of malignancy increases. CRC can metastasize (through blood or lymph) to the liver (most common site), lungs, brain, or bones. Spreading can occur because of peritoneal seeding (during surgical resection of tumor). The most common location of CRC is the rectosigmoidal region.

HEALTH PROMOTION/ DISEASE PREVENTION

- Consume a diet rich in calcium (calcium binds to free fatty acids and bile salts in the lower gastrointestinal tract).
- Consume diet low in fat and simple carbohydrates but high in fiber. Q EBP
- Receive age-specific regular colorectal cancer screening (after age 45 if at average risk; yearly fecal occult blood test; colonoscopy every 10 years; or flexible sigmoidoscopy every 5 years).
- Engage in a healthy lifestyle, including regular physical exercise and no smoking or excessive alcohol use.

DATA COLLECTION

RISK FACTORS

- Adenomatous colon polyps
- African American descent
- Inflammatory bowel disease (ulcerative colitis, Crohn's disease)
- High-fat, low-fiber diet
- Age older than 50 years; 1 in 7 new diagnoses are in adults younger than 50
- Long-term smoking
- Physical inactivity
- Heavy alcohol consumption
- Personal or family history of cancer

EXPECTED FINDINGS

- Changes in stool consistency or shape (with or without noticeable blood)
- Blood in stool (many times the only finding)
- Abdominal cramps and/or gas
- Palpable mass (elicited by provider only through abdominal palpation or digital rectal exam)
- Weight loss and fatigue
- Abdominal fullness, distention, or pain
- Sensations of bowel fullness after defecation

DIAGNOSTIC PROCEDURES

- Virtual colonoscopy can be performed using CT scan or MRI. Imaging is performed after air is injected into the colon. The procedure is otherwise noninvasive. No sedation is required.
- Fecal testing is recommended every year if the guaiac-based fecal occult blood testing or fecal immunochemical testing is used.
- Screening guidelines for individuals with polyps or a family history of CRC should be initiated at an earlier age and possibly performed more frequently.

Guaiac-based fecal occult blood testing (FOBT)

EXPECTED FINDINGS: Two positive stools within 3 days

NURSING ACTIONS: Negative results to not completely rule out the possibility of CRC.

CLIENT EDUCATION: Avoid red meat, anti-inflammatory medications, and vitamin C for 72 hr prior to testing (to prevent false positives).

Fecal immunochemical test

Stool DNA

Biopsy (endoscopic)

EXPECTED FINDINGS: Definitive diagnosis

Endoscopy: colonoscopy, sigmoidoscopy

EXPECTED FINDINGS: Visualization of polyps or lesions

CLIENT EDUCATION: Begin regular screening at age 45 (colonoscopy every 10 years, sigmoidoscopy every 5 years). At age 40 years, discuss individual risk with the provider to determine the need to screen earlier or more often. At 75 years, discuss with the provider whether to continue screenings.

Double contrast barium enema

This procedure uses the two contrasts of air and barium.

EXPECTED FINDINGS: Visualization and location of tumor

NURSING ACTIONS: Administer stimulant laxative following procedure as prescribed (facilitates evacuation of barium, which can harden in the intestine).

CBC

EXPECTED FINDINGS: Decreased hemoglobin, hematocrit

Carcinoembryonic antigen (CEA)

EXPECTED FINDINGS: Positive

CLIENT EDUCATION: Positive CEA can be indicative of many types of cancer.

CT, MRI

EXPECTED FINDINGS: Visualization and location of tumor and/or metastasis

PATIENT-CENTERED CARE

THERAPEUTIC PROCEDURES

Chemotherapy

Can be used in conjunction with surgery

Targeted medication therapy

Monoclonal antibodies
- Angiogenesis inhibitors (inhibit growth of new blood vessels to tumors): bevacizumab
- Tyrosine kinase inhibitors (decrease cell proliferation and increase cell death of certain cancers): cetuximab and panitumumab

Adjuvant therapy

Given to decrease the chance of metastases for stage II and distant metastases for type III cancers

Radiation therapy

Radiation therapy helps to minimize localized manifestations around the tumor. Radiation can also be used as a palliative measure to control pain, hemorrhage, bowel obstruction, or metastatic disease.

Surgical interventions

Colon surgery is performed using an open or laparoscopic approach. Following tumor excision, the colon might be reconnected (end-to-end anastomosis), a colostomy created (temporary or permanent), or a coloanal reservoir, or J-pouch, created temporarily.

Colon resection (colectomy): Involves removal of a portion of the colon to excise the tumor

Colectomy: Removal of the colon with a temporary or permanent colostomy or ileostomy

Abdominal–perineal (AP) resection: The tumor, sigmoid colon, rectum, and anal sphincter are removed, and the client has a permanent sigmoidostomy.

PREOPERATIVE CLIENT EDUCATION
- Understand the preoperative diet (clear liquids several days prior to surgery).
- Complete bowel prep with cathartics as prescribed.
- Understand the administration of antibiotics (neomycin, metronidazole) to eradicate intestinal flora.
- Collect data and reinforce the client's knowledge about the surgeon's description of the surgery including expected drains and possibility of colostomy.

POSTOPERATIVE NURSING ACTIONS
- Monitor the stoma (should be reddish pink, moist, small amount of blood postoperatively) and report ischemia, necrosis, or frank bleeding.
- Manage pain and instruct the client regarding PCA.
- Maintain nasogastric suction (decompression).
- Progress the diet slowly after suctioning is discontinued and monitor the client's response (bowel sounds present, no nausea or vomiting).
- Discuss possible incontinence and sexual dysfunction with the client. Ask if the client has body image concerns.
- Reinforce ostomy teaching (findings of ischemia to be reported to the provider, expected output, appliance management) if applicable. See **CHAPTER 42: GASTROINTESTINAL THERAPEUTIC PROCEDURES** for care of an ostomy.
- Management of a colostomy can be more difficult for the older adult client due to impaired vision and a decline in fine motor skills. ©

POSTOPERATIVE CLIENT EDUCATION
- Understand the care of the incision, activity limits, diet, and ostomy care, if applicable.
- Consider joining an ostomy support group, locally or online.

INTERPROFESSIONAL CARE

- Ostomy nurse referral for instruction on care of colostomy
- Referral to ostomy support group
- Referral to cancer support group as needed
- Case manager or social worker for ongoing client and family support

COMPLICATIONS

Infection, bleeding, stomal ischemia, second primary colorectal tumor, or complete intestinal obstruction.

Pancreatic cancer

Pancreatic carcinoma has vague manifestations and is usually diagnosed in late stages after liver or gall bladder involvement. Tumors are usually adenocarcinoma, originate in the pancreatic head, and grow rapidly in glandular patterns. There are approximately 57,000 new cases of pancreatic cancer. It has a high mortality rate, and the 5-year survival rates are low.

HEALTH PROMOTION/ DISEASE PREVENTION

- Encourage the client to receive hepatitis B vaccination according to scheduled recommendations
- Encourage tobacco smoke cessation. Assist with making referrals if client desires to quit. Qs

DATA COLLECTION

RISK FACTORS

- Possible inherited risk, genetic predisposition
- Older adults, male sex assigned at birth
- Ethnicity: African American
- Tobacco use (major risk factor)
- High intake of red meat (especially processed); high-fat diet
- BMI greater than 30
- History of diabetes, cirrhosis, or chronic pancreatitis

EXPECTED FINDINGS

- Boring back and abdominal pain that radiates to the back, that is sometimes relieved by sitting up and more severe at night
- Fatigue
- Anorexia, vomiting
- Pruritus

PHYSICAL FINDINGS
- Weight loss
- Palpable abdominal mass, splenomegaly
- Jaundice (late finding)
- Light or clay-colored stools
- Dark urine
- Ascites
- Pruritus (buildup of bile salt)
- Early satiety or anorexia
- Glucose intolerance
- Flatulence

DIAGNOSTIC PROCEDURES

Biopsy (percutaneous or laparoscopic)

EXPECTED FINDINGS: Presence of cancer cells QEBP

CT scan with contrast, abdominal ultrasound

EXPECTED FINDINGS: Identifies the presence of tumors or cysts

Endoscopic retrograde cholangiopancreatography (ERCP)

Provides visualization of the pancreas for diagnosis

Tumor markers

CA 19-9, CA 72-4, CA 242

Carcinoembryonic antigen (CEA)

EXPECTED FINDINGS: Positive (denotes non-specific malignancy)

OTHER LABORATORY TESTING

Blood amylase, lipase, bilirubin, and alkaline phosphatase levels are generally elevated

PATIENT-CENTERED CARE

NURSING CARE

- Care of a client who has pancreatic cancer usually focuses on palliation and not curative measures. Pain management is the priority intervention. Advise the client to ask for analgesics before the pain becomes severe.
- Monitor blood glucose and administer insulin as prescribed.
- A jejunostomy is often placed to provide enteral feedings (prevents reflux, promotes absorption). Provide nutritional support (enteral supplements, TPN).

NURSING ACTIONS: Increase feeding as tolerated, monitoring frequency of diarrhea.

THERAPEUTIC PROCEDURES

Chemotherapy, radiation

- Used to shrink tumor size. Several medications are given to improve the results.
- Administered instead of surgery in some clients; otherwise, before or after surgical intervention.
- External beam radiation used to provide pain relief, relieve obstruction of the ducts, and improves the absorption of food

Targeted therapy

Ablation, microwave therapy

Destroys pancreatic tissue by use of heat

Opioid medications

The client often reports extreme pain. High doses of opioid medications are often required.

Surgical interventions

Can be open or laparoscopic ◯EBP

Surgical interventions can be considered potentially curative or palliative.

Total pancreatectomy: Removes the entire pancreas. Whipple procedure (pancreaticoduodenectomy): Removal of the proximal head of the pancreas, duodenum, parts of the jejunum and stomach, gallbladder, and possibly the spleen. The pancreatic duct is connected to the common bile duct, and the stomach is connected to the jejunum. The surgeon may perform a splenectomy during this procedure.

NURSING ACTIONS
- Monitor NG tube and surgical drains for color and amount.
- Monitor for bloody or bile-tinged drainage, which could indicate anastomotic disruption.
- Place the client in semi-Fowler's position to facilitate lung expansion and to prevent stress on the suture line.
- Monitor blood glucose and administer insulin as needed.

CLIENT EDUCATION: Understand the support measures for pain, anorexia, weight loss, and community resources.

Palliative to relieve or prevent manifestations

Stent placement: A stent is placed to keep the bile duct open and resists compression from the surrounding cancer.

Bypass surgery: Reroutes the flow of bile from the common bile duct, bypassing the pancreas and into the small intestines.

INTERPROFESSIONAL CARE

- Case manager or social worker for continued care and possible palliative interventions
- Counselors or spiritual support personnel to assist the client and family with coping

COMPLICATIONS

Clients who have an open Whipple procedure are at risk for many complications. Intensive care is usually prescribed.

Fistulas, abscesses

Breakdown of a site of anastomosis

NURSING ACTIONS: Report drainage that is not serosanguineous from the drain, or drainage from the wound to the provider immediately. ◯s

Peritonitis

Internal leakage of corrosive pancreatic fluid

NURSING ACTIONS
- Monitor for manifestations of peritonitis (elevated fever, WBC, abdominal pain, abdominal tenderness/rebound tenderness, alteration in bowel sounds, shoulder pain).
- Administer antibiotics as prescribed.

Thromboembolism

Due to hypercoagulable state caused by release of necrotic products from the tumor, immobility postoperatively

NURSING ACTIONS
- Report findings of thromboembolism to the provider.
- Administer anticoagulants as prescribed.
- Maintain bed rest as indicated.

Liver cancer

Cancers can be primary tumors originating in the liver or metastatic cancers that spread from other organs to the liver. Liver cancer most often is the result of metastasis of other cancer types. Primary liver cancer is infrequent.

- **Hepatocellular carcinoma (HCC)** is the most frequently occurring type of primary liver cancer. Primary liver cancer can also originate in the bile duct or liver vasculature.
- **Intrahepatic cholangiocarcinoma:** Cancer that starts in the cells that line the small bile ducts

HEALTH PROMOTION AND DISEASE PREVENTION

- Avoid excessive alcohol intake.
- Encourage client to receive hepatitis B vaccination according to recommended schedules.
- Take precautions against hepatitis B and C. (Recognize that multiple sexual partners, IV drug use, and the sharing of needles all increase the risk.)

DATA COLLECTION

RISK FACTORS

- Cirrhosis
  - Alcohol-related liver disease
  - Hemochromatosis (inability to breakdown iron)
- Hepatitis B or C
- Male sex assigned at birth
- Exposure to aflatoxin (mold that grows on peanuts, corn, and grains)

EXPECTED FINDINGS

- Right upper quadrant abdominal pain that can radiate to back
- Loss of appetite
- Weakness and fatigue

PHYSICAL FINDINGS
- Edema
- Weight loss
- Enlarged liver upon palpation
- Jaundice
- Ascites
- Fever

DIAGNOSTIC PROCEDURES

Biopsy (fine-needle or brush)

Identifies the presence of cancerous cells

Alpha-fetoprotein (AFP)

EXPECTED FINDINGS: Elevated AFP: high probability of cancer (false positive: cirrhosis, hepatitis); elevated CEA along with elevated AFP can discriminate metastatic from primary cancer.

CLIENT EDUCATION: False positives are possible.

Other laboratory testing

- Alkaline phosphatase (ALP), serum aspartate aminotransferase (AST), albumin, and bilirubin: elevated
- WBCs, RBCs increased; blood glucose decreased

Imaging: contrast-enhanced ultrasound or CT scan

EXPECTED FINDINGS: Visualization of tumor biopsy

NURSING ACTIONS: Monitor for bleeding if biopsy is performed.

PATIENT-CENTERED CARE

NURSING CARE

- Observe for potential bleeding complications (frank bleeding, decreased hemoglobin and hematocrit, altered coagulation findings). Qpcc
- Encourage the client to consume small, frequent meals that are high-calorie, moderate fat.
- Reinforce fluid restrictions for clients who have ascites.
- Instruct the client on the benefits of avoiding alcohol.
- Monitor abdominal girth measurements daily (indicates increased ascites).
- Monitor for adequate nutrition (fluid and electrolytes, weight loss, anorexia).
- Monitor for worsening hepatic function (liver function tests, jaundice).
- Monitor and treat pain and abdominal discomfort.
- Provide medications as prescribed. Medications are administered sparingly (especially opioids, sedatives, and barbiturates) due to impaired liver function (reduced ability to metabolize medications).

MEDICATIONS

Targeted therapy (sorafenib)

A multi-tyrosine kinase inhibitor taken orally and used to treat advanced liver cancer.

CLIENT EDUCATION: Report bleeding, heart palpitations, or chest pain.

Hepatic arterial infusion

The direct infusion of chemotherapy via a catheter into the tumor. The client can go home with a catheter in place if continuous infusion is desired. Systemic adverse effects of chemotherapy are avoided through this delivery method. QEBP

CLIENT EDUCATION: Watch for evidence of infection at the catheter site, hepatic toxicity (jaundice, liver function tests), and immunosuppression (fatigue, decreased WBC).

> Systemically delivered chemotherapy has been found to be largely ineffective in treating tumors of the liver or prolonging life. Therefore, more direct delivery methods are used.

THERAPEUTIC PROCEDURES

Hepatic artery embolization

Using a catheter threaded through the femoral artery and up to the liver, particles are injected into the arteries that supply blood to the tumor to block blood flow. If a chemotherapeutic drug is included, this procedure is called chemoembolization. If radiation is included, this procedure is called radioembolization.

NURSING ACTIONS: Monitor for bleeding.

Ablation procedures

Can be used to destroy cancerous cells
- Radiofrequency ablation delivers an electric current directly to the tumor via thin needles. This current is converted into heat waves that kill the cancer cells.
- Percutaneous alcohol (ethanol) injections directly into the tumor mass to cause cell death.
- Cryotherapy uses liquid nitrogen injected directly into the tumor to destroy the tumor.

Chemotherapy

Useful for small, metastatic lesions

Radiation

- External: Although liver cancer cells are sensitive to radiation, the treatment cannot be used at very high doses because normal liver tissue is also easily damaged.
- Percutaneous for interstitial radiation can provide therapy at the targeted area

Surgical Interventions

Surgical resection or liver transplantation is required for long-term survival. ⓆEBP

Surgical resection: If liver cancer involves only one lobe of the liver, surgical removal can be indicated. A liver-lobe resection can result in a survival rate of up to 5 years. Most liver tumors are not resectable.

Liver transplantation: Can be an option for clients who have small primary tumors. A resection of liver from a living donor might be used, as it will grow to meet the demands of the recipient.
- Immunosuppressants that are given after the transplant can increase the risk for recurrence of cancer and for development of secondary infection.
- For interprofessional care, see **CHAPTER 83: CANCER TREATMENT OPTIONS**.

NURSING ACTIONS
- Reinforce teaching with client about diagnostic tests that are done to determine if the liver cancer has metastasized (chest x-ray, PET scan, MRI, laparoscopy).
- Monitor for altered blood glucose due to stress on the liver caused by surgery.
- Monitor for bleeding (client may require the replacement of fluids and blood as necessary).

COMPLICATIONS

- Acute graft rejection following liver transplantation
- Liver failure
- Bile duct obstruction

Kidney and renal pelvis cancer

Adenocarcinoma of the kidney, or renal cell carcinoma (RCC), is the most common form of kidney cancer. Paraneoplastic syndromes (syndromes resulting from cancer in the body) can occur with RCC. The tumor can produce hormones or prevent hormone production, causing imbalance in the body. RCC can be discovered when imaging studies or exploratory surgery are performed for other reasons.

HEALTH PROMOTION AND DISEASE PREVENTION

- Minimize exposure to chemicals (environmental).
- Encourage tobacco use cessation and provide referrals if client desires.

DATA COLLECTION

RISK FACTORS
- Von Hippel-Lindau syndrome
- Exposure to lead, asbestos, or phosphate
- Age older than 45)
- Sex assigned at birth: Males twice as often as females
- Tobacco use
- BMI greater than 30
- Hypertension
- Race: African American

EXPECTED FINDINGS
- Hematuria
- Hormonal changes
- Abdominal or flank pain (often dull, aching)
- Palpable mass
- Weight loss
- Hypertension
- Anemia

DIAGNOSTIC PROCEDURES

Urinalysis

EXPECTED FINDINGS: Hematuria (possible)

CLIENT EDUCATION
- Understand the other reasons for hematuria.
- Remember the role of the kidneys in red blood cell production.

Biopsy (percutaneous through the flank)

EXPECTED FINDINGS: Positive for cancer

NURSING ACTIONS: Maintain client activity restrictions as prescribed.

Imaging: CT, MRI, PET scans, ultrasonography, IV urography, kidney angiograms

EXPECTED FINDINGS: Identify tumor borders and presence in surrounding tissue

NURSING ACTIONS: Prepare the client for imaging.

PATIENT-CENTERED CARE

NURSING CARE

Monitor urine output and laboratory findings (BUN, serum creatinine, urinalysis) to check renal function of the unaffected kidney.

THERAPEUTIC PROCEDURES

Targeted therapy

Immunotherapy (biotherapy)

Ablation therapy for kidney cancer

- Cryoablation uses a probe to deliver cold gases to decrease tumor growth
- Microwave ablation indicated for clients who have one kidney and decreases the growth of tumor

Chemotherapy

Chemotherapy uses anti-cancer drugs administered orally or intravenously to destroy cancer cells. Kidney cancer cells are usually resistant to chemotherapy. However, chemotherapy can be used after targeted medication or immunotherapy.

Surgical interventions

Clients undergoing surgery for RCC are at increased risk for bleeding due to the highly vascular nature of RCC.

Nephrectomy is the standard of treatment for RCC.
- Ribs can be removed during surgery to allow better access to the kidney or tumor.
- Surgical entry can be transthoracic, lumbar, or abdominal. A wound drain can be placed.
- Adrenal glands are left intact, when possible.
- The unaffected kidney must be able to sustain adequate renal function.

NURSING ACTIONS: Assist with performing routine postoperative monitoring, including incision and drain care. Some clients require intensive care monitoring for the first 48 hr.
- Monitor for evidence of bleeding (hypotension, decreased urine output, altered level of consciousness). Blood can pool under the client's back.
- Monitor for adrenal insufficiency (nausea, vomiting, diarrhea, hypoglycemia, hypotension).
- Monitor hemoglobin, hematocrit, and WBC every 6 to 12 hr for first 24 to 48 hr.
- Monitor urine output to evaluate remaining kidney function (30 to 50 mL/hr).

CLIENT EDUCATION
- Avoid lifting more than 5 lb or engaging in strenuous activity.
- Understand measures to protect the function of the remaining kidney (control blood pressure, drink adequate fluids, limit NSAID use, stop smoking). Qs

Urinary bladder cancer (urothelial cancer)

- Bladder cancer begins most often in the cells that line the bladder called urothelium or transitional epithelium layer. Although bladder cancer is the name commonly used for urothelial cancers, the urothelial cells are also located in the kidney, renal pelvis, urethra, and ureters.
- Bladder cancer can be invasive (cancer cells grow outside of the transitional epithelium) or noninvasive (cancer cells remain in the transitional epithelium layer). Bladder cancer is often described based on how far it invades the bladder wall. Transitional cell carcinoma can be further classified as papillary or flat based on how it grows.

HEALTH PROMOTION AND DISEASE PREVENTION

- Use personal protective equipment (PPE) when handling chemicals, paints, fertilizers, gases, or items that contain certain environmental chemicals.
- When working with chemicals is unavoidable, shower and don clean clothing after task completion.

DATA COLLECTION

RISK FACTORS

- Occupational exposure from nitrates, dyes, rubber, or paint
- Tobacco use (smokers have twice the risk)
- Male sex assigned at birth
- Chronic urinary tract inflammation
- Age older than 55 years

CAUSES OF CHRONIC BLADDER IRRITATION: UTI, kidney and bladder stones

---

84.5 Urinary diversions

	DIVERSION	PORTAL OF EXIT	URINARY ELIMINATION
Ureterostomy	Ureters	Skin	Continuous drainage into external pouch
Ileal conduit	Ileum	Abdominal stoma	Continuous drainage into external pouch
Continent pouch (ileal reservoir, Kock pouch)	Pouch created from large intestine	Abdominal stoma	Penrose drain and catheter might be present until sutures heal. Client performs intermittent urinary catheterization.
Bladder reconstruction (neobladder)	Pouch created from small intestine	Urethra	Client performs intermittent urinary catheterization.
Ureterosigmoidostomy	Large intestine	Anus	During bowel movement

---

EXPECTED FINDINGS

- Hematuria
- Dysuria, frequency, urgency (infection or obstruction present)

DIAGNOSTIC PROCEDURES

Biopsy (cystoscopic)

EXPECTED FINDINGS: Presence of cancer

NURSING ACTIONS: Prepare the client for cystoscopy.

Bladder wash

EXPECTED FINDINGS: Presence of cancerous cells in saline wash solution (definitive diagnosis)

CLIENT EDUCATION: Saline will be instilled into the bladder, then retrieved for microscopic examination.

Imaging: CT, MRI scan

EXPECTED FINDINGS

CT scan: extent of tumor invasion

MRI: depth and spread of tumor

Urinalysis

EXPECTED FINDINGS: Microscopic or gross hematuria

CLIENT EDUCATION: Understand the other possible reasons for hematuria.

PATIENT-CENTERED CARE

THERAPEUTIC PROCEDURES

Intravesical treatments

Intravesical chemotherapy: Chemotherapy medications are put directly into the bladder. Many of these same medications are also administered systemically.

Intravesical immunotherapy: Bacillus Calmette–Guérin (BCG)
- BCG is a live virus compound commonly used to vaccinate high-risk individuals against tuberculosis.
- BCG is infused into the bladder and retained for 2 hr to prevent recurrence to superficial cancer cells.

NURSING ACTIONS Qpcc
- After the 2 hr dwell time, the urinary catheter is removed, and the client is instructed to sit to void. This position prevents urine splashing, reducing the risk of contamination.
- Provide or assist in perineal cleansing.

CLIENT EDUCATION
- Do not share a toilet with anyone for 24 hr after treatment. At that time, disinfect the toilet by pouring a 10% bleach solution in the bowl, allowing it to sit 15 min, then flushing and wiping off the toilet seat.
- If a private toilet is not possible, disinfect the toilet each time following voiding.
- Urinate in a sitting position to avoid splashes.
- If only one toilet is in the home, allow the bleach solution to sit for 15 min, then flush and clean it.
- Wash clothing and linen that comes in contact with urine for 24 hr following infusion.
- Avoid sexual intercourse for 24 hr following the infusion.

Systemic chemotherapy

Can be used alone or in combination with radiation. Chemotherapy can be given before surgery (neoadjuvant) or after surgery (adjuvant)

External beam radiation

Often used in combination with surgery. This can cause radiation cystitis.

Surgical interventions

- Surface excision, transurethral resection of bladder tumors, and partial cystectomy (removal of part of the bladder) are used to treat small, confined tumors.
- Radical cystectomy with removal of surrounding tissue or muscle is used for large, invasive, or recurrent tumors. Intensive care can be required following extensive bladder repair. Ureters are diverted to another location.
- Internal or external drains or catheters can be placed intraoperatively.
- Radical cystectomy with lymph node dissection includes the removal of other pelvic structures.
- Postoperatively, the client might have a Penrose drain, or other urinary diversions such as catheter in the stoma, pouch around the stoma, or a drainage tube in the nephrostomy.

NURSING ACTIONS
- Consult enterostomal therapy to assist with management and client/family education related to urinary diversion. Qpcc
- Monitor output from drains or catheters for expected color and amount.
- Report decreased or absent urine output in a client who has an external pouch.
- Secure the client's external drainage catheter. Notify the provider if it becomes dislodged or removed.
- Monitor urinary output in the pouch or drains.

CLIENT EDUCATION
- Self-catheterize and plan procedure at timed intervals because there is no sensation of bladder fullness (neobladder, continent pouch).
- Monitor peristomal skin for redness, excoriation, or infection (ileal conduit, continent in pouch).

INTERPROFESSIONAL CARE

- Ostomy nurse referral for instruction on care of urinary diversion or neobladder
- Referral to ostomy support group
- Counseling for clients regarding body image or sexual functioning
- Nutrition consult for clients following neobladder surgery

COMPLICATIONS

Hydronephrosis

- Inability to eliminate urine causes dilation of the renal pelvis.
- A tumor that blocks the urinary tract can prevent urinary elimination.

NURSING ACTIONS: Report decreased or absent urine output

Breast cancer

Breast cancer is the second-leading cause of cancer deaths in clients assigned female at birth in the U.S. Breast cancer in clients assigned male at birth is rare. Can present as a hard, painless mass. Gynecomastia can be present. Breast cancer can be noninvasive (in situ) or invasive (most common). Common sites of metastasis are bone, lung, brain, and liver. Q_{EBP}

NONINVASIVE BREAST CANCERS

Ductal carcinoma in situ (DCIS)
- Cancer cells are located in the duct and have not invaded surrounding tissue
- DCIS cells lack the biologic capacity to metastasize

Lobular carcinoma in situ (LCIS)
- Abnormal cell growth occurs in the milk-producing glands
- Can increase risk of developing a separate breast cancer later
- Managed with observation
- When other risk factors exist, prophylactic treatment (tamoxifen, raloxifene, or mastectomy) can be considered: cancer originates in the mammary ducts and grows in the epithelial cells lining the ducts.

INVASIVE BREAST CANCERS

Infiltrating ductal carcinoma
Can present as a lump, skin dimpling or edematous thickening and pitting of breast skin (orange peel)

Inflammatory breast cancer (IBC)
- Can present as swelling, skin redness, and breast pain
- Seldom presents as a lump and might not be present on a mammogram

OTHER TYPES OF BREAST CANCERS

Paget disease: Rare cancer that develops around the nipple

Triple-negative: Aggressive cancer in which cells lack receptors for estrogen, progesterone and human epidermal growth factor receptor 2 (HER2)

HEALTH PROMOTION AND DISEASE PREVENTION

- Foods with antioxidants and phytoestrogens are recommended for consumption (soy, whole grains, fruits and vegetables).
- Encourage mammogram screening based on scheduled recommendations.
- Maintain healthy weight.
- Engage in regular physical exercise.
- Minimize alcohol intake.
- Avoid hormone replacement therapy.

DATA COLLECTION

RISK FACTORS

- High genetic risk: Inherited mutations of BRCA1 and BRCA2
- History of previous breast cancer
- Early age at diagnosis
- Female sex assigned at birth (less than 1% of males develop breast cancer)
- First-degree relative who has breast cancer
- Females (sex assigned at birth)
  - Early menarche
  - Late menopause
  - Nulliparity or first pregnancy after age 30
- Hormone replacement therapy or hormonal contraceptives
- BMI greater than 30
- Excessive alcohol intake (possibly related to folic acid depletion)

EXPECTED FINDINGS
- Breast change (appearance, texture, presence of lumps)
- Breast pain or soreness

PHYSICAL FINDINGS
- Skin changes (peau d'orange)
- Dimpling
- Breast tumors (usually small, irregularly shaped, firm, nontender, and nonmobile)
- Nipple discharge
- Nipple retraction or ulceration
- Enlarged lymph nodes
- Male clients (sex assigned at birth) often report a mass around the areola that is hard and painless, nipple inversion, ulceration or swelling of the chest. Lymphedema and gynecomastia might be present.

DIAGNOSTIC PROCEDURES

Clients should focus on breast self-awareness, being aware of breast size, shape, and changes that occur as hormones cycle. Awareness helps clients detect changes earlier. Self-breast examination is one tool that can be used to promote breast self-awareness. Qpcc

Biopsy (open or fine-needle)

EXPECTED FINDINGS: Definitive diagnosis of cancer cell type. Sentinel lymph node biopsy can be performed during surgery.

CLIENT EDUCATION: Provide diagnosis-specific information.

Stereotactic biopsy

Nonsurgical needle biopsy for breast tissue in which affected tissue is visualized via client lying prone on special table with mammogram machine underneath.

Genetic testing

EXPECTED FINDINGS
- **BRCA1 and BRCA2**: presence of gene mutation increases breast cancer risk.
- **HER2**: presence of excess HER2 (normal gene that causes cell replication) indicates the need for targeted therapy.

CLIENT EDUCATION: Consider genetic testing for BRCA1 and BRCA2 if at risk (two first-degree relatives diagnosed with breast cancer prior to age 50 or family history of breast and ovarian cancer).

Mammography, tomosynthesis (3D mammography)

EXPECTED FINDINGS: Visualization of the lesion

CLIENT EDUCATION: Consider additional diagnostic testing.

MRI, ultrasound (US), CT scan, x-ray

EXPECTED FINDINGS: Visualization of lesions. Mammography is preferred over x-ray; MRI and US can provide better visualization of lesions for clients who have dense breasts.

NURSING ACTIONS: Prepare client for imaging.

Nuclear imaging: breast-specific gamma imaging

EXPECTED FINDINGS: Visualization of the lesion

CLIENT EDUCATION: Scanning will display the uptake of the radioactive substance injected prior to the procedure.

Positron emission mammography (PEM)

Type of PET scan

EXPECTED FINDINGS: Visualization of the lesion

CLIENT EDUCATION: PEM provides consistent images despite hormone fluctuations.

PATIENT-CENTERED CARE

THERAPEUTIC PROCEDURES

Adjuvant therapy follows surgery to decrease the risk of recurrence.

Complementary and integrative therapies

Complementary and integrative therapies can help clients who have breast cancer. These include biologically based therapies (vitamins, cancer diets, herbal remedies), prayer, guided imagery, aromatherapy, acupuncture, massage, and journaling. Encourage clients to discuss these with the provider and seek licensed practitioners to promote safety.

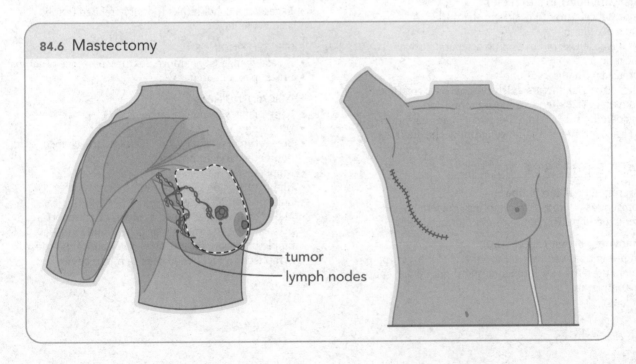

84.6 Mastectomy

tumor
lymph nodes

Hormone therapy

Most effective in cancer cells with estrogen or progesterone receptors. This type of cancer has a better prognosis.

Ovarian ablation: Luteinizing releasing hormone (LH–RH): leuprolide or goserelin
- Inhibits estrogen synthesis.
- Can be used in premenopausal clients to stop or prevent the growth of breast tumors.

Selective estrogen receptor modulators (SERMs): toremifene (tamoxifen)
- Used in clients who are at high risk for breast cancer or who have advanced breast cancer. Q EBP
- Suppress the growth of remaining cancer cells postmastectomy or lumpectomy.
- Tamoxifen has been found to increase the risk of endometrial cancer, deep-vein thrombosis, and pulmonary embolism.

Chemotherapy/radiation therapy

- Chemotherapy and/or radiation can augment or replace a mastectomy, depending on several factors (client's age, hormone status related to menopause, genetic predisposition, and staging of disease).
- Clients who undergo chemotherapy are usually given a combination of several medications (cyclophosphamide, doxorubicin, and fluorouracil).
- Radiation therapy is usually reserved for clients who had a lumpectomy or breast-conserving procedure.
  - Whole or partial breast radiation can be prescribed. Skin care is a priority concern due to radiation damage and generalized fatigue.
  - Brachytherapy with radioactive seeds can also be an option.
  - Intraoperative radiation therapy allows an intense dose of radiation to be delivered directly to the surgical site.
- Target therapy is most effective in breast cancer with HER2/neu gene. Trastuzumab, pertuzumab, and ado-trastuzumab emtansine (a) are signal transduction inhibitors. They inhibit proteins that are signals for cancer cells to grow.

Surgical interventions

Surgical procedures include lumpectomy (breast-conserving), wide excision or partial mastectomy, total mastectomy, modified radical mastectomy (lymph nodes removed), radical mastectomy (lymph nodes and muscle removed), and reconstructive surgery.

NURSING ACTIONS
- Have the client sit with the head of the bed elevated 30° when awake and support their arm on a pillow. Lying on the unaffected side can relieve pain.
- Have the client wear a sling while ambulating (to support arm).
- Avoid administering injections, taking blood pressure, or obtaining blood from the client's affected arm. Place a sign above the client's bed regarding these precautions. Q s

- Emphasize the importance of a well-fitted breast prosthesis for a client who had a mastectomy.
- Provide emotional support to the client and family.
- Encourage the client to express feelings related to perception of sexuality and body image.
- Monitor surgical drains, which can be used with lumpectomy and modified radical mastectomy surgeries.

CLIENT EDUCATION
- Care for the incision and drainage tubes. (Drains are usually left in for 1 to 3 weeks.)
- Avoid placing the arm on the surgical side in a dependent position. This position will interfere with wound healing.
- Perform early arm and hand exercises (squeezing a rubber ball, elbow flexion and extension, and hand-wall climbing) to prevent lymphedema and to regain full range of motion.
- Do not to wear constrictive clothing and avoid cuts and injuries to the affected arm.
- Conduct BSE.
- Report numbness, pain, heaviness, or impaired motor function of the affected arm to the surgeon.
- Discuss breast reconstruction alternatives with the surgeon.
  - Reconstruction can begin during the original breast removal procedure or after some healing has occurred.
  - A tissue expander (a saline-filled implant that has a port through which additional saline can be injected, gradually expanding the tissue prior to permanent implant) is often placed during the original procedure.
  - Saline or silicone implants are used for permanent placement.
  - Autologous flaps can also be used for reconstruction.
  - Nipple reconstruction can be done using tissue from the labia, abdomen, or inner thigh.
- Genetic counseling for clients who test positive for the BRCA1/BRCA2 genetic mutation includes recommendation of bilateral mastectomy and oophorectomy to prevent cancer occurrence. Clients who do not choose this option should have early, frequent, thorough screening for breast and ovarian cancer. Q TC
- Community resources are available for emotional support, particularly regarding changes in body image.
- Discuss concerns about sexuality or sexual functioning following surgery. If sexual intimacy is desired, planning to engage in sexual activity when feeling less tired can be helpful, or using physical closeness to promote intimacy during times of fatigue.

INTERPROFESSIONAL CARE

- Reach for Recovery or other support programs can assist with coping.
- Discuss options for prosthesis, dressing, and breast reconstruction.

COMPLICATIONS

Lymphedema

Swelling can occur in the arm on the side of surgery. Once it develops, it can be difficult to manage.

NURSING ACTIONS
- Reinforce teaching with client to report numbness and tingling in the affected arm which could be an indication of lymphedema.
- Monitor and report heaviness, numbness, swelling of the affected arm and the upper chest.
- Reinforce with client to avoid heavy lifting and how to apply and wear prescribed compression garments.
- Avoid obtaining venipunctures and blood pressure in the affected arm.
- Reinforce with client to perform exercise and elevate affected arm daily.

Ovarian cancer

Ovarian cancers are epithelial tumors that develop on the surface of the ovaries. The tumors grow quickly and are often in both ovaries. Metastases frequently occur before the primary ovarian malignancy is diagnosed. There is a high recurrence rate of ovarian cancer, after which it is treatable but not curable. Ovarian cancer is the leading cause of death from gynecologic cancers.

HEALTH PROMOTION AND DISEASE PREVENTION

Birth control pills and pregnancy can offer protection against ovarian cancer (reduced estrogen exposure).

DATA COLLECTION

RISK FACTORS

- Middle aged or older adult clients (age greater than 40 years; risk increases with age)
- Nulliparity or first pregnancy after 30 years of age
- Family history of ovarian, breast, or genetic mutation for hereditary nonpolyposis colon cancer (HNPCC)
- BRCA1 or BRCA2 gene mutations
- Diabetes mellitus
- Early menarche/late menopause
- Endometriosis
- Infertility

EXPECTED FINDINGS

- Abdominal pain or swelling
- Abdominal discomfort (dyspepsia, indigestion, gas, distention) Ⓠ EBP
- Abdominal mass
- Urinary frequency or urgency

DIAGNOSTIC PROCEDURES

- There is no specific test for ovarian cancer.
- Staging of ovarian cancer is determined at the time of the hysterectomy or exploratory laparotomy when the tumor is removed and examined by the pathologist.

Physical data collection

EXPECTED FINDINGS: Enlarged ovary (possible if tumor is at least 4 inches)

CLIENT EDUCATION: Understand the possible causes of an enlarged ovary.

Biopsy

EXPECTED FINDINGS: Presence of cancer cells

CLIENT EDUCATION: Biopsy is usually performed during surgery to remove the tumor.

Genetic testing

EXPECTED FINDINGS: BRCA1 and BRCA2: Presence of gene mutation increases ovarian cancer risk.

CLIENT EDUCATION: Genetic testing can be used to determine risk of developing ovarian cancer, but it is not used to diagnose or monitor treatment. Some clients who have these genetic mutations elect to have bilateral salpingo-oophorectomy to prevent ovarian cancer.

Tumor markers

EXPECTED FINDINGS
Epithelial tumor: Cancer antigen-125 (CA-125) elevated (greater than 35 units/mL)

CLIENT EDUCATION: Unexpected CA-125 findings indicate possible cancer (false positive: endometriosis, pregnancy, fibroids, and menses). More testing or surgery will likely be required.

Transvaginal ultrasound, MRI, chest x-ray, CT or PET scan

EXPECTED FINDINGS: Metastatic disease

CLIENT EDUCATION: Understand the implications of metastatic disease and offer emotional support.

PATIENT-CENTERED CARE

THERAPEUTIC PROCEDURES

Chemotherapy (traditional or intraperitoneal)

Cisplatin and carboplatin are the most common chemotherapeutic medications used for ovarian cancer.

Surgical interventions

Exploratory laparotomy can be performed to diagnose, treat, and stage ovarian tumors.

A total abdominal hysterectomy (TAH) with bilateral salpingectomy and oophorectomy (BSO) is the usual treatment for ovarian cancer. TAH with BSO also helps determine the extent of the disease as well as local and distant metastases. Staging of the cancer is done at this time.

NURSING ACTIONS

- Observe for urinary retention and difficulty voiding.
- Monitor bowel sounds. Paralytic ileus can occur due to manipulation of the bowel during surgery.
- Discuss sexuality, surgically induced menopause, and other self-image issues with the client.

CLIENT EDUCATION

- Avoid straining, driving, lifting more than 5 lb, douching, and participating in sexual intercourse until the provider gives release.
- Immediately report evidence of infection, as well as vaginal discharge that is excessive or has a foul odor.

COMPLICATIONS

Abdominal ascites, pleural effusion, and intestinal obstruction

Uterine (endometrial) cancer

Endometrial cancer is the most common gynecological cancer. There are approximately 65,000 new cases for endometrial cancer in the US each year.

HEALTH PROMOTION AND DISEASE PREVENTION

Avoid the use of unopposed estrogen (estrogen that is used without progesterone) when considering postmenopausal hormone replacement therapy.

DATA COLLECTION

RISK FACTORS

- Family history of endometrial or colorectal cancer
- Personal history of breast/ovarian cancer, or polycystic ovarian syndrome (PCOS)
- Diabetes
- Genetic mutation for HNPCC
- BMI greater than 30 (due to fat cell production of estrogen)
- Unopposed estrogen hormone replacement therapy
- Nulliparity
- Use of tamoxifen to prevent or treat breast cancer
- Late menopause (longer-term exposure to significant estrogen levels)

EXPECTED FINDINGS

- Irregular and/or postmenopausal bleeding
- Low-back, abdominal, or low pelvic pain

DIAGNOSTIC PROCEDURES

Biopsy

EXPECTED FINDINGS: Endometrial biopsy: presence of carcinoma

CLIENT EDUCATION: Biopsy is usually performed through transvaginal ultrasound.

Pathology testing for staging

EXPECTED FINDINGS: Extent, size of tumor, and metastasis

CLIENT EDUCATION: This occurs after exploratory laparotomy or hysterectomy following tumor removal.

Genetic testing

EXPECTED FINDINGS: HNPCC testing: presence of the gene

CLIENT EDUCATION: The presence of HNPCC increases the risk of carcinoma.

Tumor markers

EXPECTED FINDINGS
- Alpha-fetoprotein (AFP): elevated
- Cancer antigen-125 (CA-125): positive

CLIENT EDUCATION: Results indicate some type of carcinoma.

Transvaginal ultrasound and endometrial biopsy

Endometrial thickness and presence of carcinoma. This is the standard test for diagnosis.

Other assessments to determine metastatic cancer

Chest x-ray, intravenous pyelography, abdominal ultrasound, CT of the pelvis, MRI of the abdomen/pelvis, and liver and bone scans

PATIENT-CENTERED CARE

THERAPEUTIC PROCEDURES

Radiation therapy

Given as adjuvant therapy, usually after a hysterectomy

Chemotherapy

Often given as a palliative therapy for when cancer has recurred, or involves distant metastasis

Surgical interventions

Total hysterectomy with bilateral salpingectomy/oophorectomy is the standard treatment. The vagina is spared, allowing for sexual intercourse to continue.

- An open, laparoscopic, or vaginal approach can be used.
- A radical hysterectomy might be required. This includes removal of the pelvic lymph nodes and upper third of the vagina.

NURSING ACTIONS

- Observe for urinary retention and difficulty voiding due to proximity to the urethra (more common after vaginal hysterectomy).
- Monitor bowel sounds for paralytic ileus (more common due to manipulation of the bowel during surgery).
- Reinforce teaching with client about sexuality, surgically-induced menopause, and other self-image issues with the client. Qpcc

CLIENT EDUCATION

- Avoid straining, driving, lifting more than 5 lb, douching, and sexual intercourse until the provider gives release.
- Immediately report evidence of infection, excess vaginal discharge, or foul-smelling drainage.
- If premenopausal, consider hormone replacement therapy options.
- Explore complementary and integrative therapies, such as mind-body and biologic therapies, healing touch, herbs, vitamins, and nutrition.

Cervical cancer

Early cervical cancer is often undetected. Manifestations do not occur until the cancer has become invasive.

HEALTH PROMOTION AND DISEASE PREVENTION

- Encourage client to receive vaccination series with HPV vaccine according to recommended schedule (9 and 26 years of age [and up to 45 years of age]). Qs
- Encourage client to obtain Pap smear (with or without HPV co-testing) and pelvic exams according to screening recommendations.
- Limit the number of sexual partners.
- Use condoms during sexual intercourse.
- Avoid smoking.

DATA COLLECTION

RISK FACTORS

- Infection with high-risk HPV types (strains 16 and 18) Qebp
- Infection with HIV or other immunosuppressive disorder
- History of sexually transmitted infections
- Early sexual activity (before 18 years of age)
- Client or partner who had multiple sexual partners
- Family history of cervical cancer
- Cigarette smoking

EXPECTED FINDINGS

- Painless vaginal bleeding between menses
- Dysuria, hematuria
- Watery, blood-tinged vaginal discharge (early finding); dark, foul-smelling discharge (late finding)
- Unexplained weight loss
- Pelvic pain
- Rectal bleeding
- Leg pain or edema (late finding)

DIAGNOSTIC PROCEDURES

Simultaneous PAP test and HPV co-testing improves the accuracy of the reading.

Papanicolaou (Pap) test

EXPECTED FINDINGS: Abnormal cells

CLIENT EDUCATION

- Begin screening by 25 years of age. Frequency of screening depends on many factors (age, results, presence of a cervix).
- The Pap is a screening tool and not diagnostic. An abnormal Pap requires additional testing.

Colposcopy with biopsy

EXPECTED FINDINGS: Abnormal cells (follow-up to Pap test)

HPV typing: DNA test

EXPECTED FINDINGS: Presence of HPV on cervical cells

CLIENT EDUCATION: HPV increases the risk of cervical cancer.

Chest x-ray, MRI, CT, PET

EXPECTED FINDINGS: Metastatic/advanced disease

PATIENT-CENTERED CARE

NURSING CARE

Administer antibiotics for pelvic, vaginal, or urinary tract infections.

THERAPEUTIC PROCEDURES

Removal of the lesion

- By conization, cryotherapy, laser ablation, hysterectomy, or a loop electrosurgical excision procedure.
- Conization can be used as either a diagnostic procedure or treatment in early cancer.

CLIENT EDUCATION

- Report heavy vaginal bleeding, foul-smelling drainage, or fever to the provider. Ⓠ**PCC**
- Vaginal discharge is normal.
- Take showers rather than tub baths.
- Avoid heavy lifting, vaginal penetration, douches, and tampons for the prescribed time (typically 3 weeks).

Radiation

Brachytherapy and external radiation therapy can be options for cancer that is no longer limited to local invasion.

NURSING ACTIONS

- Monitor for skin damage, especially in the perineal area.
- Chemotherapy can be used along with radiation.

Surgical interventions

Hysterectomy: Clients who have early-stage cervical cancer might require a **simple hysterectomy** (removes the uterus and cervix) or a **radical hysterectomy** (removes the uterus, upper third of the vagina, uterosacral uterovesical ligaments, and pelvic nodes). The choice to have a hysterectomy is guided by the client's condition and desire for future childbearing. Radical hysterectomy with lymph node resection can be as effective as radiation. Care of a client following hysterectomy is found in **CHAPTER 57: DIAGNOSTIC AND THERAPEUTIC PROCEDURES FOR REPRODUCTIVE DISORDERS.**

Exenteration: Clients who have extensive cancer can require this more extensive pelvic surgery. Pelvic exenteration can include removal of all pelvic organ and lymph nodes, which requires construction of a urinary and bowel diversion, as well as a vagina.

NURSING ACTIONS

- Manage drains as well as urinary and bowel diversions.
- Monitor for body image disturbance and encourage the client to speak openly about it.
- Reinforce teaching with the client about findings of wound infection and how to care for drains that can remain after discharge.
- Instruct the client about how to care for urinary and bowel diversion.
- Instruct the client about how to care for perineal wounds and expectations regarding discharge.

CLIENT EDUCATION: Monitor vaginal bleeding. An expected finding is one saturated perineal pad every 4 hr.

COMPLICATIONS

- Fistula development can occur after pelvic exenteration.
- Kidney infections are also common secondary to the urinary diversion.

Prostate cancer

Prostate cancer is a slow-growing cancer than can develop in response to androgen (testosterone and dihydrotestosterone) and is considered the 2nd most common type of cancer in male (sex assigned at birth). Conservative treatment can be the treatment of choice for a client, based on how fast the cancer is growing, if the cancer has spread, and the client's age and life expectancy. Treatment can be delayed up to 10 years following diagnosis. Manifestations are often similar to those of benign prostatic hyperplasia. The posterior lobe or outer gland epithelium are sites of origin for most prostate cancer.

HEALTH PROMOTION AND DISEASE PREVENTION

- Consume a diet low in animal fat and include omega-3 fatty acids (fish), fruits, and vegetables.
- Engage in regular exercise.
- Encourage client to discuss prostate screening with a provider at age 50 years (average risk). Clients at higher risk might need to consider starting at age 40 years.

DATA COLLECTION

RISK FACTORS

- Age greater than 65 years (risk increases with age) Ⓖ
- Family history
- African American ethnicity
- High-fat diet
- Hereditary prostate cancer 1 (HPC1), BRCA1, or BRCA2 mutation
- Rapid growth of the prostate (benign high-grade prostatic intraepithelial neoplasia)
- Exposure to environmental toxins such as arsenic

EXPECTED FINDINGS

- Urinary manifestations: hesitancy, weak stream, urgency, frequency, nocturia
- Recurrent bladder infections
- Urinary retention
- Blood in urine and semen (late manifestation)
- Pain, particularly bone (pelvis, spine, hips, ribs)
- Unexplained weight loss

DIAGNOSTIC PROCEDURES

Digital rectal examination (DRE)

EXPECTED FINDINGS: Hard prostate with palpable irregularities

CLIENT EDUCATION: Discuss prostate screening after age 50 with a provider.

Biopsy

EXPECTED FINDINGS
- Presence of cancer.
- Staging is based on biopsy result.

CLIENT EDUCATION
- PSA, age, race, and family history are used to determine if biopsy is needed.
- Understand the diagnosis-specific information.

Prostate specific antigen (PSA)

EXPECTED FINDINGS: Elevation indicates possible prostate disease (not specific to carcinoma).

CLIENT EDUCATION
- Discuss prostate screening after age 50.
- Have the PSA determined prior to DRE to promote accuracy of results.

Transrectal ultrasonography (TRUS)

EXPECTED FINDINGS: Visualization of lesions

CLIENT EDUCATION
- Understand the possible complications and postprocedure care (extra fluids, no strenuous exercise, manifestations to report).
- An enema might be administered prior to procedure.

Urinalysis

- Expected findings: Hematuria, bacteriuria
- Client education: Understand the causes of hematuria and bacteriuria.

Bone scan, MRI CT, x-ray

Determines metastasis

PATIENT-CENTERED CARE

Active surveillance can be used to monitor the client who has prostate cancer but desires to postpone treatment. Older adult clients or clients who have less than 5 years life expectancy might opt to do this. The client's condition is monitored regularly and treatment started if the client notices a worsening of manifestations.

MEDICATIONS

Hormone therapy

Leuprolide, goserelin, triptorelin: luteinizing hormone-releasing hormone (LH-RH) agonists
- Used in advanced prostate cancer to produce chemical castration
- CLIENT EDUCATION
  - Be aware that hot flashes are an adverse effect.
  - Impotence and decreased libido can also be adverse effects.
  - Monitor for osteoporosis, which can occur due to testosterone suppression. Qs

Flutamide, bicalutamide, nilutamide: androgen receptor blocker
- Used alone or in conjunction with a LH-RH agonist
- CLIENT EDUCATION
  - Gynecomastia is a possible adverse medication effect.
  - Have liver function tests monitored frequently.

THERAPEUTIC PROCEDURES

Chemotherapy

Can be used on clients whose cancer has spread or who have had minimal improvement with other therapies.

CLIENT EDUCATION: Have routine blood tests performed to monitor for neutropenia, leukopenia, thrombocytopenia, and anemia.

Radiation

Internal (brachytherapy) or external beam (EBRT)
- External comes from a source of radiation outside the body.
- Intensity-modulated radiation uses thousands of beams and angles of varying intensity that are even more controlled to target the cancer tissues and reduce exposure of radiation to healthy tissue.
- Used as a palliative treatment or to treat cancer that has recurred.

CLIENT EDUCATION: Proctitis can occur following radiation treatment. Report rectal cramping, passing mucus or blood in the stool, or rectal urgency. Proctitis should resolve 6 weeks following surgery.

Surgical interventions

PSA levels should reduce within a few days postoperatively.
Radical prostatectomy is the treatment of choice.
- Involves the removal of the prostate gland, along with the seminal vesicles, the cuff at the bladder neck, and the regional lymph nodes.
- Open or laparoscopic surgery can be done using a suprapubic, perineal, or retropubic approach.

NURSING ACTIONS

- Provide catheter care and administer bladder antispasmodics as prescribed.
- If the suprapubic approach was used, monitor suprapubic catheter output. Catheter is usually removed when residual urine measurements are less than 75 mL.
- Provide information regarding availability of a sex therapist or intimacy counselor if needed.

CLIENT EDUCATION

- Bilateral orchiectomy might be performed as a palliative surgery to slow cancer growth by minimizing testosterone production.
- Discuss concerns about body image or sexuality.

INTERPROFESSIONAL CARE

- Case management to facilitate provider appointments and home care
- Support groups for client and family

COMPLICATIONS

- Urinary incontinence
- Erectile dysfunction

Testicular cancer

Testicular cancer is rare and most common in clients between the ages of 15 and 35 years. With early detection, testicular cancer has a 95% cure rate.

HEALTH PROMOTION AND DISEASE PREVENTION

- Perform monthly testicular self-examination is best performed during or after a bath or shower when the scrotum is relaxed. Qᴘᴄᴄ
- Move the penis to the side and examine one testicle at a time.
- Hold the testicle between the thumb and fingers of both hands and roll it gently between the fingers.
- Look and feel for any hard lumps; smooth rounded bumps; or change in size, shape, or consistency of the testicle.
- It is expected for one testicle to be larger or hang lower than the other.
- Palpation of the epididymis can feel like a lump.

Active Learning Scenario

A nurse is reinforcing teaching with a client who has a new diagnosis of prostate cancer. What information should the nurse include? Use the Active Learning Template: System Disorder to complete this item.

MEDICATIONS: Describe at least two medications and their uses.

THERAPEUTIC PROCEDURES: Describe a prostatectomy.

NURSING CARE: Describe at least three nursing actions.

Active Learning Scenario Key

Using the Active Learning Template: System Disorder

MEDICATIONS
- Hormone therapy: luteinizing hormone-releasing hormone agonists: leuprolide acetate
- Androgen receptor blocker: flutamide

THERAPEUTIC PROCEDURES: Prostatectomy is the surgical removal of the prostate gland, seminal vesicles, bladder cuff, and regional lymph nodes. It can be done by an open surgery or laparoscopic approach in the suprapubic, perineal, or retropubic area.

NURSING INTERVENTIONS
- Ask if the client has concerns about body image or sexuality.
- Offer to refer the client to a therapist or intimacy counselor, if desired.
- Provide catheter care (suprapubic or urethral). Administer bladder antispasmodics.

Ⓝ *NCLEX® Connection: Physiological Adaptation, Alterations in Body Systems*

1. A nurse is collecting data on a client who has multiple skin lesions. Which of the following findings are manifestations of malignant melanoma? (Select all that apply.)

   A. Diffuse vesicles

   B. Uniformly colored papule

   C. Area with asymmetric borders

   D. Rough, bleeding patch

   E. Irregular colored mole

2. A nurse is assisting with teaching a newly licensed nurse about leukemia and lymphoma. Sort the following findings into those associated with cute leukemia and those associated with Hodgkin's lymphoma.

   A. Reed-Sternberg cells

   B. Enlarged lymph node

   C. Ecchymosis

   D. Enlarged spleen

3. A nurse is assisting with teaching a class about lung cancer. What health promotion and disease prevention interventions should the nurse include?

4. A nurse is reinforcing teaching with a client about risk factors for gastric cancer. Which of the following risk factors should the nurse include? (Select all that apply.)

   A. Infection with *H. pylori*

   B. High intake of processed foods

   C. History of gastritis

   D. Diet high in carbohydrates

   E. BMI 18

5. A nurse is making a poster for a health fair about screening guidelines for colorectal cancer. Match the following diagnostic tests with the recommended frequency for clients starting at age 45, who are at average risk, and without family history of colorectal cancer.

A. Fecal occult blood tests	1. Every 10 years
	2. Every 5 years
B. Flexible sigmoidoscopy	3. Every year
C. Colonoscopy	

6. A nurse is reinforcing teaching with a newly licensed nurse about urinary diversions. Match the urinary diversion with the method of urinary elimination.

A. Continent pouch	1. Continuous drainage into an external pouch
B. Ureterosigmoidostomy	
C. Ureterostomy	2. During a bowel movement
	3. Intermittent catheterization

7. A nurse is assisting with the care of a client who is postoperative following a right modified radical mastectomy with axillary lymph node dissection. Which of the following actions should the nurse take? (Select all that apply.)

   A. Elevate the client's right arm on a pillow.

   B. Take blood pressure readings on the client's right arm.

   C. Begin exercises on the client's right arm 1 week after the procedure.

   D. Have the client wear a sling on the right arm when ambulating.

   E. Turn the client onto their left side when in bed.

8. A nurse is reviewing the medical record of a client. Which of the following findings are risk factors for ovarian cancer? (Select all that apply.)

   A. Previous history of endometriosis

   B. Family history of colon cancer

   C. First pregnancy at age 24

   D. First period at age 14

   E. Use of oral contraceptives for 10 years

9. A nurse is assisting with teaching a client about testicular self-examination. Which of the following client statements indicates an understanding of the teaching?

   A. "It is best to examine my testicles before bathing."

   B. "It is not necessary to report small lumps, unless they are painful."

   C. "I will examine my testicles once each month."

   D. "I will use my palms to feel for abnormalities."

Application Exercises Key

1. C, D, E. **CORRECT:** When recognizing cues, the nurse should identify that a lesion with asymmetric borders, a rough, bleeding patch, and an irregular-colored mole are manifestations of a malignant melanoma.

   Ⓝ *NCLEX® Connection: Health Promotion and Maintenance, Health Promotion/Disease Prevention*

2. **ACUTE LEUKEMIA:** C, D; **HODGKIN'S LYMPHOMA:** A, B

   When taking actions, the nurse should inform the newly licensed nurse that the presence of Reed Sternberg cells in the lymph nodes and enlarged, painless lymph nodes are findings associated with Hodgkin's lymphoma. Ecchymosis and an enlarged liver and spleen are findings associated with acute leukemia.

   Ⓝ *NCLEX® Connection: Physiological Adaptation, Alterations in Body Systems*

3. When taking actions, the nurse should include to implement measures to promote smoking cessation or to avoid smoking tobacco products. Clients should avoid exposure to second-hand smoke. Instruct the client that the safety of electronic nicotine devices is unknown, and there could be risk from inhaling the vapor of these devices. Over the counter and prescription nicotine replacement therapies are available to assist clients in smoking cessation. Clients should use protective equipment, such as a mask, and ensure proper ventilation while working in environments that can contain carcinogens or particles in the air. Clients who are at risk for lung cancer should have an annual CT scan to detect early lung cancer development.

   Ⓝ *NCLEX® Connection: Health Promotion and Maintenance, Health Promotion/Disease Prevention*

4. A, B, C. **CORRECT:** When taking actions, the nurse should reinforce with the client risk factors for the development of gastric cancer include an infection with *H. pylori*, a high intake of processed foods, and a history of gastritis. A BMI of 18 indicates underweight, however, a BMI greater than 25 is considered overweight as is a risk factor for the development of gastric cancer.

   Ⓝ *NCLEX® Connection: Health Promotion and Maintenance, Health Promotion/Disease Prevention*

5. A, 3; B, 2; C, 1

   When taking actions, the nurse should include in the poster that clients who are at average risk for colorectal cancer, without family history, should have a colonoscopy every 10 years, a flexible sigmoidoscopy every 5 years, or a fecal occult blood test every yr, starting at age 45, to screen for colorectal cancer.

   Ⓝ *NCLEX® Connection: Health Promotion and Maintenance, Health Promotion/Disease Prevention*

6. A, 3; B, 2; C, 1

   When taking action, the nurse should instruct that a ureterostomy diverts urine through the ureters and exits through the skin to an external pouch. An ureterosigmoidostomy diverts urine through the large intestine and exits through the anus. Urine is expelled with stool. A continent pouch is a pouch created by the large intestine that diverts urine through a stoma in the abdomen and is eliminated during intermittent catheterization.

   Ⓝ *NCLEX® Connection: Physiological Adaptation, Basic Pathophysiology*

7. A, D, E. **CORRECT:** When taking actions for a client following right modified radical mastectomy, the nurse should elevate the client's right arm on a pillow, support the right arm with a sling when ambulating, and position the client on their left side when in bed. These actions promote drainage of lymphatic fluid and reduces stress on the incision.

   Ⓝ *NCLEX® Connection: Physiological Adaptation, Basic Pathophysiology*

8. A, B. **CORRECT:** When analyzing cues, the nurse should identify that risk factors for ovarian cancer include previous history of endometriosis and a family history of breast, ovarian, or colon cancer are risk factors for ovarian cancer.

   Ⓝ *NCLEX® Connection: Health Promotion and Maintenance, Health Promotion/Disease Prevention*

9. C. **CORRECT:** When evaluating outcomes, the nurse should identify that the client understands to examine the testicles once each month to determine the presence of any lumps or swelling.

   Ⓝ *NCLEX® Connection: Health Promotion and Maintenance, Health Promotion/Disease Prevention*

CHAPTER 85 *Pain Management for Clients Who Have Cancer*

Management of cancer pain is necessary to optimize quality of life for a client who has cancer. Not all clients who have cancer have pain. Either the tumor or the treatment can cause cancer pain. Tumor pressure or cell invasion can cause direct tissue, bone, and nerve pain. Surgery, radiation, chemotherapy, and inactivity can also cause cancer pain.

PAIN

- Pain is subjective and can indicate tissue injury or impending tissue injury.
- Pain can have physical and emotional components.
- The reaction to pain varies from person to person. Age, sex, and culture can influence it.
- Pain can be acute or chronic.
  - **Acute pain** occurs suddenly and is short-term. Acute cancer pain can be the result of surgery.
  - **Chronic pain** can result from nerve changes and lasts longer than 3 months. Tumor growth and the effects on surrounding tissue (destruction or pressure) cause chronic cancer pain.

TYPES OF PAIN

Neuropathic
- Due to nerve damage
- Numb, tingling, shooting, burning, or radiating

Visceral/Deep
- Occurs in internal organs
- Can be difficult to identify
- Deep, sharp pain

Somatic
- Occurs in bone or connective tissues
- Localized, sharp, dull, or throbbing

DATA COLLECTION

- The most reliable indicator of pain is the client's verbal expression of pain.
- Use standard pain measures (location, quality, intensity, timing, setting, associated manifestations, aggravating or relieving factors) to check pain.
- Pain evaluation also involves observing and documenting nonverbal indicators and physiological changes.

NONVERBAL INDICATORS OF ACUTE PAIN
- Agitation, grimacing
- Elevated heart rate, respiratory rate, blood pressure
- Diaphoresis, pupil dilation
- Splinting of an area

NONVERBAL INDICATORS OF CHRONIC PAIN
- Depression
- Lethargy
- Anger
- Weakness

BARRIERS TO EFFECTIVE PAIN MANAGEMENT
- Inadequate pain evaluation
- Inadequate education with the client about analgesic use
- Health care professionals' lack of knowledge regarding pharmacological pain management
- Reluctance by the client to report pain
- Fear of addiction leading to nonadherence
- Inadequate dosing

MANAGEMENT

An interprofessional team (providers, nurses, pain management and treatment specialists) can provide optimal pain control.
- Palliative cancer pain management provides comfort and reduces pain rather than curing the cancer.
- The goal of palliative pain management is to reduce pain to improve quality of life while maintaining dignity and mental clarity.

METHODS OF PAIN MANAGEMENT: Surgery, chemotherapy, and radiation therapy can reduce pain by removing the tumor or reducing its size, which can alter pressure on adjacent tissues or organs.

NURSING ACTIONS
- Nursing care is specific to each surgery or procedure.
- Include information regarding the specific procedure or treatment.

CLIENT AND FAMILY EDUCATION Qpcc
- Include the family in care and management.
- Consider joining support groups and professional organizations (the American Cancer Society).
- **Radiation**: Perform specific skin care and avoid sun exposure.
- **Chemotherapy**: Avoid infection, and manage other adverse effects.

MEDICATIONS

Pharmacological management of pain includes NSAIDs, opioids, antidepressants, anticonvulsants, corticosteroids, and local anesthetics. Some clients who have cancer pain require a multimodal approach to pain control, in which two or more classes of analgesics are prescribed to relieve pain.

Nonopioid medications and NSAIDs

- Acetaminophen
- Ketorolac
- Aspirin (acetylsalicylic acid)
- Ibuprofen
- Celecoxib

THERAPEUTIC INTENT: For mild to moderate pain

NURSING ACTIONS

- Monitor for gastrointestinal (GI) bleeding (bloody stools, coffee-ground emesis).
- Monitor for bruising and bleeding.
- Do not administer acetaminophen to clients who have liver disease. Clients who have a healthy liver should take no more than 4 g/day. For long-term treatment, adults should take no more than 3 g/day.
- Monitor for tinnitus and hearing loss with NSAIDs.
- NSAIDs can cause cardiovascular adverse effects (heart failure, dysrhythmias).

CLIENT EDUCATION

- Take with food to prevent GI upset.
- Be alert to GI or other bleeding and bruising.
- Do not crush or chew enteric-coated products.
- Drink adequate fluids when taking NSAIDs to prevent acute renal failure due to the effect of prostaglandins on renal function.

Opioids

- Morphine
- Meperidine
- Hydromorphone
- Oxycodone
- Fentanyl (available for transdermal use as well as a lozenge/sucker, buccal film and tablets, and nasal and sublingual spray)
- Combinations, such as hydrocodone with acetaminophen, for breakthrough pain

THERAPEUTIC INTENT

- Moderate to severe pain
- Breakthrough pain

NURSING ACTIONS

- Use with caution for older adult clients.
- Manage acute severe pain with short-term (24 to 48 hr), around-the-clock administration of opioids rather than following a PRN schedule.
- The parenteral route is best for immediate, short-term relief of acute pain. The oral route is better for chronic, nonfluctuating pain.
- Monitor and intervene for adverse effects of opioid use: constipation, orthostatic hypotension, urinary retention, nausea, vomiting, and sedation.

- Monitor for respiratory depression.
- Have naloxone available to reverse effects.
- Administer stimulant laxatives to prevent opioid-induced constipation.

CLIENT EDUCATION

- Avoid driving and using hazardous equipment until the effects of the opioid are known. Qᴘᴄᴄ
- Do not take medications with alcohol.
- Prevent constipation with diet changes and stool softeners.
- Nausea can subside after a few days.
- Reduce the risk of orthostatic hypotension by rising slowly from a lying or sitting position.

Antidepressants

Tricyclic antidepressants (TCAs)

- Amitriptyline
- Desipramine
- Imipramine
- Nortriptyline

Selective norepinephrine reuptake inhibitors (SNRIs)

- Venlafaxine
- Duloxetine
- Nortriptyline

THERAPEUTIC INTENT

- Reduce depression
- Promote sleep
- Increase serotonin and norepinephrine levels to improve feelings of well-being
- Decrease neuropathic pain

NURSING ACTIONS

- Use with caution for older adult clients.
- Use with caution for young adult clients and those who are at risk for suicide, because antidepressants can increase suicide risk.
- **TCAs**
  - Do not administer to clients who have seizure disorders or a history of cardiac problems.
  - Adverse effects include dry mouth, dizziness, mental clouding, weight gain, constipation, and orthostatic hypotension.
- **SNRIs**: Adverse effects include nausea, headache, sedation, insomnia, weight gain, impaired memory, sweating, and tremors.

CLIENT EDUCATION

- Notify the provider if depression increases or if thoughts of suicide occur. Qs
- Therapeutic effects can take 2 to 3 weeks.
- Take TCAs in the evening.

Anticonvulsants

- Gabapentin
- Phenytoin
- Pregabalin
- Carbamazepine

THERAPEUTIC INTENT: Neuralgia and neuropathic pain

NURSING ACTIONS
- Monitor electrolytes.
- Monitor liver function.
- Monitor blood cell counts.
- Monitor medication levels.
- Monitor for tremors.
- Monitor for rash (life-threatening).

CLIENT EDUCATION
- Medication can cause sleepiness and dizziness.
- Avoid alcohol.
- Do not drive at the start of therapy.
- Notify the provider if rash or tremors occur.

Corticosteroids

- Prednisolone (syrup)
- Dexamethasone

THERAPEUTIC INTENT: Reduce pain by reducing swelling

NURSING ACTIONS
- Reduce dosage gradually.
- Monitor for muscle weakness, joint pain, or fever.
- Monitor glucose levels.
- Monitor for changes in behavior or confusion.

CLIENT EDUCATION
- Do not discontinue the medication suddenly.
- Take the medication with food.
- The medication weakens the immune system.
- Report any indications of infection.

Adjunctive agents: Sympatholytic agents

Clonidine

THERAPEUTIC INTENT
- Neuropathic pain
- Administered with bupivacaine in epidural or other local infusions

NURSING ACTIONS: Monitor for hypotension.

CLIENT EDUCATION: Change positions slowly, because these medications can cause orthostatic hypotension.

Adjunctive agents: Skeletal muscle relaxants

Baclofen

THERAPEUTIC INTENT: With other pain medications for muscle spasms accompanying cancer pain

NURSING ACTIONS: Monitor for seizure activity.

CLIENT EDUCATION
- Take the medication with food.
- Use caution when driving or operating machinery.
- These medications can cause drowsiness and dizziness.

Systemic local anesthetics

- Lidocaine
- Bupivacaine
- Ropivacaine

THERAPEUTIC INTENT: Administered via an infusion pump directly into the area of pain (intrathecal, intra-articular, intrapleural) to provide pain relief

NURSING ACTIONS
- Monitor for hypotension.
- Monitor for toxicity; seizures, respiratory depression, bradycardia
- Monitor for infection at the catheter insertion site.
- Evaluate pain status.
- Monitor for motor impairment and level of sedation.
- Administer with an opioid or another medication (clonidine).

CLIENT EDUCATION
- Observe the infusion site for indications of infection (redness and swelling).
- Watch for fever.
- Notify the provider of increased pain or decreased movement that can indicate a motor block.
- Care for and protect the external part of the catheter.

Topical local anesthetics

Lidocaine (patch)

THERAPEUTIC INTENT: Block generation and conduction of nerve impulses that transmit pain

NURSING ACTIONS: Monitor for pain relief and local skin reactions.

CLIENT EDUCATION: Use the medication only on intact skin.

ADMINISTRATION METHODS

Oral

- First choice for administration
- Short- and long-acting formulations available

Transdermal

Fentanyl
- Easy to administer
- Slow onset, consistent dosing
- Long duration (48 to 72 hr)

Rectal

Low WBC and platelet counts are contraindications.

Subcutaneous infusion

Morphine or hydromorphone
- Slow infusion rate (2 to 4 mL/hr)
- Requires collaboration with the RN
- Risk of infiltration
- Rapid onset

Intravenous

- Requires collaboration with the RN
- Risk of infiltration
- Rapid onset

Epidural or intrathecal

- Risk of infection, pruritus, and urinary retention
- Invasive and requires an RN to monitor and provide care, especially with increases in dosage
- More effective than IV analgesia during the immediate postoperative period

Sublingual/buccal

- Place sublingual forms under the tongue for absorption.
- Place buccal forms between the gum and cheek.
- Forms include tablets, films, and sprays.
- The client should refrain from drinking, eating, or smoking when taking the medication.

Topical/local

- Place patches directly over or adjacent to the painful area.
- Medication produces minimal systemic absorption and adverse effects.
- Lidocaine patch remains on for 12 hr, off for 12 hr.
- Monitor for local skin reactions.

ANESTHETIC INTERVENTIONS

Regional nerve blocks

Involves injecting an anesthetic agent (bupivacaine) and/or a corticosteroid directly into a nerve root to provide pain relief

- For identifying or treating an isolated area of pain; for example, an intercostal nerve block treats chest or abdominal wall pain.
- The procedure can take from 15 min to 1 hr, depending on the area receiving the block.

NURSING ACTIONS
- Measure baseline vital signs. Monitor blood pressure and vital signs during the procedure and for at least 1 hr following the procedure (follow established guidelines).
- Assist in establishing IV access before the procedure.
- Monitor for manifestations of systemic infusion (metallic taste, ringing in ears, perioral numbness, seizures).
- Check the insertion site for redness and swelling.
- Check the level of nerve block and pain.
- Protect the area of numbness from injury.

CLIENT EDUCATION
- Observe the injection site for swelling, redness, or drainage.
- Protect the area of numbness from injury and notify the provider of increased pain or manifestations of systemic infusion.

Epidural or intrathecal catheters

- Involves injecting a local anesthetic or analgesic into the epidural space (the area outside the dura mater of the spinal cord) or intrathecal space (the subarachnoid area within the spinal cord sheath that contains cerebrospinal fluid)
- Involves surgically placing an external catheter under the skin with an external port for long-term use
  - For chronic pain management
  - Allows administration of a continuous infusion or injection PRN
  - For upper abdominal pain, thoracic pain, and pain below the umbilicus

NURSING ACTIONS
- Monitor during and for at least 1 hr following insertion or injection for hypotension, anaphylaxis, muscle weakness, seizures, and dura puncture. Qs
- Monitor for respiratory depression and sedation.
- Monitor the insertion site for hematoma, infection, and leakage of cerebral spinal fluid.
- Check the level of sensory block.
- Evaluate leg strength prior to ambulating.
- Local anesthetics block the sympathetic nervous system, causing peripheral vasodilation and hypotension. This can cause reduced stroke volume, cardiac output, and peripheral resistance. Increase the rate of IV fluid infusion to compensate for the sympathetic blocking effects of regional anesthetics.

CLIENT EDUCATION
- Notify the provider of manifestations of infection (fever, swelling, redness; increase in pain or severe headache; sudden weakness of the lower extremities; decreases in bowel or bladder control).
- Notify the provider of manifestations of systemic infusion.

OTHER INVASIVE TECHNIQUES

Neurolytic ablation

Involves interrupting the nerve pathway or destroying the nerve roots that are causing pain; usually involves a CT-guided probe and injection of chemicals (phenol or ethanol)

- For example, celiac plexus nerve ablation can be effective for pancreatic, stomach, abdominal, small bowel, and proximal colon pain.
- The procedure is irreversible.
- Nerve ablation can provide relief for several months until nerve fibers regenerate.
- Nerve ablation can cause loss of sensory, motor, and autonomic function.
- Use only when noninvasive methods are ineffective.

Radiofrequency ablation

Electrical current creates heat on a probe that the provider guides to the tumor or nerves to destroy cancer cells or ablate nerve endings (for lung and bone tumors).

85.1 Case study

Part 1
Joe is a nurse in an oncology unit assisting with the care for Anne Smith. The client is postoperative following a partial mastectomy for treatment of breast cancer.

Part 2
Anne Smith has a follow-up appointment at an oncology office. The client has received oxaliplatin for treatment of breast cancer and reports numbness and tingling in fingers and toes.

Part 3
Amy, a nurse in an oncology office, is discussing treatment options with Anne Smith. The client reports experiencing pain following a partial mastectomy and requests information regarding alternatives to analgesic medications.

ALTERNATIVE APPROACHES

Use alternative approaches to pain management in addition to pain medications or other techniques. Many of these provide some pain reduction with minimal adverse effects. Qᴛᴄ

Transcutaneous electrical nerve stimulation (TENS)

Skin electrodes near or over the area of pain transmit low-voltage electrical impulses. The client regulates the voltage to achieve the perception of pins and needles or a vibrating sensation (sensory perception) rather than pain. Often used for chronic and acute postoperative pain.

NURSING ACTIONS
- Monitor electrode sites for burns and rash.
- Offer other pain medications.
- Do not use for clients who have pacemakers or cardiac dysrhythmias.
- Remove hair before applying the electrodes.

CLIENT EDUCATION
- Place the electrodes on clean, hairless, intact skin.
- Inspect the skin under the electrodes for burns or irritation.
- Do not use near the head or over the heart.

Spinal cord stimulation

Invasive technique reserved for those unresponsive to other methods. Requires a surgical procedure to place electrodes in the epidural space; the electrodes connect to an implanted or external programmed generator.

NURSING ACTIONS: Care is the same as for clients undergoing epidural anesthesia.

CLIENT EDUCATION: Program the device for maximal comfort.

Relaxation techniques and imagery Qᴇʙᴘ

Useful during a procedure or a period of increased pain
- Relaxation techniques include deep breathing, progressive relaxation, and meditation.
- Positive imagery involves visualizing a peaceful image with or without audio recordings.
- Relaxation and imagery can reduce anxiety, stress, and pain, and they can assist the client to feel more in control of the pain.

Distraction

Music, television, exercise, and family and friends can be effective distractions from pain and stress. Other distractions include repetitive actions or movements, focused breathing, or use of a visual focal point. A change of scenery can offer a distraction from pain.

Heat or cold, pressure, massage, or vibration

- Heat increases blood flow, relaxes muscles, and reduces joint stiffness.
- Cold decreases inflammation and causes local analgesia.
- Do not use heat or cold directly on skin to reduce the risk of injury. Avoid use over areas that have that have radiation damage. Qs
- Massage and vibration can cause relaxation, distraction, and increased surface circulation.

Acupuncture

Acupuncture uses vibration or electrical stimulation by inserting small needles into the skin and subcutaneous tissues at different depths to stimulate and alter nerve pathways. It can also increase the client's pain threshold.

Hypnosis

Hypnosis involves using an altered state of awareness to redirect the perception of pain. It can help induce positive imagery, reduce anxiety, and improve coping.

Peer group support

A support group helps provide emotional support for the client and family. Other benefits include the presence of a social network, availability of information, and help in strengthening coping skills.

Active Learning Scenario

An nurse manager is leading a discussion with a group of nurses on the oncology unit about alternative approaches to pain management. What information should the nurse manager include in the discussion? Use the ATI Active Learning Template: Basic Concept to complete this item.

RELATED CONTENT

- Describe four approaches.
- Describe two nursing interventions for each approach.
- Describe one instructional point for each approach.

Application Exercises

1. The nurse is reinforcing discharge teaching with the client who has a new prescription for two pain medications. Sort the following adverse effects into those that can occur with Ibuprofen or with Oxycodone.

   A. Tinnitus

   B. Respiratory depression

   C. Gastrointestinal bleeding

   D. Orthostatic hypotension

2. The nurse is assisting with the care of the client who has a prescription for gabapentin for neuropathic pain. The nurse should monitor the client for which of the following adverse effects of this medication?

   A. Constipation

   B. Urinary retention

   C. Insomnia

   D. Dizziness

3. A nurse is reinforcing teaching with a client who has chronic cancer pain and a new intrathecal catheter placed for continuous infusion of fentanyl and bupivacaine. What information should the nurse include?

4. A nurse is assisting with the care of a client who has cancer and has a prescription for transcutaneous electrical nerve stimulation (TENS) for pain management. Which of the following actions should the nurse take? (Select all that apply.)

   A. Remove hair before applying electrodes on the client's skin.

   B. Apply electrodes on the client to areas of intact skin.

   C. Place electrodes over the client's chest.

   D. Avoid administering additional pain medications to the client when using the TENS unit.

   E. Inspect the client's skin under the electrodes for burns.

5. The nurse is discussing alternative approaches to relieving pain with the client. Match the alternative therapy with the associated method.

A. Positive imagery	1. Uses an altered state of awareness to redirect the perception of pain.
B. Massage therapy	2. Small needles are inserted into the skin to stimulate and alter nerve pathways.
C. Acupuncture	3. Soft tissue is manipulated to increase surface circulation.
D. Hypnosis	4. Involves picturing a peaceful image.

Active Learning Scenario Key

Using the ATI Active Learning Template: Basic Concept
RELATED CONTENT

Transcutaneous electrical nerve stimulation (TENS)
- Monitor electrode sites for burns or rash.
- Offer pain medications.
- Do not use on clients who have pacemakers or dysrhythmias.
- Place electrodes on clean, hairless, intact skin. Inspect skin under the electrodes for burns or irritation.
- Do not use if the client is pregnant.
- Do not use near the head or over the heart.

Relaxation and imagery
- Use during a procedure or during a period of increased pain. Encourage deep breathing, progressive relaxation, meditation, or a focus on a peaceful image.
- Use with or without audio recordings.
- Reduces stress, anxiety, and pain, and promotes a feeling of control of the pain.

Application of heat or cold, pressure, massage, or vibration
- Apply heat to increase blood flow, relax muscles, and reduce joint stiffness.
- Apply cold to decrease inflammation and produce local analgesia.
- Massage can cause relaxation, distraction, and increased surface circulation.
- Do not apply heat or cold directly to skin that has radiation damage.
- Avoid further skin irritation with excessive massage or vibration.

Distraction
- Offer music.
- Encourage watching television, exercising, and activities with family and friends.
- Use repetitive actions or movements, focused breathing, a visual focal point, and a change of scenery.

Acupuncture
- Inform the client acupuncture can increase the client's pain threshold.
- Make referrals to community resources.
- Involves inserting small needles into the skin at different depths to stimulate and alter nerve pathways. This affects the pain threshold.

Hypnosis
- Inform the client that hypnosis redirects the client's perception of pain.
- Make referrals to community resources.
- Use to induce positive imagery, reduce anxiety, and improve coping.

Peer group
- Recommend referrals to community resources.
- Encourage family participation.
- Groups provide emotional support for family members and clients.
- Groups offer the presence of a social network, availability of information, and strengthening of coping skills.

Ⓝ *NCLEX® Connection: Basic Care and Comfort, Nonpharmacological Comfort Interventions*

Application Exercises Key

1. **IBUPROFEN:** A, C; **OXYCODONE:** B, D

   When taking actions, the nurse should reinforce to the client to monitor for tinnitus and gastrointestinal bleeding when taking ibuprofen for pain. The nurse should reinforce to the client to monitor for respiratory depression and orthostatic hypotension when taking oxycodone for pain.

   Ⓝ *NCLEX® Connection: Pharmacological Therapies, Pharmacological Pain Management*

2. D. **CORRECT:** When taking actions, the nurse should monitor the client for dizziness. The nurse should reinforce to the client to avoid alcohol and activities that require alertness until the medication effects are known.

   Ⓝ *NCLEX® Connection: Pharmacological Therapies, Pharmacological Pain Management*

3. When taking actions, the nurse should instruct the client to notify the provider of manifestations of infection, such as fever, swelling, and redness. The client should monitor for and report an increase in pain or severe headache, sudden weakness of the lower extremities, or decreases in bowel or bladder control. The nurse should also instruct the client to notify the provider of manifestations of systemic infusion, such as respiratory depression, hypotension, and sedation.

   Ⓝ *NCLEX® Connection: Pharmacological Therapies, Pharmacological Pain Management*

4. A, B, E. **CORRECT:** When taking actions, the nurse should remove hair before applying electrodes and place them on clean intact skin. The nurse should inspect the skin under the electrodes for burns or irritation.

   Ⓝ *NCLEX® Connection: Basic Care and Comfort, Nonpharmacological Comfort Interventions*

5. A, 4; B, 3; C, 2; D, 1

   When taking actions, the nurse should include in the discussion that hypnosis uses an altered state of awareness to redirect the perception of pain. Acupuncture uses small needles that are inserted into the skin to stimulate and alter nerve pathways. Massage therapy involves manipulation of soft tissue to increase surface circulation. Positive imagery involves picturing a peaceful image to reduce anxiety, stress, and pain.

   Ⓝ *NCLEX® Connection: Basic Care and Comfort, Nonpharmacological Comfort Interventions*

When reviewing the following chapters, keep in mind the relevant topics and tasks of the NCLEX outline.

Coordinated Care

INFORMED CONSENT: Recognize that informed consent was obtained.

Reduction of Risk Potential

POTENTIAL FOR COMPLICATIONS FROM SURGICAL PROCEDURES AND HEALTH ALTERATIONS
Identify client response to surgery or health alterations.

Assist with care for client before and after surgical procedure.

Reinforce teaching to prevent complications due to surgery or health alterations.

THERAPEUTIC PROCEDURES: Assist with the performance of a diagnostic or invasive procedure.

Physiological Adaptation

UNEXPECTED RESPONSE TO THERAPIES: Promote recovery of the client from unexpected negative response to therapy.

MEDICAL EMERGENCIES: Respond and intervene to a client life-threatening situation.

UNIT 14   NURSING CARE OF PERIOPERATIVE CLIENTS

CHAPTER 86 *Preoperative Nursing Care*

Surgery can take on many forms, including curative, palliative, cosmetic, restorative, preventative, reconstructive, diagnostic, and transplant. There are three categories of inpatient surgical procedures based on acuity: emergent, urgent, or elective. Outpatient or ambulatory surgery generally is an elective surgery that is not considered acute (cataract removal, hernia repair).

Preoperative care takes place from the time a client is scheduled for surgery until care is transferred to the operating suite. Identification of risk factors is one of the major aspects of preoperative care. Preoperative care includes thorough collection of data regarding the client's physical, emotional, and psychosocial status prior to surgery.

The Joint Commission has implemented several National Patient Safety Goals to ensure quality and safety during surgical procedures.

These goals include:

- Marking of the client's surgical site

- Pausing prior to a surgical procedure to ensure no errors are being made

- Ensuring correct procedure is performed on the correct client at the correct body area

Other actions to prevent harm include the Surgical Care Improvement Project (SCIP) which is aimed at preventing surgical complications. Team STEPPS can be used in the operative setting to increase communication, teamwork and collaboration.

RISK FACTORS

FOR SURGICAL COMPLICATIONS

- **Obstructive sleep apnea**: Airway obstruction, oxygen desaturation
- **Pregnancy**: Fetal risk with anesthesia
- **Respiratory disease**: COPD, pneumonia, asthma
- **Cardiovascular disease**: Heart failure, myocardial infarction, hypertension, dysrhythmias
- **Diabetes mellitus**: Altered blood glucose levels, delayed healing, infection, impaired circulation
- **Liver disease:** Altered medication metabolism and increased risk for bleeding
- **Kidney disease**: Altered elimination and medication excretion
- **Endocrine disorders:** Hypo/hyperthyroidism, Addison's disease, Cushing's syndrome
- **Immune system disorders**: Immunocompromised
- **Coagulation defect**: Increased risk of bleeding
- **Malnutrition**: Delayed healing
- **BMI greater than 30**: Pulmonary complications due to hypoventilation, effect on anesthesia, elimination, and wound healing
- **Some medications**: Antihypertensives, anticoagulants, NSAIDs, tricyclic antidepressants, herbal medications, over-the-counter medications
- **Substance use:** Tobacco, alcohol
- **Genetic history**: Malignant hyperthermia
- **Allergies**: Latex, anesthetic agents
- Inability to cope, lack of support system
- Disease processes involving multiple body systems
- **Older adult clients:** Possible age-related changes include the following. ©
  ○ Decreased hepatic and renal function that alters clearance of anesthetic agents and opioids
  ○ Co-morbidities (chronic disease processes, use of multiple medications)
  ○ Greater risk of adverse reactions to preoperative medications
  ○ Less physiologic reserve than younger clients, which can cause decreased immune system response and decreased wound healing
  ○ Reduction of muscle mass and amount of body water, which places older adult clients at risk for dehydration
  ○ Sensory decline (decreased eyesight, hearing loss)
  ○ Oral alterations (dentures, bridges, loose teeth) that pose problems during intubation
  ○ Perspire less, which leads to dry, itchy skin that becomes fragile and easily abraded
  ○ Decreased subcutaneous fat, which makes older adult clients susceptible to temperature changes

PREOPERATIVE DATA COLLECTION

Detailed history: Medical history, surgical history, tolerance of anesthesia, medication use, complementary or alternative practices (herbals), psychosocial history, cultural considerations, substance use (including tobacco), social support systems, genetic history, occupation, and perceptions and knowledge about surgery

Allergies: Medications, latex, contrast agents, and food products

- Allergies to banana or kiwi can indicate the client is at risk for a reaction to latex.
- Allergy to eggs or soybean oil is a contraindication to the use of propofol for anesthesia.
- Contrast media (iodine) may not always be a contraindication in clients who have a shellfish allergy. Further data collection may be needed.

Anxiety level: Regarding the procedure, support systems, and coping mechanisms

Baseline data: Head-to-toe data collection, vital signs, and oxygen saturations

Venous thromboembolism risk: Evaluation based on surgical procedure, client history, and anticipated time the client will be immobilized following surgery

DIAGNOSTIC PROCEDURES

Urinalysis: Renal function, rule out infection

Blood type and cross match: In case a blood transfusion is required. Some clients may desire an autologous donation.

CBC: Fluid status, anemia, infection/immune status

Pregnancy test: Fetal risk of anesthesia

Clotting studies: PT, INR, aPTT, platelet count

Blood electrolyte levels: Electrolyte imbalances

Blood creatinine and BUN: Renal status

ABGs: Oxygenation status

Chest x-ray: Heart and lung status

12-lead ECG: Baseline heart rhythm, dysrhythmias, history of cardiac disease; performed on all clients older than 40 years

PATIENT-CENTERED CARE

NURSING CARE

- Verify that the informed consent is accurately completed, signed, and witnessed.
- Administer enemas and/or laxatives the night before and/or the morning of the surgery for clients undergoing bowel surgery.
- Regularly check scheduled medication prescriptions. Some medications (antihypertensives, anticoagulants, antidepressants) can be withheld until after the procedure. Withhold anticoagulants at least 48 hrs before surgery.
- Determine whether autologous blood or direct blood donation from family is available if needed.
- Ensure that the client remains NPO for at least 6 hr for solid foods and 2 hr for clear liquids before surgery with general anesthesia to avoid aspiration. Note on the chart the last time the client ate or drank. Q EBP
- Perform skin preparation, which can include cleansing with antimicrobial soap. If absolutely necessary, use electric clippers or chemical depilatories to remove hair in areas that will be involved in the surgery.

86.2 Case study

Scenario introduction

0700: Amy is a nurse in a preoperative holding area caring for Anne Smith. Ms. Smith is scheduled for colon resection at 0800. Ms. Smith has a history of Crohn's disease, diabetes mellitus, transient ischemic attacks. Ms. Smith takes aspirin, 80 mg PO QD.

Scene 1

Amy: "Hello, Ms. Smith, my name is Amy. What brings you to the surgery center?"

Ms. Smith: "I am having a colon resection."

Amy: "Do you have any allergies to any medications or foods?"

Ms. Smith: "Yes, I am allergic to eggs and bananas."

Scene 2

Amy: "When was the last time you had anything to eat or drink?"

Ms. Smith: "I had dinner last night at 7 p.m. and a glass of water this morning at 6:30 a.m."

Scene 3

Amy: "I would like to check your vital signs and review your lab work results. An IV will be inserted into your arm or hand and your surgeon will be in soon to explain the procedure and obtain consent."

Ms. Smith: That is fine, thank you."

Scenario conclusion

Amy reviews the following collected information:

0700
- Allergy: Eggs, bananas
- Temp: 36° C (96.8° F)
- Heart rate 62/min
- Respirations 20/min
- Blood pressure 104/56 mm Hg (right arm supine)
- Oxygen saturation 98% on room air
- Client is awake, alert, and oriented. Bilateral breath sounds clear and present throughout. Abdomen soft, nondistended, hyperactive bowel sounds in 4 quadrants.
- BMI 16

Lab work reviewed and provider notified of results:
- Hct 37% (37% to 47%)
- Hgb 12 g/dL (12 g/dL to 16 g/dL)
- WBC 9,000/mm³ (5,000 to 10,000/mm³)
- Bleeding time 10 min (1 to 9 min)
- PT 13.5 sec (11 to 12.5 sec)
- Prealbumin 10.6 mg/dL (15 to 36 mg/dL)

- Ensure that jewelry, dentures, prosthetics, makeup, nail polish, and glasses are removed. These items can be given to the family or stored safely.
- Cover the client with a lightweight cotton blanket heated in a warmer to prevent hypothermia. Hypothermia increases the chance for surgical wound infections, alters metabolism of medication, and causes coagulation problems and cardiac dysrhythmias.
- Ensure IV access with a large-bore (18-gauge) catheter for easier infusing of IV fluids or blood products.
- Administer preoperative medications (prophylactic antimicrobials, antiemetics, sedatives) as prescribed.
  ◦ Prophylactic antibiotics are administered within 1 hr of surgical incision.
  ◦ If the client has been taking a beta blocker medication, administer the prescribed beta-blocker prior to surgery to prevent a cardiac event and possible death.
  ◦ Have the client void prior to administration.
  ◦ Monitor response to medications.
  ◦ Raise side rails following administration to prevent injury.
- Ensure that the preoperative checklist is complete.
- Confirm and verify the correct surgical site with the client and all health care team members before clearly marking the surgical site.
- Minimize client anxiety while waiting to go to surgery by using distraction techniques (watching TV, reading, listening to music).
- For clients encountering severe anxiety and panic, reassurance will be necessary and sedation medications can be given. Nonpharmacological interventions (distraction, imagery, and music therapy) can be initiated.
- Ensure that measures are taken to prevent postoperative deep-vein thromboembolism by continuing anticoagulation therapy and/or anti-embolism stockings, pneumatic compression devices, and range-of-motion exercises.

Informed consent

- Once surgery has been discussed as treatment with the client and significant other, family member, or friend, it is the responsibility of the provider to obtain consent after discussing the risks and benefits of the procedure. The nurse is not to obtain the consent for the provider in any circumstance.
- The nurse can clarify any information that remains unclear after the provider's explanation of the procedure. The nurse cannot provide any new or additional information not previously given by the provider.
- The nurse's role is to witness the client's signing of the consent form after the client acknowledges understanding of the procedure.
- The nurse should determine if the client is legally capable of providing consent.
  ◦ 18 years of age or emancipated
  ◦ Mentally capable of understanding the risks, reason, and options for surgery and anesthesia
  ◦ Free from the influence of medication that affects decision-making or judgment (opioids, benzodiazepines, sedatives)

- A legal guardian or health care surrogate can sign if the client is not capable of providing consent or if there is no family.
- Two witnesses can be required if the client is able to only sign with an "X," has vision or hearing impairments, or if there is a language barrier.
- Informed consent is required for surgical procedures, invasive procedures (biopsy, paracentesis, scopes), and any procedure requiring sedation or anesthesia, involving radiation, or that places the client at increased risk for complications.

PROVIDER RESPONSIBILITIES
- Obtain informed consent.
- To obtain informed consent, the provider must explain the following.
  ◦ Complete description of the treatment/procedure
  ◦ Description of the professionals who will be performing and participating in the treatment
  ◦ Information on the risks of anesthesia
  ◦ Description of the anticipated benefits of the treatment/procedure
  ◦ Description of the potential harm, pain, and/or discomfort that can occur
  ◦ Options for other treatments
  ◦ The right to refuse treatment

CLIENT RESPONSIBILITIES
- Give informed consent.
- To give informed consent, do the following.
  ◦ Give it voluntarily (no coercion involved).
  ◦ Receive enough information to make a decision based on an understanding of what is expected.
  ◦ Be competent and of legal age or be an emancipated minor. When the client is unable to provide consent, another authorized person must give consent.

NURSE RESPONSIBILITIES
- Witnesses informed consent.
- To witness informed consent, do the following.
  ◦ Ensure that the provider gave the client the necessary information.
  ◦ Ensure that the client understood the information and is competent to give informed consent. Qs
  ◦ Notify the provider if the client has additional questions or appears to not understand any of the information provided. (The provider is then responsible for giving clarification.)
  ◦ Observe the client sign the informed consent document.
  ◦ Document any additional reinforcement of teaching.
  ◦ Provide a trained medical interpreter (not a family member or friend) and record the use of an interpreter in the medical record.

CLIENT EDUCATION

- Understand the purpose and effects of preoperative medications that will be administered.
- Be aware of postoperative pain control techniques (medications, immobilization, patient-controlled analgesia pumps, splinting).
- Perform splinting, coughing, and deep breathing.
- Perform range-of-motion exercises and early ambulation for prevention of thrombi and respiratory complications.
- Use antiembolism stockings and pneumatic compression devices to prevent deep-vein thrombosis.
- Perform bowel and skin preparations as prescribed (cleansing enema, preoperative shower with medicated soap). Qᴘᴄᴄ
- Understand the purpose of invasive lines used in surgery and after (drains, catheters, IV lines).
- Adhere to the postoperative diet.
- Perform incentive spirometry to promote oxygenation.

- Adhere to preoperative instructions regarding medications.
  - If taking acetylsalicylic acid, stop taking it for 1 week before an elective surgery to decrease the risk of bleeding.
  - Ask the provider before taking any herbal or over-the-counter medications. Some medications can increase the risk of bleeding or adverse effects from anesthesia.
  - Medications for cardiovascular disease, pulmonary disease, seizures, diabetes mellitus, some antihypertensive medications, and eye drops for glaucoma are usually allowed prior to surgery or a procedure.
- Use a pain scale to rate pain level.
- Understand the care and restrictions relative to the surgical procedure performed.
- Avoid smoking, alcohol, or illicit drug use, which can interfere with surgical medications and increase the risk for surgical complications.

86.1 Preoperative checklist

🏥 Health Care Providers   **PREOPERATIVE CHECKLIST**

Checklist (yes, no, N/A, initials)

☐☐☐ ___ Allergies (list below)
☐☐☐ ___ Operative permit correct/signed, dated, timed
☐☐☐ ___ Authorization for treatment signed
☐☐☐ ___ Anesthesia consent/signed, dated, timed
☐☐☐ ___ Blood consent/signed, dated, timed
☐☐☐ ___ ID bracelet correct and on client
☐☐☐ ___ Blood bracelet correct and on client
☐☐☐ ___ Height and weight recorded
☐☐☐ ___ Preoperative laboratory reports on chart
☐☐☐ ___ ECG report on chart
☐☐☐ ___ Chest x-ray report on chart
☐☐☐ ___ Correct operative site marked with an X
☐☐☐ ___ MAR/home medications
☐☐☐ ___ History and physical report on chart

☐☐☐ ___ Old records with chart
☐☐☐ ___ Undergarments removed
☐☐☐ ___ Hospital gown on client
☐☐☐ ___ Operative area preparation
☐☐☐ ___ Nail polish removed
☐☐☐ ___ Indwelling urinary catheter placed
☐☐☐ ___ Body piercing removed if applicable
☐☐☐ ___ Emboli stockings/ace bandages applied
☐☐☐ ___ Contact lens/glasses removed-deposition
☐☐☐ ___ Dentures/partial plates removed-deposition
☐☐☐ ___ Valuable jewelry removed-deposition
☐☐☐ ___ Preoperative antibiotic given
☐☐☐ ___ Preoperative teaching complete by _____
☐☐☐ ___ Oxygen (detail below)

Notes

Allergies

Preoperative medications given

Preoperative vital signs

Comments

Oxygen

_____ liters per nasal cannula

_____ % per face mask

NPO since _____

Transferred to surgery per _____

   date _____ time _____

Signed _____

COMPLICATIONS

Complications during the postoperative period can be related to the medications given preoperatively.

- Other postoperative complications include respiratory complications (atelectasis, pneumonia), circulatory complications (bleeding, deep-vein thrombosis, gastrointestinal and genitourinary complications (paralytic ileus, urinary retention), inadequate wound healing, infection and sepsis; anemia; hypovolemia and possible circulatory shock; and electrolyte imbalance.
- Be alert for any allergic reactions the client has to medications.

Sedatives (benzodiazepines, barbiturates)
Respiratory depression, drowsiness, dizziness

NURSING ACTIONS
- Monitor respiratory rate and oxygen saturation.
- Administer oxygen.
- Administer a reversal agent, flumazenil.

Opioids
Respiratory depression, drowsiness, dizziness, constipation, urinary retention

NURSING ACTIONS
- Monitor respiratory rate and oxygen saturation.
- Administer oxygen.
- Administer a reversal agent, naloxone.
- Perform prescribed intermittent catheterization.

IV infusions (0.9% NaCl, lactated Ringer's)
Fluid overload, hypernatremia

NURSING ACTIONS
- Monitor I&O closely.
- Ensure the IV fluid rate of infusion is decreased.
- Administer prescribed diuretic.

Gastrointestinal medications (antiemetics, antacids, H2 receptor blockers)
Alkalosis, cardiac abnormalities (some H2 receptor blockers), drowsiness

NURSING ACTIONS
- Obtain preoperative cardiac history.
- Monitor for electrolyte abnormalities.

Active Learning Scenario

A nurse is assisting with the plan of care for a client scheduled for a surgical procedure. What potential complications should the nurse consider? Use the ATI Active Learning Template: Basic Concept to complete this item.

RELATED CONTENT: List at least three possible complications the nurse should prevent, explain the related cause, and include one intervention for each complication.

Application Exercises

1. The nurse is reviewing the client's preoperative data. Sort the following findings into the associated increased surgical risk: Delayed wound healing or Bleeding.
   A. Diabetes Mellitus
   B. Coagulation studies
   C. Aspirin use
   D. Malnutrition

2. A nurse is verifying informed consent for the client who is having a colon resection. What actions should the nurse take?

3. The nurse is reinforcing teaching with the client who is preoperative for abdominal surgery. Which of the following statements should the nurse make? (Select all that apply.)
   A. "Take your aspirin with a sip of water this morning before your surgery."
   B. "Splint the abdominal incision with a pillow when coughing and deep breathing after surgery."
   C. "You will be placed on bed rest for the first 48 hours after surgery"
   D. "You should perform calf pumping exercises after surgery."
   E. "Anti-embolism stockings are applied before surgery."

4. A preoperative nurse is caring for the client who is having a colon resection. Which of the following actions should the nurse take? (Select all that apply.)
   A. Encourage the client to void prior to receiving preoperative medications.
   B. Administer antibiotics 2 hr prior to the surgical incision.
   C. Use a disposable razor to shave hair over the surgical site.
   D. Remove nail polish on the client's finger nails.
   E. Instruct the client how to use an incentive spirometer.

5. The nurse is reviewing the client's preoperative data. Match the following findings with the associated increased surgical risk.
   A. Oral fluid intake   1. Propofol reaction
   B. Banana allergy   2. Latex reaction
   C. Egg allergy   3. Aspiration

Using the ATI Active Learning Template: Basic Concept

RELATED CONTENT

Prevent respiratory depression.
- Caused by overmedication with benzodiazepines, barbiturates, or opioids.
- Administer a prescribed reversal agent, and monitor closely.

Prevent fluid overload.
- Caused by too much IV fluids and inability to readily excrete the fluids.
- Obtain a preoperative cardiac and pulmonary history, monitor I&O closely, slow the rate of IV fluids, and administer a prescribed diuretic.

Prevent deep-vein thrombosis.
- Caused by blood stasis in lower extremities due to absent muscle contractility.
- Apply antiembolism stockings and/or pneumatic compression devices, administer prescribed anticoagulants, and reinforce range-of-motion exercises.

Prevent infection.
- Caused by micro-organisms contaminating the surgical wound.
- Administer a prescribed prophylactic antibiotic within 1 hr before the surgical incision is made.

(N) *NCLEX® Connection: Reduction of Risk Potential, Potential for Complications from Surgical Procedures and Health Alterations*

1. **DELAYED WOUND HEALING:** A, D; **BLEEDING:** B, C

   When analyzing cues, the nurse should identify that diabetes mellitus and manifestations of malnutrition, (a BMI of 16 and prealbumin level of 10.6 mg/dl), increase the client's risk for delayed wound healing. Aspirin use, an increased bleeding time, and prolonged PT, increase the client's risk for bleeding.

   (N) *NCLEX® Connection: Reduction of Risk Potential, Laboratory Values*

2. When taking actions, the nurse should ensure that the provider gave the client necessary information about the procedure and clarify any information that remains unclear. The nurse should ensure that the client understands the information and is competent to give informed consent. The nurse should notify the provider if the client has more questions or appears to not understand any of the information provided. (The provider is then responsible for giving clarification.) The nurse should document questions the client has and notify the provider. Also, the nurse should document any additional reinforcement of teaching. The nurse's role is to witness the client's signing of the consent form after the client acknowledges understanding of the procedure. The nurse should determine if the client is legally capable of providing consent: 18 years of age or emancipated, mentally capable of understanding the risks, reason, and options for surgery and anesthesia, and free from the influence of medication that affects decision-making or judgment (opioids, benzodiazepines, sedatives).

   (N) *NCLEX® Connection: Reduction of Risk Potential, Therapeutic Procedures*

3. B. **CORRECT:** When taking actions, the nurse should instruct the client to splint the abdominal incision with a pillow to cough and deep breath after the surgery to provide support and reduce discomfort.
   D. **CORRECT:** The nurse should instruct the client to perform calf pumping exercises to promote venous return and anti-embolism stockings will be applied before the surgery to reduce the risk for a deep vein thrombosis.
   E. **CORRECT:** The nurse should instruct the client to perform calf pumping exercises to promote venous return and anti-embolism stockings will be applied before the surgery to reduce the risk for a deep vein thrombosis.

   (N) *NCLEX® Connection: Reduction of Risk Potential, Therapeutic Procedures*

4. A. **CORRECT:** When taking actions, the nurse should encourage the client to void before receiving preoperative medications to reduce the risk of client injury trying to ambulate to the bathroom.
   D. **CORRECT:** The nurse should remove any nail polish present on the client's finger nails to allow monitoring of circulation and oxygenation.
   E. **CORRECT:** The nurse should instruct the client about using an incentive spirometer to reduce the risk of postoperative complications.

   (N) *NCLEX® Connection: Reduction of Risk Potential, Therapeutic Procedures*

5. A, 3; B, 2; C, 1

   When analyzing data, the nurse should identify that the client's egg allergy places them at risk for a reaction to propofol. The client's banana allergy places them at risk for a reaction to latex. The client's oral intake at 06:30 places them at risk for aspiration. The client should not drink clear liquids within 2 hrs prior to general anesthesia to reduce the risk of aspiration.

   (N) *NCLEX® Connection: Reduction of Risk Potential, Therapeutic Procedures*

CHAPTER 87

CHAPTER 87 *Postoperative Nursing Care*

Transferring a client who is postoperative from the operating suite to the postanesthesia care unit (PACU) is the responsibility of the anesthesia provider, who is an anesthesiologist or certified registered nurse anesthetist (CRNA). The circulating nurse, the anesthesiologist or CRNA will give the verbal hand-off report to the PACU nurse.

Postoperative care is usually provided initially in the PACU, where skilled nurses who are certified in advanced cardiac life support can monitor a client's recovery from anesthesia. In some instances, a client is transferred from the operating suite directly to the intensive care unit.

Initial postoperative care involves obtaining data and vital signs frequently, administering medications, managing pain, preventing complications, and determining when a client is ready to be discharged from the PACU. During the immediate postoperative stage, maintaining airway patency and ventilation and monitoring circulatory status are the priorities for care. Postoperative clients who receive general anesthesia require frequent monitoring of their respiratory status. Postoperative clients who receive epidural or spinal anesthesia require ongoing monitoring of motor and sensory function.

A client who is stable and able to breathe spontaneously is discharged to a postsurgical unit or home if an outpatient surgical procedure was performed. A client discharged home must demonstrate ability to swallow and safely ambulate to the bathroom and wheelchair with assistance. A client who had an outpatient surgery should be accompanied by a significant other, relative, or other caregiver who can receive discharge instructions and transport the client home.

RISK FACTORS FOR COMPLICATIONS

Immobility: Respiratory compromise, thrombophlebitis, pressure injury

Anemia: Blood loss, inadequate/decreased oxygenation, impaired healing factors

Hypovolemia: Tissue perfusion, deep-vein thrombosis

Hypothermia: Risk of surgical wound infection, altered absorption of medication, coagulopathy, and cardiac dysrhythmia

Cardiovascular diseases: Fluid overload, deep-vein thrombosis, dysrhythmia

Respiratory disease: Respiratory compromise

Immune disorder: Risk for infection, delayed healing

Diabetes mellitus: Gastroparesis, (delayed gastric emptying), delayed wound healing, increased risk of infection, impaired circulation, hyperglycemia

Coagulation defect: Increased risk of bleeding

Malnutrition: Delayed healing

BMI greater than 30: Respiratory compromise, postoperative nausea and vomiting, wound healing, dehiscence, evisceration

Age-related: Respiratory, cardiovascular, and renal changes necessitate specific attention to the postoperative recovery of older adults. **©**
- Older adult clients are more susceptible to cold temperatures, so additional warm blankets in the PACU can be required.
- Responses to medications and anesthetics can delay return of orientation postoperatively.
- Age-related physiologic changes (decreased liver and kidney function) can affect response to and elimination of postoperative medications. Monitor for appropriate response and possible adverse effects.
  - Older adults perspire less, which leads to dry, itchy skin that becomes fragile and easily abraded. The use of paper tape for wound dressings might be indicated, as well as precautions to protect the client's skin when lifting older adults.
  - Older adults might be at risk for delayed wound healing because of possible compromised nutrition.

DIAGNOSTIC PROCEDURES

CBC: WBC (infection/immune status), Hgb and Hct (fluid status, anemia)

Metabolic profile: Blood electrolytes (electrolyte imbalances), BUN, and creatinine (kidney function)

ABGs: Oxygenation status

Additional laboratory tests: Blood glucose, prothrombin time, INR based on procedure and associated health problems

UNIT DATA COLLECTION

Upon receiving the client from the PACU, immediately perform a full body data collection with priority given to airway, breathing, and circulation. This data collection serves as a baseline to identify changes in postoperative status.

MONITORING AND MANAGEMENT

Airway and breathing

- Monitor oxygen saturation using a pulse oximeter.
- Provide supplemental oxygen as prescribed.
- Assist with coughing and deep breathing at least every 1 hr while awake and provide a pillow or folded blanket so the client can splint as necessary for abdominal or chest incision.
- Contraindications to coughing include cosmetic, eye, or intracranial surgeries.
- Assist with the use of an incentive spirometer at least every 1 to 2 hr while awake to encourage expansion of the lungs and prevent atelectasis.

Positioning

- Reposition every 2 hr, and ambulate early and regularly.
- Do not put pillows under knees or elevate the knee gatch on the bed (decreases venous return).
- Encourage early ambulation with adequate rest periods to prevent cardiovascular disorders, deep-vein thrombosis, and pulmonary complications.

Fluid status and oral comfort

- A client who returns to the medical-surgical unit is given a prescription IV solution based on needs (hydration, electrolytes).
- Encourage ice chips and fluids as prescribed/tolerated.
- Provide frequent oral hygiene.

Pain

- If prescribed, provide continuous pain relief through the use of a patient-controlled analgesia pump. Epidural and intrathecal infusions are also used postoperatively.
- A preventative approach using around-the-clock scheduling is more effective than PRN medication delivery during the first 24 to 48 hr postoperatively.
- Monitor pain level frequently, using a standardized pain scale. Qpcc
- Encourage the client to ask for pain medication before pain gets severe.
- Monitor for manifestations of pain (an increased pulse, respirations, or blood pressure; restlessness; and wincing or moaning during movement).

- Monitor for adverse effects of opioids (respiratory depression, nausea [encourage the client to change positions slowly], urinary retention, and constipation).
- Provide analgesia 30 min before ambulation or painful procedures.
- Monitor for effectiveness of pain medication after administration.
- Incorporate nonpharmacological approaches to pain management based on client needs and preferences. These can include massage, relaxation techniques, meditation, diversion (listening to music), and noise reduction

Kidney function

- Output should equal intake within 3 days postoperatively.
- Report urinary output less than 30 mL/hr.
- Once indwelling catheter is removed, client should void within 8 hr.
- Recommend the use of a bladder scan to monitor for suspected retention of urine.

Bowel function

- Maintain the client NPO until return of gag reflex (risk of aspiration) and peristalsis (risk of paralytic ileus).
- Irrigate NG suction tubes with saline as needed to maintain patency. Do not move NG tubes in clients who are postoperative following gastric surgery (risk to incision).
- Monitor bowel sounds in all four quadrants as well as ability to pass flatus.

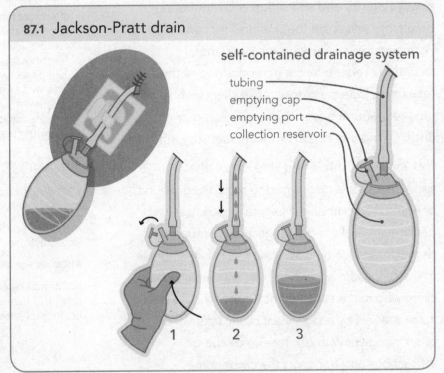

87.1 Jackson-Pratt drain

self-contained drainage system

tubing
emptying cap
emptying port
collection reservoir

1 2 3

- Advance diet as prescribed and tolerated (clear liquids to regular).
- Encourage gum chewing as a low-cost method to stimulate gastric secretions and promote the return of intestinal peristalsis.
- Administer an antiemetic for nausea and vomiting after checking bowel sounds. Place client on their side to reduce the risk of aspiration.

Thromboembolism

- Apply pneumatic compression devices and/or anti-embolism stockings.
- Reposition every 2 hr, and ambulate early and regularly.
- Administer prescribed anticoagulants or antiplatelet medications.
- Monitor extremities for calf pain, warmth, erythema, and edema.
- Promote hydration to reduce the risk of venous stasis.

Incisions and drain sites

- Monitor drainage (should progress from sanguineous to serosanguineous to serous).
- Monitor the incision site. Expected findings include pink wound edges, slight swelling under sutures/staples, and slight crusting of drainage. Report any evidence of infection, including redness, excessive tenderness, and purulent drainage.
- Monitor wound drains each time vital signs are measured. Empty closed-suction drainage collection devices as needed to maintain compression. Report increases in drainage (possible hemorrhage).
- In most instances, the surgeon will perform the first dressing change. Subsequent dressing changes can be performed by the nurse using surgical aseptic technique.
  - Use an abdominal binder as prescribed for clients who have an abdominal incision and are obese or debilitated.
- Encourage splinting with position changes, coughing, and deep breathing.
- Administer prophylactic antibiotics as prescribed.
- Remove sutures or staples in 5 to 10 days as prescribed.
- If incision is secured with wound closure tape, instruct the client to keep in place until strips fall off on their own.

Wound healing

- Encourage the client to consume a diet high in calories, protein, and vitamin C.
- If the client has diabetes mellitus, maintain appropriate glycemic control.

Reinforce discharge teaching

- Instruct the client the purpose, administration guidelines, and adverse effects of medications.
- Reinforce activity restrictions (driving, stairs, limits on weight lifting, sexual activity) with the client.
- Provide dietary guidelines, if applicable.
- Inform the client about treatment instructions (wound care, catheter care, use of assistive devices).
- Inform the client of emergency contact information.
- Advise the client to inform the surgeon if pain is unrelieved by current medication.
- Instruct the client to monitor and report any indications of infection at the surgical site to the surgeon.

87.2 Penrose drain

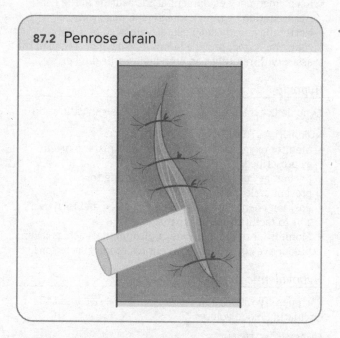

87.3 Hemovac drain

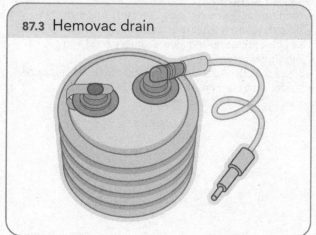

COMPLICATIONS

Airway obstruction

Swelling or spasm of the larynx or trachea, mucus in the airway, or relaxation of the tongue into the nasopharynx can cause airway obstruction, often manifesting as stridor or snoring.

NURSING ACTIONS
- Monitor for choking; noisy, irregular respirations; decreased oxygen saturation values; and cyanosis. Intervene accordingly.
- Implement a head-tilt/chin-lift maneuver to pull the tongue forward and open the airway.
- Keep emergency equipment at the bedside in the PACU (resuscitation bag, suction equipment, airways).
- Notify the anesthesiologist, elevate head of bed if not contraindicated, provide humidified oxygen, and plan to assist with reintubation with endotracheal tube.

Hypoxia

Hypoxia is evidenced by a decrease in oxygen saturation.

NURSING ACTIONS
- Monitor oxygenation status, and administer oxygen as prescribed.
- Encourage coughing and deep breathing to prevent atelectasis.
- Position client with head of bed elevated and turn every 2 hr to facilitate chest expansion.
- Monitor for manifestations of pneumonia, such as fever, productive cough, and purulent respiratory secretions.

Hypovolemic shock

Postoperative shock can result from a massive loss of circulating blood volume.

NURSING ACTIONS
- Monitor for decreased blood pressure and urinary output, increased heart and respiratory rates, narrowing of pulse pressure, and slow capillary refill.
- Administer oxygen.
- Place the client in a supine position with legs elevated.
- Assist with the administration of IV fluids and vasopressors as prescribed.

Paralytic ileus

Can occur due to the absence of GI peristaltic activity caused by abdominal surgery or other physical trauma

NURSING ACTIONS
- Monitor bowel sounds.
- Encourage ambulation.
- Advance the diet as tolerated when bowel sounds or flatus are present.
- Administer prokinetic agents (metoclopramide), as prescribed.
- The client can have an NG tube inserted to empty stomach contents.

Wound dehiscence or evisceration

- Caused by spontaneous opening of the incisional wound (dehiscence).
- Can progress to the protrusion of the internal organs through the incision (evisceration).
- Keep client NPO in case surgery is required.

NURSING ACTIONS
- Monitor risk factors (obesity, coughing, moving without splinting, poor nutritional status, diabetes mellitus, infection, hematoma, steroid use).
- If wound dehiscence or evisceration occurs, call for help, stay with the client, cover the wound with a sterile towel or dressing that is moistened with sterile saline, place in a low-Fowler's position with hips and knees bent, monitor for shock, and notify the provider immediately. Do not attempt to reinsert organs.

Deep-vein thrombosis

Caused by dehydration, stress response that leads to hypercoagulability of the blood, immobility, obesity, trauma, malignancy, history of thrombosis, hormones, and use of indwelling venous catheter

NURSING ACTIONS
- Prophylactic measures include administration of low-molecular-weight heparin, low-dose heparin, or low-dose warfarin; anti-embolism stockings; pneumatic compression devices; range-of-motion exercises; and early ambulation.
- Avoid any form of pressure behind the knee with a pillow or blanket, which can cause constriction of blood vessels and decreased venous return. Qs
- Avoid dangling the client's legs for long periods of time.
- Provide adequate hydration by assisting with the administration of IV fluids or encouraging increased oral fluid intake.

1. A nurse on a medical-surgical unit is assisting with the care of two clients who are postoperative. One client has a history of cardiovascular disease, and the other client has a history of an immune disorder. Sort the following disorders into the potential postoperative risk factors: Cardiovascular Disease or Immune Disorder.

   A. Deep-vein thrombosis

   B. Infection

   C. Fluid overload

   D. Dysrhythmia

   E. Delayed healing

2. A nurse is assisting with the plan of care for a client to reduce the risk for postoperative atelectasis. What interventions should the nurse include in the plan of care?

3. A nurse is collecting data from a client who is postoperative following abdominal surgery. Which of the following findings require action by the nurse?

   A. Urine output of 25 mL/hr

   B. Hematocrit 46%

   C. BUN 18 mg/dL

   D. Apical pulse rate 62/min

4. A nurse is assisting with the care of a client who reports postoperative nausea and vomiting. Which of the following actions should the nurse take? (Select all that apply.)

   A. Check the client for bowel sounds.

   B. Administer an antiemetic medication to the client.

   C. Restrict the client's fluids.

   D. Quickly elevate the client's head of bed.

   E. Position the client on their side.

5. A nurse is assisting with teaching a class about postoperative complications. Match the postoperative complication with the corresponding nursing intervention.

1. Airway obstruction	A. Elevate the client's legs
2. Wound evisceration	B. Administer low-molecular-weight heparin
3. Paralytic ileus	C. Insert an NG tube into the client
4. Deep-vein thrombosis	D. Bend the client's hips and knees
5. Hypovolemic shock	E. Perform head tilt/chin lift for the client

A nurse is reviewing the health records of several clients to identify postoperative complications. What information should the nurse expect to find? Use the *ATI Active Learning Template: Basic Concept* to complete this item.

RELATED CONTENT: List three possible complications. Describe one cause and one intervention for each complication.

Active Learning Scenario Key

Using the ATI Active Learning Template: Basic Concept
RELATED CONTENT

Paralytic ileus

- Caused by abdominal surgery or other physical trauma and absent gastrointestinal peristaltic activity
- Monitor bowel sounds, encourage ambulation, and insert nasogastric tube to empty stomach contents.

Wound evisceration

- Protrusion of the abdominal contents through the incisional wound of the abdominal cavity, caused by failure to splint when moving or coughing, delayed healing due to obesity or diabetes mellitus
- Call for help, cover the wound with sterile saline soaked dressings or towel, and position the client in semi-Fowler's position with hips and knees bent.

Airway obstruction

- Swelling or spasm of the larynx or trachea, mucus in the airway, or relaxation of the tongue into the nasopharynx can cause airway obstruction, often manifesting as stridor or snoring.
- Notify the anesthesiologist, provide humidified oxygen, elevate the head of the bed if not contraindicated, perform a head-tilt/chin-lift maneuver to open the airway, and plan for reintubation of the endotracheal tube.

Hypovolemic shock

- Caused by blood loss
- Monitor for decreased blood pressure and urinary output, increased heart and respiratory rates, narrowing of the pulse pressure, and slow capillary refill.
- Administer oxygen.
- Place the client in a supine position with the legs elevated.
- Assist with the administration of IV fluids and vasopressors as indicated.

Ⓝ *NCLEX® Connection: Reduction of Risk Potential, Potential for Complications from Surgical Procedures and Health Alterations*

Application Exercises Key

1. **CARDIOVASCULAR DISEASE:** A, C, D;
   IMMUNE DISORDER: B, E

   When analyzing data, the nurse should identify that deep-vein thrombosis, fluid overload, and dysrhythmias are potential postoperative risk factors in clients who have cardiovascular disease. Infection and delayed wound healing are potential postoperative risk factors for clients who have an immune disorder.

   Ⓝ *NCLEX® Connection: Reduction of Risk Potential, Potential for Complications of Diagnostic Tests/Treatments/Procedures*

2. When generating solutions, the nurse should encourage the client to use an incentive spirometer every 1 to 2 hr, splint an abdominal incision with a pillow or blanket to support the incision during coughing and deep breathing, reposition the client every 2 hr, and promote early ambulation to mobilize secretions, increase lung expansion, and reduce the risk for atelectasis.

   Ⓝ *NCLEX® Connection: Physiological Adaptation, Alterations in Body Systems*

3. A. **CORRECT:** When taking actions, the nurse should identify that a urine output less than 30 mL/hr is a manifestation of hypovolemia and requires intervention by the nurse. The nurse should report this finding to the charge nurse.

   Ⓝ *NCLEX® Connection: Basic Care and Comfort, Nutrition and Oral Hydration*

4. A, B, E. **CORRECT:** When taking actions, the nurse should check the client for bowel sounds to monitor for return of peristalsis, administer an antiemetic medication to the client to reduce the client's nausea, and position the client on their side to decrease the risk of aspiration.

   Ⓝ *NCLEX® Connection: Basic Care and Comfort, Nutrition and Oral Hydration*

5. A, 5; B, 4; C, 3; D, 2; E, 1

   When taking actions, the nurse should elevate the legs of a client who is experiencing hypovolemic shock to promote blood return to the heart. The nurse should administer low-molecular-weight heparin to reduce clot formation in a client who has a deep-vein thrombosis and insert an NG tube into a client who has a paralytic ileus to empty stomach contents. The nurse should bend the hips and knees on a client who is experiencing a wound evisceration to reduce abdominal tension and perform a head tilt/chin lift for a client who has an airway obstruction to open the client's airway.

   Ⓝ *NCLEX® Connection: Reduction of Risk Potential, Potential for Complications from Surgical Procedures and Health Alterations*

References

Alzheimer's Association Report. (2020). 2020 Alzheimer's disease facts and figures. *Alzheimer's and Dementia: The Journal of the Alzheimer's Association, 16.*

Ambrosino, N., & Vitacca, M. (2018). The patient needing prolonged mechanical ventilation: A narrative review. *Multidisciplinary Respiratory Medicine, (13)*6. https://doi.org/10.1186/s40248-018-0118-7

American Cancer Society. (2017). *Understanding your pathology report: Barrett's esophagus (with or without dysplasia).* https://www.cancer.org/treatment/understanding-your-diagnosis/tests/understanding-your-pathology-report/esophagus-pathology/barrets-esophagus.html

American Heart Association. (2022, October 31). *Understanding blood pressure readings.* https://www.heart.org/en/health-topics/high-blood-pressure/understanding-blood-pressure-readings

American Heart Association. (2022). *Managing heart failure symptoms.* https://www.heart.org/en/health-topics/heart-failure/warning-signs-of-heart-failure/managing-heart-failure-symptoms

American Heart Association. (2020). *Algorithms.* https://cpr.heart.org/en/resuscitation-science/cpr-and-ecc-guidelines/algorithms

American Pharmacists Association & Lexi-Comp, Inc. (2021). *Adult drug information handbook: A clinically relevant resource for all healthcare professionals.* Wolters Kluwer.

American Psychiatric Association Publishing. (2022). *Diagnostic and statistical manual of mental disorders: DSM-5-TR.*

Amputee Coalition. (n.d.). *Limb loss in the U.S.* https://www.amputee-coalition.org/wp-content/uploads/2020/03/LLAM-Infographic-2020.pdf

Ancheta, A. J., Bruzzese, J.-M., & Hughes, T. L. (2021). The impact of positive school climate on suicidality and mental health among LGBTQ adolescents: A systematic review. *Journal of School Nursing, 37*(2), 75–86. https://doi.org/10.1177/1059840520970847

Avital, O., & Smith, N. (2018). Uterine fibroids (leiomyoma, uterine). *CINAHL nursing guide.* EBSCO Publishing.

Balderrama, D. & Caple, C. (2018, October 5). Mechanical ventilation in the adult: Monitoring. *CINAHL nursing guide.* EBSCO Publishing.

Barnes, J.A., Eid, M.A., Creager, M.A., & Goodney, P.P. (2020). Epidemiology and risk of amputation in patients with diabetes mellitus and peripheral artery disease. *Arteriosclerosis, Thrombosis, and Vascular Biology, 40*(8):1808-1817. doi: 10.1161/ATVBAHA.120.314595

Bauman, K. & Devinsky, O. (2021). Seizure clusters: Morbidity and mortality. *Frontiers in Neurology.* doi: 10.3389/fneur.2021.636045

Berman, A., Snyder, S. & Frandsen, G. (2021). *Kozier & Erb's Fundamentals of nursing: Concepts, process, and practice* (11th ed.) e-book. Pearson.

Block, L., Ha, N., Pleak, R.R., Rosenthal, D.W. (2020). LGBTQIA+ health care: Faculty development and medical student education. *Medical Education, 54*(11),1055-1056. doi:10.1111/medu.14312

Blumlein, D., & Griffiths, I. (2022). Shock: aetiology, pathophysiology and management. *British Journal of Nursing, 31*(8), 422–428. https://doi.org/10.12968/bjon.2022.31.8.422

Boling, B., & Ashley, T. (2021). Gynecomastia. *CINAHL nursing guide.* EBSCO Publishing.

Boling, B. & Smith, N. (2018). Dumping syndrome. *CINAHL nursing guide.* EBSCO Publishing.

Boullata, J. I., Carrera, A. L., Harvey, L., Escuro, A. A., Hudson, L., Mays, A., McGinnis, C., Wessel, J. J., Bajpai, S., Beebe, M. L., Kinn, T. J., Klang, M. G., Lord, L., Martin, K., Pompeii-Wolfe, C., Sullivan, J., Wood, A., Malone, A., & Guenter, P. (2017). ASPEN safe practices for enteral nutrition therapy. *Journal of Parenteral & Enteral Nutrition, 41*(1), 15–103. https://doi.org/10.1177/0148607116673053

Burchum, J.R. & Rosenthal, L.D. (2022). *Lehne's pharmacology for nursing care* (11th ed.). Elsevier.

Cabrera, G., & Ashley, T. J. (2018). Pelvic organ prolapse. *CINAHL nursing guide.* EBSCO Publishing.

Caplan, L. R. (2022). *Stroke: Etiology, classification and epidemiology. UpToDate.* https://www.uptodate.com/contents/stroke-etiology-classification-and-epidemiology

Caple, C. & Pilgrim, J. (2017). Endoscopy: Assisting with diagnostic procedure. *CINAHL nursing guide.* EBSCO Publishing.

Centers for Disease Control and Prevention. (n.d.). *At a glance: COVID-19 vaccination schedule for most people.* https://www.cdc.gov/vaccines/covid-19/downloads/covid-19-vacc-schedule-at-a-glance-508.pdf

Centers for Disease Control and Prevention. (2019). *Document the vaccination(s).* https://www.cdc.gov/vaccines/hcp/admin/document-vaccines.html

Centers for Disease Control and Prevention. (2019). *National Center for Health Statistics: Interactive summary health statistics for adults – 2019.* https://wwwn.cdc.gov/NHISDataQueryTool/SHS_adult/index.html

Centers for Disease Control and Prevention. (2019). *Understanding the epidemic.* https://www.cdc.gov/drugoverdose/epidemic/index.html

Centers for Disease Control and Prevention. (2022, January 14). *A guide to taking a sexual history.* https://www.cdc.gov/std/treatment/sexualhistory.htm

Centers for Disease Control and Prevention. (2021). *About social determinants of health (SDOH).* https://www.cdc.gov/socialdeterminants/about.html

Centers for Disease Control and Prevention. (2022). *Acute rheumatic fever.* https://www.cdc.gov/groupastrep/diseases-hcp/acute-rheumatic-fever.html

Centers for Disease Control and Prevention. (2021, July 22). *Bacterial vaginosis.* https://www.cdc.gov/std/treatment-guidelines/bv.htm

Centers for Disease Control and Prevention. (2021, December). *COVID-19 overview and infection prevention and control priorities in non-U.S. healthcare settings.* https://www.cdc.gov/coronavirus/2019-ncov/hcp/non-us-settings/overview/index.html

Centers for Disease Control and Prevention. (2021). *What you need to know: Neutropenia and risk for infection.* https://www.cdc.gov/cancer/preventinfections/pdf/neutropenia.pdf

Centers for Disease Control and Prevention. (2022). *Chronic kidney disease initiative.* https://www.cdc.gov/kidneydisease/index.html

Centers for Disease Control and Prevention. (2022). *Chronic obstructive pulmonary disease (COPD) includes: Chronic bronchitis and emphysema.* https://www.cdc.gov/nchs/fastats/copd.htm

Centers for Disease Control and Prevention. (2022). *Flu vaccine for people with egg allergies.* https://www.cdc.gov/flu/prevent/egg-allergies.htm

Centers for Disease Control and Prevention. (2022, October 14). *Heart disease facts.* https://www.cdc.gov/heartdisease/facts.htm

Centers for Disease Control and Prevention. (2022). *Hypertension.* https://www.cdc.gov/nchs/fastats/hypertension.htm

Centers for Disease Control and Prevention. (2022). *How to report adverse events to VAERS.* https://www.cdc.gov/vaccinesafety/ensuringsafety/monitoring/vaers/reportingaes.html

Centers for Disease Control and Prevention. (2022). *Immunization schedules.* https://www.cdc.gov/vaccines/schedules/hcp/imz/adult.html#note-pneumo

Centers for Disease Control and Prevention. (2022). *Interim clinical considerations for use of COVID-19 vaccines currently approved or authorized in the United States.* https://www.cdc.gov/vaccines/covid-19/clinical-considerations/interim-considerations-us.html#contraindications

Centers for Disease Control and Prevention. (2022). *Mental health.* https://www.cdc.gov/nchs/fastats/mental-health.htm

Centers for Disease Control and Prevention. (2022). *People with certain medical conditions.* https://www.cdc.gov/coronavirus/2019-ncov/need-extra-precautions/people-with-medical-conditions.html

Centers for Disease Control and Prevention. (2022). *Stay up to date with your COVID-19 vaccines.* https://www.cdc.gov/coronavirus/2019-ncov/vaccines/stay-up-to-date.html

Centers for Disease Control and Prevention. (2022, September 1). *Stroke.* https://www.cdc.gov/stroke/index.ht

Centers for Disease Control and Prevention. (2022). *Sudden unexpected death in epilepsy: 5 things you should know about SUDEP.* https://www.cdc.gov/epilepsy/communications/features/sudep.htm

Chippa, V., Aleem, A., & Anjum, F. (2022, May 4). Post acute Coronavirus (COVID-19) syndrome. *StatPearls.* https://www.ncbi.nlm.nih.gov/books/NBK570608/

Cleveland Clinic. (2019). *Kidney infection (pyelonephritis).* https://my.clevelandclinic.org/health/diseases/15456-kidney-infection-pyelonephritis

Cleveland Clinic. (2022). *Right-sided heart failure.* https://my.clevelandclinic.org/health/diseases/21494-right-sided-heart-failure

Demir, M., Demir, F., & Aygun, H. (2021). Vitamin D deficiency is associated with COVID-19 positivity and severity of the disease. *Journal of Medical Virology, 93*(5), 2992–2999. https://doi.org/10.1002/jmv.26832

deWit, S. C., Stromberg, H. K., & Dallred, C.V. (2021). *Medical-Surgical nursing: Concepts and practice* (4th ed.). Elsevier.

Drummer, S. (2021). Prostate biopsy procedure considerations. *Urologic Nursing, 41*(5), 248–251. https://doi.org/10.7257/1053-816X.2021.41.5.248

Dudek, S.G. (2022). *Nutrition essentials for nursing practice* (9th ed.). Lippincott, Williams & Wolter.

DynaMed. (2022). *COVID-19 management.* EBSCO Information Services. https://www.dynamed. com/management/covid-19-management

DynaMed. (2022). *COVID-19: Novel coronavirus.* EBSCO Information Services. https://www. dynamed.com/condition/covid-19-novel-coronavirus

EBSCO Medical Review Board, Health Library: Evidence-Based Information. (2020). Barium enema. *Nursing Reference Center.*

EBSCO Medical Review Board, Health Library: Evidence-Based Information. (2021). Seizure disorder: Adult. *Nursing Reference Center.*

Eckler, K (ed). (2022). Pelvic organ prolapse in females: Epidemiology, risk factors, clinical manifestations, and management. *UptoDate.*

El Sayed, S. L. M., El Sayed, M. L. M., & Michael, G. C. (2020). Screening for polycystic ovarian syndrome and effect of health education on its awareness among adolescents: A Pre-Post Study. *International Journal of Nursing Education, 12*(4), 227–236.

Epilepsy Foundation. (2022a). *How to prevent SUDEP.* https://www.epilepsy.com/complications-risks/early-death-sudep/preventing-sudep

Epilepsy Foundation. (2022b). *SUDEP.* https://www.epilepsy.com/complications-risks/early-death-sudep

Ewens, B., Kemp, V., Towell-Barnard, A., & Whitehead, L. (2022). The nursing care of people with class III obesity in an acute care setting: A scoping review. *BMC Nursing, 21*(1), 1–13. https://doi.org/10.1186/s12912-021-00760-7

Fantasia, H. C., & Harris, A. L. (2020). Overview of the diagnosis and management of uterine fibroids. *Women's Healthcare: A Clinical Journal for NPs, 8*(5), 38–44.

Florence, A. M., & Fatehi, M. (2022). Leiomyoma. PubMed. *StatPearls Publishing.* https://www. ncbi.nlm.nih.gov/books/NBK538273/?msclkid=e329eb45ca4211ec9ff11e3a468d7bfd

Forcier, M., & Olson-Kennedy, J. (2021). Lesbian, gay, bisexual, and other sexual minoritized youth: Primary care. *UptoDate.*

Forcier, M., & Olson-Kennedy, J. (2020). Lesbian, gay, bisexual, and other sexual minoritized youth: Epidemiology and health concerns. *UptoDate.*

Endocrine Society. (2017). *Gender dysphoria/gender incongruence guideline resources.* https:// www.endocrine.org/clinical-practice-guidelines/gender-dysphoria-gender-incongruence

Ghanem, K., & Tuddenham, S. (n.d.). Screening for sexually transmitted infections. (A. Bloom & J. Marrazzo, Eds.). *UptoDate.*

Giruzzi N. (2020). Plenity (oral superabsorbent hydrogel). Clinical Diabetes: A publication of the American *Diabetes Association, 38*(3), 313–314. https://doi.org/10.2337/cd20-0032

Goyal, H., Kopel, J., Perisetti, A., Mann, R., Ali, A., Tharian, B., Saligram, S., & Inamdar, S. (2021). Endobariatric procedures for obesity: clinical indications and available options. *Therapeutic Advances in Gastrointestinal Endoscopy,* 1–17. https://doi. org/10.1177/2631774520984627

Grohskopf, L., Blanton, L., Ferdinands, J., Chung, J., Broder, K., Talbot, H., Morgan, R., & Fry, A. (2022). *Prevention and control of seasonal influenza with vaccines: Recommendations of the advisory committee on immunization practices, United States, 2022-23 influenza season.* https:// www.cdc.gov/mmwr/volumes/71/rr/rr7101a1.htm

Halter, M.J. (2022). *Varcarolis' foundations of psychiatric mental health nursing: A clinical approach* (9th ed.). Elsevier.

Healthy People 2030. (n.d.). *Heart disease and stroke.* https://health.gov/healthypeople/objectives-and-data/browse-objectives/heart-disease-and-stroke

Healthy People 2030. (n.d.). *Sexually transmitted infections.* https://health.gov/healthypeople/objectives-and-data/browse-objectives/sexually-transmitted-infections

Heering, H. & Balderrama, D. (2018). Mechanical ventilation: Troubleshooting. *CINAHL nursing guide.* EBSCO Publishing

Hodgens, A. & Gupta, V. (2021, November 20). *Severe acute respiratory syndrome.* StatPearls. https://www.ncbi.nlm.nih.gov/books/NBK558977/

Inserro, A. (2019). *Prevalence of hemophilia worldwide is triple that of previous estimates, new study says.* https://www.ncbi.nlm.nih.gov/books/NBK482330/?report=printable

International League Against Epilepsy. (2022). *ILAE 2017 classification of seizure types checklist.* https://www.ilae.org/guidelines/definition-and-classification/operational-classification-2017/ilae-2017-classification-of-seizure-types-checklist

Jeevannavar, J. S., Appannavar, S., & Mendigeri, S. S. (2020). Prevalence of obesity in women with polycystic ovarian syndrome: A retrospective report. *Indian Journal of Physiotherapy & Occupational Therapy, 14*(2), 84–86. https://doi.org/10.37506/ijpot.v14i2.2613

Johns Hopkins Medicine. (2022, May 17). *Electrical cardioversion.* https://www.hopkinsmedicine.org/health/treatment-tests-and-therapies/electrical-cardioversion

Johns Hopkins Medicine. (2022). *Vertebroplasty.* https://www.hopkinsmedicine.org/health/treatment-tests-and-therapies/vertebroplasty

Kaya, M. O., Pamukçu, E., & Yakar, B. (2021). The role of vitamin D deficiency on COVID-19: A systematic review and meta-analysis of observational studies. *Epidemiology and Health, 43,* e2021074. https://doi.org/10.4178/epih.e2021074

Kaynar, A.M. (2020). *Respiratory failure.* https://emedicine.medscape.com/article/167981-overview

Ker, A., Fraser, G., Lyons, A., Stephenson, C., & Fleming, T. (2020). Providing gender-affirming hormone therapy through primary care: service users' and health professionals' experiences of a pilot clinic. *Journal of Primary Health Care, 12*(1), 72–78. https://doi.org/10.1071/HC19040

Kmiec, M. M., Hou, H., Lakshmi Kuppusamy, M., Drews, T. M., Prabhat, A. M., Petryakov, S. V., Demidenko, E., Schaner, P. E., Buckey, J. C., Blank, A., & Kuppusamy, P. (2019). Transcutaneous oxygen measurement in humans using a paramagnetic skin adhesive film. *Magnetic Resonance in Medicine, 81*(2), 781–794. https://doi.org/10.1002/mrm.27445

Kornusky, J. & Caple, C. (2018). Amputation stump: Positioning and exercising. *CINAHL nursing guide.* EBSCO Publishing.

Lowdermilk, D., Perry, S.E., Cashion, K., Rhodes Alden, K. & Olshansky, E. (2020). *Maternity and women's health care* (21st ed.). Elsevier.

March, P. & Woten, M. (2022). Case management: Obesity. *CINAHL nursing guide.* EBSCO Publishing.

Mayo Clinic. (2022, May 20). *Cardioversion.* https://www.mayoclinic.org/tests-procedures/cardioversion/about/pac-20385123

Maguire, M.J., Jackson, C.F., Marson, A.G., & Nevitt, S.J. (2020). Treatments for the prevention of sudden unexpected death in epilepsy (SUDEP). *Cochrane Database of Systematic Reviews 2020,* 4. doi: 10.1002/14651858.CD011792.pub3

Mbaeyi, S., Bozio, C., Duffy, J., Rubin, L., Hariri, S., Stephens, D., & MacNeil, J. (2020). *Meningococcal vaccination: Recommendations of the advisory committee on immunization practices, United States, 2020.* https://www.cdc.gov/mmwr/volumes/69/rr/rr6909a1.htm

Medina, M. & Castillo-Pino, E. (2019). An introduction to the epidemiology and burden of urinary tract infections. *Therapeutic Advances in Urology, 11.*

Meyer, G., Boczek, U., & Bojunga, J. (2020). Hormonal gender reassignment treatment for gender Dysphoria. *Deutsches Aerzteblatt International, 117*(43), 725–732. doi:10.3238/arztebl.2020.0725

MMWR. (2021). *Sexually transmitted infections treatment guidelines.* https://www.cdc.gov/std/treatment-guidelines/STI-Guidelines-2021.pdf

Moore, J. L., Carvalho, D. Z., St Louis, E. K., Bazil, C., & Louis, E. K. S. (2021). Sleep and epilepsy: A focused review of pathophysiology, clinical syndromes, co-morbidities, and therapy. *Neurotherapeutics, 18*(1), 170–180. https://doi.org/10.1007/s13311-021-01021-w

Moran, C. I. (2021). LGBTQ Population Health Policy Advocacy. *Education for Health: Change in Learning & Practice, 34*(1), 19–21. https://doi.org/10.4103/efh.EfH_243_18

Morrell, D. J., Witte, S.R., Bello, G., Rogers, A.M., & Pauli, E.M. (2020). Nasogastric tube perforation masquerading as a delayed gastric sleeve leak. *Bariatric Times, 17*(2), 9–11.

National Institute of Health. (2021). *Clinical spectrum of SARS-CoV-2 infection.* https://www.covid19treatmentguidelines.nih.gov/overview/clinical-spectrum/

National Institute of Health. (2022). *COVID-19 treatment guidelines: Remdesivir.* https://www.covid19treatmentguidelines.nih.gov/therapies/antiviral-therapy/remdesivir/

National Institute of Health. (2022). *COVID-19 treatment guidelines.* https://www.covid19treatmentguidelines.nih.gov/management/clinical-management/clinical-management-summary/summary-hospitalized-adults-figure/

National Institutes of Health. (2021). *Sepsis.* https://www.nigms.nih.gov/education/fact-sheets/Pages/sepsis

Oliveira-Filho, J., & Mullen, M. T. (2022). *Initial assessment and management of acute stroke.* https://www.uptodate.com/contents/initial-assessment-and-management-of-acute-stroke

Oliveira-Filho, J., & Mullen, M. T. (2022). Early antithrombotic treatment of acute ischemic stroke and transient ischemic attack. *UptoDate.* https://www.uptodate.com/contents/early-antithrombotic-treatment-of-acute-ischemic-stroke-and-transient-ischemic-attack

Olson-Kennedy, J., & Forcier, M. (2020). Management of transgender and gender-diverse children and adolescents. *UptoDate.*

Pagana, K.D., Pagana, T.J., & Pagana, T.N. (2022). *Mosby's manual of diagnostic and laboratory tests* (7th ed.). Elsevier.

Pilgrm, J. & Schub, T. (2018). Epilepsy: An overview. *CINAHL nursing guide.* EBSCO Publishing.

Polsdorfer, R. (2020). Atherectomy/angioplasty of Noncoronary vessel. *EBSCO Medical Review Board, Health Library: Evidence-Based Information.*

Potter, P.A., Perry, A. G., Stockert, P. A. & Hall, A.M. (2021). *Fundamentals of nursing* (10th ed.). Elsevier.

Rhee, C., Jones, T.M., Hamad, Y., et al. (2019). Prevalence, underlying causes, and preventability of sepsis-associated mortality in US acute care hospitals. *JAMA Network Open, 2*(2), e187571. doi:10.1001/jamanetworkopen.2018.7571

Robertson, K.D., & Singh, R. (2021). Capsule endoscopy. *StatPearls*. https://www.ncbi.nlm.nih.gov/books/NBK482306/

Sandowski, S., & Maloof, M. (2019). Unique differences in screening and prevention for LGBT adolescents. Family Doctor: A Journal of the New York State Academy of Family Physicians, 7(3), 32–35.

Sarmast, S.T., Abdullahi, A.M., & Jahan, N. (2020). Current classification of seizures and epilepsies: Scope, limitations and recommendations for future action. *Cureus*, 12(9), e10549. doi: 10.7759/cureus.10549.

Schiebel, D. (2018). Frostbite. *Cinahl Information Systems*.

Shiebel, D.A. & Karkashian, A.L. (2018). Phantom limb sensation and pain. *CINAHL nursing guide*. EBSCO Publishing.

Schub, E. (2021). Sepsis and septic shock. *CINAHL nursing guide*. EBSCO Publishing.

Schub, E. & Balderrama, D. (2021). Disseminated intravascular coagulation (DIC). *CINAHL nursing guide*. EBSCO Publishing.

Schub, T. & Boling, B. (2021). Cardiac tamponade. *CINAHL nursing guide*. EBSCO Publishing.

Schub, T. & Karakashian, A.L. (2021). Bariatric surgery. *CINAHL nursing guide*. EBSCO Publishing

Schub, T. & Karakashian, A.L. (2018). Status epilepticus. *CINAHL nursing guide*. EBSCO Publishing.

Schub, T. & March, P. (2018). Colonoscopy. *CINAHL nursing guide*. EBSCO Publishing.

Shebl, E., Mirabile, V.S., & Burns, B. (2022, May 4). Respiratory failure. *StatPearls*. https://www.ncbi.nlm.nih.gov/books/NBK526127/

Simon, P., Grajo, L., & Dirette, D. P. (2021). The role of occupational therapy in supporting the needs of older adults who identify as lesbian, gay, bisexual, and/or transgender (LGBT). *Open Journal of Occupational Therapy (OJOT)*, 9(4), 1–9. https://doi.org/10.15453/2168-6408.1742

Sison, S. M., Sivakumar, G. K., Caufield-Noll, C., Greenough, W. B., Oh, E. S., & Galiatsatos, P. (2021). Mortality outcomes of patients on chronic mechanical ventilation in different care settings: A systematic review. *Heliyon*, 7(2), e06230. https://doi.org/10.1016/j.heliyon.2021.e06230

Smith, N., & Karakashian, A. (2018). Uterine prolapse. *CINAHL nursing guide*, EBSCO Publishing.

Stromberg, H.K. (2021). *Medical-surgical nursing: Concepts and practice* (4th ed.). Elsevier.

Stromberg, H.K. (2023). *Medical surgical nursing: Concepts and practice* (5th ed.). Elsevier.

Tangpricha, V., & Safer, J. (2020). Transgender men: Evaluation and management [Review of Transgender men: Evaluation and management]. *UptoDate*.

The Joint Commission. (2022). *Emergency department.* https://www.jointcommission.org/measurement/measures/emergency-department/

Thein, A., Pereira, J., Nitchingham, A. & Caplan, G. (2020). A call to action for delirium research: Meta-analysis and regression of delirium associated mortality. *BMC Geriatrics*, 20. https://doi.org/10.1186/s12877-020-01723-4

Thomas, N. D., & Leon, R. (2021). Future directions of care management: Care management in a world of many cultures. *Generations*, 45(1), 1–11.

U.S. Department of Health and Human Services. (n.d.). *Reduce the proportion of emergency department visits with a longer wait time than recommended: Data methodology and measurement.* https://health.gov/healthypeople/objectives-and-data/browse-objectives/health-care-access-and-quality/reduce-proportion-emergency-department-visits-longer-wait-time-recommended-ahs-09/data-methodology

U.S. Department of Health and Human Services. (n.d.). *Healthy People 2030: Building a healthier future for all.* https://health.gov/healthypeople

U.S. Department of Health and Human Services. (n.d). *Healthy People 2030: Social determinants of health.* https://health.gov/healthypeople/objectives-and-data/social-determinants-health

U.S. Food and Drug Administration. (2019). *Plenity.* https://www.accessdata.fda.gov/cdrh_docs/pdf18/DEN180060.pdf

U.S. Food and Drug Administration. (December 4, 2020). *FDA approves weight management drug for patients aged 12 and older.* https://www.fda.gov/drugs/news-events-human-drugs/fda-approves-weight-management-drug-patients-aged-12-and-older

Vallerand, A.H. & Sanoski, C.A. (2021). *Davis's drug guide for nurses* (17th ed). F.A. Davis.

Venes, D. (2021). *Taber's Cyclopedic Medical Dictionary.* (24th ed.). F. A. Davis.

Venkatesh, B., Schlapbach, L., Mason, D., Wilks, K., Seaton, R., Lister, P., Irwin, A., Lane, P., Redpath, L., Gibbons, K., Ergetu, E., & Rice, M. (2021). Impact of 1-hour and 3-hour sepsis time bundles on patient outcomes and antimicrobial use: A before and after cohort study. *The Lancet Regional Health, Western Pacific, 18,* 100305. https://doi.org/10.1016/j.lanwpc.2021.100305

WPATH World Professional Association for Transgender Health. (2022). *Standards of care.* https://www.wpath.org/publications/soc

Yunusa, I., Helou, M., & Alsahali, S. (2020). Pimavanserin: A novel antipsychotic with potentials to address an unmet need of older adults with dementia-related psychosis. *Frontiers in Pharmacology, 11.* https://www.ncbi.nlm.nih.gov/pmc/articles/PMC7054448/

STUDENT NAME _____

CONCEPT_____ REVIEW MODULE CHAPTER_____

Related Content

(E.G., DELEGATION,
LEVELS OF PREVENTION,
ADVANCE DIRECTIVES)

Underlying Principles

Nursing Interventions

WHO? WHEN? WHY? HOW?

STUDENT NAME _____

PROCEDURE NAME _____ REVIEW MODULE CHAPTER_____

Description of Procedure

Indications

CONSIDERATIONS

Nursing Interventions (pre, intra, post)

Interpretation of Findings

Client Education

Potential Complications

Nursing Interventions

STUDENT NAME _____

DEVELOPMENTAL STAGE _____ REVIEW MODULE CHAPTER_____

EXPECTED GROWTH AND DEVELOPMENT

Physical Development	Cognitive Development	Psychosocial Development	Age-Appropriate Activities

Health Promotion

Immunizations	Health Screening	Nutrition	Injury Prevention

STUDENT NAME _____

MEDICATION _____ REVIEW MODULE CHAPTER_____

CATEGORY CLASS_____

PURPOSE OF MEDICATION

Expected Pharmacological Action

Therapeutic Use

Complications

Medication Administration

Contraindications/Precautions

Nursing Interventions

Interactions

Client Education

Evaluation of Medication Effectiveness

STUDENT NAME _____

SKILL NAME_____ REVIEW MODULE CHAPTER_____

Description of Skill

Indications

CONSIDERATIONS

Nursing Interventions (pre, intra, post)

Outcomes/Evaluation

Client Education

Potential Complications

Nursing Interventions

STUDENT NAME _____

DISORDER/DISEASE PROCESS _____ REVIEW MODULE CHAPTER_____

Alterations in Health (Diagnosis)

Pathophysiology Related to Client Problem

Health Promotion and Disease Prevention

ASSESSMENT

SAFETY CONSIDERATIONS

Risk Factors

Expected Findings

Laboratory Tests

Diagnostic Procedures

PATIENT-CENTERED CARE

Nursing Care

Medications

Client Education

Complications

Therapeutic Procedures

Interprofessional Care

STUDENT NAME _____

PROCEDURE NAME _____ REVIEW MODULE CHAPTER_____

Description of Procedure

Indications

CONSIDERATIONS

Nursing Interventions (pre, intra, post)

Outcomes/Evaluation

Client Education

Potential Complications

Nursing Interventions

Concept Analysis

STUDENT NAME _____

CONCEPT ANALYSIS_____

Defining Characteristics

Antecedents

(WHAT MUST OCCUR/BE IN PLACE FOR CONCEPT TO EXIST/FUNCTION PROPERLY)

Negative Consequences

(RESULTS FROM IMPAIRED ANTECEDENT — COMPLETE WITH FACULTY ASSISTANCE)

Related Concepts

(REVIEW LIST OF CONCEPTS AND IDENTIFY, WHICH CAN BE AFFECTED BY THE STATUS OF THIS CONCEPT — COMPLETE WITH FACULTY ASSISTANCE)

Exemplars